Fish Parasites: Pathobiology and Protection, 2nd Edition

Fish Parasites: Pathobiology and Protection, 2nd Edition

Edited by

Patrick T.K. Woo

University of Guelph, Canada

and

Kurt Buchmann

University of Copenhagen, Denmark

CABI

CABI is a trading name of CAB International

CABI
Nosworthy Way
Wallingford
Oxfordshire OX10 8DE
UK

Tel: +44 (0)1491 832111
E-mail: info@cabi.org
Website: www.cabi.org

CABI
200 Portland Street
Boston
MA 02114
USA

Tel: +1 (617)682-9015
E-mail: cabi-nao@cabi.org

A catalogue record for this book is available from the British Library, London, UK.

ISBN-13: 9781800628724 (hardback)
9781800628731 (ePDF)
9781800628748 (ePub)

DOI: 10.1079/9781800628748.0000

Commissioning Editor: Jamie Lee
Editorial Assistant: Emma McCann
Production Editor: Shankari Wilford

Typeset by Straive, Pondicherry, India
Printed and bound in the UK by CPI Group (UK) Ltd, Croydon, CR0 4YY

Contents

Contributors

Julie D. Alexander, Department of Microbiology, 226 Nash Hall, Oregon State University, Corvallis, OR 97331, USA. E-mail: julie.alexander@oregonstate.edu.

Stephen D. Atkinson, Department of Microbiology, 226 Nash Hall, Oregon State University, Corvallis, OR 97331, USA. E-mail: stephen.atkinson@oregonstate.edu. ORCID: 0000-0002-7180-6672.

Annemariè Avenant-Oldewage, Department of Zoology, University of Johannesburg, PO Box 524, Auckland Park, Johannesburg, South Africa. E-mail: aoldewage@uj.ac.za. ORCID: 0000-0001-8820-7679.

Miguel Bao, Institute of Marine Research, PO Box 1870 Nordnes, NO-5817 Bergen, Norway. E-mail: miguel.bao-dominguez@hi.no.

Paola Beraldo, Section of Animal and Veterinary Sciences, Department of Agricultural, Food, Environmental and Animal Sciences, University of Udine, Via Sondrio 2, 33100 Udine, Italy. E-mail: paola.beraldo@uniud.it. ORCID: 0000-0002-5806-4109.

Stephen A. Bullard, Southeastern Cooperative Fish Parasite and Disease Laboratory, School of Fisheries, Aquaculture, and Aquatic Sciences, College of Agriculture, Auburn University, Auburn, AL, 36849, USA; and Department of Zoology, School for Environmental Sciences and Development, North-West University, Private Bag X6001, Potchefstroom 2520, South Africa. E-mail: Ash.Bullard@auburn.edu. ORCID: 0000-0001-6681-7724.

Kurt Buchmann, Laboratory of Aquatic Pathobiology, Department of Veterinary and Animal Sciences, Faculty of Health and Medical Sciences, University of Copenhagen, Frederiksberg C, Denmark. E-mail: kub@sund.ku.dk. ORCID: 0000-0002-2747-237X.

Ryan B. Carnegie, Virginia Institute of Marine Science, William & Mary, PO Box 1346, Gloucester Point, VA 23062, USA. E-mail: carnegie@vims.edu.

Anindo Choudhury, Division of Natural Sciences, St. Norbert College, 100 Grant Street, De Pere, WI 54115, USA. E-mail: anindo.choudhury@snc.edu. ORCID: 0000-0001-7553-4179.

Paolo Cipriani, Institute of Marine Research, PO Box 1870 Nordnes, NO-5817 Bergen, Norway. E-mail: paolo.cipriani@hi.no.

Nilanjana Das, Department of Microbiology, 226 Nash Hall, Oregon State University, Corvallis, OR 97331, USA. E-mail: dasni@oregonstate.edu. ORCID: 0009-0007-3162-2346.

Harry W. Dickerson, Department of Infectious Diseases, College of Veterinary Medicine, University of Georgia, Athens, GA 30602, USA. E-mail: hwd@uga.edu.

Itziar Estensoro, Instituto de Acuicultura Torre de la Sal, Consejo Superior de Investigaciones Científicas (CSIC), Torre de la Sal, s/n, 12595 Ribera de Cabanes, Castellón, Spain. E-mail: itziar.estensoro@csic.es. ORCID: 0000-0002-6218-2191.

Mark D. Fast, Professor, Department of Pathology and Microbiology, Atlantic Veterinary College, University of Prince Edward Island, 550 University Avenue, Charlottetown, Prince Edward Island, Canada C1A 4P3. E-mail: mfast@upei.ca. ORCID: 0000-0002-6382-8193.

Margarita P. González-Gómez, Escuela de Medicina Veterinaria, Facultad de Medicina Veterinaria, Universidad San Sebastián, Sede de la Patagonia, Lago Panguipulli 1390, Puerto Montt, Chile. E-mail: margarita.gonzalez@uss.cl. ORCID: 0000-0003-0382-0736.

Matt J. Griffin, Thad Cochran National Warmwater Aquaculture Center, College of Veterinary Medicine and Mississippi Agricultural and Forestry Experiment Station, Mississippi State University, Stoneville, MS 38756, USA; and Department of Pathobiology and Population Medicine, College of Veterinary Medicine, Mississippi State University, Mississippi State, MS 39762, USA. E-mail: griffin@cvm.msstate.edu. ORCID: 0000-0002-7920-3446.

Sascha L. Hallett, Department of Microbiology, 226 Nash Hall, Oregon State University, Corvallis, OR 97331, USA. E-mail: sascha.hallett@oregonstate.edu. ORCID: 0000-0002-8112-8203.

Hanna Hartikainen, School of Life Sciences, University of Nottingham, University Park, Nottingham NG7 2RD, UK. E-mail: hanna.hartikainen@nottingham.ac.uk. ORCID: 0000-0002-1533-261X.

Jemma Hudson, School of Science, RMIT University, Melbourne, Victoria 3000, Australia. E-mail: s3988903@student.rmit.edu.au.

Kate S. Hutson, Cawthron Institute, 98 Halifax St East, The Wood Nelson, New Zealand 7010. Adjunct at: Centre for Sustainable Tropical Fisheries and Aquaculture, College of Science and Engineering, James Cook University, 150 Angus Smith Drive, Townsville, QLD 4811, Australia. E-mail: kate.hutson@cawthron.org.nz. ORCID: 0000-0003-2408-3990.

Anssi Karvonen, Department of Biological and Environmental Science, University of Jyväskylä, PO Box 35, FI-40010 Jyväskylä, Finland. E-mail: anssi.t.karvonen@jyu.fi. ORCID: 0000-0002-2731-3344.

Lester H. Khoo, Director Aquatic Diagnostic Laboratory, Thad Cochran National Warmwater Aquaculture Center, College of Veterinary Medicine, Mississippi State University, Stoneville, MS 38756, USA; and Department of Pathobiology and Population Medicine, College of Veterinary Medicine, Mississippi State University, Mississippi State, MS 39762, USA. E-mail: khoo@cvm.msstate.edu. ORCID: 0000-0002-1436-9795.

Ruth S. Kirk, School of Life Sciences, Pharmacy and Chemistry, Kingston University London, Kingston upon Thames, Surrey KT1 2EE, UK. E-mail: Ruth.Kirk@kingston.ac.uk. ORCID: 0000-0003-3739-2530.

Roman Kuchta, Institute of Parasitology, Biology Centre of the Academy of Sciences of the Czech Republic, Branišovská 31, 370 05 České Budějovice, Czech Republic. E-mail: krtek@paru.cas.cz. ORCID: 0000-0002-4219-6924.

Arne Levsen, Institute of Marine Research, PO Box 1870 Nordnes, NO-5817 Bergen, Norway. E-mail: arne.levsen@hi.no.

Jan Lovy, US Geological Survey, Western Fisheries Research Center, 6505 NE 65th Street, Seattle, WA 98115, USA. Email: jl4825@cornell.edu. ORCID: 0000-0003-2704-0822.

Sandra L. Marín, Instituto de Acuicultura y Medio Ambiente, Universidad Austral de Chile Sede Puerto Montt, Los Pinos s/n Pelluco, Puerto Montt, Chile. E-mail: smarin@uach.cl. ORCID: 0000-0002-2892-1536.

Dylan Michaud, Pacific Biological Station, Fisheries and Oceans, Canada, 3190 Hammonds Road, Nanaimo, British Columbia, Canada, V9T 6N7. E-mail: dylan.michaud@dfo-mpo.gc.ca. ORCID: 0000-0003-3277-8127.

Barbara F. Nowak, Institute for Marine and Antarctic Studies, University of Tasmania, Hobart, Launceston, Tasmania 7250, Australia; and School of Science, RMIT University, Melbourne, Victoria 3000, Australia. E-mail: b.nowak@utas.edu.au. ORCID: 0000-0002-0347-643X

Kazuo Ogawa, Meguro Parasitological Museum, Shimomeguro, Meguro-ku, Tokyo 153-0064, Japan. E-mail: ogawak@kiseichu.org.

Oswaldo Palenzuela, Instituto de Acuicultura Torre de la Sal, Consejo Superior de Investigaciones Científicas (CSIC), Torre de la Sal, s/n, 12595 Ribera de Cabanes, Castellón, Spain. E-mail: oswaldo.palenzuela@csic.es. ORCID: 0000-0001-7702-6098.

M. Carla Piazzon, Instituto de Acuicultura Torre de la Sal, Consejo Superior de Investigaciones Científicas (CSIC), Torre de la Sal, s/n, 12595 Ribera de Cabanes, Castellón, Spain. E-mail: carla.piazzon@csic.es. ORCID: 0000-0002-4949-8984.

Hamish Rodger, PFHS Ltd, Kinvara, Co. Galway, H91 F8XF, Ireland. E-mail: hamish.rodger@patogen.no.

T. Graham Rosser, Department of Comparative Biomedical Sciences, College of Veterinary Medicine, Mississippi State University, Mississippi State, MS 39762, USA. E-mail: graham.rosser@msstate.edu. ORCID: 0000-0001-6180-8802.

Tomáš Scholz, Institute of Parasitology, Biology Centre of the Academy of Sciences of the Czech Republic, Branišovská 31, 370 05 České Budějovice, Czech Republic. E-mail: tscholz@paru.cas.cz. ORCID: 0000-0002-6340-3750.

Ariadna Sitjà-Bobadilla, Instituto de Acuicultura Torre de la Sal, Consejo Superior de Investigaciones Científicas (CSIC), Torre de la Sal, s/n, 12595 Ribera de Cabanes, Castellón, Spain. E-mail: ariadna.sitja@csic.es. ORCID: 0000-0002-7473-3413.

David J. Speare, Department of Pathology and Microbiology, Atlantic Veterinary College, University of Prince Edward Island, 550 University Avenue, Charlottetown, Prince Edward Island, Canada C1A 4P4. E-mail: speare@upei.ca. ORCID: 0000-0003-2304-9010.

Justin M. Stilwell, Department of Pathobiology and Population Medicine, College of Veterinary Medicine, Mississippi State University, Mississippi State, MS 39762, USA. Email: justin.stilwell@msstate.edu. ORCID: 0000-0002-8177-9823.

Micah B. Warren, Southeastern Cooperative Fish Parasite and Disease Laboratory, School of Fisheries, Aquaculture, and Aquatic Sciences, College of Agriculture, Auburn University, Auburn, AL, 36849, USA. E-mail: brett.warren@auburn.edu. ORCID: 0000-0002-5008-4826.

Lisa King Wolf, School of Life Sciences, University of Nottingham, University Park, Nottingham NG7 2RD, UK. E-mail: lisa.kingwolf@nottingham.ac.uk. ORCID: 0009-0002-0718-903X.

Ian D. Whittington† (deceased), formerly of The South Australian Museum and Australian Centre for Evolutionary Biology and Biodiversity, The University of Adelaide, Adelaide, Australia.

Patrick T.K. Woo, Department of Integrative Biology, College of Biological Science, University of Guelph, Guelph, Ontario, Canada N1G 2W1. E-mail: pwoo@uoguelph.ca.

Preface

Finfish is the primary source of animal protein for humans in many developing and even in developed countries as it is more readily available and less expensive than land-based meat. It is easy to digest and a good source of many essential minerals and vitamins. Fish is now considered an important component of a well-balanced diet for humans. Parasitic infections challenge cultured and wild fish stocks and with ongoing climate change pathogens often cause increased fish morbidity/mortality. A few parasites may even challenge food accessibility and security for humans. Consequently, an up-to-date comprehensive book is needed to help meet these ongoing challenges.

The present volume, *Fish Parasites: Pathobiology and Protection*, 2nd edition (FPPP.2), focuses on protozoan and metazoan parasites that cause disease and/or mortality in economically important captive and wild fish populations. Parasites for inclusion in FPPP.2 are selected by the editors and the criteria used are on the jacket of FPPP.2. These same criteria were initially used in the 1st edition of *Fish Parasites: Pathobiology and Protection* (FPPP.1). An updated book is warranted as a significant volume of research has been conducted since the publication of FPPP.1 in 2012. This may partly be due to increased concerns on fish biosecurity and fish as a component in food security for humans. These concerns are increasing, especially given the effects that ongoing climate change has, and will have, on the biology of fish and infectious pathogens.

The aims and format of FPPP.2 are the same as those in FPPP.1. As in previous books on 'fish health', the basic premise in FPPP.2 is that: 'No single author can hope to write these volumes with any authority, hence I [we in FPPP.2] have chosen well qualified international recognized experts to write the chapters' (*Preface* in *Fish Diseases and Disorders, Volume I: Protozoan and Metazoan Infections*, 1995).

FPPP.2 is interdisciplinary, and it has 22 chapters authored by research scientists from 13 countries in six continents. Eighteen chapters are either updated or rewritten by their original contributors and the remaining chapters are by new experts. We are delighted to welcome our 16 new contributors and are very grateful for the continuing support of authors from FPPP.1. Other major changes in the current volume include deletion of two chapters from FPPP.1 ('*Miamiensis avidus* and Related Species' and '*Anguillicoloides crassus*'). These are replaced with reviews on *Tetracapsuloides bryosalmonae* and *Caligus rogercresseyi* which have increasing impacts on fish health and production. Also, each chapter in FPPP.2 has an abstract, at least five main sections (with appropriate subsections) and conclusions with suggestions for future research:

- Introduction: e.g. morphology and biology of the pathogen, geographical distribution, its impact(s) on fish production.
- Diagnosis of infection: e.g. parasitological, serological, molecular confirmation.

- Pathobiology: e.g. gross pathology, histopathology, disease mechanism, pathophysiology, factors that enhance or reduce parasite multiplication.
- Protective and control strategies: e.g. innate and adaptive immunities including chemotherapy and immunochemotherapy, selective breeding of pathogen-tolerant and/or pathogen-resistant fish, environmental modification(s) to reduce pathogen transmission.
- Conclusions with suggestions for future research, which may include changes and/or adaptations of pathogens and fish to the ongoing climate change.

The principal audience of FPPP.2 is scientists in universities and the aquaculture sector (e.g. fish health consultants, scientists and managers of private and government fish health laboratories). It is also appropriate for training fish health specialists and students who are conducting research on diseases of aquatic organisms.

The secondary audience is scientists with expertise in related disciplines (e.g. molecular biology, immunology, epidemiology, ecology, fish biology) so that they may be able to initiate their own programmes and/or collaborate with fish health scientists. With the ongoing climate change we expect this secondary audience to increase as fish health becomes a more challenging problem which will require interdisciplinary research. Studies on fish health in wild populations may also be used by ecologists as important indicators of current and/or future problems in the aquatic ecosystem.

Patrick T.K. Woo and Kurt Buchmann

1 *Neoparamoeba perurans*

Barbara F. Nowak[1,2]*, Jemma Hudson[2] and Hamish Rodger[3]
[1]Institute for Marine and Antarctic Studies, University of Tasmania, Hobart, Australia; [2]School of Science, RMIT University, Melbourne, Australia; [3]PFHS Ltd, Kinvara, Ireland

Abstract

Amoebic gill disease (AGD) is a potentially fatal disease of farmed and wild marine fish. The causative agent, *Neoparamoeba perurans*, is a ubiquitous free-living amoeba found from polar to subtropical marine environments. *Neoparamoeba* spp. are characterized by the presence of one or more eukaryotic symbionts. *N. perurans* colonizes fish gills, and the signs of subsequent disease include epithelial hyperplasia of the gills with epithelial desquamation and oedema, an increase in mucous cells and decreased chloride cell numbers. Major risk factors include high salinity (lower threshold: 20–25 ppt) and above-average temperatures (lower threshold: 4–8°C). PCR is required for definitive diagnosis, though gross gill scores in farms are a standard measure of disease severity. Affected fish show a reduction in maximum rate of O_2 uptake. Freshwater bathing remains the main commercial treatment. Since first reports of the disease >40 years ago, AGD has become prevalent worldwide in salmonid aquaculture.

1.1. Introduction[1]

Neoparamoeba perurans Young, Crosbie, Adams, Nowak et Morrison, 2007 is a marine amoeba (Amoebozoa, Dactylopodida) which colonizes fish gills resulting in outbreaks of amoebic gill disease (AGD) in fish farmed in the marine environment (Young *et al.*, 2007, 2008a). The transmission is horizontal. Experimental AGD infections are achieved either by cohabitation with infected fish or by exposure to amoebae isolated from the gills of fish affected by AGD (for review, see Hudson and Nowak, 2021). Exposure to the lowest concentration of amoebae tested, which was 0.1 amoebae/l of water, caused AGD in naïve Atlantic salmon (*Salmo salar*) (Bridle *et al.*, 2021). There is a positive correlation between the number of amoebae in the water and the severity of the lesions (Zilberg *et al.*, 2001; Morrison *et al.*, 2004). Other members of this genus are free-living amoebae, ubiquitous in the marine environment (Page, 1974, 1983) and have been cultured from marine sediments, water and marine invertebrates both from fish-farming and non-farming areas, ranging from polar to subtropical climate zones (Page, 1973; Crosbie *et al.*, 2003, 2005; Mullen *et al.*, 2005; Dyková *et al.*, 2007; Moran *et al.*, 2007). Mass mortality of American lobster (*Homarus americanus*) in Western Long Island Sound, which resulted in the collapse of the fishery, was partly attributed to *Neoparamoeba pemaquidensis*, which was identified on the basis of small-subunit ribosomal RNA (SSU rRNA) fragments having 98% identity with *N. pemaquidensis* from the gills

*Email: B.Nowak@utas.edu.au

(eds P.T.K. Woo and K. Buchmann)
DOI: 10.1079/9781800628748.0001

of Atlantic salmon (Mullen *et al.*, 2005). It was also proposed that *Paramoeba invadens*, which is a pathogen of sea urchins (Jones and Scheibling, 1985), is a junior synonym of *N. pemaquidensis* (see Mullen *et al.*, 2005).

Presence of one or more endosymbionts (parasomes) is the main characteristic of all paramoebae (Page, 1987; Dyková *et al.*, 2003). Co-evolution of the amoeba and their endosymbiont was suggested in phylogenetic studies (Young *et al.*, 2014; Sibbald *et al.*, 2017). Furthermore, metabolic and cellular interdependence was shown in genome analysis of *N. pemaquidensis* (Tanifuji *et al.*, 2017). The two main genera of paramoebae are differentiated by microscales covering the cell membrane which are present in the genus *Paramoeba* but absent in *Neoparamoeba* (Page, 1987). The lack of molecular data from *Paramoeba* spp. means that it is important to continue to differentiate those two genera (Young *et al.*, 2014; Kudryavtsev *et al.*, 2021). Based on morphological and ecological heterogeneity of paramoebae, a recent review retained all the genera to ensure the preservation of taxonomic diversity in publications (Kudryavtsev *et al.*, 2021).

There is limited information about the biology of *N. perurans*. Using PCR tests, *N. perurans* DNA has been detected in water from cages containing farmed Atlantic salmon affected by AGD in Tasmania and from fresh water used to bathe fish on the same farm (Bridle *et al.*, 2010). It was not detected in water from another salmon farm that was not affected by AGD at the sampling time, or in other areas further away from salmon farms (Bridle *et al.*, 2010). Negative results may have been due to the low sensitivity of the technique as small volumes of water were used (50 ml). Amoebae concentration in sea water was highest in Tasmania in early autumn months and in surface water samples with a mean of 4.7 ± 2.0 cells/l and a range from 0 to 62.3 cells/l (Wright *et al.*, 2015) with salinity mediating *N. perurans* depth distribution during intermittent halocline development (Wright *et al.*, 2017a). A survey using PCR in Norway detected *N. perurans* DNA in water, biofilm, plankton, filter-feeding organisms and wild fish during episodes of clinical AGD in farmed salmon (Hellebø *et al.*, 2017). The environmental samples were positive, most likely as a result of spread of the amoebae through water, emphasizing the need for early detection for intervention to reduce infection pressure and spread of the parasite within farms. *N. perurans* DNA was detected in net biofouling organisms (*Ectopleura larynx*), sea lice (*Lepeophtheirus salmonis*) and cleaner fish (*Cyclopterus lumpus*, *Labrus bergylta*) in Ireland in pens with salmon affected by clinical AGD (H. Rodger, 2013, unpublished results) and at least 20 different wild and farmed fish species globally (Oldham *et al.*, 2016; Kim *et al.*, 2017; Rodger, 2019). AGD was first reported more than 40 years ago in coho salmon (*Oncorhynchus kisutch*) farmed in Washington State, USA and *Paramoeba pemaquidensis* was proposed as the disease agent (Kent *et al.*, 1988). This species was transferred (together with *Paramoeba aestuarina*) to genus *Neoparamoeba* due to the absence of microscales on the surface of the trophozoites (Page, 1987; Dyková *et al.*, 2000). *N. pemaquidensis* was repetitively isolated by *in vitro* culture from gills of infected coho salmon and Atlantic salmon from different locations, including the USA and Australia (Kent *et al.*, 1988; Dyková *et al.*, 1998). Another species, *Neoparamoeba branchiphila*, was described based on cultures from the gills of AGD-affected Atlantic salmon in Tasmania (Dyková *et al.*, 2005). A molecular study that was to determine if both or one of these species caused AGD resulted in the description of *N. perurans* (see Young *et al.*, 2007).

N. perurans (Fig. 1.1) is the only species associated with AGD lesions on the gills of fish (Young *et al.*, 2008a; Crosbie *et al.*, 2010a; Bustos *et al.*, 2011). The other two species of *Neoparamoeba* have not been found (using *in situ* hybridization) in histological sections of gills of fish affected by

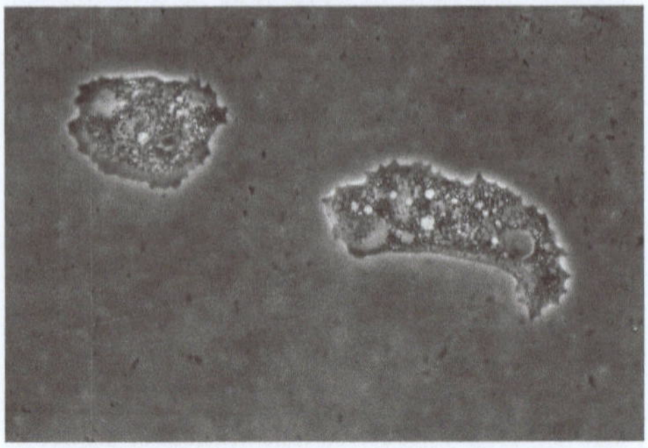

Fig. 1.1. Amoebae isolated from the gills of Atlantic salmon affected by AGD. The amoebae were later confirmed to be *Neoparamoeba perurans* using PCR. (Photo, Dr Philip Crosbie.)

AGD. While experimental exposure to *N. perurans* isolated from the gills of affected salmon caused AGD in naïve Atlantic salmon (Young *et al.*, 2007; Crosbie *et al.*, 2010a), cultured *N. pemaquidensis* or *N. branchiphila* or other species of amoebae previously isolated from Atlantic salmon gills, including *Platyamoeba* sp., *Nolandella* sp. and *Pseudoparamoeba* sp., did not (Nowak *et al.*, 2004a; Morrison *et al.*, 2005; Vincent *et al.*, 2007; English *et al.*, 2021). However, it is possible that the presence of other amoebae may contribute to dysbiosis and gill diseases (Nowak and Archibald, 2018; English *et al.*, 2019). This was not supported by the results of an experimental exposure to *Nolandella* sp. and *Pseudoparamoeba* sp., which did not increase the severity of *N. perurans*-induced AGD (English *et al.*, 2021).

AGD was reported during the 1980s from farmed coho salmon in Washington State in the USA (Kent *et al.*, 1988) and from Atlantic salmon in Tasmania, Australia (Munday, 1986; Munday *et al.*, 1990). The disease affects fishes farmed in the marine environment (Kent *et al.*, 1988; Dyková *et al.*, 1998; Young *et al.*, 2007, 2008a; Crosbie *et al.*, 2010a; Kim *et al.*, 2017; Rodger 2019), and they include coho salmon (*O. kisutch*), Atlantic salmon (*S. salar*), rainbow trout (*Oncorhynchus mykiss*), Chinook salmon (*Oncorhynchus tshawytscha*), turbot (*Scophthalmus maximus*), sea bass (*Dicentrarchus labrax*), ayu (*Plecoglossus altivelis*), black seabream (*Acanthopagrus schlegelii*), rock bream (*Oplegnathus fasciatus*), grey mullet (*Mugil cephalus*), olive flounder (*Paralichthys olivaceus*) and halibut (*Hippoglossus hippoglossus*). It has been suggested that some salmonids may be more resistant to AGD than others (Munday *et al.*, 2001); however, this is difficult to resolve given the difficulty of running experimental infections in exactly the same environmental conditions and using comparable fish from different species. Despite surveys of large numbers of wild fishes near salmon farms affected by AGD in Tasmania (Nowak *et al.*, 2004b), only one individual wild fish has ever been found with *Neoparamoeba* sp. on its gills (Adams *et al.*, 2008). This fish, a blue warehou (*Seriolella brama*), was from a cage containing infected Atlantic salmon (Adams *et al.*, 2008). *N. perurans* has a cosmopolitan distribution in temperate marine waters (Kudryavtsev *et al.*, 2021) and some genetic variability has been found between geographical isolates, in particular between Tasmanian and other isolates (Johnson-Mackinnon *et al.*, 2019) as well as between earlier European isolates (Ireland 1997 and Norway 2006) and more recent European isolates (Hansen *et al.*, 2019). AGD has been reported from the west coast of the USA, Australia, Chile, New Zealand, Japan, South Africa, Ireland, Scotland, Norway, Canada, South Korea, France, Spain and the Faroe Islands (Table 1.1; Rodger and McArdle, 1996; Young *et al.*, 2007; Nylund *et al.*, 2008; Steinum *et al.*, 2008; Crosbie *et al.*, 2010a; Bustos *et al.*, 2011; Kim *et al.*, 2017; Marcos-López and Rodger, 2020).

If the infected fish are not treated, AGD can cause mortalities of over 50% affected fish (Munday *et al.*, 1990). Mortalities have been reported in farmed fish in the USA, Tasmania, Ireland, Scotland, Norway, Japan and Chile (Kent *et al.*, 1988; Rodger and McArdle, 1996; Palmer *et al.*, 1997; Nylund *et al.*, 2008; Steinum *et al.*, 2008; Crosbie *et al.*, 2010a; Bustos *et al.*, 2011). At the time of writing, the only countries farming marine-stage salmon that have not reported AGD are Iceland and Russia. While the outbreaks in some of the geographical locations AGD was reported from have been sporadic, AGD is the most significant health problem in Atlantic salmon farmed in Tasmania where it contributes up to 20% of production costs (Munday *et al.*, 2001), mostly due to the cost of freshwater bathing. AGD has also been reported regularly from the USA, UK, Norway and Chile, where it can contribute to significant mortalities of Atlantic salmon (Douglas-Helders *et al.*, 2001a; Nowak *et al.*, 2010; Bustos *et al.*, 2011) as well as associated farm management and treatment costs (Rodger, 2014; Shinn *et al.*, 2015).

One of the main risk factors for the disease outbreaks is high salinity (Munday *et al.*, 1990; Clark and Nowak, 1999; Nowak, 2001; Adams and Nowak, 2003; Bustos *et al.*, 2011). Outbreaks in Ireland (Palmer *et al.*, 1997) and Chile (Bustos *et al.*, 2011) have occurred in years with unusually low rainfall. In experimental AGD infections mortalities are greater at salinities of 37–40 ppt than 35 ppt and below (Nowak, 2001). In Tasmania and Ireland, salmon farmed at sites with a strong influx of fresh water following heavy rain were less affected by AGD (Munday *et al.*, 1993). This may be due to the sensitivity of the amoeba to low salinity as it is a marine species. There was a reduced survival of amoebae isolated

Table 1.1. Geographic distribution of AGD in farmed and wild fish. NR, not recorded.

Location	Host	Mortality	Temperature (°C)/ Salinity (ppt)	Method of detection	Reference
Tasmania, Australia	Atlantic salmon (*Salmo salar*)	Up to 50%	12–20/NR	*In situ* hybridization, PCR	Munday (1986); Young *et al.* (2008a)
	Rainbow trout (*Oncorhynchus mykiss*)	Up to 50%	12–20/NR	*In situ* hybridization	Munday *et al.* (1990); Young *et al.* (2008a)
Chile	Atlantic salmon (*S. salar*)	NR	NR/NR	Indirect fluorescent antibody technique (IFAT)	Nowak *et al.* (2002)
		Up to 53.8%	9–12/27.9–32.8	*In situ* hybridization, PCR	Bustos *et al.* (2011)
	Rainbow trout (*O. mykiss*)	NR	NR/NR	PCR	Rozas *et al.* (2012)
	Coho salmon (*Oncorhynchus kisutch*)	NR	NR/NR	PCR	Rozas *et al.* (2012)
British Columbia, Canada	Atlantic salmon (*S. salar*)	NR	NR/NR	NR	ICES (2016)
France	Atlantic salmon (*S. salar*)	NR	NR/NR	Histology	Findlay *et al.* (1995); Rodger and McArdle (1996)
	Brown trout (*Salmo trutta*)	NR	NR/NR	NR	Munday *et al.* (2001)
Faroe Islands	Atlantic salmon (*S. salar*)	0	NR/NR	NR	Oldham *et al.* (2016)
Ireland	Atlantic salmon (*S. salar*)	Up to 10%	12–17/NR	*In situ* hybridization	Rodger and McArdle (1996); Young *et al.* (2008a)
Japan	Ayu (*Plecoglossus altivelis*)	49.4%	14/NR	*In situ* hybridization, PCR	Crosbie *et al.* (2010a)
Korea	Coho salmon (*O. kisutch*)	~70%	15–17/33	PCR	Kim *et al.* (2016)
	Olive flounder (*Paralichthys olivaceus*)	NR	NR/NR	Histology, transmission election microscopy (TEM)	Kim *et al.* (2005)
	Black seabream (*Acanthopagrus schlegelii*)	60%	13–14/33	PCR	Kim *et al.* (2017)
	Rock bream (*Oplegnathus fasciatus*)	10%	13–14/33	PCR	Kim *et al.* (2017)
	Grey mullet (*Mugil cephalus*)	6.7%	11–17/33	PCR	Kim *et al.* (2017)
	Atlantic salmon (*S. salar*)	80%	13/NR	PCR	Kim *et al.* (2024)

Mediterranean	Sea bass (*Dicentrarchus labrax*)	NR	NR/NR	TEM	Dykova *et al*. (2000)
New Zealand	Chinook salmon (*Oncorhynchus tshawytscha*)	NR	NR/NR	PCR	Young *et al*. (2008a)
Norway	Atlantic salmon (*S. salar*)	Up to 82%	7–14/>30	Reverse transcriptase (RT) PCR	Nylund *et al*. (2008); Steinum *et al*. (2008)
	Corkwing wrasse (*Symphodus melops*)	NR	NR/NR	PCR	VKM (2014)
	Ballan wrasse (*Labrus bergylta*)	NR	NR/NR	PCR	VKM (2014)
	Rainbow trout (*O. mykiss*)	NR	NR/NR	PCR	VKM (2014)
Scotland	Atlantic salmon (*S. salar*)	Up to 70%	1.5–13.5/NR	*In situ* hybridization	Young *et al*. (2008a)
	Halibut (*Hippoglossus hippoglossus*)	<0.01%	12/NR	RT PCR	Rodger (2019)
	Horse mackerel (*Trachurus trachurus*)	0	NR/NR	PCR	Stagg *et al*. (2015)
Spain	Atlantic salmon (*S. salar*)	NR	NR/NR	Histology	Rodger and McArdle (1996)
	Turbot (*Scophthalmus maximus*)	Up to 20%	NR/22	Histology	Dykova *et al*. (1995, 1998)
South Africa	Atlantic salmon (*S. salar*)	~5%	15/NR	*In situ* hybridization, PCR	Mouton *et al*. (2014)
	Turbot (*S. maximus*)	~5%	14–16.7/NR	*In situ* hybridization	Mouton *et al*. (2014)
Washington, USA	Atlantic salmon (*S. salar*)	Up to 21.85%	8.9–10.3/NR	PCR	Douglas-Helders *et al*. (2001a); Young *et al*. (2008a)
	Coho salmon (*O. kisutch*)	~25%	9–11/30	Histology	Kent *et al*. (1988)

from the gills of AGD-affected salmon when the amoebae were exposed for 6 days to 15 ppt salinity compared to survival at 27 or 38 ppt (Douglas-Helders *et al.*, 2005). Collins *et al.* (2019) reported growth in culture of the amoeba at salinities between 25 and 50 ppt at 15°C, that amoebae numbers were sustained at 4°C and considered that lower temperature and salinity thresholds for growth lie between 4 and 8°C and 20 and 25 ppt, respectively. Pseudocyst formation for *N. perurans* was reported by Lima *et al.* (2017) as a short-term strategy to abrupt salinity variation.

Complex gill disease (CGD), which has been reported in farmed Atlantic salmon in Norway, Scotland, Canada and Ireland, can include AGD (Herrero *et al.*, 2018). CGD is a multifactorial condition causing gill pathology and can involve a range of pathogens, including parasites, viruses and bacteria (Herrero *et al.*, 2018). For example, salmon gill pox virus, the microsporidian *Desmozoon lepeophtherii* and *Candidatus* Branchiomonas cysticola were reported in CGD cases in Atlantic salmon (Herrero *et al.*, 2018).

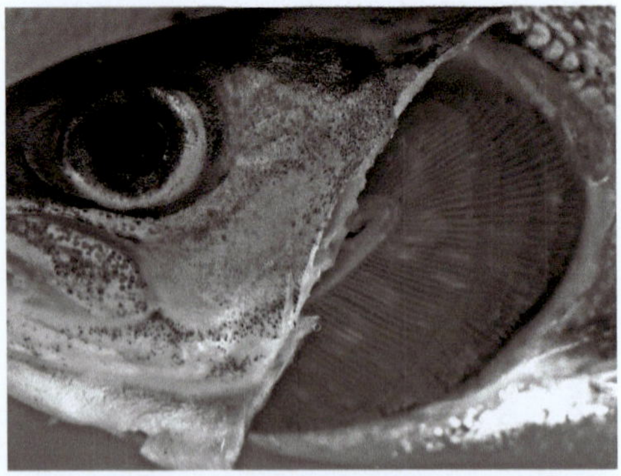

Fig. 1.2. Gross gill lesions characteristic of Atlantic salmon affected by AGD. (Photo, Dr Benita Vincent.)

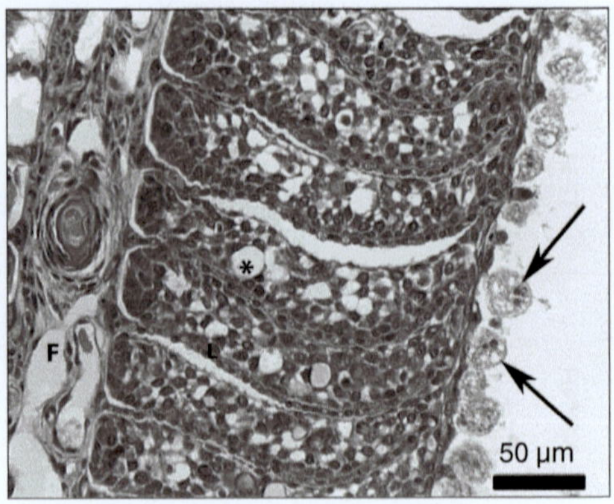

Fig. 1.3. Gill lesions typical of AGD, showing hyperplasia of epithelial and mucous cells leading to lamellar fusion. Numerous amoebae are present between gill filaments. Arrows indicate two examples of amoebae showing nucleus and endosymbiont; F, filament; L, lamella; *, mucous cell. (Photo, Karine Cadoret.)

1.2. Diagnosis of the Infection: Clinical Signs of the Disease

While respiratory distress and lethargy have been reported in AGD-affected fish, behavioural changes are not used to diagnose infection. Salmon farmers in Tasmania determine the severity of AGD by the presence of white gross lesions on the gills (Fig. 1.2) as they are a good indicator of AGD in fish farmed in areas enzootic for AGD (Adams *et al.*, 2004) when gill checks are done by an experienced person (Clark and Nowak, 1999). The gill patches represent hyperplastic lesions (Fig. 1.3), which can lead to lamellar fusion, often affecting whole filaments (Adams *et al.*, 2004). A standardized gross gill score methodology has been developed based on severity of lesions across 26 gill surfaces – both sides of all gill arches (Taylor *et al.*, 2007, 2016). A scoring system has been assessed for cases of complex or multifactorial gill disease (Fridman *et al.*, 2021).

Amoebae are usually present in the histological sections (Adams and Nowak, 2003; Dyková *et al.*, 2003, 2008). The parasite can be distinguished as a member of one of the two genera *Paramoeba* or *Neoparamoeba* on the basis of the presence of endosymbionts (Dyková *et al.*, 2003; Adl *et al.*, 2005); however, more detailed identification (to genus and species level) requires either PCR or *in situ* hybridization (Table 1.2 and Fig. 1.4; Young *et al.*, 2007, 2008a,b). This is due to the lack of morphological differences (even ultrastructural) between species of *Neoparamoeba* (see Dyková *et al.*, 2005; Young *et al.*, 2007). While immunofluorescence antibody test and immune-dot blot were used to confirm the presence of the parasite (Howard *et al.*, 1993; Douglas-Helders *et al.*, 2001b), the polyclonal antibodies used were not species specific (Morrison *et al.*, 2004). PCR of gill swabs has been developed

Table 1.2. Molecular methods for detection of *Neoparamoeba perurans*.

Method	Primers	Sample type	Reference
In situ hybridization	TGA CYG GTT CTT TCG RGA GCT G	Formalin-fixed, paraffin-embedded gills	Young *et al.* (2007)
PCR	Forward: 5′-ATC TTG ACY GGT TCT TTC GRG A-3′ Reverse: 5′-ATA GGT CTG CTT ATC ACT YAT TCT-3′	Gill/live culture	Young *et al.* (2008b)
	Forward: 5′-CTT ACT AGA CTT TCA CTA TTA CAC-3′ Reverse: 5′-TCT AAG CAG AAC GAA CTT TC-3′	Gill	Rozas *et al.* (2011)
Real-time PCR, SYBR green-based	QNperF3: 5′-GTT TAC ATA TTA TGA CCC ACT-3′ QNperR3: 5′-TAA ACC CAA TAG GTC TGC-3′	Gill swabs/sea water	Bridle *et al.* (2010)
Real-time TaqMan PCR	Peru forward: GTT CTT TCG GGA GCT GGG AG Peru reverse: GAA CTA TCG CCG GCA CAA AAG	Formalin-fixed, paraffin-embedded gills	Fringuelli *et al.* (2012)
	NP1: 5′-AAA AGA CCA TGC GAT TCG TAA AGT-3′ NP2: 5′-CAT TCT TTT CGG AGA GTG GAA ATT-3′	Gill	Downes *et al.* (2015)
CFX Connect PCR Detection system	QNperR3: 5′-TAA ACC CAA TAG GTC TGC-3′	Gill/gill swabs/sea water	Bridle *et al.* (2015); Wright *et al.* (2015)
RT qPCR	Pspp-forward: TTG TCA GAG GTG AAA TTC TTG GAT T Pspp-probe: ATG AAA GAC GAA CTT CTG Pspp-reverse: TGA AAA CAT CTT TGG CAA ATG C	Gill	Steigen *et al.* (2018)
LAMP	F3: 5′-TGA GTG ATA AGC AGA CCT ATT G-3′ B3: 5′-TTC GCA GAA GTT CGT CTT-3′	Gill swabs	Cano *et al.* (2019)
Salmonid 18S rDNA blocking PCR	1391F: 5′-TCG TCG GCA GCG TCA GAT GTG TAT AAG AGA CAG GTA CAC ACC GCC CGT C-3′ EukBr: 5′-GTC TCG TGG GCT CGG AGA TGT GTA TAA GAG ACA GTG ATC CTT CTG CAG GTT CAC CTA C-3′	Gill swabs	Patchett *et al.* (2024)

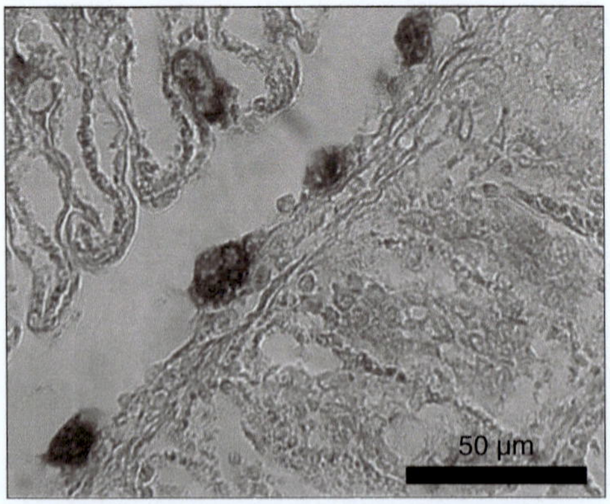

Fig. 1.4. *In situ* hybridization showing that all amoebae in the field of view are positive for *Neoparamoeba perurans*. (Photo, Karine Cadoret.)

and validated (Young *et al.*, 2008b; Bridle *et al.*, 2010). The advantages of this method are high sensitivity and specificity for the parasite and non-terminal sampling (Young *et al.*, 2008b). There was a positive correlation between the severity of the gross gill lesions and quantitative real-time PCR (qPCR) of gill swabs for *N. perurans* (see Bridle *et al.*, 2010), which further validates it as a diagnostic method. Downes *et al.* (2017) demonstrated that there were variations in detection sensitivities using PCR and that gill swabs had higher detection rates than gill samples. Type of gill swab affected sensitivity of detection (Fernandez-Senac *et al.*, 2020). PCR swabbing could detect *N. perurans* infection at least 3 weeks prior to any gross gill pathologies (Downes *et al.*, 2015) and is the preferred routine method for monitoring the pathogen in Norway and Scotland, in addition to gross gill scores (Boerlage *et al.*, 2022). In addition to fresh smear microscopy for characteristic amoebae on gills, point-of-care tests such as loop-mediated isothermal amplification (LAMP) assays have been developed targeting the parasite 18S rRNA (Cano *et al.*, 2019), although they are not yet in commercial use. Patchett *et al.* (2024) demonstrated improved sensitivity of *N. perurans* detection in gill swabs using a host 18S rDNA blocking assay. Propidium monoazide treatment of cultured amoebae prior to PCR has also been shown to distinguish between viable and non-viable cells, though this has not yet been applied to samples from infected fish (Wynne *et al.*, 2024).

Paramoeba and *Neoparamoeba* have eukaryotic endosymbionts (parasomes) in the trophozoites when examined under the light microscope (Fig. 1.3; Adl *et al.*, 2005). These endosymbionts, *Perkinsela amoebae*-like organisms (PLOs), are members of the order Kinetoplastida and are closely related to the fish parasite, *Ichthyobodo necator*, based on SSU rRNA gene sequence from different strains of *Neoparamoeba* (see Dyková *et al.*, 2003). The endosymbionts can be easily seen in smears (Zilberg *et al.*, 1999) and histological sections (Dyková and Novoa, 2001). The diagnosis of AGD is based on gill histopathology when amoebae possessing one or more endosymbiotic PLOs are detected in close association with hyperplastic epithelial-like cells with lamellar fusion and vesicle formation (Fig. 1.3; Dyková and Novoa, 2001; Adams and Nowak 2003; Dyková *et al.*, 2003, 2008).

1.3. External/Internal Lesions

Gills are the only organ affected, and most fish species develop white raised lesions on their gills (Fig. 1.2). The lesions usually start from the base of filaments, spread through the gill arch and often coalesce into a big lesion. In Atlantic salmon the dorsal area of the gills is usually more affected than the ventral area (Adams and Nowak, 2001). Macroscopic lesions in Atlantic salmon show good agreement with histological changes during the progression of AGD (Adams *et al.*, 2004).

In Atlantic salmon farmed in Tasmania, AGD was detected in histological sections at 13 weeks post-transfer to the marine environment, while gross signs were not detected until a week later (Adams and Nowak, 2003), whereas in Ireland gross AGD lesions can be detected within 6 weeks of transfer to sea (authors' experience). Increased intensity of lesions was associated with increased salinity (cessation of halocline) and higher water temperatures (Adams and Nowak 2003; Oldham *et al.*, 2016). Natural infections in farmed Atlantic salmon start with colonization of gills by amoeba and localized cellular changes, including epithelial desquamation and oedema. This is followed by initial focal epithelial hyperplasia and finally squamation-stratification of epithelium and an increase in the numbers of mucous cells within the lesions (Adams and Nowak, 2003). Formation of fully enclosed interlamellar vesicles in the advanced lesion is most likely a result of the proliferative character of this disease and may help with trapping and killing of amoebae (Adams and Nowak, 2001). Reinfection of salmon on the farm is evident 2 weeks after commercial freshwater bathing, with the severity of the lesions increasing 4 weeks post-bathing when gross pathology appears (Adams and Nowak, 2004). The lesion development is identical to the initial infection of the naïve fish (Adams and Nowak, 2004). Lesion characteristics and disease progression are the same in the laboratory challenges as that on farms. The disease usually progresses faster in a laboratory challenge, particularly when gill-isolated amoebae are added directly to the water in the tank containing naïve salmon, with morbidity occurring within 4 weeks at 15°C (Crosbie *et al.*, 2010b).

Reduced numbers of chloride cells and increased numbers of mucous cells (Munday *et al.*, 1990; Nowak and Munday, 1994; Zilberg and Munday, 2000; Powell *et al.*, 2001; Adams and Nowak, 2003; Roberts and Powell 2003, 2005) and formation of fully enclosed interlamellar vesicles (Adams and Nowak, 2001) were reported within AGD lesions. Inflammatory cells, identified on the basis of their morphology as neutrophils and macrophages, are present in the interlamellar cysts (Adams and Nowak, 2001). Cells positive for major histocompatibility complex (MHC) class II were present in higher numbers in AGD lesions (Morrison *et al.*, 2006a), while immunoglobulin (Ig)-positive cells occurred in low numbers similar to those in uninfected Atlantic salmon (Gross, 2007). While eosinophils were claimed to be the primary infiltrating cells in AGD lesions (Lovy *et al.*, 2007), this might have been due to the moribund state of salmon used for the ultrastructural study and not AGD, as there was no evidence of eosinophilia at the transcriptional level (Young *et al.*, 2008c).

1.4. Pathophysiology

The behaviour of fish dying of AGD and the fact that the disease causes severe gill lesions suggest that fish respiration would be affected (Kent *et al.*, 1988; Munday *et al.*, 1990; Rodger and McArdle, 1996). However, this was not supported in some physiological studies (Powell *et al.*, 2000; Fisk *et al.*, 2002; Leef *et al.*, 2005a, 2007). There were no differences in the rate of O_2 uptake between infected and control fish (Powell *et al.*, 2000). Arterial PO_2 and pH were significantly lower in the infected fish whereas PCO_2 was significantly higher in infected fish compared with controls prior to hypoxia (Powell *et al.*, 2000). The respiratory acidosis could have been due to increased mucus secretion observed during AGD (Powell *et al.*, 2000). Despite respiratory acidosis in AGD-affected fish, environmental hypoxia down to 25% of oxygen saturation did not result in respiratory failure in those fish (Powell *et al.*, 2000). Atlantic salmon with clinical AGD showed increased amplitude and rate of opercular movements (Fisk *et al.*, 2002).

This discrepancy between the presence of gill lesions and apparent lack of effects on respiration could be at least partly due to the fact that survival in AGD-affected Atlantic salmon following even minor surgical procedures such as dorsal aorta cannulation is relatively poor (Leef *et al.*, 2005a,b) and the fish used in most of the studies that did not report respiratory effects underwent surgery before the experiments. The lack of AGD effect on fish respiration could also be explained by cardiovascular or respiratory adjustments that can compensate for the reduction in gill surface area (Powell *et al.*, 2008).

In contrast, Hvas *et al.* (2017) demonstrated numerous physiological disturbances in salmon infected with *N. perurans* with a drastic reduction in maximum rate of O_2 uptake and a decrease in haematocrit and haemoglobin levels, suggesting that the previously used methods were inadequate to show effects of AGD. Furthermore, the severity of lesion was greater in this study (Hvas *et al.*, 2017) than in the previous experiments (Leef *et al.*, 2005a,b).

Changes in heart morphology in AGD-affected fish were reported (Powell *et al.*, 2002); however, there were no changes in lactate dehydrogenase activity in the ventricle suggesting that at least some of the heart functions were not affected. However, there was an overall thickening of the muscularis compactum in the ventricle of fish that had a history of heavy AGD (Powell *et al.*, 2002). AGD-affected Atlantic salmon had lower cardiac output and higher systemic vascular resistance than control fish (Leef *et al.*, 2005a,b, 2007). AGD-associated cardiac dysfunction appeared to be specific to Atlantic salmon, which would explain the higher susceptibility of this species compared with both brown and rainbow trout (Leef *et al.*, 2005b). While Atlantic salmon, brown trout (*Salmo trutta*) and rainbow trout had similar dorsal aortic pressure, cardiac output and systemic vascular resistance values, only AGD-affected salmon had significantly elevated systemic vascular resistance compared with the non-affected controls (Leef *et al.*, 2005a,b). Cardiac output was also approximately 35% lower in affected fish (Leef *et al.*, 2005a,b).

Numbers of chloride cells were reduced in AGD-affected fish in the lesions (Adams and Nowak, 2001) and in the intralamellar space (Chang *et al.*, 2019), suggesting that osmoregulation might be affected. This is further reflected by reduced succinate dehydrogenase activity and greater whole-body net efflux of ions (Powell *et al.*, 2001; Roberts and Powell, 2003). While there is some evidence of osmoregulatory problems in fish with AGD (Munday *et al.*, 2001; Powell *et al.*, 2005), it occurs only in severely affected fish, most likely those that are becoming moribund (Powell *et al.*, 2008). Osmoregulatory problems in AGD-affected fish may be because of the fish dying and not a cause of mortality due to AGD.

One of the main responses in AGD lesions is epithelial hyperplasia (Adams and Nowak, 2001). This morphological change is confirmed by an increase of proliferating cell nuclear antigen (PCNA) and interleukin-1β in the gill epithelium (Adams and Nowak, 2003; Bridle *et al.*, 2006a) and downregulation of the p53 tumour suppressor gene in the gills of Atlantic salmon experimentally infected with *N. perurans* (see Morrison *et al.*, 2006b). Other gene expression changes observed in the gills of infected fish may be due to changes in the types and ratios of cell populations in lesions. Despite different experimental conditions, including duration of infection and controls used, some of the changes in gene regulation were consistent in two experimental AGD infections (Table 1.3). The upregulation of anterior gradient 2-like protein could be a result of an increased number of mucous cells in lesions (Morrison and Nowak, 2005). Similarly, the downregulation of Na/K ATPase in AGD-affected fish or AGD lesions could reflect the reduction in numbers of chloride cells in AGD lesions (Adams and Nowak, 2001). Significant downregulation of immune genes was observed in the gills, and particularly in the gill lesions, of AGD-affected Atlantic salmon (Young

Table 1.3. Consistent changes in gene expression in Atlantic salmon from two separate experimental infections with *Neoparamoeba perurans*, shown as fold change.

	Fold change	
Genes	Whole gill versus infected naïve fish up to 8 days post-infection (hours post-infection in parentheses) (Morrison *et al.*, 2006b)	Lesion area versus normal gill area of the same individual 36 days post-infection (Young *et al.*, 2008c)
Upregulated genes		
Differentially regulated trout protein	2.31 (114–189)	2.82
Anterior gradient 2-like protein[a]	2.0–2.57 (0–189)	2.15–2.52
Downregulated genes		
TIMP-2 (tissue inhibitor of metalloproteinases)	7.67 (189)	2.32
Brain protein 44	2.36 (189)	2.12
Guanine nucleotide-binding protein	2.15 (189)	2.63–3.57
β_2-Microglobulin	3.08 (114)	2.06–2.56
Na/K ATPase	2.32 (44)	3.12–6.10

[a]Anterior gradient 2 expression was confirmed by qPCR (Morrison *et al.*, 2006b).

et al., 2008c). Similarly, a transcriptome study of AGD-affected gills revealed downregulation of genes involved in antigen processing and presentation through MHC-I/MHC-II complexes, the phosphatidylinositol 3′-kinase (PI3K)-Akt signalling pathway and the nuclear factor-κB (NF-κB) signalling pathway, while upregulated genes were from the C-type lectin and Toll-like receptor pathways and the Wnt and NOD signalling pathways (Botwright *et al.*, 2022). Upregulation of genes related to mucin secretion and cell proliferation and downregulation of pro-inflammatory and pro-apoptotic genes were associated with AGD severity, with mucin-5 and interleukin-4/13 considered key molecules during AGD (Marcos-López *et al.*, 2018). Investigation of AGD in salmon gill and serum, at a proteomic level, across various subclinical and clinical time points has provided insight into protein expression in very early disease stages (McCormack *et al.*, 2021) demonstrating a lack of a robust classical immune response before 7 days post-infection in the gill (Marcos-López and Rodger, 2020). Conversely, some of the proteins differentially expressed in serum initially exhibited a positive immune response with some immune suppression evident at later stages. Taken together, the pro-immune trend in serum and the diversity of downregulated proteins in the gill may indicate a local pathogen-derived suppression of host immune response (McCormack *et al.*, 2021).

Haemoglobin subunit β was downregulated both at gene (36 days post-infection; Young *et al.*, 2008c) and protein (21 days post-infection; E. Lowe and B.F. Nowak, 2009, unpublished results) levels in AGD-affected Atlantic salmon. This might be due directly to respiratory changes, or alternatively it could be related to changes in the level of antimicrobial peptides derived from β subunit of haemoglobin, which have been described from channel catfish (*Ictalurus punctatus*) infected with *Ichthyophthirius multifiliis* (see Ullal *et al.*, 2008). These peptides were reported to have parasiticidal properties against *I. multifiliis*, *Tetrahymena pyriformis* and *Amyloodinium ocellatum* (see Ullal *et al.*, 2008; Ullal and Noga, 2010).

An increase in standard and metabolic rates has been reported in AGD-affected fish (Powell *et al.*, 2008). This effect was related to the severity of infection. AGD can affect swimming performance of Atlantic salmon, particularly in repeated tests, possibly due to the inability of the infected salmon to recover from the previous test (Powell *et al.*, 2008).

1.5. Protective/Control Strategies

Freshwater bathing (Fig. 1.5) has been used by the salmon industry in Tasmania on a regular basis with frequency depending on severity of AGD as determined by gross gill checks. In the past, three to four freshwater baths during the full marine salmon production cycle were used (Clark and Nowak, 1999). Later the bathing frequency at least doubled, possibly partly due to an increased biomass of salmon in sea cages. Bathing frequency is driven by infection intensity; however, now it is conducted at a lower gill score than previously as the infection proceeds more rapidly and hence requires earlier treatment. Salmon farms in Scotland, Norway and Ireland now routinely use fresh water (either naturally sourced or produced by reverse osmosis on boats or pontoons) for bath treatments in pens or in well-boats. Freshwater bathing involved moving affected fish to an empty production cage with a liner filled with oxygenated fresh water (usually hyperoxic, at least at the beginning of the bath) or more recently freshwater barges/well-boats have been used (Figs 1.6 and 1.7) that often have reverse osmosis units on board to provide fresh water. The bath takes approximately 2–4 h from the time when the last fish entered the bath, but duration depends on the fish size with the larger salmon (over 3 kg) bathed for a shorter time. AGD in turbot has also been treated with freshwater bathing (Nowak *et al.*, 2002). The life cycle of ayu requires the fish to be moved from the marine hatchery to freshwater grow-out during the production cycle, which resolves AGD in the surviving fish (Crosbie *et al.*, 2010a).

Freshwater treatment is successful in removing most of the amoebae from the gills of infected fish; however, reinfection can occur within a few weeks, particularly in summer when the water temperature is high (Parsons *et al.*, 2001; Adams and Nowak, 2004). While a shorter freshwater bath to detach amoebae from the gills was suggested (Wright *et al.*, 2018a), it appears that a longer bath is necessary to kill *N. perurans*.

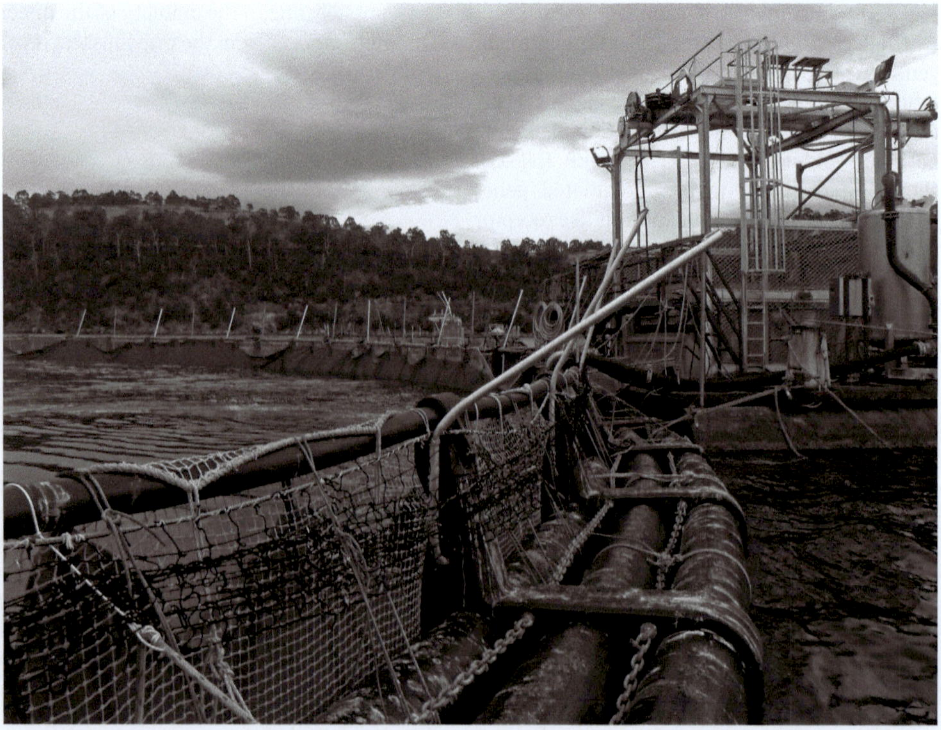

Fig. 1.5. Freshwater bathing on an Atlantic salmon farm in Tasmania. Note liner inside the mesh cage.

Atlantic salmon experimentally exposed for 2 h to used bath water were AGD-positive after 20 days, but an exposure to used bath water after a 4 h bath resulted in slower AGD development and less severe AGD signs (Taylor *et al.*, 2021). Additionally, limited access to fresh water in some salmon-farming areas and a high number of cages requiring bathing can restrict salmon production. Even very low salinity of the bath water can affect bathing efficacy. Bathing in soft water (19.3–37.4 mg $CaCO_3$/l) is more beneficial than bathing in hard water (173–236.3 mg $CaCO_3$/l) (Roberts and Powell, 2003). Freshwater bathing (up to 2 h in a hyperoxic bath) has no demonstrable adverse effects on Atlantic salmon, including no significant effect on blood plasma ions, acid–base and respiratory variables (Powell *et al.*, 2001). Alterations in bathing procedure or an alternative treatment may be required to achieve the total removal of the amoebae from the gills of fish (Parsons *et al.*, 2001).

While freshwater bathing is effective, it is however a short-term solution that is labour-intensive, expensive and requires access to fresh water. A range of alternative experimental treatments were tested. Bath treatments ranged from using disinfectants (hydrogen peroxide, chlorine dioxide and chloramine T) to parasiticides such as levamisole and bithionol (Clark and Nowak, 1999; Zilberg *et al.*, 2000; Munday and Zilberg, 2003; Harris *et al.*, 2004, 2005; Powell *et al.*, 2005; Florent *et al.*, 2007a; Martinsen *et al.*, 2018). In some trials, chemicals were added to the freshwater bath. Generally new treatments would be more useful if they could be applied directly to fish in sea water so that there would no longer be need for freshwater bathing. Sometimes *in vitro* results were promising but the treatment was not effective *in vivo*; for example, 15 min exposure to low temperature (3°C) reduced attachment of *N. perurans in vitro* but did not reduce AGD (Hudson *et al.*, 2022). Some experimental results suggested that a treatment should work well, but the field studies based on the experimental results did not confirm this. For example, levamisole (1.25 mg/l) added to the freshwater bath reduced mortality of AGD-affected Atlantic salmon under laboratory

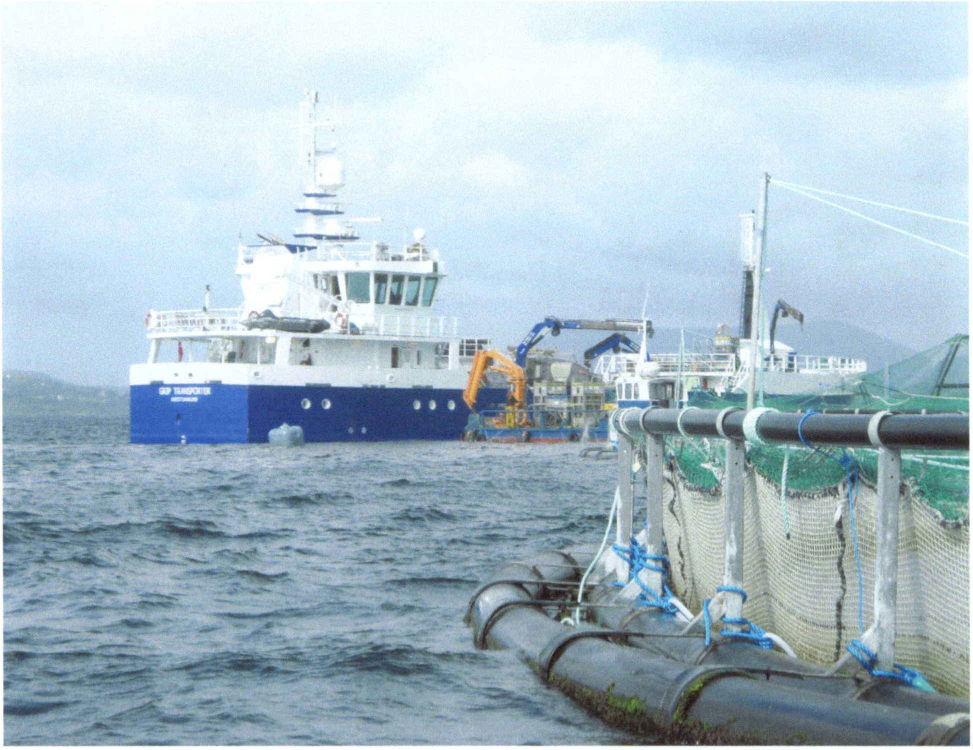

Fig. 1.6. Well-boat conducting freshwater bath treatments at marine Atlantic salmon pens (Ireland).

conditions (Zilberg *et al.*, 2000) but 2.5–5.0 mg/l did not have any effect on: (i) the time between bathings; (ii) the number of lesions; or (iii) the number of amoebae in histological lesions (Clark and Nowak, 1999). Levamisole was ineffective in a seawater bath at concentrations below 50 mg/l. At the effective concentration (results comparable to freshwater bath) it caused high fish mortality (Munday and Zilberg, 2003). Oral treatments included bithionol and mucolytic agents (Roberts and Powell, 2005; Florent *et al.*, 2007b, 2009). While some of these treatments gave promising results in laboratory challenges, particularly l-cysteine (a mucolytic agent) and bithionol (Roberts and Powell, 2005; Florent *et al.*, 2007a,b), they are not used commercially possibly due to their higher costs. Hydrogen peroxide has been used on salmon farms with no access to fresh water despite the low margin of safety at higher water temperatures (Adams *et al.*, 2012; Rodger, 2014; Martinsen *et al.*, 2018; Wynne *et al.*, 2019). Bath treatments with fresh water or hydrogen peroxide can lead to physical trauma, crowding stress and to subsequent manifestations of other systemic diseases, and these plus other mechanical or thermal bath treatments for sea lice have led to these methods being one of the priority health and welfare challenges for marine salmon in Norway and the UK (Persson *et al.*, 2022; Wiese *et al.*, 2023; Sommerset *et al.*, 2024).

Novel fish-farming systems have been used to control parasitic diseases. For example, snorkel cages based on a controlled and limited surface access, which can vary environmental conditions (e.g. salinity), were developed to control sea lice infections (Wright *et al.*, 2017b). Elevated AGD score was observed in fewer salmon in the seawater and freshwater snorkel cages; in particular, there was a decrease by 65% in salmon positive for *N. perurans* in the freshwater snorkel cage (Wright *et al.*, 2018b). While reduced AGD lesions were observed in the salmon in snorkel cages, the cages may require particular environmental conditions and the effect on AGD may be related to other factors (Wright *et al.*, 2017b).

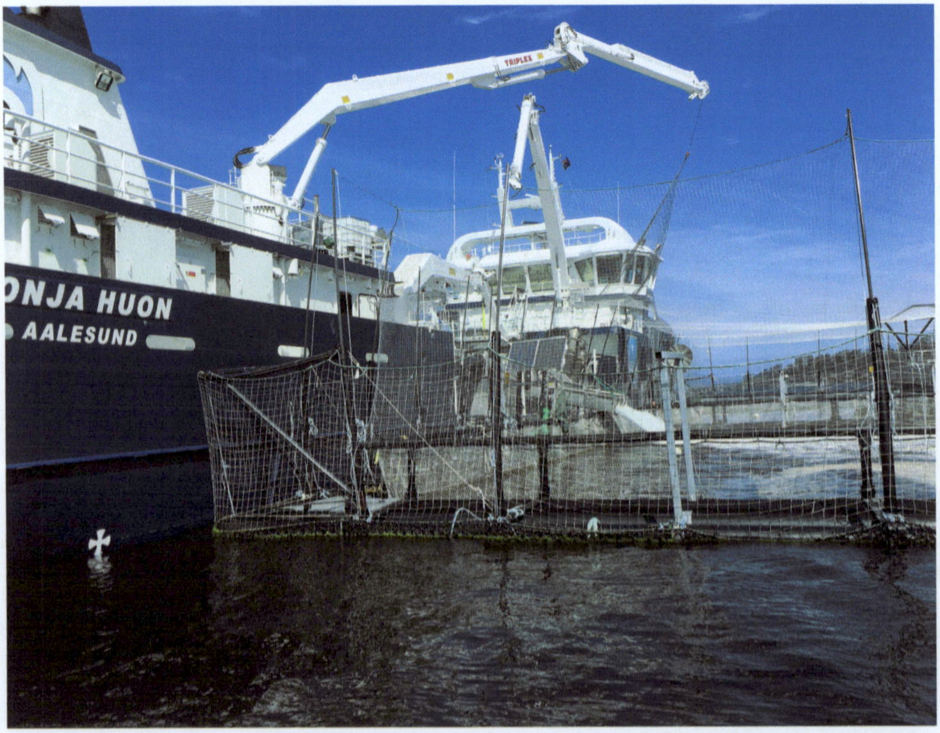

Fig. 1.7. Farmed Atlantic salmon crowded in a pen adjacent to the well-boat in preparation for transfer to wells for freshwater treatment (Australia).

Offshore farming or recirculating aquaculture systems are two other options to reduce the impact of AGD. Offshore farming moves the fish further away from the coastal environment where *N. perurans* is prevalent and it could reduce parasitic infections including impact of AGD (Sokołowska and Nowak, 2020). Significant reduction of parasitic infections was shown for ranched southern bluefin tuna, *Thunnus maccoyii*, when the fish were moved further from the coast (Kirchhoff *et al.*, 2011). Parasites, such as blood fluke, *Cardicola* spp. and sea lice (*Caligus chiastos*), were absent from the offshore ranched tuna, possibly as a result of the increased distance between the bottom of the pen and the ocean floor, increased currents and reduced encounters with wild fish (Kirchhoff *et al.*, 2011). Offshore farming of Atlantic salmon is under development in a number of countries (Kristiensen *et al.*, 2017).

The innate immune response appears to be suppressed in infected fish. Atlantic salmon kidney phagocyte respiratory burst was suppressed 8 and 11 days post-infection in a laboratory challenge (Gross *et al.*, 2004a, 2005). However, it is possible that these results were size specific as most experiments with Atlantic salmon are done using smaller smolt. The large Atlantic salmon smolt (>350 g) cohort had significantly lower loads of *N. perurans* and reduced AGD gill scores compared to the smaller smolt (<200 g) (Smith *et al.*, 2022a). Upregulation of immune genes was observed in large smolts, suggesting size-dependent resistance to AGD in AGD-naïve Atlantic salmon (Smith *et al.*, 2022a).

Innate immunity is considered important for protection against AGD (Findlay and Munday, 1998) and thus immunostimulants should have a role in reducing the impact of AGD on the salmon industry. Experimental injection with CpGs (DNA motifs characteristic for bacteria) increased protection against AGD by 38% (Bridle *et al.*, 2003). This suggested that immunostimulants could contribute to the successful management of AGD. However, there were no consistent effects detected in laboratory or field experiments involving Atlantic salmon fed β-glucans or other commercially available immunostimulants (Zilberg *et al.*, 2000; Nowak *et al.*, 2004a; Bridle *et al.*, 2005).

Both increased survival and reduced gill pathology have been used to measure resistance to AGD in experimental studies. Resistance to AGD was described in Atlantic salmon as a result of previous exposure (Table 1.4) or prolonged exposure (Bridle *et al.*, 2005; Vincent *et al.*, 2008) at low water temperatures. This resistance to subsequent infections suggests vaccination may be a successful way to manage AGD. Experimental vaccines tested ranged from live or killed amoebae (with or without adjuvant) to DNA vaccine (Zilberg and Munday, 2001; Morrison and Nowak, 2005; Cook *et al.*, 2008). The live or killed vaccines were applied by bath (Morrison and Nowak, 2005) or anal intubation or intraperitoneal injection (Zilberg and Munday, 2001). DNA vaccine was injected intramuscularly (Cook *et al.*, 2008). Recombinant protein r22C03 together with Freund Complete Adjuvant were injected interperitoneally as a recombinant vaccine (Valdenegro-Vega *et al.*, 2015). None of the experimental vaccinations provided significant and consistent protection against infection (Zilberg and Munday, 2001; Morrison and Nowak, 2005; Cook *et al.*, 2008; Valdenegro-Vega *et al.*, 2015).

So far there is no evidence of an effective innate (Bridle *et al.*, 2006a,b; Morrison *et al.*, 2007) or acquired (Findlay and Munday, 1998; Gross *et al.*, 2004b; Morrison *et al.*, 2006b; Vincent *et al.*, 2006, 2009; Valdenegro-Vega *et al.*, 2015) immune response to AGD. Based on a transcriptional response study of AGD-affected Atlantic salmon it was suggested that *N. perurans* can evade the host immune response by disrupting the molecular mechanisms essential for activation of effector T-cell mediated responses (Young *et al.*, 2008c). However, the mechanism of this disruption is still unclear. A comparison of the transcriptomes of virulent and avirulent *N. perurans* isolates suggested that elongation factor and cathepsin were potential vaccine targets (Smith *et al.*, 2022b). An interaction between host and *N. perurans* cathepsin B was identified in another study, providing an opportunity for development of a vaccine or novel treatments against AGD (Botwright *et al.*, 2022).

Selective breeding for AGD resistance has been one of the components of Atlantic salmon industry selective breeding programmes in Tasmania. Knowledge of the actual resistance mechanism is not essential for the success of selection for resistance (Guy *et al.*, 2006). A significant heritable component in AGD resistance, measurable through gross gill scores, was demonstrated in an Atlantic salmon population in Tasmania (Taylor *et al.*, 2007, 2009a,b). The selection trait for AGD resistance utilized in the Tasmanian Atlantic salmon industry breeding programme is gill score at the population-average freshwater bathing threshold (Taylor, 2010). There was no relationship between resistance to AGD and specific anti-*Neoparamoeba* antibody titre in both natural and experimental infections (Vincent *et al.*, 2008; Taylor *et al.*, 2009a,b, 2010; Villavedra *et al.*, 2010). It therefore appears that resistance to AGD in Atlantic salmon is most likely multifactorial and under polygenic control (Taylor, 2010). Genomic selection for AGD resistance in Atlantic salmon has indicated heritable characteristics ($h^2 \sim 0.25$–0.30) in two regions of chromosome 18 (Robledo *et al.*, 2018). Quantitative trait locus (QTL) regions on chromosomes ssa04, ssa09 and ssa13 in Atlantic salmon were linked with AGD resistance (Boison *et al.*, 2019).

Other health management strategies used on salmon farms can include: (i) reducing stocking density; (ii) frequent removal of mortalities; (iii) net fouling management; and (iv) fallowing of sites. Lower Atlantic salmon stocking density significantly improved survival of the fish in an experimental AGD challenge, with morbidity starting after 23 days for salmon stocked at 5.0 kg/m^3 and after 29 days for salmon stocked at 1.7 kg/m^3 (Crosbie *et al.*, 2010b). AGD prevalence was greater in Atlantic salmon farmed in 60 m cages (stocked at 1.7 kg/m^3) than 80 m cages (stocked at 0.7 kg/m^3) at the beginning of a field experiment (Douglas-Helders *et al.*, 2004). This is consistent with anecdotal information from salmon farms in Tasmania where cages with lower stocking densities require less frequent freshwater bathing (Nowak, 2001). One salmon company in Tasmania uses reduced stocking density in summer (summer average 5–6 kg/m^3 with summer maximum at 8 kg/m^3; and winter average 7–8 kg/m^3 with winter maximum at 12 kg/m^3). Removal of dead fish can contribute to reduction of the risks of AGD outbreaks. The amoebae can not only survive on the gills of

Table 1.4. Experimental evidence for resistance to subsequent AGD infections following previous exposures. (Adapted from Gross, 2007; Vincent, 2008).

		Findlay and Munday (1998)			
	Findlay *et al*. (1995)	Trial 1	Trial 2	Gross *et al*. (2004a)	Vincent *et al*. (2006)
Treatment groups	FW[a] maintained[b]/ FW bathed/SW[a] maintained; naïve	FW bathed[b]; naïve	FW maintained/×2 FW bath/×1 FW bath; naïve	FW bathed/SW maintained[b]/ FW maintained; naïve	FW bathed[b]; naïve
Infection method	Cohabitation	Cohabitation	Cohabitation	Inoculation (3300 cells/l)	Inoculation (500 cells/l)
Salinity (ppt)	Unknown	Unknown	Unknown	36	35
Temperature (°C)	14	14	14	17	12/16
First exposure (weeks)	4	4	4	2	4
FW bath (h)	None	2	2	4	24
Resolution (weeks)	4	4	4	4	5
Second exposure (weeks)	4	4	4	4	5
Assessment of infection	Gross gill score	Gross gill score	Gross gill score	Cumulative mortality, histology	Cumulative mortality, histology

[a]FW, fresh water; SW, sea water.
[b]Treatment protected from subsequent infection.

dead fish for up to 30 h but also colonize salmon gills post-mortem, therefore dead salmon can be a reservoir of the pathogen (Douglas-Helders *et al.*, 2000).

Cage netting and associated fouling were suggested to be reservoirs of amoebae (Nowak, 2001; Tan *et al.*, 2002). There was a negative relationship between the number of net changes and the prevalence of AGD infection (Clark and Nowak, 1999). However, Atlantic salmon in cages treated with copper-based antifouling paint had significantly greater prevalence of AGD infection (Douglas-Helders *et al.*, 2003a,b). This is in contrast to the results of *in vitro* toxicity tests. Six days' exposure to copper sulfate concentrations (ranging from 10 to 100,000 μM) at 20°C significantly reduced survival of gill-isolated amoebae under *in vitro* conditions (Douglas-Helders *et al.*, 2005). This discrepancy could be due to the antifouling paint affecting AGD prevalence through other mechanisms than its toxicity to the amoeba. Cnidarian biofouling organisms (such as *E. larynx*) which are washed into the water column when cleaning nets have been shown to contribute to gill histopathology (Østevik *et al.*, 2021) and co-challenge trials with these and *N. perurans* to assess whether susceptibility to AGD is increased did not indicate increased gill pathology (Bloecher *et al.*, 2018).

Fallowing has not been fully investigated as a management strategy. Atlantic salmon from cages that were rotated to other farm sites fallowed for 4–97 days needed fewer freshwater baths and had greater biomass at the end of the trial than fish grown in stationary cages (Douglas-Helders *et al.*, 2004). While towing cages was considered by the industry as a potential way to reduce infection through increased water flow, a short-term towing experiment did not show any effect on AGD prevalence (Douglas-Helders *et al.*, 2004).

Most experimental studies on AGD were initially based on mixed-sex diploid Atlantic salmon farmed in Tasmania. However, salmon industries increasingly rely on all-female stock and triploid fish to provide whole-year market supply and avoid early maturation. Triploid Atlantic salmon appeared to be more sensitive to AGD on the farms (Nowak, 2001). In an experimental infection the survival of triploid fish was significantly lower and mortality occurred earlier than in diploid Atlantic salmon (Powell *et al.*, 2008). However, this difference was not related to the severity of gill lesions as on day 28 post-infection the triploid fish had a lower percentage of gill filaments affected by AGD than diploid fish (Powell *et al.*, 2008). Furthermore, current research uses Atlantic salmon selectively bred for AGD resistance (Smith *et al.*, 2022a), which may explain discrepancies in results between earlier and later studies. Genetic differences between Atlantic salmon used in AGD studies may result in other inconsistencies in the results of AGD research; for example, most of the initial AGD studies were done in Tasmania using salmon originating from the Philip River in Canada which are genetically different from Atlantic salmon farmed and used for research in Europe (Lubieniecki *et al.*, 2010).

1.6. Conclusions and Suggestions for Future Studies

While AGD has been continuously affecting Tasmanian salmon producers, now it has become an emerging disease on a global scale. There are increased reports of new geographic locations and hosts for AGD, which is not surprising as *N. perurans* is a cosmopolitan species. The increase of AGD outbreaks may be related to the intensification of aquaculture (Nowak, 2007) or global climate change (Nowak *et al.*, 2010), or to an increased awareness of the disease and improved diagnostic tests.

The presence of the eukaryotic endosymbiont is one of the characteristics of this species and the genus, as well as for the members of the genus *Paramoeba*. SSU rRNA gene phylogenies of *Neoparamoeba* sp. and its endosymbiont (PLO) strongly supported co-evolution of the amoeba and the endosymbiont (Dyková *et al.*, 2008). However, the role of the endosymbiont, in particular its contribution to pathogenicity of different isolates, is still unclear and warrants further investigation.

Co-infections with other parasites were described in some AGD outbreaks (Dyková *et al.*, 2010; Nowak *et al.*, 2010; Bustos *et al.*, 2011); however, their significance is unclear. CGD continues to be a major challenge for marine salmon farms with AGD being a part of the complex disease picture in some, but not all, of the cases (Herrero *et al.*, 2018; Jones and Price, 2022). *Uronema marinum* was isolated from gills of a salmon affected by AGD and on rare occasions was seen in histological sections from AGD-affected salmon gills, however its contribution to the gill pathology is unknown (Dyková *et al.*, 2010). Ectoparasites such as the sea louse *L. salmonis* were suggested to be involved in the AGD infection of farmed Atlantic salmon in the USA (Nowak *et al.*, 2010) and co-infection of *N. perurans* and *Caligus rogercresseyi* was reported in Atlantic salmon in Chile (Bustos *et al.*, 2011). The role of bacteria was evaluated in experimental challenges and in the field (Bowman and Nowak, 2004; Embar-Gopinath *et al.*, 2005, 2006). Exposure to bacteria *Winogradskyella* sp. before exposure to *N. perurans* significantly increased the percentage of affected gill filaments, but the salmon exposed to the amoeba alone still got infected (Embar-Gopinath *et al.*, 2006). Gill microbiome dysbiosis was suggested as a contributor to the development of AGD (Nowak and Archibald, 2018; Slinger *et al.*, 2020) and local environment and environmental change highlighted as a significant factor (Nowak and Archibald, 2018; O'Halloran *et al.*, 2022). A holistic approach to AGD is essential, including taking into account the host, the amoeba, its eukaryotic endosymbiont *Perkinsela* sp., and the bacteria that interact with each of these organisms, including gill microbiome and amoeba microbiome (Nowak and Archibald, 2018). Comparative genomic and transcriptomic frameworks and well-designed experimental infections are needed to investigate these interactions. Improved understanding of the relationship between the amoeba and other organisms may improve management of this disease (Botwright *et al.*, 2022).

While our knowledge of *N. perurans* and AGD has increased significantly since they were first reported, there are still many unanswered questions about the pathogen and the disease. As the disease is increasingly affecting fish farmed in the marine environment and is one of the more significant emerging diseases in mariculture, further research is necessary to improve our ability to manage AGD.

Acknowledgements

B.F.N. is grateful to her research students (Honours, Masters and PhD) who worked on AGD as well as research and technical staff who significantly contributed to our knowledge and understanding of AGD. She would like to thank Dr Phil Crosbie, Dr Mark Adams, Dr Benita Vincent, Dr Andrew Bridle, Dr Dina Zilberg and Dr Melanie Leef for their helpful comments on drafts of the original chapter. All authors are grateful to the salmon industry for providing information on current management strategies. Thanks to Dr Benita Vincent, Dr Philip Crosbie and Karine Cadoret for providing photographs used in this chapter. Financial support for the original chapter, in the 1st edition of *Fish Parasites: Pathobiology and Protection* (2012), was provided by the Australian Research Council (ARC)/National Health and Medical Research Council (NHMRC) Network for Parasitology and the Australian Academy of Science.

Note

[1] Figures 1.5, 1.6 and 1.7, and Tables 1.1, 1.2 and 1.3, are the author's own.

References

Adams, M.B. and Nowak, B.F. (2001) Distribution and structure of lesions in the gills of Atlantic salmon, *Salmo salar* L., affected with amoebic gill disease. *Journal of Fish Diseases* 24, 535–542.

Adams, M.B. and Nowak, B.F. (2003) Amoebic gill disease (AGD): sequential pathology in cultured Atlantic salmon (*Salmo salar* L.). *Journal of Fish Diseases* 26, 601–614.

Adams, M.B. and Nowak, B.F. (2004) Experimental amoebic gill disease of Atlantic salmon, *Salmo salar* L.: further evidence for the primary pathogenic role of *Neoparamoeba* sp., (Page, 1987). *Journal of Fish Diseases* 27, 105–113.

Adams, M.B., Ellard, K. and Nowak, B.F. (2004) Gross pathology and its relationship with histopathology of amoebic gill disease (AGD) in farmed Atlantic salmon, *Salmo salar* L. *Journal of Fish Diseases* 27, 151–161.

Adams, M.B., Villavedra, M. and Nowak, B.F. (2008) An opportunistic detection of amoebic gill disease (AGD) in blue warehou (*Seriolella brama* Günther) collected from an Atlantic salmon (*Salmo salar* L.) production cage in south eastern Tasmania. *Journal of Fish Diseases* 31, 713–717.

Adams, M.B., Crosbie, P.B.B. and Nowak, B.F. (2012) Preliminary success using hydrogen peroxide to treat Atlantic salmon, *Salmo salar* L., affected with experimentally induced amoebic gill disease (AGD). *Journal of Fish Diseases* 35, 839–848.

Adl, S.M., Simpson, A.G.B., Farmer, M.A., Anderson, R.A., Anderson, O.R. *et al.* (2005) The new higher level classification of eukaryotes with emphasis on the taxonomy of protists. *Journal of Eukaryotic Microbiology* 52, 399–455.

Bloecher, N., Powell, M., Hytterød, S., Gjessing, M., Wiik-Nielsen, J. *et al.* (2018) Effects of cnidarian biofouling on salmon gill health and development of amoebic gill disease. *PLoS One* 13, e0199842.

Boerlage, A.S., Ashby, A., Eze, J.I., Gunn, G.J. and Reeves, A. (2022) Field evaluation of diagnostic sensitivity (DSe) and specificity (DSp) of common tests for amoebic gill disease (AGD) and complex gill disease (CGD) in cultured Atlantic salmon (*Salmo salar*) in Scotland using Bayesian latent class models. *Preventive Veterinary Medicine* 204, 105654.

Boison, S.A., Gjerde, B., Hillestad, B., Makvandi-Nejad, S. and Moghadam, H.K. (2019) Genomic and transcriptomic analysis of amoebic gill disease resistance in Atlantic salmon (*Salmo salar* L.). *Frontiers in Genetics* 10, 68.

Botwright, N.A., Mohamed, A.R., Slinger, J., Lima, P.C. and Wynne, J.W. (2022) Host–parasite interaction of Atlantic salmon (*Salmo salar*) and the ectoparasite *Neoparamoeba perurans* in amoebic gill disease. *Frontiers in Immunology* 12, 672700. DOI: 10.3389/fimmu.2021.672700.

Bowman, J. and Nowak, B. (2004) Salmonid gill bacteria and their relationship to amoebic gill disease (AGD). *Journal of Fish Diseases* 27, 483–492.

Bridle, A.R., Butler, R. and Nowak, B.F. (2003) Immunostimulatory CpG oligodeoxynucleotides increase resistance against amoebic gill disease in Atlantic salmon, *Salmo salar* L. *Journal of Fish Diseases* 26, 367–371.

Bridle, A.R., Carter, C.G., Morrison, R.N. and Nowak, B.F. (2005) The effects of beta-glucan administration on macrophage respiratory burst activity and Atlantic salmon (*Salmo salar* L.) challenged with amoebic gill disease (AGD) – evidence of inherent resistance. *Journal of Fish Diseases* 28, 347–356.

Bridle, A.R., Morrison, R.N. and Nowak, B.F. (2006a) The expression of immune-regulatory genes in rainbow trout, *Oncorhynchus mykiss*, during an amoebic gill disease (AGD) infection. *Fish and Shellfish Immunology* 20, 346–364.

Bridle, A., Morrison, R., Cupit Cunningham, P.M. and Nowak, B. (2006b) Quantitation of immune response gene expression and cellular localisation of interleukin-1β mRNA in Atlantic salmon, *Salmo salar* L., affected by amoebic gill disease (AGD). *Veterinary Immunology and Immunopathology* 114, 121–134.

Bridle, A.R., Crosbie, P.B.B., Cadoret, K. and Nowak, B.F. (2010) Rapid detection and quantification of *Neoparamoeba perurans* in the marine environment. *Aquaculture* 301, 56–61.

Bridle, A.R., Davenport, D., Crosbie, P.B.B., Polinski, M. and Nowak, B.F. (2015) *Neoparamoeba perurans* loses virulence during clonal culture. *International Journal for Parasitology* 45(9–10), 575–578. DOI: 10.1016/j.ijpara.2015.04.005.

Bridle, A.R., Hill, T., Smith, A., Crosbie, P. and Nowak, B.F. (2021) Experimental exposure to low concentrations of *Neoparamoeba perurans* induces amoebic gill disease in Atlantic salmon. *Journal of Fish Diseases* 44(7), 1025–1031. DOI: 10.1111/jfd.13363.

Bustos, P.A., Young, N.D., Rozas, M.A., Bohle, H.M., Ildefonso, R.S. *et al.* (2011) Amoebic gill disease (AGD) in Atlantic salmon (*Salmo salar*) farmed in Chile. *Aquaculture* 310(3–4), 281–288. DOI: 10.1016/j.aquaculture.2010.11.001.

Cano, I., McCullough, R., Mulhearn, B., Gunning, S., Waine, A. *et al.* (2019) Non-lethal loop-mediated amplification assay as a point-of-care diagnostics tool for *Neoparamoeba perurans*, the causative agent of amoebic gill disease. *Journal of Fish Diseases* 43, 779–790.

Chang, Y., Hamlin-Wright, H., Monaghan, S., Herath, T., Baily, J. *et al.* (2019) Changes in distribution, morphology and ultrastructure of chloride cell in Atlantic salmon during an AGD infection. *Journal of Fish Diseases* 42, 1433–1446.

Clark, A. and Nowak, B.F. (1999) Field investigations of amoebic gill disease in Atlantic salmon, *Salmo salar* L., in Tasmania. *Journal of Fish Diseases* 22, 433–443.

Collins, C., Hall, M., Fordyce, M.J. and White, P. (2019) Survival and growth *in vitro* of *Paramoeba perurans* populations cultured under different salinities and temperatures. *Protist* 170, 153–167.

Cook, M., Elliott, N., Campbell, G., Patil, J., Holmes, B. *et al.* (2008) *Amoebic Gill Disease (AGD) Vaccine Development Phase II – Molecular Basis of Host–Pathogen Interactions in Amoebic Gill Disease.* Aquafin Cooperative Research Centre for Sustainable Aquaculture of Finfish project 3.4.4 (2) (Fisheries Research and Development Corporation project 2004/217). Commonwealth Scientific and Industrial Research Organisation (CSIRO), Hobart, Tasmania, Australia, 85 pp.

Crosbie, P.B.B., Nowak, B.F. and Carson, J. (2003) Isolation of *Neoparamoeba pemaquidensis* Page, 1987 from marine and estuarine sediments in Tasmania. *Bulletin of the European Association of Fish Pathologists* 23, 241–244.

Crosbie, P.B.B., Macload, C., Forbes, S. and Nowak, B. (2005) Distribution of *Neoparamoeba* sp. in sediments around marine finfish farming sites in Tasmania. *Diseases of Aquatic Organisms* 67, 61–66.

Crosbie, P.B.B., Ogawa, K., Nakano, D. and Nowak, B.F. (2010a) Amoebic gill disease in hatchery-reared ayu, *Plecoglossus altivelis* (Temminck and Schlegel), in Japan is caused by *Neoparamoeba perurans*. *Journal of Fish Diseases* 33, 455–458.

Crosbie, P.B.B., Bridle, A.R., Leef, M.J. and Nowak, B.F. (2010b) Effects of different batches of *Neoparamoeba perurans* and fish stocking densities on the severity of amoebic gill disease in Atlantic salmon, *Salmo salar* L. *Aquaculture Research* 41, e505–e516.

Douglas-Helders, M., Nowak, B., Zilberg, D. and Carson, J. (2000) Survival of *Paramoeba pemaquidensis* on dead salmon: implications for management of cage hygiene. *Bulletin of the European Association of Fish Pathologists* 20, 167–169.

Douglas-Helders, M., Saksida, S., Raverty, S. and Nowak, B.F. (2001a) Temperature as a risk factor for outbreaks of amoebic gill disease in farmed Atlantic salmon (*Salmo salar*). *Bulletin of the European Association of Fish Pathologists* 21, 114–116.

Douglas-Helders, M., Carson, J., Howard, T. and Nowak, B. (2001b) Development and validation of a new dot blot test for the detection of *Paramoeba pemaquidensis* (Page) in fish. *Journal of Fish Diseases* 24, 273–280.

Douglas-Helders, M., Tan, C.F.K., Carson, J. and Nowak, B.F. (2003a) Effects of copper-based antifouling treatment on the presence of *Neoparamoeba pemaquidensis* Page 1987 on nets and gills of reared Atlantic salmon (*Salmo salar*). *Aquaculture* 221, 13–22.

Douglas-Helders, M., O'Brien, D.P., McCorkell, B.E., Zilberg, D., Gross, A. *et al.* (2003b) Temporal and spatial distribution of paramoebae in the water column – a pilot study. *Journal of Fish Diseases* 26, 231–240.

Douglas-Helders, G.M., Weir, I.J., O'Brien, D.P., Carson, J. and Nowak, B.F. (2004) Effects of husbandry on prevalence of amoebic gill disease and performance of reared Atlantic salmon (*Salmo salar* L.). *Aquaculture* 241, 21–30.

Douglas-Helders, M., Nowak, B. and Butler, R. (2005) The effect of environmental factors on the distribution of *Neoparamoeba pemaquidensis* in Tasmania. *Journal of Fish Diseases* 28, 583–592.

Downes, J.K., Henshilwood, K., Collins, E.M., Ryan, A., O'Connor, I. *et al.* (2015) A longitudinal study of amoebic gill disease on a marine Atlantic salmon farm utilising a real-time PCR assay for the detection of *Neoparamoeba perurans*. *Aquaculture Environment Interactions* 7, 239–251.

Downes, J.K., Rigby, M.L., Taylor, RS., Maynard, B.T., MacCarthy, E. *et al.* (2017) Evaluation of non-destructive molecular diagnostics of the detection of *Neoparamoeba perurans*. *Frontiers in Marine Science* 4, 61. DOI: 10.3389/fmars.2017.00061.

Dyková, I. and Novoa, B. (2001) Comments on diagnosis of amoebic gill in turbot (*Scophthalmus maximus*). *Bulletin of the European Association of Fish Pathologists* 21, 40–44.

Dykova, I., Figueras, A. and Novoa, B. (1995) Amoebic gill infection of turbot, *Scophthalmus maximus*. *Folia Parasitologica (Praha)* 42(2), 91–96.

Dyková, I., Figueras, A., Novoa, B. and Casal, J.F. (1998) *Paramoeba* sp., an agent of amoebic gill disease of turbot *Scophthalmus maximus*. *Diseases of Aquatic Organisms* 33, 137–141.

Dyková, I., Figueras, A. and Peric, Z. (2000) *Neoparamoeba* Page 1987: light and electron microscopic observations on six strains of different origin. *Diseases of Aquatic Organisms* 43, 217–223.

Dyková, I., Fiala, I., Lom, J. and Lukeš, J. (2003) *Perkinsiella amoebae*-like endosymbionts of *Neoparamoebae* spp., relatives of the kinetoplastid *Ichthyobodo*. *European Journal of Protistology* 39, 37–52.

Dyková, I., Nowak, B.F., Crosbie, P.B.B., Fiala, I., Pecková, H. *et al.* (2005) *Neoparamoeba branchiphila* n. sp. and related species of genus *Neoparamoeba* Page, 1987: morphological and molecular characterisation of selected strains. *Journal of Fish Diseases* 28, 49–64.

Dyková, I., Nowak, B., Pecková, H., Fiala, I., Crosbie, P. and Dvořáková, H. (2007) Phylogeny of *Neoparamoeba* strains isolated from marine fish and invertebrates as inferred from SSU rDNA sequences. *Diseases of Aquatic Organisms* 74, 57–65.

Dyková, I., Fiala, I. and Pecková, H. (2008) *Neoparamoeba* spp. and their eukaryotic endosymbionts similar to *Perkinsela amoebae* (Hollande, 1980): coevolution demonstrated by SSU rRNA gene phylogenies. *European Journal of Protistology* 44, 269–277.

Dyková, I., Tyml, T., Kostka, M. and Pecková, H. (2010) Strains of *Uronema marinum* (Scuticociliatia) co-isolated with amoebae of the genus *Neoparamoeba*. *Diseases of Aquatic Organisms* 89, 71–77.

Embar-Gopinath, S., Butler, R. and Nowak, B. (2005) Influence of salmonid gill bacteria on development and severity of amoebic gill disease. *Diseases of Aquatic Organisms* 67, 55–60.

Embar-Gopinath, S., Crosbie, P. and Nowak, B.F. (2006) Concentration effects of *Winogradskyella* sp. on the incidence and severity of amoebic gill disease. *Diseases of Aquatic Organisms* 73, 43–47.

English, C.J., Tyml, T., Botwright, N., Barnes, A.C., Wynne, J.W. *et al.* (2019) A diversity of amoebae colonise the gills of farmed Atlantic salmon (*Salmo salar*) with amoebic gill disease (AGD). *European Journal of Protistology* 67, 27–45.

English, C.J., Botwright, N.A., Adams, M.B., Barnes, A.C., Wynne, J.W. *et al.* (2021) Immersion challenge of naïve Atlantic salmon with cultured *Nolandella* sp. and *Pseudoparamoeba* sp. did not increase the severity of *Neoparamoeba perurans*-induced amoebic gill disease (AGD). *Journal of Fish Diseases* 44, 149–160. DOI: 10.1111/jfd.13319.

Fernandez-Senac, C., Fridman, S., Sokolowska, J., Monaghan, S.J., Garzon, T. *et al.* (2020) A comparison of the use of different swab materials for optimal diagnosis of amoebic gill disease (AGD) in Atlantic salmon (*Salmo salar* L.). *Journal of Fish Diseases* 43, 1463–1472.

Findlay, V.L. and Munday, B.L. (1998) Further studies on acquired resistance to amoebic gill disease (AGD) in Atlantic salmon, *Salmo salar* L. *Journal of Fish Diseases* 21, 121–125.

Findlay, V., Helders, M., Munday, B.L. and Gurney, R. (1995) Demonstration of resistance to reinfection with *Paramoeba* sp. by Atlantic salmon, *Salmo salar* L. *Journal of Fish Diseases* 18, 639–642.

Fisk, D.M., Powell, M.D. and Nowak, B.F. (2002) The effect of amoebic gill disease and hypoxia on survival and metabolic rate of Atlantic salmon (*Salmo salar*). *Bulletin of the European Association of Fish Pathologists* 22, 190–194.

Florent, R.L., Becker, J. and Powell, M.D. (2007a) Evaluation of bithionol as a bath treatment for amoebic gill disease caused by *Neoparamoeba* spp. *Veterinary Parasitology* 144, 197–207.

Florent, R.L., Becker, J. and Powell, M.D. (2007b) Efficacy of bithionol as an oral treatment for amoebic gill disease in Atlantic salmon *Salmo salar* (L.). *Aquaculture* 270, 15–22.

Florent, R.L., Becker, J. and Powell, M.D. (2009) Further development of bithionol therapy as a treatment for amoebic gill disease in Atlantic salmon, *Salmo salar*. *Journal of Fish Diseases* 32, 391–400.

Fridman, S., Tsairidou, S., Jayasuriya, N., Sobolewska, H., Hamilton, A. *et al.* (2021) Assessment of marine gill disease in farmed Atlantic salmon (*Salmo salar*) in Chile using a novel total gross gill scoring system: a case study. *Microorganisms* 9(12), 2605. DOI: 10.3390/microorganisms9122605.

Fringuelli, E., Gordon, A.W., Rodger, H., Welsh, M.D. and Graham, D.A. (2012) Detection of *Neoparamoeba perurans* by duplex quantitative Taqman real-time PCR in formalin-fixed, paraffin-embedded Atlantic salmonid gill tissues. *Journal of Fish Diseases* 35(10), 711–724. DOI: 10.1111/j.1365-2761.2012.01395.x.

Gross, K.A. (2007) Interactions between *Neoparamoeba* spp. and Atlantic salmon (*Salmo salar* L.) immune system components. PhD thesis, University of Tasmania, Launceston, Tasmania, Australia.

Gross, K., Morrison, R.N., Butler, R. and Nowak, B.F. (2004a) Atlantic salmon (*Salmo salar* L.) previously infected with *Neoparamoeba* sp. are not resistant to re-infection and have suppressed macrophage function. *Journal of Fish Diseases* 27, 47–56.

Gross, K., Carson, J. and Nowak, B.F. (2004b) The presence of anti-*Neoparamoeba* sp. antibodies in Tasmanian cultured Atlantic salmon (*Salmo salar* L.). *Journal of Fish Diseases* 27, 81–88.

Gross, K.A., Powell, M.D., Butler, R., Morrison, R.N. and Nowak, B.F. (2005) Changes in the innate immune response of Atlantic salmon (*Salmo salar*) exposed to experimental infection with *Neoparamoeba* sp. *Journal of Fish Diseases* 28, 293–299.

Guy, D.R., Bishop, S.C., Brotherstone, S., Hamilton, A., Roberts, R.J. *et al.* (2006) Analysis of the incidence of infectious pancreatic necrosis mortality in pedigreed Atlantic salmon, *Salmo salar* L., populations. *Journal of Fish Diseases* 29, 637–647.

Hansen, H., Botwright, N.A., Cook, M.T., Douglas, A., Downes, J. *et al.* (2019) Genetic diversity among geographically distant isolates of *Neoparamoeba perurans*. *Diseases of Aquatic Organisms* 137, 81–87. DOI: 10.3354/dao03433.

Harris, J.O., Powell, M.D., Attard, M. and Green, T.J. (2004) Efficacy of chloramines-T as a treatment for amoebic gill disease (AGD) in marine Atlantic salmon (*Salmo salar* L.) *Aquaculture Research* 35, 1448–1456.

Harris, J.O., Powell, M.D., Attard, M.G. and Dehayr, L. (2005) Clinical assessment of chloramines-T and freshwater treatments for the control of gill amoebae in Atlantic salmon, *Salmo salar* L. *Aquaculture Research* 36, 776–784.

Hellebø, A., Stene, A. and Aspehaug, V. (2017) PCR survey for *Paramoeba perurans* in fauna, environmental samples and fish associated with marine farming sites for Atlantic salmon (*Salmo salar* L.). *Journal of Fish Diseases* 40, 661–670.

Herrero, A., Thompson, K.D., Ashby A., Rodger, H.D. and Dagleish, M.P. (2018) Complex gill disease: an emerging syndrome in farmed Atlantic salmon (*Salmo salar* L.). *Journal of Comparative Pathology* 163, 23–28.

Howard, T.S., Carson, J. and Lewis, T. (1993) Development of a model of infection for amoebic gill disease. In: Valentine, P. (ed.) *Salmon Enterprises of Tasmania (SALTAS) Research and Development Seminar*. SALTAS, Hobart, Tasmania, Australia, pp. 103–111.

Hudson, J. and Nowak, B.F. (2021) Experimental challenge models and *in vitro* models to investigate efficacy of treatments and vaccines against amoebic gill disease. *Microorganisms* 9(4), 710. DOI: 10.3390/microorganisms9040710.

Hudson, J., Adams, M., Jantawongsri, K., Dempster, T. and Nowak, B.F. (2022) Evaluation of low temperature and salinity as a treatment of Atlantic salmon against amoebic gill disease. *Microorganisms* 10(2), 202. DOI: 10.3390/microorganisms10020202.

Hvas, M., Karlsbakk, E., Mæhle, S., Wright, D.W. and Oppedal, F. (2017) The gill parasite *Paramoeba perurans* compromises aerobic scope, swimming performance and ion balance in Atlantic salmon. *Conservation Physiology* 5, cox066. DOI: 10.1093/conphys/cox066.

ICES (2016) *Interim Report of the Working Group on Pathology and Diseases of Marine Organisms (WGPDMO)*. ICES CM 2016/SSGEPI:07; 17–20 February 2016, Virginia, USA. International Council for the Exploration of the Sea, Copenhagen, p. 18.

Johnson-Mackinnon, J.C., Crosbie, P.B.B., Karlsbakk, E., Marcos-Lopez, M., Paley, R. *et al.* (2019) Multilocus sequence typing (MLST) and random polymorphic DNA (RAPD) comparisons of geographic isolates of *Neoparamoeba perurans*, the causative agent of amoebic gill disease. *Pathogens* 8(4), 244. DOI: 10.3390/pathogens8040244.

Jones, G.M. and Scheibling, R.E. (1985) *Paramoeba* sp. (Amoebida, Paramoebaidae) as the possible causative agent of sea-urchin mass mortality in Nova Scotia. *Journal of Parasitology* 71, 559–565.

Jones, S.R.M. and Price, D. (2022) Elevated seawater temperature and infection with *Neoparamoeba perurans* exacerbate complex gill disease in farmed Atlantic salmon (*Salmo salar*) in British Columbia, Canada. *Microorganisms* 10, 1039. DOI: 10.3390/microorganisms10051039.

Kent, M.L., Sawyer, T.K. and Hedrick, R.P. (1988) *Paramoeba pemaquidensis* (Sarcomastigophora: Paramoebidae) infestation of the gills of coho salmon *Oncorhnychus kisutch* reared in sea water. *Diseases of Aquatic Organisms* 5, 163–169.

Kim, D.H., Joo, M.S., Woo, S.J., Son, K.T., Hong, W.S. *et al.* (2024) The first report on *Saprolegnia parasitica* and *Neoparamoeba perurans* isolated from Atlantic salmon (*Salmo salar*) reared in Korea. *Microbiology Research* 15(2), 1016–1027. DOI: 10.3390/microbiolres15020067.

Kim, H.J., Cho, J.B., Lee, H.K., Huh, M.D. and Kim, K.H. (2005) *Neoparamoeba* sp. infection on gills of olive flounder, *Paralichthys olivaceus* in Korea. *Journal of Fish Pathology* 18, 125–131.

Kim, W.S., Kong, K.H., Kim, J.O., and Oh, M.J. (2016) Amoebic gill infection in coho salmon *Oncorhynchus kisutch* farmed in Korea. *Diseases of Aquatic Organisms* 121(1), 75–78. DOI: 10.3354/dao03037.

Kim, W.S., Kong, K.H., Kim, J.O., Jung, S.J., Kim, J.H., and Oh, M.J. (2017) Amoebic gill disease outbreak in marine fish cultured in Korea. *Journal of Veterinary Diagnostic Investigation* 29, 357–361.

Kirchhoff, N.T., Rough, K. and Nowak, B.F. (2011) Moving cages further offshore: effects on southern bluefin tuna, *T. maccoyii*, parasites, health and performance. *PLoS One* 6(8), e23705. DOI: 10.1371/journal.pone.0023705.

Kristiansen, D., Aksnes, V., Su, B., Lader, P. and Bjelland, H.V. (2017) Environmental description in the design of fish farms at exposed locations. *Proceedings of ASME 2017 36th Conference on Ocean, Offshore and Arctic Engineering OMAE 2017*, Trondheim, Norway. DOI: 10.1115/OMAE2017-61531.

Kudryavtsev, A., Volkova, E. and Voytinsky, F. (2021) A checklist of Amebozoa species from marine and brackish-water biotopes with notes on taxonomy, species concept and distribution patterns. *Protistology* 15(4), 220–273.

Leef, M.J., Harris, J.O. and Powell, M.D. (2005a) Respiratory pathogenesis of amoebic gill disease (AGD) in experimentally infected Atlantic salmon *Salmo salar*. *Diseases of Aquatic Organisms* 66, 205–213.

Leef, M.J., Harris, J.O., Hill, J. and Powell, M.D. (2005b) Cardiovascular responses of three salmonid species affected with amoebic gill disease (AGD). *Journal of Comparative Physiology B – Biochemical Systemic and Environmental Physiology* 175, 523–532.

Leef, M.J., Harris, J.O. and Powell, M.D. (2007) Metabolic effects of amoebic gill disease (AGD) and chloramine-T exposure in seawater-acclimated Atlantic salmon *Salmo salar*. *Disease of Aquatic Organisms* 78, 37–44.

Lima, P.C., Taylor, R.S. and Cook, M. (2017) Pseudocyst formation in the marine parasitic amoeba *Neoparamoeba perurans*: a short-term survival strategy to abrupt salinity variation. *Journal of Fish Diseases* 40, 1109–1113.

Lovy, J., Becker, J.A., Speare, D.J., Wadowska, D.W., Wright, G.M. and Powell, M.D. (2007) Ultrastructural examination of the host cellular response in the gills of Atlantic salmon, *Salmo salar*, with amoebic gill disease. *Veterinary Pathology* 44, 663–671.

Lubieniecki, K.P., Jones, S.L., Davidson, E.A., Park, J., Koop, B.F. *et al.* (2010) Comparative genomic analysis of Atlantic salmon, *Salmo salar*, from Europe and North America. *BMC Genetics* 11, 105. DOI: 10.1186/1471-2156-11-105.

Marcos-López, M. and Rodger, H.D. (2020) Amoebic gill disease and host response in Atlantic salmon (*Salmo salar* L.): a review. *Parasite Immunology* 42, e12766.

Marcos-López, M., Calduch-Giner, J.A., Mirimim, L., MacCarthy, E., Rodger, H.D. *et al.* (2018) Gene expression analysis of Atlantic salmon gills reveals mucin 5 and interleukin 4/13 as key molecules during amoebic gill diseases. *Scientific Reports* 8, 13689.

Martinsen, K.H., Thorisdottir, A. and Lillehammer, M. (2018) Effect of hydrogen peroxide as treatment for amoebic gill disease in Atlantic salmon (*Salmo salar* L.) in different temperatures. *Aquaculture Research* 49, 1733–1739. DOI: 10.1111/are.13627.

McCormack, M., Dillon, E., O'Connor, I. and MacCarthy, E. (2021) Investigation of the initial host response of naïve Atlantic salmon (*Salmo salar*) inoculated with *Paramoeba perurans*. *Microorganisms* 9, 746.

Moran, D.M., Anderson, O.R., Dennett, M.R., Caron, D.A. and Gast, R.J. (2007) A description of seven Antarctic marine Gymnamoebae including a new subspecies, two new species and a new genus: *Neoparamoeba aestuarina antarctica* n. subsp., *Platyamoeba oblongata* n. sp., *Platyamoeba contorta* n. sp. and *Vermistella antarctica* n. gen. n. sp. *Journal of Eukaryotic Microbiology* 54, 169–183.

Morrison, R.N. and Nowak, B.F. (2005) Bath treatment of Atlantic salmon (*Salmo salar*) with amoebae antigens fails to affect survival to subsequent amoebic gill disease (AGD) challenge. *Bulletin of the European Association of Fish Pathologists* 25, 155–160.

Morrison, R.N., Crosbie, P.B.B. and Nowak, B.F. (2004) The induction of laboratory-based amoebic gill disease (AGD) revisited. *Journal of Fish Diseases* 27, 445–449.

Morrison, R.N., Crosbie, P., Adams, M.B., Cook M.T. and Nowak, B.F. (2005) Cultured gill derived *Neoparamoeba pemaquidensis* fail to elicit AGD in Atlantic salmon (*Salmo salar*). *Diseases of Aquatic Organisms* 66, 135–144.

Morrison, R.N., Koppang, E.O., Hordvik, I. and Nowak, B.F. (2006a) MHC class II$^+$ cells in the gills of salmon experimentally infected with amoebic gill disease. *Veterinary Immunology and Immunopathology* 109, 297–303.

Morrison, R.N., Cooper, G.A., Koop, B.F., Rise, M.L., Bridle, A.R. *et al.* (2006b) Transcriptome profiling of the gills of amoebic gill disease (AGD)-affected Atlantic salmon (*Salmo salar* L.) – a role for the tumor suppressor protein p53 in AGD-pathogenesis? *Physiological Genomics* 26, 15–34.

Morrison, R.N., Zou, J., Secombes, C.J., Scapigliatti, G., Adams, M.B. and Nowak, B.F. (2007) Molecular cloning and expression analysis of tumor necrosis factor-α in amoebic gill disease (AGD)-affected Atlantic salmon (*Salmo salar* L.). *Fish and Shellfish Immunology* 23, 1015–1031.

Mouton, A., Crosbie, P., Cadoret, K. and Nowak, B. (2014) First record of amoebic gill disease caused by *Neoparamoeba perurans* in South Africa. *Journal of Fish Diseases* 37(4), 407–409. DOI: 10.1111/jfd.12133.

Mullen, T.E., Nevis, K.R., O'Kelly, C.J., Gast, R.J. and Frasca, S. (2005) Nuclear small-subunit ribosomal RNA gene-based characterisation, molecular phylogeny and PCR detection of the *Neoparamoeba* from western Long Island Sound lobster. *Journal of Shellfish Research* 24, 719–731.

Munday, B.L. (1986) Diseases of salmonids. In: Humphrey, J.D. and Langdon, J.S. (eds) *Proceedings of the Workshop on Diseases of Australian Fish and Shellfish*. Department of Agriculture and Rural Affairs, Benalla, Victoria, Australia, pp. 127–141.

Munday, B.L. and Zilberg, D. (2003) Efficacy of, and toxicity associated with, the use of levamisole in seawater to treat amoebic gill disease. *Bulletin of the European Association of Fish Pathologists* 23, 3–6.

Munday, B.L., Foster, C.K., Roubal, F.R. and Lester, R.J.G. (1990) Paramoebic gill infection and associated pathology of Atlantic salmon, *Salmo salar*, and rainbow trout, *Salmo gairdneri*, in Tasmania. In: Perkins, F.O. and Cheng, T.C. (eds) *Pathology in Marine Science*. Academic Press, London, pp. 215–222.

Munday, B.L., Lange, K., Foster, C., Lester, R.J.G. and Handlinger, J. (1993) Amoebic gill disease of sea-caged salmonids in Tasmanian waters. *Tasmanian Fisheries Research* 28, 14–19.

Munday, B.L., Zilberg, D. and Finlay, V. (2001) Gill disease of marine fish caused by infection with *Neoparamoeba pemaquidensis*. *Journal of Fish Diseases* 24, 497–507.

Nowak, B. (2001) Qualitative evaluation of risk factors for amoebic gill disease in cultured Atlantic salmon. In: Rodgers, C.J. (ed.) *Risk Analysis in Aquatic Animal Health*. World Organisation for Animal Health, Paris, pp. 158–154.

Nowak, B.F. (2007) Parasitic diseases in marine cage culture – an example of experimental evolution of parasites? *International Journal for Parasitology* 37, 581–588.

Nowak, B.F. and Archibald, J.M. (2018) Opportunistic but lethal: the mystery of Paramoebae. *Trends in Parasitology* 34(5), 404–419. DOI: 10.1016/j.pt.2018.01.004.

Nowak, B.F. and Munday, B.L. (1994) Histology of gills of Atlantic salmon during the first few months following transfer to sea water. *Bulletin of the European Association of Fish Pathologists* 14(3), 77–81.

Nowak, B.F., Powell, M.D., Carson, J. and Dykova, I. (2002) Amoebic gill disease in the marine environment. *Bulletin of the European Association of Fish Pathologists* 22, 144–147.

Nowak, B., Morrison, R., Crosbie, P., Adams, M., Butler, R. *et al.* (2004a) *Host-Pathogen Interactions in Amoebic Gill Disease*. Aquafin Cooperative Research Centre (Australia); Fisheries Research and Development Corporation (Australia); Tasmanian Aquaculture and Fisheries Institute University of Tasmania, Launceston, Australia.

Nowak, B.F., Dawson, D., Basson, L., Deveney, M. and Powell, M.D. (2004b) Gill histopathology of wild marine fish in Tasmania – potential interactions with gill health of cultured Atlantic salmon (*Salmo salar* L.). *Journal of Fish Diseases* 27, 709–717.

Nowak, B.F., Bryan, J. and Jones, S. (2010) A role of sea lice *Lepeophtheirus salmonis* in the epidemiology of amoebic gill disease caused by *Neoparamoeba perurans*? *Journal of Fish Diseases* 33, 683–687.

Nylund, A., Watanabe, K., Nylund, S., Karlsen, M., Sather, P.A. *et al.* (2008) Morphogenesis of salmonid gill poxvirus associated with proliferative gill disease in farmed Atlantic salmon (*Salmo salar*) in Norway. *Archives of Virology* 153, 1299–1309.

O'Halloran, E., Mooney, R., Rodgers, K. and Henriquez, F.L. (2022) Microbial interactions that contribute to gill disease in aquaculture. *Parasitologia* 2, 266–291.

Oldham, T.M., Rodger, H. and Nowak, B.F. (2016) Incidence and distribution of amoebic gill disease (AGD) – an epidemiological review. *Aquaculture* 457, 35–42. DOI: 10.1016/j.aquaculture.2016.02.013.

Østevik, L., Stormoen, M., Nødtvedt, A., Alarcón, M., Lie, K-I. *et al.* (2021) Assessment of acute effects of *in situ* net cleaning on gill health of farmed Atlantic salmon (*Salmo salar* L.). *Aquaculture* 545, 737203.

Page, F.C. (1973) *Paramoeba*: a common marine genus. *Hydrobiologia* 41, 183–188.

Page, F.C. (1974) *Rosculus ithacus* Hawes, 1963, Amoebida, Flabellulidea and the amphizoic tendency in amoebae. *Acta Protozoologica* 13, 143–154.

Page, F.C. (1983) *Marine Gymnamoebae*. Institute of Terrestrial Ecology, Culture Centre of Algae and Protozoa, Cambridge, 54 pp.

Page, F.C. (1987) The classification of 'naked' amoebae of phylum Rhizopoda. *Archives of Protistenkunde* 133, 199–217.

Palmer, R., Carson, J., Ruttledge, M., Drinan, E. and Wagner, T. (1997) Gill disease associated with *Paramoeba*, in sea reared Atlantic salmon in Ireland. *Bulletin of the European Association of Fish Pathologists* 17, 112–114.

Parsons, H., Powell, M., Fisk, D. and Nowak, B. (2001) Effectiveness of commercial freshwater bathing as a treatment against amoebic gill disease in Atlantic salmon. *Aquaculture* 195, 205–210.

Patchett, A.L., Rigby, M.L. and Wynne, J.W. (2024) Improved 18S rDNA profiling of parasite communities in salmonid tissues using a host blocking primer. *Parasitology Research* 123(2), 124. DOI:10.1007/s00436-024-08136-x.

Persson, D., Nødtvedt, A., Aunsmo, A. and Stormoen, M. (2022) Analysing mortality patterns in salmon farming using daily cage registrations. *Journal of Fish Diseases* 45, 335–347.

Powell, M., Fisk, D. and Nowak, B. (2000) Effects of graded hypoxia on Atlantic salmon (*Salmo salar* L.) infected with amoebic gill disease (AGD). *Journal of Fish Biology* 57, 1047–1057.

Powell, M.D., Parsons, H.J. and Nowak, B.F. (2001) Physiological effects of freshwater bathing of Atlantic salmon (*Salmo salar*) as a treatment for amoebic gill disease. *Aquaculture* 199, 259–266.

Powell, M.D., Nowak, B.F. and Adams, M. (2002) Cardiac morphology in relation to amoebic gill disease history in Atlantic salmon (*Salmo salar* L.). *Journal of Fish Diseases* 25, 209–215.

Powell, M.D., Attard, M., Harris, J., Roberts, S.D. and Leef, M.J. (2005) *Why Fish Die – Treatment and Pathophysiology of AGD*. University of Tasmania, Launceston, Tasmania, Australia.

Powell, M.D., Leef, M.J., Roberts, S.D. and Jones, M.A. (2008) Neoparamoebic gill infections: host response and physiology of salmonids. *Journal of Fish Biology* 73, 2161–2183.

Roberts, S.D. and Powell, M.D. (2003) Reduced total hardness of fresh water enhanced the efficacy of bathing as a treatment against amoebic gill disease in Atlantic salmon, *Salmo salar* L. *Journal of Fish Diseases* 26, 591–599.

Roberts, S.D. and Powell, M.D. (2005) Oral l-cysteine ethyl ester (LCEE) reduces amoebic gill disease (AGD) in Atlantic salmon *Salmo salar*. *Diseases of Aquatic Organisms* 66, 21–28.

Robledo, D., Matika, O., Hamilton, A. and Houston, R.D. (2018) Genome-wide association and genomic selection for resistance to amoebic gill disease in Atlantic salmon. *G3: Genes, Genomes, Genetics* 8, 1195–1203. DOI: 10.1534/g3.118.200075.

Rodger, H.D. (2014) Amoebic gill disease (AGD) in farmed salmon (*Salmo salar*) in Europe. *Fish Veterinary Journal* 14, 16–26.

Rodger, H.D. (2019) Amoebic gill disease in farmed halibut (*Hippoglossus hippoglossus*) in the United Kingdom. *Veterinary Record Case Reports* 7, e000797. DOI: 10.1136/vetreccr-2018-000797.

Rodger, H.D. and McArdle, J.F. (1996) An outbreak of amoebic gill disease in Ireland. *Veterinary Record* 139, 348–349.

Rozas, M., Bohle, H., Ildefonso, R.S. and Bustos, P. (2011) Development of PCR assay for detection of *Neoparamoeba perurans* and comparison of histological diagnosis. *Bulletin of the European Association of Fish Pathologists* 31(6), 211–218.

Rozas, M., Bohle, H., Grothusen, H. and Bustos, P. (2012) Epidemiology of amoebic gill disease (AGD) in Chilean salmon industry between 2007 and 2010. *Bulletin of the European Association of Fish Pathologists* 32(5), 181–188.

Shinn, A.P., Pratoomyot, J., Bron, J.E., Paladini, G., Brooker, E.E. and Brooker, A.J. (2015) Economic costs of protistan and metazoan parasites to global mariculture. *Parasitology* 142, 196–270.

Sibbald, S.J., Cenci, U., Colp, M., Eglit, Y., O'Kelly, C.J. and Archibald, J.M. (2017) Diversity and evolution of *Paramoeba* spp. and their kinetoplastid endosymbionts. *Journal of Eukaryotic Microbiology* 64, 598–607. DOI: 10.1111/jeu.12394.

Slinger, J., Adams, M.B. and Wynne, J.W. (2020) Bacteriomic profiling of branchial lesions induced by *Neoparamoeba perurans* challenge reveals commensal dysbiosis and an association with *Tenacibaculum dicentrarchi* in AGD-affected Atlantic salmon (*Salmo salar* L.). *Microorganisms* 8, 1189.

Smith, A.J., Adams, M.B., Crosbie, P.B.B., Nowak, B.F. and Bridle, A.R. (2022a) Size-dependent resistance to amoebic gill disease in naïve Atlantic salmon (*Salmo salar*). *Fish and Shellfish Immunology* 122, 437–445. DOI: 10.1016/j.fsi.2022.02.035.

Smith, A.J., Crosbie, P.B.B., Nowak, B.F. and Bridle, A.R. (2022b) Comparative transcriptome profiling of virulent and avirulent isolates of *Neoparamoeba perurans*. *Scientific Reports* 12(1), 11. DOI: 10.1038/s41598-022-09806-5.

Sokołowska, J. and Nowak, B.F. (2020) Amoebiosis (*Neoparamoeba perurans*). In: Woo, P.T.K., Leong, J.-A. and Buchmann, K. (eds) *Climate Change and Infectious Fish Diseases*. CABI International, Wallingford, UK, pp. 303–318.

Sommerset, I., Wiik-Nielsen, J., Moldal, T., Oliveira, V.H.S., Svendsen, J.C. *et al.* (2024) *Norwegian Fish Health Report 2023*. Norwegian Veterinary Institute Report #8b/2024. Norwegian Veterinary Institute Ås, Norway. Available at: https://www.vetinst.no/rapporter-og-publikasjoner/rapporter/2024/fishhealthreport-2023/_/attachment/inline/bb455bc6-1daa-4f9e-b855-e07ed1274663:889eac6a944fd63d13ed5b4d6dfac01cae645d39/FHR%202023%20Engelsk%20utgave_web.pdf (accessed 21 November 2025).

Stagg, H.E.B., Hall, M., Wallace, I.S., Pert, C.C., Garcia Perez, S. and Collins, C. (2015) Detection of *Paramoeba perurans* in Scottish marine wild fish populations. *Bulletin of the European Association of Fish Pathologists* 35, 217–226.

Steigen, A., Nylund, A., Plarre, H., Watanabe, K., Karlsbakk, E. and Brevik, O. (2018) Presence of selected pathogens on the gills of five wrasse species in western Norway. *Diseases of Aquatic Organisms* 128(1), 21–35. DOI: 10.3354/dao03198.

Steinum, T., Kvellestad, A., Rønneberg, L.B., Nilsen, H., Asheim, A. *et al.* (2008) First case of amoebic gill disease (AGD) in Norwegian seawater farmed Atlantic salmon, *Salmo salar* L., and phylogeny of the causative amoeba using 18S cDNA sequences. *Journal of Fish Diseases* 31, 205–214.

Tan, C., Nowak, B.F. and Hodson, S.L. (2002) Biofouling as a reservoir of *Neoparamoeba pemaquidensis* (Page 1970), the causative agent of amoebic gill disease in Atlantic salmon. *Aquaculture* 210, 49–58.

Tanifuji, G., Cenci, U., Moog, D., Dean, S., Nakayma, T. *et al.* (2017) Genome sequencing reveals metabolic and cellular interdependence in an amoeba–kinetoplastid symbiosis. *Scientific Reports* 7, 11688. DOI: 10.1038/s41598-017-11866-x.

Taylor, R.S. (2010) Assessment of resistance to amoebic gill disease in the Tasmanian Atlantic salmon selective breeding population. PhD thesis, University of Tasmania, Launceston, Tasmania, Australia.

Taylor, R.S. (2016) *Gill Score Guide – Amoebic Gill Disease (AGD) Management Training Document.* Tassal Pty, Hobart, Tasmania, Australia.

Taylor, R.S., Wynne, J.W., Kube, P.D. and Elliott, N.G. (2007) Genetic variation of resistance to amoebic gill disease in Atlantic salmon (*Salmo salar*) assessed in a challenge system. *Aquaculture* 272, S94–S99.

Taylor, R.S., Kube, P.D., Muller, W.J. and Elliott, N.G. (2009a) Genetic variation of gross gill pathology and survival of Atlantic salmon (*Salmo salar* L.) during natural amoebic gill disease challenge. *Aquaculture* 294, 172–179.

Taylor, R.S., Muller, W.J., Cook, M.T., Kube, P.D. and Elliott, N.G. (2009b) Gill observations in Atlantic salmon (*Salmo salar*, L.) during repeated amoebic gill disease (AGD) field exposure and survival challenge. *Aquaculture* 290, 1–8.

Taylor, R.S., Crosbie, P.B. and Cook, M.T. (2010) Amoebic gill disease resistance is not related to the systemic antibody response of Atlantic salmon (*Salmo salar*, L.). *Journal of Fish Diseases* 33, 1–14.

Taylor, R.S., Slinger, J., Stratford, C., Rigby, M., and Wynne, J.W. (2021) Evaluation of the infectious potential of *Neoparamoeba perurans* following freshwater bathing treatments. *Microorganisms* 9(5), 967. DOI: 10.3390/microorganisms9050967.

Ullal, A.J. and Noga, E.J. (2010) Antiparasitic activity of the antimicrobial peptide Hb beta P-1, a member of the beta-haemoglobin peptide family. *Journal of Fish Diseases* 33, 657–664.

Ullal, A.J., Litaker, R.W. and Noga, E.J. (2008) Antimicrobial peptides derived from hemoglobin are expressed in epithelium of channel catfish (*Ictalurus punctatus*, Rafinesque). *Developmental and Comparative Immunology* 32, 1301–1312.

Valdenegro-Vega, V.A., Cook, M., Crosbie, P., Bridle, A.R. and Nowak, B.F. (2015) Vaccination with recombinant protein (*r*22C03), a putative attachment factor of *Neoparamoeba perurans*, against AGD in Atlantic salmon (*Salmo salar*) and implications of a co-infection with *Yersinia ruckeri*. *Fish and Shellfish Immunology* 44(2), 692–602. DOI: 10.1016/j.fsi.2015.03.016.

Villavedra, M., To, J., Lemke, S., Birch, D., Crosbie, P. *et al.* (2010) Characterisation of an immunodominant, high molecular weight glycoprotein on the surface of infectious *Neoparamoeba* spp., causative agent of amoebic gill disease (AGD) in Atlantic salmon. *Fish and Shellfish Immunology* 29, 946–955.

Vincent, B.N. (2008) Amoebic gill disease of Atlantic salmon: resistance, serum antibody response and factors that may affect disease severity. PhD thesis, University of Tasmania, Launceston, Tasmania, Australia.

Vincent, B.N., Morrison, R.N. and Nowak, B.F. (2006) Amoebic gill disease (AGD)-affected Atlantic salmon *Salmo salar* L. are resistant to subsequent AGD challenge. *Journal of Fish Diseases* 29, 549–559.

Vincent, B.N., Adams, M.B., Crosbie, P.B.B., Nowak, B.F. and Morrison, R.N. (2007) Atlantic salmon (*Salmo salar* L.) exposed to cultured gill-derived *Neoparamoeba branchiphila* fail to develop amoebic gill disease (AGD). *Bulletin of the European Association of Fish Pathologists* 27, 112–115.

Vincent, B.N., Nowak, B.F. and Morrison, R.N. (2008) Detection of serum anti-*Neoparamoeba* spp. antibodies in amoebic gill disease affected Atlantic salmon. *Journal of Fish Biology* 73, 429–435.

Vincent, B.N., Adams, M.B., Nowak, B.F. and Morrison, R.N. (2009) Cell surface carbohydrate antigen(s) of wild type *Neoparamoeba* spp. are immunodominant in sea-cage cultured Atlantic salmon (*Salmo salar* L.) affected by amoebic gill disease (AGD). *Aquaculture* 288, 153–158.

VKM (2014) *Risk Assessment of Amoebic Gill Disease*. VKM Report 2014:11. Norwegian Scientific Committee for Food Safety (VKM), Oslo, p. 3. Available at: https://vkm.no/download/18.7e19596115dabec04172a6b/1501851063568/Risk%20assessment%20of%20amoebic%20gill%20disease.pdf (accessed 4 December 2025).

Wiese, T.R., Haskell, M., Jarvis, S., Rey-Planellas, S. and Turnbull, J. (2023) Concerns and research priorities for Scottish farmed salmon welfare – an industry perspective. *Aquaculture* 566, 739235.

Wright, D.W., Nowak, B.F., Oppedal, F., Bridle, A.R. and Dempster, T. (2015) Depth distribution of the amoebic gill disease agent, *Neoparamoeba perurans*, in salmon sea-cages. *Aquaculture Environment Interactions* 7, 67–74. DOI: 10.3354/aei00137.

Wright, D.W., Nowak, B., Oppedal, F., Bridle, A. and Dempster, T. (2017a) Free-living *Neoparamoeba perurans* depth distribution is mostly uniform in salmon cages, but reshaped by stratification and potentially extreme fish crowding. *Aquaculture Environment Interactions* 9, 269–279. DOI: 10.3354/aei00233.

Wright, D.W., Stien, L.H., Dempster, T., Vågseth, T., Nola, V. *et al.* (2017b) 'Snorkel' lice barrier technology reduced two co-occurring parasites, the salmon louse (*Lepeophtheirus salmonis*) and the amoebic gill disease causing agent (*Neoparamoeba perurans*), in commercial salmon sea-cages. *Preventive Veterinary Medicine* 140, 97–105. DOI: 10.1016/j.prevetmed.2017.03.002.

Wright, D.W., Nowak, B., Oppedal, F., Crosbie, P., Stien, L.H., and Dempster, T. (2018a) Repeated sublethal freshwater exposures reduce the amoebic gill disease parasite, *Neoparamoeba perurans*, on Atlantic salmon. *Journal of Fish Diseases* 41(9), 1403–1410. DOI: 10.1111/jfd.12834.

Wright, D.W., Geitung, L., Karlsbakk, E., Stien, L.H., Dempster, T. *et al.* (2018b) Surface environment modification in Atlantic salmon sea-cages: effects on amoebic gill disease, salmon lice, growth and welfare. *Aquaculture Environment Interactions* 10, 255–265. DOI: 10.3354/aei00269.

Wynne, J.W., Stratford, C., Slinger, J., Samsing, F., Rigby, M. *et al.* (2019) The interaction between temperature and dose on the efficacy and biochemical response of Atlantic salmon to hydrogen peroxide treatment for amoebic gill disease. *Journal of Fish Diseases* 43, 39–48.

Wynne, J.W., Rigby, M.L., Maynard, B. and Taylor, R.S. (2024) Improved environmental detection of *Neoparamoeba perurans* using sensitive RNA-based qPCR. *Journal of Fish Diseases* 47(2), e13879. DOI: 10.1111/jfd.13879.

Young, N.D., Crosbie, P.B.B., Adams, M.B., Nowak, B.F. and Morrison, R.N. (2007) *Neoparamoebae perurans* n. sp., an agent of amoebic gill disease of Atlantic salmon (*Salmo salar*). *International Journal for Parasitology* 37, 1469–1481.

Young, N.D., Dyková, I., Snekvik, K., Nowak, B.F. and Morrison, R.N. (2008a) *Neoparamoeba perurans* is a cosmopolitan aetiological agent of amoebic gill disease. *Diseases of Aquatic Organisms* 78, 217–223.

Young, N.D., Dyková, I., Nowak, B.F. and Morrison, R.N. (2008b) Development of a diagnostic PCR to detect *Neoparamoeba perurans*, agent of amoebic gill disease (AGD). *Journal of Fish Diseases* 31, 285–295.

Young, N.D., Cooper, G.A., Nowak, B.F., Koop, B.F. and Morrison, R.N. (2008c) Coordinated down-regulation of the antigen processing machinery in the gills of amoebic gill disease-affected Atlantic salmon (*Salmo salar*). *Molecular Immunology* 45, 1469–1481.

Young, N.D., Dyková, I., Crosbie, P.B., Wolf, M., Morrison, R.N. *et al.* (2014) Support for the coevolution of *Neoparamoeba* and their endosymbionts, *Perkinsela amoebae*-like organisms. *European Journal of Protistology* 50, 509–523. DOI: 10.1016/j.ejop.2014.07.004.

Zilberg, D. and Munday, B.L. (2000) Pathology of experimental amoebic gill disease in Atlantic salmon (*Salmo salar* L.) and the effect of pre-maintenance of fish in seawater on the infection. *Journal of Fish Diseases* 23, 401–407.

Zilberg, D. and Munday, B.L. (2001) Response of Atlantic salmon (*Salmo salar* L.) to *Paramoeba* antigens administered by a variety of routes. *Journal of Fish Diseases* 24, 181–183.

Zilberg, D., Nowak, B., Carson, J. and Wagner, T. (1999) Simple gill smear staining for diagnosis of amoebic gill disease. *Bulletin of the European Association of Fish Pathologists* 19, 186–189.

Zilberg, D., Findlay, V.L., Girling, P. and Munday, B.L. (2000) Effects of treatment with levamisole and glucans on mortality rates in Atlantic salmon (*Salmo salar* L.) suffering from amoebic gill disease. *Bulletin of the European Association of Fish Pathologists* 20, 23–27.

Zilberg, D., Gross, A. and Munday, B.L. (2001) Production of salmonid amoebic gill disease by exposure to *Paramoeba* sp. harvested from the gills of infected fish. *Journal of Fish Diseases* 24, 79–82.

2 *Amyloodinium ocellatum*

Paola Beraldo*
Department of Agricultural, Food, Environmental and Animal Sciences, University of Udine, Italy

Abstract

Amyloodinium ocellatum, a triphasic dinoflagellate parasite, is a significant threat to captive fish resulting in substantial economic losses in temperate and tropical aquaculture, especially in lagoon-based and land-based systems. Amyloodiniosis, or marine velvet disease, results in high morbidity and up to 100% mortality under certain farming conditions (e.g. parasite load, fish species and season). Current knowledge includes significant biological and epidemiological data on *A. ocellatum*, diagnostic methods and effective therapeutic protocols which may not be eco-friendly. While a few studies provide valuable insights, comprehensive knowledge concerning parasite–host interactions and the diverse physiological responses in different hosts remains incomplete. Genomic characterization is lacking, and further efforts are needed to identify critical genes involved in its life-cycle stages and virulence. Also, the development of effective vaccines against amyloodiniosis and pharmacological therapies is warranted.

2.1. Introduction

Amyloodinium ocellatum is an ectoparasitic protozoan belonging to the phylum Dinoflagellata. Dinoflagellates are unicellular organisms commonly found in both freshwater and marine ecosystems. There are approximately 2000 species in the phylum, of which 140 species are parasites of invertebrates (Drebes, 1984). Six genera parasitize fish (Noga and Levy, 2006), and of these, *Amyloodinium*, *Ichthyodinium* and *Piscinoodinium* can cause high fish mortality.

A. ocellatum is the only species in the genus *Amyloodinium* (class Dinophyceae, order Peridiniales, family Thoracosphaeraceae) and is an obligate ectoparasitic protozoan of marine and brackish-water fish. In tropical and temperate regions, it is the only dinoflagellate capable of infecting both bony fish and elasmobranchs (Lawler, 1980), and it has been isolated in aquatic organisms belonging to four phyla: Chordata, Arthropoda (Aravindan *et al.*, 2007; Massimo, 2019), Mollusca (de Souza, 2015) and Platyhelminthes (Colorni, 1994). Indeed, *A. ocellatum* is able to utilize various marine organisms (including crustaceans and platyhelminths) for its survival (Colorni, 1994; Massimo, 2019).

The parasitic dinoflagellate *A. ocellatum* exhibits a direct, triphasic life cycle (Fig. 2.1) which can be completed within a week, dependent on environmental temperature.

*Email: paola.beraldo@uniud.it

 Fish Parasites: Pathobiology and Protection, 2nd Edition (eds P.T.K. Woo and K. Buchmann)
DOI: 10.1079/9781800628748.0002

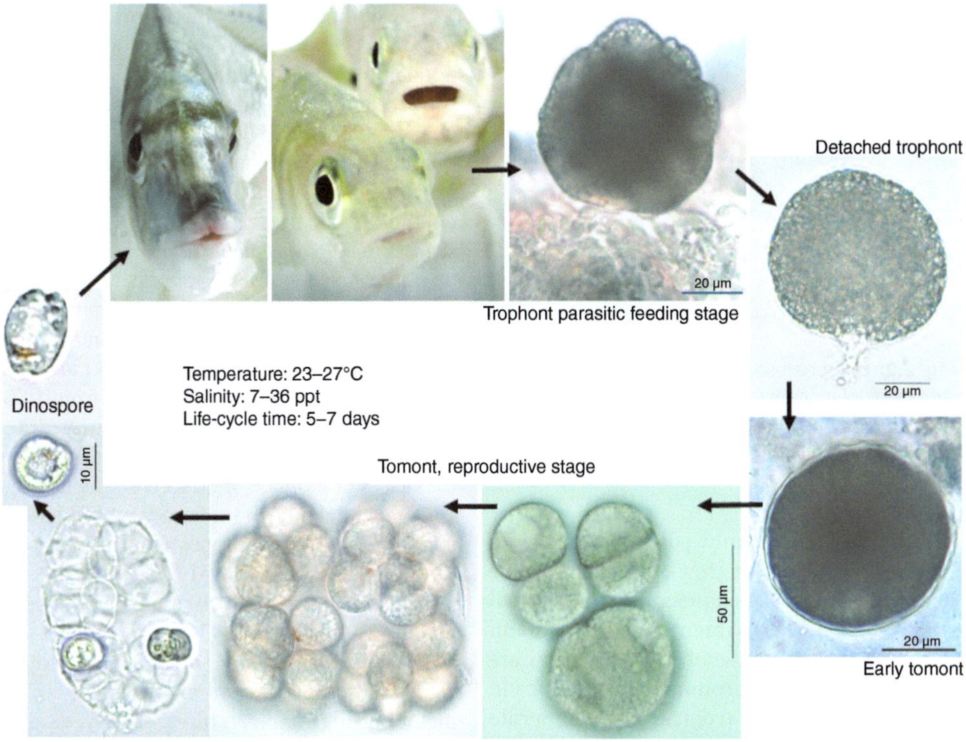

Fig. 2.1. Representation of *Amyloodinium ocellatum* life cycle. (Original from P. Beraldo.)

The parasitic trophont is sessile and attaches to the gill and skin epithelium of the host using rhizoids. Depending on the parasitic load and host species, trophonts are found in the eyes, on the fins and throughout the oropharyngeal cavity (Kuperman and Matey, 1999; Cruz-Lacierda *et al.*, 2004; Noga, 2010; Byadgi *et al.*, 2019a). Although never definitively elucidated, the stomopode is the apparatus through which the trophont assimilates nutrients from the host (Lom and Lawler, 1973; Noga and Levy, 2006). After the feeding phase (2–6 days), the trophont detaches from the fish by retracting its rhizoids and transforms into a tomont, encysting on inert substrates to initiate the reproductive stage. Within 2–4 days, a single tomont can potentially produce several dozen dinospores, depending on the trophic resources accumulated during the vegetative phase (Paperna, 1984). The dinospore is the motile, infective stage of the parasite and has two flagella, one transverse and one longitudinal, that enable it to swim in the water. It moves with whirling motions alternated by sudden sprints in random directions, helping it to find a new host. Once it locates a host, it adheres within a few minutes and transforms into a trophont (Fig. 2.2). If temperature and salinity are favourable (i.e. 23–27°C and 30–35 ppt, respectively), the life cycle can be completed in 5–7 days.

A. ocellatum is the aetiological agent of amyloodiniosis, also known as marine velvet disease or oodiniasis, due to its previous classification as *Oodinium ocellatum*. This parasitic disease can have an extremely rapid and severe course (12–24 h), sometimes with lethal outcomes (100% fish mortality) due to compromised respiratory function, as the gills are the primary site of infection (Lawler, 1980; Beraldo *et al.*, 2017). However, mortality, morbidity and prevalence rates can vary significantly depending on the type of farming (typically in land-based and lagoon grow-out), parasitic load, fish species, immunological status and environmental conditions (Kuperman *et al.*, 2001; Saraiva *et al.*, 2011; Bahri, 2012; Beraldo *et al.*, 2017; Moreira *et al.*, 2017; Oidtmann *et al.*, 2024).

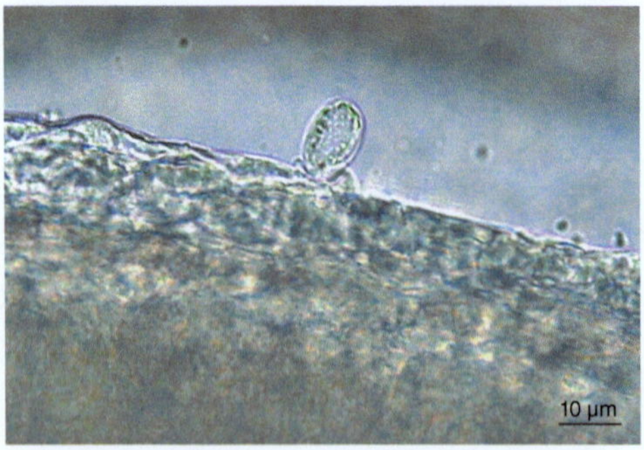

Fig. 2.2. European sea bass gills, showing an *Amyloodinium ocellatum* dinospore newly transformed into a trophont in the adhering phase on the gill epithelium. (Author's own image.)

A. ocellatum mainly poses a problem in land-based and lagoon grow-out systems, while its impact in sea-cage aquaculture is minimal (Rigos *et al.*, 1998; Diamant, 2001; Oidtmann *et al.*, 2024). Outbreaks of amyloodiniosis are influenced by the environmental conditions in aquaculture sites in tropical and temperate regions, such as in southern Europe and southern Asia (Francis-Floyd and Floyd, 2011; Soares *et al.*, 2012; Li *et al.*, 2021; Oidtmann *et al.*, 2024). These fish-rearing systems typically use untreated sea water, which provides a direct entry point for dinospores. Moreover, fish farms are usually located near the coast; therefore, waves and strong winds can easily transport dinospores in aerosols and fish-eating birds can spread infected fish. The impact of *A. ocellatum* infestations in European sea bass is particularly significant in Italy, where there are currently no licensed drugs (Oidtmann *et al.*, 2024). In amyloodiniosis cases, cumulative mortality is higher in fish up to 300 g in lagoon-based and land-based grow-out in Italy compared to Spain. *A. ocellatum* prevalence reaches 100% in Italian lagoon grow-out sites; however, disease manifestation is contingent upon environmental conditions and the host's immunological status. In contrast, land-based Italian sites exhibit a prevalence of approximately 20–30%, with infections typically limited to facilities employing sea water rather than borehole water. Although rare, *A. ocellatum* infections among juvenile fish within hatcheries can be highly detrimental.

A significant review by Shinn *et al.* (2015) examined major global marine and brackish aquaculture production sectors, highlighting the economic consequences of key parasite species, including *A. ocellatum*, which can limit production. They reported cases of amyloodiniosis in several commercially important species, including milkfish (*Chanos chanos*), sharpsnout seabream (*Diplodus puntazzo*), turbot (*Scophthalmus maximus*), bullseye pufferfish (*Sphoeroides annulatus*) and Nile tilapia (*Oreochromis niloticus*). For the latter species, the estimated economic loss, based on moderate (20%) and high (50%) mortality rates, could range from US$7 million to US$17 million (market value in 2000) (Shinn *et al.*, 2015). In addition to the costs due to the loss of biomass, indirect costs such as feed consumed, labour and treatments must also be included. An Italian European sea bass farm was forced to shut down in 2017 following an amyloodiniosis outbreak which resulted in the loss of about 63,000 juveniles (100% mortality). This outbreak occurred under a combination of adverse environmental and management factors, including high temperatures, stormy weather, poorly oxygenated brackish water from a nearby coastal lake, naïve fish to *A. ocellatum* and inexperienced staff (Beraldo *et al.*, 2017; Byadgi *et al.*, 2019a).

2.2. Pathobiology

The pathogenicity of *A. ocellatum* is attributed to the adhesion of trophonts via rhizoids to the epithelial cells of the gills, oropharyngeal cavity and skin (including the eyes and nostrils), coupled with multiple cellular necrosis induced by feeding activity through the stomopode (Noga, 1987) (Fig. 2.3).

The clinical pattern caused by *A. ocellatum* is directly proportional to the area of branchial and skin epithelium colonized and damages caused by the parasite. A single trophont can colonize multiple epithelial cells simultaneously (Fig. 2.4), which, coupled with the constant swimming activities of the fish, causes cellular degeneration and necrosis. Death of the host can occur within 12–48 h when the parasitic load is very high (e.g. over 200 trophonts/primary lamella).

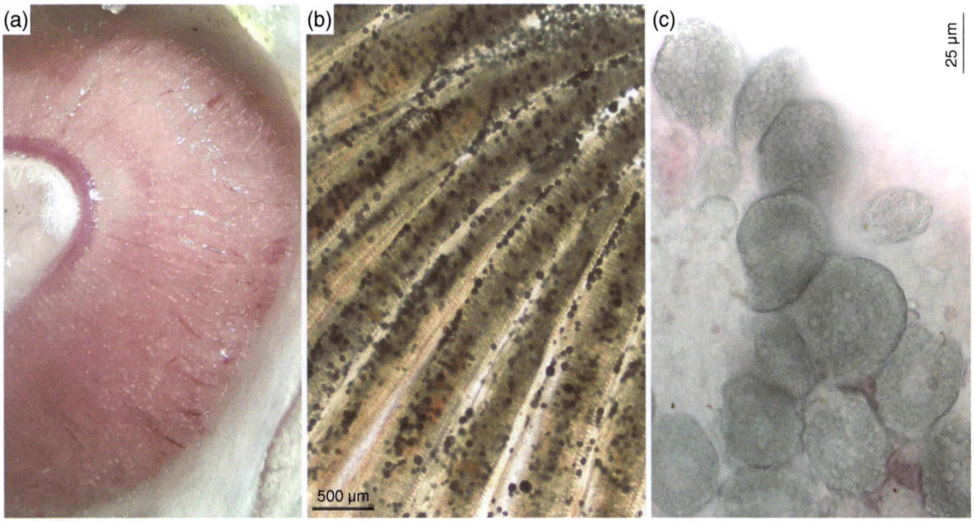

Fig. 2.3. Severe amyloodiniosis in European sea bass gills. (a) Numerous trophonts (whitish spots), filiform haemorrhages, anaemia and oedematous aspect of the gills; (b) microscopic examination showing the aspect of primary infested lamella (trophonts appear in black); (c) magnification of the previous image showing different sized trophonts on the primary lamellae, depending on the trophic resources accumulated during the vegetative phase. (Author's own image.)

Amyloodiniosis, especially in severe infestations, causes behavioural changes including jerky movements, flashing to relieve itching on the body, surface swimming near water inlets and dyspnoea. Anorexia is frequently associated with prolonged infestations as a possible consequence of stress and decrease of neuropeptide Y (Nozzi *et al.*, 2016). In some fish species, a granular, almost velvety appearance of the skin (hence the name 'marine velvet disease') induced by trophonts colonizing this site can be observed. Nevertheless, in European sea bass (*Dicentrarchus labrax*), regardless of the parasitic load, this skin appearance is not observed and the skin rarely presents noteworthy lesions. This may delay early diagnosis and leave fish to die rapidly from hypoxia (Beraldo *et al.*, 2017).

A. ocellatum induces moderate to intense tissue reactions, characterized in the gills by haemorrhages and branchial anaemia, epithelial hyperplasia, inflammation and necrosis, the severity of which depends on the parasitic load.

Nevertheless, mortality occurs even in subclinical or mild infestation, potentially from osmoregulatory dysfunction, anoxia and the subsequent onset of secondary infections due to severe epithelial damage (Lawler, 1980; Noga, 2012; Ragab *et al.*, 2022). The potential role of toxins in these abrupt mortalities cannot be excluded, considering the phylogenetic proximity of *A. ocellatum* to toxin-producing dinoflagellate genera responsible for mass mortality in wild and reared fish and molluscs. Based on *in vitro* studies on gilthead seabream (*Sparus aurata*) cell cultures, Moreira *et al.* (2022) confirmed life stage-specific compounds secreted by *A. ocellatum* can induce cell death. These compounds have haemolytic activities via a mechanism similar to that of karlotoxins.

Environmental factors, including water temperature, salinity and dissolved oxygen concentration, are significantly correlated with disease severity (Kuperman and Matey, 1999; Kuperman *et al.*, 2001; Pereira *et al.*, 2011; Saraiva *et al.*, 2011; Massimo *et al.*, 2022). The production of viable and infective dinospores occurs within few days at temperatures between 23 and 27°C and salinities of 10 to 60 ppt. Substantial deviations from these parameters lead to a progressive reduction of reproductive stages, often with development of non-viable dinospores (Paperna, 1984; Beraldo *et al.*,

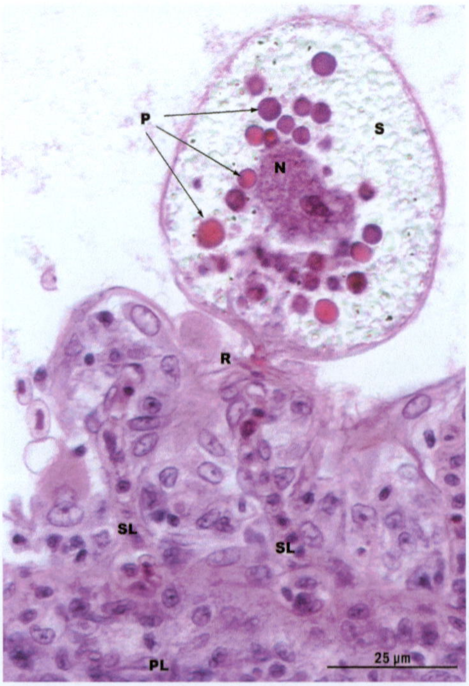

Fig. 2.4. European sea bass gills, showing an *Amyloodinium ocellatum* trophont simultaneously attached to multiple epithelial cells of three secondary lamellae. N, nucleus; P, protein granules; R, rhizoids; S, starch granules; SL, secondary lamellae; PL, primary lamellae. Haematoxylin and eosin stain. (Author's own image.)

2021). Nevertheless, severe outbreaks of amyloodiniosis have been documented under extreme aquaculture conditions (salinity 7 ppt and temperature 36°C, or salinity 46 ppt and temperature 40°C) (Kuperman and Matey, 1999; Beraldo *et al.*, 2017), demonstrating the remarkable biological plasticity of this dinoflagellate. Fish mortalities are more commonly observed during warmer months (especially between July and August in Europe), when water temperatures are high (e.g. above 28°C) and dissolved oxygen concentrations are low. These abiotic conditions indirectly enhance the negative impact of *A. ocellatum* (Massimo *et al.*, 2022). Atmospheric events such as storms or typhoons can facilitate the dispersal of dinospores via aerosols and contaminate nearby aquaculture facilities (Roberts-Thomson *et al.*, 2006; Dequito *et al.*, 2015; Beraldo *et al.*, 2017).

2.2.1. Histopathology

The histopathology in amyloodiniosis is dependent on the parasite density. In the early stages or mild infections (with no more than 10 trophonts/primary lamella), minimal lesions are observed (Fig. 2.5a). However, mild epithelial hyperplasia may occasionally occur around the attachment site of individual trophonts, sometimes accompanied by epithelial cell degeneration. Conversely, in more severe infections (100–200 trophonts/primary lamella), severe and multifocal epithelial degeneration of the oropharyngeal cavity (including pseudobranchs and nostrils), characterized by hydropic changes in the gill epithelial and chloride cells, along with necrosis and oedema, occurs. In European sea bass and other species, there is pronounced hyperplasia of the gill epithelium (Fig. 2.5b), particularly in the distal third of the primary lamellae, associated with the presence of synechiae (Kuperman *et al.*, 2001; Cruz-Lacierda *et al.*, 2004; Saraiva *et al.*, 2011; Guerra-Santos *et al.*, 2012; Vivanco-Aranda *et al.*, 2018; Byadgi *et al.*, 2019a).

Epithelial hyperplasia is also evident in pseudobranchs, the pharynx and the branchial arches. In the gill lamella the inflammatory cells are difficult to appreciate, but along the filaments lymphocytes, macrophages and mast cells are observable (Paperna, 1980; Guerra-Santos *et al.*, 2012; Vivanco-Aranda *et al.*, 2018; Massimo *et al.*, 2022). The same inflammatory response may occur in the buccal cavity and pharynx, whose epithelium is rich in mucous cells, while rodlet cells are often scattered throughout the gill epithelium, particularly at the base of the secondary lamellae (Beraldo and Massimo, 2022). Multiple anchoring of trophonts on the gill epithelium also causes rupture of the pillar cells and formation of aneurysms or microhaemorrhages in the lamellae, resulting in gill anaemia (Fig. 2.3). In European sea bass, the inflammatory response caused by moderate to severe infestation of *A. ocellatum* can be classified as hyperplastic parasitic branchitis, without any skin lesions.

2.2.2. Diagnosis of infection

The conventional diagnostic approach is microscopic detection/identification of trophonts in

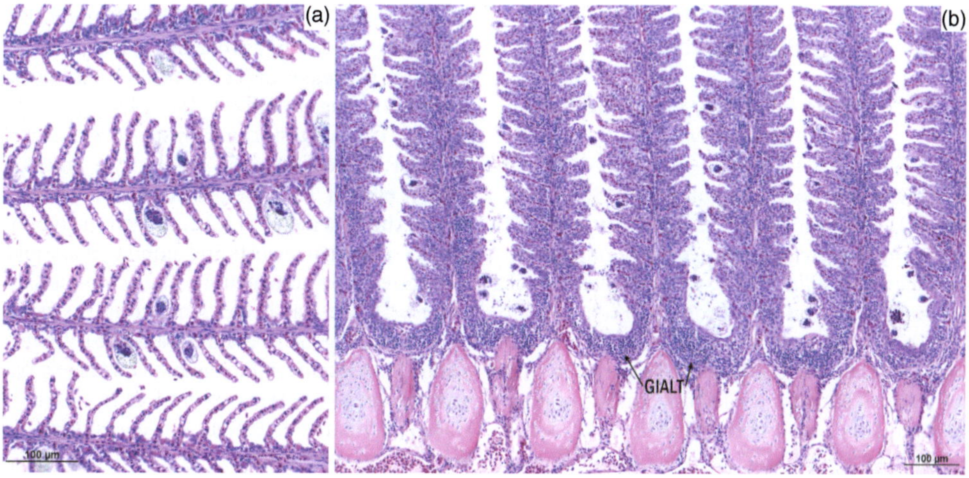

Fig. 2.5. European sea bass gills. (a) Few trophonts are attached to gill epithelium in early *Amyloodinium ocellatum* infection, showing no evident lesions. Haematoxylin and eosin stain. (b) Severe and diffuse gill hyperplasia as consequence of heavy infections, showing the activated GIALT. Haematoxylin and eosin stain. (Author's own image.)

fresh wet mounts of skin scrapings and branchial biopsies after observing clinical signs in affected fish (Fig. 2.3b and c). This approach is easy, immediate and reliable.

However, recent development of immunological and molecular techniques allows routine screening for subclinical infections or monitoring of aquatic environments prior to the introduction of sensitive fish species. Early-stage amyloodiniosis is clinically discrete with no clinical signs, but it can progress rapidly and lead to high mortality and thereby to significant economic losses (Cruz-Lacierda *et al.*, 2004; Soares *et al.*, 2012; Beraldo *et al.*, 2017).

Molecular approaches (e.g. PCR, loop-mediated isothermal amplification (LAMP)) have proven effective in specifically detecting *A. ocellatum* (Picón-Camacho *et al.*, 2013; Bessat and Fadel, 2018), even when the parasite is present in very low numbers (Levy *et al.*, 2007). A promising rapid quantitative real-time PCR (qPCR)-based analytical method has been developed to quantify *A. ocellatum* dinospores (Zhuang *et al.*, 2025), released from tomonts, in the rearing systems. Dinospores are exceedingly difficult to collect and quantify compared to trophonts within host tissues. This novel method employs the primer pair ITS-F3/ITS-R3 (conserved internal transcribed spacer (ITS) region within the *A. ocellatum* genome) for qPCR assays, demonstrating its suitability for evaluating the population dynamics of *A. ocellatum* and predicting the onset of disease in farms.

Molecular diagnosis of *A. ocellatum* employs primers AO18SF (5′-GACCTTGCCCGAGAGGG-3′) and AO18SR (5′-GGTGTTAAGATTCACCA-CACTTTCC-3′) to amplify a 248 bp segment of the 3′ end of the large-subunit ribosomal RNA (LSU rDNA) gene (Levy *et al.*, 2007; Byadgi *et al.*, 2019a). Sequence alignment using CLUSTALw has shown that the sequenced *A. ocellatum* is conserved across various geographic isolates from the Mediterranean Sea (DQ490256.1), the Red Sea (DQ490257.1), Fujian, China (KU761581.1 and KR057921.1) and Southern Mississippi, USA (JX905204.1) (Byadgi *et al.*, 2019a).

The ELISA method can measure specific antibody titres against *A. ocellatum* in fish recovering from natural or experimentally induced amyloodiniosis (Smith *et al.*, 1992; Cobb *et al.*, 1998a; Cecchini *et al.*, 2001; Byadgi *et al.*, 2019b; Massimo, 2019). It can also be used for surveillance of protective immunity levels in susceptible or experimentally vaccinated populations.

2.3. Protective and Control Strategies

2.3.1. Innate immunity and adaptive immunity

Some wild fish species, as gulf killifish (*Fundulus grandis*), American eel (*Anguilla rostrata*) and sailfin molly (*Poecilia latipinna*), have natural resistance to *A. ocellatum* due to their thick mucus layer and/or tolerance to chronic hypoxia (Lawler, 1977). *A. ocellatum* parasitizes the gill or skin epithelium; consequently, host recognition and defence mechanisms are localized in the mucus, epithelial cells and extracellular fluid of the epithelium (Noga, 2012). Various mediators secreted by immune cells contribute to robust humoral immunity, regulate immune mechanisms and maintain host homeostasis. Fish produce innate antimicrobial substances, including histone-like proteins (HLPs) (Noga *et al.*, 2001, 2002) and antimicrobial peptides (AMPs) such as piscidins, hepcidin and haemoglobin-derived peptides (HbβP-1), which provide broad-spectrum or specific protection against *A. ocellatum* (Ullal *et al.*, 2008). Hepcidin is a crucial regulator of iron metabolism in fish, playing an essential role in their physiology by supporting respiration, growth and immune function, and it is generally upregulated by bacterial and parasitic infection (Byadgi *et al.*, 2019a; Yang *et al.*, 2022). Hepcidin significantly contributes to host defence in infected European sea bass and may serve as a marker related to *A. ocellatum* infection (Byadgi *et al.*, 2019a). Related to this, the observed upregulation of haemopexin in the liver of infested gilthead seabream implies a crucial role for iron transport and metabolism during disease progression, potentially linked to the development of haemorrhages (Soares *et al.*, 2025).

Vertebrate innate immunity relies on germline-encoded pathogen pattern recognition receptors (PRRs) to recognize conserved microbial components (pathogen-associated molecular patterns (PAMPs)) on both pathogenic and non-pathogenic organisms, leading to a coordinated immune response (Boltaña *et al.*, 2011). Current knowledge regarding the recognition of PAMPs in *A. ocellatum* indicates that Toll-like receptors (TLRs) serve as key mediators of innate immunity against this dinoflagellate. Although no activation of TLR1, TLR2, TLR4 and TLR9 has been observed in European sea bass infested gills, an increase in TLR9 mRNA has been detected in the anterior kidney (Byadgi *et al.*, 2019a). This suggests that parasite DNA, serving as PAMP, is recognized by TLR9 in the anterior kidney, even if this host–pathogen interaction should be clarified. TLR22, which has only been described in teleosts and amphibians, could recognize or be activated also by ectoparasites. Indeed, TLR22 has been identified as a significant immune gene in the antiparasitic response against *A. ocellatum* in Japanese yellowtail (*Seriola quinqueradiata*) (Reyes-Becerril *et al.*, 2015). However, the role of TLR as anti-parasite in fish is still largely unknown.

A. ocellatum pathogenicity elicits a strong innate immune response, including apoptosis and pro-inflammatory gene upregulation (Byadgi *et al.*, 2019a, 2021; Zhang *et al.*, 2022; Li *et al.*, 2024). While interleukin-1β (IL-1β) and tumour necrosis factor-α (TNF-α) were unexpectedly absent in European sea bass gill tissue, potentially due to host susceptibility or leucopoietic damage, other pro-inflammatory markers (interleukin-8 (IL-8), cyclooxygenase-2 (COX-2), CC1) were upregulated, indicating a host response. IL-8 suggests neutrophil recruitment, and CC chemokines may contribute to wound healing (Byadgi *et al.*, 2019a, 2021). In European sea bass, in contrast, increases in intestinal levels of IL-1β and TNF-α were observed (Nozzi *et al.*, 2016).

Tissue damage, hypoxia and other factors trigger the intrinsic apoptosis pathway, as evidenced by the upregulation of pro-apoptotic genes following infection with *A. ocellatum*. Notably, there is a significant upregulation of caspase-3 and caspase-9 in the gills and anterior kidney of infected fish (Byadgi *et al.*, 2019a; Zhang *et al.*, 2022). Apoptotic cell death plays a crucial role in maintaining host homeostasis, and the timely removal of damaged cells is essential for reducing inflammation. However, despite the activation of apoptotic pathways in European sea bass, this response is insufficient to limit infection and trophonts still survive in the host (Byadgi *et al.*, 2019a).

A. ocellatum, similar to other protozoa, can stimulate the host immune response, leading to the release of pro-inflammatory cytokines and enzymes such as inducible nitric oxide synthase (iNOS). Immunolabelling of infested gill tissue from European sea bass revealed macrophages mainly within hyperplastic epithelial foci (Fig. 2.6a) (Byadgi *et al.*, 2019a; Massimo *et al.*, 2022).

Evidently, innate immunity constitutes the initial protective barrier against *A. ocellatum*, and its function is inherently connected to the transition towards adaptive immunity. Resistance to natural or experimental amyloodiniosis in fish is associated with the production of antibodies (Noga *et al.*, 1991; Smith *et al.*, 1992; Cobb *et al.*, 1998a; Cecchini *et al.*, 2001; Massimo, 2019). Fish that survive infections develop immunity, which is evident through the agglutination and immobilization of dinospores by antisera, as well as the presence of antibodies in the serum. Massimo *et al.* (2022) confirmed the fish capability to develop specific immunity against *A. ocellatum* by labelling plasma cells and macrophages with an anti-immunoglobulin M (IgM) polyclonal antibody in infested European sea bass (Fig. 2.6b).

Despite the absence of changes in some genes related to adaptive immunity (major histocompatibility complexes MHC-I and MHC-II, IgM) (Byadgi *et al.*, 2019a) in natural infested European sea bass, the significant high expression of immunoglobulin T (IgT) in gills and head kidney and the activation of branchial lymphoid tissue indicate an active role for mucosal immunity with the activation of gill-associated lymphoid tissue (GIALT).

Although fish that survive natural infestations or are immunized with *A. ocellatum* develop adaptive immune responses, no vaccines against this dinoflagellate are currently available (Smith *et al.*, 1993; Cobb *et al.*, 1998b).

Recent research has investigated the induction of innate and adaptive immunity-related gene expression and antibody titres in European sea bass vaccinated with inactivated, fragmented dinospores (Byadgi *et al.*, 2019b). Specifically, the protective efficacy of an intra-coelomic vaccine, with or without adjuvant, was evaluated through *A. ocellatum* challenge trials at 1 and 6 months post-vaccination. Injection of a vaccine with adjuvant conferred protection at 30 days post-vaccination but did not protect fish at 6 months. The limited *A. ocellatum*-specific IgM synthesis in vaccinated fish (using ELISA) may be from the cellulose-based antigen, instead of antigenic proteins, or the non-mucosal administration route, which contrasts with the natural ectoparasite exposure. However, gene expression analysis of head kidney and gill tissues showed upregulation of innate immune genes (IL-8 and hepcidin) and adaptive immune genes (IgM and IgT) following vaccination. The observed gene expression patterns at 1 month post-vaccination suggested that both humoral and cell-mediated immunity contribute to, or synergistically mediate, early pathogen clearance during *A. ocellatum* infection (Byadgi *et al.*, 2019b).

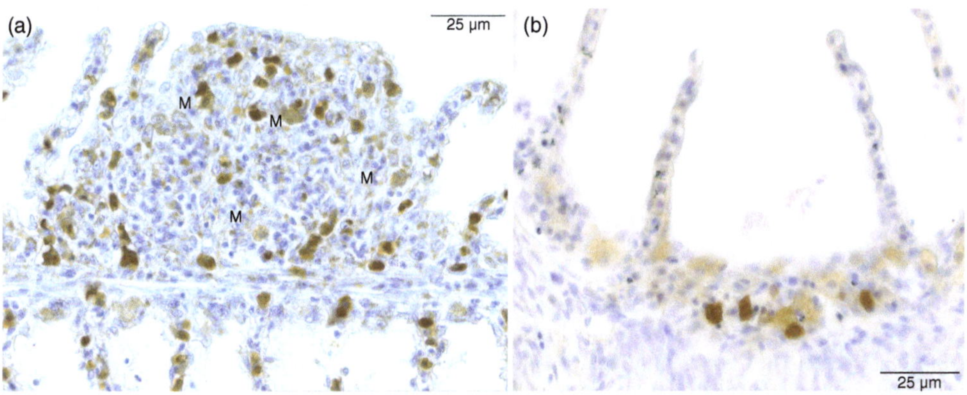

Fig. 2.6. Immunohistochemical staining of *Amyloodinium ocellatum*-infected European sea bass gills. (a) iNOS immunoreactivity of red blood cells, but also macrophage-like cells (M) which are mainly localized in hyperplastic epithelial foci. (b) IgM immunoreactivity at 30 days post-infestation; note plasma cells or IgM-bearing macrophages mainly located in the pockets between primary lamellae. (Author's own image.)

Another study explored a European sea bass vaccine using hydrophilic extracts from *A. ocellatum* tomonts, showing promising initial immune modulation (Soares *et al.*, 2025). However, the lack of standardized *A. ocellatum* dinospore/trophont production seems to hinder this research for amyloodiniosis prevention.

2.3.2. Chemotherapies and prophylaxis

Numerous studies have been undertaken to control amyloodiniosis in diverse fish species (Oestmann and Lewis, 1996a; Fajer-Ávila *et al.*, 2003; Benetti *et al.*, 2008; Noga, 2012; Kumar *et al.*, 2015; Virgula *et al.*, 2017; Bessat and Fadel, 2018; Sousa *et al.*, 2024; Soares *et al.*, 2025) but, despite these efforts, no effective and legal chemotherapy is available. Consequently, current management strategies primarily focus on disease control rather than eradication.

Unfortunately, the exponential reproductive rate of *A. ocellatum* during warmer seasons requires early detection and timely therapeutic intervention. The dinospore is the most sensitive parasitic stage to chemotherapy, whereas trophonts and tomonts are relatively resistant. To date, copper sulfate remains the most widely used treatment to control disease outbreaks, due to the proven dinosporicidal efficacy of the copper ion (Noga, 2010; Francis-Floyd and Floyd, 2011; Virgula *et al.*, 2017; Owatari *et al.*, 2020; Dhayanithi *et al.*, 2022; Moreira *et al.*, 2024). Furthermore, copper sulfate is inexpensive and readily available because it is widely used as an algicide and fungicide. The addition of copper sulfate at 0.75–1 g/m^3 for about 2 weeks to ponds/tanks kills dinospores while tomonts and trophonts are not very susceptible. The free copper ion is unstable in sea water; therefore, its levels require close monitoring using a copper test kit. In contrast, chelated copper exhibits greater stability in water, although its monitoring can be more challenging (Noga, 2010) and the bioavailable concentration is also reduced, which limits the effectiveness against pathogens (Lieke *et al.*, 2020). Careful monitoring is also crucial because certain fish species are sensitive to copper and may exhibit toxicity at concentrations necessary for pathogen control (Cardeilhac and Whitaker, 1988). Alternatively, in European sea bass trials, positive outcomes were obtained by reducing salinity to 10 ppt with freshwater influx and employing a lower copper sulfate concentration (0.1 ppm) (Sousa *et al.*, 2024).

Nevertheless, copper sulfate is not licensed for amyloodiniosis treatment in farmed fish in Europe and other countries, due to its potential negative effects on the environment and food safety.

Freshwater baths can induce rapid detachment of trophonts from skin and gills, providing an eco-friendly disease control method. It is not a conclusive treatment as not all trophonts detach. Exposure for 1–2 min in treatment tanks is recommended, with subsequent transfer of the fish to other tanks to prevent encystment of detached tomonts and restart of their reproductive phase when salinity is restored (above 4 ppt). However, fresh water is not readily available to most marine fish farms, therefore this treatment is useful to control outbreaks in aquaria, and some fish species cannot tolerate a sudden osmotic shock. Rapid detachment of trophonts in fresh water from the skin and gills is a useful method to collect them for experimental purposes (Beraldo *et al.*, 2021), but it is better not to prolong the treatment (no more than 1–2 min) since the absence of salt in the water is lethal for *A. ocellatum*.

Formalin (125–250 ppm for 1 h and repeated over several days if necessary) (Noga, 2010) and other chemical treatments (hydrogen peroxide at 75 and 150 mg/l for 30 min, repeated after 6 days) (Montgomery-Brock *et al.*, 2001) exhibit limited efficacy in controlling amyloodiniosis. This is because these treatments induce the detachment of the trophont from the fish, leading to its rapid encystment and adherence to substrates within the rearing system. Therefore, treatment in quarantine tanks is advisable, or alternatively, the treatment strategy should target the dinospores and be maintained until most of them have hatched from tomonts and been inactivated.

Alternative treatments can be applied to limit the impact of amyloodiniosis. Chloroquine diphosphate (5–10 mg/l), an antimalarial drug employed in human medicine, is effective and less toxic than copper sulfate as a dinosporicide in immersion treatments (Kumar *et al.*, 2015); furthermore, it exhibits prophylactic potential when administered orally (Lewis *et al.*, 1988). However, the substantial cost of chloroquine and its unauthorized status for aquaculture species limit its practical application. Similarly, 2′,4′-dihydroxychalcone and tomatine have been investigated *in vitro* against *A. ocellatum* dinospores, but their very high costs make their usage prohibitive under practical fish farm conditions, although they are effective (Tedesco *et al.*, 2020). Future studies should investigate the effects of these compounds on fish (e.g. growth, development, longevity).

The aquaculture industry faces a significant threat from amyloodiniosis and there is an urgent need for an economical, environmentally benign and effective control strategy. Conventional chemical treatments pose ecotoxicological risks to the environment and aquatic life, while eco-sustainable alternatives (e.g. plant compounds and *Artemia salina* nauplii as bioremediation) are either economically unviable for widespread use in aquaculture or remain limited to experimental studies (Oestmann *et al.*, 1995; Kumar *et al.*, 2015; Tedesco *et al.*, 2020). Recent innovative research, however, has revealed that galvanized materials offer an effective means of mitigating *A. ocellatum* reinfestation. The significant reduction in parasite load observed with galvanized iron mesh and plates strongly suggests that the release of zinc ions exerts a substantial anti-*A. ocellatum* effect, indicating a promising avenue for disease management (Luo *et al.*, 2024).

Prophylactic strategies are paramount for effective disease management to avert catastrophic outbreaks characterized by high mortality rates. The crucial measures to implement for limiting the introduction and dissemination of *A. ocellatum* vary depending on the aquaculture production site (hatchery, land-based facility, lagoon, sea cage, aquarium). Biosecurity measures should include:

- treatment of incoming water when feasible (mechanical filtration, ultraviolet irradiation, ozonation);
- parasitological examination and quarantine of newly introduced fish coupled with preventive therapies;
- maintenance of adequate hygiene standards for facilities and equipment, including the implementation of periodic sanitary fallowing (letting the pond or tank bottom dry in the sun before introducing new fish in the rearing site);
- paying attention to the characteristics of the site where the farm is located (e.g. endemicity of amyloodiniosis) and weathering, which are important aspects influencing presence of the parasite;
- systematic parasitological monitoring, particularly during the summer months in endemic areas; and
- regulating the water temperature and salinity during the periods of highest risks, if practicable.

Increased fish welfare, as well as enhanced immune-related and overall health, may help prevent amyloodiniosis or help fish recover from infection. An alternative approach is to prophylactically stimulate the general health and immune response of the fish to prevent disease. A promising alternative to promote growth performance and to increase immune resistance in fish is the use of functional feed additives (such as amino acids, polyunsaturated fatty acids and different kinds of 'biotics') (Reyes-Becerril *et al.*, 2008; Buentello *et al.*, 2010; Lieke *et al.*, 2020) also, in addition to chemotherapeutic agents.

Immunoprophylactic strategies would be highly advantageous for the aquaculture of fish species in lagoon/land-based rearing systems, as they could prevent fish losses and diminish the reliance on unauthorized chemotherapeutic treatments. The development of a protective vaccine for fish against *A. ocellatum* could be a realistic outcome for the future. Starting with an 'omics' approach, parasite antigens can be evaluated as potential candidates for the production of recombinant vaccines (Byadgi *et al.*, 2019a, 2020).

2.4. Maintenance and Propagation of *Amyloodinium ocellatum* in the Laboratory

The parasites used in most host/parasite studies were obtained from infected fish by bathing them in fresh water (Beraldo *et al.*, 2021). This process causes trophonts to detach from the gills and skin and rapidly transform into tomonts. Maintaining them in culture allows for the recovery of dinospores, which can be used in both *in vitro* and *in vivo* studies.

A key limitation in research is the lack of a system that enables the parasite to be produced consistently and in large quantities. The trophont stage is particularly interesting to study because it interacts directly with the host, but it is also the most difficult to obtain without bacterial or host contamination. Alternatively, 'early-tomontized' trophonts can be easily obtained in large numbers through controlled *A. ocellatum* infestation, often without the need to sacrifice the fish, and with minimal bacterial or host contamination.

Cell culture is a crucial technique widely used to investigate host–pathogen interactions. However, only a few fish cell lines have been developed for studying parasitic infections and potential treatment strategies that could benefit research on parasitic diseases (Li *et al.*, 2024). All life-cycle stages of *A. ocellatum* were successfully propagated on catfish (*Clarias batrachus*) gill cells (G1B). Infections in fish from *in vitro* cultures were comparable to those observed in natural hosts, regarding cytopathology and development (Noga, 1987). Subsequently, a system for culturing *A. ocellatum* was developed using aggregates of red drum (*Sciaenops ocellatus*) dorsal fin cells, which improved *in vitro* culture conditions (Oestmann and Lewis, 1996b). Recently, a new cell line derived from the gill tissues of yellowfin seabream (*Acanthopagrus latus*) (ALG) has been established. *A. ocellatum* can effectively infect this cell monolayer and complete an entire life cycle *in vitro*. Moreover, the *in vitro* gill cell monolayer closely mimics the *in vivo* host response of *A. latus* to *A. ocellatum* infection. This newly developed cell line shows great promise as a valuable tool for studying *A. ocellatum* and host interactions.

However, it is expensive (purchase of the cell line and its maintenance) and laborious to produce just a small number of dinospores.

To overcome these challenges, Beraldo *et al.* (2021) developed a hibernation protocol for *A. ocellatum* by allowing the parasite to be preserved at the tomont stage (at 16 ± 0.5°C in an incubator) under controlled artificial conditions for several months. This approach ensures a steady supply of dinospores for research, such as studying motility (during exposure to medicine or chemicals), conducting experimental infections, testing vaccines and coating ELISA plates. It is essential to maintain the parasite in sterile salt water (30 ppt) with antibiotics to prevent microbial contamination and to sustain the viability of both tomonts and dinospores. Hibernated tomonts have been shown to remain viable for more than 6 months, and they produce dinospores at temperatures between 20 and 25°C. It is advisable to renew the parasite stock every 6 months by obtaining new tomonts from controlled infected fish.

2.5. Conclusions and Suggestions for Future Studies

Amyloodiniosis poses a significant threat to fish health (up to 100% mortality within a few days) and can cause substantial economic losses, particularly in lagoon-based and land-based farms located in geographical areas with temperate and tropical climates. Climate change (e.g. temperature variations, ocean acidification, alterations in marine currents, salinity shifts and harmful algal blooms are already occurring) will have a major impact on aquaculture (Cascarano *et al.*, 2021). Among these, temperature is expected to have the most profound effect on aquaculture systems, as it influences the well-being of farmed fish, propagation of the parasite population and the emergence of diseases.

Rising temperatures influence parasites by increasing their reproductive rates, expanding their geographic distribution and potentially leading to more mortality outbreaks. Currently, sea surface temperatures in the Mediterranean range from 24 to 30°C, with the eastern basin being warmer. This temperature range is unlikely to pose a significant threat to *A. ocellatum*, given its high plasticity regarding temperature but also salinity. However, elevated temperatures can impair host health due to thermal stress and decrease dissolved oxygen levels in the water, thereby exacerbating the impact of the parasite.

Furthermore, challenges also induced by climate changes underscore the urgent need to deepen our understanding of *A. ocellatum* and its interactions with hosts across all aspects of its biology.

Currently, it is crucial to expand knowledge regarding the interaction mechanisms of *A. ocellatum* with its host and the host's response, particularly concerning the vegetative (trophont) and dinospore stages. While some studies have begun to provide valuable insights (Byadgi *et al.*, 2020; Moreira *et al.*, 2022; Zhang *et al.*, 2022), further efforts are required to obtain a comprehensive gene expression profile of *A. ocellatum* dinospores and trophonts, thereby aiding in the identification of genes critical for its life cycle and virulence. Contemporary 'omics' approaches will facilitate the comprehension of stage-specific functions and genes associated with pathogenesis, potentially paving the way for the development of effective vaccines against amyloodiniosis and targeted pharmacological therapies.

The development of a prophylactic vaccination system, potentially via immersion, should be a primary objective, employing both classical and modern vaccinology approaches. This would enable a reduction in the impact of the disease in aquaculture settings with a higher risk of amyloodiniosis.

Further histopathological investigations across diverse fish species would be valuable to compare the lesion and inflammatory responses to *A. ocellatum* infestation under controlled conditions of equivalent parasite load and host age. Precisely characterizing the inflammatory pattern elicited in different hosts of this parasite would be highly helpful.

Finally, the improvement of highly specific and sensitive infection detection systems would be advisable for effective biosecurity and management this disease and for minimizing the use of chemotherapeutics.

References

Aravindan, N., Chaganti, K. and Aravindan, S. (2007) Protozoan parasites in commercially important shrimp species from northeast coast of Andhra Pradesh, India. *Journal of Experimental Zoology India* 10(1), 9–20.

Bahri, S. (2012) Protozoan and myxozoan infections in wild gilthead seabream (*Sparus aurata* L.) from North Lake of Tunis, Tunisia. *Acta Parasitologica* 57, 114–121. DOI: 10.2478/s11686-012-0021-x.

Benetti, D.D., Orhun, M.R., Sardenberg, B., O'Hanlon, B., Welch, A. *et al.* (2008) Advances in hatchery and grow-out technology of cobia *Rachycentron canadum* (Linnaeus). *Aquaculture Research* 39, 701–711. DOI: 10.1111/j.1365-2109.2008.01922.x.

Beraldo, P. and Massimo, M. (2022) Amyloodiniosis. In: Kibenge, F.S.B., Baldisserotto, B. and Chong, R.S.-M. (eds) *Aquaculture Pathophysiology, Volume I: Finfish Diseases*. Academic Press, Cambridge, Massachusetts, pp. 475–483. DOI: 10.1016/B978-0-12-812211-2.00038-X.

Beraldo, P., Byadgi, O., Massimo, M., Bulfon, C., Volpatti, D. and Galeotti, M. (2017) Grave episodio di amyloodiniosi in giovanili di branzino (*Dicentrarchus labrax*): analisi dei determinanti di malattia e rilievi anatomopatologici. In: *Atti del convegno, XXIII Convegno nazionale S.I.P.I.* Società Italiana di Patologia Ittica, Lecce, Italy, p. 30.

Beraldo, P., Massimo, M. and Galeotti, M. (2021) *Amyloodinium ocellatum*. In: Sitjà-Bobadilla, A., Bron, J.E., Wiegertjes, G. and Piazzon, C. (eds) *Fish Parasites: A Handbook of Protocols for their Isolation, Culture and Transmission*. 5m Books, Great Easton, UK. DOI: 10.52517/9781789181531.004.

Bessat, M. and Fadel, A. (2018) Amyloodiniosis in cultured *Dicentrarchus labrax*: parasitological and molecular diagnosis, and an improved treatment protocol. *Diseases of Aquatic Organisms* 129, 41–51. DOI: 10.3354/dao03237.

Boltaña, S., Roher, N., Goetz, F.W. and MacKenzie, S.A. (2011) PAMPs, PRRs and the genomics of gram negative bacterial recognition in fish. *Developmental and Comparative Immunology* 35(12), 1195–1203. DOI: 10.1016/j.dci.2011.02.010.

Buentello, J.A., Neill, W.H. and Gatlin III, D.M. (2010) Effects of dietary prebiotics on the growth, feed efficiency and non-specific immunity of juvenile red drum *Sciaenops ocellatus* fed soybean-based diets. *Aquaculture Research* 41, 411–418. DOI: 10.1111/j.1365-2109.2009.02178.x.

Byadgi, O., Beraldo, P., Volpatti, D., Massimo, M., Bulfon, C. and Galeotti, M. (2019a) Expression of infection-related immune response in European sea bass (*Dicentrarchus labrax*) during a natural outbreak from a unique dinoflagellate *Amyloodinium ocellatum*. *Fish and Shellfish Immunology* 84, 62–72. DOI: 10.1016/j.fsi.2018.09.069.

Byadgi, O., Volpatti, D., Massimo, M., Bulfon, C., Galeotti, M. and Beraldo, P. (2019b) *Amyloodinium ocellatum* vaccine-induced modulation of immune genes expression in European sea bass (*Dicentrarchus *labrax*). In: *Book of Abstracts of the 19th International Conference on Diseases of Fish and Shellfish*. European Association of Fish Pathologists, Porto, Portugal, p. 220.

Byadgi, O., Marroni, F., Dirks, R., Massimo, M., Volpatti, D. *et al.* (2020) Transcriptome analysis of *Amyloodinium ocellatum* tomonts revealed basic information on the major potential virulence factors. *Genes* 11, 1252. DOI: 10.3390/genes11111252.

Byadgi, O., Massimo, M., Dirks, R.P., Pallavicini, A., Bron, J.E. *et al.* (2021) Innate immune-gene expression during experimental amyloodiniosis in European seabass (*Dicentrarchus labrax*). *Veterinary Immunology and Immunopathology* 234, 110217. DOI: 10.1016/j.vetimm.2021.110217.

Cardeilhac, P.T. and Whitaker, B.R. (1988) Copper treatments: uses and precautions. *Veterinary Clinics of North America: Small Animal Practice* 18, 435–448. DOI: 10.1016/S0195-5616(88)50041-4.

Cascarano, M.C., Stavrakidis-Zachou, O., Mladineo, I., Thompson, K.D., Papandroulakis, N. and Katharios, P. (2021) Mediterranean aquaculture in a changing climate: temperature effects on pathogens and diseases of three farmed fish species. *Pathogens* 10(9), 1205. DOI: 10.3390/pathogens10091205.

Cecchini, S., Saroglia, M., Terova, G. and Albanesi, F. (2001) Detection of antibody response against *Amyloodinium ocellatum* (Brown, 1931) in serum of naturally infected European sea bass by an enzyme-linked immunosorbent assay (ELISA). *Bulletin of the European Association of Fish Pathologists* 21, 104–108.

Cobb, C.S., Levy, M.G. and Noga, E.J. (1998a) Acquired immunity to amyloodiniosis is associated with an antibody response. *Diseases of Aquatic Organisms* 34(2), 125–133. DOI: 10.3354/dao034125.

Cobb, C.S., Levy, M.G. and Noga, E.J. (1998b) Development of immunity by the tomato clownfish *Amphiprion frenatus* to the dinoflagellate parasite *Amyloodinium ocellatum*. *Journal of Aquatic Animal Health* 10, 259–263. DOI: 10.1577/1548-8667(1998)010<0259:DOIBTT>2.0.CO;2.

Colorni, A. (1994) Hyperparasitism of *Amyloodinium ocellatum* (Dinoflagellida: Oodinidae) on *Neobenedenia melleni* (Monogenea: Capsalidae). *Diseases of Aquatic Organisms* 19, 157–159. DOI: 10.3354/dao019157.

Cruz-Lacierda, E.R., Maeno, Y., Pineda, A.J.T. and Matey, V.E. (2004) Mass mortality of hatchery-reared milkfish (*Chanos chanos*) and mangrove red snapper (*Lutjanus argentimaculatus*) caused by *Amyloodinium ocellatum* (Dinoflagellida). *Aquaculture* 236, 85–94. DOI: 10.1016/j.aquaculture.2004.02.012.

de Souza, N.A. (2015) Resposta metabólica da ostra *Crassostrea gigas* na presença do parasita *Amyloodinium ocellatum*. Master's thesis, University of the Algarve, Faro, Portugal. Available at: https://sapientia.ualg.pt/entities/publication/77271106-15ba-458a-9bb4-6b91a1258714 (accessed 18 May 2025).

Dequito, A.Q.D., Cruz-Lacierda, E.R. and Corre Jr, V.L. (2015) A case study on the environmental features associated with *Amyloodinium ocellatum* (Dinoflagellida) occurrences in a milkfish (*Chanos chanos*) hatchery. *AACL Bioflux* 8, 390–397.

Dhayanithi, N.B., Sudhagar, A., Kumar, T.T.A. and Lal, K.K. (2022) Study on amyloodiniosis outbreak in captive-bred percula clownfish (*Amphiprion percula*) and improved control regimens. *Journal of Parasitic Diseases* 46, 1103–1109. DOI: 10.1007/s12639-022-01530-1.

Diamant, A. (2001) Cross-infections between marine cage-cultured stocks and wild fish in the northern Red Sea: is the environment at risk? In: *Risk Analysis in Aquatic Animal Health. Proceedings of an International Conference, Paris, France, 8–10 February, 2000*. Office International des Épizooties, Paris, pp. 202–208.

Drebes, G. (1984) Life cycle and host specificity of marine parasitic dinophytes. *Helgolinder Meeresunters* 37, 603–622.

Fajer-Ávila, E.J., Abdo-de la Parra, I., Aguilar-Zarate, G., Contreras-Arce, R., Zaldívar-Ramírez, J. and Betancourt-Lozano, M. (2003) Toxicity of formalin to bullseye puffer fish (*Sphoeroides annulatus* Jenyns, 1843) and its effectiveness to control ectoparasites. *Aquaculture* 223, 41–50. DOI: 10.1016/S0044-8486(03)00166-2.

Francis-Floyd, R. and Floyd, M.R. (2011) *Amyloodinium ocellatum, An Important Parasite of Cultured Marine Fish*. SRAC Publication No. 4705. Southern Regional Aquaculture Center, Stoneville, Mississippi, 11 pp.

Guerra-Santos, B., Albinati, R.C.B., Moreira, E.L.T., Lima, F.W.M., Azevedo, T.M.P. *et al.* (2012) Parameters hematological and histopathologic alterations in cobia (*Rachycentron canadum* Linnaeus, 1766) com amyloodiniose. *Pesquisa Veterinária Brasileira* 32, 1184–1190. DOI: 10.1590/S0100-736X2012001100019.

Kumar, P.R., Nazar, A.K.A., Jayakumar, R., Tamilmani, G., Sakthivel, M. *et al.* (2015) *Amyloodinium ocellatum* infestation in the broodstock of silver pompano *Trachinotus blochii* (Lacepede, 1801) and its therapeutic control. *Indian Journal of Fisheries* 62(1), 131–134.

Kuperman, B.I. and Matey, V.E. (1999) Massive infestation by *Amyloodinium ocellatum* (Dinoflagellida) of fish in a highly saline lake, Salton Sea, California, USA. *Diseases of Aquatic Organisms* 39, 65–73. DOI: 10.3354/dao039065.

Kuperman, B.I., Matey, V.E. and Hurlbert, S.H. (2001) Parasites of fish from the Salton Sea, California, USA. *Hydrobiologia* 466, 195–208. DOI: 10.1023/A:1014555904968.

Lawler, A.R. (1977) Dinoflagellate (*Amyloodinium*) infestation of pompano. In: Sindermann, C.J. (ed.) *Disease Diagnosis and Control in North American Marine Aquaculture*. Elsevier, Amsterdam, pp. 257–264.

Lawler, A.R. (1980) Studies on *Amyloodinium ocellatum* (Dinoflagellata) in Mississippi Sound: natural and experimental hosts. *Gulf Research Reports* 6, 403–413. DOI: 10.18785/grr.0604.08.

Levy, M.G., Poore, M.F., Colorni, A., Noga, E.J., Vandersea, M.W. and Litaker, R.W. (2007) A highly specific PCR assay for detecting the fish ectoparasite *Amyloodinium ocellatum*. *Diseases of Aquatic Organisms* 73, 219–226. DOI: 10.3354/dao073219.

Lewis, D.H., Wenxing, W., Ayers, A. and Arnold, R. (1988) Preliminary studies on the use of chloroquine as a systemic chemotherapeutic agent for amyloodinosis in red drum (*Sciaenops ocellatus*). *Contributions in Marine Science* 30(supplement), 183–189.

Li, Z., Jiang, B., Zhong, Z., Li, S., He, R. *et al.* (2021) Treatment of amyloodiniosis in golden pompano (*Trachinotus ovatus*) by copper sulfate. *South China Fisheries Science* 17, 108–114. DOI: 10.12131/20200260.

Li, Z., Zhuang, J., Chen, J., Cao, J., Han, Q. (2024) Establishment of a gill cell line from yellowfin seabream (*Acanthopagrus latus*) for studying *Amyloodinium ocellatum* infection of fish. *Journal of Fish Diseases* 47, e13923. DOI: 10.1111/jfd.13923.

Lieke, T., Meinelt, T., Hoseinifar, S.H., Pan, B., Straus, D.L. and Steinberg, C.E.W. (2020) Sustainable aquaculture requires environmental-friendly treatment strategies for fish diseases. *Reviews in Aquaculture* 12, 943–965. DOI: 10.1111/raq.12365.

Lom, J. and Lawler, A. (1973) An ultrastructural study on the mode of attachment in dinoflagellates invading gills of Cyprinodontidae. *Protistologica* 9, 293–309.

Luo, Z., Zhong, Z., Li, Z., Zhuang, J., Li, H. *et al.* (2024) Galvanized material is a promising approach to control *Amyloodinium ocellatum* infection in fishes. *Aquaculture* 578, 740045. DOI: 10.1016/j.aquaculture.2023.740045.

Massimo, M. (2019) New perspectives in the control of *Amyloodinium ocellatum* infection in reared sea bass (*Dicentrarchus labrax*). PhD thesis, University of Udine, Udine, Italy.

Massimo, M., Volpatti, D., Galeotti, M., Bron, J.E. and Beraldo, P. (2022) News insights into the host–parasite interactions of amyloodiniosis in European sea bass: a multi-modal approach. *Pathogens* 11, 62. DOI: 10.3390/pathogens11010062.

Montgomery-Brock, D., Sato, V.T., Brock, J.A. and Tamaru, C.S. (2001) The application of hydrogen peroxide as a treatment for the ectoparasite *Amyloodinium ocellatum* (Brown 1931) on the Pacific threadfin *Polydactylus sexfilis*. *Journal of the World Aquaculture Society* 32, 250–254. DOI: 10.1111/j.1749-7345.2001.tb01103.x.

Moreira, M., Herrera, M., Pousão-Ferreira, P., Navas Triano, J.I. and Soares, F. (2017) Stress effects of amyloodiniosis in gilthead sea bream *Sparus aurata*. *Diseases of Aquatic Organisms* 127, 201–211. DOI: 10.3354/dao03199.

Moreira, M., Soliño, L., Marques, C.L., Laizé, V., Pousão-Ferreira, P. *et al.* (2022) Cytotoxic and hemolytic activities of extracts of the fish parasite dinoflagellate *Amyloodinium ocellatum*. *Toxins* 14, 467. DOI: 10.3390/toxins14070467.

Moreira, M., Costas, B., Rodrigues, P.M., Lourenço-Marques, C., Sousa, R. *et al.* (2024) Amyloodiniosis in aquaculture: a review. *Reviews in Aquaculture* 16, 1042–1068. DOI: 10.1111/raq.12883.

Noga, E.J. (1987) Propagation in cell culture of the dinoflagellate *Amyloodinium*, an ectoparasite of marine fishes. *Science, USA* 236, 1302–1304.

Noga, E.J. (2010) *Fish Disease: Diagnosis and Treatment*, 2nd edn. Wiley-Blackwell, Ames, Iowa.

Noga, E.J. (2012) *Amyloodinium ocellatum*. In: Woo, P.T.K. and Buchmann, K. (eds) *Fish Parasites: Pathobiology and Protection*, 1st edn. CAB International, Wallingford, UK, pp. 19–29. DOI: 10.1079/9781845938062.0019.

Noga, E.J. and Levy, M.G. (2006) Phylum dinoflagellata. In: Woo, P.T.K. (ed.) *Fish Diseases and Disorders. Volume 1: Protozoan and Metazoan Infections.* CAB International, Wallingford, UK, pp. 16–45. DOI: 10.1079/9780851990156.0016.

Noga, E.J., Smith, S.A. and Landsberg, J.A. (1991) Amyloodiniosis in cultured hybrid striped bass (*Morone saxatilis* × *M. chrysops*) in North Carolina. *Journal of Aquatic Animal Health* 3, 294–297. DOI: 10.1577/1548-8667(1991)003<0294:AICHSB>2.3.CO;2.

Noga, E.J., Fan, Z. and Silphaduang, U. (2001) Histone-like proteins from fish are lethal to the parasitic dinoflagellate *Amyloodinium ocellatum*. *Parasitology* 123, 57–65. DOI: 10.1017/S0031182001007971.

Noga, E.J., Fan, Z.Q. and Silphaduang, U. (2002) Host site of activity and cytological effects of histone like proteins on the parasitic dinoflagellate *Amyloodinium ocellatum*. *Diseases of Aquatic Organisms* 52, 207–215. DOI: 10.3354/dao052207.

Nozzi, V., Strofaldi, S., Piquer, I.F., di Crescenzo, D., Olivotto, I. and Carnevali, O. (2016) *Amyloodinum ocellatum* in *Dicentrarchus labrax*: study of infection in salt water and freshwater aquaponics. *Fish and Shellfish Immunology* 57, 179–185. DOI: 10.1016/j.fsi.2016.07.036.

Oestmann, D.J. and Lewis, D.H. (1996a) Effects of 3,N-methylglucamine lasalocid on *Amyloodinium ocellatum*. *Diseases of Aquatic Organisms* 24, 179–184. DOI: 10.3354/dao024179.

Oestmann, D.J. and Lewis, D.H. (1996b) Improved cell culture propagation of *Amyloodinium ocellatum*. *Diseases of Aquatic Organisms* 24, 173–178. DOI: 10.3354/dao024173.

Oestmann, D.J., Lewis, D.H. and Zettler, B.A. (1995) Clearance of *Amyloodinium ocellatum* dinospores by *Artemia salina*. *Journal of Aquatic Animal Health* 7, 257–261. DOI: 10.1577/1548-8667(1995)007<0257:CCOAOD>2.3.CO;2.

Oidtmann, B.C., Mladineo, I., Cook, A., Beraldo, P., Palenzuela, O. *et al.* (2024) Main parasitic infections in gilthead seabream and European seabass aquaculture: risk factors from stakeholders' perspective. *Aquaculture International* 32, 4275–4302. DOI: 10.1007/s10499-023-01374-3.

Owatari, M.S., Sterzelecki, F.C., da Silva, C.S., Magnotti, C., Mouriño, J.L.P. and Cerqueira, V.R. (2020) Amyloodiniosis in farmed *Sardinella brasiliensis* (Steindachner, 1879): case report of successful therapeutic control with copper sulfate. *Parasitology International* 76, 102091. DOI: 10.1016/j.parint.2020.102091.

Paperna, I. (1980) *Amyloodinium ocellatum* (Brown, 1931) (Dinoflagellida) infestations in cultured marine fish at Eilat, Red Sea: epizootiology and pathology. *Journal of Fish Diseases* 3, 363–372. DOI: 10.1111/j.1365-2761.1980.tb00421.x.

Paperna, I. (1984) Reproduction cycle and tolerance to temperature and salinity of *Amyloodinium ocellatum* (Brown, 1931) (Dinoflagellida). *Annales de Parasitologie Humaine et Comparee* 59, 7–30.

Pereira, J.C., Abrantes, I., Martins, I., Barata, J., Frias, P. and Pereira, I. (2011) Ecological and morphological features of *Amyloodinium ocellatum* occurrences in cultivated gilthead seabream *Sparus aurata* L.: a case study. *Aquaculture* 310, 289–297. DOI: 10.1016/j.aquaculture.2010.11.011.

Picón-Camacho, S.M., Thompson, W.P., Blaylock, R.B. and Lotz, J.M. (2013) Development of a rapid assay to detect the dinoflagellate *Amyloodinium ocellatum* using loop-mediated isothermal amplification (LAMP). *Veterinary Parasitology* 196(3), 265–271. DOI: 10.1016/j.vetpar.2013.04.010.

Ragab, R.H., Elgendy, M.Y., Sabry, N.M., Sharaf, M.S., Attia, M.M. *et al.* (2022) Mass kills in hatchery-reared European seabass (*Dicentrarchus labrax*) triggered by concomitant infections of *Amyloodinium ocellatum* and *Vibrio alginolyticus*. *International Journal of Veterinary Science and Medicine* 10, 33–45. DOI: 10.1080/23144599.2022.2070346.

Reyes-Becerril, M., Tovar-Ramírez, D., Ascencio-Valle, F., Civera-Cerecedo, R., Gracia-López, V. and Barbosa-Solomieu, V. (2008) Effects of dietary live yeast *Debaryomyces hansenii* on the immune and antioxidant system in juvenile leopard grouper *Mycteroperca rosacea* exposed to stress. *Aquaculture* 280, 39–44. DOI: 10.1016/j.aquaculture.2008.03.056.

Reyes-Becerril, M., Ascencio-Valle, F., Alamillo, E., Hirono, I., Kondo, H. *et al.* (2015) Molecular cloning and comparative responses of Toll-like receptor 22 following ligands stimulation and parasitic infection in yellowtail (*Seriola lalandi*). *Fish and Shellfish Immunology* 46, 323–333. DOI: 10.1016/j.fsi.2015.06.020.

Rigos, G., Christophilogiannis, P., Giahnishi, M., Andriopoulou, A., Koutsodimoy, M. *et al.* (1998) *Amyloodinium occelatum* infestation on sharpsnout sea bream, *Puntazzo puntazzo* Cetti [*Diplodus puntazzo*]. *Bulletin of the European Association of Fish Pathologists* 18, 198–200.

Roberts-Thomson, A., Barnes, A., Fielder, D.S., Lester, R.J.G. and Adlard, R.D. (2006) Aerosol dispersal of the fish pathogen, *Amyloodinium ocellatum*. *Aquaculture* 257, 118–123. DOI: 10.1016/j.aquaculture.2006.02.058.

Saraiva, A., Jerónimo, D. and Cruz, C. (2011) *Amyloodinium ocellatum* (Chromalveolata: Dinoflagellata) in farmed turbot. *Aquaculture* 320, 34–36. DOI: 10.1016/j.aquaculture.2011.07.034.

Shinn, A.P., Pratoomyot, J., Bron, J.E., Paladini, G., Brooker, E.E. and Brooker, A.J. (2015) Economic costs of protistan and metazoan parasites to global mariculture. *Parasitology* 142, 196–270. DOI: 10.1017/S0031182014001437.

Smith, S.A., Levy, M.G. and Noga, E.J. (1992) Development of an enzyme-linked immunosorbent assay (ELISA) for the detection of antibody to the parasitic dinoflagellate *Amyloodinium ocellatum* in *Oreochromis aureus*. *Veterinary Parasitology* 42, 145–155. DOI: 10.1016/0304-4017(92)90110-u.

Smith, S.A., Noga, E.J., Levy, M.G. and Gerig, T.M. (1993) Effect of serum from tilapia *Oreochromis aureus* immunized with the dinospore *Amyloodinium ocellatum* on the motility, infectivity and growth of the parasite in cell culture. *Diseases of Aquatic Organisms* 15, 73–80. DOI: 10.3354/dao015073.

Soares, F., Quental-Ferreira, H., Moreira, M., Cunha, E., Ribeiro, L. and Pousão-Ferreira, P. (2012) First report of *Amyloodinium ocellatum* in farmed meagre (*Argyrosomus regius*). *Bulletin of the European Association of Fish Pathologists* 32, 30–33.

Soares, F., Moreira, M., Sousa, R. and Lourenço-Marques, C. (2025) Amyloodiniosis in semi-intensive aquaculture. In: De-Simone, S.G. and Lechuga, G.C. (eds) *Exploring the World of Parasites*. IntechOpen, London. DOI: 10.5772/intechopen.1007867.

Tedesco, P., Beraldo, P., Massimo, M., Fioravanti, M.L., Volpatti, D. *et al.* (2020) Comparative therapeutic effects of natural compounds against *Saprolegnia* spp. (Oomycota) and *Amyloodinium ocellatum* (Dinophyceae). *Frontiers in Veterinary Science* 6, 83. DOI: 10.3389/fvets.2020.00083.

Ullal, A.J., Litaker, R.W. and Noga, E.J. (2008) Antimicrobial peptides derived from hemoglobin are expressed in epithelium of channel catfish (*Ictalurus punctatus*, Rafinesque). *Developmental and Comparative Immunology* 32, 1301–1312. DOI: 10.1016/j.dci.2008.04.005.

Virgula, J.C., Cruz-Lacierda, E.R., Estante, E.G. and Corre Jr, V.L. (2017) Copper sulfate as treatment for the ectoparasite *Amyloodinium ocellatum* (Dinoflagellida) on milkfish (*Chanos chanos*) fry. *AACL Bioflux* 10, 365–371.

Vivanco-Aranda, M., del Río-Zaragoza, O.B., Lechuga-Sandoval, C.E., Viana, M.T. and Rombenso, A.N. (2018) Health response in yellowtail *Seriola dorsalis* exposed to an *Amyloodinium ocellatum* outbreak. *Ciencias Marinas* 44, 267–277. DOI: 10.7773/cm.v44i4.2858.

Yang, L.-G., Wang, Y., Xu, W.-B., Qin, B., Ying, N. *et al.* (2022) Transcriptome analysis of greenfin horse-faced filefish (*Thamnaconus septentrionalis*) gills in response to *Amyloodinium ocellatum* (AO) infection. *Fishes* 7, 252. DOI: 10.3390/fishes7050252.

Zhang, D., Mohammed, H., Ye, Z., Rhodes, M.A., Thongda, W. *et al.* (2022) Transcriptomic profiles of Florida pompano (*Trachinotus carolinus*) gill following infection by the ectoparasite *Amyloodinium ocellatum*. *Fish and Shellfish Immunology* 125, 171–179. DOI: 10.1016/j.fsi.2022.05.017.

Zhuang, J., Li, Z., Cao, J., Luo, Z., Wang, B. *et al.* (2025) A quantitative real-time PCR assay for rapid detection and quantification of *Amyloodinium ocellatum* parasites in seawater samples. *Aquaculture* 595, 741651. DOI: 10.1016/j.aquaculture.2024.741651.

3 *Cryptobia (Trypanoplasma) salmositica*

Patrick T.K. Woo*
Department of Integrative Biology, University of Guelph, Canada

Abstract

This chapter reviews *Cryptobia salmositica*, its pathobiology and proof-of-concept strategies against *Cryptobia* and cryptobiosis. The haemoflagellate infects *Oncorhynchus* on the west coast of North America. It is normally transmitted indirectly by the freshwater leech, *Piscicola salmositica*; however, its ectoparasitic stage allows direct transmission. Salmonid cryptobiosis occurs in streams, hatcheries and sea cages. Anorexia, abdominal distension and anaemia indicate the disease; but microscopic and/or serological examinations of blood are needed for confirmation. *Cryptobia* secretes metalloprotease which causes clinical disease, histopathology and generalized inflammation. Hypoxaemia stimulates leptin-A1 secretion which contributes to anorexia. Cryptobiosis retards fish growth and metabolism. *Cryptobia* has cortisol receptors and uses cortisol as a 'reproductive activating factor'. Rapid parasite multiplications deplete plasma cortisol which is not produced at peak parasitaemia because of hypothalamic–pituitary–interrenal axis dysfunction. The immune system takes over as cortisol is depleted and recovered fish are protected. Two vaccines and a monoclonal antibody are also protective. Isometamidium chloride is therapeutic against cryptobiosis. *Oncorhynchus* can breed/develop immunity at 20°C.

3.1. Introduction

3.1.1. The parasite

Cryptobia spp. are parasitic flagellates (class Kinetoplastea, subclass Metakinetoplastina, order Parabodonida) of invertebrates and vertebrates, and they have worldwide distribution. There are at least 52 nominal species, most of which are not known to cause disease (Woo, 2003). The pathogenic species are relatively well studied as they cause disease and/or mortality in marine and freshwater fishes. They are either haematozoic (in the blood system) or non-haematozoic (on gills or in the digestive system) parasites. Scientists in Europe prefer to assign the haematozoic species to the genus *Trypanoplasma* and the non-haematozoic species to the genus *Cryptobia*; however, many North American workers do not believe there is sufficient evidence for the separation into two genera and this has been discussed extensively earlier (Woo, 1994, 2006). Briefly, Woo (1987a, 1994) agrees there are similarities and differences between haematozoic and non-haematozoic species, and a close relationship between the two groups. Consequently, he divided the genus *Cryptobia* into two subgenera: (i) subgenus *Trypanoplasma*

*Email: pwoo@uoguelph.ca

 Fish Parasites: Pathobiology and Protection, 2nd Edition (eds P.T.K. Woo and K. Buchmann)
DOI: 10.1079/9781800628748.0003

for haematozoic species; and (ii) subgenus *Cryptobia* for non-haematozoic species. The pathogenic haematozoic species include: *Cryptobia (Trypanoplasma) bullock* (in flatfishes), *Cryptobia (Trypanoplasma) salmositica* (in salmonids) and *Cryptobia (Trypanoplasma) borreli* (in cyprinids); while the non-haematozoic species that cause disease in fishes are *Cryptobia (Cryptobia) iubilans* (in the digestive system) and *Cryptobia (Cryptobia) branchialis* (on the gills). In general, non-haematozoic *Cryptobia* spp. of fishes are transmitted directly between hosts while blood-sucking invertebrates are vectors of haematozoic species.

The research cited in this chapter was interdisciplinary and the parasite, *C. (T.) salmositica*, was cloned (Woo, 1979). It was isolated from an infected leech (*Piscicola salmositica*) that was attached to an infected salmon in British Columbia, Canada. This chapter includes relevant information on the parasite (Section 3.1), its pathobiology (Sections 3.2, 3.3 and 3.4), strategies against cryptobiosis (Section 3.5) and conclusions (Section 3.6) with suggestions (Section 3.7) for future research.

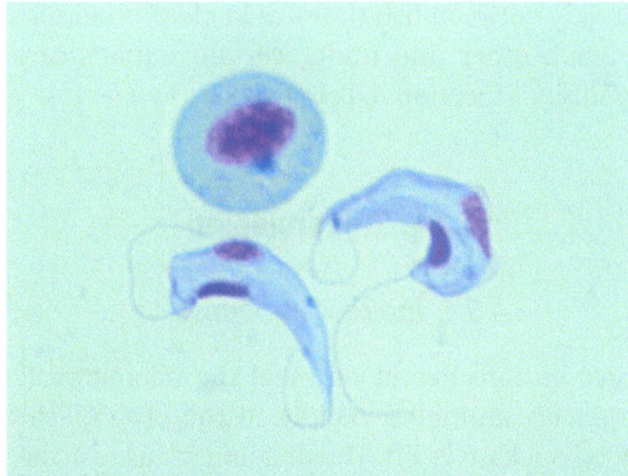

Fig. 3.1. *Cryptobia salmositica* with a red blood cell from a fish with microcytic and hypochromic anaemia; note the red blood cell is not oval and there is reduced haemoglobin (×1150). (From Woo, 1987a; courtesy of *Advances in Parasitology*.)

3.1.2. *Cryptobia (Trypanoplasma) salmositica*

The parasite (Fig. 3.1) was first described from coho salmon (*Oncorhynchus kisutch*) in Washington State, USA (Katz, 1951). It is not host specific and has since been reported in all species of Pacific salmon (*Oncorhynchus* spp.) and in seven species of sculpins (*Cottus* spp.) which inhabit freshwater streams/rivers from California (USA) to British Columbia (Canada) and to south-western Alaska. Although it causes cryptobiosis in most species of salmonids it is not known to cause disease in sculpins in the wild, and they are considered the natural reservoir hosts of the pathogen (Woo, 2003). Further studies with experimentally infected laboratory-raised sculpins are needed to confirm the absence of disease and elucidation of the protective mechanism (Section 3.7; proposal #1).

C. salmositica is an elongated organism which is longer than a red blood cell. Its body measurements are based on air-dried blood smears stained with Giemsa's stain (mean (range)): (i) body length 14.9 (6.0–25.0) μm; (ii) body width 2.5 (1.3–4.0) μm; (iii) anterior flagellum 16.1 (6.5–27.0) μm; (iv) posterior free flagellum 9.0 (4.0–17.0) μm; (v) kinetoplast length 2.0–9.0 μm; (vi) kinetoplast width 0.5–2.0 μm; (vii) nucleus length 1.5–3.5 μm; (viii) nucleus width 1.0–2.5 μm; (ix) ratio of anterior flagellum to body length 1.07 (0.40–1.95); (x) ratio of posterior flagellum to body length 0.61 (0.25–1.15); and (xi) ratio of anterior flagellum to posterior free flagellum 1.97 (0.6–3.7) (Katz, 1951).

The ultrastructure of *C. salmositica* is similar to those of other *Cryptobia* spp. However, the blood form of *C. salmositica* has a functional contractile vacuole (with systole and diastole stages) and its lumen has electron-dense filamentous materials (Paterson and Woo, 1983). Contractile vacuoles have not been found in other haematozoic species (Vickerman, 1971; Brugerolle *et al.*, 1979). In *C. salmositica*, the vacuole is located at the base of the flagellar pocket and is associated with the post-flagellar pit (Paterson and Woo, 1983).

As indicated earlier, *C. salmositica* causes cryptobiosis in salmonids and the pathogen has been reported from all species of Pacific *Oncorhynchus*. Outbreaks of cryptobiosis with high fish mortalities have occurred in freshwater hatcheries and in sea-cage cultures on the west coast of North America (Section 3.1.4). The parasite is normally transmitted indirectly by blood-sucking leeches (Section 3.1.3) in freshwater streams and rivers; however, it can also be transmitted directly between fish that are in close proximity to each other and under certain aquaculture conditions (Section 3.1.3).

3.1.3. Transmission

3.1.3.1. Indirect transmission

After an infective blood meal the haematozoic *Cryptobia* multiplies rapidly in the crop of the blood-sucking leech. The dividing parasite accumulates in large numbers either in the crop and/or in the proboscis sheath of the leech, and they are transmitted to fish when the infected leech feeds again (Woo, 1994).

The freshwater leech, *P. salmositica*, is the only known natural vector for *C. salmositica* and it occurs in streams and rivers on the west coast of North America. Leeches hatch in late summer/early autumn from cocoons before the salmon return to fresh water from the sea (Becker and Katz, 1965b, 1966; Bower and Margolis, 1984b). It is assumed the leeches initially pick up the *C. salmositica* by feeding on infected resident fishes (including sculpins). Briefly, once the parasite is ingested by the leech it multiplies, and large numbers of dividing parasites are in the crop of the leech 7–8 days after an infective blood meal. The flagellate is always infective to fish and *C. salmositica* are not in the proboscis sheath of the infected leech (Becker and Katz, 1965a). Further studies on its development in the leech are suggested, as S. Li and P.T.K. Woo (1995, unpublished results) found numerous *C. salmositica* in the proboscis sheaths of *P. salmositica* removed from infected salmon. The *Cryptobia* from the proboscis sheaths were infective and caused disease when inoculated into rainbow trout (*Oncorhynchus mykiss*).

3.1.3.2. Direct transmission

In experimentally infected fish the parasite first multiplied in the blood of infected sockeye salmon fry (*Oncorhynchus nerka*) and later in the infection it was also found on the body surface. It was suggested the parasite passed through blisters caused by the dissociation of connective tissues near the abdominal pore. If heavily infected fish and uninfected fish were held together in dip nets for brief periods out of water, the eventual fish mortality due to cryptobiosis ranged from 64 to 89% in fish maintained in fresh water and was 94% in fish maintained in sea water (Bower and Margolis, 1983). This mode of transmission may occur in hatcheries, for example when fish are periodically brought together during grading and/or weighing or when fish are transferred from pond to pond.

Woo and Wehnert (1983) independently demonstrated the parasite in the mucus on the body surface of adult rainbow trout about 6 weeks after experimental infection. These ectoparasitic flagellates were infective when inoculated into fish. Also, in three repeated experimental studies 67–80% of uninfected trout became infected in about 20 weeks if they were allowed to mix freely with infected trout in the same tank. The percentage of infected trout was lower if the two groups of fish were separated by a wire screen with the water flowing from the infected to uninfected fish.

C. salmositica has at least two proteases: a cysteine protease (49, 60, 66 and 97 kDa); and a metalloprotease (200 kDa). These have been isolated and purified (Fig. 3.2). The 200 kDa metalloprotease is a histolytic enzyme (Fig. 3.3) and is an important virulent factor (Zuo and Woo, 1997a, d, 1998a). It is likely involved in direct transmission of the parasite; initially by causing lesions in the skin so that the parasite can become ectoparasitic and in entry of the parasite (e.g. via the mucous membrane) in uninfected fish. As indicated earlier (Section 3.1.2), the parasite has a functional contractile vacuole (Paterson and Woo, 1983) which allows the ectoparasitic parasite to osmoregulate when fish are in hypo-osmotic environments (e.g. in fresh water). Also, a copious amount of mucous is secreted by the infected fish and may also help the parasite to survive in the hypo-osmotic environment. Woo and Wehnert (1983) suggested the ectoparasitic form was carried in mucous strands in the water column, and the parasite entered uninfected fish either through lesions on the body surface or it penetrated (with the help of the metalloprotease) the mucous membrane of the gills and/or the oral cavity.

3.1.4. Impacts of cryptobiosis

In the Fraser River drainage, British Columbia, Canada, the prevalence of *C. salmositica* in salmon

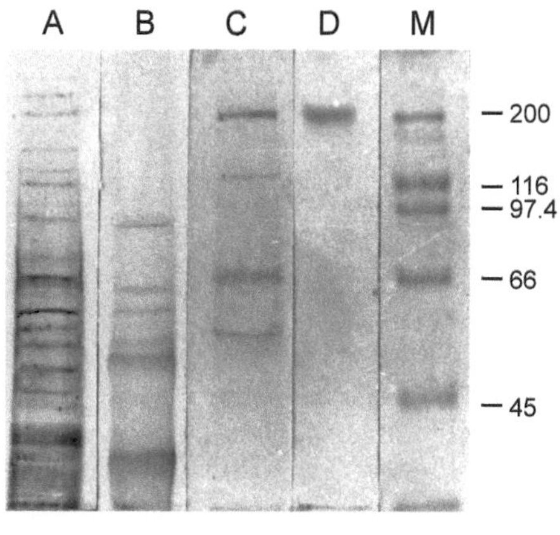

Fig. 3.2. Purified cysteine protease and metalloprotease from *Cryptobia salmositica*. Lane A, crude parasite lysate; lane B, partially purified cysteine protease from diethylaminoethyl (DEAE)-agarose column; lane C, metalloprotease from DEAE-agarose column; lane D, purified metalloprotease from Sephacryl S-300 column; lane M, molecular-weight markers (kDa). (From Woo, 2003; courtesy of *Journal of Fish Diseases*. The figure was modified (addition of lane B on cysteine protease) in 2003 to a figure on metalloprotease in Zuo and Woo, 1997d; courtesy of *Diseases of Aquatic Organisms*.)

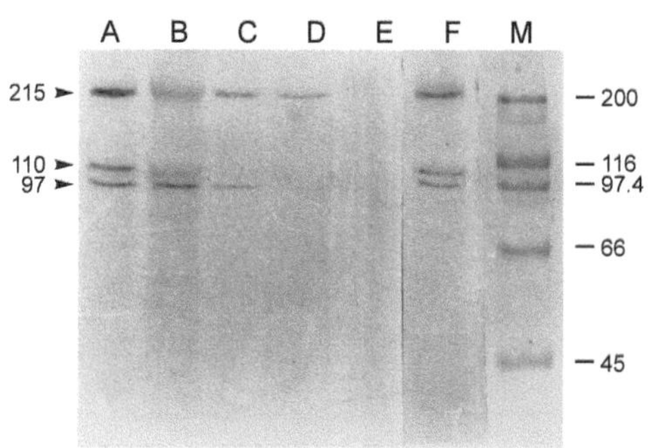

Fig. 3.3. *In vitro* degradation of collagen type V by purified metalloprotease from *Cryptobia salmositica*. Lanes A–E, collagen incubated with metalloprotease for 0, 2, 5, 6 and 8 h, respectively; lane F, collagen + phosphate-buffered saline at 8 h; lane M, molecular-weight markers (kDa). (From Zuo and Woo, 1997d; courtesy of *Diseases of Aquatic Organisms*.)

returning to fresh water to spawn was low in September but increased to about 100% by December and January. Also, returning salmon had detectable infections within 5 days in fresh water and the longer the fish were in fresh water the higher were their parasitaemias (Bower and Margolis, 1984b). These increases were related to increased numbers of infected leeches in the streams in November (Becker and Katz, 1965b, 1966; Bower and Margolis, 1984b).

Putz (1972) indicated that *C. salmositica* was more pathogenic to coho salmon (*O. kisutch* with 100% mortality) than to Chinook salmon (*Oncorhynchus tshawytscha*) in the USA. However, Bower and Margolis (1985) found 100% mortality in Chinook salmon while coho salmon from some stocks in Canada did not die from the infection (0% mortality). The difference is probably due to the genetics of the fish. For example, sockeye salmon (*O. nerka*) from the Fulton River stock (British Columbia, Canada) suffered high mortality when injected with a low dose (about 100 parasites per fish), while the Weaver Creek stock of sockeye salmon (British Columbia) had no mortality even when injected with about a million parasites per fish (Bower and Margolis, 1984a). Mortality of infected sockeye salmon is consistent within the same fish stock and to different parasite isolates (Bower and Margolis, 1985).

The parasite is considered a lethal pathogen of salmon in many semi-natural and intensive salmon culture facilities on the Pacific coast of North America (Bower and Thompson, 1987). In the USA, the prevalence of the parasite in downstream migrants of salmon ranged from 3 to 21% in some streams (Becker and Katz, 1966). It is most likely the prevalence would be lower if more fish were examined and from more streams. Experimental studies showed that presmolt salmon infected in fresh water retained their infection and with no reduction in mortality after they were transferred to salt water (Bower and Margolis, 1985). Consequently, the disease may be quite a significant cause of fish loss due to mortality in the sea; however, no field studies had been conducted to test the validity of this suggestion.

There had been a few reported serious outbreaks of the disease in juvenile salmon held in freshwater hatcheries in Washington State, USA. These include three outbreaks in Chinook salmon in three localities between 1972 and 1973 (Wood, 1979). Also, P.F. Chapman (Department of Fisheries, State of Washington, USA, 1993, personal communication) described outbreaks of the disease in Chinook salmon in hatcheries in Washington State which began in December 1992 and peaked in February 1993. Infected fish had the typical clinical signs (anaemia, splenomegaly and ascites) of the disease (Section 3.2.1) and 65,000 fish were involved, with peak mortality of 0.1%/day in February. In one hatchery the mortality of adult Chinook brood stock brought into the hatchery (for breeding purposes) was about 50%. Chapman noted that cryptobiosis had occurred in the same hatcheries in the past but they were not as severe. The drug isometamidium chloride (Samorin®) was effective against the haemoflagellate in experimentally infected juvenile Chinook salmon (Ardelli and Woo, 2001b) and in naturally infected mature Chinook salmon (Chen *et al.*, 2011). Untreated control fish died from the infection (Section 3.5.4).

Outbreaks of the disease had also occurred in fish held in sea cages. In 1997 the parasite caused significant morbidity/mortality in smolts and pre-harvest Chinook salmon in a hatchery on Vancouver Island, Canada. There was a small mortality spike (about 1%) in post-smolts in the first 10–15 weeks after fish were transferred to salt water. However, re-emergence of the disease with significant morbidity and mortality occurred later in the pre-harvest fish. Another outbreak in the pre-harvest Chinook salmon occurred in the same hatchery in 2001. Large numbers of *Cryptobia* were in the blood and ascites fluid of moribund fish, and clinical signs (Section 3.2.1) were evident in many fish. Fish mortality varied between cages and ranged from 3.3 to 24.9%. Briefly, the parasite was detected in the blood of some fish (while in fresh water in the hatchery) before they were transferred to sea cages in August–September 1999. Parasites from moribund fish in sea cages were morphologically similar to *C. salmositica* and caused clinical disease in experimentally infected rainbow trout (Woo, 2006).

Significant mortalities due to cryptobiosis were also associated with post-spawning rainbow trout in a hatchery in California, USA (Wales and Wolf, 1955). The authors suggested that many of the post-spawning trout died from a combined effect of *Cryptobia* and *Saprolegnia parasitica*. In field studies conducted in the 1980s adult salmon returning from the Pacific Ocean had detectable infections as early as 5 days after they returned to fresh water in the Fraser River, British Columbia, Canada. The parasitaemias were very high in many fish at spawning, and numerous fish had died before they spawned (Bower and Margolis, 1984b). In the Soleduck hatchery (Washington State, USA) about 50% of spring Chinook salmon brood stock brought in from streams annually died from cryptobiosis (L. Peck, Department of Fisheries, State of Washington, USA, 1994, personal communication). Outbreak of the disease in brood stock had occurred in a hatchery on the Rogue River in Oregon, USA (C. Banner, Oregon Department of Fisheries and Wildlife, Oregon State, USA, 2004, personal communication). Mortality was over 50% and moribund fish had massive numbers of parasites in the blood (Fig. 3.4). No leeches were found on infected fish and total mortality was similar in both male and female fish.

Currie and Woo (2007, 2008) conducted experimental studies on the infection in sexually mature rainbow trout. They showed infected sexually mature females were more susceptible than sexually mature males. All infected females had exophthalmia (Section 3.2.1) while none of the males showed this clinical sign, although both males and females were anaemic. Most infected females with eggs died before or shortly after spawning and none of the infected males died. Infected males initially increased milt production and sperm concentration after infection; however, this declined as the disease progressed. Also, parasitaemias were higher in

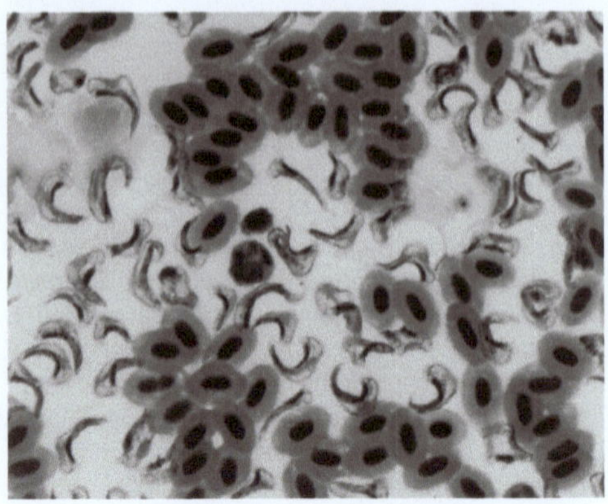

Fig. 3.4. Blood smear from a sexually mature spring Chinook salmon naturally infected with *Cryptobia salmositica*. (Courtesy of Craig Banner, Oregon Department of Fish and Wildlife, USA.)

females than in males. Fresh plasma from both sexually mature females and males significantly increased the *in vitro* multiplication of the parasite, and plasma from females was better than plasma from males. The addition of 17 β-oestradiol (at physiological level or higher) did not enhance *in vitro* multiplication of the *Cryptobia*.

3.1.5. Cortisol: 'reproductive activating factor' for *Cryptobia*

As handling and transportation of rainbow trout elevated cortisol level up to 57 ng/ml (Barton, 2000), P.T.K. Woo (2008, unpublished results) postulated this 'stress hormone' might have roles on *Cryptobia* and cryptobiosis. He conducted a simple in *vitro* study by adding cortisol (10 ng/ml) to the culture medium to produce a cortisol-enriched medium. The parasite multiplied rapidly in the cortisol-enriched culture medium with numbers consistently higher than those with no additional cortisol. Similar results were obtained when the experiment was repeated (P.T.K. Woo, 2008, unpublished results). A more robust study (Li *et al.*, 2013) confirmed rapid parasite multiplications and the parasite numbers in cortisol-enriched media (10–50 ng/ml) were significantly higher than parasite numbers in control media (no additional cortisol). The synthetic glucocorticoid, dexamethasone (Dex), also significantly stimulated rapid parasite replications with numbers higher than in controls. However, mifepristone (RU486), a synthetic steroid that has anti-glucocorticoid receptor (GR) properties, when added (100 ng/ml) to either cortisol- or Dex-enriched media inhibited the stimulatory effects of either glucocorticoid. The dose effect of glucocorticoid (cortisol or Dex) on *Cryptobia* multiplication indicates a novel relationship in which the 'stress hormone' in the host is used by the parasite to enhance its replication. The authors also suggested cortisol exerts its effect on GR-like proteins in/on *C. salmositica* as it does to vertebrate cells. This was the first demonstration of a functional steroid hormone receptor in/on a protozoan.

An antibody produced against GR proteins rapidly agglutinated living *Cryptobia* (about 20 parasites per clump). Also, confocal microscopy with immunohistofluorescence visually confirmed GRs on the plasma membrane and in the parasite cytoplasm (Li and Woo, 2014). The addition of mifepristone (50 ng/ml) was more effective in inhibiting parasite replication in cultures with 7000 parasites/ml than in those with 14,000 parasites/ml. However, mifepristone concentration of 100 ng/ml was more effective than 50 ng/ml in inhibiting parasite multiplication in cultures with 14,000 parasites/ml. These studies indicate the number of binding sites on and in *Cryptobia* is finite and confirms cortisol is a 'reproductive activating factor' ('raf') for the parasite.

Future studies (Section 3.7; proposal #2) should be conducted on the relationships between cortisol and pathogens. The proposal has two components: the first is to test the hypothesis that cortisol may also be a 'raf' for other pathogens, while the second component is to elucidate the uptake mechanism and subsequent activities of the cortisol in *Cryptobia*.

3.1.6. Relationships between cortisol and *Cryptobia* in fish

The cortisol levels in stressed rainbow trout range between 30 and 200 ng/ml (Barton, 2000; Schreck, *et al.*, 2001; Norris and Hobbs, 2006) and these are within the levels (70–650 ng/ml) in sexually mature female *Oncorhynchus* spp. (Caldwell *et al.*, 1991; Kubokawa *et al.*, 1999; Carruth *et al.*, 2000; Koldkjær *et al.*, 2004; McConnachie *et al.*, 2012). Amounts of cortisol in most of these studies were 'total plasma cortisol', and 'free' hormone that would be available to *Cryptobia* in sexually mature fish would be lower. The amount of 'free cortisol' in mature rainbow trout is about 45% of the total plasma cortisol in females and only 22% in males. This difference in the percentage of 'free cortisol' in the plasma of male and female trout would explain the lower parasitaemias in infected male trout and the higher efficacy of female plasma to stimulate *in vitro* multiplication of *Cryptobia* (Currie and Woo 2007).

It is suggested here that cortisol plays significant and complex roles in cryptobiosis. Briefly, production of this 'stress hormone' increases after infection and cortisol acts as a 'raf' (Section 3.1.5) resulting in rapid *Cryptobia* multiplication. Multiple generations of parasites continue to deplete the cortisol in the blood and at peak parasitaemia (about 4–6 weeks post-infection (pi)) the amount of cortisol becomes low because it is also not produced due to hypothalamic–pituitary–interrenal (HPI) axis dysfunction (Section 3.4). As cortisol is deleted the replication rate of *Cryptobia* slows down, and this also lowers the immunodepressive role of cortisol (Faught and Schaal, 2024). However, the high parasite load continues to stimulate the immune system which controls the infection and fish recover from cryptobiosis (Section 3.5.3). Some infected fish may still die as mortality depends on numerous factors including the genetics of the fish (Section 3.1.4).

Cortisol as a 'raf' may not be unique to cryptobiosis. Consequently, a component in proposal #2 (Section 3.7) is to test the hypothesis that cortisol may also be a 'raf' in other pathogens.

3.2. Clinical Signs and Diagnosis of Salmonid Cryptobiosis

3.2.1. Clinical signs

C. salmositica is in the blood soon after infection and it multiplies readily by longitudinal binary fission (Woo, 1978). The severity of the disease, peak parasitaemia, appearance of the clinical signs and mortality are related to numerous abiotic and biotic factors which include: (i) the size of the parasite inoculum; (ii) water temperature; (iii) fish diets; (iv) size and strain/species of the fish; and (v) the genetics and sexual maturity of the fish (e.g. Woo, 1979; Woo *et al.*, 1983; Bower and Margolis, 1985; Thomas and Woo, 1990b; Li and Woo, 1991; Li *et al.*, 1996; Chin *et al.*, 2002, 2004a; Currie and Woo, 2008).

Infected fish produce copious amounts of mucus on the body surface, are lethargic, and remain at the bottom of the tank during the acute phase of the disease. Briefly, the parasitaemia peaks at about 4–8 weeks after infection (acute phase of the disease), and as indicated earlier this is dependent on the dosage of the inoculum and size and genetics of the fish. The severity of the anaemia (microcytic and hypochromic) in trout is directly related to the parasitaemia (Woo, 1979). Another consistent clinical sign is anorexia; its onset is at 3–5 weeks pi and this is also partly influenced by water temperature (Thomas and Woo, 1992; Chin *et al.*, 2004b). The most consistent clinical signs of the disease are the anaemia and anorexia, and both are most evident at peak parasitaemia. Other clinical signs of the disease include: (i) exophthalmia (Fig. 3.5); (ii) general oedema; (iii) abdominal distension with ascites; and (iv) a positive anti-globulin reaction (or positive Coombs' test) of red cells (e.g. Woo, 1979; Li and Woo, 1995; Thomas and Woo, 1988).

3.2.2. Diagnosis of infection

3.2.2.1. Parasitological techniques

Clinical signs can be used for preliminary diagnosis of the disease, and the infection can be confirmed by examination of blood and/or ascites under a microscope. During the acute phase of the disease parasites are easily detected when freshly collected blood or ascites is examined under the compound microscopic (wet mount technique). The identity and morphology of the parasite can be confirmed by examination of air-dried Giemsa-stained smears (Woo, 1969) and/or by using a DNA probe which is specific for *C. salmositica* (Li and Woo, 1996).

The haematocrit centrifuge technique (HCT) (Woo, 1969), which was initially described to detect low numbers of trypanosomes in animals including humans (Woo, 1970), was

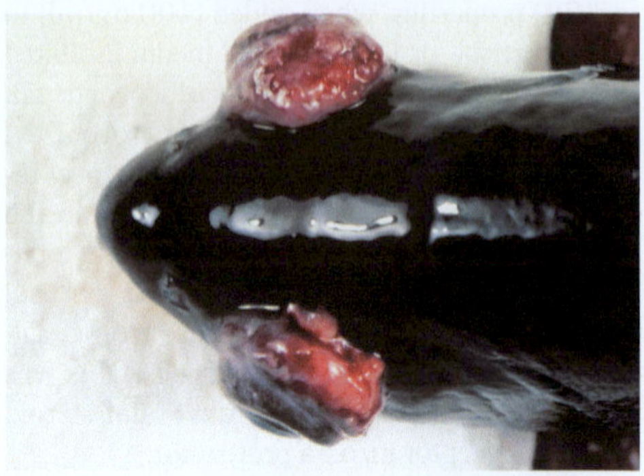

Fig. 3.5. Dorsal view of obvious exophthalmia in a rainbow trout experimentally infected with *Cryptobia salmositica*. (From Woo and Poynton, 1995; courtesy of CAB International.)

modified to detect *Cryptobia* infections (Woo and Wehnert, 1983). It is used routinely to detect *Cryptobia* in the blood either before the acute phase of the disease or during the chronic phase of the infection as it is much more sensitive and less time-consuming than the wet mount technique. Briefly, haematocrit tubes with freshly collected blood are centrifuged cold (5–10°C) for about 5 min at 13,000 *g* (Woo and Wehnert, 1983; Bower and Margolis, 1984a). The parasite becomes very sluggish and dies if the blood is not kept cold (about 10°C) at all times. After centrifugation, the junction of the plasma and packed red cell is examined under a compound microscope (Woo, 1969). The sensitivity of the technique is relatively high, detecting infections when there are about 75 *Cryptobia*/ml of blood (Bower and Margolis, 1984a). However, its sensitivity could be increased if more than one capillary tube of centrifuged blood was examined, as was shown with pathogenic mammalian trypanosomes (Woo and Rogers, 1974).

3.2.2.2. Immunological techniques

Both cell-mediated and humoral assays have been developed to detect *C. salmositica* infections and the techniques are quite sensitive.

Cell-mediated techniques include: (i) delayed-type hypersensitivity (DTH – skin test) reactions; (ii) the macrophage migration inhibition (MMI – head kidney cells) assay (Thomas and Woo, 1990a); and (iii) the respiratory burst (RB – head kidney cells) assay (Mehta and Woo, 2002). Both MMI and RB cannot be used routinely as they require killing the fish; however, DTH is a non-lethal technique, and it only involves intradermal injection of sonicated parasite antigen and determining the increase in skin thickness 72 h later; it is relatively sensitive and is positive at 2 weeks pi.

Serological (detection of either antibodies or parasite antigens in the blood) assays include using the complement-fixing antibody test (*in vitro* immune lysis test on live *Cryptobia*) and the indirect haemagglutination test using sonicated parasite antigens (Jones and Woo, 1987), the microscopic immune-substrate-enzyme technique (MISET) and the immunofluorescent antibody technique (IFAT) on whole parasites (Woo, 1990). Both MISET and IFAT are equally sensitive (about 1–2 weeks pi) in detecting specific antibodies against *C. salmositica*; however, MISET is preferred because it does not require a fluorescent microscope and the slide can be stored for extended periods after it has been examined.

An antibody-capture ELISA (enzyme-linked immunosorbent assay) is also available to detect *C. salmositica* infections in salmonids. It is sensitive and can also be used on blood blotted on to filter paper and stored at −20°C (Sitja-Bobadilla and Woo, 1994). Finally, Verity and Woo (1996) developed an antigen-capture ELISA using a monoclonal antibody. The antibody (designated mAb-007) was produced against a major *C. salmositica* surface polypeptide (47 kDa) and the technique detected infections in experimentally infected rainbow trout (inoculated with either the virulent or avirulent strains of *C. salmositica*) as early as 1 week pi. This antigen-capture ELISA can detect as little as 0.5 μg/ml of *C. salmositica* antigen in a cell lysate. However, the technique is not species specific as it reacts with the 47 kDa polypeptide from *C. bullock* and *Cryptobia catostomi*. The technique may be useful for detection of *Cryptobia* infections in naturally infected fishes.

3.3. Pathology

The anaemia and anorexia are very consistent clinical signs, and their severities are directly related to parasitaemia (Woo, 1979); consequently they are most severe at peak parasitaemia (acute phase of the disease) which is usually 4–8 weeks pi, this period depending on numerous abiotic and biotic factors (Section 3.2.1). There are obvious lesions in haemopoietic tissues during the acute phase in rainbow trout. Severity of the anaemia and histopathological lesions (see below) are directly related to the parasitaemia in the blood and to the extravascular localization of the parasite (Bahmanrokh and Woo, 2001). If an infected fish survives the disease the blood values return to near pre-infection levels during the chronic phase of the infection (Li and Woo, 1991). The other contributing factors to the anaemia include: (i) haemodilution; (ii) splenomegaly; and (iii) haemolysis (Woo, 1979; Laidley *et al.*, 1988; Thomas and Woo, 1988).

Haemolysis is a major contributing cause of the anaemia; it is the result of secretion of a 'haemolysin' by the parasite that is also released when the parasite is lysed by complement-fixing antibodies produced by the host. The 'haemolysin' lyses red cells directly while other released antigens (from lysed parasites) form immune complexes with antibodies to coat red blood cells. These result in intravascular and/or extravascular haemolysis (Thomas and Woo, 1988). Red blood cells from infected trout are anti-globulin positive (or Coombs' positive), and these red cells are lysed when incubated with fresh trout complement. However, in infected fish haemolytic activity of serum complement is significantly lowered (Section 3.4) partly because it is used by complement-fixing antibodies to control the infection (Thomas and Woo, 1989b). The antigen(s) is also secreted by the pathogenic strain when it is cultured (Thomas and Woo, 1989a; Woo and Thomas, 1992).

A 200 kDa metalloprotease (glycoprotein) has been identified, isolated and purified (Fig. 3.2) from the pathogenic *C. salmositica*. The optimal activity of the purified enzyme is at pH 7.0 (Zuo and Woo, 1997a,d, 1998a). It has high proteolytic activities against azocasein, haemoglobin, fibrinogen and gelatin, but low activity against albumin. It is inhibited by metal-chelating agents and zinc ions, but it is activated by calcium ions (Zuo and Woo, 1997d, 1998a). The purified enzyme also lyses red blood cells under *in vitro* conditions (Zuo and Woo, 2000) by digesting proteins in erythrocyte membranes (Zuo and Woo, 1997d). Hence, it is an important contributing factor to the anaemia and is the 'haemolysin' that was identified earlier as an important cause of the anaemia (Thomas and Woo, 1988, 1989a). The metalloprotease also digests collagen (Fig. 3.3), and it readily degrades different collagens (types I, IV and V) and laminin (Zuo and Woo, 1997d). The protease is secreted by the parasite during an infection (Zuo and Woo, 1997c) and in culture (Zuo and Woo, 1998a). In cultures, its secretion is significantly increased in the presence of either type I or IV collagen and/or their breakdown products (Zuo and Woo, 1998b). Since the metalloprotease is secreted by the pathogen it contributes to the development of the disease and histopathological lesions (see below) in infected fish. This confirms that the severity of the disease in *Oncorhynchus* spp. is directly related to parasitaemia (Woo, 1979).

The histopathology includes: (i) focal haemorrhages; (ii) congestion of blood vessels; (iii) occlusion of capillaries with parasites; and (iv) changes in kidney glomeruli (Putz, 1972). Bahmanrokh and Woo (2001) conducted a sequential study in experimentally infected juvenile rainbow trout and showed the histopathology was a generalized inflammatory reaction, and lesions were in connective tissues and the reticulo-endothelial systems. Lesions were seen first in the liver, gills and spleen at about 1–2 weeks pi. Endovasculitis and mononuclear infiltration occurred at 3 weeks pi and these were followed by tissue necrosis and extravascular localization of parasites at 4 weeks pi. Extensive necrosis of tissues was related directly to high parasitaemias and extravascular localization of flagellates. Necrosis in the liver and kidney, depletion of haematopoietic tissues, and anaemia were probably responsible for mortality of fish during the acute phase of the disease. In some fish regeneration and replacement of necrotic tissues with normal structures were noticeable in haematopoietic and reticular tissues at 7–9 weeks pi and these were associated with reduced parasitaemias in the blood (recovery or chronic phase of the disease).

3.4. Pathophysiology

During the acute phase of the disease the haemolytic activity of serum complement is significantly lowered in infected trout (Thomas and Woo, 1989b), and this would contribute to the immunodepression and increased susceptibility to secondary infections (Jones *et al.*, 1986; Thomas and Woo, 1992). In infected rainbow trout the haemolytic levels of complement are about 20% of pre-infected levels and this persists throughout the infection (Thomas and Woo, 1989b). Low complement decreases phagocytic activity and antigen presentation by macrophages and hence contributes to immunodepression. Anorexia also contributes to the immunodepression (Thomas and Woo, 1992) and is also correlated with the anaemia during acute disease (MacDonald *et al.*, 2014).

In addition, plasma thyroxine (T3 and T4), protein and glucose are reduced along with depletion of liver glycogen (Laidley *et al.*, 1988).

The metabolism and swimming performance of infected juvenile rainbow trout are also significantly reduced especially during the acute phase of the disease (Kumaraguru *et al.*, 1995), and the bioenergetic cost of the disease in juvenile fish is considerable. These are contributing factors to the retarded growth of juvenile fish as there are significant reductions in food consumption, dry weight and energy gained, energy concentration and gross conversion efficiency. However, the attenuated vaccine strain (Section 3.5.3) has no detectable bioenergetic cost to juvenile fish (Beamish *et al.*, 1996).

Infected trout with high parasitaemias have low levels of cortisol as it is used up or bound to cortisol receptors on and in the *Cryptobia* (Sections 3.1.4 and 3.1.5). The pathogen likely also suppresses production of cortisol by inhibiting the HPI axis. To test this suggestion, the response of the HPI axis and the amount of cortisol produced were determined in *Cryptobia*-injected trout and 'stressed' uninfected fish that were 'air exposure in saline' fish ('aesf'). Fish were sampled at 4 and 6 weeks pi (peak parasitaemias). While both groups had similar initial resting cortisol levels, the infected fish had lower plasma adrenocorticotropic hormone (ACTH) than 'aesf'. Infected fish had higher mRNA levels of brain pre-optic corticotrophin-releasing factor (CRF), pituitary CRF receptor type 1 and other endocrine factors. The infected fish also had lower plasma cortisol compared to the 'air exposure in saline' stressor. Super fusion of the head kidney tissues from infected fish led to significantly lower ACTH-stimulated cortisol release rates than in control fish. These novel findings show that trout infected with *Cryptobia* had complex changes in the transcriptional activity of both central and peripheral regulators of the HPI axis and a reduction in the interrenal capacity to synthesize/secrete cortisol (Madison *et al.*, 2013).

The anaemia and large numbers of parasites occluding small blood vessels would combine to reduce oxygen delivery to tissues and vital organs. Part of this is manifested as an increase in susceptibility of infected fish to environmental hypoxia. This would be an important contributing factor to fish mortality under some conditions, especially when dissolved oxygen is reduced as a result of overcrowding, or in slow water flow or during algal blooms (Woo and Wehnert, 1986).

Anorexia is another consistent clinical sign of the disease (Section 3.2.1) and contributes to the immunodepression in infected fish during acute disease (Thomas and Woo, 1992); however, it is also beneficial to the host because anorexia decreases plasma protein by reducing protein intake (Li and Woo, 1991). Reduction in plasma protein lowers parasite multiplication which in turn reduces the parasitaemia, and a lower parasitaemia decreases the severity of the disease and fish mortality. As the infection progresses anorexia strengthens the feeding hierarchy within groups of fish; that is, it exacerbates the difference between dominant and subordinate fish (Chin *et al.*, 2004a). It is also positively correlated with reduction in oxygen-carrying capacity during acute disease. There are also increases in CRF and urotensin 1 (U1) mRNA but these are not correlated with food intake. Interleukin-1β mRNA levels in the head kidney and spleen are significantly reduced in infected fish. Consequently, it is suggested hypoxaemia is probably a mediator of anorexia in cryptobiosis (MacDonald *et al.*, 2014).

As indicated earlier (Section 3.2.1), anorexia is most evident during the acute phase of the disease and contributes to the immunodepression in cryptobiosis (Thomas and Woo, 1992). As a result of the immunodepression fish are more susceptible to secondary infections and their ability to mount a protective response (via vaccination) is also significantly reduced (Jones *et al.*, 1986). If the infected fish survive the acute disease, the anaemia and anorexia gradually subside as the parasitaemia is reduced (chronic phase of the disease) due to the development of protective humoral (e.g. Jones and Woo, 1987; Li and Woo, 1995; Feng and Woo, 1997a) and cell-mediated (e.g. Thomas and Woo, 1990a; Feng and Woo, 1996a; Mehta and Woo, 2002) immune responses to the pathogen.

There are close relationships between food intake, oxygen-carrying capacity and liver leptin-A1 gene expression, including leptin-A1 in plasma, in *Cryptobia*-infected rainbow trout (MacDonald *et al.*, 2014). *Cryptobia*-infected fish at high parasitaemias are anaemic, which significantly reduces oxygen-carrying capacity of the blood and food intake However, the major conclusion of the study with pair-fed but uninfected fish indicated hypoxemia and not feed restriction stimulates leptin-A1 secretion in infected trout.

3.5. Protective and Control Strategies

Most parasitic (protozoan and metazoan) infections in fishes are usually controlled using chemotherapy. Chemical treatments are necessary under certain circumstances (e.g. during disease outbreaks); however, the use of chemicals is becoming more restrictive due to many factors which include increasing concerns over food safety and environmental pollution. Woo (e.g. 1987b, 1992, 2001, 2007) has always been interested in the immune response of fish to parasites and exploiting it (both innate and adaptive components) as part of an overall control strategy against parasites. The following section shows that this approach is possible, and it is hoped that these proof-of-concept strategies developed using *C. salmositica* are considered and modified/refined for use on other piscine parasites.

3.5.1. Serological

Fish that have recovered from cryptobiosis are protected from the pathogen and their antisera have high titres of agglutinating, neutralizing and complement-fixing antibodies (e.g. Jones and Woo, 1987; Thomas and Woo, 1990b; Sitja-Bobadilla and Woo, 1994; Li and Woo, 1995; Feng and Woo, 1997a; Ardelli and Woo, 2002; Mehta and Woo, 2002). Also, intraperitoneal implantation of cortisol lowers antibody production and increases parasitaemia in rainbow trout. *In vitro* studies (P.T.K. Woo, 2008, unpublished results; Li, *et al.* 2013; Li and Woo, 2014) show the pathogen uses cortisol ('stress hormone') produced by the fish as a 'raf' (Section 3.1.5). Mortality of infected cortisol-implanted fish was higher than in infected fish or uninfected cortisol-implanted fish (Woo *et al.*, 1987). Also, both antisera from recovered fish and the monoclonal antibody mAb-001 (see below) are therapeutic and prophylactic against the parasite in fish (Feng and Woo, 1997b). Titres of complement-fixing antibodies in recovered and vaccinated fish rise significantly after *C. salmositica* challenge (e.g. Li and Woo, 1995; Ardelli and Woo, 1997, 2002; Feng and Woo, 1998c; Mehta and Woo, 2002), and this classical anamnesis response also confirms that the protection is in part due to humoral response in recovered and vaccinated fish.

A murine immunoglobulin G1 (IgG1) monoclonal antibody (mAb-001) was produced against the 200 kDa glycoprotein (Feng and Woo, 1996b). The epitope (designated Cs-gp200) consists of carbohydrate determinants and conformational polypeptide with internal disulfide bonds. It is hydrophilic and is secreted by the parasite (Feng and Woo, 1998a). Cs-gp200 has its asparagine-bound *N* glycosidically linked to a hybrid-type carbohydrate chain with the minimum length of a chitobiose core unit. It has a phosphatidylinositol residue which anchors the conformational polypeptide (with disulfide bonds) to the surface of the pathogen. The molecule is extensively post-translationally modified (Feng and Woo, 1998b). Cs-gp200 has high mannose components and it appears as a doublet in the pathogenic strain and as a single band in the vaccine strain (Feng and Woo, 2001).

The antibody mAb-001 is therapeutic when injected intraperitoneally into infected fish – it significantly lowered the parasitaemias in fish and this was similar to the effects of the inoculation of antisera from fish that had recovered from cryptobiosis (Fig. 3.6). Also, the antibody was prophylactic against *C. salmositica* (Feng and Woo, 1997b); however, it did not fix complement to lyse the parasite but agglutinated it. *In vitro* exposure of the parasite to mAb-001 reduced its survival and infectivity when inoculated back into fish (Feng and Woo, 1996b). Under *in vitro* conditions the parasite normally consumed oxygen; however, its aerobic respirations and mobility were inhibited when it was exposed to sodium azide. These activities were restored on washing even after prolonged exposure (24 h) to the metabolic poison; attempts to show it had glycolytic enzymes were not successful (Thomas *et al.*, 1992), however using more refined techniques it was later shown that the parasite indeed had glycolytic enzymes sequestered in microbodies called glycosomes (Ardelli *et al.*, 2000). In another metabolic study it was confirmed that parasite multiplication and aerobic respiration were totally inhibited in the presence of mAb-001 (Hontzeas *et al.*, 2001).

Also, the antibody neutralizes 100% of the histolytic activities of the metalloprotease and about 80% of the enzymatic activities of the

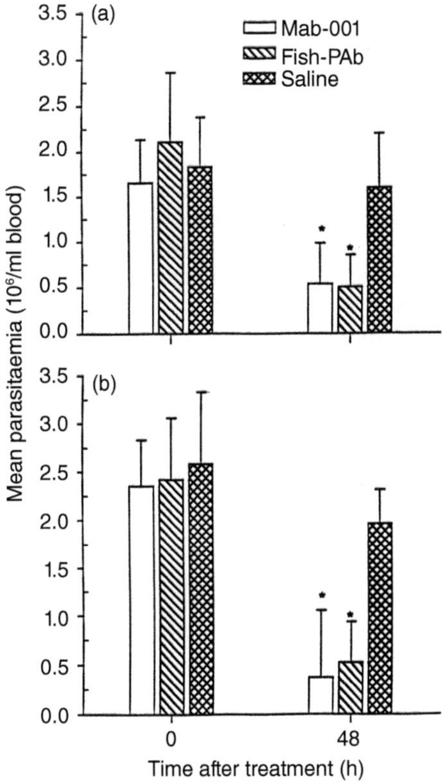

Fig. 3.6. Parasitaemias (mean ± SE) in rainbow trout 48 h after injection of antibodies: (a) fish infected with 2000 parasites; (b) fish infected with 20,000 parasites. MAb-001, fish injected with monoclonal antibody (mAb-001); Fish-PAb, fish injected with antiserum from a recovered fish; Saline, fish injected with cold-blooded vertebrate Ringer's saline; *, significantly lower ($P < 0.05$) than prior to injection of antibodies. (From Feng and Woo, 1997b; courtesy of *Diseases of Aquatic Organisms*).

cysteine protease under *in vitro* conditions (Zuo *et al.*, 1997). Consequently, mAb-001 has two main effects in cryptobiosis: (i) the neutralization of the metalloprotease which forms the basis of the metalloprotease-DNA vaccine (Section 3.5.3); and (ii) inhibition of the metabolism of the parasite which is manifested in inhibition of aerobic respiration and parasite multiplication. These inhibitory effects would contribute to its therapeutic and prophylactic properties in fish against the pathogen (Feng and Woo, 1997b); however, further studies are needed to confirm this suggestion.

3.5.2. Innate (natural) immunity

Two forms of natural immunity have been shown to occur in fish against *C. salmositica* and both are humoral related: (i) resistance to infection by a fish (pathogen-resistant fish); and (ii) the absence of disease in an infected fish (pathogen-tolerant fish). Besides these humoral immune responses there is also an innate cell-mediated response, and this is evident soon after infection (Chin and Woo, 2005). The nitroblue tetrazolium slide assay (Anderson *et al.*, 1992) was used to detect activated peripheral phagocytes in the blood of experimentally infected Atlantic salmon (*Salmo salar* L.) (Chin and Woo, 2005). However, the importance of peripheral phagocytes in innate protection against *Cryptobia* needs further studies and elucidation.

3.5.2.1. Cryptobia-resistant fish

Some hatchery-raised brook charr (*Salvelinus fontinalis*) with no prior exposure to the parasite or its antigens cannot be infected with *C. salmositica*; this is innate resistance to infection. The resistance is inherited by progeny and is controlled by a single dominant Mendelian locus. Briefly, *Cryptobia*-infected brook charr are homozygous recessive while the *Cryptobia*-resistant fish are either homozygous or heterozygous dominant for the locus (Forward *et al.*, 1995). Fresh plasma from *Cryptobia*-resistant brook charr lyses the parasite via the alternative pathway of complement activation under *in vitro* conditions (Forward and Woo, 1996). Consequently, we can now pre-select and breed *Cryptobia*-resistant brook charr by testing the freshly collected plasma from the brood fish for cryptobiocidal effects. There is no detectable difference in the immune responses of both *Cryptobia*-tolerant and *Cryptobia*-resistant brook charr to antigenic stimulations including to a commercially available bacterial vaccine (Ardelli and Woo, 1995).

3.5.2.2. Cryptobia-tolerant fish

Parasitaemias in some infected brook charr are just as high as those in *Oncorhynchus* spp.; however, they do not have clinical signs (e.g. anaemia, anorexia) associated with cryptobiosis – these are *Cryptobia*-tolerant fish (Ardelli *et al.*,

1994). These brook charr do not have the disease because the metalloprotease secreted by *C. salmositica* is neutralized by the α_2-macroglobulin (a natural anti-protease) in the blood. The amount of α_2-macroglobulin is higher in brook charr than in rainbow trout prior to infection and remains relatively high (about 40% of initial α_2-macroglobulin) even at peak parasitaemia, while that in trout drops to about 12% (Zuo and Woo, 1997a,b). Parasitaemias in infected rainbow trout and brook charr peak at 4–6 weeks pi and decline as antibodies are produced; however, the parasitaemia fluctuates in rainbow trout (e.g. Woo, 1979) while that in infected *Cryptobia*-tolerant charr declines rapidly after peak parasitaemia. Since *Cryptobia*-tolerant charr do not suffer from clinical disease, the immune system readily controls the infection and charr recover more rapidly than trout from the infection (Ardelli and Woo, 1995).

An obvious option to control cryptobiosis is to consider producing *Cryptobia*-tolerant salmon, perhaps using the CRISPR/Cas9 (clustered regularly interspaced short palindromic repeats/CRISPR-associated protein 9) system (Section 3.7; proposal #3). It is expected these modified salmon will maintain high levels of α_2-macroglobulin in their blood to neutralize the metalloprotease secreted by the pathogen – this will eliminate or at least reduce the severity of the disease in salmon. Since the disease is absent or less severe the fish immune system can more effectively control the infection. This proposal is a novel approach to the management of an infectious disease and needs further research and discussions. Obvious important 'downsides' to consider would include the acceptance of modified fish for human consumption. Also, should these fish escape from hatcheries they would breed with the 'wild' population, which might not be acceptable. However, the latter point could be overcome with further research on biosecurity. One important advantage is that no further human intervention (e.g. vaccination, chemotherapy) is required once the modified fish is produced.

3.5.3. Adaptive (acquired) immunity

Two distinctly different experimental vaccines (a live attenuated vaccine and a metalloprotease-DNA vaccine) have been developed to protect fish from the pathogen and disease. Susceptible fish inoculated with the attenuated *Cryptobia* vaccine are protected from infection when challenged with the pathogen. The second experimental vaccine (metalloprotease-DNA vaccine) does not prevent infection in vaccinated fish after they are challenged with the pathogen. However, antibodies produced in metalloprotease-DNA vaccinated fish neutralize the disease-causing factor (metalloprotease) secreted by the pathogen so that the vaccinated fish does not suffer from cryptobiosis. The vaccinated fish essentially turns the pathogenic *Cryptobia* into a non-pathogenic flagellate as in the case of the *Cryptobia*-tolerant brook charr (Section 3.5.2) and the antibody also (like mAb-001) inhibits parasite respiration and multiplication (Section 3.5.1).

3.5.3.1. Live vaccine

The pathogen was attenuated after prolonged *in vitro* culture and the strain was cloned. It is maintained in tissue culture medium and has remained avirulent since its attenuation in 1990. The strain produces a low infection in rainbow trout, does not cause disease, circulates in the blood for at least 6 months and is protective when the fish is challenged with the pathogen (Woo and Li, 1990). A single injection of the vaccine protects fish, and all vaccinated fish are protected from disease when challenged. Consequently, the strain is also used routinely as an experimental vaccine to study the development and mechanism of protective immunity in salmonids and the pathobiology of the disease. As indicated earlier (Section 3.4), the vaccine has no detectable bioenergetic cost to juvenile trout, and it protects various species of juvenile and adult salmonids from the pathogen (e.g. Sitja-Bobadilla and Woo, 1994; Li and Woo, 1995; Ardelli and Woo, 1997, 2002; Feng and Woo, 1997a, 1998c; Mehta and Woo, 2002; Chin *et al.*, 2004a,b).

Rainbow trout vaccinated while in fresh water and transferred to sea water are also protected on challenge (Li and Woo, 1997), and a single dose of the vaccine protects them for at least 24 months (Li and Woo, 1995). Vaccinated fish are only partially protected if they are challenged at 2 weeks post-vaccination (pv) while all vaccinated fish are protected at 3 weeks pv

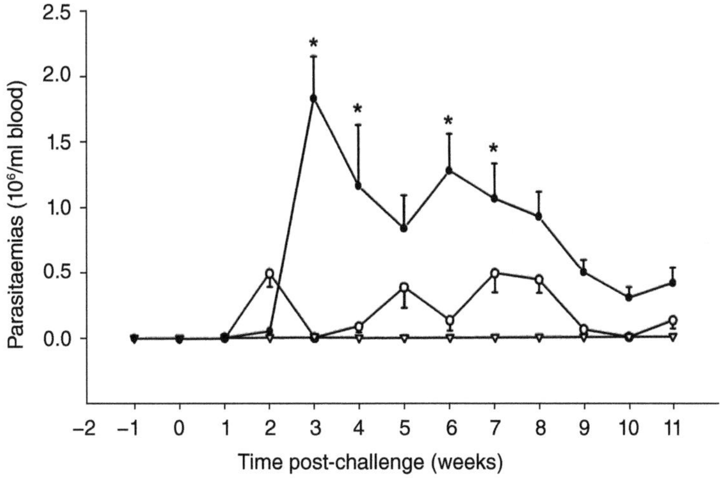

Fig. 3.7. Parasitaemias (mean ± SE) in vaccinated (10,000 attenuated *Cryptobia salmositica*) rainbow trout experimentally challenged with the pathogenic *C. salmositica*. Open triangles, vaccinated fish challenged at 3 weeks post-vaccination (pv); open circles, vaccinated fish challenged at 2 weeks pv; solid circles, control fish challenged at 3 weeks after inoculation with Ringer's saline; *, significantly higher at $P \leq 0.05$. (Redrawn from Li and Woo, 1995; courtesy of *Veterinary Immunology and Immunopathology*.)

(Fig. 3.7). Protection is via the production of complement-fixing antibodies (Fig. 3.8) and under *in vitro* conditions activated macrophages from head kidneys of vaccinated fish have enhanced phagocytosis and show antibody-independent and antibody-dependent cytotoxicity. Also, in the presence of antiserum, macrophages are very efficient in engulfing living parasites (Fig. 3.9). Moreover, the complement-fixing antibody titres (e.g. Li and Woo, 1995) and cell-mediated response (e.g. Mehta and Woo, 2002) in vaccinated fish rise significantly soon after parasite challenge (classical secondary responses). Humoral and cell-mediated immunity are involved in the protective mechanism in both vaccinated and recovered fish (e.g. Li and Woo, 1995; Ardelli and Woo, 1997, 2002; Mehta and Woo, 2002; Feng and Woo, 1996a).

3.5.3.2. Metalloprotease-DNA vaccine

As discussed earlier, the metalloprotease is the main disease-causing agent and this 200 kDa glycoprotein can be neutralized either by a natural anti-protease (α_2-macroglobulin) in *Cryptobia*-tolerant brook charr (Zuo and Woo, 1997a,b,c) or by an antibody (mAb-001) against the 200 kDa glycoprotein (Zuo *et al.*, 1997). The monoclonal antibody mAb-001 agglutinates the parasite and reduces its survival and infectivity (Feng and Woo, 1996b). Neutralization of the metalloprotease secreted by the pathogen and inhibition of the pathogen's multiplication and metabolic activities (Section 3.5.1) by specific antibodies are the main functions of the DNA vaccine.

Briefly, the metalloprotease (histolytic enzyme) and cysteine protease (metabolic enzyme) genes of *C. salmositica* were sequenced (Jesudhasan *et al.*, 2007a,b) and inserted into plasmid vectors (pEGFP-N) to produce a metalloprotease-plasmid vaccine and a cysteine-plasmid vaccine (Tan *et al.*, 2008). Rainbow trout and Atlantic salmon injected intramuscularly with the metalloprotease-plasmid vaccine consistently had lower packed cell volume (as metalloprotease was secreted into the blood) than control fishes (fishes inoculated either with plasmid alone or with the cysteine-plasmid vaccine) at 2–4 weeks pv. However, the packed cell volume in metalloprotease-vaccinated fishes returned to normal by 5 weeks pv – this was because the metalloprotease (secreted by the vaccine) was neutralized as antibodies were produced by the fish. Agglutinating antibodies against *C. salmositica* were detected 5–7 weeks pv in the blood (but not before 5 weeks pv) in metalloprotease-vaccinated trout. However, no

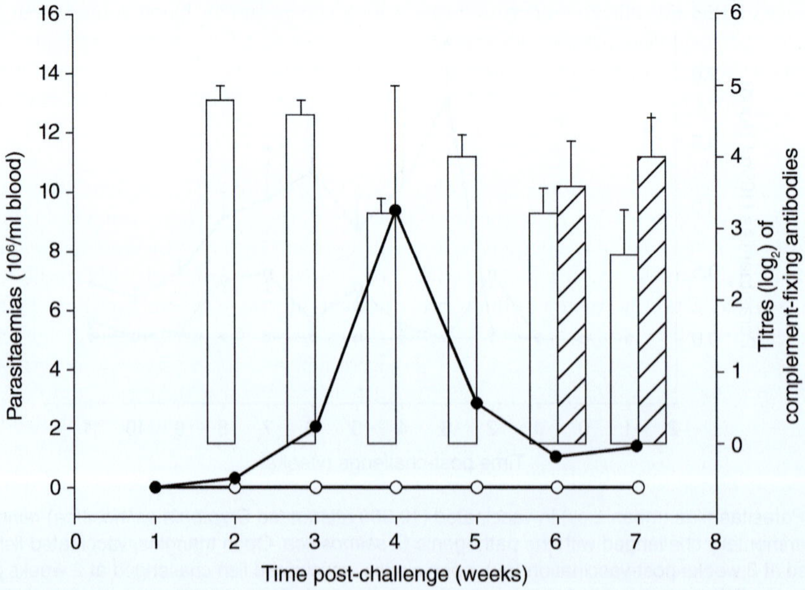

Fig. 3.8. Parasitaemias (line graph; mean ± SE) and complement-fixing antibodies (bar graph; mean ± SE) in infected controls (solid circles and bars with diagonal lines) and in vaccinated rainbow trout (open circles and open bars) challenged with 100,000 pathogenic *Cryptobia salmositica* at 4 weeks after vaccination. (From Li and Woo, 1995; courtesy of *Veterinary Immunology and Immunopathology*.)

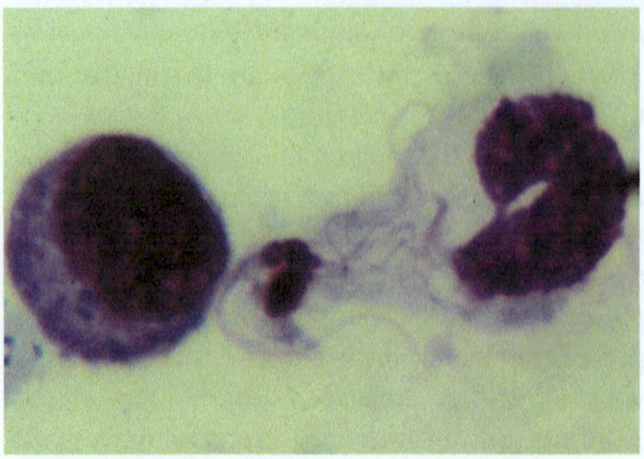

Fig. 3.9. Peritoneal macrophage in ascites of an experimentally infected rainbow trout, showing *Cryptobia salmositica* in the process of being engulfed. (From Woo, 1979; courtesy of *Experimental Parasitology*).

agglutinating antibodies were detected in either the cysteine-plasmid-injected fish or the plasmid-alone-injected fish. On challenge with the pathogen the metalloprotease-vaccinated trout had: (i) lower parasitaemia; (ii) delayed peak parasitaemia; and (iii) faster recovery than control infected fish. Further studies are needed to refine this very promising approach, and this would include determination of dosages and longevity of protection. In a review on the use of DNA vaccines in aquatic organisms, Kurath (2008) confirms that this is the 'first published demonstration of protective effects of a fish parasite DNA vaccine in fish'.

3.5.4. Chemotherapy and immunochemotherapy

Chemotherapy is essentially differential toxicity of the administered chemical; that is, the drug is more toxic to the target organism than it is to host tissues. Severity of the side effects of chemotherapy is dependent partly on tissue damage and adverse reactions by the host to the chemical. However, the drug can be directed more specifically to the pathogen if it is conjugated to an antibody against the target organism (immunochemotherapy). This will obviously increase the cost of treatments and is generally not meant for routine use. It may, however, be a useful tool under certain circumstances as it reduces the drug dosage and its side effects. In cryptobiosis, it can be used to treat infected brood fish as about 50% of brood fish die from cryptobiosis annually in some hatcheries on the west coast of North America (Section 3.1.4). It is expected side effects and accumulation of drug residues in host tissues are reduced in immunochemotherapy, and this may also lower the risk of the development of drug resistance by the pathogen. Reduction in drug residue in host tissues is also an important consideration if treated animals are for human consumption.

3.5.4.1. Chemotherapy

A combination of antibiotics (penicillin, streptomycin and amphotericin B) affects the viability of the parasite under *in vitro* conditions; however, this combination does not modulate the infection in infected fish (Thomas and Woo, 1991). According to Chapman (1994) the main cryptobiocidal factor in the combination is amphotericin B. Crystal violet, a triphenylmethane dye, is also cryptobiocidal and under *in vitro* conditions low concentrations of this dye inhibit parasite multiplication, reduce its infectivity to fish and cause ultrastructural lesions on mitochondrial and nuclear membranes (Ardelli and Woo, 1998). However, its therapeutic dose is too toxic (74% mortality) in juvenile trout (B.F. Ardelli and P.T.K. Woo, 1997, unpublished results).

Isometamidium chloride (Samorin) is widely used against trypanosomiasis in domestic animals in tropical Africa (e.g. Kinabo *et al.*, 1989), and it is also used as a prophylactic drug against bovine trypanosomiasis (e.g. Kinabo and Bogan, 1987). In fish, isometamidium chloride (1.0 mg/kg body weight) peaks in the blood 2–3 weeks after intramuscular injection (Ardelli and Woo, 2000). The drug is therapeutic against *C. salmositica* in experimentally infected rainbow trout during pre- and post-clinical phases of the disease. However, it is not effective during acute disease partly as it is believed the drug 'modifies' surface epitopes of the parasite so that parasites are not lysed by complement-fixing antibodies (Ardelli and Woo, 1999). All infected juvenile Chinook salmon injected with a single dose (1.0 mg/kg) survived the disease while 100% of untreated fish died with massive parasitaemias. The drug also had prophylactic protection and there was no evidence it affected fish growth, food consumption, blood complement levels or haematocrit values (Ardelli and Woo, 2001b).

Mortality of naturally infected Chinook salmon brood stock at the Soleduck State Hatchery (Washington State, USA) injected with isometamidium chloride (2.0 mg/kg body weight) was significantly lower than of control fish (injected with sterile deionized water). Progenies of drug-treated fish also survived better than those of control fish (injected with sterile deionized water) at the eyed-embryo and first-feeding stages. Also, no developmental abnormalities were detected in the progeny of drug-injected fish at 78 days after the first-feeding stage (Chen *et al.*, 2011). Isometamidium chloride was also effective in infected Atlantic salmon, and at a higher dose (2.5 mg/kg) the infection was eliminated in about 30% of adult fish and the parasitaemias were significantly reduced in the remaining fish (Ardelli and Woo, 2001b).

Isometamidium chloride accumulates rapidly in the kinetoplast of the parasite (Ardelli and Woo, 2001a) and causes condensation of its kinetoplast DNA, formation of vacuoles and swelling of the mitochondrial cristae (Fig. 3.10). The parasite normally undergoes aerobic respiration (Thomas *et al.*, 1992; Hontzeas *et al.*, 2001); however, it also has glycolytic enzymes sequestered in microbodies called glycosomes (Ardelli *et al.*, 2000). The *in vitro* oxygen consumption and carbon dioxide production by the parasite decrease significantly after drug exposure, and there are very significant increases in secretion of glycolytic products (lactate and pyruvate) as the parasite switches from aerobic respiration to glycolysis after its mitochondrion is damaged by the drug (Ardelli and Woo, 2001a). Also, *in vitro* exposure to sublethal dosages of the drug reduces infectivity of the parasite to fish and changes the surface glycoprotein antibody-receptor sites of the parasite (Ardelli and Woo, 1999). This alteration of surface epitopes by the drug would explain the protection of some parasites from lysis by complement-fixing antibodies when the treatment was administered to rainbow trout with acute infections.

3.5.4.2. Immunochemotherapy

Isometamidium chloride was conjugated to polyclonal antibodies (from 'recovered' fish) and to the monoclonal antibody (mAb-001). On

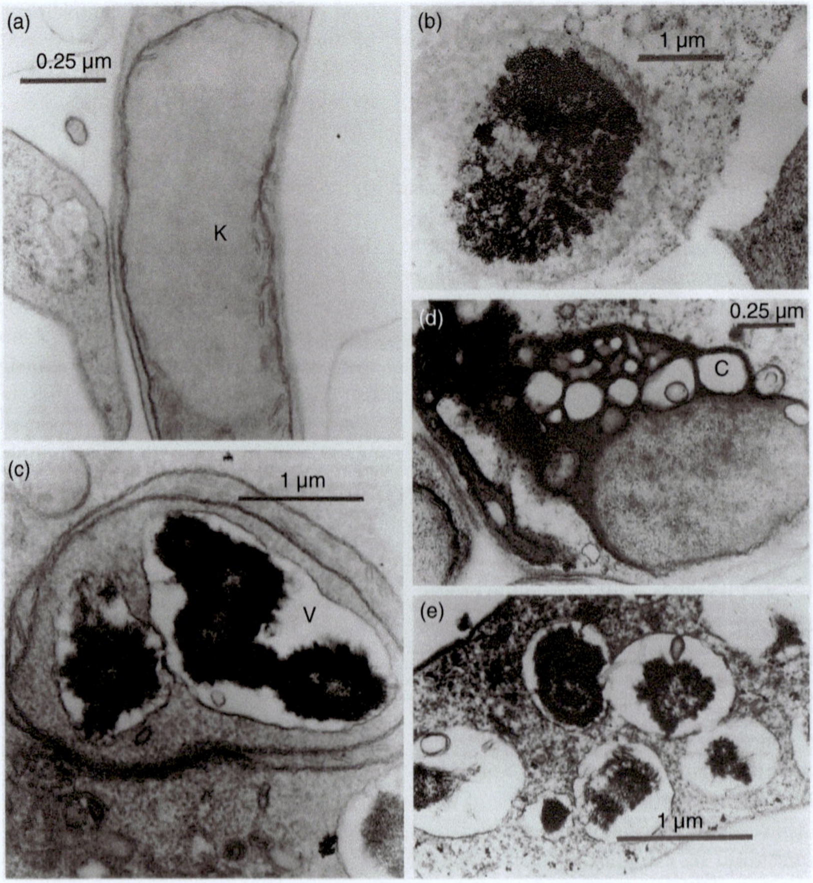

Fig. 3.10. Micro-lesions in *Cryptobia salmositica* (transmission electron microscopy) after *in vitro* exposure to the drug, isometamidium chloride. (a) Normal kinetoplast – not exposed to the drug; (b) condensation of DNA in kinetoplast after drug exposure; (c) vacuole formation in kinetoplast after drug exposure; (d) swelling of cristae after drug exposure; (e) vacuole formation in cytoplasm after drug exposure. C, cristae; K, kinetoplast; V, vacuole. (From Ardelli and Woo, 2001a; courtesy of *Journal of Parasitology*.)

in vitro exposure the conjugated drug was on the entire parasite while the unconjugated drug accumulated only in the kinetoplast (Ardelli and Woo, 2001c). Before drug conjugation both antibodies agglutinated living parasites, but the antibodies reacted differently after drug conjugation. The polyclonal antibodies-conjugated drug (PAIC) lysed most of the parasite under *in vitro* conditions and it no longer agglutinated the parasite. In contrast, the mAb-001-conjugated drug did not lyse *C. salmositica* but agglutinated it. After *in vitro* exposure to PAIC the infectivity of the parasite was significantly lowered. The number of infected juvenile Chinook salmon and their parasitaemias at 7 weeks pi were significantly lower in fish injected with PAIC-exposed parasites than in those exposed to drug alone or to polyclonal antibodies alone or to drug plus polyclonal antibody without conjugation (Table 3.1). Also, fish survival in the PAIC group was higher than in the other groups. Preliminary studies indicate the drug–antibody conjugate is also effective when injected into infected fish. These results are encouraging, and further studies are needed (e.g. to determine dosages needed for effective treatment and refinement of the approach, which would include stage of infection and species of salmonids).

Table 3.1. Infectivity of cultured *Cryptobia salmositica* to Chinook salmon after *in vitro* exposure to isometamidium chloride conjugated to anti-*C. salmositica* polyclonal antibodies. (Author's own table.)

Time after infection (weeks)	Group 1	Group 2	Group 3	Group 4	Group 5
	PAIC[a]	Isometamidium	PAI[a]	Antibody	Untreated controls
1	1/10[b]	7/10	0/10	0/10	8/10
	0.30 ± 0.95[c]	1.80 ± 2.78	0	0	6.60 ± 4.72
2	1/10	6/10	2/10	0/10	10/10
	0.30 ± 0.95	8.10 ± 5.28	1.80 ± 3.91	0	48 750 ± 45 814
3	2/10	7/10	2/10	0/10	10/10
	0.50 ± 1.27	33 250 ± 38 207	1950 ± 4310	0	35 625 ± 29 978
4	2/10	8/10	3/10	3/10	10/10
	0.30 ± 0.675	302 000 ± 254 142	2500 ± 5270	5558 ± 16 665	5 487 500 ± 5 439 838
5	2/10	10/10	4/10	4/9	10/10
	0.60 ± 1.58	9 395 000 ± 16 925 911	54 740 ± 112 499	556 944 ± 1 500 001	3 175 000 ± 3 639 196
6	1/10	10/10	4/10	4/10	10/10
	3750 ± 11 858	13 475 000 ± 15 298 624	503 750 ± 1 030 810	2 600 000 ± 5 577 465	3 243 750 ± 5 416 196
7	1/10	10/10	4/10	4/10	10/10
	11 250 ± 35 575	18 305 000 ± 52 500 000	928 860 ± 1 326 575	44 383 334 ± 129 150 260	27 051 250 ± 56 209 714

[a]PAIC, polyclonal antibodies-conjugated drug; PAI, drug plus polyclonal antibodies without conjugation.
[b]Number of infected fish/number of fish inoculated.
[c]Mean parasitaemia ± SD; determined by HCT or haemocytometer.

3.5.5. Environmental modification: higher temperature tolerance in salmon and in leech vector

3.5.5.1. Water temperature

The parasite becomes sluggish and does not survive if infected blood is left at room temperature (about 20°C) for any length of time. Experimentally infected juvenile rainbow trout lost their infections or there was no fish mortality when the water temperature was slowly raised from about 10°C to 20°C (Woo *et al.*, 1983; Bower and Margolis, 1985). Consequently Woo (1987a) suggested that modification(s) of this approach might be useful for protecting fish under certain circumstances. Bower and Evelyn (1988) showed infected juvenile sockeye salmon acclimatized to 20°C survived a *Cryptobia* infection while all infected fish maintained at 10°C died from the disease. Also, 60 of temperature-acclimatized infected fish survived a parasite challenge at 10°C while 95 of infected non-temperature-acclimatized fish died.

Selective breeding of rainbow trout over an extended period produced fish with higher temperature tolerance and their progenies (F_1 and F_2 generations) retained the higher temperature tolerance (Ineno *et al.*, 2005, 2018). Gonen *et al.* (2024) also concluded that selective breeding of Atlantic salmon could produce fish with higher temperature tolerance and that this trait would be inherited by progenies. In a recent review of 168 published articles on upper thermal limits (UTLs) of five *Oncorhynchus* species, Mayer *et al.* (2023) found 'considerable variations in UTLs among species, within species and across life stages' and suggested these variations might be due, in part, to the method used. Also, fish with identical UTLs had variations 'within species; UTL was higher for populations historically encountering higher temperatures' (Mayer *et al.*, 2023). This suggests the environment may gradually modify the UTL which is inherited. Since the genes for higher temperature tolerance (HTT genes) are already in salmonid genomes, the CRISPR/Cas9 system would more efficiently enhance the frequencies and/or expressions of HTT genes in salmon (Section 3.7; proposal #4).

3.5.5.2. Vector control

P. salmositica is the only known vector of the pathogen (Section 3.1.3). This freshwater leech is not host specific and is present in cold, fast-flowing rivers and streams (Becker and Katz, 1965a,c). Since leech cocoons and adult *P. salmositica* are susceptible to drying and freezing, draining areas is a method to control leeches in hatcheries where cocoons are deposited or where large numbers of leeches are present (Bower and Thompson, 1987). Also, adult leeches are susceptible to chlorine (Bower *et al.*,1985), hence the chemical can be considered for controlling leeches under certain conditions. Leeches would likely have reduced survival and/or transmission ability at higher water temperatures.

3.6. Conclusions

C. salmositica infects all species of Pacific salmon and sculpins on the west coast of North America. It is normally transmitted indirectly by the freshwater leech, *P. salmositica*, in streams and rivers; however, direct transmission between fish can occur under certain aquaculture conditions. Salmonids in freshwater hatcheries, streams/rivers and sea cages have experienced high fish mortality due to cryptobiosis. Although the parasite is pathogenic to salmon it is not known to cause disease in naturally infected sculpins. However, this assumption needs confirmation using experimentally infected laboratory-raised sculpins (Section 3.7; proposal #1).

Cortisol ('stress hormone') in fish plasma stimulates rapid *Cryptobia* multiplication. It acts as a 'raf' as cortisol receptors are on and in the parasite. In an infected fish at peak parasitaemia, the hormone in the plasma is low or depleted as no cortisol is produced because of HPI axis dysfunction. Low level of plasma cortisol reduces the rate of *Cryptobia* multiplication, as well as lowering the immunodepressive role of the hormone. This allows the immune system to take control of the infection, and some fish recover from the disease. Future studies will include the mechanisms of cortisol uptake and its utilization by *Cryptobia* and test the hypothesis that cortisol may also be used by other pathogens as a 'raf' (Section 3.7; proposal #2).

Metalloprotease secreted by *Cryptobia* and numerous other factors contribute to severity of the disease. These factors include: (i) the size of the parasite inoculums; (ii) water temperature; (iii) fish diets; (iv) size and strain/species of the fish; and (v) the genetics and sexual maturity of the fish. Clinical signs of the disease include anaemia, anorexia, abdominal distension with ascites and exophthalmia. Severity of cryptobiosis, appearance of the clinical signs and mortality are related to parasitaemias, and the disease-causing factor is a secreted 200 kDa metalloprotease which is a histolytic enzyme. Hypoxia in infected fish due to the anaemia stimulates infected fish to secrete leptin-A1 which contributes to anorexia. As indicated earlier, *Cryptobia* depletes plasma cortisol and cryptobiosis causes dysfunction of the HPI axis, so no new cortisol is produced. Bioenergetic costs of cryptobiosis retard the growth, metabolism and swimming performance of juvenile salmonids; however, the attenuated protective *Cryptobia* strain has no such effects and does not cause disease. The histopathology indicates the disease is a generalized inflammatory reaction, and lesions are in connective tissues and the reticulo-endothelial systems. During acute infections the immune system is depressed, the fish are more susceptible to secondary infections and they do not respond to vaccination.

Salmonids that survived the infection are protected from the pathogen. Humoral (neutralizing antibodies, complement-fixing antibodies, etc.) and cell-mediated (cell-mediated cytotoxicity, enhanced phagocytosis, etc.) immunity are involved in the protection against cryptobiosis. Several protective strategies have been developed to protect salmonids, and these proof-of-concept strategies include the exploitation of innate breeding of *Cryptobia*-resistant brook charr and the possibility of producing *Cryptobia*-tolerant salmon using the CRISPR/Cas9 system (Section 3.7; proposal #3). Two experimental vaccines (an attenuated live *Cryptobia* strain and the metalloprotease-DNA vaccine) and a monoclonal antibody (mAb-001) protect salmonids from *Cryptobia* and cryptobiosis.

Isometamidium chloride is therapeutic against *Cryptobia*/cryptobiosis in experimentally and naturally infected juvenile and mature salmonids. The drug does not affect fish growth or development. Attaching an antibody against *Cryptobia* to the drug increases its effectiveness.

In laboratory studies *Oncorhynchus* can survive and develop protective immunity against *Cryptobia* at 20°C if the water temperature is gradually increased. Over an extended period salmonids can be bred to survive and breed at higher temperatures, and their progenies (F_1 and F_2 generations) retain high temperature tolerance. Future study using the CRISPR/Cas9 system (Section 3.7; proposal #4) is suggested as this biotechnology method may more efficiently enhance gene expressions for higher temperature tolerance.

Further studies of these tested strategies under field conditions are suggested. It is also hoped that some of these proof-of-concept strategies against *Cryptobia* and cryptobiosis would be considered and be adapted or modified against other pathogens.

3.7. Suggestions for Future Research

- *Proposal #1*: Sculpins are considered reservoir hosts of *C. salmositica* (Sections 3.1.3 and 3.1.4). A robust study using laboratory-raised sculpins is warranted to examine the *Cryptobia*–sculpin relationships. This study should include: (i) susceptibility of sculpins to *Cryptobia*; (ii) course of infection; (iii) haematology; (iv) innate and acquired immune responses; and (v) longevity of infected sculpins.
- *Proposal #2*: Test the hypothesis that cortisol is also used by other pathogens as a 'raf' as by *Cryptobia* (Sections 3.1.4 and 3.1.5). The second component of this proposal should include elucidating the mechanism of cortisol uptake and its utilization by *Cryptobia*.

  The CRISPR/Cas9 system is used to add and/or alter genetic material at specific DNA sites in cells (Tavakoli, *et al.*, 2021). It is an appropriate technique to consider for proposals #3 and #4 – to enhance the frequencies/expressions of 'useful' genes in salmonid genomes. If successful, no further human interventions will be needed to protect juvenile salmon from cryptobiosis in freshwater hatcheries (proposal #3) and heat-related mortality in freshwater streams as climate change continues (proposal #4).
- *Proposal #3*: *Oncorhynchus* already has genes to produce α_2-macroglobulin to neutralize the metalloprotease secreted by *Cryptobia*; however, infected *Oncorhynchus* cannot maintain high enough levels of α_2-macroglobulin to control cryptobiosis. The CRISPR/Cas9 system may be able to enhance frequencies and/or expressions of these genes in salmonids so that additional α_2-macroglobulin will be secreted and maintained to neutralize the secreted metalloprotease, as in infected *Cryptobia*-tolerant brook charr (Section 3.5.2).
- *Proposal #4*: The ongoing climate change will continue to increase global temperatures and acidification of water, which result in reduced dissolved oxygen. Water temperatures will rise, especially in shallow, cold freshwater streams where salmon spawn and eggs develop, hatch and grow into juveniles. Experimental studies indicate that juvenile *Oncorhynchus* spp. can, over an extended period, adapt to breed at 20°C and their progenies retain the higher temperature tolerance (Section 3.5.5). Consequently, the CRISPR/Cas9 system may be a more efficient system to enhance frequencies and/or expressions of HTT alleles. Higher temperature tolerance fish will survive but their growth/longevity may be affected by other abiotic changes, which need to be addressed.

Acknowledgements

The review in this chapter is largely based on one component of the author's interdisciplinary research programme on parasitic flagellates in terrestrial and aquatic organisms. The programme has had continuous financial support (>40 years) from the Natural Science and Engineering Research Council, Canada and *ad hoc* research grants from other sponsors which include the AquaNet Networks of Centres of Excellence and the Department of Fisheries and Oceans, Canada. He is extremely grateful for invaluable contributions from and discussions with highly talented/motivated graduate students, postdoctoral fellows and colleagues who, over the years, have joined him in this delightful and exciting venture.

References

Anderson, D.P., Moritamo, T. and Grooth, R. (1992) Neutrophil, glass-adherent, nitroblue tetrazolium assay gives early indication of immunization effectiveness in rainbow trout. *Veterinary Immunology and Immunopathology* 30, 419–429.

Ardelli, B.F. and Woo, P.T.K. (1995) Immune response of *Cryptobia*-resistant and *Cryptobia*-susceptible *Salvelinus fontinalis* to an *Aeromonas salmonicida* vaccine. *Diseases of Aquatic Organisms* 23, 33–38.

Ardelli, B.F. and Woo, P.T.K. (1997) Protective antibodies and anamnestic response in *Salvelinus fontinalis* to *Cryptobia salmositica* and innate resistance of *Salvelinus namaycush* to the hemoflagellate. *Journal of Parasitology* 83, 943–946.

Ardelli, B.F. and Woo, P.T.K. (1998) The *in vitro* effects of crystal violet on the pathogenic haemoflagellate *Cryptobia salmositica* Katz 1951. *Parasite* 5, 27–36.

Ardelli, B.F. and Woo, P.T.K. (1999) The therapeutic use of isometamidium chloride against *Cryptobia salmositica* in rainbow trout (*Oncorhynchus mykiss*). *Diseases of Aquatic Organisms* 37, 195–203.

Ardelli, B.F. and Woo, P.T.K. (2000) An antigen-capture enzyme-linked immunosorbent assay (ELISA) to detect isometamidium chloride in *Oncorhynchus* spp. *Diseases of Aquatic Organisms* 39, 231–236.

Ardelli, B.F. and Woo, P.T.K. (2001a) The *in vitro* effects of isometamidium chloride (Samorin) on the piscine hemoflagellate *Cryptobia salmositica* (Kinetoplastida, Bodonina). *Journal of Parasitology* 87, 194–202.

Ardelli, B.F. and Woo, P.T.K. (2001b) Therapeutic and prophylactic effects of isometamidium chloride (Samorin) against the haemoflagellate *Cryptobia salmositica* in chinook salmon (*Oncorhynchus tshawytscha*). *Parasitology Research* 87, 18–26.

Ardelli, B.F. and Woo, P.T.K. (2001c) Conjugation of isometamidium chloride to antibodies and the use of the conjugate against the haemoflagellate, *Cryptobia salmositica*: an immuno-chemotherapeutic strategy. *Journal of Fish Diseases* 24, 439–451.

Ardelli, B.F. and Woo, P.T.K. (2002) Experimental *Cryptobia salmositica* (Kinetoplastida) infections in Atlantic salmon, *Salmo salar* L.: cell-mediated and humoral immune responses against the pathogenic and vaccine strains of the parasite. *Journal of Fish Diseases* 25, 265–274.

Ardelli, B.F., Forward, G.M. and Woo, P.T.K. (1994) Brook charr (*Salvelinus fontinalis*) and cryptobiosis: a potential salmonid reservoir host for *Cryptobia salmositica* Katz 1951. *Journal of Fish Diseases* 17, 567–577.

Ardelli, B.F., Witt, J.D.S. and Woo, P.T.K. (2000) The identification of glycosomes and metabolic end products in pathogenic and nonpathogenic strains of *Cryptobia salmositica* (Kinetoplastida). *Diseases of Aquatic Organisms* 42, 41–51.

Bahmanrokh, M. and Woo, P.T.K. (2001) Relationships between histopathology and parasitaemias in *Oncorhynchus mykiss* infected with *Cryptobia salmositica*, a pathogenic haemoflagellate. *Diseases of Aquatic Organisms* 46, 41–45.

Barton, B.A. (2000) Salmonid fishes differ in their cortisol and glucose responses to handling and transport stress. *North American Journal of Aquaculture* 62, 12–18.

Beamish, F.W.H., Sitja-Bobadilla, A., Jebbink, J.A. and Woo, P.T.K. (1996) Bioenergetic cost of cryptobiosis in fish: rainbow trout (*Oncorhynchus mykiss*) infected with *Cryptobia salmositica* and with an attenuated live vaccine. *Diseases of Aquatic Organisms* 25, 1–8.

Becker, C.D. and Katz, M. (1965a) Transmission of the haemoflagellate *Cryptobia salmositica* Katz 1951, by a rhynchobdellid leech vector. *Journal of Parasitology* 51, 95–99.

Becker, C.D. and Katz, M. (1965b) Infections of the haemoflagellate *Cryptobia salmositica* Katz 1951, in freshwater teleosts of the Pacific coast. *Transactions of the American Fisheries Society* 94, 327–333.

Becker, C.D. and Katz, M. (1965c) Distribution, ecology and biology of the salmonid leech, *Piscicola salmositica* Meyer 1946 (Rhynchobdella, Piscicolidae). *Journal of the Fisheries Research Board of Canada* 22, 1175–1195.

Becker, C.D. and Katz, M. (1966) Host relationships of *Cryptobia salmositica* (Protozoa, Mastigophora) in Washington hatchery stream. *Transactions of the American Fisheries Society* 95, 196–202.

Bower, S.M. and Evelyn, T.P.T. (1988) Acquired and innate resistance to the haemoflagellate *Cryptobia salmositica* in sockeye salmon (*Oncorhynchus nerka*). *Developmental and Comparative Immunology* 12, 749–760.

Bower, S.M. and Margolis, L. (1983) Direct transmission of the haemoflagellate *Cryptobia salmositica* among Pacific salmon (*Oncorhynchus* spp.). *Canadian Journal of Zoology* 61, 1242–1250.

Bower, S.M. and Margolis, L. (1984a) Detection of infection and susceptibility of different Pacific salmon stocks (*Oncorhynchus* spp.) to the haemoflagellate *Cryptobia salmositica*. *Journal of Parasitology* 70, 273–278.

Bower, S.M. and Margolis, L. (1984b) Distribution of *Cryptobia salmositica*, a haemoflagellate of fishes in British Columbia and the seasonal pattern of infection in a coastal river. *Canadian Journal of Zoology* 62, 2512–2518.

Bower, S.M. and Margolis, L. (1985) Effects of temperature and salinity on the course of infection with the haemoflagellate *Cryptobia salmositica* in juvenile Pacific salmon (*Oncorhynchus* spp.). *Journal of Fish Diseases* 8, 25–33.

Bower, S.M. and Thompson, A.B. (1987) Hatching of the Pacific salmon leech (*Piscicola salmositica*) from cocoons exposed to various treatments. *Aquaculture* 66, 1–8.

Bower, S.M., Margolis, L. and MacKay, R.J. (1985) Potential usefulness of chlorine for controlling Pacific salmon leeches, *Piscicola salmositica* in hatcheries. *Canadian Journal of Fisheries and Aquatic Sciences* 42, 1986–1993.

Brugerolle, C., Lom, J., Nohynkova, E. and Joyon, L. (1979) Comparison et evolution des structures cellulaires chez plusieurs especes de bodonides et cryptobiides appartenant aux genres *Bodo*, *Cryptobia* et *Trypanoplasma* (Kinetoplastida, Mastigophora). *Protistologica* 15, 197–221.

Caldwell, C.A., Kattesh, H.G. and Strange, R.J. (1991) Distribution of cortisol among its free and protein-bound fractions in rainbow trout (*Oncorhynchus mykiss*): evidence of control by sexual maturation. *Comparative Biochemistry and Physiology* 99A, 593–595.

Carruth, L.L., Dores, R.M., Maldonado, T.A., Norris, D.O., Rut, T. and Jones, R.E. (2000) Elevation of plasma cortisol during the spawning migration of landlocked kokanee salmon (*Oncorhynchus nerka kennerlyi*). *Comparative Biochemistry and Physiology* 127C, 123–131.

Chapman, P.F. (1994) Effects of amphotericin B, penicillin, and streptomycin on cultures of *Cryptobia salmositica*. *Journal of Aquatic Animal Health* 6, 215–219.

Chen, M.F., Cheng, Y.W., Popochock, D., Russell, B., Kerwin, J. *et al.* (2011) Isometamidium chloride reduces mortality of adult Chinook salmon due to *Cryptobia salmositica*. *North American Journal of Aquaculture* 73, 304–310.

Chin, A. and Woo, P.T.K. (2005) Innate cell-mediated immune response and peripheral leukocyte populations in Atlantic salmon, *Salmo salar* L., to a live *Cryptobia salmositica* vaccine. *Parasitology Research* 95, 299–304.

Chin, A., Eldridge, M., Glebe, B.D. and Woo, P.T.K. (2002) *Salmo salar* and *Cryptobia salmositica*: variations in susceptibility and humoral response in families of Atlantic salmon to the pathogen. Presented at *AquaNet II, Annual General Meeting*, 2002, Moncton, New Brunswick, Canada (abstract).

Chin, A., Glebe, B. and Woo, P.T.K. (2004a) Humoral response and susceptibility of five full-sib families of Atlantic salmon (*Salmo salar* L) to the haemoflagellate, *Cryptobia salmositica* Katz 1951. *Journal of Fish Diseases* 27, 471–481.

Chin, A., Guo, F.C., Bernier, N.J. and Woo, P.T.K. (2004b) Effect of *Cryptobia salmositica*-induced anorexia on feeding behavior and immune response in juvenile rainbow trout, *Oncorhynchus mykiss*. *Diseases of Aquatic Organisms* 58, 17–26.

Currie, J.L.M. and Woo, P.T.K. (2007) Susceptibility of sexually mature rainbow trout, *Oncorhynchus mykiss* to experimental cryptobiosis caused by *Cryptobia salmositica*. *Parasitology Research* 101, 1057–1067.

Currie, J.L.M. and Woo, P.T.K. (2008) Effects of the pathogenic haemoflagellate, *Cryptobia salmositica* on brood fish, *Oncorhynchus mykiss*. *Environmental Biology of Fishes* 83, 355–365.

Faught, E and Schaal, M.J.M (2024) Molecular mechanisms of the stress-induced regulation of the inflammatory response in fish. *General and Comparative Endocrinology* 345, 114387. DOI: 10.1016/j.ygcen.2023.114387.

Feng, S. and Woo, P.T.K. (1996a) Cell-mediated immune response and T-like cells in thymectomized *Oncorhynchus mykiss* (Walbaum) infected with or vaccinated against the pathogenic hemoflagellate *Cryptobia salmositica* Katz 1951. *Parasitology Research* 82, 604–611.

Feng, S. and Woo, P.T.K. (1996b) Biological characterization of a monoclonal antibody against a surface membrane antigen on *Cryptobia salmositica* Katz 1951. *Journal of Fish Diseases* 19, 137–143.

Feng, S. and Woo, P.T.K. (1997a) Complement fixing antibody production in thymectomized *Oncorhynchus mykiss* (Walbaum), vaccinated against or infected with the pathogenic haemoflagellate *Cryptobia salmositica*. *Folia Parasitologica* 44, 188–194.

Feng, S. and Woo, P.T.K. (1997b) The therapeutic and prophylactic effects of a protective monoclonal antibody (MAb-001) against the pathogenic haemoflagellate *Cryptobia salmositica* Katz 1951. *Diseases of Aquatic Organisms* 28, 211–219.

Feng, S. and Woo, P.T.K. (1998a) Characterization of a 200 kDa glycoprotein (Cs-gp2000) on the pathogenic piscine haemoflagellate *Cryptobia salmositica*. *Diseases of Aquatic Organisms* 32, 41–48.

Feng, S. and Woo, P.T.K. (1998b) Biochemical characterization of an epitope on the surface membrane antigen (Cs-gp200) of the pathogenic piscine hemoflagellate *Cryptobia salmositica* Katz 1951. *Experimental Parasitology* 88, 3–10.

Feng, S. and Woo, P.T.K. (1998c) The *in vitro* and *in vivo* effects of rabbit anti-thymocyte serum on circulating leucocytes and production of complement fixing antibodies in thymectomized *Oncorhynchus mykiss* (Walbaum) infected with *Cryptobia salmositica* Katz 1951. *Journal of Fish Diseases* 21, 241–248.

Feng, S. and Woo, P.T.K. (2001) Cell membrane glycoconjugates on virulent and avirulent strains of the pathogenic haemoflagellate *Cryptobia salmositica* Katz. *Journal of Fish Diseases* 24, 23–32.

Forward, G.M. and Woo, P.T.K. (1996) An *in vitro* study on the mechanism of innate immunity in *Cryptobia*-resistant brook charr (*Salvelinus fontinalis*) against *Cryptobia salmositica*. *Parasitology Research* 82, 238–241.

Forward, G.M., Ferguson, M.M. and Woo, P.T.K. (1995) Susceptibility of brook charr, *Salvelinus fontinalis* to the pathogenic haemoflagellate, *Cryptobia salmositica*, and the inheritance of innate resistance by progenies of resistant fish. *Parasitology* 111, 337–345.

Gonen, S., Benfey, T.J. and Garbar, A.F. (2024) The genomic architecture of high temperature tolerance in a year class of Atlantic salmon. *Aquaculture* 578, 740020. DOI: 10.1016/j.aquaculture.2023.740020.

Hontzeas, N., Feng, S. and Woo, P.T.K. (2001) Inhibitory effects of a monoclonal antibody (Mab-001) on *in vitro* oxygen consumption and multiplication of the pathogenic haemoflagellate, *Cryptobia salmositica* Katz. *Journal of Fish Diseases* 24, 391–398.

Ineno, T., Tsuchida, S., Kanada, M, and Watabe, S. (2005) Thermal tolerance of a rainbow trout, *Oncorhynchus mykiss* strain selected by high temperature breeding. *Fisheries Science* 71, 767–775.

Ineno, T., Tarnaki, K., Yamada, K., Kodama, K., Ischida, S. *et al.* (2018) Thermal tolerance of a thermally selected strain of rainbow trout, *Oncorhynchus mykiss* and the pedigree of its F1 and F2 generations indicated by their critical thermal maxima. *Fisheries Science* 84, 671–679.

Jesudhasan, P.R.R., Tan, C.W. and Woo, P.T.K. (2007a) A metalloproteinase gene from the pathogenic piscine hemoflagellate, *Cryptobia salmositica*. *Parasitology Research* 100, 899–904.

Jesudhasan, P.R.R., Tan, C.W., Hontzeas, N. and Woo, P.T.K. (2007b) A cathepsin L-like cysteine proteinase gene from the pathogenic piscine hemoflagellate, *Cryptobia salmositica*. *Parasitology Research* 100, 881–886.

Jones, S.R.M. and Woo, P.T.K. (1987) The immune response of rainbow trout *Salmo gairdneri* Richardson to the haemoflagellate *Cryptobia salmositica* Katz 1951. *Journal of Fish Diseases* 10, 395–402.

Jones, S.R.M., Woo, P.T.K. and Stevenson, R.M.W. (1986) Immunosuppression in *Salmo gairdneri* Richardson caused by the haemoflagellate, *Cryptobia salmositica* (Katz, 1951). *Journal of Fish Diseases* 9, 431–438.

Katz, M. (1951) Two new hemoflagellates (genus *Cryptobia*) from some western Washington teleosts. *Journal of Parasitology* 37, 245–250.

Kinabo, L.D.B. and Bogan, J.A. (1987) Binding of isometamidium to calf thymus DNA and lipids: pharmacological implications. *Journal of Veterinary Pharmacology and Therapeutics* 10, 357–362.

Kinabo, L.D.B., Bogan, J.A., McKellar, Q.A. and Murray, M. (1989) Relay bioavailability and toxicity of isometamidium residues: a model for human risk assessment. *Veterinary and Human Toxicology* 31, 417–421.

Koldkjær, P., Pottinger, T.G., Perry, S.F. and Cossins, A.R. (2004) Seasonality of the red blood cell stress response in rainbow trout (*Oncorhynchus mykiss*). *Journal of Experimental Biology* 207, 357–367.

Kubokawa, K., Watanabe, T., Yoshioka, M. and Iwata, M. (1999) Effects of acute stress on plasma cortisol, sex steroid hormone and glucose levels in male and female sockeye salmon during the breeding season. *Aquaculture* 172, 335–349.

Kumaraguru, A.K., Beamish, F.W.H. and Woo, P.T.K. (1995) Impact of a pathogenic haemoflagellate, *Cryptobia salmositica* on the metabolism and swimming performance of rainbow trout, *Oncorhynchus mykiss* (Walbaum). *Journal of Fish Diseases* 18, 297–305.

Kurath, G. (2008) Biotechnology and DNA vaccines for aquatic animals. *Revue Scientifique et Technique* 27, 175–196.

Laidley, C.W., Woo, P.T.K. and Leatherland, J.F. (1988) The stress response of rainbow trout to experimental infection with the blood parasite, *Cryptobia salmositica* Katz, 1951. *Journal of Fish Biology* 32, 253–261.

Li, S. and Woo, P.T.K. (1991) Anorexia reduces the severity of cryptobiosis in *Oncorhynchus mykiss*. *Journal of Parasitology* 77, 467–471.

Li, S. and Woo, P.T.K. (1995) Efficacy of a live *Cryptobia salmositica* vaccine, and the mechanism of protection in vaccinated *Oncorhynchus mykiss* (Walbaum) against cryptobiosis. *Veterinary Immunology and Immunopathology* 48, 343–353.

Li, S. and Woo, P.T.K. (1996) A species specific *Cryptobia salmositica* (Kinetoplastida) DNA probe and its uses in salmonid cryptobiosis. *Diseases of Aquatic Organisms* 25, 11–16.

Li, S. and Woo, P.T.K. (1997) Vaccination of rainbow trout, *Oncorhynchus mykiss* (Walbaum) against cryptobiosis: efficacy of the vaccine in fresh and sea water. *Journal of Fish Diseases* 20, 369–374.

Li, M. and Woo, P.T.K. (2014) Glucocorticoid receptors on and in a unicellular organism, *Cryptobia salmositica*. *International Journal for Parasitology* 44, 205–210.

Li, S., Cowey, C.B. and Woo, P.T.K. (1996) The effects of dietary ascorbic acid on *Cryptobia salmositica* infection and on vaccination against cryptobiosis in *Oncorhynchus mykiss*. *Diseases of Aquatic Organisms* 24, 11–16.

Li, M., Leatherland, J.F. and Woo, P.T.K. (2013) Cortisol and dexamethasone increase the *in vitro* multiplication of the haemoflagellate, *Cryptobia salmositica*, possibly by interaction with a glucocorticoid receptor-like protein. *International Journal for Parasitology* 43, 353–360.

MacDonald, L.E. Alderman, S.L., Kramer, S., Woo, P.T.K and Bernier, N.J. (2014) Hypoxemia induced leptin secretion: a mechanism for the control of food intake in diseased fish. *Journal of Endocrinology* 221, 441–455.

Madison, B.N., Woo, P.T.K. and Bernier, N.J. (2013) Duress without stress: *Cryptobia* infection on HPI axis dysfunction in rainbow trout. *Journal of Endocrinology* 218, 289–297.

Mayer, N.B., Hinch, S.G. and Eliason, E.J. (2023) Thermal tolerance in Pacific salmon; a systematic review of species populations, life stages and methodologies. *Fish and Fisheries* 25, 283–302. DOI: 10.1111/faf.12808.

McConnachie, S.H., Cook, K.V., Patterson, D.A., Gilmour, K.M., Hinch, S.G. *et al.* (2012) Consequences of acute stress and cortisol manipulation on the physiology, behavior, and reproductive outcomes of female Pacific salmon on spawning grounds. *Hormones and Behavior* 62, 67–76.

Mehta, M. and Woo, P.T.K. (2002) Acquired cell-mediated protection in rainbow trout, *Oncorhynchus mykiss* against the haemoflagellate, *Cryptobia salmositica*. *Parasitology Research* 88, 956–962.

Norris, D.O. and Hobbs, S.L. (2006) The HPA axis and functions of corticosteroids in fishes. In: Reinecke, M., Zaccone, G. and Kapoor, B.G. (eds) *Fish Endocrinology*, Vol. 2. Science Publishers, Enfield, New Hampshire, pp. 721–765.

Paterson, W.B. and Woo, P.T.K. (1983) Electron microscopic observations of the bloodstream form of *Cryptobia salmositica* Katz, 1951 (Kinetoplastida, Bodonina). *Journal of Protozoology* 39, 431–437.

Putz, R.E. (1972) Biological studies on the hemoflagellates *Cryptobia cataractae* and *Cryptobia salmositica*. *Technical Paper Bureau of Sport Fisheries and Wildlife* 63, 3–25.

Schreck, C.B., Contreras-Sanchez, W. and Fitzpatrick, M.S. (2001) Effects of stress on fish reproduction, gamete quality, and progeny. *Aquaculture* 197, 3–24.

Sitja-Bobadilla, A. and Woo, P.T.K. (1994) An enzyme-linked immunosorbent assay (ELISA) for the detection of antibodies against the pathogenic haemoflagellate, *Cryptobia salmositica* Katz, and protection against cryptobiosis in juvenile rainbow trout, *Oncorhynchus mykiss* (Walbaum) inoculated with a live vaccine. *Journal of Fish Diseases* 17, 399–408.

Tan, C.W., Jesudhasan, R.R.R. and Woo, P.T.K. (2008) Towards a metalloprotease-DNA vaccine against piscine cryptobiosis caused by *Cryptobia salmositica*. *Parasitology Research* 102, 265–275.

Tavakoli, K., Pour-Aboughadareh, A., Kianersi, F., Poczai, P., Etminan, A. *et al.* (2021) Applications of CRISPR-Cas9 as an advanced genome editing system in life sciences. *BioTech* 10(3), 14. DOI: 10.3390/biotech10030014.

Thomas, P.T. and Woo, P.T.K. (1988) *Cryptobia salmositica*: *in vitro* and *in vivo* study on the mechanism of anaemia in infected rainbow trout, *Salmo gairdneri* Richardson. *Journal of Fish Diseases* 11, 425–431.

Thomas, P.T. and Woo, P.T.K. (1989a) An *in vitro* study on the haemolytic components of *Cryptobia salmositica*. *Journal of Fish Diseases* 12, 89–393.

Thomas, P.T. and Woo, P.T.K. (1989b) Complement activity in *Salmo gairdneri* Richardson infected with *Cryptobia salmositica* and its relationship to the anaemia in cryptobiosis. *Journal of Fish Diseases* 12, 395–397.

Thomas, P.T. and Woo, P.T.K. (1990a) *In vivo* and *in vitro* cell-mediated immune responses of *Oncorhynchus mykiss* (Walbaum) against *Cryptobia salmositica* Katz, 1951 (Sarcomastigophora, Kinetoplastida). *Journal of Fish Diseases* 13, 423–433.

Thomas, P.T. and Woo, P.T.K. (1990b) Dietary modulation of humoral immune response and anaemia in *Oncorhynchus mykiss* (Walbaum) infected with *Cryptobia salmositica* Katz, 1951. *Journal of Fish Diseases* 13, 435–446.

Thomas, P.T. and Woo, P.T.K. (1991) *In vitro* and *in vivo* effects of antimicrobial agents on viability of *Cryptobia salmositica* (Sarcomastigophora: Kinetoplastida). *Diseases of Aquatic Organisms* 10, 7–11.

Thomas, P.T. and Woo, P.T.K. (1992) Anorexia in *Oncorhynchus mykiss* (Walbaum) infected with *Cryptobia salmositica* (Sarcomastigophora, Kinetoplastida), its onset and contribution to the immunodepression. *Journal of Fish Diseases* 15, 443–447.

Thomas, P.T., Ballantyne, J.S. and Woo, P.T.K. (1992) *In vitro* oxygen consumption and motility of *Cryptobia salmositica*, *Cryptobia bullocki* and *Cryptobia catostomi*. *Journal of Parasitology* 78, 747–749.

Verity, C.K. and Woo, P.T.K. (1996) Characterization of a monoclonal antibody against the 47 kDa antigen of *Cryptobia salmositica* Katz and its use in an antigen-capture enzyme-linked immunosorbent assay for detection of parasite antigen in infected rainbow trout, *Oncorhynchus mykiss* (Walbaum). *Journal of Fish Diseases* 19, 91–109.

Vickerman, K. (1971) Morphological and physiological considerations of extracellular blood protozoa. In: Fallis, A.M. (ed.) *Physiology and Ecology of Parasites*. Toronto University Press, Toronto, Ontario, Canada, pp. 59–91.

Wales, J.H. and Wolf, H. (1955) Three protozoan diseases of trout in California. *California Fish and Game* 41, 183–187.

Woo, P.T.K. (1969) The haematocrit centrifuge for the detection of trypanosomes in blood. *Canadian Journal of Zoology* 47, 921–923.

Woo, P.T.K. (1970) The haematocrit centrifuge technique for the diagnosis of African trypanosomiasis. *Acta Tropica* 27, 384–386.

Woo, P.T.K. (1978) The division process of *Cryptobia salmositica* in experimentally infected rainbow trout (*Salmo gairdneri*). *Canadian Journal of Zoology* 56, 1514–1518.

Woo, P.T.K. (1979) *Trypanoplasma salmositica*: experimental infections in rainbow trout, *Salmo gairdneri*. *Experimental Parasitology* 47, 36–48.

Woo, P.T.K. (1987a) *Cryptobia* and cryptobiosis in fishes. *Advances in Parasitology* 26, 199–237.

Woo, P.T.K. (1987b) Immune response of fish to protozoan infections. *Parasitology Today* 3, 186–188.

Woo, P.T.K. (1990) MISET: an immunological technique for the serodiagnosis of *Cryptobia salmositica* (Sarcomastigophora, Kinetoplastida) infection in *Oncorhynchus mykiss*. *Journal of Parasitology* 76, 389–393.

Woo, P.T.K. (1992) Immunological responses of fish to parasitic organisms. *Annual Review of Fish Diseases* 2, 339–366.

Woo, P.T.K. (1994) Flagellate parasites of fishes. In: Kreier, J.P. (ed.) *Parasitic Protozoa*, 2nd edn, Vol. VIII. Academic Press, London, pp. 1–80.

Woo, P.T.K. (2001) Cryptobiosis and its control in North American fishes. *International Journal for Parasitology* 31, 566–574.

Woo, P.T.K. (2003) *Cryptobia* (*Trypanoplasma*) *salmositica* and salmonid cryptobiosis. *Journal of Fish Diseases* 26, 627–646.

Woo, P.T.K. (2006) Diplomonadida (Phylum Parabasalia) and Kinetoplastea (Phylum Euglenozoa). In: Woo, P.T.K. (ed.) *Fish Diseases and Disorders, Volume 1: Protozoan and Metazoan Infections*, 2nd edn. CAB International, Wallingford, UK, pp. 116–153.

Woo, P.T.K. (2007) Protective immunity in fish against protozoan diseases. *Parassitologia* 49, 185–191.

Woo, P.T.K. and Li, S. (1990) *In vitro* attenuation of *Cryptobia salmositica* and its use as a live vaccine against cryptobiosis in *Oncorhynchus mykiss*. *Journal of Parasitology* 76, 752–755.

Woo, P.T.K. and Poynton, S.L. (1995) Diplomonadida, Kinetoplastida and Amoebida (Phylum Sarcomastigophora). In: Woo, P.T.K. (ed.) *Fish Diseases and Disorders, Volume 1: Protozoan and Metazoan Infections*. CAB International, Wallingford, UK, pp. 27–96.

Woo, P.T.K. and Rogers, D.J. (1974) A statistical study of the sensitivity of the haematocrit centrifuge technique in the detection of trypanosomes in blood. *Transactions of the Royal Society of Tropical Medicine and Hygiene* 68, 319–326.

Woo, P.T.K. and Thomas, P.T. (1992) Comparative *in vitro* studies on virulent and avirulent strains of *Cryptobia salmositica* Katz, 1951 (Sarcomastigophora, Kinetoplastida). *Journal of Fish Diseases* 15, 261–266.

Woo, P.T.K. and Wehnert, S.D. (1983) Direct transmission of a haemoflagellate, *Cryptobia salmositica* Katz, 1951 (Kinetoplastida, Bodonina) between rainbow trout under laboratory conditions. *Journal of Protozoology* 39, 334–337.

Woo, P.T.K. and Wehnert, S.D. (1986) *Cryptobia salmositica*, susceptibility of infected trout, *Salmo gairdneri*, to environmental hypoxia. *Journal of Parasitology* 72, 392–396.

Woo, P.T.K., Wehnert, S.D. and Rodgers, D. (1983) The susceptibility of fishes to haemoflagellates at different ambient temperatures. *Parasitology* 87, 385–392.

Woo, P.T.K., Leatherland, J.F. and Lee, M.S. (1987) *Cryptobia salmositica*: cortisol increases the susceptibility of *Salmo gairdneri* Richardson to experimental cryptobiosis. *Journal of Fish Diseases* 10, 75–83.

Wood, J.W. (1979) *Diseases of Pacific Salmon: Their Prevention and Treatment*, 3rd edn. State of Washington, Department of Fisheries, Hatchery Division, Olympia, Washington.

Zuo, X. and Woo, P.T.K. (1997a) Proteases in pathogenic and nonpathogenic hemoflagellates, *Cryptobia* spp. (Sarcomastigophora: Kinetoplastida) of fishes. *Diseases of Aquatic Organisms* 29, 57–65.

Zuo, X. and Woo, P.T.K. (1997b) Natural antiproteases in rainbow trout, *Oncorhynchus mykiss*, and brook charr, *Salvelinus fontinalis*, and the *in vitro* neutralization of fish alpha2-macroglobulin by the metallo-protease from the pathogenic haemoflagellate, *Cryptobia salmositica*. *Parasitology* 114, 375–382.

Zuo, X. and Woo, P.T.K. (1997c) The *in vivo* neutralization of proteases from *Cryptobia salmositica* by α2-macroglobulin in the blood of rainbow trout, *Oncorhynchus mykiss* and brook charr, *Salvelinus fontinalis*. *Diseases of Aquatic Organisms* 29, 67–72.

Zuo, X. and Woo, P.T.K. (1997d) Purified metalloprotease from the pathogenic haemoflagellate, *Cryptobia salmositica*, and its *in vitro* proteolytic activities. *Diseases of Aquatic Organisms* 30, 177–185.

Zuo, X. and Woo, P.T.K. (1998a) Characterization of purified metallo- and cysteine proteases from the pathogenic haemoflagellate, *Cryptobia salmositica* Katz 1951. *Parasitology Research* 84, 492–498.

Zuo, X. and Woo, P.T.K. (1998b) *In vitro* secretion of metalloprotease (200 kDa) by the pathogenic piscine haemoflagellate, *Cryptobia salmositica* Katz, and stimulation of protease production by collagen. *Journal of Fish Diseases* 21, 249–255.

Zuo, X. and Woo, P.T.K. (2000) *In vitro* haemolysis of piscine erythrocytes by purified metalloprotease from the pathogenic haemoflagellate, *Cryptobia salmositica* Katz. *Journal of Fish Diseases* 23, 227–230.

Zuo, X., Feng, S. and Woo, P.T.K. (1997) The *in vitro* inhibition of proteases from *Cryptobia salmositica* Katz by a monoclonal antibody (MAb-001) against a glycoprotein on the pathogenic haemoflagellate. *Journal of Fish Diseases* 20, 419–426.

4 *Ichthyophthirius multifiliis*

Harry W. Dickerson*
College of Veterinary Medicine, University of Georgia, Athens, Georgia, USA

Abstract

The obligate parasitic ciliate *Ichthyophthirius multifiliis* has been the subject of applied and basic research for over 100 years because of its worldwide distribution, its ability to infect the skin and gills of a broad and diverse spectrum of freshwater fish species, and its economic importance to fish farmers and aquarists. Outbreaks of ichthyophthiriasis (commonly referred to as 'ich', or 'white spot disease') occur in feral and farm-raised fishes. Strategies to control *I. multifiliis* include water management as well as drug and chemical treatments. Fish surviving an infection develop immunity, and a significant amount of research on the mechanisms of immune protection has been carried out with the goal of developing vaccines. A commercial vaccine is not currently available. Acquired immunity to *I. multifiliis* has contributed to a basic understanding of mucosal immunity in teleost fishes.

4.1. Introduction

The ciliate, *Ichthyophthirius multifiliis* Fouquet, 1876, is an obligate parasite that infects the epithelia of skin and gills and is one of the most common protozoan pathogens of freshwater fishes. It has significant economic impact and infects a broad spectrum of wild and cultured fish species in most parts of the world. *I. multifiliis* also has been used as a model for elucidating the mechanisms of teleost cutaneous immunity (Dickerson and Clark, 1998; Gonzalez *et al.*, 2007b; von Gersdorff Jorgensen, 2016; Shiota *et al.*, 2021). This chapter provides an overview of the biology of the parasite, host pathophysiology and immunity, as well as treatment and prevention of infection.

I. multifiliis is a holotrichous ciliate, class Oligohymenophora, subclass Hymenostomata, order Hymenostomatida, suborder Ophryoglenina, family Ichthyophthiridae (Canella and Rocchi-Canella, 1976; Corliss, 1979; Wright and Lynn, 1995; Van Den Bussche *et al.*, 2000; Lynn, 2008); it and other species in the suborder Ophryoglenina are characterized by the presence of the organelle of Lieberkühn (Canella and Rocchi-Canella, 1976; Lynn *et al.*, 1991). The entire surface of the organism is covered by motile membrane-bound cilia which are responsible for its progressive motility in the water as well as its movement within the host's epithelium (Ewing and Kocan, 1992). Like most other ciliate genera in the order Hymenostomatida (e.g. the free-living ciliates *Tetrahymena* and *Paramecium*),

*Email: hwd@uga.edu

 Fish Parasites: Pathobiology and Protection, 2nd Edition (eds P.T.K. Woo and K. Buchmann)

DOI: 10.1079/9781800628748.0004

it has a somatic macronucleus and up to four germ-line micronuclei, which are transcriptionally inactive (Peshkov and Tikhomirova, 1968; Hauser, 1973; Nanney, 1980; Matthews, 1996). Although direct visual evidence of sexual conjugation, which occurs in free-living ciliates, has not been found, the macronuclear genome contains genes for conjugation (Chi *et al.*, 2013; MacColl *et al.*, 2015). Also, comparisons of single-nucleotide polymorphisms found in the genomes of field isolates suggest mating at some point in the life cycle (MacColl *et al.*, 2015). Additional evidence for the existence of sex in *I. multifiliis* includes the identification of a gene for an ancestral gamete fusion protein, HAP2/GCS1 (Pinello *et al.*, 2017; Pinello and Clark, 2022), and its expression during the free-swimming theront stage.

4.2. Life Cycle and Parasite Stages

The direct life cycle of the parasite is comprised of three stages: (i) infective theront; (ii) obligate, fish-associated trophont; and (iii) water-borne reproductive tomont (Fig. 4.1). Some authors add a fourth stage: the protomont, which refers to the parasite after it leaves the fish and before it secretes the gelatinous cyst (Li *et al.*, 2023). All stages are ciliated and motile. The theront is oblong (pyriform) in shape, approximately 40 μm in length (Fig 4.2), with a distinctive caudal cilium (see Fig. 4.6 below) (Maclennon, 1942; Kheisin and Mosevich, 1969; Canella and Rocchi-Canella, 1976; Kozel, 1986; Geisslinger, 1987). When the pelagic theront encounters a susceptible host, it rapidly penetrates the surface epithelia of the skin, gill and other surface mucosa (Kong *et al.*, 2024) through ciliary action and the use of the perforatorium, a specialized membrane-cortical structure on the anterior of the cell (Maclennon, 1935; Ewing and Kocan, 1992; Buchmann and Nielsen, 1999). The theront is positively phototactic, a function postulated to be attributed to the organelle of Lieberkühn (Wahli and Meier, 1991; Matthews, 2005). Also, the theront is positively chemotactic to components of fish tissue, including immunoglobulin and mucus (Lom and Cerkasova, 1974; Buchmann and Nielsen, 1999). It has been proposed that the parasite approaches and enters the epithelium of the skin through the goblet cells (Buchmann and Nielsen, 1999). After entry into the host the theront rapidly

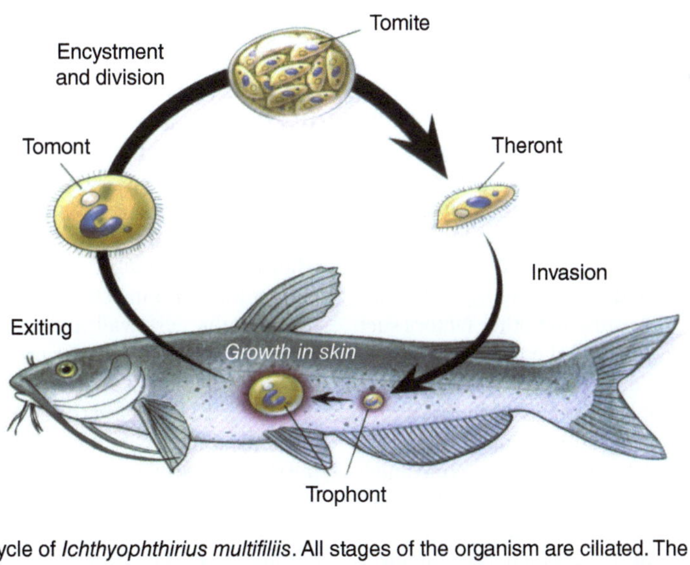

Fig. 4.1. Life cycle of *Ichthyophthirius multifiliis*. All stages of the organism are ciliated. The free-swimming theront penetrates through the mucus and invades the epithelia of the skin, gill and other surface mucosa. Upon entering the host it transforms into the trophont, which feeds and grows up to 800–1000 μm in size. The trophont actively moves within the epithelium. The parasite exits the fish as the mature tomont (some authors refer to the exiting tomont as a protomont), which secretes a protective cyst and divides within it to form 500–1000 daughter cells (tomites). Tomites differentiate into invasive theronts, which bore through the cyst wall and enter the water. (Figure used with permission from Dickerson and Clark, 1998.)

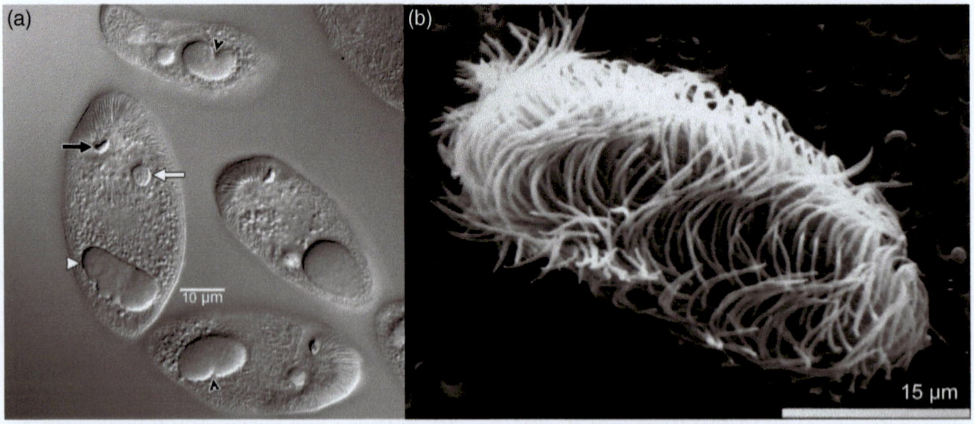

Fig. 4.2. *Ichthyophthirius multifiliis* theronts. (a) The large macronucleus (white arrowhead), smaller micronucleus (white arrow) and organelle of Lieberkühn (black arrow) are visible. The typical indented shape of the macronucleus is indicated in several theronts (black arrow heads). Note that surface cilia are not evident in this micrograph. Differential interference contrast image. (b) The entire surface of the theront is covered with cilia as seen in this micrograph. The caudal cilium is not evident. Scanning electron microscope image. (Photograph and Art by Jane Noe. © 2010 University of Georgia Research Foundation, Inc.)

(within several minutes) differentiates into a feeding trophont, which involves the formation of a functional cytostome and vestibular apparatus (Maclennon, 1935; Canella and Rocchi-Canella, 1976). *I. multifiliis* is endoparasitic within the epithelium of the host (Matthews, 2005).

The trophont changes from the rigid theront (pyriform shape) to a polymorphic cellular form propelled by ciliary action between epithelial cells and within tissue spaces created as it feeds in epithelia (Fig. 4.3). The trophont grows rapidly, increasing in size to 200–800 μm, which relates to the duration of feeding (Maclennon, 1942). The parasite remains on the fish for a variable number of days, depending on the ambient water temperature and other factors such as the immune status of the fish. Typically, at a temperature of 25°C, it feeds for a period of 5–7 days. The trophont develops and grows within the epithelium, penetrating no deeper than the basal germinal cell layer, which lies immediately adjacent to the underlying dermis (Chapman, 1984; Dickerson, 2009). At maturity the parasite leaves the fish, which presumably is triggered by cell volume, size, development and other unknown factors (Maclennon, 1937, 1942; Ewing *et al.*, 1986; Ewing and Kocan, 1992; Aihua and Buchmann, 2001; Matthews, 2005).

Once it leaves the host and is back in the water the motile organism, now referred to as a tomont (or protomont), swims for approximately 1 h after which it attaches to any available substrate (e.g. vegetation, inorganic material and other surfaces) by means of a translucent proteinaceous cyst produced by extrusion of the contents of its cortical mucocysts (Ewing *et al.*, 1983). The tomont remains ciliated and rotates within the cyst. It undergoes symmetrical cell divisions and amitotic nuclear divisions at approximately 1 h intervals doubling the number of daughter cells, which are called tomites (Hauser, 1973; Dickerson, 2006). These cells differentiate into infective theronts, which bore through the cyst wall and leave progressively through the perforation(s) created by the first theronts that exit. It takes several minutes for all of the theronts to leave the cyst. The number of theronts produced by each tomont depends on the size of the cell when it leaves the fish and the number of cell divisions within the cyst. Cell division in the tomont is referred to as palintomy because there is no growth between subsequent divisions (Lynn, 2008). Typically, 500–1000 parasites are produced following nine to ten divisions. It has been suggested that adhesion of tomonts to substrate in the immediate environment of a susceptible host population facilitates

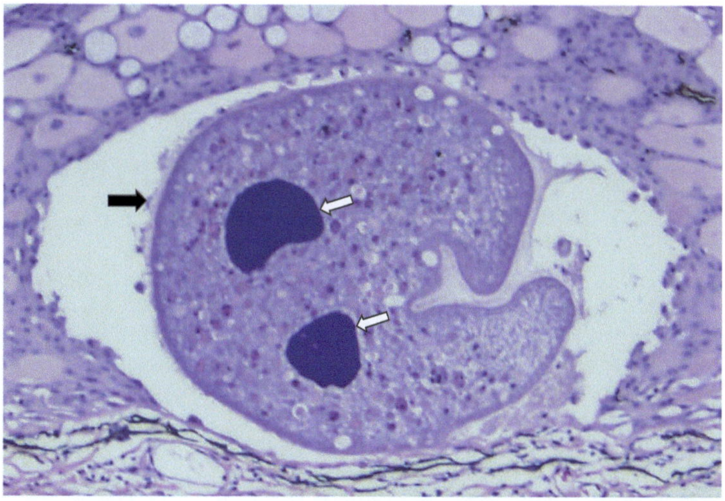

Fig. 4.3. *Ichthyophthirius multifiliis* trophont within the epidermis of a channel catfish. The parasite is motile due to action of surface cilia (black arrow) and creates a tissue space within which it feeds on cells and cellular debris that are processed in food vacuoles in the cytoplasm. The polymorphic shape of the trophont with its folded cell membrane is evident, and in this image the single, large 'horseshoe'-shaped nucleus appears as two parts (white arrows) due to the angle of the section. Numerous alarm cells (larger cells, many have visible nuclei) and goblet cells (smaller cells without visible nuclei and lighter cytoplasm) are visible in the surrounding epithelium that covers the trophont. Inflammatory cells (neutrophils, macrophages and lymphocytes) are present immediately below the parasite in the dermis. Haemotoxylin and eosin-stained paraffin thin section, light microscope image, 100× magnification. (Photograph and Art by Alvin Camus. © 2010 University of Georgia Research Foundation, Inc.)

subsequent infection of the same population, particularly in riparian systems with rapidly flowing water (Matthews, 2005). The life cycle is completed in approximately 16–18 h at 22–25°C. Development of the different stages is temperature dependent, which makes the total length of the life cycle inversely related to temperature. A detailed description of the life cycle and the individual stages with extensive reference to the literature is available (Matthews, 2005; Dickerson, 2006).

Endosymbiotic bacteria are present in the cytoplasm of *I. multifiliis* theronts and trophonts (Sun *et al.*, 2009) (Fig. 4.4). Two classes of bacteria have been identified, Sphingobacteriales and rickettsial alphaproteobacteria, which are found in laboratory isolates as well as parasites collected from fish naturally infected in the wild. The rickettsial alphaproteobacteria in *I. multifiis* consist of three subclades of *Candidatus* Megaira: namely, C, D and polyxenophilia (Zaila *et al.*, 2017). The mechanisms by which *Ca.* Megaira enters *I. multifiliis* are unknown, as are the means of its transmission in the host. The role that *Ca.* Megaira plays in *I. multifiliis* biology and virulence is also unknown. Endosymbiotic bacteria are relatively common in free-living ciliates (Fokin, 2004) and have been previously described at the structural level in *I. multifiliis* as well (Roque *et al.*, 1967; Lobo-da-Cunha and Azevedo, 1988; Matthews, 2005).

4.3. Transmission and Geographical Distribution

Naturally occurring epizootic outbreaks of ichthyophthiriasis (commonly referred to as 'ich', or 'white spot disease') have occurred on most continents in populations of feral and farm-raised fishes (Paperna, 1972; Nigrelli *et al.*, 1976; Valtonen and Keränen, 1981; Wahli and Meier, 1987; Wurtsbaugh and Tapia, 1988; Bragg, 1991; Buchmann *et al.*, 1995; Rintamaki-Kinnunen and Valtonen, 1997; Traxler *et al.*, 1998; Scholz, 1999; Kim *et al.*, 2002; Thila-

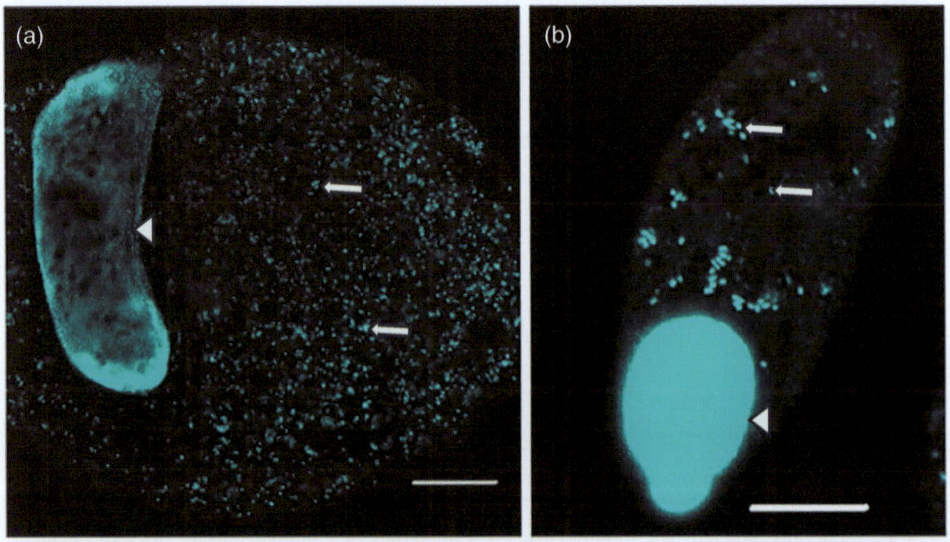

Fig. 4.4. Endosymbiotic bacteria in *Ichthyophthirius multifiliis*. Confocal images of an *I. multifiliis* G13 tomont and theront stained with DAPI (4′,6-diamidino-2-phenylindole; blue). (a) DAPI-stained tomont showing the macronucleus (white arrowhead) and endosymbionts (white arrows). Bar = 100 µm. (b) DAPI-stained theront showing the macronucleus (white arrowhead), micronucleus (which appears merged with macronucleus in micrograph) and endosymbionts (white arrows). Bar = 10 µm. (Figure used with permission from Sun *et al*., 2009.)

karatne *et al.*, 2003; Molnar, 2006; Piazza *et al.*, 2006; Lemos *et al.*, 2007; Jalali *et al.*, 2008; Maceda-Veiga *et al.*, 2009; Qin *et al.*, 2024). Low-level infections can occur in natural habitats. The direct life cycle of *I. multifiliis* is conducive to producing explosive outbreaks in dense fish populations, which is often when fish are raised under intense aquaculture. In a 12-month study of pond-reared rainbow trout (*Oncorhynchus mykiss*) in an *I. multifiliis*-endemic region of Turkey, a positive correlation of ambient water temperature and mean intensity of parasite load was clearly demonstrated (Ogut *et al.*, 2005). Outbreaks have been reported to occur in channel catfish (*Ictalurus punctatus*) at ambient temperatures as low as 6–12°C (Bodensteiner *et al.*, 2000) and in rainbow trout at 14–18°C (Ogut *et al.*, 2005), although epizootics are more prevalent at higher temperatures; i.e. 24–28°C. *I. multifiliis* does not usually survive temperatures above 30°C (Dickerson, 2006); however, a South-East Asian isolate apparently can live at 34°C (Bauer and Iunchis, 2001). How the parasite overwinters is not known, but it has been postulated that low numbers of trophonts survive on fish for months in a near-dormant state at low temperatures (Noe and Dickerson, 1995). The parasite is transmitted from fish to fish by infective theronts in the water.

4.4. Diagnosis of Infection and Appearance of Lesions

When exposed to theronts, fish become agitated, hyperactive, and rub their gill opercula and flanks against available surfaces. This behaviour is referred to as 'flashing' and is presumably in response to the intense irritation elicited as the parasite bores into the skin and gills and feeds in the tissues. It is a common clinical sign of *I. multifiliis* infection, but it should be noted that any irritant in the water can cause a similar behavioural response.

As the parasite feeds and grows within the skin and gills damage to the epithelia interferes with normal gaseous exchange, and infected individuals become starved of oxygen and acidotic. As a behavioural response, fish in ponds swim to the surface and rest at the edges in shallow water to gain access to dissolved oxygen and minimize expended energy. Fish in aquaria initially swim near the surface but eventually sink to the bottom as they weaken due to oxygen depletion in their tissues. Within 3–4 days (at 22–25°C) numerous trophonts appear as vesicular lesions (approximately 0.5–1.0 mm in diameter) disseminated in the skin over the entire surface of the fish (Fig. 4.5). Heavy infections in the gill cause extensive disruption of epithelia and capillary haemorrhage with subsequent loss of physiological function. Severely infected fish die within 5–7 days, which is during the first period of the initial parasite exposure and growth of trophonts. Less severe infections (i.e. those that do not kill fish in the first period of growth) are usually diagnosed by 'flashing' behaviour and the presence of white spots in the skin, each of which contains one to four parasites surrounded by hyperplastic epithelial cells (Chapman, 1984; Dickerson, 2006).

Definitive diagnosis of an *I. multifiliis* infection is made by microscopic detection of the parasite in biopsies or tissues taken at necropsy. To prepare specimens for microscopic examination in the field, place skin and mucus scrapings, small pieces of gill lamellae and/or small tail clippings on a glass slide, add several drops of water and place a coverslip over the specimen. Tissues should be taken from either live fish as a biopsy or as soon as possible following the death of the fish. It is not necessary to fix or stain the tissue. In unstained preparations the large trophont in skin and gill tissues is easily detected with a low-power objective lens (4×–10× magnification). The large 'horseshoe'-shaped nucleus is a pathognomonic diagnostic indicator for *I. multifiliis*. It is usually fairly easy to find the parasite due to its ciliary activity and movement in the tissue. In heavily infected fish the parasite moves freely within the damaged epithelium, presumably due to the naturally loose structure of fish epithelium, which is loosened further by physical and/or enzymatic activity of the feeding parasite.

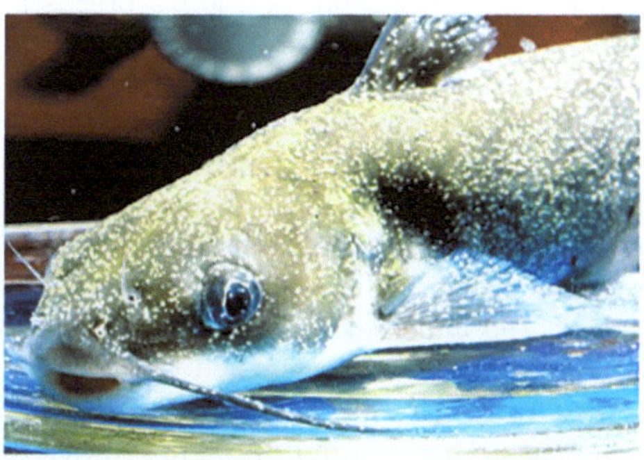

Fig. 4.5. Channel catfish infected with *Ichthyophthirius multifiliis*. Trophonts are within vesicular lesions that appear as 'white spots' in the skin. Most vesicles contain a single organism, but in heavy infections multiple parasites can occur within the same vesicles due to coalescence of the lesions. (Figure used with permission from Clark and Dickerson, 1997.)

In haematoxylin and eosin-stained histological thin sections of formalin-fixed skin and gills, large parasites are visible within the epithelia under a compound microscope with 50×–100× objective lenses (see Figs 4.3 and 4.7b below). The macronucleus, cytoplasmic food vacuoles and surface cilia are usually visible. The parasite lies within an interstitial tissue space, which contains cellular debris and proteinaceous tissue fluid. The epithelium immediately surrounding the parasite is hyperplastic; the epithelial cells are degenerating, appear hydropic and necrotic with pyknotic nuclei. The epithelium contains an infiltration of lymphocytes and other inflammatory cells including macrophages and neutrophils (see below). The degree of inflammatory response and tissue damage depends on the number of invading parasites and severity of infection; the response varying from mild to severe. The underlying stratum spongiosum and stratum compactum of the dermis appear oedematous and also contain inflammatory cells. The parasites invade the basal epithelium of the gill lamellae. Gill epithelial cells proliferate in the immediate vicinity of the parasite as well as over the entire gill lamellae (see Fig. 4.7b below). Large trophonts often reside within multiple adjacent lamellae. In severe infections, the entire interlamellar space becomes occluded with hyperplastic epithelium and the tissue takes on a 'clubbed appearance' (Hines and Spira, 1974c). Hyperplasia and excess mucus production in the gills interfere with gaseous exchange (Dickerson, 2006). The lesions in primary and secondary lamellae of the gills are comparable in all species of fish that have been studied (Bu *et al.*, 2025). The parasite also invades the surface epithelia of the ocular membrane, and studies in trout have shown an increase in mucus cell density and epithelial cell proliferation at this site (Kong *et al.*, 2024). Environmental DNA and RNA released into the water from the parasite and host could provide a non-invasive means to diagnose and evaluate early disease in infected fish (Duan *et al.*, 2025).

4.5. Local and Systemic Pathophysiology

4.5.1. Local response to *Ichthyophthirius multifiliis* infection

The pathophysiological effects of chronic and acute *I. multifiliis* infection (ichthyophthiriasis) are attributed to cellular damage and subsequent inflammatory responses in the skin and gills. Expression of the potent inflammatory mediator interleukin-1β (IL-1β) is upregulated in the skin of carp (*Cyprinus carpio*) within 36 h of parasite exposure (Gonzalez *et al.*, 2007a). In rainbow trout both IL-1β and tumour necrosis factor-α (TNF-α) are significantly increased at 4 days (Sigh *et al.*, 2004a). The cells in skin and gills responsible for production of IL-1β have not been identified, but macrophages, epithelial cells and fibroblasts have been suggested as sources (Sigh *et al.*, 2004a).

The physical integrity of the epithelia is compromised during invasion by theronts and growth of trophonts within the skin and gills, and massive infections with large numbers of parasites can kill the host within 12 h after infection (Ewing *et al.*, 1985; Ventura and Paperna, 1985; Matthews, 1994). Although challenge with fewer theronts (less than 15,000/15–40 g fish) does not usually overwhelm the host at initial infection, subsequent rounds of infection increase the numbers of parasites and susceptible fish are overcome by synchronized waves of theronts (Wang *et al.*, 2002; Swennes *et al.*, 2006; Gonzalez *et al.*, 2007a). Variations in virulence among *I. multifiliis* isolates are determined by differential growth rates on the fish that modulate subsequent infection and immunity (Swennes *et al.*, 2006). The macroscopic and microscopic lesions resulting from parasite invasion and feeding are described in Section 4.4.

4.5.2. Systemic response to *Ichthyophthirius multifiliis* infection

Severe ichthyophthiriasis leads to significant damage of the skin and gill epithelia, which impedes gaseous exchange resulting in acidosis, oxygen depletion and loss of energy reserves, indicating significant disruption of osmoregulatory mechanisms. In carp, a drop in the serum levels of Na^+, K^+ and Mg^{2+} ions, and a rise in blood urea nitrogen, occurs (Hines and Spira, 1973b, 1974a,c). A differential shift occurs in blood leucocytes, with infected fish developing a lymphocytopenia and neutrophilia (Hines and Spira, 1974a). *I. multifiliis* infection elicits changes in the natural microbiota of the gills and intestinal tract (Bu *et al.*, 2025).

4.6. Protective Control Strategies: Immune Response and Vaccine Strategies

Immunity to *I. multifiliis* was described as early as 1910 (Bushkiel, 1910), and a significant amount of increasing research on the phenomenology of the response and the mechanisms of immune protection has been conducted over the past 50 years. An overview of this appears in several comprehensive reviews (Buchmann *et al.*, 2001; Matthews, 2005; Dickerson, 2006; Dickerson and Findly, 2014; von Gersdorff Jorgensen, 2017; Wang *et al.*, 2019). Research has been driven by the need to develop a protective vaccine against this economically important parasite as well as the desire to understand the mechanisms of the long-lasting protection that is elicited following infection. Further, *I. multifiliis* provides an excellent system to study host–pathogen interactions and mucosal immunity in an early vertebrate model (Dickerson and Clark, 1998; Christoffersen *et al.*, 2017; Shiota *et al.*, 2021).

A basic understanding of immunity to *I. multifiliis* infection has emerged that includes both innate and adaptive immune mechanisms. For more detailed information on innate and systemic immunity against *I. multifiliis*, the reader is referred to the following comprehensive reviews on the subject: Dickerson and Findly (2014); von Gersdorff Jorgensen (2017); Wang *et al.* (2019).

4.6.1. Local innate immunity

The mucosal surfaces of the skin and gills serve as a natural barrier to *I. multifiliis* infection. This protection is mediated by physical factors that include the surface mucus barrier, the glycocalyx and the underlying epithelial cells, as well as constitutively expressed proteins and induced cellular and humoral elements of the inflammatory response (Dickerson, 2009).

In carp the leucocyte response to *I. multifiliis* infection in the skin and gills has been described in detail (Hines and Spira, 1973a; Cross and Matthews, 1993b). The study of Cross and Matthews complements the early classic research of Hines and Spira, providing a comprehensive description of the cellular changes in the skin epithelium at both the microscopic and the ultrastructural levels. Tissue lesions and cellular responses in the caudal tail fin were described at sequential time points following challenge in both naïve and immunized fish (Cross and Matthews, 1993b). Within 1 day of exposure of naïve fish to theronts, neutrophils infiltrate the skin and appear within non-vascularized areas of the dermis near the parasite. Increased expression of the chemokines CXCa, CXCR1 and CXCR2 in the skin also occurs at this time and is probably responsible for the early influx of neutrophils (Gonzalez *et al.*, 2007a). Studies in zebrafish (*Danio rerio*) showed that neutrophils increase by over threefold at 24 h after infection with *I. multifiliis* (von Gersdorff Jorgenen, 2016). By 2–3 days, these inflammatory cells reach and surround the trophont in the epidermis. At 5–6 days, many leucocytes (eosinophils, neutrophils and basophils) are associated with the parasite in the epidermis and in the dermis directly below it. At this point, the cellular response is predominated by eosinophils, but lymphocytes are also present, primarily in the dermis.

In immune fish, eosinophilic granular cells (EGCs) and macrophages are the predominant leucocytes at days 5–7 following challenge, and they surround the parasite and are in tissue sites from which the parasite has exited (Cross and Matthews, 1993b; Cross, 1994).

The increased expression of CXCa, CXCR1, CXCR2, IL-1β and TNF-α over the course of *I. multifiliis* infection suggests that these molecules play a role in the recruitment of leucocytes to the skin (Sigh *et al.*, 2004a; Gonzalez *et al.*, 2007a). Necrotic granulocytic cells, cellular membranes and released granules surround the ciliated parasites, which remain motile and show no visible signs of damage (Cross and Matthews, 1993b). The necrotic remains of leucocytes are visible in cytoplasmic food vacuoles of the feeding trophonts (Matthews, 2005), suggesting that inflammatory cells serve as a nutrient source for the feeding organisms. In fact, it has been suggested that their continual ingestion might explain the relatively low inflammatory cell response associated with larger trophonts (Ventura and Paperna, 1985). Enzymes released from degranulated inflammatory cells probably play a role in the inflammatory response (Matthews, 1994). Tissue breakdown and cellular damage also could be caused by enzymes such as phosphatases and non-specific esterases secreted by the parasite itself (Kozel, 1986; Lobo-da-Cunha and Azevedo, 1990). In grass carp (*Ctenopharyngodon idella*), mRNA expression studies in the skin and gills have shown upregulation of genes encoding tumour necrosis factor 6 (TNF-6) and transforming growth factor-β (TGF-β)-activated kinase, molecules which are involved in Toll-like receptor (TLR) transduction (Zhao *et al.*, 2013). Direct comparisons of local innate immune responses between the skin and gills have not been done, but the cellular response in gills appears similar to that seen in skin.

4.6.2. Systemic innate immunity

In carp, a differential shift in circulating leucocytes occurs during parasite infection with fish developing an initial lymphopenia and neutrophilia (Hines and Spira, 1973a). Circulating neutrophils increase in number (up to fivefold) during the acute phase of the infection (Hines and Spira, 1973a). Natural cytotoxic cells (NCCs), first described in channel catfish, have been postulated to play a role in non-specific protection against *I. multifiliis* (Graves *et al.*, 1984, 1985). Following *I. multifiliis* infection in channel catfish, NCCs from the head kidney move into circulation (Graves *et al.*, 1985).

In rainbow trout, *I. multifiliis* infection elicits a decrease in gene expression of complement factor C3 in the head kidney at 24 h (Sigh *et al.*, 2004b). In the spleen, gene expression of complement factor C3 is significantly raised at day 26. In trout injected with live theronts, C3 gene expression in the spleen was upregulated at day 28 (von Gersdorff Jorgensen *et al.*, 2008). In infected trout major histocompatibility complex class II (MHC-II) gene expression is depressed at 48 h in the spleen. Extra-hepatic expression of C3 is postulated to be the result of circulating macrophages (Sigh *et al.*, 2004b). The early gene expression (48 h) of immunoglobulin M (IgM), MHC-II and complement factor C3 in skin, followed by later systemic expression (4 days) of these genes in the head kidney and spleen, suggests that a local immune response to *I. multifiliis* is initiated first, followed later by a systemic response (Sigh *et al.*, 2004b). In rainbow trout, the expression of cytokines IL-1β and TNF-α in the head kidney and spleen remains elevated at 26 days (Sigh *et al.*, 2004a).

Plasma lysozyme activity increased following the injection of live theronts into the peritoneal (coelomic) cavity of rainbow trout suggesting that systemic expression of non-specific components of innate immunity may be elicited following exposure to the parasite (Alishahi and Buchmann, 2006). The injection of live theronts also elicited upregulation of genes encoding acute-phase proteins in the liver (Alishahi and Buchmann, 2006).

4.6.3. Local adaptive immunity

It is well established that naïve fish surviving infection become resistant to a subsequent challenge and that antibodies are important effectors of immune protection (Hines and Spira, 1974b; Wahli and Meier, 1985; Houghton and Matthews, 1986; Clark *et al.*, 1987; Dickerson and Clark, 1996; Lin *et al.*, 1996). Although both serum and mucus antibodies are elicited against the parasite, specific antibodies in the mucus and epithelia of the skin and gills are most likely responsible for protection (Lin *et al.*, 1996; Xu *et al.*, 2002; Maki and Dickerson, 2003; Sigh *et al.*, 2004b; Zhao *et al.*, 2008; Findly *et al.*, 2013).

For many years it was unclear if teleosts had a mucosal immune system analogous to that in mammals. It is now well established that a mucosal immune system exists in fish, but fundamental gaps in knowledge remain regarding the sites of induction and differentiation of B and T cells involved in the mucosal antibody response (Zhao *et al.*, 2008; Dickerson, 2009; Dickerson and Findly, 2014). *I. multifiliis* serves as a useful model to explore the mechanisms of local adaptive immunity because it naturally infects only surface epithelia and elicits the production of specific antibodies at these sites (Dickerson and Clark, 1998; Xu *et al.*, 2002; Maki and Dickerson, 2003; Zhao *et al.*, 2008). Acquired protective immunity against *I. multifiliis* is present for at least 2 years in channel catfish held under laboratory conditions, and research indicates that memory B cells are present in the skin of immune fish (Zhao *et al.*, 2008; Findly *et al.*, 2013). Studies in a fish fin model in ginbuna crucian carp (*Carassius auratus langsdorfii*) have shown that T cells ($CD4^+$ and $CD8\alpha^+$) are the first to populate fin sites in response to theront and trophont antigens, suggesting that T cells migrate to local sites of infection before B cells (Shiota *et al.*, 2021).

I. multifiliis infection elicits the expression in skin of several genes relevant to adaptive immunity, including those encoding IgM and MHC-II (Sigh *et al.*, 2004b). IgM is the primary functional antibody found in fish and is found in mucus, although at a much lower concentration than in sera (Bradshaw *et al.*, 1971; Zilberg and Klesius, 1997; Maki and Dickerson, 2003). In trout and other species (e.g. zebrafish), immunoglobulin T (IgT) isotype antibody in skin appears to function similarly to immunoglobulin A (IgA) in mammals (Zhang *et al.*, 2010; Buchmann, 2020). In channel catfish in which IgT has not been shown to occur, however, mucosal antibody appears to be structurally and functionally similar to serum antibody.

4.6.4. Systemic adaptive immunity

Serum antibodies are produced in response to infection, but their role as effectors of immunity is questionable because they do not appear to reach surface epithelia under normal physiological conditions (Lobb and Clem, 1981; Lin *et al.*, 1996). For example, although acquired protection is abrogated following treatment of *I. multifiliis*-immune fish with corticosteroids, serum antibody concentrations remain unchanged (Houghton and Matthews, 1986). In passive immunity experiments carried out in channel catfish using protective immobilizing mouse monoclonal antibodies, it was shown that protection was conferred only by immunoglobulin G (IgG) antibodies, which can reach parasites located in the skin. In contrast, immobilizing mouse IgM antibodies and *I. multifiliis*-immune catfish serum antibodies, which are much larger molecules, do not reach surface tissues or confer protection following adaptive transfer (Lobb and Clem, 1981; Lin *et al.*, 1996; Clark and Dickerson, 1997). These findings suggest that serum antibodies are minimally involved (if at all) in protection due to their physiological confinement to the blood. It is possible, however, that serum antibodies reach parasites embedded in the skin and gills when blood enters tissues following inflammation and physical disruption of the epithelia. Inflammatory responses elicited by parasites result in the influx of phagocytes into mucosal tissues, and antigens released from the parasite are probably taken up, processed and presented by these cells to B and T cells in the skin and/or lymphoid tissues in the spleen and head kidney. Plasma cells producing *I. multifiliis*-specific antibodies are found in the skin as well as the head kidney (Zhao *et al.*, 2008; Findly *et al.*, 2013).

Regardless of whether antibodies in the blood play a role in protection, their presence is diagnostic of *I. multifiliis* infection, and they can be used to monitor previous exposure to the parasite. One of the earliest *in vitro* assays used to measure the immune response to the parasite was immobilization, which detects serum antibodies that bind surface antigens on ciliary membranes causing the cilia to adhere together with resultant loss of synchronous beating and cessation of swimming, i.e. immobilization (Fig. 4.6) (Hines and Spira, 1974b; Clark *et al.*, 1987, 1988; Cross, 1993; Cross and Matthews, 1993a). Immobilization is serotype specific depending on the immobilization antigen (i-antigen) displayed on the parasite's surface (Dickerson *et al.*, 1993). To date five serotypes exist (designated A–E), but 17 i-antigen genes have been identified in the *I. multifiliis* genome (Coyne *et al.*, 2011). Thus, it is likely that more serotypes will be characterized as additional isolates are studied (Dickerson and Findly, 2014). Several reviews and publications are available on i-antigens of *I. multifiliis* (Figs 4.6 and 4.7) (Clark and Forney, 2003; Matthews, 2005; Dickerson, 2006; Xu *et al.*, 2009b). I-antigens play a role in eliciting protective immunity and have been targeted for vaccine production (see below).

4.6.5. Vaccine development

The elicitation of acquired protective immunity following natural infection by *I. multifiliis* suggests that the creation of a vaccine is feasible. Attempts to develop vaccines against the parasite were initiated almost as soon as it was discovered that fish surviving an infection become immune to subsequent challenge (Bushkiel, 1910; Butcher, 1941; Bauer, 1953; Beckert and Allison, 1964; Hines and Spira, 1974b). The use of vaccines is considered an economical and environmentally effective means to protect fish and would be of great benefit for the prevention of *I. multifiliis* infections in farm-raised and aquarium fish.

(a)

(b)

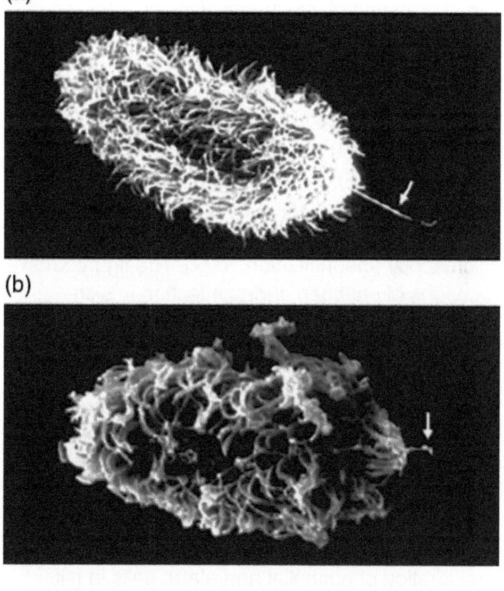

Fig. 4.6. Antibody immobilization. (a) Normal theront. (b) Theront immobilized by mouse monoclonal antibody (IgG). The cilia in the immobilized theront appear thickened and fused. Note the caudal cilium (white arrows), which in the immobilized theront appears to be folded back on itself. Antibodies bind to surface antigens on the cilia resulting in immobilization. Scanning electron microscope image, theronts are approximately 40 μm in size. (Photograph and Art by Jane Noe. © 2010 University of Georgia Research Foundation, Inc.)

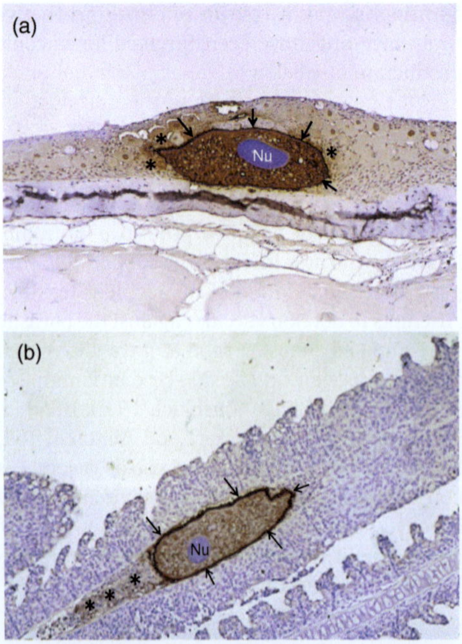

Fig. 4.7. Immunohistochemical *in situ* labelling of i-antigen associated with *Ichthyophthirius multifiliis* trophonts in channel catfish skin and gill. *I. multifiliis* trophonts in paraffin sections were fixed and incubated with mouse anti-i-antigen IgG monoclonal antibody (G3-61) followed by rabbit anti-mouse IgG conjugated to horseradish peroxidase. The sections were post-stained with haematoxylin and eosin and examined by light microscopy (magnification 100×). The figure shows locations of i-antigen during infection in skin (a) and gill (b). I-antigen is associated with the parasite surface membrane (arrows) and cytoplasm as shown by intense dark brown staining. It also appears to be released into tissues as indicated by lighter areas of brown staining (asterisks) adjacent to the trophonts, where it is available to be taken up by phagocytes initiating adaptive immune responses. In gill tissue, antigen appears to trail behind the parasite. Also note proliferation of epithelial and alarm cells in gill section (b). Nu, macronucleus. (Figure used with permission from Dickerson and Findly, 2014.)

Extensive vaccine research has been conducted in different fish species (Buchmann *et al.*, 2001; Matthews, 2005; Dickerson, 2006; Dickerson and Findly, 2014; von Gersdorff Jorgensen, 2017). To date, the most effective means of immunization is to expose fish to controlled surface infections (Parker, 1965; Areerat, 1974; Hines and Spira, 1974b; Burkart *et al.*, 1990) or to inject live parasites (theronts) into the peritoneal region of the coelomic cavity (Dickerson *et al.*, 1985; Burkart *et al.*, 1990; Dickerson and Clark, 1996; Buchmann *et al.*, 2001; Wang and Dickerson, 2002; Xu *et al.*, 2004; Alishahi and Buchmann, 2006; Xu *et al.*, 2008). The fact that the injection of parasites elicits strong mucosal immunity and that surface infection elicits production of systemic antibodies suggests that there is 'cross-talk' between the systemic and mucosal components of the fish immune system (Dickerson, 2009; Dickerson and Findly, 2014).

Also, vaccines consisting of inactivated parasites (theronts and trophonts) or subunit components (cilia, membrane proteins, recombinant proteins and purified i-antigens) confer varying degrees of protection under laboratory conditions (Parker, 1965; Areerat, 1974; Beckert, 1975; Burkart *et al.*, 1990; Wang and Dickerson, 2002; Wang *et al.*, 2002; Xu *et al.*, 2008, 2009a; von Gersdorff Jorgensen, 2017). I-antigens injected with Freund's adjuvant into the peritoneal (coelomic) cavity elicit good protection only against challenge by parasites bearing homologous i-antigens on their surface (Wang *et al.*, 2002). In contrast, fishes immunized by injection with or exposure to live theronts are protected against different immobilization serotypes, which suggests that other antigens exist in addition to the i-antigens (Leff *et al.*, 1994; Jarrett, 1997). These cross-reactive antigens have not yet been identified (Swennes *et al.*, 2007).

Since i-antigens elicit protective immunity against homologous *I. multifiliis* immobilization serotypes and limited serotypes exist in nature, it is possible that these antigens could be used as a subunit vaccine. Because *I. multifiliis* is an obligate parasite and cannot be grown in culture, the difficulty to produce large amounts of antigen is a major obstacle to commercial vaccine development. To address this problem, genes encoding i-antigens were transformed and expressed in the free-living and easily cultured ciliate *Tetrahymena pyriformis* with the idea that this organism could be used to produce sufficient amounts of antigen for a vaccine (Gaertig *et al.*, 1999). I-antigen genes have also been expressed in other cell types including the bacterium *Escherichia coli*, COS-7 mammalian cells and baculovirus (He *et al.*, 1997; Lin *et al.*, 2002; von Gersdorff Jorgensen *et al.*, 2017). Although work is ongoing, a vaccine using recombinant i-antigens and other possible protective *I. multifiliis* antigens has not yet been developed for field use (He *et al.*, 1997; Wang and Dickerson, 2002; von Gersdorff Jorgensen *et al.*, 2017). In DNA vaccine studies using i-Ag 52B cDNA, a specific antibody immune response was elicited, but protection upon challenge was not achieved (von Gersdorff Jorgensen *et al.*, 2012). A degree of protection was elicited, however, in studies using three different *I. multifiliis* recombinant i-antigens (von Gersdorff Jorgensen *et al.*, 2017).

Methods to present antigens either orally or through the skin and gills by immersion have been investigated but an oral or immersion vaccine against *I. multifiliis* has not yet been developed (Burkart *et al.*, 1990; Wang *et al.*, 2002; Xu *et al.*, 2004).

Studies have indicated that cross-reactive antigens from other organisms, including *Tetrahymena*, elicit a degree of protection against *I. multifiliis* (Goven *et al.*, 1981; Wolf and Markiw, 1982; Dickerson *et al.*, 1984; Ling *et al.*, 1993; Buchmann *et al.*, 1999; Sigh and Buchmann, 2002). Although common antigens on different parasites and ciliate species are possible, it appears that the protection is more likely attributed to an innate immune response against heterologous molecules, which allows sufficient time for the fish to develop an adaptive response against the parasite (Dickerson and Clark, 1994; Matthews, 1994, 2005). Nevertheless, it is becoming evident that elicitation of both innate and adaptive immune responses is required for an effective vaccine against *I. multifiliis*.

4.7. Protective Control Strategies: Chemotherapy and Husbandry Practices

The most effective way to eliminate ichthyophthiriasis is to prevent introduction of the parasite (Brown and Gratzek, 1980). This is accomplished through good husbandry practices that include quarantine and prophylactic treatment of new fish before introduction into a pond or aquarium system. Because the periodicity of the life cycle of *I. multifiliis* is inversely related to temperature, fish should be isolated in water of elevated temperature to reduce the time necessary to keep them under observation. At 25–30°C the parasite develops within 3–5 days and trophonts will become easily detectable. It is not always possible to isolate fish before bringing them into a water system, however, and the introduction of parasites and initiation of devastating epizootic outbreaks is always a threat. Breeding fish that are naturally resistant to *I. multifiliis* infection is a potential long-term approach to limiting ichthyophthiriasis in aquaculture. Preliminary research has been undertaken to identify genetic markers and genes in rainbow trout that might be associated with variable parasite resistance among individuals during infection (Jaafar *et al.*, 2020). Quantitative trait loci (QTLs) have been validated in trout by selecting male spawners carrying genetic resistance markers. Fertilization of outbred eggs with sperm from these males resulted in resistant fish with lowered susceptibility to *I. multifiliis* infection (Buchmann *et al.*, 2022).

Several methods have been developed for the treatment of *I. multifiliis*. These include water management strategies as well as drug and chemical treatments, which have been reviewed (Matthews, 2005; Picon-Camacho *et al.*, 2012; von Gersdorff Jorgensen, 2017). If logistically possible, daily or semi-daily removal of fish from infected aquaria and transfer to clean water and aquaria is an effective way to eliminate the parasite. The combination of chemical treatment and microfiltration of water has been shown to be more efficacious than treatment with chemicals alone (Heinecke and Buchmann, 2009). Sodium chloride treatments have been used for many years (Cross, 1972), and the addition of NaCl to water at the concentration of 4–5 g/l is effective against theronts (Selosse and Rowland, 1990; Aihua and Buchmann, 2001; Miron *et al.*, 2004). In addition to its detrimental effect on the parasite, salt may also have an ameliorative effect on the osmotic stress elicited by epithelial damage caused by the parasite (Cross, 1972; Dickerson, 2006).

Treatment with chemicals and drugs is warranted, especially if the majority of fish in the population are not severely infected and do not appear moribund. A number of chemicals are available, and many can be used on fish not intended for human consumption (Cross, 1972; Hoffman, 1999). Chemicals that can be used in food fish are limited (Matthews, 2005; Dickerson, 2006). Formalin is the only chemical currently permitted for use in the USA. A recommended treatment is the addition of formaldehyde at a concentration of 25 ppm for 10 days, with water changes every other day. Higher concentrations of 100–250 ppm can be used for up to 1 h (Brown and Gratzek, 1980). It is suggested that formalin is effective as an early treatment to prevent transmission of the parasite from fish to fish during the early stages of an outbreak, but that it is less effective against severe and extensive infections (Matthews, 2005).

Malachite green, which has proven to be an effective drug against the parasite, is now prohibited for use on food fish in the USA and the European Union. The water-soluble, zinc-free oxalate salt is effective against theronts at a concentration of 0.1 ppm for 3–4-day periods with subsequent water changes and re-treatment until the parasite has been eliminated. A non-water-soluble form has been shown to be effective against trophonts located in the skin and gills when administered orally and is less toxic to the fish than the water-soluble chemical (Schmahl *et al.*, 1992).

Many chemicals and drugs have been tested or used for the treatment of *I. multifiliis* including copper sulfate (Straus, 1993; Straus *et al.*, 2009), potassium permanganate (Straus and Griffin, 2002), chloramine T (Cross, 1972), sodium percarbonate, garlic (Buchmann *et al.*, 2003), sodium percarbonate (Heinecke and Buchmann, 2009) and others (Matthews, 2005; von Gersdorff Jorgensen, 2017). Bronopol has been shown to be efficacious in the control of *I. multifiliis* infection in rainbow trout (Shinn *et al.*, 2003). Efficacy and toxicity vary among fish species and water quality (Straus and Griffin, 2002; Straus *et al.*, 2009). Numerous medicinal plants and phytochemicals have also been tested for efficacy against *I. multifiliis* infection with some success, but their large-scale use remains limited in aquaculture (von Gersdorff Jorgensen, 2017; Ozil, 2023).

4.8. Conclusions and Suggestions for Further Study

I. multifiliis has been the subject of applied and basic research for over 100 years (Bushkiel, 1910); a fact attributed to its wide-ranging distribution throughout the world, its ability to infect a broad and diverse spectrum of freshwater fish species, and its economic importance to fish farmers and aquarists.

Also, *I. multifiliis* has emerged as a useful model system for the study of innate and acquired immunity against pathogenic parasites of fish (Buchmann *et al.*, 2001; Matthews, 2005; Dickerson, 2006; Dickerson and Findly, 2014; von Gersdorff Jorgensen, 2017; Wang *et al.*, 2019). Although an obligate parasite, it can be passaged from fish to fish in laboratory aquaria, and because of its relatively large size (40–800 μm) it is easily observed, collected and manipulated under laboratory conditions. It parasitizes the epithelia of the skin, gills and other surfaces (i.e. ocular membrane and nasal pharynx), which facilitates *in vivo* observations of its activity and quantification of infection. *I. multifiliis* has disadvantages as an experimental model, however, because it cannot be grown in culture under axenic conditions (Hurley, 1999; Li *et al.*, 2023) and viable samples cannot be stored by cryopreservation (Beeler, 1981; Everett *et al.*, 2002). With these disadvantages it is extremely difficult, if not impossible, to carry out forward or reverse genetic screens to identify phenotypic mutants in this system. Further, the inability for long-term cryogenic storage makes it difficult to carry out longitudinal studies on isolates collected from temporally and geographically disparate outbreaks, as well as comparison of virulence. Thus, the development of effective methods for *in vitro* growth and cryopreservation is critically needed.

Despite these shortcomings, stage-specific transcriptional profiling of expressed genes has been carried out (Abernathy *et al.*, 2009, 2011; Cassidy-Hanley *et al.*, 2011), and an annotated version of the near-complete macronuclear genome sequence of *I. multifiliis* is also available (Coyne *et al.*, 2011; https://ich.ciliate.org/, accessed 13 November 2025). Whole-genome sequencing led directly to the identification and characterization of endosymbionts in *I. multifiliis* (Sun *et al.*, 2009; Zaila *et al.*, 2017) and opens the door to many avenues for future research. For instance, it is now possible to identify genes encoding potentially important proteins such as enzymes, diagnostic markers and protective vaccine antigens (Coyne *et al.*, 2011). On the other hand, this may allow the discovery of safer and more effective drugs to control infection. On a more basic level, genomic studies may uncover new insights into the biology of host invasion and parasite growth, as well as advance our understanding of the parasite's population genetic structure (MacColl *et al.*, 2015; Pekmezci *et al.*, 2022; Yang *et al.*, 2023).

Despite advances in identifying and characterizing protective antigens (such as the i-antigens) and moderate success with protective vaccination in the laboratory using live, inactivated and subunit vaccines (Buchmann *et al.*, 2001; Wang and Dickerson, 2002; Wang *et al.*, 2002; Xu *et al.*, 2008, 2009a), a practical field vaccine against *I. multifiliis* is still not available. Because it cannot be easily cultured, the first commercial vaccines for *I. multifiliis* will probably come from the development of inexpensive means to produce recombinant protective antigens (von Gersdorff Jorgensen *et al.*, 2012, 2017). Thus, further research is needed to create new protein expression systems, such as *Tetrahymena thermophila* (Gaertig *et al.*, 1999; Clark *et al.*, 2001; Bednenko *et al.*, 2018; Watanabe *et al.*, 2024), or to enhance the capabilities of existing systems, such as *E. coli* (Lin *et al.*, 2002; von Gersdorff Jorgensen *et al.*, 2017). Alternatively, the use of nucleic acid vaccines may hold promise as well (von Gersdorff Jorgensen *et al.*, 2012; Xu *et al.*, 2019, 2020).

Regardless of the approach, successful immunization will require effective methods of vaccine delivery, preferably though oral or immersion routes, and adjuvant formulations that stimulate and enhance long-lasting mucosal immunity in the skin and gills. Research should also be continued on elucidating the mechanisms of innate and adaptive immunity including: (i) the sites of antigen presentation and induction; (ii) antibody production and secretion in epithelia; (iii) trafficking of immune cells; and (iv) immune memory.

References

Abernathy, J.W., Xu, D., Li, P., Klesius, P., Kucuktas, H. and Liu, Z. (2009) Transcriptomic profiling of *Ichthyophthirius multifiliis* reveals polyadenylation of the large subunit ribosomal RNA. *Comparative Biochemistry and Physiology, Part D* 4, 179–186.

Abernathy, J., Xu, D., Peatman, E., Kucuktas, H., Klesius, P. and Liu, Z. (2011) Gene expression profiling of a fish parasite *Ichthyophthirius multifiliis*: insights into development and senescence-associated avirulence. *Comparative Biochemistry and Physiology, Part D* 6, 382–392.

Aihua, L. and Buchmann, K. (2001) Temperature- and salinity-dependent development of a Nordic strain of *Ichthyophthirius multifiliis* from rainbow trout. *Journal of Applied Ichthyology* 17, 273–276.

Alishahi, M. and Buchmann, K. (2006) Temperature-dependent protection against *Ichthyophthirius multifiliis* following immunization of rainbow trout using live theronts. *Diseases of Aquatic Organisms* 72, 269–273.

Areerat, S. (1974) The immune response of channel catfish, *Ictalurus punctatus* Rafinesque, to *Ichthyophthirius multifiliis*. MSc thesis, Auburn University, Auburn, Alabama.

Bauer, O.N. (1953) The immune response of channel catfish *Ictalurus punctatus* Rafinesque to *Ichthyophthirius multifiliis* Fouquet. *Doklady Novaia Serviia, SSSR* 93, 377–379.

Bauer, O.N. and Iunchis, O.N. (2001) A new genus of parasitic ciliata from tropical fishes. *Parazitologiia* 35, 142–144.

Beckert, H. (1975) Observations on the biology of *Ichthyophthirius multifiliis* Fouquet, 1876. Its susceptibility to ethoxyquin, and some immunological responses of channel catfish, *Ictalurus punctatus*, to this parasite. PhD thesis, University of Southwestern Louisiana, Lafayette, Louisiana.

Beckert, H. and Allison, R. (1964) Some host responses of white catfish to *Ichthyophthirius multifiliis*. *Proceedings of the Southeastern Association of Game Fish Commissioners* 18, 438–441.

Bednenko, J., Harriman, R., Marien, L., Nguyen, H.M., Agrawal, A. *et al.* (2018) A multiplatform strategy for the discovery of conventional monoclonal antibodies that inhibit the voltage-gated potassium channel Kv1.3. *mAbs* 10(4), 636–650.

Beeler, C.R. (1981) Controlling cooling rates with a variable vacuum in a Dewar flask. *Cryobiology* 18, 79–81.

Bodensteiner, L.R., Sheehan, R.J., Wills, P.S., Brandenburg, A.M. and Lewis, W.M. (2000) Flowing water: an effective treatment for ichthyophthiriasis. *Journal of Aquatic Animal Health* 12, 209–219.

Bradshaw, C.M., Richard, A.S. and Sigel, M.M. (1971) IgM antibodies in fish mucus. *Proceedings of the Society of Experimental and Biological Medicine* 136, 1122–1124.

Bragg, R.R. (1991) Health status of salmonids in river systems in natal. I. Collection of fish and parasitological examination. *The Onderstepoort Journal of Veterinary Research* 58, 59–62.

Brown, E.E. and Gratzek, J.B. (1980) *Fish Farming Handbook. Food, Bait, Tropicals and Goldfish*. AVI Publishing, Westport, Connecticut.

Bu, X., Peng, X., Huang, L., Zhao, Y., Jiao, J. *et al.* (2025) Effect of ectoparasite *Ichthyopththirius multifiliis* on the histopathology and gill and gut microbiota of goldfish (*Carassius auratus*). *Frontiers in Veterinary Science* 2025, 1539446.

Buchmann, K. (2020) Immune response to *Ichthyophthirius multifiliis* and role of IgT. *Parasite Immunology* 42, e12675.

Buchmann, K. and Nielsen, M.E. (1999) Chemoattraction of *Ichthyophthirius multifiliis* (ciliophora) theronts to host molecules. *International Journal for Parasitology* 29, 1415–1423.

Buchmann, K., Uldal, A. and Lyholt, H.C. (1995) Parasite infections in Danish trout farms. *Acta Veterinaria Scandinavica* 36, 283–298.

Buchmann, K., Lindenstrom, T. and Sigh, J. (1999) Partial cross protection against *Ichthyophthirius multifiliis* in *Gyrodactylus derjavini* immunized rainbow trout. *Journal of Helminthology* 73, 189–195.

Buchmann, K., Sigh, J., Nielsen, C.V. and Dalgaard, M. (2001) Host responses against the fish parasitizing ciliate *Ichthyophthirius multifiliis*. *Veterinary Parasitology* 100, 105–116.

Buchmann, K., Jensen, P.B. and Kruse, K.D. (2003) Effects of sodium percarbonate and garlic extract on *Ichthyophthirius multifiliis* theronts and tomocysts: *in vitro* experiments. *North America Journal of Aquaculture* 65, 21–24.

Buchmann, K., Nielsen, T., Mathiessen, H., Marana, M.H.., Duan, Y. *et al.* (2022) Validation of two QTL associated with lower *Ichthyopthirius multifiliis* infection and delayed-time-to-death in rainbow trout. *Aquaculture Reports* 23, 101078.

Burkart, M.A., Clark, T.G. and Dickerson, H.W. (1990) Immunization of channel catfish, *Ictalurus punctatus* Rafinesque, against *Ichthyophthirius multifiliis* (Fouquet): killed versus live vaccines. *Journal of Fish Diseases* 13, 401–410.

Bushkiel, A.L. (1910) Beitrage zur kenntnis des *Ichthyophthirius multifiliis*. *Archiv für Protistenkunde* 21, 61–102.

Butcher, A.D. (1941) Outbreaks of white spot or ichthyophthiriasis (*Ichthyophthirius multifiliis* Fouquet, 1876) at the hatcheries of Ballarat fish acclimatization society with notes on laboratory experiments. *Proceedings of the Royal Society of Victoria* 53, 126–144.

Canella, M.F. and Rocchi-Canella, I. (1976) Biologie des Ophryoglenina (cilies hymenostermes, histophages). *Annals of the University of Ferrara (N.S. Sect. III)* 3(Suppl. 2), 1–510.

Cassidy-Hanley, D., Cordonnier-Pratt, M., Pratt, L., Devine, C., Hossain, M. *et al.* (2011) Transcriptional profiling of stage specific gene expression in the parasitic ciliate *Ichthyophthirius multifiliis*. *Molecular and Biochemical Parasitology* 178, 29–39.

Chapman, G.B. (1984) Ultrastructural aspects of the host–parasite relationship in ichthyophthiriasis. *Transactions of the American Microscopical Society* 103, 364–375.

Chi, J., Mahe, F., Loidl, J., Logsdon, J. and Dunthorn, M. (2013) Meiosis gene inventory of four ciliates reveals the prevalence of synaptonemal complex-independent crossover pathway. *Molecular Biology and Evolution* 31(3), 660–672.

Christoffersen, T.B., Kania, P.W., von Gersdorff Jorgensen, L. and Buchmann, K. (2017) Zebrafish *Danio rerio* as a model to study the immune response against infection with *Ichthyophthirius multifiliis*. *Journal of Fish Diseases* 40, 847–852.

Clark, T.G. and Dickerson, H.W. (1997) Antibody-mediated effects on parasite behaviour: evidence of a novel mechanism of immunity against a parasitic protist. *Parasitology Today* 13(12), 470–480.

Clark, T. and Forney, J. (2003) Free-living and parasitic ciliates. In: Craig, A. and Sherf, A. (eds) *Antigenic Variation*. Academic Press (Elsevier Science Ltd), London, pp. 375–402.

Clark, T.G., Dickerson, H.W., Gratzek, J.B. and Findly, R.C. (1987) *In vitro* response of *Ichthyophthirius multifiliis* to sera from immune channel catfish. *Journal of Fish Biology* 31, 203–208.

Clark, T.G., Dickerson, H.W. and Findly, R.C. (1988) Immune response of channel catfish to ciliary antigens of *Ichthyophthirius multifiliis*. *Developmental and Comparative Immunology* 12, 581–594.

Clark, T.G., Gao, Y., Gaertig, J., Wang, X and Cheng, G. (2001) The i-antigens of *Ichthyophthirius multifiliis* are GPI-anchored proteins. *Journal of Eukaryotic Microbiology* 48(3), 332–337.

Corliss, J. (1979) *The Ciliated Protozoa: Characterization, Classification, and Guide to the Literature*. Pergamon Press, Oxford, UK.

Coyne, R.S., Hannick, L., Shanmugam, D., Hostetler, J.B., Brami, D. *et al.* (2011) Comparative genomics of the pathogenic ciliate *Ichthyophthirius multifiliis*, its free-living relatives and a host species provide insights into adoption of a parasitic lifestyle and prospects for disease control. *Genome Biology* 12, R100.

Cross, D.G. (1972) A review of methods to control ichthyophthiriasis. *The Progressive Fish-Culturist* 34, 165–170.

Cross, M.L. (1993) Antibody binding following exposure of live *Ichthyophthirius multifiliis* (Ciliophora) to serum from immune carp *Cyprinus carpio*. *Diseases of Aquatic Organisms* 17, 159–164.

Cross, M.L. (1994) Localized cellular-responses to *Ichthyophthirius multifiliis* – protection or pathogenesis. *Parasitology Today* 10, 364–368.

Cross, M.L. and Matthews, R.A. (1993a) *Ichthyophthirius multifiliis* Fouquet (Ciliophora): the localization of sites immunogenic to the host *Cyprinus carpio* (L.). *Fish and Shellfish Immunology* 3, 13–24.

Cross, M.L. and Matthews, R.A. (1993b) Localized leukocyte response to *Ichthyophthirius multifiliis* establishment in immune carp *Cyprinus carpio* L. *Veterinary Immunology and Immunopathology* 38, 341–358.

Dickerson, H.W. (2006) *Ichthyophthirius multifiliis* and *Cryptocaryon irritans* (phylum Ciliophora). In: Woo, P.T.K. (ed.) *Fish Diseases and Disorders, Volume 1: Protozoan and Metazoan Infections*, 2nd edn. CAB International, Wallingford, Oxon, pp. 55–72.

Dickerson, H.W. (2009) The biology of teleost mucosal immunity. In: Giacomo, Z., Perriere, C., Mathis, A. and Kapoor, B.G. (eds) *Fish Defenses, Volume 2: Pathogens, Parasites and Predators*. Science Publishers, Enfield, New Hampshire, pp. 1–42.

Dickerson, H.W. and Clark, T.G. (1994) Vaccination against ich. *Aquaculture* 127, 278–280.

Dickerson, H. and Clark, T. (1996) Immune response of fishes to ciliates. *Annual Review of Fish Diseases* 6, 107–120.

Dickerson, H. and Clark, T. (1998) *Ichthyophthirius multifiliis*: a model of cutaneous infection and immunity in fishes. *Immunological Reviews* 166, 377–384.

Dickerson, H. and Findly, R.C. (2014) Immunity to *Ichthyophthirius* infections in fish: a synopsis. *Developmental and Comparative Immunology* 43, 290–299.

Dickerson, H.W., Brown, J., Dawe, D.L. and Gratzek, J.B. (1984) *Tetrahymena pyriformis* as a protective antigen against *Ichthyophthirius multifiliis* infection – comparisons between isolates and ciliary preparations. *Journal of Fish Biology* 24, 523–528.

Dickerson, H.W., Lohr, A.L. and Gratzek, J.B. (1985) Experimental intraperitoneal infection of channel catfish, *Ictalurus punctatus* (Rafinesque) with *Ichthyophthirius multifiliis* (Fouquet). *Journal of Fish Diseases* 8, 139–142.

Dickerson, H.W., Clark, T.G. and Leff, A.A. (1993) Serotypic variation among isolates of *Ichthyophthirius multifiliis* based on immobilization. *Journal of Eukaryotic Microbiology* 40, 816–820.

Duan, Y., Marana, M.H., Jensen, H.M., Henard, C. and von Gersdorff Jorgensen, L. (2025) Implementing an environmental DNA/RNA-based approach to non-invasively investigate disease caused by *Ichthyophthirius multifiliis*. *Aquaculture Reports* 40, 102562.

Everett, K.D., Knight, J.R. and Dickerson, H.W. (2002) Comparing tolerance of *Ichthyophthirius multifiliis* and *Tetrahymena thermophila* for new cryopreservation methods. *Journal of Parasitology* 88, 41–46.

Ewing, M.S. and Kocan, K.M. (1992) Invasion and development strategies of *Ichthyophthirius multifiliis*, a parasitic ciliate of fish. *Parasitology Today* 8, 204–208.

Ewing, M.S., Kocan, K.M. and Ewing, S.A. (1983) *Ichthyophthirius multifiliis*: morphology of the cyst wall. *Transactions of the American Microscopical Society* 102, 122–128.

Ewing, M.S., Kocan, K.M. and Ewing, S.A. (1985) *Ichthyophthirius multifiliis* (Ciliophora) invasion of gill epithelium. *Journal of Protozoology* 32, 305–310.

Ewing, M.S., Lynn, M.E. and Ewing, S.A. (1986) Critical periods in development of *Ichthyophthirius multifiliis* (Ciliophora) populations. *Journal of Protozoology* 33, 388–391.

Findly, R.C., Zhao, X., Noe, J., Camus, A.C. and Dickerson, H.W. (2013) B cell memory following infection and challenge of channel catfish with *Ichthyophthirius multifiliis*. *Developmental and Comparative Immunology* 39, 302–311.

Fokin, S.I. (2004) Bacterial endocytobionts of Ciliophora and their interactions with the host cell. *International Review of Cytology* 236, 181–249.

Gaertig, J., Gao, Y., Tishgarten, T., Clark, T. and Dickerson, H. (1999) Surface display of a parasite antigen in the ciliate *Tetrahymena thermophila*. *Nature Biotechnology* 17, 462–465.

Geisslinger, M. (1987) Observations on the caudal cilium of the tomite of *Ichthyophthirius multifiliis* Fouquet 1876. *Journal of Protozoology* 341, 180–182.

Gonzalez, S.F., Buchmann, K. and Nielsen, M.E. (2007a) Real-time gene expression analysis in carp (*Cyprinus carpio* L.) skin: inflammatory responses caused by the ectoparasite *Ichthyophthirius multifiliis*. *Fish and Shellfish Immunology* 22, 641–650.

Gonzalez, S.F., Chatziandreou, N., Nielsen, M.E., Li, W., Rogers, J. *et al.* (2007b) Cutaneous immune responses in the common carp detected using transcript analysis. *Molecular Immunology* 44, 1664–1679.

Goven, B.A., Dawe, D.L. and Gratzek, J.B. (1981) *In vitro* demonstration of serological cross-reactivity between *Ichthyophthirius multifiliis* Foquet and *Tetrahymena pyriformis* Lwoff. *Developmental and Comparative Immunology* 5, 283–289.

Graves, S.S., Evans, D.L., Cobb, D. and Dawe, D.L. (1984) Nonspecific cytotoxic cells in fish (*Ictalurus punctatus*) I. Optimum requirements for target cell lysis. *Developmental and Comparative Immunology* 8, 293–302.

Graves, S.S., Evans, D.L. and Dawe, D.L. (1985) Mobilization and activation of nonspecific cytotoxic cells (NCC) in the channel catfish (*Ictalurus punctatus*) infected with *Ichthyophthirius multifiliis*. *Comparative Immunology Microbiology and Infectious Diseases* 8, 43–51.

Hauser, M. (1973) Acetomyosin-like filaments in the dividing macronucleus of the ciliated protozoon *Ichthyophthirius multifiliis*. *Chromosoma* 44, 49–71.

He, J., Yin, Z., Xu, G., Gong, Z., Lam, T.J. and Sin, Y.M. (1997) Protection of goldfish against *Ichthyophthirius multifiliis* by immunization with a recombinant vaccine. *Aquaculture* 158, 1–10.

Heinecke, R.D. and Buchmann, K. (2009) Control of *Ichthyophthirius multifiliis* using a combination of water filtration and sodium percarbonate; dose–response studies. *Aquaculture* 288, 32–35.

Hines, R.S. and Spira, D.T. (1973a) Ichthyophthiriasis in the mirror carp. II. Leukocyte response. *Journal of Fish Biology* 5, 527–534.

Hines, R.S. and Spira, D.T. (1973b) *Ichthyophthirius multifiliis* (Fouquet) in the mirror carp, *Cyprinus carpio* L. I. Course of infection. *Journal of Fish Biology* 5, 385–392.

Hines, R.S. and Spira, D.T. (1974a) Ichthyophthiriasis in the mirror carp *Cyprinus carpio* (L.). IV. Physiological dysfunction. *Journal of Fish Biology* 6, 365–371.

Hines, R.S. and Spira, D.T. (1974b) Ichthyophthiriasis in the mirror carp *Cyprinus carpio* (L.). V. Acquired immunity. *Journal of Fish Biology* 6, 373–378.

Hines, R.S. and Spira, D.T. (1974c) Ichthyophthiriasis in the mirror carp *Cyprinus carpio* L. III. Pathology. *Journal of Fish Biology* 6, 189–196.

Hoffman, G. (1999) *Parasites of North American Fishes*. Comstock Publishing Associates, Ithaca, New York.

Houghton, G. and Matthews, R.A. (1986) Immunosuppression of carp (*Cyprinus carpio* L.) to ichthyophthiriasis using the corticosteroid triamcinolone acetonide. *Veterinary Immunology and Immunopathology* 12, 413–419.

Hurley, L. (1999) *Ichthyopthirius multifiliis* Fouquet: development and assessment of *in vitro* systems for long term maintenance. Thesis, University of Plymouth, Plymouth, UK. Available at: https://pearl.plymouth.ac.uk/bms-theses (accessed 13 November 2025).

Jaafar, R., Odegard, J., Mathiessen, H. Karami, A.M., Marana, M.H. *et al.* (2020) Quantitative trait loci (QTL) associated with resistance of rainbow trout *Oncorhynchus mykiss* against the parasitic ciliate *Ichthyophthirius multifiliis*. *Journal of Fish Diseases* 43, 1591–1602.

Jalali, B., Barzegar, M. and Nezamabadi, H. (2008) Parasitic fauna of the spiny eel, *Mastacembelus mastacembelus* Banks et Solander (Teleostei: Mastacembelidae) in Iran. *Iranian Journal of Veterinary Research* 9, 158–161.

Jarrett, L.C. (1997) The immune response of channel catfish against different immobilization serotypes of *Ichthyophthirius multifiliis*. MSc thesis, University of Georgia, Athens, Georgia.

Kheisin, E.M. and Mosevich, T.N. (1969) Particuliarities of surface structures in the parasitic ciliate *Ichthyophthirius multifiliis*. *Tsitologiia* 11, 689–694.

Kim, J.H., Hayward, C.J., Joh, S.J. and Heo, G.J. (2002) Parasitic infections in live freshwater tropical fishes imported to Korea. *Diseases of Aquatic Organisms* 52, 169–173.

Kong, W., Ding, G., Cheng, G., Yang, P. and Xu, Z. (2024) Mucosal immune responses to *Ichthyophthirius multifiliis* in the ocular mucosa of rainbow trout (*Oncorhynchus mykiss*, Walbaum), an ancient teleost fish. *Marine Life Science and Technology* 6, 266–279.

Kozel, T.R. (1986) Scanning electron microscopy of theronts of *Ichthyophthirius multifiliis*: their penetration into host tissue. *Transactions of the American Microscopical Society* 105, 357–364.

Leff, A.A., Yoshinaga, T. and Dickerson, H.W. (1994) Cross immunity in channel catfish against two immobilization serotypes of *Ichthyophthirius multifiliis*. *Journal of Fish Diseases* 17, 429–432.

Lemos, J.R.G., Tavares-Dias, M., De Aquino Sales, R.S., Nobre Filho, G.D.R. and Fim, J.D.I. (2007) Parasites in gills of farmed *Brycon amazonicus* (Characidae, Bryconinae) in stream channels of Turumamirim, Amazonas State, Brazil. *Acta Scientiarum Biological Sciences* 29, 217–222.

Li, M., Gomes, G.B., Zhao, W., Hu, G., Huang, K. *et al.* (2023) Cultivation of fish ciliate parasites: progress and prospects. *Reviews in Aquaculture* 15, 142–162.

Lin, T.L., Clark, T.G. and Dickerson, H. (1996) Passive immunization of channel catfish (*Ictalurus punctatus*) against the ciliated protozoan parasite *Ichthyophthirius multifiliis* by use of murine monoclonal antibodies. *Infection and Immunity* 64, 4085–4090.

Lin, Y., Cheng, G., Wang, X. and Clark, T.G. (2002) The use of synthetic genes for the expression of ciliate proteins in heterologous systems. *Gene* 288, 85–94.

Ling, K.H., Sin, Y.M. and Lam, T.J. (1993) Protection of goldfish against some common ectoparasitic protozoans using *Ichthyophthirius multifiliis* and *Tetrahymena pyriformis* for vaccination. *Aquaculture* 116, 303–314.

Lobb, C.J. and Clem, L.W. (1981) The metabolic relationship of the immunoglobulins in fish serum, cutaneous mucus, and bile. *Journal of Immunology* 127, 1525–1529.

Lobo-da-Cunha, A. and Azevedo, C. (1988) Association between xenosomes and glycogen in the cytoplasm of the ciliate *Ichthyophthirius multifiliis*. *Endocytobiosis and Cell Research* 5, 225–231.

Lobo-da-Cunha, A. and Azevedo, C. (1990) Enzyme cytochemistry of the alveolar sacs and golgian-like cisternae in the ciliate *Ichthyophthirius multifiliis*. *Journal of Protozoology* 37, 206–211.

Lom, J. and Cerkasova, A. (1974) Host finding in invasive stages of *Ichthyophthirius multifiliis*. *Journal of Protozoology* 21, 457.

Lynn, D.H. (2008) *The Ciliated Protozoa: Characterization, Classification, and Guide to the Literature*. Springer, Heidelberg, Germany.

Lynn, D.H., Frombach, S., Ewing, M.S. and Kocan, K.M. (1991) The organelle of Lieberkühn as a synapomorphy for the Ophryoglenina (Ciliophora: Hymenostomatida). *Transactions of the American Microscopical Society* 110, 1–11.

MacColl, E., Therkelsen, M.D., Sherpa, T., Ellerbrock, H., Johnston, L.A. *et al.* (2015) Molecular genetic diversity and characterization of conjugation genes in the fish parasite *Ichthyophthirius multifiliis*. *Molecular Phylogenetics and Evolution* 86, 1–7.

Maceda-Veiga, A., Salvado, H., Vinyoles, D. and De Sostoa, A. (2009) Outbreaks of *Ichthyophthirius multifiliis* in redtail barbs *Barbus haasi* in a Mediterranean stream during drought. *Journal of Aquatic Animal Health* 21, 189–194.

Maclennon, R.F. (1935) Observations on the life cycle of *Ichthyophthirius*, a ciliate parasitic on fish. *Northwestern Scientist* 9, 12–14.

Maclennon, R.F. (1937) Growth in the ciliate *Ichthyophthirius*. I. Maturity and encystment. *Journal of Experimental Zoology* 76, 423–440.

Maclennon, R.F. (1942) Growth in the ciliate *Ichthyophthirius*. II. Volume. *Journal of Experimental Zoology* 91, 1–13.

Maki, J.L. and Dickerson, H.W. (2003) Systemic and cutaneous mucus antibody responses of channel catfish immunized against the protozoan parasite *Ichthyophthirius multifiliis*. *Clinical and Diagnostic Laboratory Immunology* 10, 876–881.

Matthews, R.A. (1994) *Ichthyophthirius multifiliis* Fouquet 1876: infection and protective responses within the fish host. In: Pike, A.W. and Lewis, J.W. (eds) *Parasitic Diseases of Fish*. Samara Publishing, Cardigan, UK, pp. 17–42.

Matthews, R.A. (1996) *Ichthyophthirius*: observations on the life-cycle and indications of a possible sexual phase. *Folia Parasitologica* 43, 203–208.

Matthews, R.A. (2005) *Ichthyophthirius multifiliis* Fouquet and ichthyophthiriosis in freshwater teleosts. *Advances in Parasitology* 59, 159–241.

Miron, D.S., Silva, L.V.F., Golombieski, J.I. and Baldisserotto, B. (2004) Efficacy of different salt (NaCl) concentrations in the treatment of *Ichthyophthirius multifiliis*-infected silver catfish, *Rhamdia quelen*, fingerlings. *Journal of Applied Aquaculture* 14, 155–161.

Molnar, K. (2006) Some remarks on parasitic infections of the invasive *Neogobius* spp. (Pisces) in the Hungarian reaches of the Danube River, with a description of *Goussia szekelyi* sp. n. (Apicomplexa: Eimeriidae). *Journal of Applied Ichthyology* 22, 395–400.

Nanney, D.L. (1980) *Experimental Ciliatology: An Introduction to Genetic and Developmental Analysis in Ciliates*. Wiley, New York.

Nigrelli, R.F., Pokorny, K.S. and Ruggieri, G.D. (1976) Notes on *Ichthyophthirius multifiliis*, a ciliate parasitic on fresh-water fishes, with some remarks on possible physiological races and species. *Transactions of the American Microscopical Society* 95, 607–613.

Noe, J.G. and Dickerson, H.W. (1995) Sustained growth of *Ichthyophthirius multifiliis* at low temperature in the laboratory. *Journal of Parasitology* 81, 1022–1024.

Ogut, H., Akyol, A. and Alkahn, M.Z. (2005) Seasonality of *Ichthyophthirius multifiliis* in the trout (*Onchorynchus mykiss*) farms of the eastern Black Sea region of Turkey. *Turkish Journal of Fisheries and Aquatic Sciences* 5, 23–27.

Ozil, O. (2023) Antiparasitic activity of medicinal plants against protozoan parasite *Ichthyopththirius multifiliis*. *Israeli Journal of Aquaculture – Bamidgeh* 75(2), 1–9.

Paperna, I. (1972) Infection by *Ichthyophthirius multifiliis* of fish in Uganda. *The Progressive Fish-Culturist* 34, 162–164.

Parker, J.C. (1965) Studies on the natural history of *Ichthyophthirius multifiliis* Fouquet 1876, an ectoparasitic ciliate of fish. PhD thesis, University of Maryland, College Park, Maryland.

Pekmezci, G.Z., Yildirim, A., Duzlu, O., Simsek, E., Balta, F. *et al.* (2022) Genetic diversity of *Ichthyophthirius multifiliis* (Fouquet, 1876) infecting farmed rainbow trout (*Oncorhynchus mykiss* Walbaum, 1792) in Turkey. *Journal of Fish Diseases* 45, 1109–1115.

Peshkov, M.A. and Tikhomirova, L.A. (1968) Ultra-fine structure of the nuclear apparatus of *Ichthyophthirius multifiliis* at the cystal stage in protomites. *Doklady Novaia Serviia* 183, 451–452.

Piazza, R.S., Martins, M.L., Guiraldelli, L. and Yamashita, M.M. (2006) Parasitic diseases of freshwater ornamental fishes commercialized in Florianopolis, Santa Catarina, Brazil. *Boletim do Instituto de Pesca (Sao Paulo)* 32, 51–57.

Picon-Camacho, S.M., Marcos-Lopez, M., Bron, J.E. and Shinn, A.P. (2012) An assessment of the use of drug and non-drug interventions in the treatment of *Ichthyophthirius multifiliis* Fouquet, 1876, a protozoan parasite of freshwater fish. *Parasitology* 139, 149–190.

Pinello, J.F. and Clark, T.G. (2022) HAP2-mediated gamete fusion: lessons from the world of unicellular eukaryotes. *Frontiers in Cellular and Developmental Biology* 9, 807313.

Pinello, J.F., Lai, A.L., Millet, J.K., Cassidy-Hanley, D., Freed, J.H. and Clark, T.G. (2017) Structure–function studies link class II viral fusogens with the ancestral gamete fusion protein HAP2. *Current Biology* 27(5), 651–660.

Qin, T., Hu, G., Cheng, J., Chen, F., Fu, P. *et al.* (2024) Investigation of Ichthyophthirius *multifiliis* infection in fish from natural water bodies in the Lhasa and Nagqu regions of Tibet. *International Journal for Parasitology: Parasites and Wildlife* 23, 100894.

Rintamaki-Kinnunen, P. and Valtonen, E.T. (1997) Epizootiology of protozoans in farmed salmonids at northern latitudes. *International Journal for Parasitology* 27, 89–99.

Roque, M., De Puytorac, P. and Lom, J. (1967) L'architecture buccale et la stomatogenese d'*Ichthophthirius multifiliis* Fouquet, 1876. *Protistologica* 3, 79–89.

Schmahl, G., Ruider, S., Mehlhorn, H., Schmidt, H. and Ritter, G. (1992) Treatment of fish parasites. 9. Effects of a medicated food containing malachite green on *Ichthyophthirius multifiliis* Fouquet, 1876 (Hymenostomatida, Ciliophora) in ornamental fish. *Parasitology Research* 78, 183–192.

Scholz, T. (1999) Parasites in cultured and feral fish. *Veterinary Parasitology* 84, 317–335.

Selosse, P.M. and Rowland, S.J. (1990) Use of common salt to treat ichthyophthiriasis in Australian warm-water fishes. *The Progressive Fish-Culturist* 52, 124–127.

Shinn, A.P., Wootten, R., Cote, I. and Sommerville, C. (2003) Efficacy of selected oral chemotherapeutants against *Ichthyophthirius multifiliis* (Ciliophora: Ophyroglenidae) infecting rainbow trout *Oncorhynchus mykiss*. *Diseases of Aquatic Organisms* 55, 17–22.

Shiota, K., Sukeda, M., Prakash, H., Kondo, M., Nakanishi, T. *et al.* (2021) Local immune responses to two stages of *Ichthyophthirius multifiliis* in ginbuna crucian carp. *Fish and Shellfish Immunology* 118, 19–24.

Sigh, J. and Buchmann, K. (2002) Comparative analysis of cross-reactivity between *Ichthyophthirius* and *Tetrahymena*. *Bulletin of the European Association of Fish Pathologists* 22, 37–44.

Sigh, J., Lindenstrom, T. and Buchmann, K. (2004a) Expression of pro-inflammatory cytokines in rainbow trout (*Oncorhynchus mykiss*) during an infection with *Ichthyophthirius multifiliis*. *Fish and Shellfish Immunology* 17, 75–86.

Sigh, J., Lindenstrom, T. and Buchmann, K. (2004b) The parasitic ciliate *Ichthyophthirius multifiliis* induces expression of immune relevant genes in rainbow trout, *Oncorhynchus mykiss* (Walbaum). *Journal of Fish Diseases* 27, 409–417.

Straus, D.L. (1993) Prevention of *Ichthyophthirius multifiliis* infestation in channel catfish fingerlings by copper sulphate treatment. *Journal of Aquatic Animal Health* 5, 152–154.

Straus, D.L. and Griffin, B.R. (2002) Efficacy of potassium permanganate in treating ichthyophthiriasis in channel catfish. *Journal of Aquatic Animal Health* 14, 145–148.

Straus, D.L., Hossain, M.M. and Clark, T.G. (2009) Copper sulfate toxicity to two isolates of *Ichthyophthirius multifiliis* relative to alkalinity. *Diseases of Aquatic Organisms* 83, 31–36.

Sun, H.Y., Noe, J., Barber, J., Coyne, R.S., Cassidy-Hanley, D. *et al.* (2009) Endosymbiotic bacteria in the parasitic ciliate *Ichthyophthirius multifiliis*. *Applied and Environmental Microbiology* 75, 7445–7452.

Swennes, A.G., Noe, J.G., Findly, R.C. and Dickerson, H.W. (2006) Differences in virulence between two serotypes of *Ichthyophthirius multifiliis*. *Diseases of Aquatic Organisms* 69, 227–232.

Swennes, A.G., Findly, R.C. and Dickerson, H.W. (2007) Cross-immunity and antibody responses to different immobilisation serotypes of *Ichthyophthirius multifiliis*. *Fish and Shellfish Immunology* 22, 589–597.

Thilakaratne, I., Rajapaksha, G., Hewakopara, A., Rajapakse, R. and Faizal, A.C.M. (2003) Parasitic infections in freshwater ornamental fish in Sri Lanka. *Diseases of Aquatic Organisms* 54, 157–162.

Traxler, G.S., Richard, J. and McDonald, T.E. (1998) *Ichthyophthirius multifiliis* (Ich) epizootics in spawning sockeye salmon in British Columbia, Canada. *Journal of Aquatic Animal Health* 10, 143–151.

Valtonen, E.T. and Keränen, A. (1981) Ichthyophthiriasis of atlantic salmon, *Salmo salar* L. at the Montta hatchery in Northern Finland in 1978–1979. *Journal of Fish Diseases* 4, 405–411.

Van Den Bussche, R.A., Hoofer, S.R., Drew, C.P. and Ewing, M.S. (2000) Characterization of histone h3/h4 gene region and phylogenetic affinity of *Ichthyophthirius multifiliis* based on h4 DNA sequence variation. *Molecular and Phylogenetic Evolution* 14, 461–468.

Ventura, M.T. and Paperna, I. (1985) Histopathology of *Ichthyophthirius multifiliis* infections in fishes. *Journal of Fish Biology* 27, 185–203.

Von Gersdorff Jørgensen, L. (2016) Infection and immunity against *Ichthyophthirius multifiliis* in zebrafish (*Danio rerio*). *Fish and Shellfish Immunology* 57, 335–339.

Von Gersdorff Jorgensen, L. (2017) The fish parasite Ichthyophthirius *multifiliis* – host immunity, vaccines, and novel treatments. *Fish and Shellfish Immunology* 67, 586–595.

Von Gersdorff Jorgensen, L., Nemli, E., Heinecke, R.D., Raida, K.M. and Buchmann, K. (2008) Immune-relevant genes expressed in rainbow trout following immunization with live vaccine against *Ichthyophthirius multifiliis*. *Diseases of Aquatic Organisms* 80, 189–197.

Von Gersdorff Jorgensen, L., Sigh, J., Kania, P., Holten-Andersen, L., Buchmann, K. *et al.* (2012) Approaches towards DNA vaccination against a skin ciliate parasite in fish. *PLoS One* 7 (11), e48129.

Von Gersdorff Jorgensen, L., Kania, P.W., Rasmussen, K.J., Mattsson, A.H., Schmidt, J. *et al.* (2017) Rainbow trout (*Oncorhynchus mykiss*) immune response towards a recombinant vaccine targeting the parasitic ciliate *Ichthyophthirius multifiliis*. *Journal of Fish Diseases* 40, 1815–1821.

Wahli, T. and Meier, W. (1985) Ichthyophthiriasis in trout: investigation of natural defence mechanisms. In: Ellis, A.E. (ed.) *Fish and Shellfish Pathology*. Academic Press, London, pp. 347–352.

Wahli, T. and Meier, W. (1987) Occurrence and significance of *Ichthyophthirius multifiliis* in Switzerland. *Schweizer Archiv für Tierheilkunde* 129, 205–213.

Wahli, T. and Meier, W. (1991) Affinity of *Ichthyophthirius multifiliis* theronts to light and/or fish. *Journal of Applied Ichthyology* 7, 244–249.

Wang, Q., Yu, Y., Zhang, X. and Xu, Z. (2019) Immune responses of fish to *Ichthyophthirius multifiliis* (Ich): a model for understanding immunity against protozoan parasites. *Developmental and Comparative Immunology* 93, 93–102.

Wang, X. and Dickerson, H.W. (2002) Surface immobilization antigen of the parasitic ciliate *Ichthyophthirius multifiliis* elicits protective immunity in channel catfish (*Ictalurus punctatus*). *Clinical and Diagnostic Laboratory Immunology* 9, 176–181.

Wang, X., Clark, T.G., Noe, J. and Dickerson, H.W. (2002) Immunisation of channel catfish, *Ictalurus punctatus*, with *Ichthyophthirius multifiliis* immobilisation antigens elicits serotype-specific protection. *Fish and Shellfish Immunology* 13, 337–350.

Watanabe, Y., Asada, M., Inokuchi, M., Kotake, M. and Yoshinaga, T. (2024) Target protein expression on *Tetrahymena thermophila* cell surface using the signal peptide and GPI anchor sequences of the immobilization antigen of *Cryptocaryon irritans*. *Molecular Biotechnology* 66, 1907–1918.

Wolf, K. and Markiw, M.E. (1982) Ichthyophthiriasis: immersion immunization of rainbow trout (*Salmo gairdneri*) using *Tetrahymena thermophila* as a protective immunogen. *Canadian Journal of Fisheries and Aquatic Sciences* 39, 1772–1775.

Wright, A.D. and Lynn, D.H. (1995) Phylogeny of the fish parasite *Ichthyophthirius* and its relatives *Ophryoglena* and *Tetrahymena* (Ciliophora, Hymenostomatia) inferred from 18S ribosomal RNA sequences. *Molecular and Biological Evolution* 12, 285–290.

Wurtsbaugh, W.A. and Tapia, R.A. (1988) Mass mortality of fishes in Lake Titicaca (Peru–Bolivia) associated with the protozoan parasite *Ichthyophthirius multifiliis*. *Transactions of the American Fisheries Society* 117, 213–217.

Xu, D.H., Klesius, P.H. and Shelby, R.A. (2002) Cutaneous antibodies in excised skin from channel catfish, *Ictalurus puctatus* Rafinesque, immune to *Ichthyophthirius mutlfiliis*. *Journal of Fish Diseases* 25, 45–52.

Xu, D.H., Klesius, P.H. and Shelby, R.A. (2004) Immune responses and host protection of channel catfish, *Ictalurus punctatus* (Rafinesque), against *Ichthyophthirius multifiliis* after immunization with live theronts and sonicated trophonts. *Journal of Fish Diseases* 27, 135–141.

Xu, D.H., Klesius, P.H. and Shoemaker, C.A. (2008) Protective immunity of Nile tilapia against *Ichthyophthirius multifiliis* post-immunization with live theronts and sonicated trophonts. *Fish and Shellfish Immunology* 25, 124–127.

Xu, D.H., Klesius, P.H. and Shoemaker, C.A. (2009a) Effect of immunization of channel catfish with inactivated trophonts on serum and cutaneous antibody titers and survival against *Ichthyophthirius multifiliis*. *Fish and Shellfish Immunology* 26, 614–618.

Xu, D.H., Panangala, V.S., Van Santen, V.L., Dybvig, K., Abernathy, J.W. *et al.* (2009b) Molecular characteristics of an immobilization antigen gene of the fish-parasitic protozoan *Ichthyophthirius multifiliis* strain ars-6. *Aquaculture Research* 40, 1884–1892.

Xu, D.H., Zhang, D., Shoemaker, C. and Beck, B. (2019) Immune response of channel catfish (*Ictalurus punctatus*) against *Ichthyophthirius multifiliis* post vaccination using DNA vaccines encoding immobilization antigens. *Fish and Shellfish Immunology* 24, 308–317.

Xu, D.H., Zhang, D., Shoemaker, C. and Beck, B. (2020) Dose effects of a DNA vaccine encoding immobilization antigen on immune response of channel catfish against *Ichthyophthirius multifiliis*. *Fish and Shellfish Immunology* 106, 1031–1041.

Yang, H., Tu, X., Xiao, J., Hu, J. and Gu, Z. (2023) Investigations on white spot disease reveal high genetic diversity of the fish parasite, *Ichthyophthirius multifiliis* (Fouquet, 1876) in China. *Aquaculture* 562, 738804.

Zaila, K.E., Doak, T.G., Ellerbrock, H., Tung, C.-H., Martins, M.L. *et al.* (2017) Diversity and universality of endosymbiotic *Rickettsia* in the fish parasite *Ichthyophthirius multifiliis*. *Frontiers in Microbiology* 8, 189.

Zhang, Y.A., Salinas, I., Li, J., Parra, D., Bjork, S. *et al.* (2010) IgT, a primitive immunoglobulin class specialized in mucosal immunity. *Nature Immunology* 11, 827–835.

Zhao, F., Li, Y.-W., Pan, H.-J., Wu, S.-Q., Shi., C.-B. *et al.* (2013) Grass carp (*Ctenopharyngodon idella)* TRAF6 and TAK1: molecular cloning and expression analysis after *Ichthophthirius multifiliis* infection. *Fish and Shellfish Immunology* 34, 1514–1523.

Zhao, X., Findly, R.C. and Dickerson, H.W. (2008) Cutaneous antibody-secreting cells and B cells in a teleost fish. *Developmental and Comparative Immunology* 32, 500–508.

Zilberg, D. and Klesius, P.H. (1997) Quantification of immunoglobulin in the serum and mucus of channel catfish at different ages and following infection with *Edwardsiella ictaluri*. *Veterinary Immunology and Immunopathology* 58, 171–180.

5 *Perkinsus marinus* and *Haplosporidium nelsoni*

Ryan B. Carnegie*
Virginia Institute of Marine Science, William & Mary, Gloucester Point, Virginia, USA

Abstract
Perkinsus marinus and *Haplosporidium nelsoni* are parasitic protozoans which cause ecological and economically significant diseases in the eastern oyster, *Crassostrea virginica*. Both were described from the USA in the last century, *P. marinus* in the Gulf of Mexico and *H. nelsoni* along the mid-Atlantic coast, and both have been the subject of intensive study for over 65 years. This chapter reviews the biology and ecology of these pathogens, their detection, impacts on hosts, methods for control, and highlights the potential importance of the *P. marinus–H. nelsoni–C. virginica* system as a model for understanding the evolution of marine diseases.

5.1. Introduction

Perkinsus marinus and *Haplosporidium nelsoni* are the two most important pathogens of the eastern oyster (*Crassostrea virginica*) along the Atlantic and Gulf of Mexico coasts of the USA. *H. nelsoni*, a pathogen introduced from Asia, decimated oyster populations in the mid-Atlantic region in the 1950s (Andrews, 1966; Ford and Haskin, 1982); *P. marinus* has probably always been present along the south Atlantic and Gulf coasts, but prolonged drought conditions in the mid-Atlantic region in the late 1980s allowed the pathogen to increase in abundance and expand its range into areas where low salinity had previously prevented its occurrence (Burreson and Ragone Calvo, 1996; Ford, 1996; Ford and Smolowitz, 2007). These two pathogens have devastated ecologically and commercially important oyster populations as far north as New England and Nova Scotia, Canada, but especially in Chesapeake Bay and Delaware Bay. *P. marinus* is the primary pathogen of *C. virginica* in the Gulf of Mexico (Soniat, 1996), where *H. nelsoni* is absent.

5.1.1. *Perkinsus marinus*

P. marinus, a Dinozoa, is in the family Perkinsidae. It is primarily a parasite of the eastern oyster *C. virginica*, occurring in eastern oyster populations throughout the Gulf of Mexico and along the Atlantic coast from Florida to Maine (Burreson *et al.*, 1994; Ford and Smolowitz, 2007). It also infects additional hosts including the pleasure oyster (*Crassostrea corteziensis*) and the palmate oyster (*Saccostrea palmula*) on the Pacific coast of

*Email: carnegie@vims.edu

DOI: 10.1079/9781800628748.0005

Mexico (Cáceres-Martínez *et al.*, 2008, 2012), and the mangrove cupped oyster (*Crassostrea rhizophorae*) on the coast of Brazil (da Silva *et al.*, 2013). Geographical distribution and seasonal cycle are controlled by temperature, with the parasite proliferating most rapidly at water temperatures over 25°C (Andrews, 1965). Local distribution is mainly controlled by salinity. *P. marinus* is most pathogenic at salinity greater than 12 ppt, but it can survive in its host at salinities as low as 1 or 2 ppt for extended periods (Ragone Calvo and Burreson, 1993).

P. marinus cells are generally 2–10 μm in diameter, spherical in shape, and characterized by a single nucleus displaced to the cell margin by a large vacuole (Fig. 5.1). Parasites occur in the connective tissue of all organs and in the gut epithelium. *P. marinus* cells are released from the host in faeces or upon death and decomposition of the host. Transmission is direct from oyster to oyster (Chu, 1996) and occurs primarily at the time of maximum host mortality (Ragone Calvo *et al.*, 2003b). Thus, oysters become infected in the autumn and host mortality peaks in August/September 1 or 2 years later, concurrent with maximum infection prevalence and intensity. The portal of entry is not well understood, but it may be via the gut with infection facilitated by host haemocytes that phagocytose the parasite in the gut lumen and carry it across the gut epithelium (Alvarez *et al.*, 1992). *P. marinus* cells are often phagocytosed by host haemocytes, but they survive and multiply within haemocytes, eventually causing the host cell to burst, releasing parasites into the tissue, where the phagocytosis/multiplication/cell death cycle is repeated. Within the host, *P. marinus* cells are spread in host haemocytes via the haemolymph.

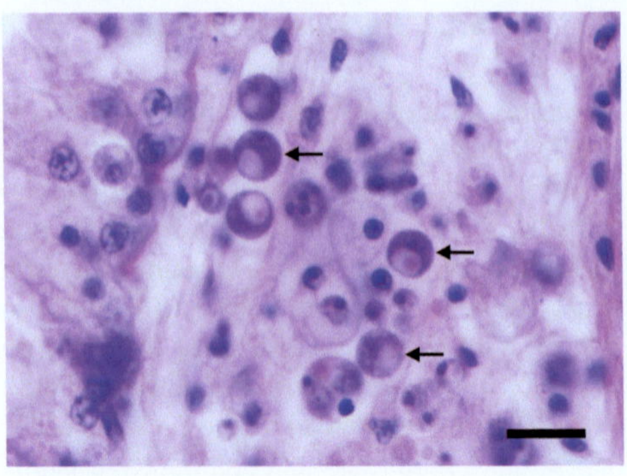

Fig. 5.1. *Perkinsus marinus* cells (arrows) showing vacuole and displaced nucleus with prominent nucleolus. Paraffin histology; bar = 10 μm. (Author's own image.)

5.1.2. *Haplosporidium nelsoni*

H. nelsoni is a member of the phylum Cercozoa, family Haplosporidiidae, which is characterized by spores with an orifice covered by an external lid or internal flange of wall material. The phylum consists of only four genera and about 40 species but contains a number of important pathogens of molluscs. *H. nelsoni* infects the Pacific oyster (*Crassostrea gigas*) in Asia, Europe and the west coast of the USA, and *C. virginica* along the east coast of North America from Florida to Nova Scotia, Canada; it is absent from the Gulf of Mexico. Initial observations of the multinucleate plasmodia in oysters from Delaware Bay in 1957 led to the acronym 'MSX' for Multinucleate Sphere X (unknown). The parasite was not formally described until 9 years after its discovery (Haskin *et al.*, 1966), and the MSX acronym was ingrained in the literature in the interim.

Unlike *P. marinus*, *H. nelsoni* is very sensitive to salinity below 10 ppt where it is eliminated from oysters after about 10 days at temperatures above 20°C (Andrews, 1983; Ford, 1985; Ford and Haskin, 1988). It survives at salinities above 10 ppt, but it is only seriously pathogenic at salinities above 12–15 ppt. Thus, significant oyster mortality occurs primarily in the higher-salinity portions of major east coast estuaries and in coastal bays.

H. nelsoni has two life stages: (i) multinucleate plasmodia; and (ii) spores. Plasmodia (Fig. 5.2a and b) occur in the connective tissue or epithelium of all tissues and range from 5 to over 50 μm in diameter. They may contain 30 nuclei or more. Sporulation occurs only in digestive tubule epithelium (Fig. 5.3a) and primarily in first-year oysters less than 30 mm in shell height (Barber *et al.*, 1991; Burreson, 1994). Spores are about 7 μm in length with an external lid covering the spore orifice (Fig. 5.3b). The complete life cycle of *H. nelsoni* is unknown. Direct transmission trials with both plasmodia and spores have been unsuccessful, and the suspected intermediate host has not been identified (Haskin and Andrews, 1988). Based on

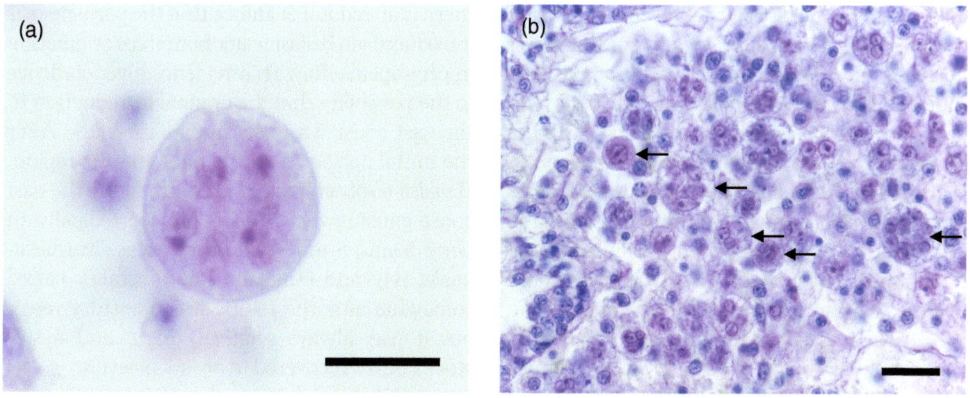

Fig. 5.2. *Haplosporidium nelsoni* multinucleate plasmodia. (a) Plasmodium in oyster haemolymph. Paraffin histology; bar = 10 μm. (b) Plasmodia (arrows) in gill connective tissue, surrounded by oyster haemocytes. Note diverse appearance, in shape and size, of parasite nuclei. Paraffin histology; bar = 20 μm. (Author's own image.)

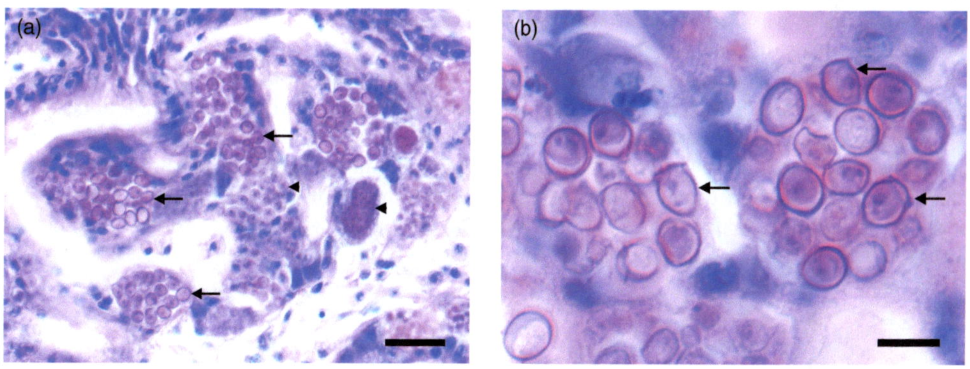

Fig. 5.3. *Haplosporidium nelsoni* spores. (a) Digestive gland tubule with several sporocysts, some with mature spores (arrows), others in earlier stages of development (arrowheads). Paraffin histology; bar = 20 μm. (b) Mature spores, with lid covering operculum apparent in some (arrows). Paraffin histology; bar = 10 μm. (Author's own image.)

evidence from sentinel oysters deployed in spring, oysters become infected as water temperature rises above 17°C; the infection period continues through the summer. Initial infections are in the palp or gill epithelium, but the actual mechanism of infection is unknown. Infections develop rapidly, with peak oyster mortality in early August only about 3 months after infection (Andrews, 1966). Sporulation can occur at any time of year. Spores are released in faeces or upon death and decomposition of the host; fate of spores in the environment is unknown.

5.1.3. Impact of the diseases on oyster production

P. marinus was first observed in oysters in the Gulf of Mexico after reports of significant oyster mortality that was blamed on the oil industry (Andrews, 1988). However, subsequent reports of *P. marinus*-related oyster mortality in Chesapeake Bay, where there is no oil industry, led to the conclusion that this parasite and not the oil industry was the cause of mortality in the Gulf of Mexico. Historically, *P. marinus* has caused significant oyster mortality in the Gulf of

Mexico and in Chesapeake Bay, especially during drought years. In Chesapeake Bay annual oyster mortality from *P. marinus* averaged about 20% prior to 1985, and this was manageable by industry (Andrews, 1988). Disaster struck in the 1950s with catastrophic oyster mortality from *H. nelsoni* in Delaware Bay beginning in 1957 and in Chesapeake Bay beginning in 1959 (Fig. 5.4). Within a few years 95% of the oyster populations were lost in high-salinity areas of both estuaries (Andrews, 1966; Ford and Haskin, 1982). There is compelling evidence from molecular studies that *H. nelsoni* is an introduced pathogen (Burreson *et al.*, 2000). *H. nelsoni* is a natural parasite of the Pacific oyster (*C. gigas*) in Asia, where it is not a significant pathogen because prevalence is very low. The parasite was introduced to California with importation of juvenile *C. gigas* from Japan over an 80-year period beginning in 1902 (Friedman, 1996). Exactly how the parasite was introduced to the east coast of the USA is unclear, but there were importations of *C. gigas* from Asia or the west coast of the USA beginning in the 1930s (Burreson *et al.*, 2000). However, a ballast water introduction cannot be ruled out as there was much shipping traffic between Asia and the east coast of the USA during and after World War II. *H. nelsoni* appeared in Nova Scotia, Canada in 2002, and there is anecdotal evidence that the parasite was introduced via ballast water from ships originating in Chesapeake Bay. This evidence gives credence to the possibility that the original introduction to the east coast was also via ballast water. After the initial epizootics in the mid-Atlantic region, *H. nelsoni* spread north and south along the east coast causing oyster mortality periodically in Long Island Sound and other areas. In Chesapeake Bay and Delaware Bay mortality varied somewhat after the 1960s due to wet/dry years, but it was always relatively high, and oyster stocks never recovered to pre-MSX levels.

In Chesapeake Bay the 1970s were relatively wet years and disease pressure abated somewhat (Fig. 5.4). 1980 and 1981 were very dry and *H. nelsoni* intensified again. Consecutive drought years from 1985 to 1988 along the US east coast, with concomitant salinity increase, coupled with warm winters, allowed *H. nelsoni* to increase in abundance and to move up estuaries into naïve oyster populations. However, perhaps more important, the drought caused a similar increase in the abundance and distribution of *P. marinus*. Prior to the late 1980s *P. marinus* was not known to occur in the upper Chesapeake Bay or north of the mouth of Chesapeake Bay along the east coast. Drought conditions, with concomitant warm winters, provided

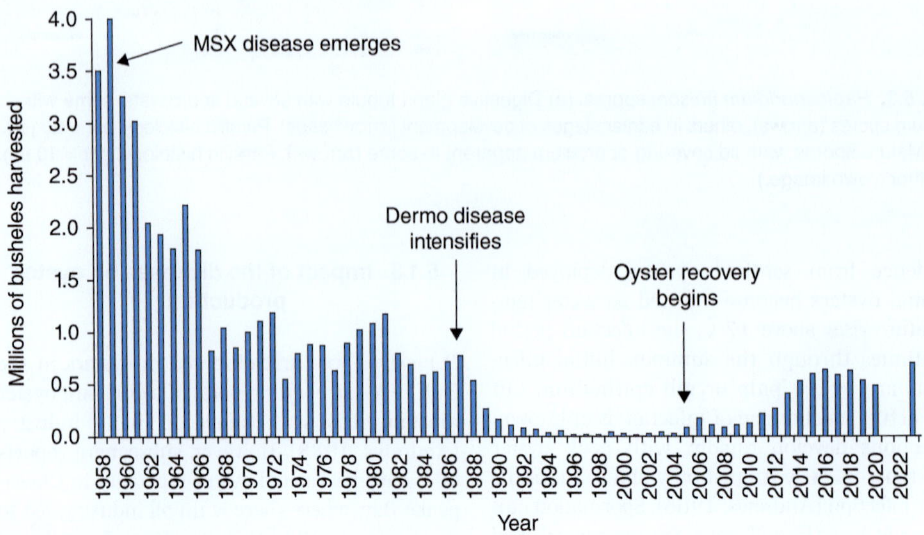

Fig. 5.4. Annual oyster harvest in Virginia, 1958–2023. (Data courtesy of the Virginia Marine Resources Commission.)

favourable conditions for *P. marinus* and the parasite spread throughout Chesapeake Bay and north into Delaware Bay, either naturally or by intentional movement of oysters. Oyster populations in these areas were naïve to *P. marinus* and mortality was high (Burreson and Ragone Calvo, 1996). Because *P. marinus* is tolerant of low salinity the parasite was not affected when climate conditions returned to normal and it continues to cause significant mortality throughout its range during dry years. Along with overharvesting and habitat degradation, the combination of *P. marinus* and *H. nelsoni* has reduced oyster populations to about 1% of what they were in the 1940s in both Delaware Bay and Chesapeake Bay, though they have begun to recover in recent years (Fig. 5.4).

5.2. Pathobiology

5.2.1. *Perkinsus marinus* detection

There are no clinical signs that are diagnostic for *P. marinus*. The pathogen causes a warm-season general wasting disease resulting in oysters with thin, watery tissue (Fig. 5.5a); however, this syndrome can also be caused by other pathogens or conditions.

The preferred diagnostic technique depends on the purpose of the study. For routine surveillance, where *P. marinus* is the only common species of *Perkinsus* in an area, Ray's fluid thioglycollate medium (RFTM) culture assay is the method of choice (Ray, 1966a). This technique is not species specific, but it is sensitive, inexpensive and relatively fast. Briefly, infected oyster tissue is cultured for 5 days in the culture medium with antibiotics, macerated on a glass slide, stained with Lugol's iodine and examined using a compound microscope. *P. marinus* cells appear as blue-black spheres (Fig. 5.5b). Histopathological analysis is also acceptable, but it is less sensitive than RFTM diagnosis and may miss low-intensity infections. In histopathology, *P. marinus* cells are spherical with a large vacuole that displaces the nucleus to the margin of the cell (Fig. 5.1). Species-specific molecular diagnostics, conventional and quantitative PCR protocols (Audemard *et al.*, 2004; Gauthier *et al.*, 2006; De Faveri *et al.*, 2009) and *in situ* hybridization assays (Reece *et al.*, 2008) have been developed to detect *P. marinus*, and these are useful for confirming species identification, myriad research applications, and aquaculture biosecurity applications in which the PCR assays in particular are widely used. The preferred PCR assays, both conventional and quantitative, target the internal transcribed spacer (ITS) region of the ribosomal RNA gene complex, which is well characterized across *Perkinsus* species. The *in situ* hybridization assay targets the large-subunit (LSU) ribosomal RNA distributed on ribosomes in the parasite cell cytoplasm.

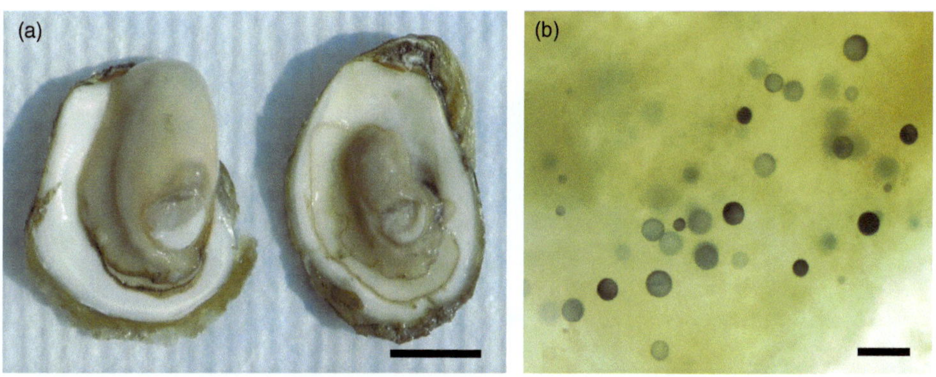

Fig. 5.5. Diagnosis of *Perkinsus marinus* infections. (a) Healthy oyster on the left, compared with watery, thin tissue of emaciated oyster on the right, often typical of *P. marinus* infection. Bar = 30 mm. (b) Diagnosis by RFTM. *P. marinus* cells typically appear as black spheres when stained with Lugol's iodine. Bar = 20 μm. (Author's own image.)

5.2.2. *Haplosporidium nelsoni* detection

There are no reliable clinical signs for diagnosis of *H. nelsoni* as mortality is so rapid, usually 2–3 months after infection, that dead oysters can appear otherwise healthy. This is unlike the wasting disease often associated with *P. marinus*.

Histopathological analysis has long been the preferred method for diagnosis of *H. nelsoni* because it allows determination of life-cycle stages and host reactions. The presence of ~7 µm-long spores restricted to the epithelium of the digestive diverticula (Fig. 5.3a) is diagnostic for *H. nelsoni*. If spores are absent and only multinucleate plasmodia are present, diagnosis using histology can be problematic because plasmodia of all haplosporidians are similar and there is one other species, *Haplosporidium costale*, which partially overlaps in distribution with *H. nelsoni*. Both species are present in high-salinity coastal bays where salinity is greater than about 25 ppt and mixed plasmodial infections of the two species have been reported (Stokes and Burreson, 2001). If spores are present the two species are readily distinguishable by location of sporulation: (i) epithelium of the digestive diverticula in *H. nelsoni*; and (ii) throughout the visceral connective tissue in *H. costale*. In addition, spores of *H. costale* (about 4 µm in length) are much smaller than those of *H. nelsoni*. In major estuaries such as Delaware Bay and Chesapeake Bay, where salinity is less than about 25 ppt, *H. costale* is absent, so the presence of plasmodia in these areas can reliably be attributed to *H. nelsoni*. DNA-based diagnostic techniques, both PCR and *in situ* hybridization assays, are available for *H. nelsoni* and *H. costale* (Stokes *et al.*, 1995; Stokes and Burreson, 1995, 2001; Wilbur *et al.*, 2012; Piesz *et al.*, 2022), so histopathological identification can be confirmed using these molecular techniques. PCR assays target small-subunit (SSU) ribosomal genes, and the *in situ* hybridization assay targets SSU ribosomal RNA expressed in parasite cell ribosomes as for *P. marinus*.

5.2.3. Internal lesions

There are no external lesions on the mantle or gill surface of oysters infected with either *P. marinus* or *H. nelsoni*. Internally, *P. marinus* can cause significant disruption of the stomach or intestine epithelium architecture, which probably interferes with digestion (Fig. 5.6a), and also focal lesions in the vesicular connective tissue and/or gonad (Fig. 5.6b). Host haemocyte accumulation in the infected region (haemocytosis) is common with both pathogens (Fig. 5.6b), and *P. marinus* cells are readily phagocytosed by host haemocytes, although they are not killed. There is little phagocytosis of *H. nelsoni*

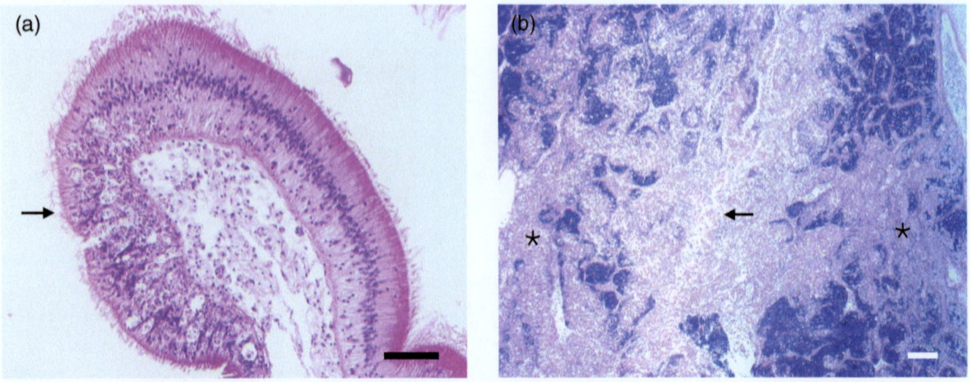

Fig. 5.6. Lesions caused by *Perkinsus marinus* in oyster tissue. (a) Stomach epithelium architecture destroyed (arrow) by proliferation of *P. marinus* cells. Note the contrast with normal epithelium to the right of the image. Paraffin histology; bar = 50 µm. (b) Massive lesion in male gonad, the darkly basophilic masses at the margin of the image being mature sperm. Note the areas of heavy proliferation of *P. marinus* cells and infiltration of oyster haemocytes (asterisks), with a broad area of necrosis (arrow) at the centre. Paraffin histology; bar = 200 µm. (Author's own image.)

plasmodia, probably because they are as large as or larger than the host haemocytes. The large size of *H. nelsoni* plasmodia causes mechanical disruption of tissues and metaplasia of infected epithelium.

5.2.4. *Perkinsus marinus* pathophysiology

As noted above, parasitism by *P. marinus* produces a wasting disease in *C. virginica*. Initial infections seem to occur primarily in digestive tract epithelia and may occur anywhere from the stomach of an oyster to its rectum. Lytic secretions of *P. marinus* cells disrupt columnar epithelial tissues, an effect that is compounded by infiltrating haemocytes (Mackin, 1951). As an infection progresses the epithelial pathology becomes more extensive, and consequently, epithelial contributions to digestion and nutrition are increasingly compromised. In healthy oysters contributions by the epithelium include: (i) the sorting of food particles in the stomach, to ensure that only the smallest particles enter the ducts of the digestive diverticula; (ii) mixing of particles with digestive enzymes in the stomach; and (iii) enzymatic digestion and nutrient absorption in the mid-gut and rectum (Langdon and Newell, 1996). Parasite sequestration of nutrients, of course, further impacts oyster nutrition (Choi *et al.*, 1989). Even light infections reduce growth (Menzel and Hopkins, 1955), so infections that are primarily epithelial may none the less have energetic costs. Heavier infections bring more serious reductions in growth and in reproductive output. Paynter and Burreson (1991) observed that *P. marinus* infections in waters of moderate salinity (12–15 ppt) reduced oyster growth by 60%. In waters of higher salinity (16–20 ppt), growth was reduced by 80%. Adverse effects on reproduction are focused primarily on late gametogenesis in the spring and early summer and include a reduction in fecundity but not egg size or quality. Kennedy *et al.* (1995) found no decrease in oocyte diameters or lipid investments with increasing *P. marinus* infection intensity, but they did observe a decrease in 'reproductive index' (calculated as the average gonad width ÷ body area × 100). Even moderate infections reduced the reproductive index by half. Dittman *et al.* (2001) similarly found that gonadal indices (defined as 'the proportion of the cross-sectional visceral mass area occupied by the gonad'), condition index and the percentage of gametogenic tissue decreased with increasing intensity of *P. marinus* infection. The heaviest infections in an oyster population nearing peak gametogenic development reduced: (i) the mean gonadal index by more than half; (ii) the mean condition index by a third; and (iii) the mean percentage of gametogenic tissue by two-thirds. Our own observations are that the most intense early-season infections can entirely abolish reproduction.

Interestingly, *P. marinus* infection in one season, provided it is not so intense as to be lethal, does not significantly limit oyster reproduction the next summer. Even when infection reduces the winter glycogen storage that would normally fuel gametogenesis in the spring, such compromised oysters may instead rely on energy assimilated from feeding on the spring phytoplankton bloom to produce gametes (Kennedy *et al.*, 1995; Dittman *et al.*, 2001).

In oysters that are unable to resist *P. marinus*, parasite cells breach the basement membrane of the epithelium and reach the connective tissues and haemolymph spaces, thus allowing infections to become systemic. As *P. marinus* numbers increase in connective tissues, parasite proteases produce widening areas of host tissue liquefaction. Haemocytosis continues, but haemocytes are unable to destroy phagocytosed parasite cells, and rupture from the proliferation of the parasite. Haemocytes, parasite cells and debris can occlude haemolymph vessels and impede circulation (Mackin, 1951). This pathology probably combines with nutrient depletion, which ultimately causes death (Ford and Tripp, 1996).

It is not known if oysters with advanced systemic infections recover. Some do recover from more serious epithelial infections, as indicated by healing epithelium observed in some oysters examined in late winter. Such individuals may have been saved by falling water temperatures in autumn: *P. marinus* is most lethal at water temperatures greater than 25°C, and below 15–20°C the metabolic rate of *P. marinus* is reduced (Chu and La Peyre, 1993; Ford and Tripp, 1996). None the less, it is clear that many oysters, while lightly infected, can resist *P. marinus* proliferation and disease for years. The nature of this resistance remains unclear. Significant lytic activity is a hallmark of *P. marinus* infection (Mackin, 1951), and serine proteases secreted by *P. marinus* are key agents of this lysis (La Peyre *et al.*, 1995). They may suppress oyster haemocyte migration, lysozyme activity and agglutination (Garreis *et al.*, 1996). *C. virginica* counters parasite proteolytic activity by having protease inhibitors in its plasma (Oliver *et al.*, 1999; Xue *et al.*, 2006, 2009). General protease inhibition (Oliver *et al.*, 2000) and expression and activity of a specific inhibitory protein (La Peyre *et al.*, 2010) are higher in oysters selectively bred for *P. marinus* resistance, which indicates that these proteins may play an important role in suppressing parasite multiplication. *P. marinus* may also be capable of modulating, or interfering with, the production of reactive oxygen species by oyster haemocytes (Anderson, 1999). Resisting superoxide and hydrogen peroxide that have been produced (Schott *et al.*, 2003) may be a key to parasite survival in haemocytes after phagocytosis. Variation among oysters in ability to counter this activity may also contribute to variation in resistance to *P. marinus* but this has not been studied.

5.2.5. *Haplosporidium nelsoni* pathophysiology

Unlike the more chronic *P. marinus* infections, *H. nelsoni* infections are typically acute. *H. nelsoni*-caused mortality in a susceptible oyster population may exceed 60% within just 3 months of parasite exposure (Ragone Calvo *et al.*, 2003b). The parasite first colonizes gill epithelium, or occasionally gut epithelium, of the oyster (Ford and Haskin, 1982). The host haemocyte response to focal infection of the gills by *H. nelsoni* plasmodia is often intense (Ford and Tripp, 1996) and typically exceeds the response to similar numbers of *P. marinus* infecting gut epithelium. Haemocytes infiltrating gill tissues can be so numerous that the fine plical architecture of a normal oyster gill is obliterated. Systemic *H. nelsoni* infections reduce oyster clearance rates and condition, the latter of which is directly proportional to the amount of glycogen stored in tissues and partly a product of feeding. These reductions have been attributed to impairment of ciliary function in affected gills (Newell, 1985). Focal to multifocal epithelial infections, which were not studied by Newell (1985), presumably cause similar impairment and physiological effects. Barber *et al.* (1988a) found that gill epithelial infection by *H. nelsoni* reduced the oyster condition index by 13% and fecundity by 35% relative to uninfected oysters. Glycogen in oyster tissues was reduced by 22% (Barber *et al.*, 1988b).

H. nelsoni-resistant oysters, if they become infected at all, can contain the parasite within gill epithelia. In more susceptible oysters *H. nelsoni* penetrates the base of the epithelium and colonizes connective tissues to become systemic. As *H. nelsoni* proliferates in connective tissues and reaches the digestive diverticula, physical damage can include 'mechanical disruption and lysis of tissues ... metaplasia of digestive tubule epithelium, and fibrosis' (Ford and Tripp, 1996). Physiological consequences deepen, with condition index, fecundity and glycogen reduced more sharply (Barber *et al.*, 1988a,b), and with protein levels also depressed in haemolymph (Ford, 1986) and tissues (Barber *et al.*, 1988b). Death is probably caused by the impact of *H. nelsoni* on the metabolic condition of the host. The most susceptible oysters, however, die so quickly that significant pathology and reduction in metabolic condition may not be obvious. This has prompted speculation that a parasite toxin may contribute to mortality (Ford and Tripp, 1996).

5.3. Protection

Adaptive immunity is not known in oysters or other molluscs, so they cannot be immunized against either *P. marinus* or *H. nelsoni*. The primary means of protection against these pathogens is selective breeding. As early as the 1960s, scientists working with *H. nelsoni* in Delaware Bay began observing increased resistance to *H. nelsoni* parasitism produced from survivors of earlier outbreaks (Haskin and Ford, 1979). These positive results justified investment in breeding programmes for *H. nelsoni* resistance, and aquaculturists in the mid-Atlantic region of the USA continue to cultivate descendants of these early disease-resistant strains. Since the 1980s, resistance to *P. marinus* has also been incorporated into breeding programmes (Ragone Calvo *et al.*, 2003a; Allen *et al.*, 2021). Genetic resistance does not confer complete protection: some oysters will still develop *H. nelsoni* infections, and most will become infected by *P. marinus* in parasite-enzootic waters. None the less, fewer infections develop to lethal intensities, and because resistant oysters have also been selected for rapid growth, enough oysters survive to marketable size for oyster aquaculture to be profitable despite disease.

Promotion of genetic resistance to disease is now being applied to the management and restoration of wild oyster populations. While lower salinities in upper parts of estuaries provide some mitigation of parasitism, infection pressure on wild oyster populations in higher-salinity waters must be intense. Decades of this pressure have produced more resistant oyster populations. This is especially clear with respect to *H. nelsoni*. In Delaware Bay, major epizootics swept the estuary, purging the most susceptible oysters from the population. Today the parasite is rarely observed histologically, even though PCR data indicate it remains abundant in the environment (Ford *et al.*, 2009). In Chesapeake Bay, a long-term study (1960 to the present) of naïve sentinel oysters annually deployed to the *H. nelsoni*- and *P. marinus*-enzootic York River reveals *H. nelsoni* levels to be relatively high, yet levels in wild oysters have been declining (Carnegie and Burreson, 2011) (Fig. 5.7), an indication that Chesapeake Bay populations too are increasingly resistant. Resistance to *P. marinus* has been slower to develop, for reasons that are not obvious. Despite continued intense disease caused by *P. marinus* in particular, oyster populations have rebounded across much of Chesapeake Bay, particularly where they have been protected from harvest (Schulte *et al.*, 2009). In light of these observations, protection of brood stock oysters in sanctuaries from harvest is being incorporated into management plans for the Chesapeake Bay oyster population. It is hoped that these sanctuaries will maximize the possibility that resistant oysters will reproduce, pass on their genes and thus improve the resistance of the population.

Pathogen control through interference with parasite life cycles or transmission was once reasonably effective for *P. marinus*, which has a simple, direct life cycle. In the 1950s, a distance

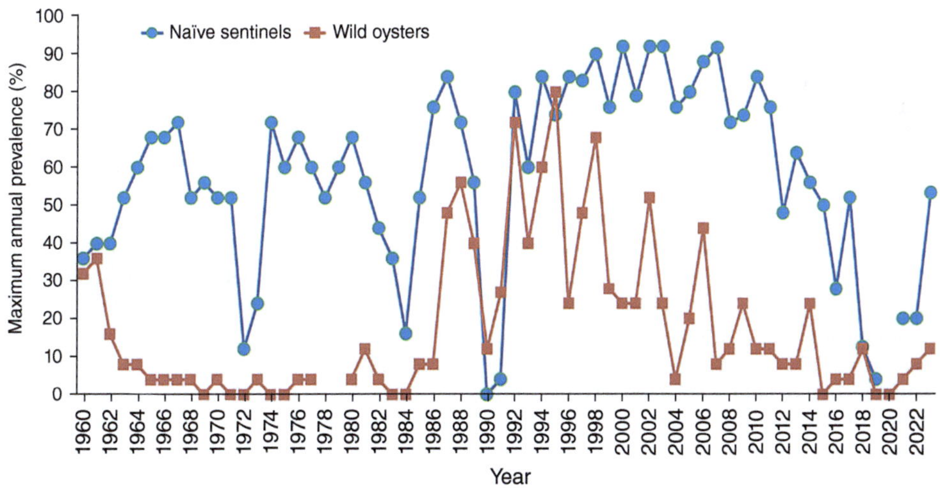

Fig. 5.7. Maximum annual prevalence of *Haplosporidium nelsoni* in naïve sentinel oysters deployed each spring to the *H. nelsoni*-enzootic York River, Virginia, USA, and in wild oysters from Wreck Shoal, an *H. nelsoni*-enzootic reef in the nearby James River. After colonizing Wreck Shoal during the initial epizootic in the 1960s, *H. nelsoni* was generally absent from Wreck Shoal until the droughts of the 1980s. Oysters at Wreck Shoal have become increasingly resistant to *H. nelsoni* since the mid-1990s. The recent (2012–2022) decrease in maximum *H. nelsoni* prevalence in the sentinels is unlikely to be due to reduced salinities but may be due to changes in the distribution or abundance of an intermediate host. (Author's own image.)

of 40–50 ft (12–15 m) from sources of *P. marinus* accomplished a reduction in transmission efficiency (Andrews, 1965). Culturists planting small oysters, called seed, extensively on Chesapeake Bay bottom were advised to avoid foci of infection like natural reefs and pilings, and to intensively clean and then fallow beds before planting new seed to slow recolonization by *P. marinus*. With intensification of *P. marinus* parasitism in the 1980s (Burreson and Andrews, 1988; Burreson and Ragone Calvo, 1996) came a great increase in *P. marinus* abundance, and dispersal distances are now in kilometres (McCollough *et al.*, 2007). Control of *P. marinus* infections by reducing transmission in this manner is no longer practical.

The unresolved life cycle of *H. nelsoni* limits options for its control. The environmental source of this parasite remains a mystery. Manipulating oyster densities and fallowing beds yield no benefit for management. The absence of a relationship between oyster population size and location and *H. nelsoni* infection pressure remains key evidence pointing towards the existence of an intermediate host for this parasite (Haskin and Andrews, 1988).

Neither *P. marinus* nor *H. nelsoni* is fully pathogenic at salinities below 10 ppt. The former can withstand long periods of lower salinity, but its disease impact on oyster hosts is reduced. The latter is intolerant of even short periods of salinity below 10 ppt, which may purge it from estuarine systems (Ford and Tripp, 1996). Establishing aquaculture farms in waters of relatively lower salinity reduces parasite effects, but lower salinities also reduce the growth rate of *C. virginica* (Shumway, 1996), and very low salinities produced by serious floods that periodically affect these areas can kill oysters (Galtsoff, 1964). For these reasons and also because oysters are more flavourful when bred in more saline waters, this strategy of disease mitigation is not widely pursued.

Immersion of *C. virginica* for short periods (e.g. 2 weeks) in water of low salinity (below 10 ppt) does have potential for treatment of *H. nelsoni* infections (Ford, 1992). While use of disease-resistant seed has largely obviated such strategies in aquaculture, even resistant seed is occasionally found to harbour *H. nelsoni* at 10–20% prevalence. Eventual mortality due to *H. nelsoni* parasitism may be avoided by the immersion method. Such treatment would not be effective for *P. marinus* infections, however, as even longer periods at lower salinities (e.g. 8 weeks at 6 ppt; Ragone Calvo and Burreson, 1993) have not been shown to reduce infection.

The nature and scale of oyster aquaculture, with oysters maintained in large arrays of cages or floats in open waters, does not lend itself to the use of chemotherapeutants. Application of chemicals to oysters in wild populations is out of the question. None the less, chemotherapeutants may have utility in small, closed systems, where seed or valuable brood stock are being held. *P. marinus* was originally thought to have fungal affinities, so the earliest study of chemotherapeutant potential focused on the antimycotic cycloheximide. It suppressed *P. marinus* infections and extended the lives of infected oysters, but parasite proliferation resumed when cycloheximide treatment was discontinued (Ray, 1966b). Subsequent research produced similar findings with cycloheximide, but found other anticoccidial compounds (amprolium, malachite green and sulfadimethoxine) to be ineffective (Calvo and Burreson, 1994). Antibiotics bacitracin (Faisal *et al.*, 1999) and triclosan (Chu *et al.*, 2008) have been shown to slow the proliferation of *P. marinus* in oyster tissues.

5.4. Conclusions and Suggestions for Future Research

P. marinus and *H. nelsoni* are as relevant today as they ever have been. There are two reasons for this. The first is our continued inability to effectively control these pathogens, genetic progress notwithstanding. In drought years, even relatively resistant oyster populations may be seriously impacted by *H. nelsoni* parasitism, and annual mortality due to *P. marinus* can exceed 70% (Mann *et al.*, 2009). The second is our renewed interest in oysters. As keystone estuarine species by virtue of their role in benthic–pelagic coupling and the habitat their reefs provide, they are recognized as essential to the ecological restoration of many coastal ecosystems in the eastern and southern USA (Coen *et al.*, 2007). Because of their potential as aquaculture species, which is already being realized in places, we expect them to be central to the economic restoration of many coastal communities. Many of these communities have been in decline since the collapse of oyster and other fisheries decades ago. Diseases caused by *H. nelsoni* and *P. marinus* loom as major impediments to both types of restoration.

Critical gaps in our understanding of these pathogens remain. The most obvious is the *H. nelsoni* life cycle. Resolving the life cycle of *H. nelsoni* may explain the 'irregular' and generally low activity of *H. nelsoni* in polyhaline coastal lagoons (Andrews and Castagna, 1978) and the continued absence of *H. nelsoni* from the Gulf of Mexico coast. It may allow the development of biosecurity guidelines to help ensure that the latter remains the case.

More generally, an understanding of the molecular and cellular bases of pathogenesis is non-existent for *H. nelsoni*, and nearly so in *P. marinus*. Genes and proteins such as the natural resistance-associated macrophage protein (Nramp) and superoxide dismutases that may relate to intrahaemocytic survival of *P. marinus* have begun to be characterized (e.g. Robledo *et al.*, 2004; Fernández-Robledo *et al.*, 2008), but questions remain as to how these molecules relate to observed variability in parasite virulence (Bushek and Allen, 1996). Our appreciation of the potential interplay between *P. marinus* proteases and the protease inhibitors expressed by *C. virginica* is only marginally more advanced (see references above). Further work to characterize these molecules and others integral to host–parasite interactions and pathogenesis will be beneficial. This work should extend to a characterization of genetic diversity and to the relative roles of genetics and environmental influences in determining disease outcomes. We may hope that biomarkers for oyster resistance can be identified for use in oyster breeding programmes. Biomarkers for parasite virulence may eventually be used to gauge disease risk.

Finally, we should embrace the view of interactions of *C. virginica* and its parasites as dynamic, not static, and attempt to understand the nature and causes of this dynamism. The great intensification of oyster disease in Chesapeake Bay, especially that caused by *P. marinus*, in the mid-1980s is perhaps the most striking example (Burreson and Andrews, 1988). Others include: (i) the cycling of *P. marinus* in the Gulf of Mexico in connection with El Niño–Southern Oscillation cycles (Soniat *et al.*, 2005); (ii) the progression of *P. marinus* northward from Chesapeake Bay beginning in 1990 (Ford, 1996); and (iii) the decline of *H. nelsoni* impacts in the mid-Atlantic, especially notable in Delaware Bay (Ford *et al.*, 2009). While climate impacts are clearly at work, other influences must be considered. The generally increasing *H. nelsoni* pressure in Chesapeake Bay (Fig. 5.7) suggests an environment increasingly favourable for this parasite. While this may be partly attributable to increasingly milder winter water temperatures (Preston, 2004), it is also the case that a more eutrophic Chesapeake Bay (Kemp *et al.*, 2005) has seen changes in benthic community structure, with smaller, short-lived, opportunistic species of various phyla increasingly favoured (Holland *et al.*, 1987; Long and Seitz, 2009). One of the opportunistic species that has increased in abundance may be the intermediate host for *H. nelsoni*.

In viewing the oyster–parasite system as dynamic, we should also strive to understand the evolutionary forces shaping it. In the Gulf of Mexico, *P. marinus* and *C. virginica* must each act as agents of selection upon the other. In the Atlantic, *H. nelsoni* joins the system, interacting not only with *C. virginica* but, presumably, competing with *P. marinus* as well (Fig. 5.8). How

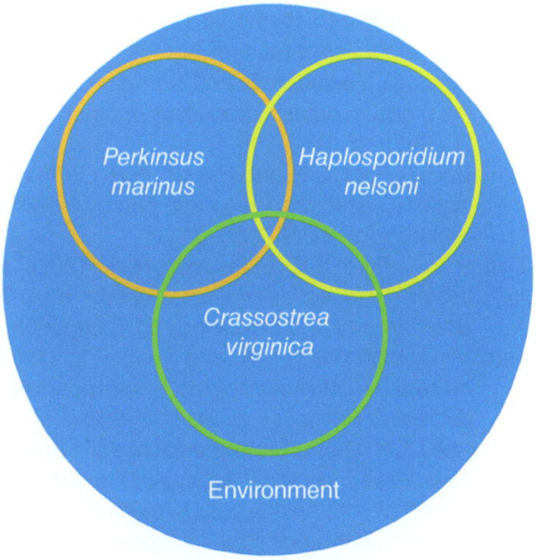

Fig. 5.8. Venn diagram illustrating interactions among oyster host *Crassostrea virginica* and parasites *Haplosporidium nelsoni* and *Perkinsus marinus*, with the environment influencing the entire system. (Author's own image.)

selection operates in this system needs to be studied as it has relevance to considerations of host resistance versus susceptibility, and pathogen virulence. We may hypothesize, for example, that decreasing *H. nelsoni* levels in wild oysters (Ford *et al.*, 2009) are a result of parasite-imposed selection for increasing disease resistance. More intriguing is the possibility that *H. nelsoni* may have acted as an agent of selection upon *P. marinus*: as hypothesized by Carnegie *et al.* (2021), selecting for increased virulence in *P. marinus* as a strategy for ensuring transmission from oysters decreased in longevity and density by introduced *H. nelsoni*. Gene flow (dispersal of host and parasite genotypes) is important, and so is genetic drift: *P. marinus* abundance contracts to very low levels, particularly at more northern latitudes, in the spring, when it becomes nearly undetectable in oysters (Burreson and Ragone Calvo, 1996). Marrying an evolutionary approach to understanding *C. virginica–P. marinus–H. nelsoni* interactions to the basic molecular and cellular pathobiology would be a most interesting and important direction for future research.

References

Allen, S.K. Jr, Small, J.M. and Kube, P.D. (2021) Genetic parameters for *Crassostrea virginica* and their application to family-based breeding in the mid-Atlantic, USA. *Aquaculture* 538, 736578.

Alvarez, M.R., Friedl, F.E., Hudson, C.M. and O'Neill, R.L. (1992) Uptake and tissue distribution of abiotic particles from the alimentary tract of the American oyster: a simulation of intracellular parasitism. *Journal of Invertebrate Pathology* 59, 290–294.

Anderson, R.S. (1999) *Perkinsus marinus* secretory products modulate superoxide anion production by oyster (*Crassostrea virginica*) haemocytes. *Fish and Shellfish Immunology* 9, 51–60.

Andrews, J.D. (1965) Infection experiments in nature with *Dermocystidium marinum* in Chesapeake Bay. *Chesapeake Science* 6, 60–67.

Andrews, J.D. (1966) Oyster mortality studies in Virginia. V. Epizootiology of MSX, a protistan pathogen of oysters. *Ecology* 47, 19–31.

Andrews, J.D. (1983) *Minchinia nelsoni* (MSX) infections in the James River seed-oyster area and their expulsion in spring. *Estuarine and Coastal Shelf Science* 16, 255–269.

Andrews, J.D. (1988) Epizootiology of the disease caused by the oyster pathogen *Perkinsus marinus* and its effects on the oyster industry. *American Fisheries Society Special Publication* 18, 47–63.

Andrews, J.D. and Castagna, M. (1978) Epizootiology of *Minchinia costalis* in susceptible oysters in seaside bays of Virginia's Eastern Shore, 1959–1976. *Journal of Invertebrate Pathology* 32, 124–138.

Audemard, C., Reece, K.S. and Burreson, E.M. (2004) Real-time PCR for detection and quantification of the protistan parasite *Perkinsus marinus* in environmental waters. *Applied Environmental Microbiology* 70, 6611–6618.

Barber, B.J., Ford, S.E. and Haskin, H.H. (1988a) Effects of the parasite MSX (*Haplosporidium nelsoni*) on oyster (*Crassostrea virginica*) energy metabolism. I. Condition index and relative fecundity. *Journal of Shellfish Research* 7, 25–31.

Barber, B.J., Ford, S.E. and Haskin, H.H. (1988b) Effects of the parasite MSX (*Haplosporidium nelsoni*) on oyster (*Crassostrea virginica*) energy metabolism. II. Tissue biochemical composition. *Comparative Biochemistry and Physiology* 91A, 603–608.

Barber, R.D., Kanaley, S.A. and Ford, S.E. (1991) Evidence for regular sporulation by *Haplosporidium nelsoni* (MSX) (Ascetospora Haplosporidiidae) in spat of the American oyster, *Crassostrea virginica*. *Journal of Protozoology* 38, 305–306.

Burreson, E.M. (1994) Further evidence of regular sporulation by *Haplosporidium nelsoni* in small oysters, *Crassostrea virginica*. *Journal of Parasitology* 80, 1036–1038.

Burreson, E.M. and Andrews, J.D. (1988) Unusual intensification of Chesapeake Bay oyster diseases during recent drought conditions. In: *Proceedings of the Oceans '88 Conference 1988*, 31 October–2 November 1988, Baltimore, Maryland. Marine Technology Society and the Institute of Electrical and Electronic Engineers, New York, pp. 799–802.

Burreson, E.M. and Ragone Calvo, L.M. (1996) Epizootiology of *Perkinsus marinus* disease of oysters in Chesapeake Bay, with emphasis on data since 1985. *Journal of Shellfish Research* 15, 17–34.

Burreson, E.M., Alvarez, R.S., Martinez, V.V. and Macedo, L.A. (1994) *Perkinsus marinus* (Apicomplexa) as a potential source of oyster *Crassostrea virginica* mortality in coastal lagoons of Tabasco, Mexico. *Diseases of Aquatic Organisms* 20, 77–82.

Burreson, E.M., Stokes, N.A. and Friedman, C.S. (2000) Increased virulence in an introduced pathogen: *Haplosporidium nelsoni* (MSX) in the eastern oyster *Crassostrea virginica*. *Journal of Aquatic Animal Health* 12, 1–8.

Bushek, D. and Allen, S.K. Jr (1996) Host–parasite interactions among broadly distributed populations of the eastern oyster *Crassostrea virginica* and the protozoan *Perkinsus marinus*. *Marine Ecology Progress Series* 139, 127–141.

Cáceres-Martínez, J., Vásquez-Yeomans, R., Padilla-Lardizábal, G. and del Río-Portilla, M.A. (2008) *Perkinsus marinus* in pleasure oyster *Crassostrea corteziensis* from Nayarit, Pacific coast of Mexico. *Journal of Invertebrate Pathology* 99, 66–73.

Cáceres-Martínez, J., García Ortega, M., Vásquez-Yeomans, R., de Jesús Pineda García, T., Stokes, N.A. and Carnegie, R.B. (2012) Natural and cultured populations of the mangrove oyster *Saccostrea palmula* from Sinaloa, Mexico, infected by *Perkinsus marinus*. *Journal of Invertebrate Pathology* 110, 321–325.

Calvo, G.W. and Burreson, E.M. (1994) *In vitro* and *in vivo* effects of eight chemotherapeutants on the oyster parasite *Perkinsus marinus* (Mackin, Owen, and Collier). *Journal of Shellfish Research* 13, 101–107.

Carnegie, R.B. and Burreson, E.M. (2011) Declining impact of an introduced pathogen: *Haplosporidium nelsoni* in the oyster *Crassostrea virginica* in Chesapeake Bay. *Marine Ecology Progress Series* 432, 1–15.

Carnegie, R.B., Ford, S.E., Crockett, R.K., Kingsley-Smith, P.R., Bienlien, L.M. *et al.* (2021) A rapid phenotype change in the pathogen *Perkinsus marinus* was associated with a historically significant marine disease emergence in the eastern oyster. *Scientific Reports* 11, 12872.

Choi, K.-S., Wilson, E.A., Lewis, D.H., Powell, E.N. and Ray, S.M. (1989) The energetic cost of *Perkinsus marinus* parasitism in oysters: quantification of the thioglycollate method. *Journal of Shellfish Research* 8, 125–131.

Chu, F.-L.E. (1996) Laboratory investigations of susceptibility, infectivity and transmission of *Perkinsus marinus* in oysters. *Journal of Shellfish Research* 15, 57–66.

Chu, F.-L.E. and La Peyre, J.F. (1993) *Perkinsus marinus* susceptibility and defense-related activities in eastern oysters *Crassostrea virginica*: temperature effects. *Diseases of Aquatic Organisms* 16, 223–234.

Chu, F.-L.E., Lund, E.D. and Podbesek, J.A. (2008) Effects of triclosan on the oyster parasite, *Perkinsus marinus* and its host, the eastern oyster, *Crassostrea virginica*. *Journal of Shellfish Research* 27, 769–773.

Coen, L.D., Brumbaugh, R.D., Bushek, D., Grizzle, R., Luckenbach, M.W. *et al.* (2007) Ecosystem services related to oyster restoration. *Marine Ecology Progress Series* 341, 303–307.

da Silva, P.M., Vianna, R.T., Guertler, C., Ferreira, L.P., Santana, L.N. *et al.* (2013) First report of the protozoan parasite *Perkinsus marinus* in South America, infecting mangrove oysters *Crassostrea rhizophorae* from the Paraíba River (NE, Brazil). *Journal of Invertebrate Pathology* 113, 96–103.

De Faveri, J., Smolowitz, R.M. and Roberts, S.B. (2009) Development and validation of a real-time quantitative PCR assay for the detection and quantification of *Perkinsus marinus* in the eastern oyster, *Crassostrea virginica*. *Journal of Shellfish Research* 28, 459–464.

Dittman, D.E., Ford, S.E. and Padilla, D.K. (2001) Effects of *Perkinsus marinus* on reproduction and condition of the eastern oyster, *Crassostrea virginica*, depend on timing. *Journal of Shellfish Research* 20, 1025–1034.

Faisal, M., La Peyre, J., Elsayed, E. and Wright, D.C. (1999) Bacitracin inhibits the oyster pathogen *Perkinsus marinus in vitro* and *in vivo*. *Journal of Aquatic Animal Health* 11, 130–138.

Fernández-Robledo, J.A., Schott, E.J. and Vasta, G.R. (2008) *Perkinsus marinus* superoxide dismutase 2 (PmSOD2) localizes to single-membrane subcellular compartments. *Biochemical and Biophysical Research Communications* 375, 215–219.

Ford, S.E. (1985) Effects of salinity on survival of the MSX parasite *Haplosporidium nelsoni* (Haskin, Stauber and Mackin) in oysters. *Journal of Shellfish Research* 2, 85–90.

Ford, S.E. (1986) Comparison of hemolymph proteins from resistant and susceptible oysters, *Crassostrea virginica*, exposed to the parasite *Haplosporidium nelsoni* (MSX). *Journal of Invertebrate Pathology* 47, 283–294.

Ford, S.E. (1992) Avoiding the transmission of disease in commercial culture of molluscs, with special reference to *Perkinsus marinus* (Dermo) and *Haplosporidium nelsoni* (MSX). *Journal of Shellfish Research* 11, 539–546.

Ford, S.E. (1996) Range extension by the oyster parasite *Perkinsus marinus* into the northeastern United States: response to climate change? *Journal of Shellfish Research* 15, 45–56.

Ford, S.E. and Haskin, H.H. (1982) History and epizootiology of *Haplosporidium nelsoni* (MSX), an oyster pathogen, in Delaware Bay, 1957–1980. *Journal of Invertebrate Pathology* 40, 118–141.

Ford, S.E. and Haskin, H.H. (1988) Comparison of *in vitro* salinity tolerance of the oyster parasite *Haplosporidium nelsoni* (MSX) and hemocytes from the host, *Crassostrea virginica*. *Comparative Biochemistry and Physiology* 90A, 183–187.

Ford, S.E. and Smolowitz, R. (2007) Infection dynamics of an oyster parasite in its newly expanded range. *Marine Biology* 151, 119–133.

Ford, S.E. and Tripp, M.R. (1996) Diseases and defense mechanisms. In: Kennedy, V.S., Newell, R.I.E. and Eble, A.F. (eds) *The Eastern Oyster Crassostrea virginica*. Maryland Sea Grant College, College Park, Maryland, pp. 581–660.

Ford, S.E., Allam, B. and Xu, Z. (2009) Using bivalves as particle collectors with PCR detection to investigate the environmental distribution of *Haplosporidium nelsoni*. *Diseases of Aquatic Organisms* 83, 159–168.

Friedman, C.S. (1996) Haplosporidan infections of the Pacific oyster, *Crassostrea gigas* (Thunberg), in California and Japan. *Journal of Shellfish Research* 15, 597–600.

Galtsoff, P.S. (1964) The American oyster *Crassostrea virginica* Gmelin. *Fishery Bulletin* 64, 1–480.

Garreis, K.A., La Peyre, J.F. and Faisal, M. (1996) The effects of *Perkinsus marinus* extracellular products and purified proteases on oyster defense parameters *in vitro*. *Fish and Shellfish Immunology* 6, 581–597.

Gauthier, J.D., Miller, C.R. and Wilbur, A.E. (2006) TaqMan® MGB real-time PCR approach to quantification of *Perkinsus marinus* and *Perkinsus* spp. in oysters. *Journal of Shellfish Research* 25, 619–624.

Haskin, H.H. and Andrews, J.D. (1988) Uncertainties and speculations about the life cycle of the eastern oyster pathogen *Haplosporidium nelsoni* (MSX). *American Fisheries Society Special Publication* 18, 5–22.

Haskin, H.H. and Ford, S.E. (1979) Development of resistance to *Minchinia nelsoni* (MSX) mortality in laboratory-reared and native oyster stocks in Delaware Bay. *Marine Fisheries Review* 41, 54–63.

Haskin, H.H., Stauber, L.A. and Mackin, J.A. (1966) *Minchinia nelsoni* sp. n. (Haplosporida, Haplosporidiidae): causative agent of the Delaware Bay oyster epizootic. *Science* 153, 1414–1416.

Holland, A.F., Shaughnessy, A.T. and Hiegel, M.H. (1987) Long-term variation in mesohaline Chesapeake Bay macrobenthos: spatial and temporal patterns. *Estuaries* 10, 227–245.

Kemp, W.M., Boynton, W.R., Adolf, J.E., Boesch, D.F., Boicourt, W.C. *et al.* (2005) Eutrophication of Chesapeake Bay: historical trends and ecological interactions. *Marine Ecology Progress Series* 303, 1–29.

Kennedy, V.S., Newell, R.I.E., Krantz, G.E. and Otto, S. (1995) Reproductive capacity of the eastern oyster *Crassostrea virginica* infected with the parasite *Perkinsus marinus*. *Diseases of Aquatic Organisms* 23, 135–144.

Langdon, C.J. and Newell, R.I.E. (1996) Digestion and nutrition in larvae and adults. In: Kennedy, V.S., Newell, R.I.E. and Eble, A.F. (eds) *The Eastern Oyster Crassostrea virginica*. Maryland Sea Grant College, College Park, Maryland, pp. 231–269.

La Peyre, J.F., Schafhauser, D.Y., Rizkalla, E.H. and Faisal, M. (1995) Production of serine proteases by the oyster pathogen *Perkinsus marinus* (Apicomplexa) *in vitro*. *Journal of Eukaryotic Microbiology* 42, 544–551.

La Peyre, J.F., Xue, Q.-G., Itoh, N., Li, Y. and Cooper, R.K. (2010) Serine protease inhibitor cvSI-1 potential role in the eastern oyster host defense against the protozoan parasite *Perkinsus marinus*. *Developmental and Comparative Immunology* 34, 84–92.

Long, W.C. and Seitz, R.D. (2009) Hypoxia in Chesapeake Bay tributaries: worsening effects on macrobenthic community structure in the York River. *Estuaries and Coasts* 32, 287–297.

Mackin, J.G. (1951) Histopathology of infection of *Crassostrea virginica* (Gmelin) by *Dermocystidium marinum* Mackin, Owen and Collier. *Bulletin of Marine Science of the Gulf and Caribbean* 1, 72–87.

Mann, R., Southworth, M., Harding, J.M. and Wesson, J.A. (2009) Population studies of the native eastern oyster, *Crassostrea virginica* (Gmelin, 1791) in the James River, Virginia, USA. *Journal of Shellfish Research* 28, 193–220.

McCollough, C.B., Albright, B.W., Abbe, G.R., Barker, L.S. and Dungan, C.F. (2007) Acquisition and progression of *Perkinsus marinus* infections by specific-pathogen-free juvenile oysters (*Crassostrea virginica* Gmelin) in a mesohaline Chesapeake Bay tributary. *Journal of Shellfish Research* 26, 465–477.

Menzel, R.W. and Hopkins, S.H. (1955) The growth of oysters parasitized by the fungus *Dermocystidium marinum* and by the trematode *Bucephalus cuculus*. *Journal of Parasitology* 41, 333–342.

Newell, R.I.E. (1985) Physiological effects of the MSX parasite *Haplosporidium nelsoni* (Haskin, Stauber & Mackin) on the American oyster *Crassostrea virginica* (Gmelin). *Journal of Shellfish Research* 5, 91–95.

Oliver, J.L., Lewis, T.D., Faisal, M. and Kaattari, S.L. (1999) Analysis of the effects of *Perkinsus marinus* protease on plasma proteins of the eastern (*Crassostrea virginica*) and Pacific oyster (*Crassostrea gigas*). *Journal of Invertebrate Pathology* 74, 173–183.

Oliver, J.L., Gaffney, P.M., Allen, S.K. Jr, Faisal, M. and Kaattari, S.L. (2000) Protease inhibitory activity in selectively bred families of eastern oysters. *Journal of Aquatic Animal Health* 12, 136–145.

Paynter, K.T. and Burreson, E.M. (1991) Effects of *Perkinsus marinus* infection in the eastern oyster, *Crassostrea virginica*: II. Disease development and impact on growth rate at different salinities. *Journal of Shellfish Research* 10, 425–431.

Piesz, J.L., Scro, A.K., Corbett, R., Markey Lundgren, K., Smolowitz, R. and Gomez-Chiarri, M. (2022) Development of a multiplex qPCR for the quantification of three protozoan parasites of the eastern oyster *Crassostrea virginica*. *Diseases of Aquatic Organisms* 151, 111–121.

Preston, B.L. (2004) Observed winter warming of the Chesapeake Bay estuary (1949–2002): implications for ecosystem management. *Environmental Management* 34, 125–139.

Ragone Calvo, L.M. and Burreson, E.M. (1993) Effect of salinity on infection progression and pathogenicity of *Perkinsus marinus* in the eastern oyster, *Crassostrea virginica*. *Journal of Shellfish Research* 12, 1–7.

Ragone Calvo, L.M., Calvo, G.W. and Burreson, E.M. (2003a) Dual disease resistance in a selectively bred eastern oyster, *Crassostrea virginica*, strain tested in Chesapeake Bay. *Aquaculture* 220, 69–87.

Ragone Calvo, L.M., Dungan, C.F., Roberson, B.S. and Burreson, E.M. (2003b) Systematic evaluation of factors controlling *Perkinsus marinus* transmission dynamics in lower Chesapeake Bay. *Diseases of Aquatic Organisms* 56, 75–86.

Ray, S.M. (1966a) A review of the culture method for detecting *Dermocystidium marinum*, with suggested modifications and precautions. *Proceedings of the National Shellfisheries Association* 54, 55–69.

Ray, S.M. (1966b) Cycloheximide: inhibition of *Dermocystidium marinum* in laboratory stocks of oysters. *Proceedings of the National Shellfisheries Association* 56, 31–36.

Reece, K.S., Dungan, C.F. and Burreson, E.M. (2008) Molecular epizootiology of *Perkinsus marinus* and *P. chesapeaki* infections among wild oysters and clams in Chesapeake Bay, USA. *Diseases of Aquatic Organisms* 82, 237–248.

Robledo, J.-A.F., Courville, P., Cellier, M.F.M. and Vasta, G.R. (2004) Gene organization and expression of the divalent cation transporter Nramp in the protistan parasite *Perkinsus marinus*. *Journal of Parasitology* 90, 1004–1014.

Schott, E.J., Pecher, W.T., Okafor, F. and Vasta, G.R. (2003) The protistan parasite *Perkinsus marinus* is resistant to selected reactive oxygen species. *Experimental Parasitology* 105, 232–240.

Schulte, D., Burke, R.P. and Lipcius, R.N. (2009) Unprecedented restoration of a native oyster metapopulation. *Science* 325, 1124–1128.

Shumway, S.E. (1996) Natural environmental factors. In: Kennedy, V.S., Newell, R.I.E. and Eble, A.F. (eds) *The Eastern Oyster Crassostrea virginica*. Maryland Sea Grant College, College Park, Maryland, pp. 467–513.

Soniat, T.M. (1996) Epizootiology of *Perkinsus marinus* disease of eastern oysters in the Gulf of Mexico. *Journal of Shellfish Research* 15, 35–43.

Soniat, T.M., Klinck, J.M., Powell, E.N. and Hofmann, E.E. (2005) Understanding the success and failure of oyster populations: climatic cycles and *Perkinsus marinus*. *Journal of Shellfish Research* 24, 83–93.

Stokes, N.A. and Burreson, E.M. (1995) A sensitive and specific DNA probe for the oyster pathogen *Haplosporidium nelsoni*. *Journal of Eukaryotic Microbiology* 42, 350–357.

Stokes, N.A. and Burreson, E.M. (2001) Differential diagnosis of mixed *Haplosporidium costale* and *Haplosporidium nelsoni* infections in the eastern oyster, *Crassostrea virginica*, using DNA probes. *Journal of Shellfish Research* 20, 207–213.

Stokes, N.A., Siddall, M.E. and Burreson, E.M. (1995) Detection of *Haplosporidium nelsoni* (Haplosporidia: Haplosporidiidae) in oysters by PCR amplification. *Diseases of Aquatic Organisms* 23, 145–152.

Wilbur, A.E., Ford, S.E., Gauthier, J.D. and Gomez-Chiarri, M. (2012) Quantitative PCR assay to determine prevalence and intensity of MSX (*Haplosporidium nelsoni*) in North Carolina and Rhode Island oysters *Crassostrea virginica*. *Diseases of Aquatic Organisms* 102, 107–118.

Xue, Q.-G., Waldrop, G.L., Schey, K.L., Itoh, N., Ogawa, M. *et al.* (2006) A novel slow-tight binding serine protease inhibitor from eastern oyster (*Crassostrea virginica*) plasma inhibits perkinsin, the major extracellular protease of the oyster protozoan parasite *Perkinus marinus*. *Comparative Biochemistry and Physiology Part B: Biochemistry and Molecular Biology* 145, 16–26.

Xue, Q.-G., Itoh, N., Schey, K.L., Cooper, R.K. and La Peyre, J.F. (2009) Evidence indicating the existence of a novel family of serine protease inhibitors that may be involved in marine invertebrate immunity. *Fish and Shellfish Immunity* 27, 250–259.

6 *Loma salmonae* and Related Species

Jan Lovy[1]* and David J. Speare[2]
[1]*US Geological Survey, Western Fisheries Research Center, Seattle, Washington, USA;* [2]*Atlantic Veterinary College, University of Prince Edward Island, Charlottetown, Canada*

Abstract

Loma salmonae is a microsporidium that infects Pacific salmon and causes a gill inflammatory syndrome known as microsporidial gill disease of salmon. This disease has been mostly associated with netpen-farmed Chinook salmon (*Oncorhynchus tshawytscha*) in British Columbia, Canada. Clinical, diagnostic, pathological aspects of disease, as well as approaches for disease avoidance in salmon aquaculture are discussed. A laboratory infection model in rainbow trout was used to determine life cycle-stages, transmission dynamics, pathophysiology, influence of temperature, and to test therapeutics applicable to aquaculture. This experimental model has been informative on various approaches of disease control, including the development of a promising vaccine. In addition to improving fish health in salmon farming in North America, this *L. salmonae* model will be applicable to other microsporidial diseases that may be encountered in emerging aquaculture regions.

6.1. Introduction

'Microsporidial gill disease of salmon' (MGDS), caused by the xenoma-forming intracellular pathogen *Loma salmonae*, has become increasingly recognized in recent years from many parts of the world. The disease most commonly affects the gills, and to a lesser extent other systemic organs, of farmed and wild salmonids in both freshwater and marine environments. Although, in general, microsporidian infections of animals are difficult to treat, or are refractory to most treatment regimes, research into the pathobiology of *L. salmonae* has now begun to yield insight into how this disease might be managed. Although *L. salmonae* appears to have a near global distribution, it has its greatest economic effect on the commercial marine cage culture of Pacific salmon, notably Chinook salmon (*Oncorhynchus tshawytscha*), in and around coastal British Columbia, Canada (Constantine, 1999). In this region, the microsporidium can also be found in wild salmon (Kent *et al*., 1998), a likely source of infection for farmed Chinook salmon. Here, since the early 1990s MGDS has become an endemic seasonal problem, arising in late summer and early autumn; the disease is recognized by the presence of slow-moving, top-swimming fish, which exhibit laboured respiratory efforts reflecting the underlying multifocal chronic inflammatory branchitis (gill inflammation) which is the disease's hallmark lesion (Kent and Speare, 2005). Much of the research introduced in this chapter has its applications aimed at this

*Email: jl4825@cornell.edu

DOI: 10.1079/9781800628748.0006

sector of aquaculture, but the approaches are probably pertinent to other scenarios where *L. salmonae* may be a problem, and, to a degree yet to be determined, other related microsporidial diseases of farmed fish, such as gill and visceral infections of *Loma morhua* in farm-reared Atlantic cod (*Gadus morhua*).

Microsporidians have long been identified as significant pathogens of invertebrates and vertebrates. Their relationship to fungi (Keeling and Fast, 2002), and their abilities to cause disease in mammals, notably in humans suffering from immunosuppression, has sparked interest in: (i) their intracellular biology; (ii) their modes of transmission; (iii) their relationship to other organisms; and (iv) treatment and control measures (Williams, 2009). Despite intensive efforts to find clinical management techniques to control microsporidians causing disease in humans, there has been little substantive progress (Bacchi *et al.*, 2002). Treatment regimens tend to be prolonged; prognosis tends to be guarded (Costa and Weiss, 2000); and prevention methods remain elusive. Hampering progress, *in vitro* approaches, which could be used to better understand intracellular biology, are only rarely successful for microsporidia (Bigliardi *et al.*, 2000; Williams, 2009). Many questions remain and, in this case, a comparative medicine approach has not provided useful starting points.

Microsporidians are well recognized as pathogens of fish, and this has provided an extensive background of published reports and reviews describing: (i) infections; (ii) host ranges of different microsporidians; and (iii) ultrastructural descriptions of various stages although often limited to the spore stage (Lom and Nilsen, 2003). Potentially germane to this chapter, there have been several reports of microsporidians within the genus *Loma* affecting various non-salmonid aquaculture species; this is succinctly outlined by Casal *et al.* (2009) in their paper on *Loma psittica* in the Amazonian freshwater puffer fish (*Colomesus asellus*). Previously, there have been only sporadic published reports geared towards examining the clinical and economic consequences of these diseases, pathophysiological consequences of infection, or evidence-based findings in the areas of disease prevention and treatment. Treatment and management programmes devised for *L. salmonae* may provide starting templates or approaches for a myriad of emerging related microsporidial diseases of cultured fish. For example, as will be noted elsewhere in this chapter, systemic *L. morhua* affecting cod has proven to be a limiting factor in the establishment and growth of cod aquaculture, particularly in eastern North America. In contrast to the relative ease of establishing *L. salmonae* infection models in salmonids, developing a repeatable and reliable *L. morhua*/cod infection model has been challenging and, in particular, non-infected controls are difficult to source (Frenette *et al.*, 2017). The recognition of widespread *Pseudoloma neurophilia* in research colonies of zebrafish (*Danio rerio*) is having a significant effect on the reliability of zebrafish as a research model as 'disease-free' status is very difficult to achieve (Murray *et al.*, 2011; Sanders *et al.*, 2012). The value, therefore, of studying the pathogenesis and control of *L. salmonae* has applications beyond those originally anticipated.

The history of MGDS in farmed salmon dates to the late 1980s, although recognition and description of *L. salmonae* as a salmon parasite and putative pathogen predates this by several years (Morrison and Sprague, 1983; Hauck, 1984; Poynton, 1986). The first report of *L. salmonae* as a cause of disease in salmon cultivated in marine netpens appeared in 1989 (Speare and Ferguson, 1989); it described a 1987 clinical case arising off the coast of British Columbia which involved a group of 40 g coho salmon (*Oncorhynchus kisutch*) smolts, recently transferred from a hatchery setting to a marine netpen grow-out environment. Dying in large numbers, they were found to have a severe gill disease related to the diatom *Corethron hystrix* and an interstitial branchitis caused by xenomas of *L. salmonae*. Since that time, as a disease of notable economic consequence, *L. salmonae* has established itself as an endemic disease of marine-cultured Pacific salmon (notably Chinook salmon), becoming known as MGDS, and has been found in salmonid culture elsewhere in the world (Bruno *et al.*, 1995; Gandhi *et al.*, 1995). The disease is typically present in late summer and early autumn along coastal British Columbia. Mortality rates depend on infection severity and can vary from a low of 2.4% to over 30% (Kent and Speare, 2005). In contrast to its initial report MGDS is most often seen affecting salmon that are nearing market weight, in their second summer of marine culture and thus of high commercial value. Estimating the costs of disease is a difficult process, and this data is often not reported for aquaculture. A study on one farm site, reported in 1999, experienced a 12% mortality rate from MGDS. Within one production season, this translated to lost productivity (direct costs from mortality) due to MGDS that approached CAN$315,000 and indirect costs related to changes in feed conversion efficiency valued at CAN$1,470,000 (Constantine, 1999). Unfortunately, total production numbers were not provided for this particular farm and more recent data on disease costs has not become available.

MGDS is not generally reported from Chinook salmon during early rearing in freshwater hatcheries, although early on it was suspected that hatchery fish carried latent infections that gave rise to MGDS epidemics after the smolt were transferred from freshwater hatcheries to marine sea cages. Stress of transfer was believed to be the trigger for recrudescence. This theory of latency and recrudescence has largely given way to a widely held alternative hypothesis implicating wild salmon in the marine environment as reservoir sources of the parasite. This is supported by the finding of *L. salmonae* in wild salmon in the marine environment and the fact that Chinook salmon in marine sea cages are often most severely impacted in their second year in sea water. Under the wild fish reservoir hypothesis, strategies of screening juveniles prior to transfer to marine netpen sites, previously considered as a key management tool against MGDS, is therefore of less importance than understanding the dynamics of a 'spillover and amplification' scenario whereby a farmed population acquires its initial infection from transfer from wild reservoirs. As reviewed by Becker and Speare (2007), several studies have addressed the transmission dynamics of *L. salmonae* within carefully controlled laboratory settings to help elucidate factors (host, pathogen or environmental) that affect the horizontal transmission of this pathogen (Mustafa *et al.*, 2000; Becker *et al.*, 2005a, 2006).

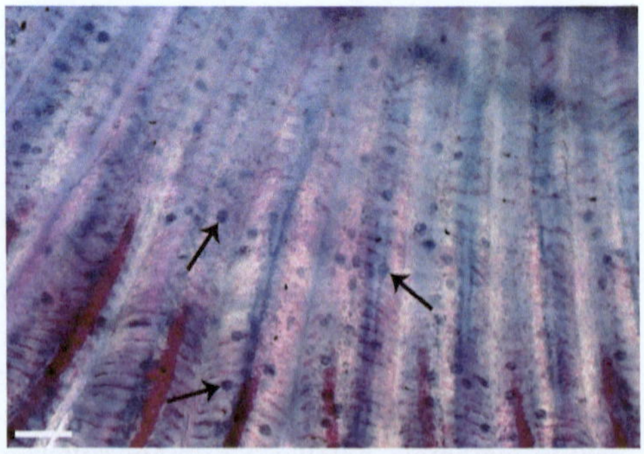

Fig. 6.1. A wet mount of rainbow trout (*Oncorhynchus mykiss*) gills 6 weeks after experimental infection with *Loma salmonae*. Xenomas (arrows) are found throughout the tissue. Bar = 200 μm. (Author's own image.)

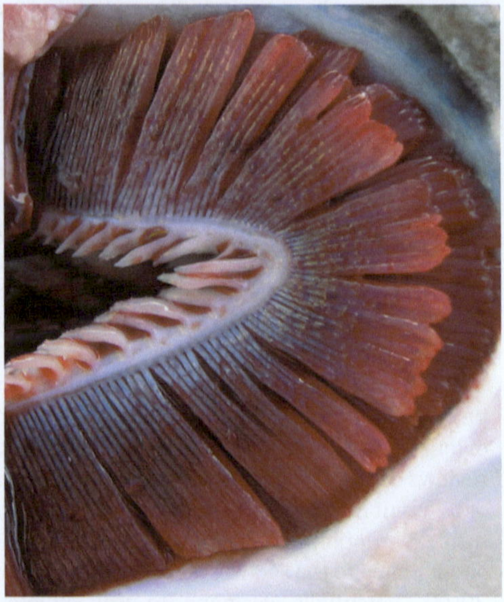

Fig. 6.2. The gills of a farmed Chinook salmon (*Oncorhynchus tshawytscha*) clinically affected with microsporidial gill disease caused by *Loma salmonae*. The rupture of xenomas causes a multifocal haemorrhagic cystic branchitis. (Author's own image.)

6.2. Pathobiology

6.2.1. Diagnosis

It is not difficult to diagnose MGDS: the clinical, gross and subgross signs (Figs 6.1 and 6.2), when taken together, are distinctive (Constantine, 1999). Fish will swim lethargically at the surface, often close to the net walls, darken in colour, and exhibit laboured respiration and inappetence. The gills show random or coalescing patches of redness from congestion and white patches of hyperplasia; filament fusion may be grossly apparent on larger fish (Figs 6.1 and 6.2). White- to cream-coloured pin-head-sized xenomas have a random multifocal distribution across all regions of the gill arch; xenomas when fully formed are just large enough to be detected by the naked eye and may be more visible, because of the contrast of white on red, in areas of congestion. In a region where MGDS is endemic, these signs can be used as a definitive non-lethal diagnosis. The presence of xenomas is made more distinct under a dissecting microscope; examining gill whole mounts permits a better assessment of the degree and nature of gill changes (hyperplasia) in the vicinity of xenomas and helps to determine whether other pathogens or foreign bodies (particularly harmful diatoms) are present. Microscopic wet mounts will aid in determining the presence of the xenomas in the gills, for example if they occur in the filament arteries or in gill lamellae (Fig. 6.1). Lightly pressing on a gill whole mount can disrupt the xenomas sufficiently to permit visualization and measurement of spores.

Histopathology approaches are an effective means to more critically evaluate the host response to xenomas, and this diagnostic modality can also be used to stage the infection (e.g. detecting smaller 'pre-xenoma' stages or detection of spores which may be retained in the gills after xenomas have ruptured). Detection of spores is aided by the birefringent nature of the microsporidial spore walls (Tiner, 1988), and in our experience we find this characteristic for approximately 40% of the spores. Special histology stains are also useful to identify spores within tissue sections, with Luna and Gram stains being the most useful (Peterson *et al.*, 2011). Luna stains spores brick red, as it is believed to stain chitin, though Luna also stains granules within eosinophils, eosinophilic granule cells and erythrocytes, and thus stained host-cell granules must be carefully interpreted to prevent their confusion with microsporidian spores. A tissue Gram stain can be useful, as microsporidia frequently stain as Gram-positive. Standard operating procedures for monitoring the development of *L. salmonae* infections during experiments, along with spore isolation procedures, have been summarized by Jones and McConnachie (2021). This information should aid in the standardization of *L. salmonae* studies across different laboratories.

Confirming a species of microsporidia in a diagnosis had historically been based on host, tissue tropism, and morphological characters including spore size, coils in the polar tube, and developmental aspects of merogony and sporogony. For unusual case presentations or for confirming *L. salmonae* in new host species, genetic sequencing could complement a diagnosis. Microsporidia-specific primers for amplification of the ribosomal RNA (rDNA) and elongation factor-1α (EF-1α) genes are reported (Vossbrinck *et al.*, 2004, 2014; Brown *et al.*, 2010). The internal transcribed spacer (ITS) region of the rDNA is particularly useful for detecting intraspecific variations and highlighting species differences, since this non-coding region evolves at a faster rate than the coding regions of the rDNA. This has been particularly useful for the identification of *L. morhua* in cod (Frenette *et al.*, 2017). Additionally, specific labelling of tissue sections for *L. salmonae* is possible via *in situ* hybridization or various methods based on the application of monoclonal antibodies (Speare *et al.*, 1998c; Sanchez *et al.*, 1999, 2001b).

6.2.2. External and internal lesions

Although not accompanied by evidence of pathological host response, early stages of *L. salmonae* can be found in the lamina propria of the intestinal tract; the parasite is found subsequently in the cardiac subendocardium, as revealed using *in situ* hybridization studies (Sanchez *et al.*, 2000, 2001a,d), although the mode of the parasite migration is unknown. Lesions visible with routine microscopy and staining are not detected until spore-filled xenomas are formed (and rupture) in the gills and to a much lesser extent in other organs.

The lesions can be divided into two major stages, the first includes the parasite growth and replication phase that occurs within xenomas. In this stage the lesion per se is the xenoma: an infected host cell that is induced to undergo severe hypertrophy to accommodate the developing parasite (Figs 6.3 and 6.4). The second stage is when the xenomas rupture, thereby releasing spores into tissue, causing an inflammatory response that leads to tissue damage. The rupture of xenomas causes a multifocal haemorrhagic cystic branchitis.

6.2.2.1. Formation of xenomas in gills

The target cell type for *L. salmonae* is either a pillar cell, an endothelial cell or an infected leucocyte that migrates through the basement membrane

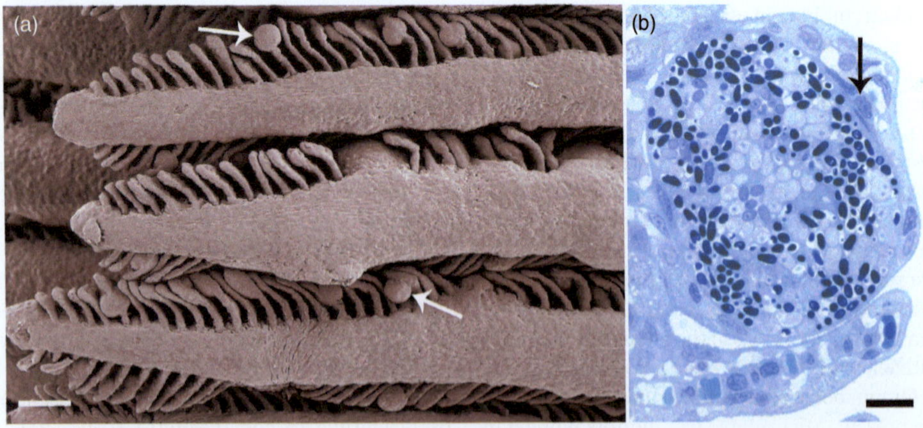

Fig. 6.3. Rainbow trout (*Oncorhynchus mykiss*) gills 6 weeks post-infection with *Loma salmonae*. (a) A scanning electron micrograph showing the tissue compression caused by multifocal xenomas (arrows) within the lamellae. Coloured post image capture; bar = 100 μm. (b) A high-resolution light micrograph showing localization of a xenoma within the gill lamellae in close association with a pillar cell (arrow). Staining with toluidine blue; bar = 10 μm. (Author's own image.)

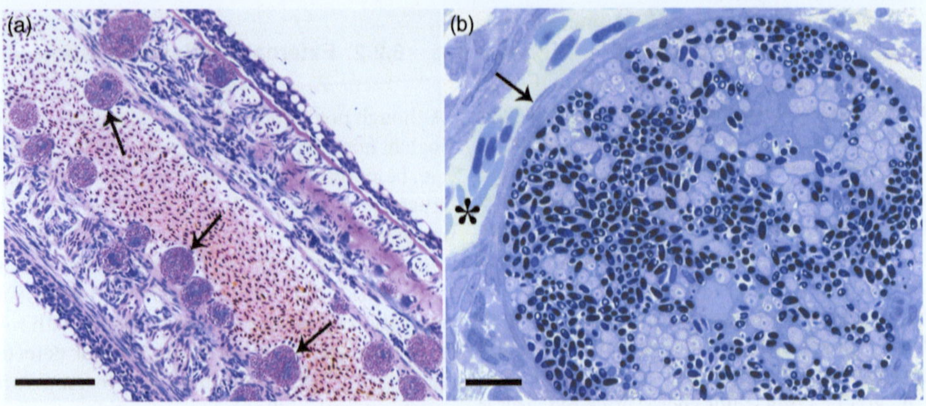

Fig. 6.4. Gills from farmed Chinook salmon (*Oncorhynchus tshawytscha*) clinically affected with microsporidial gill disease. (a) A section through a gill filament artery showing numerous xenomas (arrows) attached to the blood vessel wall and protruding into the artery lumen. Staining with haematoxylin and eosin; bar = 500 μm. (b) A high-resolution light micrograph showing a xenoma localized beneath the endothelium (arrow) of the filament artery (the artery lumen is indicated by *). Staining with toluidine blue; bar = 10 μm. (Author's own image.)

of a blood vessel and localizes among, or within, pillar and endothelial cells (Rodriguez-Tovar *et al.*, 2002). Several hypotheses (Rodriguez-Tovar *et al.*, 2002) have been put forward to help describe the cellular interactions that permit a circulating leucocyte to cooperatively transfer the immature parasite into another cell which is permissive for the final maturation of the parasite–cell assembly into the characteristic xenoma. Xenomas can occur within the gill lamellae, where xenomas are found closely associated with pillar cells (Fig. 6.3), or in the gill filament, most frequently within endothelial cells lining arteries and arterioles (Fig. 6.4). Xenomas which rupture within the lamellae often lead to lamellar fusion caused by proliferation of epithelial cells and influx of inflammatory cells. The lamellar lesions tend to be less severe than lesions in the gill filament; in the former location it is likely that the majority of spores will be released into the environment whereas those in the filament will probably become trapped thereby provoking a prolonged host response.

A fascinating but poorly understood area is the relationship between the parasite and the fish host cell that leads to the development of the xenoma (Williams, 2009); theoretically this may involve inhibition of host-cell apoptosis by the parasite. Extending the lifespan of the host cell permits the extended development cycle of the parasite to be completed. Development of the parasite within the xenoma (advancing through merogonial and sporogonial stages), followed by the formation of sporoblasts and lastly spores, is common for *L. salmonae* and many other microsporidia. Through the exploitation of an *in vivo* model and sequential ultrastructural examination of *L. salmonae* development within xenomas, a new hypothesis has emerged on how some microsporidia exploit host cellular functions, particularly autophagy, to facilitate their development from meronts to sporonts (Lovy *et al.*, 2006b). Autophagy, an intracellular process for eliminating unwanted cytoplasmic elements through degradation, is a common response to the presence of intracellular organisms and injured organelles. Products destined for degradation are enclosed within host endoplasmic reticulum. This forms an autophagosome which subsequently fuses with a lysosome. Degraded proteins are recycled back into the cell. Meronts of *L. salmonae* within xenomas are enclosed by host endoplasmic reticulum membranes as might occur in the first stages of autophagy; however, subsequent degradation of the parasite does not occur, but rather the parasite adapts host endoplasmic reticulum membranes for the development of an outer parasite membrane and the limiting membrane of the parasitophorous vacuole (PV). With the parasites enclosed in the former endoplasmic reticulum lumen, containing proteins not freely available in the cytoplasm, development to mature spores occurs (Lovy *et al.*, 2006b). If this process is common among microsporidia it may represent an interesting pathway by which parasites exploit host-cell processes and host-cell structures for their own development. As is the case for highly 'reduced' parasites which offer few targets for chemotherapeutic agents, further research into how these parasites utilize host-cell machinery may provide insights into classes of promising chemotherapeutic compounds.

Intracellular localization within the xenoma benefits the developing parasite by helping it to evade host immune responses. *L. salmonae* forms xenomas in the gills of rainbow trout that persist from 4 to 8 weeks, and the xenomas in Chinook salmon persist for an even longer period (Ramsay *et al.*, 2002). The intact xenomas elicit, at best, a muted immune response, and the parasite seems to remain well hidden from the host response within the confines of the host cell throughout its development. In *L. salmonae*, intact xenomas are limited by only the xenoma plasma membrane, as this species does not have a thick xenoma wall as in other microsporidian species such as those of the genus *Glugea*, which has a thick collagenous barrier around the limiting membrane of the xenoma (Lovy *et al.*, 2009a). In *L. salmonae*, although intact xenomas elicit a minimal inflammatory response, there is a fibroblast response which is one or two cell layers thick. This may come about as a result of concentric local tissue damage from compression caused by these massively hypertrophied cells (Fig. 6.4). Nevertheless, an unusual feature of the surrounding fibroblasts is the formation of desmosomes with neighbouring fibroblasts, which appears to more efficiently encapsulate the xenomas. The fibroblastic response is not observed in all xenomas, and often they are only bound by a plasma membrane with minimal response around the periphery. During the late stages of xenoma maturation some phagocytic cells such as neutrophils and macrophages begin to surround the xenoma; this response is thought to be caused by a weak antigenic signal leaking from the xenoma (Rodriguez-Tovar *et al.*, 2003b). Matured xenomas, containing a high proportion of mature spores, also have spores everting their polar tube and piercing host cells around the perimeter of the xenoma. The stimulus to trigger the apparently premature germination of spores within xenomas is unknown. Spore germination within mature xenomas could hypothetically be a method for the parasite to induce or initiate destruction of the xenoma to free other non-germinated pathogenic spores. Small breaches of the xenoma wall caused by everted polar tubes may cause leaking of antigenic signal and subsequent recruitment of inflammatory cells that further enhance xenoma-wall destruction (Rodriguez-Tovar *et al.*, 2003b). This is also supported by the presence of an inflammatory infiltrate mainly dominated by neutrophils that leads to the eventual loss of the xenoma plasma membrane and liberation of spores into the gill tissue (Lovy *et al.*, 2007b). Autoinfection seems plausible, as nearby host cells are penetrated by the germinating spores, though development of new xenomas in these sites has not been documented.

6.2.2.2. Host response subsequent to xenoma rupture

Destruction of the xenoma membrane liberates spores into the surrounding gill tissue and this leads to an inflammatory response that sequentially demonstrates hallmarks of acute reaction (suppurative) transitioning to a chronic reaction (granulomatous). Interestingly, *L. morhua* affecting Atlantic cod causes a typical granulomatous inflammation within the gill but forms a very different host response within the non-gill organs. *L. morhua* causes severe systemic infections and the degrading, mature xenomas elicit a strong walling-off response, as opposed to the diffuse inflammatory response as seen in salmonids. The response in cod consists of the development of a thick wall of macrophages with an epithelioid-like transformation recognized by large numbers of desmosomes (Fig. 6.5). This response is commonly seen in the spleen and heart of cod; a similar response is absent in splenic and cardiac xenomas in salmonids, suggesting that the cod's immune response may rely more on macrophage encapsulation of foreign agents. These differences may also be explained by species-related differences in the immune system. Whereas the major histocompatibility complex (MHC) class II is conserved in most jawed vertebrates, including salmon, Atlantic cod have lost the genes for and associated with MHC-II, while greatly expanding loci within MHC-I pathways (Star *et al.*, 2011). Further, when compared to other teleosts, the pattern recognition receptor family of Toll-like receptors (TLR) have been greatly lost in some forms, while expanded in others (Solbakken *et al.*, 2016). These differences in immune responses and pathogen recognition may at least partially explain these differences between salmon and cod in their response to *L. salmonae*.

The host-cell response towards ruptured xenomas begins with neutrophils, but these are subsequently replaced by macrophages and lymphocytes (Lovy *et al.*, 2007b). Neutrophils are highly phagocytic and within lesions it is typical to see them containing either single or multiple mature spores within a phagosome. However, there is no evidence of spore degradation

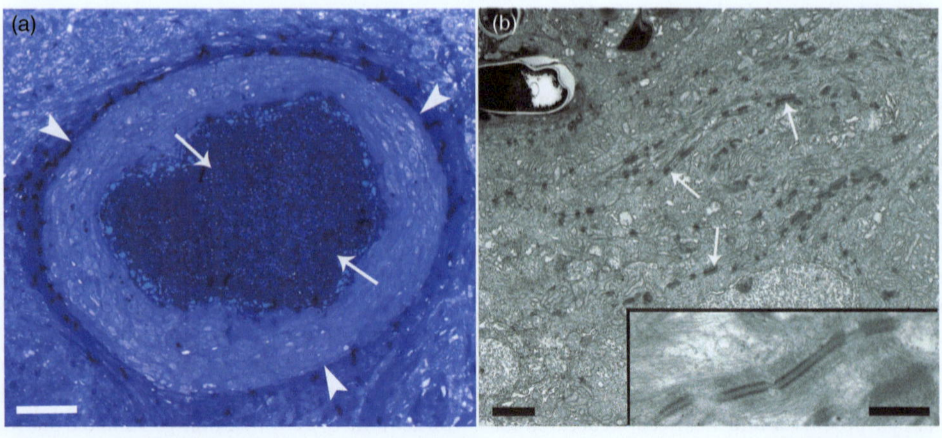

Fig. 6.5. A degraded xenoma of *Loma morhua* within the heart of Atlantic cod (*Gadus morhua*). (a) A high-resolution light micrograph showing the strong 'walling-off' response to a degrading xenoma (arrows), with an approximately 10-cell-layer thick encapsulation of epithelioid macrophages (arrowheads). Staining with toluidine blue; bar = 50 µm. (b) A transmission electron micrograph showing the abundance of desmosomes (arrows) between epithelioid macrophages. Bar = 2 µm. Inset shows details of the epithelioid macrophage desmosomes. Bar = 500 nm. (Author's own image.)

within neutrophils (Fig. 6.6), which suggests that neutrophils are either unable to degrade the thick exospores/endospores or that the parasite is inhibiting neutrophil functions. It is curious to see such a strong chemotactic and phagocytic response by neutrophils to the spores, especially given the subsequent inability of the neutrophils to degrade them. This raises the possibility that the parasite is using the neutrophil as a method to protect itself and ensure intact spores make it into the environment. In mammals, a strong neutrophil response leads to the development of pustules, and the fate of neutrophils is often to be released out of the body through exudates. The neutrophil response in fish with MGDS is heavy enough to cause swelling of the gill filament and epithelial oedema (Lovy *et al.*, 2007b), which can lead to subepithelial blisters full of red blood cells, neutrophils and spores (Fig. 6.7). It is possible that the neutrophils containing intact spores will be released into the environment, making it possible for spores within the gill filament to be released through the exudate. Neutrophils may also be involved in the dissemination of the infection, as it is believed that a leucocyte is responsible for carrying the parasite to the gills during the early stages of infection.

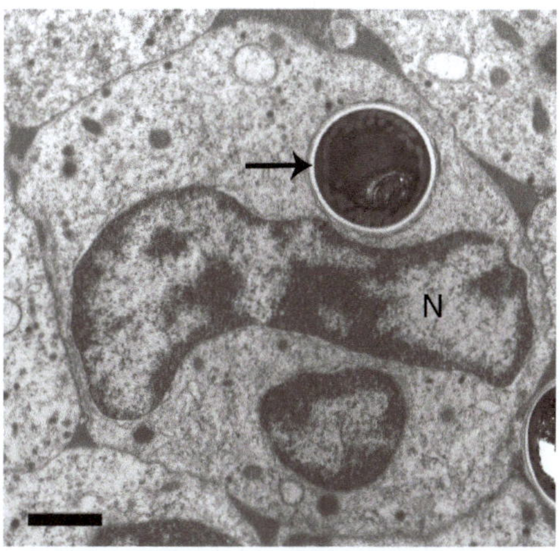

Fig. 6.6. A neutrophil with a segmented nucleus (N) containing a spore of *Loma salmonae* (arrow) showing no evidence of lysosomal fusion or degradation; host species, Chinook salmon (*Oncorhynchus tshawytscha*). Bar = 1 μm. (Author's own image.)

6.2.2.3. Chronic responses and tissue regeneration

Subsequent to the neutrophil-rich response early after xenoma rupture, macrophages initially arrive in small numbers relative to neutrophils and in chronic inflammatory lesions they become more abundant. In contrast to neutrophils, macrophages are efficiently able to degrade the spores (Fig. 6.8), and chronic inflammatory lesions contain mostly macrophages with degenerated spores.

In addition to phagocytic cells and lymphocytes, cells that resemble Langerhans cells can also be found in areas of acute and chronic inflammation. These cells have peri-centriolar racket-shaped granules containing lattice-structured material structurally similar to Birbeck granules which are characteristic for human Langerhans cells (Lovy *et al.*, 2006a). Although Langerhans cells in mammals are dendritic cells in the epidermis, work indicates that these cells in salmonids are typically residents of lymphoid tissues, predominantly found in the spleen and to a lesser extent within the kidney (Lovy *et al.*, 2008b); Langerhans-like cells in salmonids mount systemic responses and can be found within inflammatory

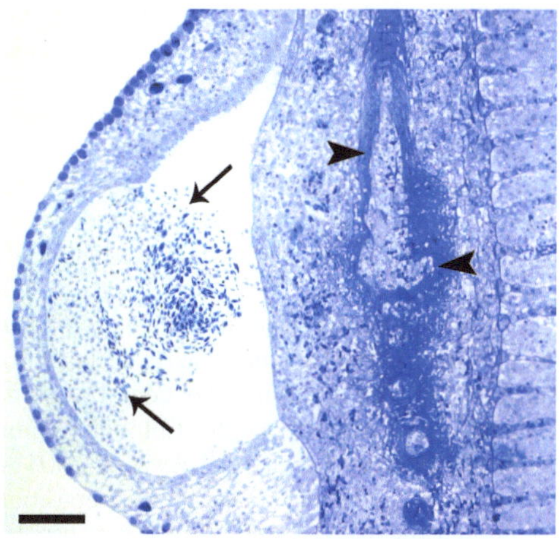

Fig. 6.7. A high-resolution light micrograph of a farmed Chinook salmon (*Oncorhynchus tshawytscha*) gill with clinical microsporidial gill disease, showing an inflammatory response around the filament artery (arrowheads) causing deposition of fibrin in the adjacent tissue and subepithelial oedema leading to a blister containing red blood cells, neutrophils and spores (arrows). Bar = 100 μm. (Author's own image.)

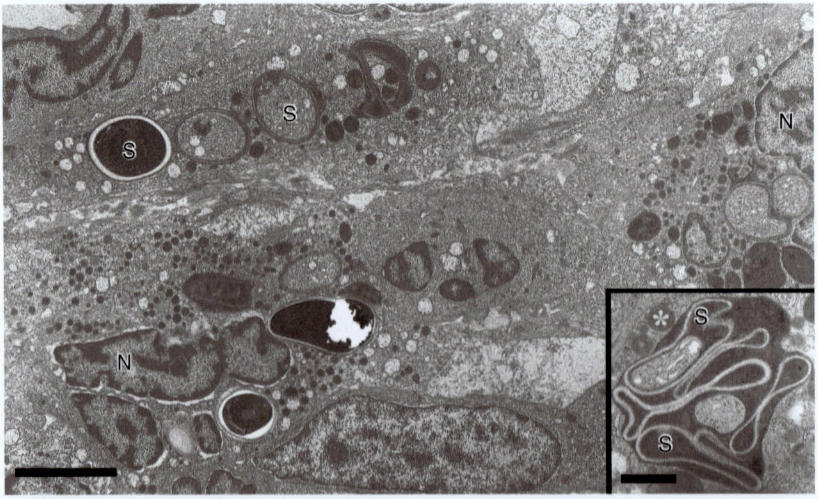

Fig. 6.8. Transmission electron micrograph of a chronic inflammatory lesion within the gill filament of a Chinook salmon (*Oncorhynchus tshawytscha*) with clinical microsporidial gill disease, demonstrating three macrophages (N, macrophage nuclei) containing *Loma salmonae* spores in various stages of degradation. Bar = 4 μm. Inset shows degenerated spores (S) and secondary lysosomes (*) within the cytoplasm of the macrophages. Bar = 600 nm. (Author's own image.)

lesions. These cells may represent a primitive dendritic cell lineage, forming a key component of the antigen-processing and -presenting system necessary for induction of cell-mediated immunity in salmonids (Lovy *et al.*, 2009b, 2010). Based on their presence within *L. salmonae*-induced lesions and given the cell-mediated response that develops in salmonid hosts within 4 weeks following infection (Speare *et al.*, 1998c; Rodriguez-Tovar *et al.*, 2006a), further work into the properties and functions of these cells could be beneficial.

The endothelial-tropic nature of *L. salmonae* results in vascular pathology being a significant part of the tissue reaction subsequent to xenoma rupture, particularly in farmed Chinook salmon clinically affected with MGDS (Lovy *et al.*, 2007b). Arterial damage is evidenced by the deposition of fibrin within blood vessel walls and perivascular connective tissue, and the degree of tissue oedema (Fig. 6.7). *Loma*-induced perivasculitis causes marked alterations to the integrity of the gill vasculature, often accompanied by thrombosis in acute inflammatory lesions and neovascularization in chronic lesions. It is likely that in MGDS-affected Chinook salmon, the presence of xenomas, the associated inflammatory response and the formation of thrombi, when combined, is sufficiently severe to alter the course of normal blood flow; vascular remodelling noted late in the disease may be a physiological response to blood flow deficiency. Thrombosis is common in fish with clinical MGDS, sometimes resulting in full obstruction of arteries and arterioles (Fig. 6.9). During xenoma rupture and associated inflammation, the thrombocyte response appears to be a crucial step in early blood vessel repair; neovascularization as a later-onset response coincides with other markers of chronic inflammatory lesions such as the presence of macrophages and lymphocytes. A future area of study could be to assess whether the use of treatment drugs aimed at limiting thrombogenesis could reduce mortalities during the pivotal xenoma-rupture stage of MGDS.

Healing of gills following xenoma rupture is an interesting area of study; as inflammation begins to subside, the first evidence of lamellar regeneration appears and this progresses until the gill shows little or no anatomical evidence of prior infection (Fig. 6.10). The regenerative capacity of the gill has not been thoroughly studied to date, but it remains fascinating that fish gills can quickly regenerate. *L. salmonae* in

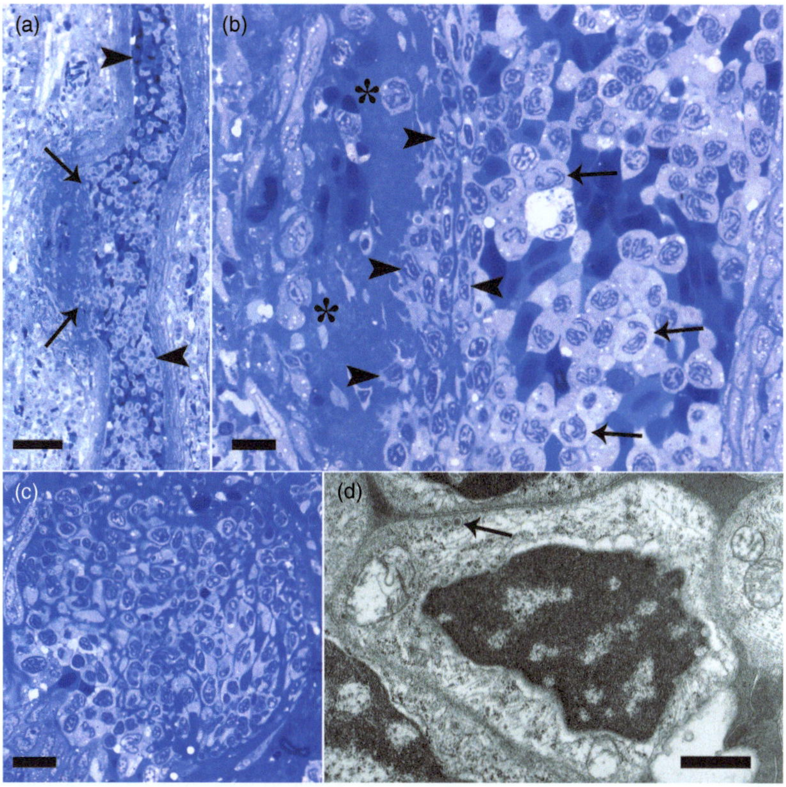

Fig. 6.9. Arterial thrombosis in gills of farmed Chinook salmon (*Oncorhynchus tshawytscha*) with clinical microsporidial gill disease. (a) A major filament artery (arrowheads) with endothelial damage (arrows). Bar = 50 μm. (b) A higher magnification of the damaged endothelial area from (a) showing an aggregation of thrombocytes (arrowheads) and deposition of fibrin (*) in the damaged area. Also notice the abundance of neutrophils (arrows) within the lumen of the artery. Bar = 10 μm. (c) A thrombus fully occluding the luminal space of a filament arteriole. Staining with toluidine blue; bar = 10 μm. (d) A transmission electron micrograph showing an activated thrombocyte with abundant microtubules and granules (arrow) within the cytoplasm. Bar = 1 μm. (Author's own image.)

rainbow trout would be an excellent model to better understand the regenerative capacity of gill lamellae after disease and to better understand host and environmental factors that could modify recovery rates. In a recent review of gill regeneration in fish it was noted that most of the studies of gill regeneration have been conducted on gills where filaments are transected, whereas little study has been done on gills more extensively and randomly damaged during disease (Jonz, 2024). Given the multifocal nature of the xenoma distribution during *L. salmonae* infections, and the time frame of development and dissolution, an opportunity exists to use the *Loma* model to study gill recovery following lamellar damage within the homeostatic domain (rather than the terminal growth domain) of gill filaments. This would serve as an interesting comparison point to the filament resection–regeneration model currently being proposed to approximate the various branchitis conditions in aquaculture (Ghanizadeh-Kazerouni *et al.*, 2024). Noting that *L. salmonae* infection is often a chronically debilitating disease, furthering our knowledge of how we might modulate gill recovery from infection could be an important approach to reducing the economic effect of *L. salmonae* in commercial facilities.

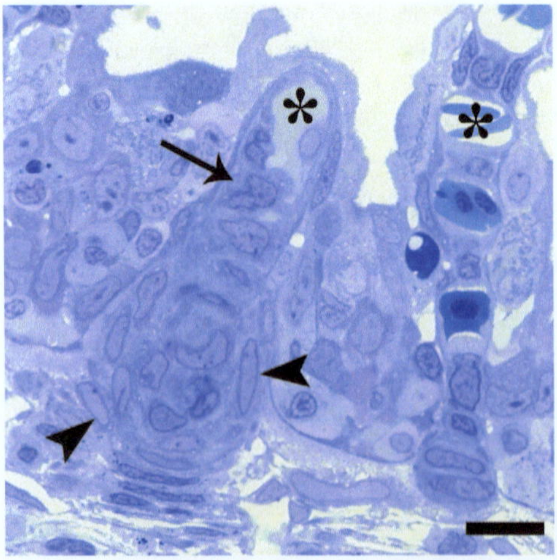

Fig. 6.10. High-resolution light micrograph of a regenerating gill lamella from a rainbow trout (*Oncorhynchus mykiss*) recovering from infection with *Loma salmonae*. An aggregation of non-differentiated cells is observed at the base of the lamella (arrowheads), and a newly formed pillar cell (arrow) is developing its attachments to the basement membrane in the blood vessel lumen (*). Notice the normal structure of the gill lamellae on the right side of the micrograph. Bar = 10 μm. (Author's own image.)

6.2.3. Pathophysiology

6.2.3.1. Haematology

Although the anatomical pathology of the gill during MGDS has been the subject of intensive study, much work remains to be completed to gain a better understanding of the systemic pathophysiological responses of salmonids during MGDS as this may yield vital clues as to treatment geared towards physiological support of fish with MGDS. The remarkably intense inflammatory response noted in the gills is accompanied in the kidney, and to a lesser extent in the spleen, by an increase in myeloid production with a degree of early asynchrony in which immature cells outnumber mature cells. There is a progressive decrease in leucocrit during the course of infection (Powell *et al.*, 2006) suggesting that consumption of white blood cells directed towards gill inflammation exceeds systemic production capacity. No changes were noted in the haematocrit. Assessment of whole-body net ion flux suggests that, despite MGDS causing considerable gill damage, the gill remains able to defend plasma electrolyte concentrations (Powell *et al.*, 2006); however, it remains to be tested whether, under *L. salmonae* challenge, infected fish can deal with dramatic osmoregulatory issues such as changes in environmental salinity or pH. This may be of interest in the context of the wild salmon fishery, particularly given the recent concerns of high mortality levels of infected wild salmon returning to freshwater rivers and streams to spawn (Bowerman *et al.*, 2016). It could also become of interest in the aquaculture industry if MGDS becomes a hatchery disease as survival of infected smolt subsequent to transport to marine sites could be impacted.

Although the ionoregulatory capacity of MGDS-affected fish remains in place, much work remains to be completed to fully understand the oxygen exchange disruptions caused by MGDS. In a key study, it has been shown that whereas rainbow trout with MGDS increase their routine metabolic rate, the opposite is true for brook trout (*Salvelinus fontinalis*) (Powell *et al.*, 2005). Furthermore, the maximum post-exercise metabolic rate for infected rainbow trout exceeds that of controls, whereas it remains the same in brook trout (Powell *et al.*, 2005). These may be important factors when we consider the effects incurred by handling/sorting/treating of fish with MGDS and the relative cost-effective value of providing supplemental oxygen during MGDS outbreaks. Studies by Powell and Gamperl (2016) provide interesting insights into the oxygen exchange and physiological stability of Atlantic cod with *L. morhua*. Cardiac function and metabolic capacity were both negatively affected by up to 40%. However, affected fish showed the ability to compensate for this by enhanced tissue oxygen extraction and increased capacity for anaerobic metabolism. The authors note that these findings are a good example of the ability of fish to compensate for disease-related changes to cardiorespiratory physiology and this is a reasonable cautionary note to consider whenever these types of studies are performed. Although a physiological change might be noted during an infection trial, this does not necessarily mean that the actual impact on fish health or performance will be to the same degree. Furthermore, this would mean that levels of infection do not necessarily correlate in a linear fashion with symptomology.

6.2.3.2. Effects of MGDS on growth indices

Despite assumptions that diseases of fish limit their growth and/or feed conversion efficiency, there are relatively few studies that have identified the extent to which this actually occurs. In studies with rainbow trout, it has been shown that the specific growth rate (SGR) of fish begins to decline coincident with the dissolution of xenomas (Speare *et al.*, 1998c), a temporal pattern which had been anticipated due to the degree of host response that is elicited by xenoma rupture. Prior to xenoma rupture, growth rates of infected and control fish were identical; the period of SGR reduction persisted for 6 weeks during which all xenomas ruptured from the gills. Significant differences in biomass, stemming from reduced growth rates, were detected by week 9 post-infection. SGR of infected fish recovered to match those of control fish by week 10 post-infection (Speare *et al.*, 1998c). A follow-up study demonstrated that SGR reductions were correlated with both a marked reduction in appetite (reduced by 33–46%) and an impairment in feed conversion efficiency (efficiency reduced by 50–95%); compared with appetite reduction, changes in feed conversion efficiency had a later onset and continued for several weeks after appetite had recovered (Ramsay *et al.*, 2004). Based on the timing of changes to appetite, and conversion efficiency relative to changes in SGR, it can be shown that appetite suppression has the greatest negative impact on fish growth, whereas feed conversion impairment, occurring later in the course of MGDS, was more likely linked to diversion of energy into repair of gill tissue rather than somatic growth. A degree of compensatory growth and increased food intake was also noted in the weeks following recovery from MGDS (Ramsay *et al.*, 2004). These results suggest that continuing to feed fish during MGDS outbreaks is likely to be wasteful; however, towards the end of MGDS it would be of benefit to provide increased access to rations, despite the diminished conversion indices, to allow for gill recovery and compensatory growth. In practice, this should be used cautiously, since not all fish in a population would be equally impacted, and though MGDS is seasonal, it should not be assumed that there is always synchronous disease development.

Using an *L. morhua* infection model in Atlantic cod confirms the significance of a systemic microsporidian infection on growth characteristics of teleosts and further demonstrates the potential for brood stock selection to minimize this effect. In the *L. morhua* model, the spleen, as well as the gill, are the most significant target organs for xenoma development; the growth of cod, as monitored through fillet mass, was reduced by 14% and body condition was adversely affected in some affected families of cod (Frenette *et al.*, 2020).

6.2.3.3. Regulatory effects of water temperature

Given the role of temperature in the metabolism of fish and parasites, it is anticipated that the seasonality and temporal course of MGDS will be heavily influenced by water temperature. However, this relationship has yet to be fully utilized in treatment and control protocols. For example, an understanding of the relationship of disease development with water temperature might suggest allowing harvest of susceptible populations of fish ahead of forecasted outbreaks. The summer and early autumn pattern of MGDS has been reported for Pacific salmon in marine netpens in Washington State, USA (Kent *et al.*, 1989), in British Columbia, Canada (Speare *et al.*, 1989), and in earlier reports of *L. salmonae* affecting other salmonid species in fresh water (Markey *et al.*, 1994; Bader *et al.*, 1998), although it has also been postulated that factors other than water temperature, such as seasonal variation in mineral content of water supplies and season per se, may be critical determinant factors (Markey *et al.*, 1994). Perhaps a more important reason to understand the thermal regulatory biology of *L. salmonae* is to help design timing strategies for the use of antimicrosporidial treatments, given that some of these may only be effective on certain stages of the pathogen.

The preferred water temperature for *L. salmonae* is between 13 and 17°C (Beaman and Speare, 1999; Becker *et al.*, 2003; Becker and Speare, 2004b) and within this range, compared with temperatures slightly outside this range (11 and 19°C), survival of the parasite through to xenoma formation is optimized. At water temperatures below 11°C or above 20°C xenoma formation is sharply inhibited (Beaman and

Speare, 1999) and parasite development is abrogated before reaching the gills (Sanchez *et al.*, 2000); the potential for the parasite to continue its life cycle once water temperatures increase to permissive ranges has been demonstrated with a quiescent period of over 4 weeks (Beaman and Speare, 1999). Through the preferred temperature range of 13–17°C, the rate of development of xenomas relative to water temperature has been effectively modelled; the rate of development follows temperature through a polynomial relationship: Xenoma onset (days) = 33.4 (T) + 0.954 (T^2), where T is degrees Celsius. This can be further simplified through a thermal unit (TU) model that corrects for a 'no development temperature' (NDT) of 7°C below which parasite development halts (Beaman and Speare, 1999). Xenomas can be predicted to form once 260–304 TUs have been logged; working backwards from the time of MGDS outbreaks, one can extrapolate the exposure window and from this construct a treatment protocol (Speare *et al.*, 1999b) for subsequent years. In the Pacific Northwest, based on MGDS outbreaks noted in late August and early September, and further by examining ocean water-temperature data from the sea-cage sites, the TU value of 280 points to a period in June where fish are most likely to be acquiring their initial infections with *L. salmonae*. Accordingly, a treatment window constructed during June, well in advance of the first evidence of MGDS (based on detection of xenomas), is likely to be critical for the success of any chemotherapeutic approach to this disease. A more thorough review of the role of water temperature as a disease control method, and the role of increasing coastal water temperatures brought about by climate change, has recently been published (Speare, 2021).

6.3. Protective and Control Strategies

6.3.1. Protecting against exposure to spores

Strict avoidance of exposure to *L. salmonae* can only be achieved with land-based cultivation where control of water sources is possible and where the farm has a closed population and with diligent screening of incoming stock. Since salmon are the main reservoirs for *L. salmonae*, water from a drilled well is unlikely to be contaminated with *Loma* spores and lake water may also be expected to be *Loma*-free if the lake does not contain a salmonid population. Ultraviolet (UV) treatment of incoming water can block horizontal transmission of MGDS (Becker and Speare, 2004a) even in situations anticipated to result in high spore loading of incoming water. The use of recirculation technologies will be of value as it limits the volume of water that may be needed. However, recirculation systems can exacerbate an outbreak by retaining infective spores within the system and particularly so if the recirculation system is used to elevate and maintain water temperature into the range favoured by the parasite (13–17°C) (Beaman and Speare, 1999). Coupling recirculation with the use of UV is therefore suggested.

Avoidance approaches, although suitable to salmon hatcheries and other land-based operations, are not practical for marine netpens. It is expected that salmon in marine netpens will be exposed to spores that are carried in the water column, and it is common for juvenile wild salmon to enter netpens, especially when pit lamps are used to alter perceived daylength. MGDS has been transmitted in fresh and salt water, and the ease of cohabitation transmission has been demonstrated (Shaw *et al.*, 1998; Becker *et al.*, 2003). Remarkably, the brief cohabitating presence of even one moderately infected fish is sufficient to broadly introduce *L. salmonae* into a naïve population (Becker *et al.*, 2005b).

As discussed by Shaw *et al.* (1999), early suggestions, based on the observations of *L. salmonae* spores in the ovaries of sexually mature Chinook salmon, support the concerns that MGDS may also be transmitted either vertically, or congenitally, from brood stock to offspring. This has yet to be substantiated. However, for those culture situations where this is suspected to be the reason for persistent multigenerational problems with MGDS, control may prove difficult based on the limited success of iodophor treatments even when iodophor concentrations used are much higher than industry standards for other diseases (Shaw *et al.*, 1999), attesting to the resilience inherent to spore structures.

6.3.2. Marketing ahead of losses

The seasonal nature of MGDS provides an opportunity to develop production and marketing strategies ahead of MGDS outbreaks. A general goal of marketing fish prior to late summer or early autumn is a reasonable strategy, although it is also feasible to use water temperature history, a thermal model (Beaman and Speare, 1999) and sequential screening of fish to more precisely predict MGDS losses.

6.3.3. Use of more resistant strains/related species

To date, experimental transmission models for *L. salmonae* have been developed for rainbow trout, Chinook salmon, coho salmon (using the typical strain of *L. salmonae* OA) and brook trout (using a variant strain *L. salmonae* SV). The typical (OA) and variant (SV) strains originated from material collected from British Columbia in the autumn of 2000 from farmed Chinook salmon with MGDS. These distinct strains with unique host tropisms were identified after passage of this infective material in rainbow trout and brook trout (Sanchez *et al.*, 2001c; Lovy *et al.*, 2004). Successful modes of infection range from oral delivery of spores or infectious gill material, intraperitoneal injection of semi-purified spore suspensions, to through cohabitation with infected donor fish. Within the permissive host range, there are marked differences between species with respect to susceptibility as demonstrated by Ramsay *et al.* (2002), with Chinook and coho salmon developing far greater numbers of gill xenomas following a standard oral challenge as compared with rainbow trout; rainbow trout are more vulnerable than brook trout to the typical OA strain of *L. salmonae*, but the opposite is true when the SV strain is used (Speare and Daley, 2003). *L. salmonae* infections leading to xenomas have not been established in non-salmonid species (Shaw *et al.*, 2000c).

In addition to differences in susceptibility between salmonid species it is interesting to note that, despite the intracellular nature of microsporidians, the organ and tissue distribution of xenomas as well as the period of xenoma persistence within host tissues vary somewhat between susceptible species (Ramsay *et al.*, 2002). In rainbow trout, xenomas develop almost exclusively within the gill (Speare *et al.*, 1998a), where they grow at quantifiable rates within gill pillar cells (Rodriguez-Tovar *et al.*, 2003a, 2004) and persist for 4–5 weeks regardless of water temperature (Becker and Speare, 2004b). In contrast, in Chinook salmon, although the gill remains by far the most significant location for xenomas, they can also be present in the heart, spleen and occasionally in other locations (Kent *et al.*, 1995). Although the pillar cell appears to be the preferred/required host cell in rainbow trout, it appears that non-pillar endothelial cells in the gill and endothelial cells in other organs are also permissive for xenoma development in Chinook salmon (Kent *et al.*, 1995; Ramsay *et al.*, 2002). Further, in Chinook salmon, although some xenomas rupture in 4–5 weeks as with rainbow trout, others persist for several months (Ramsay *et al.*, 2002). These differences in tropism likely account for the increased pathogenicity in Chinook salmon compared to rainbow trout.

Interesting work by Shaw *et al.* (2000b), who assessed three strains of Chinook salmon in British Columbia, points to the feasibility of selecting strains of fish with enhanced natural resistance to MGDS. Their work showed that although fish strain did not affect prevalence of infection, it did confer a significant effect on the intensity of infection and subsequent mortality. Although the mechanism of this strain-specific resistance was not fully deduced, these authors later investigated species-specific natural resistance and found that macrophages of Atlantic salmon, a species that appears to have natural resistance to *L. salmonae* (Shaw *et al.*, 2000c), have a significantly higher phagocytic response to spores of *L. salmonae* compared with the highly susceptible Chinook salmon (Shaw *et al.*, 2001). Rainbow trout, although susceptible to *L. salmonae*, typically develop far fewer xenomas compared to Chinook or coho salmon (Ramsay *et al.*, 2002), and brook trout are far less susceptible than rainbow trout (Shaw *et al.*, 2000c; Sanchez *et al.*, 2001c; Speare and Daley, 2003). The mechanism(s) behind these species variations remains to be fully elucidated although Sanchez *et al.* (2001a) demonstrated in Atlantic salmon that the parasite successfully enters the lamina propria of the intestine, is transported to the heart (potentially reaching the subendocardial macrophages) but fails to subsequently reach the gill. The infection stalls in the heart and the parasite life cycle does not proceed to sporogony. These findings suggest that macrophage-mediated destruction of the parasite within the subendocardial macrophages, or during the translocation from heart to gill, may be key limiting steps.

6.3.4. Site fallowing

Massive numbers of spores are expected to be shed over at least a 4-week period during an MGDS epizootic from a netpen stocked with salmon at commercial densities. However, very little is currently known about the physical characteristics of these spores (e.g. settling and dispersion rates, the extracorporeal viability of spores) under a range of environmental conditions. Shaw *et al.* (2000a) demonstrated that spore survival at cool temperatures (4°C) can exceed 3 months, but before fallowing policies can be considered, further work is clearly required to examine variables such as temperature, salinity and microenvironmental conditions in sediment.

The emergence of Integrated Multitrophic Aquaculture (IMTA) systems is an example of a technological advance that might offer some benefits connected to reduction of pathogens at farmed sites. Briefly, an IMTA approach to a marine aquaculture site will involve the simultaneous production of a 'fed species' such as salmon, along with high-value aquaculture species such as bivalves which will make use of various outputs from the salmon operation to enhance their production. A salmon farm surrounded by an extensive mussel cultivation would be an example most likely to arise in Canada (Ridler *et al.*, 2007). Mussel cultivation could continue even when the salmon site is fallowed, and this could provide mitigative services for fish diseases by reducing pathogen loads at the farm site. With specific reference to *L. salmonae*, the spores released from infected gills fall into a size range of 2–6 μm and this is an excellent particle size for efficient filtration by mussels. Although promising, research has shown that IMTA has the potential to allow *L. salmonae* to be persistent through a fallowing period. Specifically, although mussels are very efficient at removing *Loma* spores from the water column, the spores are retained by the mussels for several weeks and are subsequently expelled in a viable state capable of reinfecting target salmonids (McConnachie *et al.*, 2013).

The importance of year-class separation is highlighted by Kent *et al.* (1999) and Ramsay *et al.* (2002) who showed that in both Chinook and coho salmon, and to a lesser extent in rainbow trout (Ramsay *et al.*, 2001, 2002), xenoma clearance runs for an extended period and fish remain infective for prolonged periods. Furthermore, Ramsay *et al.* (2001) demonstrated that even with rainbow trout (a species in which branchial xenomas tend to clear relatively quickly) fish will remain potentially infective (have infective spores in their viscera) for over 20 weeks. This 'duration of potential infectivity' is expected to be much longer in Chinook and coho salmon compared with rainbow trout.

6.3.5. Antiparasitic treatments

In vitro screening of antimicrosporidial compounds has faced a historical roadblock due to inabilities to establish *L. salmonae* within a cell culture system. This roadblock, generally and to a variable degree, is also a factor in the slow progress made in finding anti-microsporidia agents. Consequently, this remains an important potential future goal. In its absence, refined, standardized *in vivo* models for MGDS (Speare *et al.*, 1998a), with quantifiable outcomes including prevalence and infection intensity (Beaman and Speare, 1999) or survival analysis (Ramsay *et al.*, 2003), have been developed for a range of antiparasitic agents against MGDS. In general, it is unlikely that anti-infective chemotherapeutic strategies will have much effect on *L. salmonae* once it has reached the spore-laden xenoma stage; therefore, it will be critical to use the TU model previously described to predict the timing for effective application of promising chemotherapeutic agents.

A high degree of efficacy has been demonstrated with orally administered fumagillin (Kent and Dawe, 1994), albendazole (Speare *et al.*, 1999a) and the cationic ionophore monensin (Speare *et al.*, 2000). These treatments resulted in a 70% decrease in the numbers of xenomas forming in treated versus untreated fish. This degree of reduction is likely to translate into a marked reduction in gill pathology and perhaps reduce the disease into a subclinical form. Monensin, a sodium ionophore that is selectively active on post-Golgi endosome and Golgi subcompartments (Dinter and Berger, 1998) which, in microsporidia, may have a key function in the development of the coiled polar tube (Vavra and Larsson, 1999), to date has proven to be the most effective treatment drug, achieving a xenoma reduction rate up to 93% while having no untoward effects on fish growth rates and feed conversion efficacy (Speare *et al.*, 2000; Becker *et al.*, 2002). Early, rather than later, treatment of MGDS is highlighted by the loss of efficacy of monensin when treatment is not given during the earliest stages of infection (Becker *et al.*, 2002). Some drugs, notably quinine hydrochloride, are effective only in delaying the rate of onset of xenomas (Speare *et al.*, 1998d).

There has been some very encouraging and surprising early work showing the opportunities for using cell culture systems for *L. salmonae*. Based on the development of *Loma* xenomas within the gill pillar cells (cells that form the intralamellar vascular channels – pillar channels), it was generally felt that a cell culture system based on teleost endothelial cells, or gill pillar cells, might be the cell line of choice for *L. salmonae*. However, and unexpectedly, work with a rainbow trout gill epithelial cell line (RTG-1) has shown that this cell line can support the growth of this microsporidian (McConnachie *et al.*, 2015). Spores obtained from infected rainbow trout gills were harvested and semi-purified, then subsequently plated on to RTG-1 cells. This led to the development of hypertrophic RTG-1 cells after 3 days and subsequent evidence of spore production within a PV. By 10 days post-inoculation, mature spore-filled xenomas were detected. Notably, this is several weeks faster than would be expected within the gills of experimentally infected fish where 4 weeks is considered a minimum length of time. This marks the first evidence of a fully formed, spore-filled teleost microsporidian xenoma (with spore production happening within a PV) developing within a cell culture system. Given this finding, and the speed at which fully developed spores are produced, this suggests that further refinement of this system could facilitate rapid screening of a large number of potential therapeutic agents – particularly those that may interfere with critical early stages of *L. salmonae* such that production of spore-filled xenomas is blocked.

6.3.6. Immune response, immunomodulation and vaccination

The possibility of developing a vaccine for MGDS was foreshadowed through the observation that recovered fish demonstrate a remarkably strong resistance to reinfection, even when rechallenged with massive numbers of infective spores. This effective resistance also occurs when the initial spore exposure is at water temperatures that do not permit xenomas to form in the gills (Speare *et al.*, 1998b; Kent *et al.*, 1999; Beaman *et al.*, 1999). Additionally, in cod, Frenette *et al.* (2020) have demonstrated the potential for enhancing natural immunity to microsporidian infection through careful selection of brood stock, which further supports the idea that enhancing immunity to *Loma* holds potential for minimizing the related disease condition.

Vaccine prototypes based on killed whole-spore preparations of either the virulent or low-virulence strain of *L. salmonae* have been shown to be effective, with rainbow trout developing a strong protective cell-mediated immune response within 3 weeks following vaccination (Sanchez *et al.*, 2001a; Rodriguez-Tovar *et al.*, 2006a,b). Acquired immunity appears to block the ability of the parasite to transfer from the subendocardial macrophages to the gill pillar cells (Sanchez *et al.*, 2001a), a transfer that is probably mediated by intracellular transport (Rodriguez-Tovar *et al.*, 2002). Protection arising from exposure to these spore-based vaccine prototypes is exceptionally robust and, even without the use of adjuvants, protection exceeds 8 months (Speare *et al.*, 2007). Dexamethasone, known to diminish the innate immune responses to *L. salmonae*, does not diminish the functional protective immunity acquired by *L. salmonae* vaccination (Lovy *et al.*, 2008a). Although rainbow trout and Chinook salmon develop effective immune responses against *L. salmonae*, the vaccine in brook trout appears to be less effective (Speare and Daley, 2003) and in the laboratory they can be sequentially reinfected many times.

Given the interesting results stemming from the use of the low-virulence *L. salmonae* variant as a vaccine candidate, further work was done on more distantly related microsporidia to determine whether they could also become vaccine candidates. *Glugea* spp. were of particular interest given the massive xenomas that they produce and the enhanced spore harvest that this facilitates. Towards this goal, a vaccine study using *Glugea hertwigi* spores and *Glugea anomala* spores showed that viable spores and a killed-spore vaccine preparation markedly reduced the numbers of xenomas on the gills of trout experimentally exposed to *L. salmonae* following vaccine administration. The protective effect of the *Glugea* vaccines was similar to the protective effect arising from *L. salmonae* vaccines (Harkness *et al.*, 2013). The spore-based prototype vaccine against *L. salmonae* represents the first example of a vaccine developed against a microsporidial disease (Speare *et al.*, 2007). Vaccination could therefore be considered for microsporidial diseases of fish and other vertebrates.

Another protective strategy is to boost the immune response to protect fish from disease. There is a growing repository of papers demonstrating the efficacy of glucans containing β-1,3 and β-1,6 glycosidic linkages (known as β-glucans) against a wide range of pathogens affecting farmed fish. Administration of β-glucan through intraperitoneal injection or with oral delivery in feed can markedly reduce the severity of MGDS in experimental trials (Guselle *et al.*, 2006, 2010), although the efficacy is only noted when used early in the course of infection (Guselle *et al.*, 2007). Given the present-day concerns over the use of drugs in aquaculture (Burridge *et al.*, 2010), immune stimulation is likely to be the treatment protocol of choice adopted by the aquaculture industry. There is also potential to use this alongside vaccination for a potential boost in efficacy, though this has not been directly tested.

Based on the temporal pathobiology of MGDS, in which lesions in the gill arise only after xenomas rupture and host inflammatory responses are initiated, it appeared useful to examine the potential therapeutic role of anti-inflammatory agents. Previous work by Davis (1994) supported this idea, and showed that catfish with proliferative gill disease, caused by the myxozoan *Henneguya ictaluri*, developed less severe gill lesions when treated with indomethacin, a non-steroidal anti-inflammatory drug that downregulates the manufacture of prostaglandins by inhibiting cyclooxygenase (inducible and constitutive). If the use of indomethacin for MGDS in salmonids is to be further explored, then it may help to consider the target species. Rainbow trout and Chinook salmon both are affected with inflammatory lesions during the rupture of xenomas, though Chinook salmon are more likely to suffer from vascular pathology, including fibrin deposition around blood vessels and thrombosis. It would be beneficial to understand if indomethacin may reduce inflammatory lesions or reduce vascular pathology which is a common sign in Chinook salmon dying from MGDS (Lovy *et al.*, 2007b). Lovy *et al.* (2007a) demonstrated gastric ulceration and skin lesions as a severe side effect of indomethacin treatment, particularly at higher dosages. These results suggest that if anti-inflammatory agents are considered for use in fish, then mucosal-protective precautions similar to those used for mammalian treatment regimens must be taken into consideration.

6.4. Conclusions and Potential Future Studies

MGDS is a recurrent problem for the aquaculture production of Pacific salmon, and to a lesser degree in other cultivated species. Through the development of a quantifiable *in vivo* model of MGDS, subsequent research has elucidated much about the life cycle and transmission of the parasite along with the role of temperature in modulating the infection. Several promising drug treatments including immunostimulants have been evaluated in the laboratory, and a prototype spore-based vaccine has been developed and tested successfully under laboratory conditions. Much remains to be understood with respect to the dynamics of infection, transmission and subsequent amplification of the disease at farm sites. The reason(s) for MGDS striking salmon as they reach market weight is unclear. These important questions could be more fully understood through ongoing surveillance programmes aimed at identifying the MGDS status of salmon during their first and second year at marine sites. With our knowledge of the regulating role of water temperature on infection, and observations of the efficacy of several treatment approaches (administered during the early phases of infection), the stage is set for field trial evaluations.

Considering that MGDS is mainly a problem with Pacific salmon raised in netpens in British Columbia, Canada, it is noteworthy to understand how this industry will adjust to the announcement that British Columbia will ban netpen rearing of salmon by 2029 (Mather, 2024). A similar move away from netpen aquaculture has occurred in Washington State in the USA (Clark *et al.*, 2017). This aims to replace salmon netpen aquaculture with closed-containment and inshore aquaculture systems that rely on recirculation aquaculture technology. At first glance, this shift in production systems will aid in preventing the introduction of *L. salmonae* into farms because of the higher control of biosecurity, i.e. wild Pacific salmon are common hosts for this agent and are the main reservoirs. Considering the direct life cycle of *L. salmonae*, the environmentally resistant spores and the ability to massively multiply spore numbers just within passage of a single host, these closed-production intensive systems will pose new challenges to the control of MGDS. To avoid issues with *L. salmonae* and prevent its introduction into closed recirculation systems, strengthening efforts in biosecurity related to farm practices, sea water and fish sources could aid in ensuring that no reservoirs or vectors for *L. salmonae* exist. As previously discussed in this chapter, UV treatment may be applied to incoming water sources if spores are believed to be in a water source. Maintaining high biosecurity is a good method to avoid MGDS, though other closed production systems have struggled to remain free of microsporidia. This has best been seen in the zebrafish industry with the microsporidium *P. neurophilia*. Despite high biosecurity efforts, *P. neurophilia* is the most reported pathogen in zebrafish facilities, (reviewed by Caballero-Huertas *et al.*, 2021). Some challenges in preventing *P. neurophilia* introduction in systems include inadequate screening methods in fish and ease of horizontal and vertical transmission. Often the lack of apparent clinical signs related to *P. neurophilia* has added to the difficulty in preventing its spread. Improved biosecurity including quarantine of new stock combined with sensitive detection approaches will aid in reducing future spread/introductions of this microsporidium. Testing quarantined or newly introduced populations with the most sensitive diagnostic techniques will aid in detecting asymptomatic or early infections. For example, real-time PCR has been shown to be highly effective at detecting early stages of infection which would be missed by using histology alone (Schuster *et al.*, 2022).

In closed aquaculture systems, temperature mitigation may become an important management strategy to overcome MGDS if the microsporidian becomes introduced. The most beneficial temperature threshold includes using waters that are 11°C or cooler to constrain development of MGDS. Trade-offs for disease avoidance and optimal growth rates should be considered, as growth rates for Chinook salmon are better at 16 and 20°C compared to 12°C (Araújo *et al.*, 2023). Though temperature manipulation can also include warming waters beyond the permissive temperature range of 20°C, this may be less advisable for most Pacific salmon species as these high temperatures can introduce sublethal temperature stress that can exacerbate other infectious agents as well as reduce the performance of fish in the system. As the use of intensive recirculation systems in the production of salmon in British Columbia is expected to rise, there will be opportunities in fish health to recommend design practices within land-based systems to ensure adequate disease management for issues such as MGDS.

In the USA, there is desire to develop a sustainable offshore aquaculture industry to offset seafood import costs (Fujita *et al.*, 2023). Offshore aquaculture has many benefits; though with lower biosecurity, it will be possible to introduce unwanted pathogens from wild fish reservoirs. With the high diversity of microsporidial species found in wild fish, these could pose fish health risks for this developing industry. For example, as Atlantic bluefin tuna (*Thunnus thynnus*) aquaculture is developing in the Spanish Mediterranean, a novel microsporidium (*Glugea thunni*) has emerged as a potential disease of concern (López-Verdejo *et al.*, 2022). The biology and life cycle of *L. salmonae* in MGDS will serve as an excellent foundation and model for understanding other microsporidia in emerging aquaculture regions. Vaccination against MGDS clearly holds significant promise and developing methods to generate commercial quantities of spores (for killed whole-spore preparations) could advance this approach. The exciting finding of cross-protection between the microsporidia species *Glugea* spp. and *L. salmonae* (Harkness *et al.*, 2013) suggests that perhaps vaccines target a common antigen present in various microsporidial species, opening the possibility of a more broadly appliable microsporidia vaccine. Alternatively, work to identify candidate genes for DNA-based vaccines could be beneficial despite the cautionary note of the historical challenges encountered in developing effective vaccines against parasitic diseases.

Disclaimer

Any use of trade, firm or product names is for descriptive purposes only and does not imply endorsement by the US Government.

References

Araújo, B.C., Miller, M.R., Walker, S.P. and Symonds, J.E. (2023) The influence of temperature on performance, biological indices, composition, and nutrient retention of juvenile Chinook salmon (*Oncorhynchus tshawytscha*) reared in freshwater. *Comparative Biochemistry and Physiology Part A: Molecular & Integrative Physiology* 280, 111412.

Bacchi, C.J., Weiss, L.M., Lane, S. and Wittner, M. (2002) Novel synthetic polyamines are effective in the treatment of experimental microsporidiosis, an opportunistic AIDS-associated infection. *Antimicrobial Agents and Chemotherapy* 46, 55–61.

Bader, J.A., Shotts, E.B., Steffens, W.L. and Lom, J. (1998) Occurrence of *Loma* cf. *salmonae* in brook, brown and rainbow trout from Buford trout hatchery, Georgia, USA. *Diseases of Aquatic Organisms* 34, 211–216.

Beaman, H.J., and Speare, D.J. (1999) Regulatory effects of water temperature on *Loma salmonae* (Microspora) development in rainbow trout. *Journal of Aquatic Animal Health* 11, 237–245.

Beaman, H.J., Speare, D.J., Brimacombe, M. and Daley, J. (1999) Evaluating protection against *Loma salmonae* generated from primary exposure of rainbow trout, *Oncorhynchus mykiss* (Walbaum) outside of the xenoma-expression temperature boundaries. *Journal of Fish Diseases* 22, 445–450.

Becker, J.A. and Speare, D.J. (2004a) Ultraviolet light control of horizontal transmission of *Loma salmonae*. *Journal of Fish Diseases* 27, 177–180.

Becker, J.A. and Speare, D.J. (2004b) Impact of water temperature shift on xenoma clearance and recovery time during a *Loma salmonae* (Microsporidia) infection in rainbow trout *Oncorhynchus mykiss*. *Diseases of Aquatic Organisms* 58, 185–191.

Becker, J.A. and Speare, D.J. (2007) Transmission of the microsporidian gill parasite, *Loma salmonae*. *Animal Health Research Reviews* 8, 59–68.

Becker, J.A., Speare, D.J., Daley, J. and Dick, P. (2002) Effects of monensin dose and treatment time on xenoma reduction in microsporidial gill disease in rainbow trout, *Oncorhynchus mykiss* (Walbaum). *Journal of Fish Diseases* 25, 673–680.

Becker, J.A., Speare, D.J. and Dohoo, I.R. (2003) Effect of water temperature and flow rate on the transmission of microsporidial gill disease caused by *Loma salmonae* in rainbow trout *Oncorhynchus mykiss*. *Fish Pathology* 38, 105–112.

Becker, J.A., Speare, D.J. and Dohoo, I.R. (2005a) Influence of feeding ratio and size on susceptibility to microsporidial gill disease caused by *Loma salmonae* in rainbow trout, *Oncorhynchus mykiss* (Walbaum). *Journal of Fish Diseases* 28, 173–180.

Becker, J.A., Speare, D.J. and Dohoo, I.R. (2005b) Effects of the number of infected fish and acute exposure period on the horizontal transmission of *Loma salmonae* (Microsporidia) in rainbow trout, *Oncorhynchus mykiss*. *Aquaculture* 244, 1–9.

Becker, J.A., Speare, D.J. and Dohoo, I.R. (2006) Interaction of water temperature and challenge model on xenoma development rates for *Loma salmonae* (Microspora) in rainbow trout, *Oncorhynchus mykiss* (Walbaum). *Journal of Fish Diseases* 29, 139–145.

Bigliardi, E., Bernuzzi, A.M., Corona, S., Gatti, S., Scaglia, M. and Sacchi, L. (2000) *In vitro* efficacy of nikkomycin Z against the human isolate of the microsporidian species *Encephalitozoon hellem*. *Antimicrobial Agents and Chemotherapy* 44, 3012–3016.

Bowerman, T., Keefer, M.L. and Caudill, C.C. (2016) Pacific salmon prespawn mortality: patterns, methods, and study design considerations. *Fisheries* 41, 738–749.

Brown, A.M.V., Kent, M.L. and Adamson, M.L. (2010) Low genetic variation in the salmon and trout parasite *Loma salmonae* (Microsporidia) supports marine transmission and clarifies species boundaries. *Diseases of Aquatic Organisms* 91, 35–46.

Bruno, D.W., Collins, R.O. and Morrison, C.M. (1995) The occurrence of *Loma salmonae* (Protozoa: Microspora) in farmed rainbow trout, *Oncorhynchus mykiss* Walbaum, in Scotland. *Aquaculture* 133, 341–344.

Burridge, L., Weis, J.S., Cabello, F., Pizarro, J. and Bostick, K. (2010) Chemical use in salmon aquaculture: a review of current practices and possible environmental effects. *Aquaculture* 306, 7–23.

Caballero-Huertas, M., Soto, M. and Ribas, L. (2021) Reviewing *Pseudoloma neurophilia* infections in the popular zebrafish model. *Reviews in Aquaculture* 13, 1816–1827.

Casal, G., Matos, E., Teles-Grilo, M.L. and Azevedo, C. (2009) Morphological and genetical description of *Loma psittica* sp. n. isolated from the Amazonian fish species *Colomesus psittacus*. *Parasitology Research* 105, 1261–1271.

Clark, D., Lee, K., Murphy, K. and Windrope, A. (2017) *Cypress Island Atlantic Salmon Net Pen Failure: An Investigation and Review*. Washington Department of Natural Resources, Olympia, Washington.

Constantine, J. (1999) *Estimating the Cost of Loma salmonae to B.C. Aquaculture*. Animal Health Branch, Ministry of Agriculture and Food, British Columbia, Canada.

Costa, S.F. and Weiss, L.M. (2000) Drug treatment of microsporidiosis. *Drug Resistance Updates* 3, 384–399.

Davis, S.W. (1994) Effect of indomethacin on the development of proliferative gill disease. *Journal of Aquatic Animal Health* 6, 122–125.

Dinter, A. and Berger, E.G. (1998) Golgi-disturbing agents. *Histochemistry and Cell Biology* 109, 571–590.

Frenette, A.P., Eydal, M., Hansen, H., Burt, M.D.B. and Duffy, M.S. (2017) Integrative approach for the reliable detection and specific identification of the microsporidium *Loma morhua* in Atlantic cod (*Gadus morhua*). *Journal of Eukaryotic Microbiology* 64, 67–77.

Frenette, A.P., Harrold, T., Bentzen, P., Paterson, I.G., Malenfant, R.M. *et al.* (2020) *Loma morhua* infections in Atlantic cod (*Gadus morhua*) reveal relative parasite resistance and differential effects on host growth among family lines. *Aquaculture* 522, 745111.

Fujita, R., Brittingham, P., Cao, L., Froehlich, H., Thompson, M. and Vorhees, T. (2023) Toward an environmentally responsible offshore aquaculture industry in the United States: ecological risks, remedies, and knowledge gaps. *Marine Policy* 147, 105351.

Gandhi, S., Locatelli, L. and Feist, S.W. (1995) Occurrence of *Loma* sp. (Microsporidia) in farmed rainbow trout (*Oncorhynchus mykiss*) at a farm site in south west England. *Bulletin of the European Association of Fish Pathologists* 15, 58–60.

Ghanizadeh-Kazerouni, E., Wilson, J.M., Jones, S.R.M. and Brauner, C.J. (2024) Characteristics of a gill resection–regeneration model in freshwater laboratory-reared Atlantic salmon (*Salmo salar*). *Aquaculture* 579, 740210.

Guselle, N.J., Markham, R.J.F. and Speare, D.J. (2006) Intraperitoneal administration of β-1,3/1,6-glucan to rainbow trout, *Oncorhynchus mykiss* (Walbaum), protects against *Loma salmonae*. *Journal of Fish Diseases* 29, 375–381.

Guselle, N.J., Markham, R.J.F. and Speare, D.J. (2007) Timing of intraperitoneal administration of β-1,3/1,6-glucan to rainbow trout (*Oncorhynchus mykiss*) affects protection against the microsporidian *Loma salmonae*. *Journal of Fish Diseases* 29, 1–8.

Guselle, N.J., Speare, D.J. and Markham, R.J.F. (2010) Efficacy of intraperitoneally and orally administered ProVale, a yeast β-(1,3)/(1,6)-d-glucan product, in inhibiting xenoma formation by the Microsporidian *Loma salmonae* on rainbow trout gills. *North American Journal of Aquaculture* 72, 65–72.

Harkness, J.E., Guselle, N.J. and Speare, D.J. (2013) Demonstrated efficacy of a pilot heterogenous whole-spore-vaccine against microsporidial gill disease in rainbow trout. *Clinical and Vaccine Immunology* 20, 1483–1484.

Hauck, A.K. (1984) A mortality and associated tissue reactions of chinook salmon, *Oncorhynchus tshawytscha* (Walbaum), caused by the microsporidian *Loma* sp. *Journal of Fish Diseases* 7, 217–229.

Jones, S.R.M. and McConnachie, S.H. (2021) *Loma salmonae*. In: Sitja-Bobadilla, A., Bron, J.E., Wiegertjes, G.F. and Piazzon, M.C. (eds) *Fish Parasites: A Handbook of Protocols for Their Isolation, Culture and Transmission*. 5m Books, Great Easton, UK, pp. 95–109.

Jonz, M.G. (2024) Cell proliferation and regeneration in the gill. *Journal of Comparative Physiology B* 194, 583–593.

Keeling, P.J. and Fast, N.M. (2002) Microsporidia: biology and evolution of highly reduced intracellular parasites. *Annual Reviews in Microbiology* 56, 93–116.

Kent, M.L. and Dawe, S.C. (1994) Efficacy of fumagillin DCH against experimentally induced *Loma salmonae* (Microspora) infections in chinook salmon *Oncorhynchus tshawytscha*. *Diseases of Aquatic Organisms* 20, 231–233.

Kent, M.L. and Speare, D.J. (2005) Review of the sequential development of *Loma salmonae* (Microsporidia) based on experimental infections with rainbow trout (*Oncorhynchus mykiss*) and chinook salmon (*O. tshawytscha*). *Folia Parasitologia* 52, 1–6.

Kent, M.L., Elliot D.G., Groff, J.M. and Hedrick R.P. (1989) *Loma salmonae* (Protozoa: Microspora) infections in seawater reared coho salmon *Oncorhynchus kisutch*. *Aquaculture* 60, 211–222.

Kent, M.L., Dawe, S.C. and Speare, D.J. (1995) Transmission of *Loma salmonae* (Microsporea) to chinook salmon in seawater. *Canadian Veterinary Journal* 36, 98–101.

Kent, M.L., Traxler, G.S., Kieser, D., Richard, J., Dawe S.C. *et al.* (1998) Survey of salmonid pathogens in ocean-caught fishes in British Columbia, Canada. *Journal of Aquatic Animal Health* 10, 211–219.

Kent, M.L., Dawe, S.C. and Speare, D.J. (1999) Resistance to reinfection in chinook salmon *Oncorhynchus tshawytscha* to *Loma salmonae* (Microsporidia). *Diseases of Aquatic Organisms* 37, 205–208.

Lom, J. and Nilsen, F. (2003) Fish microsporidia: fine structural diversity and phylogeny. *International Journal for Parasitology* 33, 107–127.

López-Verdejo, A., Montero, F.E., de la Gándara, F., Gallego, M.A., Ortega, A. *et al.* (2022) A severe microsporidian disease in cultured Atlantic bluefin tuna (*Thunnus thynnus*). *IMA Fungus* 13, 5.

Lovy, J., Wadowska, D.W., Wright, G.M. and Speare, D.J. (2004) Morphological characterization and notes on the life cycle of a newly discovered variant of *Loma salmonae* (Putz, Hoffman & Dunbar) from a natural infection of Chinook salmon, *Oncorhynchus tshawytscha* (Walbaum). *Journal of Fish Diseases* 27, 609–616.

Lovy, J., Wright, G.M. and Speare, D.J. (2006a) Morphological presentation of a dendritic-like cell within the gills of chinook salmon infected with *Loma salmonae*. *Developmental and Comparative Immunology* 30, 259–263.

Lovy, J., Wright, G.M., Wadowska, D.W. and Speare, D.J. (2006b) Ultrastructural morphology suggesting a new hypothesis for development of microsporidians seen in *Loma salmonae* infecting the gills of trout. *Journal of Fish Biology* 68, 450–457.

Lovy, J., Wright, G.M. and Speare, D.J. (2007a) Pathological effects caused by chronic treatment of rainbow trout with indomethacin. *Journal of Aquatic Animal Health* 19, 94–98.

Lovy, J., Wright, G.M. and Speare, D.J. (2007b) Ultrastructural examination of the host inflammatory response within gills of netpen reared chinook salmon (*Oncorhynchus tshawytscha*) with microsporidial gill disease. *Fish and Shellfish Immunology* 22, 131–149.

Lovy, J., Speare, D.J., Stryhn, H. and Wright, G.M. (2008a) Effects of dexamethasone on host innate and adaptive immune responses and parasite development in rainbow trout *Oncorhynchus mykiss* infected with *Loma salmonae*. *Fish and Shellfish Immunology* 26, 1–10.

Lovy, J., Wright, G.M. and Speare D.J. (2008b) Comparative cellular morphology suggesting the existence of resident dendritic cells within immune organs of salmonids. *The Anatomical Record* 291, 456–462.

Lovy, J., Kostka, M., Dykova, I., Arsenault, G., Peckova, H. *et al.* (2009a) Phylogeny and morphology of *Glugea hertwigi* from rainbow smelt *Osmerus mordax* found in Prince Edward Island, Canada. *Diseases of Aquatic Organisms* 86, 235–243.

Lovy, J., Savidant, G.P., Speare, D.J. and Wright, G.M. (2009b) Langerin CD/207 positive dendritic-like cells in the haemopoietic tissues of salmonids. *Fish and Shellfish Immunology* 27, 365–368.

Lovy, J., Wright, G.M., Speare, D.J., Tyml, T. and Dykova, I. (2010) Comparative ultrastructure of Langerhans-like cells in spleens of ray-finned (Actinopterygii) fishes. *Journal of Morphology* 271, 1229–1239.

Markey, P.T., Blazer, V.S., Ewing, M.S. and Kocan, K.M. (1994) *Loma* sp. in salmonids from the eastern United States: associated lesions in rainbow trout. *Journal of Aquatic Animal Health* 6, 318–328.

Mather, C. (2024) Phasing out open net-pen salmon farming in British Columbia. *Science Advances* 10, eadt4568.

McConnachie, S.H., Guselle, N.J. and Speare, D.J. (2013) Retention of viable microsporidial (*Loma salmonae*) spores within the blue mussel (*Mytilus edulis*): use of an experimental model probing pathogen transfer within a multi-trophic aquaculture setting. *Aquaculture* 376–379, 1–5.

McConnachie, S.H., Sheppard, J., Wright, G.M. and Speare, D.J. (2015) Development of the microsporidian parasite, *Loma salmonae*, in a rainbow trout gill epithelial cell line (RTG-1): evidence of xenoma development *in vitro*. *Parasitology* 142, 326–331.

Morrison, C.M. and Sprague, V. (1983) *Loma salmonae* (Putz, Hoffman and Dunbar, 1965) in the rainbow trout, *Salmo gairdneri* Richardson, and *L. fontinalis* sp. nov. (Microsporida) in the brook trout, *Salvelinus fontinalis* (Mitchill). *Journal of Fish Diseases* 6, 345–353.

Murray, K.N., Dreska, M., Nasiadka, A., Rinne, M., Mathews, J.L. *et al.* (2011) Transmission, diagnosis, and recommendations for control of *Pseudoloma neurophilia* infections in laboratory zebrafish (*Danio rerio*) facilities. *Comparative Medicine* 61, 322–329.

Mustafa, A., Speare, D.J., Daley, J., Conboy, G.A. and Burka, J.F. (2000) Enhanced susceptibility of sea water cultured rainbow trout to the microsporidian *Loma salmonae* during a primary infection with the 'sea louse' *Lepeophtheirus salmonis*. *Journal of Fish Diseases* 23, 337–341.

Peterson, T.S., Spitsbergen, J.M., Feist, S.W. and Kent, M.L. (2011) Luna stain, an improved selective stain for detection of microsporidian spores in histologic sections. *Diseases of Aquatic Organisms* 95, 175–180.

Powell, M.D. and Gamperl, A.K. (2016) Effects of *Loma morhua* (Microsporidia) infection on the cardiorespiratory performance of Atlantic cod *Gadus morhua* (L). *Journal of Fish Diseases* 39, 189–204.

Powell, M.D., Speare, D.J., Daley, J. and Lovy, J. (2005) Differences in metabolic response to *Loma salmonae* infection in juvenile rainbow trout *Oncorhynchus mykiss* and brook trout *Salvelinus fontinalis*. *Diseases of Aquatic Organisms* 67, 233–237.

Powell, M.D., Speare, D.J. and Becker, J.A. (2006) Whole body net ion fluxes, plasma electrolyte concentrations and haematology during a *Loma salmonae* infection in juvenile rainbow trout, *Oncorhynchus mykiss* (Walbaum). *Journal of Fish Diseases* 29, 727–735.

Poynton, S.L. (1986) Distribution of the flagellate *Hexamita salmonis* Moore, 1922 and the microsporidian *Loma salmonae* Putz, Hoffman and Dunbar, 1965 in brown trout, *Salmo trutta* L. and rainbow trout, *Salmo gairdneri* Richardson, in the River Itchen (UK) and three of its fish farms. *Journal of Fish Biology* 29, 417–429.

Ramsay, J.M., Speare, D.J., Sanchez, J.G. and Daley, J. (2001) The transmission potential of *Loma salmonae* (Microspora) in the rainbow trout, *Oncorhynchus mykiss* (Walbaum), is dependent upon the method and timing of exposure. *Journal of Fish Diseases* 24, 453–460.

Ramsay, J.M., Speare, D.J., Dawe, S.C. and Kent, M.L. (2002) Xenoma formation during microsporidial gill disease of salmonids caused by *Loma salmonae* is affected by host species (*Oncorhynchus tshawytscha*, *O. kisutch*, *O. mykiss*) but not by salinity. *Diseases of Aquatic Organisms* 48, 125–131.

Ramsay, J.M., Speare, D.J., Becker, J.A. and Daley, J. (2003) *Loma salmonae*-associated xenoma onset and clearance in rainbow trout, *Oncorhynchus mykiss* (Walbaum): comparisons of *per os* and cohabitation exposure using survival analysis. *Aquaculture Research* 34, 1329–1335.

Ramsay, J.M., Speare, D.J. and Daley, J. (2004) Timing of changes in growth rate, feed intake and feed conversion in rainbow trout, *Oncorhynchus mykiss* (Walbaum), experimentally infected with *Loma salmonae* (Microspora). *Journal of Fish Diseases* 27, 425–429.

Ridler, N., Wowchuk, M., Robinson, B., Barrington, K., Chopin, T. *et al.* (2007) Integrated multi-trophic aquaculture (IMTA): a potential strategic choice for farmers. *Aquaculture Economics and Management* 11, 99–110.

Rodriguez-Tovar, L.E., Wright, G.M., Wadowska, D.W., Speare, D.J. and Markham, R.J.F. (2002) Ultrastructural study of the early development and localization of *Loma salmonae* in the gills of experimentally infected rainbow trout. *Journal of Parasitology* 88, 244–254.

Rodriguez-Tovar, L.E., Wadowska, D.W., Wright, G.M., Groman, D.B., Speare, D.J. and Whelan, D.S. (2003a) Ultrastructural evidence of autoinfection in the gills of Atlantic cod *Gadus morhua* infected with *Loma* sp. (phylum Microsporidia). *Diseases of Aquatic Organisms* 57, 227–230.

Rodriguez-Tovar, L.E., Wright, G.M., Wadowska, D.W., Speare, D.J. and Markham, R.J.F. (2003b) Ultrastructural study of the late stages of *Loma salmonae* development in the gills of experimentally infected rainbow trout. *Journal of Parasitology* 89, 464–474.

Rodriguez-Tovar, L.E., Speare, D.J., Markham, R.J.F. and Daley, J. (2004) Predictive modelling of post-onset xenoma growth during microsporidial gill disease (*Loma salmonae*) of salmonids. *Journal of Comparative Pathology* 131, 330–333.

Rodriguez-Tovar, L.E., Becker, J.A., Markham, R.J.F. and Speare, D.J. (2006a) Induction time for resistance to microsporidial gill disease caused by *Loma salmonae* following vaccination of rainbow trout (*Oncorhynchus mykiss*) with a spore-based vaccine. *Fish and Shellfish Immunology* 21, 170–175.

Rodriguez-Tovar, L.E., Markham, R.J.F., Speare, D.J. and Sheppard, J. (2006b) Cellular immunity in salmonids infected with the microsporidian parasite *Loma salmonae* or exposed to non-viable spores. *Veterinary Immunology and Immunopathology* 114, 72–83.

Sanchez, J.G., Speare, D.J. and Markham, R.J.F. (1999) Nonisotopic detection of *Loma salmonae* in rainbow trout (*Oncorhynchus mykiss*) gills by *in situ* hybridization. *Veterinary Pathology* 36, 610–612.

Sanchez, J.G., Speare, D.J. and Markham, R.J.F. (2000) Normal and aberrant tissue distribution of *Loma salmonae* (Microspora) within rainbow trout (*Oncorhynchus mykiss*) following experimental infection at water temperatures within and outside of the xenoma-expression temperature boundaries. *Journal of Fish Diseases* 23, 235–242.

Sanchez, J.G., Speare, D.J. and Markham, R.J.F. (2001a) Altered tissue distribution of *Loma salmonae*: effects of natural and acquired resistance. *Journal of Fish Diseases* 24, 33–40.

Sanchez, J.G., Speare, D.J., Markham, R.J.F. and Jones, S.R.M. (2001b) Experimental vaccination of rainbow trout against *Loma salmonae* using a live low-virulence variant of *L. salmonae*. *Journal of Fish Biology* 59, 427–441.

Sanchez, J.G., Speare, D.J., Markham, R.J.F. and Jones, S.R.M. (2001c) Isolation of a *Loma salmonae* variant: biological characteristics and host range. *Journal of Fish Biology* 59, 427–441.

Sanchez, J.G., Speare, D.J., Markham, R.J.F., Wright, G.M. and Kibenge, F.S.B. (2001d) Localization of the initial developmental stages of *Loma salmonae* in rainbow trout (*Oncorhynchus mykiss*). *Veterinary Pathology* 38, 540–546.

Sanders, J.L., Watral, V., Kent, M.L. (2012) Microsporidiosis in zebrafish research facilities. *Institute for Laboratory Animal Research Journal* 53, 106–113.

Schuster, C.J., Kreul, T.G., Al-Samarrie, C.E., Peterson, J.T., Sanders, J.L. and Kent, M.L. (2022) Progression of infection and detection of *Pseudoloma neurophilia* in zebrafish *Danio rerio* Hamilton by PCR and histology. *Journal of Fish Diseases* 45, 1463–1475.

Shaw, R.W., Kent, M.L. and Adamson, M.L. (1998) Modes of transmission of *Loma salmonae* (Microsporidia). *Diseases of Aquatic Organisms* 33, 151–156.

Shaw, R.W., Kent, M.L. and Adamson, M.L. (1999) Iodophor treatment is not completely efficacious in preventing *Loma salmonae* (Microsporidia) transmission in experimentally challenged chinook salmon, *Oncorhynchus tshawytscha* (Walbaum). *Journal of Fish Diseases* 22, 311–313.

Shaw, R.W., Kent, M.L. and Adamson, M.L. (2000a) Viability of *Loma salmonae* (Microsporidia) under laboratory conditions. *Parasitology Research* 86, 978–981.

Shaw, R.W., Kent, M.L. and Adamson, M.L. (2000b) Innate susceptibility differences in chinook salmon *Oncorhynchus tshawytscha* to *Loma salmonae* (Microsporidia). *Diseases of Aquatic Organisms* 43, 49–53.

Shaw, R.W., Kent, M.L., Brown, A.M.V., Whipps, C.M. and Adamson, M.L. (2000c) Experimental and natural host specificity of *Loma salmonae* (Microsporidia). *Diseases of Aquatic Organisms* 40, 131–136.

Shaw, R.W., Kent, M.L. and Adamson, M.L. (2001) Phagocytosis of *Loma salmonae* (Microsporidia) spores in Atlantic salmon (*Salmo salar*), a resistant host, and chinook salmon (*Oncorhynchus tshawytscha*), a susceptible host. *Fish and Shellfish Immunology* 11, 91–100.

Speare, D.J. (2021) Microsporidiosis (*Loma salmonae*). In: Woo, P.T.K., Leong, J.-A. and Buchman, K. (eds) *Climate Change and Infectious Fish Diseases*. CAB International, Wallingford, UK, pp. 369–380.

Speare, D.J. and Daley, J. (2003) Failure of vaccination in brook trout *Salvelinus fontinalis* against *Loma salmonae* (Microspora). *Fish Pathology* 38, 27–28.

Speare, D.J. and Ferguson, H.W. (1989) Clinical and pathological features of common gill diseases of cultured salmonids in Ontario. *Canadian Veterinary Journal* 30, 882–887.

Speare, D.J., Brackett, J. and Ferguson, H.W. (1989) Sequential pathology of the gills of coho salmon with a combined diatom and microsporidian gill infection. *Canadian Veterinary Journal* 30, 571–576.

Speare, D.J., Arsenault, G.J. and Buote, M.A. (1998a) Evaluation of rainbow trout as a model species for studying the pathogenesis of the branchial microsporidian *Loma salmonae*. *Contemporary Topics in Laboratory Animal Science* 37, 55–58.

Speare, D.J., Beaman, H.J., Jones, S.R.M., Markham, R.J.F. and Arsenault, G.J. (1998b) Induced resistance in rainbow trout to gill disease associated with the microsporidian gill parasite *Loma salmonae*. *Journal of Fish Diseases* 21, 93–100.

Speare, D.J., Daley, J., Markham, R.J.F., Sheppard, J., Beaman, H.J. and Sanchez, G.J. (1998c) *Loma salmonae*-associated growth rate suppression in rainbow trout (*Oncorhynchus mykiss*) occurs during early-onset xenoma dissolution as determined by *in situ* hybridization and immunohistochemistry. *Journal of Fish Diseases* 21, 345–354.

Speare, D.J., Ritter, G. and Schmidt, H. (1998d) Quinine hydrochloride treatment delays xenoma formation and dissolution in rainbow trout challenged with *Loma salmonae*. *Journal of Comparative Pathology* 119, 459–465.

Speare, D.J., Athanassopoulou, F., Daley, J. and Sanchez, J.G. (1999a) A preliminary investigation of alternatives to fumagillin for the treatment of *Loma salmonae* infection in rainbow trout. *Journal of Comparative Pathology* 121, 241–248.

Speare, D.J., Beaman, H.J. and Daley, J. (1999b) Effect of water temperature manipulation on a thermal unit predictive model for *Loma salmonae*. *Journal of Fish Diseases* 22, 277–283.

Speare, D.J., Daley, J., Dick. P., Novilla, M. and Poe, S. (2000) Ionophore-mediated inhibition of xenoma expression in trout challenged with *Loma salmonae* (Microspora). *Journal of Fish Diseases* 23, 231–233.
Speare, D.J., Markham, R.J.F. and Guselle, N.J. (2007) Development of an effective whole-spore vaccine using a low-virulence strain of *Loma salmonae* to protect against microsporidial gill disease in rainbow trout (*Oncorhynchus mykiss*). *Clinical and Vaccine Immunology* 14, 12–18.
Star, B., Nederbragt, A.J., Jentoft, S., Grimholt, U., Malmstrøm, M. *et al.* (2011) The genome sequence of Atlantic cod reveals a unique immune system. *Nature* 477(7363), 207–210.
Solbakken, M.H., Tørresen, O.K., Nederbragt, A.J., Seppola, M., Gregers, T.F. *et al.* (2016) Evolutionary redesign of the Atlantic cod (*Gadus morhua* L.) Toll-like receptor repertoire by gene losses and expansions. *Scientific Reports* 6, 25211.
Tiner, J.D. (1988) Birefringent spores differentiate *Encephalitozoon* and other microsporidia from coccidian. *Veterinary Pathology* 25, 227–230.
Vavra, J. and Larsson, J.I.R. (1999) Structure of the microsporidia. In: Wittner, M. and Weiss, L.M. (eds) *The Microsporidia and Microsporidiosis*. American Society for Microbiology, Washington, DC, pp. 7–84.
Vossbrinck, C.R., Andreadis, T.G., Vavra, J. and Becnel, J.J. (2004) Molecular phylogeny and evolution of mosquito parasitic microsporidia (Microsporidia: Amblyosporidae). *Journal of Eukaryotic Microbiology* 51, 88–95.
Vossbrinck, C.R., Debrunner-Vossbrinck, B.A. and Weiss, L.M. (2014) Phylogeny of the Microsporidia. In: Weiss, L.M. and Becnel, J.J. (eds) *Microsporidia Pathogens of Opportunity*. Wiley, Ames, Iowa, pp. 203–220.
Williams, B.A.P. (2009) Unique physiology of host–parasite interactions in microsporidia infections. *Cellular Microbiology* 11, 1551–1560.

7 *Tetracapsuloides bryosalmonae*

Hanna Hartikainen[1]*, Lisa King Wolf[1], Nilanjana Das[2] and Sascha L. Hallett[2]
[1]*School of Life Sciences, University of Nottingham, UK;*
[2]*Department of Microbiology, Oregon State University, USA*

Abstract

Tetracapsuloides bryosalmonae is a significant member of Malacosporea, the less speciose class of the cnidarian subphylum Myxozoa Grasse, 1970. This freshwater endoparasite is transmitted via malacospores from bryozoans and causes proliferative kidney disease in salmonid fishes. Due to the highly temperature-sensitive development of disease and transmission dynamics, *T. bryosalmonae* continues to be an emerging threat to both wild and farmed salmonid populations in the northern hemisphere. The parasite can persist and disperse through its propagation in clonal bryozoans that fragment and travel downstream as resistant statoblasts that can attach to migratory birds, e.g. *Anas* species, that traverse continents. Unique among myxozoans, *T. bryosalmonae* infection can induce at least partial immunity and thereby reduce the severity of reinfection and enhance survival in endemic environments.

7.1. Introduction

7.1.1. Description

Tetracapsuloides bryosalmonae is a malacosporean myxozoan and the causative agent of proliferative kidney disease (PKD) of wild and farmed salmonid fishes. PKD is characterized by severe kidney swelling and mortality, and the development of chronic infections in permissive fish hosts recovered from clinical PKD. Although recognized as 'PKX' since the early 20th century, the myxozoan aetiology was only attributed much later (Kent and Hedrick, 1985). The life cycle was resolved when freshwater bryozoans were identified as invertebrate hosts in 1999 (Anderson *et al.*, 1999), enabling formal characterization of the parasite. Today, PKD is considered one of the most serious emerging, temperature-dependent parasitic diseases of salmonids in Europe and North America (Okamura *et al.*, 2011), with its severity and distribution increasingly driven by and predicted to rise with water temperatures (Bettge *et al.*, 2009; Borgwardt *et al.*, 2020; Ros *et al.*, 2021).

T. bryosalmonae produces infectious malacospores, with two phenotypically distinct forms: fish malacospores and bryozoan malacospores (Fig. 7.1), named according to the host in which they develop. Fish malacospores possess two polar capsules, whereas bryozoan malacospores have four (Feist *et al.*, 2015). Bryozoan malacospores

*Email: hanna.hartikainen@nottingham.ac.uk

 Fish Parasites: Pathobiology and Protection, 2nd Edition (eds P.T.K. Woo and K. Buchmann)

DOI: 10.1079/9781800628748.0007

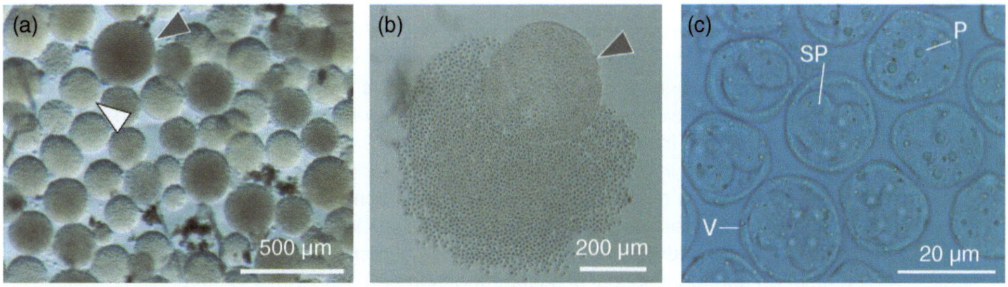

Fig. 7.1. *Tetracapsuloides bryosalmonae* stages in bryozoan host. (a) Parasite sacs dissected from bryozoans, showing sacs full of mature malacospores (black arrowhead) and sacs with maturing malacospores (white arrowhead); (b) one sac ruptured under coverslip, most malacospores are fully mature (arrowhead indicates sac wall); (c) malacospores released from the ruptured sac, with different focal plane revealing sporoplasms (SP), polar capsules (P) and valve cells (V). (Author's own image.)

are spherical, tetra-radially symmetric (Fig. 7.1c) and larger (approx. 19 µm diameter) than the subspherical fish malacospores (measurements in tissue: typically 12–14 µm in height, 6–8 µm in width) (Kent *et al.*, 2000). The structure of bryozoan malacospores has been described in detail (McGurk *et al.*, 2005; Morris and Adams, 2007; Feist *et al.*, 2015); they consist of eight valve cells, four capsulogenic cells, four polar capsules and two sporoplasms. The polar tubule is tightly coiled within each polar capsule (nematocyst), typically forming five to seven coils (Canning *et al.*, 2000), arranged in a transverse or oblique orientation. In fish malacospores, four coils at the anterior end of the spore are described (Kent *et al.*, 2000). Unlike many myxosporean actinospores that develop in annelids, malacospores lack embellishments such as caudal style processes on the valve cells.

7.1.2. Transmission

The complex life cycle of *T. bryosalmonae* obligately involves both fish and freshwater bryozoan hosts (Fig. 7.2, within Box 7.1). No direct transmission between fish hosts or bryozoan hosts takes place, although the parasite can spread along the asexually reproducing and expanding bryozoan host colony. Meiosis during sporogenesis marks bryozoans as the primary hosts of the parasite (Canning *et al.*, 2000). Box 7.1 provides additional information on the bryozoan–parasite interactions and biology, relevant for understanding *T. bryosalmonae* persistence and epidemiology.

Malacospores released from fish into water infect freshwater bryozoans during their suspension-feeding activities and presumably invade this host via the exposed epidermis on the tentacular crown or in the gut (reviewed in Hartikainen and Okamura, 2015). Malacosporean trophic stages, consisting of single cells, grow within the body wall (Canning *et al.*, 2008) and in association with the coelom (Morris and Adams, 2006). These covert parasite stages are immature and not transmissible to fish, pose little virulence in the bryozoan host (Tops *et al.*, 2009; Hartikainen and Okamura, 2015) and expand into new host tissue during growth.

It is important to note that *T. bryosalmonae* can also invade developing statoblasts during the infection in bryozoans (Hartikainen *et al.*, 2013; Abd-Elfattah *et al.*, 2014a). Statoblasts are the highly resistant, dormant resting stages of bryozoans (Box 7.1) and by hiding inside these stages, *T. bryosalmonae* can survive harsh conditions, including desiccation and freezing. This has importance for the persistence and dispersal of *T. bryosalmonae*, because the covert infection stage allows the parasite, at least theoretically, to persist in bryozoan populations even without reinfection from the fish host. Covert infections have also been recorded in bryozoan larval stages, suggesting a systemic presence of parasite stages in infected colonies (I. Fontes, Zürich, 2018, personal communication) (Fig. 7.2).

The development of a covert infection into an overt infection produces malacospores infectious to fish. Covert infection accrues no significant virulence in the bryozoan host, whereas overt infections are virulent and cause reduced

Box 7.1. Phylactolaemate bryozoans as hosts for *Tetracapsuloides bryosalmonae*

Freshwater bryozoans are colonial suspension-feeding animals that use their tentacular crowns, or lophophores, to capture algae, bacteria and other suspended food particles from water. They are sessile and can form dense stands in suitable conditions. Bryozoans grow via budding of genetically identical zooids in the colony, which in many species can fragment and reattach to establish new colonies.

Bryozoans are common in rivers, ponds and lakes, and some are considered a fouling species, growing abundantly on undisturbed artificial substrate and in piping (Wood and Marsh, 1999). Colonies can be readily found on the undersides of rocks, among submerged tree roots and on artificial substrates. They require an abundant supply of suspended food and often thrive in eutrophic conditions.

Bryozoans survive adverse conditions via production of resistant resting stages, statoblasts. Statoblasts are chitinous, seed-like structures that can be produced in large numbers (Fig. 7.2). Statoblasts are adapted to dispersal (gas-filled floats, hooks and spines to attach to floating debris and e.g. bird feathers) and for persistence (firmly attached to surfaces (sessoblasts) to avoid being washed away from a suitable habitat).

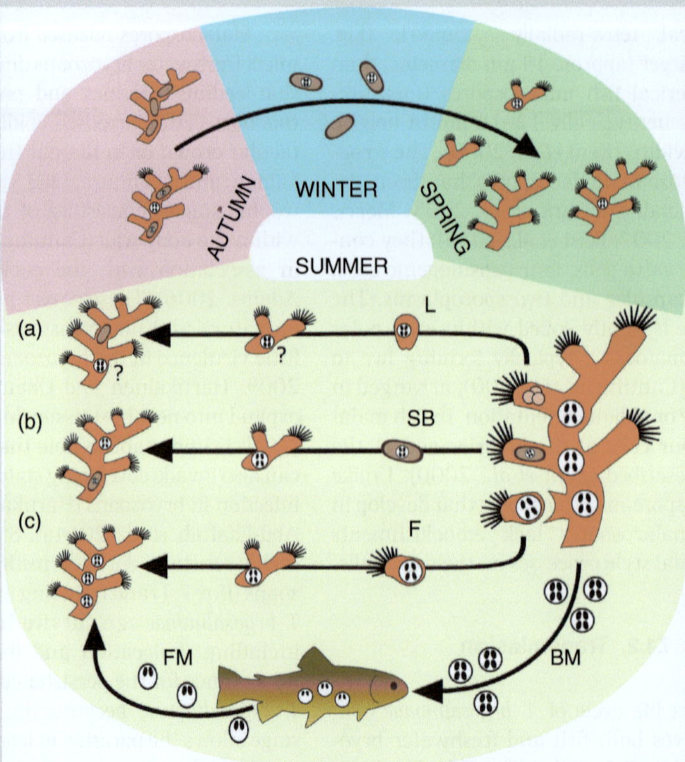

Fig. 7.2. Transmission of *Tetracapsuloides bryosalmonae* and infection dynamics across two-host life cycles. In the autumn, statoblasts are produced within bryozoan colonies, which overwinter and hatch in spring. In summer the bryozoans propagate sexually, via larval production (a), but most asexually, by frequently produced statoblasts (b), and via colony fragmentation (c). The parasite can infect all these offspring types via covert infections (indicated by a malacospore icon where known). Development of overt infections within colonies, their release to water and encounter with fish result in infection and possible Proliferative Kidney Disease (PKD). Competent fish hosts shed spores into water which infect bryozoans. FM, fish malacospore; BM, bryozoan malacospore; L, larvae; SB, statoblast; F, fragment. (Figure created by F. Melzer, University of Nottingham, used with permission.)

Continued

Box 7.1. Continued.

Warmer waters and abundance of substrates for colonization increase bryozoan biomass. The temperature dependence of both the bryozoan host and the parasite impose a clear seasonal pattern on PKD outbreaks, with peak spore release from bryozoans typically occurring during late spring/early summer, and clinical infections becoming evident in late summer/autumn, depending on yearly temperature variation.

growth (Tops *et al.*, 2009), castration of the statoblast production in the overtly infected part of the bryozoan colony and morphological change (Hartikainen *et al.*, 2013). Overtly infected colonies can be recognized by eye as notably 'clumpier', lacking the usual long zooids and branches, and appear stunted, with 'curled over' tips of the zooids (Fig. 7.3).

Overt infections derive from aggregated presaccular amoeboid cells within the bryozoan metacoel, which differentiate into a sac-lined structure, where sporogenesis occurs (Gruhl and Okamura, 2015). Coelomocytes in the bryozoan coelomic fluid (Schwaha *et al.*, 2016) often precede the appearance of sacs. The fluid inside the bryozoan coelomic cavity moves rapidly due to ciliary action, and the parasite sacs can be readily observed 'whirling' around with the coelomic fluid. In opaque host species (e.g. fredericellids collected from the wild), the parasite sacs are readily observed during dissection under a stereomicroscope at 20× magnification. *T. bryosalmonae* sacs are distinctly spherical, of various sizes (asynchronous development, but often >350 μm in size) and typically number three to 15 in an infected branch (although there can be many more).

The malacospores mature within the sacs, which typically burst inside the bryozoan colony, turning the coelomic fluid into a spore soup. A single average-sized sac can produce several thousand spores, and unlike the slow release of only a few malacospores at a time with fish urine, infected bryozoans release large numbers of spores into water, creating temporal and spatial infection hot spots in the environment (Carraro *et al.*, 2017). Spores likely exit via a pore in the tentacular sheath area and remain infectious to fish for <24 h (De Kinkelin *et al.*, 2002). A single bryozoan malacospore can elicit infection and subsequent PKD in a susceptible host salmonid (McGurk *et al.*, 2006).

On contact with a fish, the polar tubule is rapidly extruded from the polar capsule and one or both of the motile sporoplasms exit the spore, possibly guided by the tubule (Feist *et al.*, 2015). The main entry point of the parasite are epidermal mucous cells (e.g. skin, gills) (Morris *et al.*, 2000). Following invasion, the sporoplasms initiate intracellular development and likely migrate through the vascular system of the fish host. Once localized primarily within the interstitial tissue of the posterior kidney, the parasite transitions into a proliferative trophic stage, consisting of amoeboid, uninucleate cells. These cells undergo repeated rounds of binary fission and budding, forming multinucleate plasmodial stages that colonize renal interstitium (Fig. 7.4a). These forms exhibit no overt tissue differentiation as observed during sacculogenesis in bryozoan hosts. This phase represents the pre-sporogonic proliferation stage, during which parasite biomass expands significantly within host tissue.

As development proceeds, the parasite shifts into early sporogonic stages (Fig. 7.4b), characterized by the formation of capsulogenic and sporoplasmic cell lineages within a syncytial envelope. These cells differentiate internally, with capsulogenic cells producing the polar capsules and sporoplasmic cells forming the infective content of the eventual spore. In permissive (compatible or active) hosts, the mature spores are released with urine and infect bryozoan hosts (Hedrick *et al.*, 2004).

7.1.3. Host range and parasite diversity

All salmonid fishes are considered susceptible to infection by *T. bryosalmonae*, with infections having been documented in 16 species. Northern pike (*Esox lucius*) represents the only non-salmonid fish susceptible to the parasite (Seagrave *et al.*, 1981; Bucke *et al.*, 1991; Morris *et al.*, 2000). Morbidity and mortality are typically most pronounced among farmed and hatchery

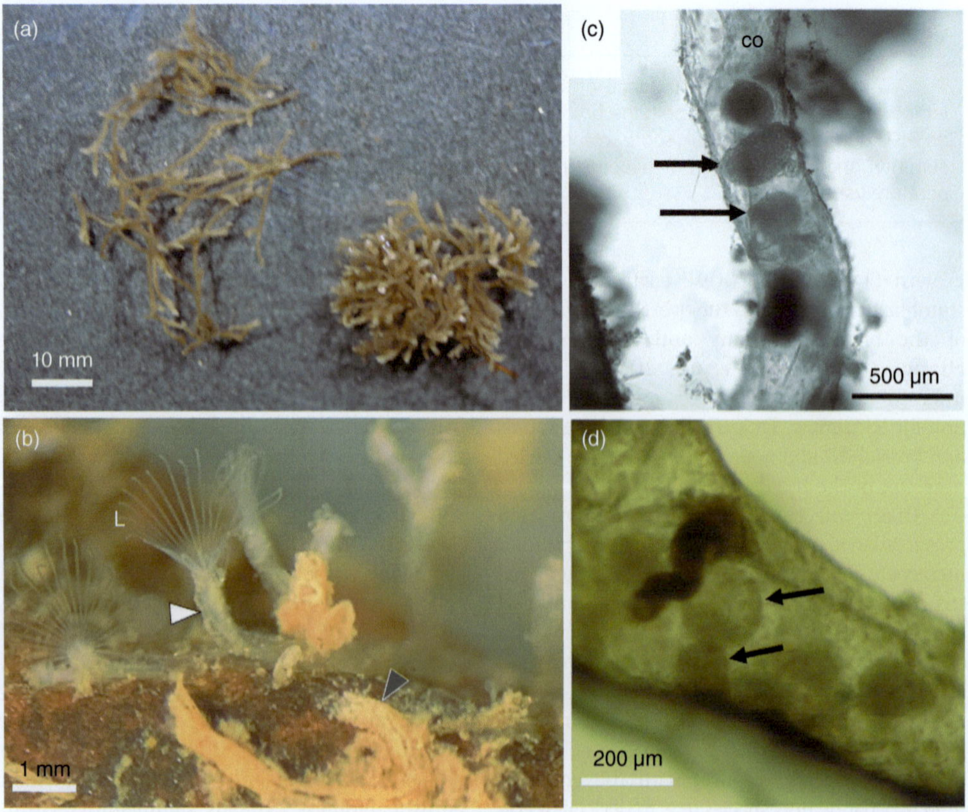

Fig. 7.3. Visual signs of *Tetracapsuloides bryosalmonae* infection in freshwater bryozoans. (a) Uninfected (on left) and infected (on right) *Fredericella sultana* colonies, showing morphology difference; (b) *Fredericella borealis* grown in laboratory, showing the development of translucent zooids in the laboratory (white arrowhead) compared to zooids grown in the field, which are encrusted with sediment (black arrowhead). A circular lophophore is extended for feeding (L); sac stages within coelom (co) in (c) *F. borealis* and in (d) *F. sultana*, visible in laboratory-grown colonies (indicated by black arrow). (Author's own image.)

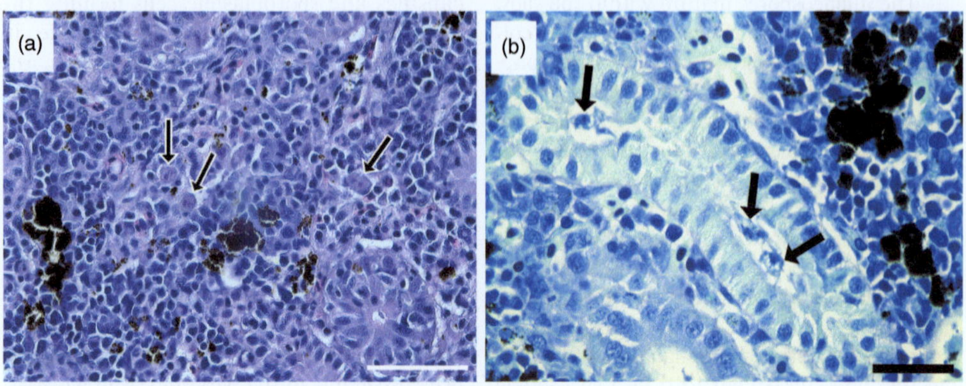

Fig. 7.4. Histology of the posterior kidney in rainbow trout (*Oncorhynchus mykiss*) with developmental stages of *Tetracapsuloides bryosalmonae* (North American strain). (a) Pre-sporogonic stages in the renal interstitium (arrows). Haematoxylin and eosin stain; bar = 100 µm. (b) Intraluminal sporogonic stages (arrows). Giemsa stain; bar = 20 µm. (Author's own image.)

populations of rainbow trout (*Oncorhynchus mykiss*) and wild brown trout (*Salmo trutta*) in Europe (Feist and Bucke, 1993), and rainbow trout and Chinook salmon (*Oncorhynchus tshawytscha*) in North American hatcheries (Hedrick *et al.*, 1984). Outbreaks have also been documented among cultured and wild Atlantic salmon (*Salmo salar*) (Sterud *et al.*, 2007). While clinical PKD develops in most salmonids, exceptions include limited or no observable clinical signs among infected brook trout (*Salvelinus fontinalis*) and European whitefish (*Coregonus lavaretus*) (Feist and Bucke, 1993; Sobociński *et al.*, 2018).

It is not clear if all susceptible host species are competent, facilitating the completion of the parasite life cycle. Confirmation requires evidence of parasite transmission to a bryozoan host in order to distinguish between dead-end and competent hosts. Fish-to-bryozoan transmission has been assessed for naturally infected brown, brook and rainbow trout, grayling (*Thymallus thymallus*) and northern pike (Grabner and El-Matbouli, 2008). Infections developed only in bryozoan colonies cohabitated with brook and brown trout (Grabner and El-Matbouli, 2008), confirming these species as competent hosts in the European context.

Two genetically distinct strains originating from Europe and North America have been proposed based on ITS1 (internally transcribed spacer region 1) (Henderson and Okamura, 2004) and COI (cytochrome oxidase subunit 1) (Hutchins *et al.*, 2021) sequences. It is now known that mature spore formation and completion of the parasite's life cycle is achieved in locally adapted host–parasite pairings (Das *et al.*, 2026). For instance, spore development in rainbow trout infected with the European parasite strain rarely advances beyond pre-sporogonic proliferation, and surviving fish typically clear the infection within 15 weeks (Schmidt-Posthaus *et al.*, 2012). In contrast, infections with the North American strain in native rainbow and steelhead trout (resident and anadromous *O. mykiss*, respectively) consistently progress to the intraluminal sporogonic stage with visible polar capsules. The presence of mature spores in rainbow trout urine (Hedrick *et al.*, 2004) and successful parasite transmission from steelhead trout to *Fredericella borealis* Wood, 2022 (Das *et al.*, 2026) have since confirmed *O. mykiss* as a competent host in the region. Locally adapted host–parasite pairings show longer duration of subclinical infections and a prolonged presence of intraluminal stages in the kidney (Das *et al.*, 2026), with spore shedding evident for up to 5 years post-infection in European brown trout (Soliman *et al.*, 2018). It is currently not known whether further genomic signatures of local adaptation could explain differences in disease severity and spore development observed among various Pacific salmon species (Arkush and Hedrick, 1990).

7.1.4. Bryozoan host range

Overt *T. bryosalmonae* infections have been observed in several species of freshwater bryozoans, including *Plumatella emarginata* and *Fredericella sultana* in the UK and Europe (Longshaw *et al.*, 1999), and *Pectinatella magnifica*, *Cristatella mucedo*, *Plumatella rugosa* and *F. borealis* in North America (Anderson *et al.*, 1999; Okamura *et al.*, 2001; Das *et al.*, 2026). We note that older literature may refer to *Fredericella indica* Annandale, 1909 from northern temperate zones; however, the species name for specimens from this geographic is now *F. borealis* Wood, 2022. *F. indica* remains in use for specimens from the Indian subcontinent (Wood, 2022). The parasite has also been detected molecularly in *Plumatella fruticosa* within a recirculating aquaculture system enzootic for PKD in the Czech Republic (Syrová *et al.*, 2020). Fredericellid species are considered the predominant hosts for *T. bryosalmonae* (Hartikainen and Okamura, 2015), and bryozoan-to-fish transmission studies have confirmed the roles of *F. sultana* and *F. borealis* as competent hosts of the European and North American parasite strains (Feist *et al.*, 2001; Das *et al.*, 2026).

7.1.5. Geographical distribution

T. bryosalmonae exhibits a cosmopolitan distribution across temperate freshwater ecosystems of the northern hemisphere, closely mirroring the biogeography of its salmonid hosts and bryozoan vectors (Henderson and Okamura, 2004; Sudhagar *et al.*, 2020). In Europe, its presence is well documented across a broad latitudinal range, from Scandinavia through Central Europe to the Mediterranean basin. Countries with established records include the UK, Germany, Switzerland, France, the Czech Republic, Norway, Sweden, Denmark, Wales, Italy, Netherlands, Spain, Iceland, Estonia and Poland. The parasite is also endemic to North America, with confirmed infections in native and introduced salmonids across British Columbia and Newfoundland in Canada, and Alaska, Washington, Oregon, California, Montana and Michigan (Fusianto *et al.*, 2024) in the USA. Recent findings of PKD in more northerly regions (e.g. Iceland: Kristmundsson *et al.*, 2023; Baltic: Lauringson *et al.*, 2021; Alaska: Gorgoglione *et al.*, 2020; Finland: Vasemägi *et al.*, 2017) suggest an apparent range expansion. However, a possible alternative scenario is that the new records reflect temperature-driven increase in disease severity and mortality, rather than dispersal and movement of the parasite to new locations. This remains to be confirmed and requires molecular phylogenetic insights to *T. bryosalmonae* evolutionary history.

7.1.6. Impact

T. bryosalmonae infection that progresses to PKD has negatively impacted captive and free-ranging salmonid populations across the northern hemisphere. In aquaculture, the parasite is responsible for substantial economic losses, particularly in rainbow trout farming, steelhead production and Atlantic salmon hatcheries in Europe (Clifton-Hadley and Bucke, 1986). Today in the UK, it is estimated that at least 300,000 fish in inland rainbow trout aquaculture incur the severest grades of PKD over several months. Pre-exposure methods developed since the 1980s (manipulated exposure and recovery that affords protection from disease; see Section 7.3.1) have reduced the burden of mortality, but the renal pathology still compromises fish growth, feed conversion efficiency and overall health, necessitating increased husbandry inputs and often culminating in elevated culling.

In the USA, aquaculture and hatcheries accrue PKD-related losses, although the economic impact of this disease is not well documented. Cultivation of first-summer Chinook and coho salmon in California hatcheries has been noted to be impacted even in some of the earliest work on PKD (Hedrick *et al.*, 1984). In Oregon, only four occurrences of *T. bryosalmonae* infections were recorded prior to 2020, all occurring in the state's fish hatcheries between 1994 and 2001 (S. Bjork, Oregon Department of Fish and Wildlife, Fish Health Section, 2020, personal communication). However, in the summers of 2020/2021, a PKD outbreak in a hatchery on the McKenzie River caused an epizootic loss of juvenile rainbow and steelhead trout and Chinook salmon (>0.1–5.2% per day) (A. Reed, Oregon Department of Fish and Wildlife, Fish Health Section, 2020, personal communication). The outbreaks followed a 68-year history of the hatchery with no previous PKD outbreaks.

In wild populations, *T. bryosalmonae* infection contributes to population-level declines across an increasing number of countries, with evidence for mass mortality events (reviewed in Ros *et al.*, 2022). While young-of-the-year (YOY) and parr are most severely affected, adult fish can also experience PKD-related impacts (Bailey *et al.*, 2017a; Arndt *et al.*, 2019). For instance, YOY brown trout densities have been reported to be over 90% lower in PKD-affected rivers compared to unaffected ones (Schager *et al.*, 2007) and epidemiological modelling suggests similar trends (Carraro *et al.*, 2017).

The 2016 Yellowstone River fish kill was the most severe documented outbreak of PKD in a wild fish population (Hutchins *et al.*, 2021), causing catastrophic short-term losses. Tens of thousands of primarily mountain whitefish (*Prosopium williamsoni*) died along a 183 km stretch of the river during a period of sustained high water temperatures (>21°C) and low flows. Histological and molecular analyses confirmed severe PKD pathology, with infection prevalence exceeding 90% in affected fish. While trout species were also infected, mountain whitefish experienced the highest mortality, reflecting species-specific susceptibility. Retrospective molecular testing revealed the parasite was present as early as 2012, and follow-up surveys in 2017 and 2018 detected ongoing infections without comparable mortality, indicating that PKD is endemic and can cause episodic mass mortality under certain conditions.

7.2. Pathobiology

7.2.1. Clinical signs

External clinical signs of PKD commonly include pallor and anaemia of the gills, abdominal distension and exophthalmos, occasionally with cutaneous darkening (Clifton-Hadley *et al.*, 1987a). Internal pathology is characterized by pronounced renal swelling, ascites, liver pallor and splenic enlargement (Hedrick *et al.*, 1993). Behavioural signs such lethargy, anorexia, abnormal swimming and respiratory distress typically emerge during peak parasite proliferation and coincide with worsening clinical condition (El-Matbouli and Hoffmann, 1994; Kent, 2014). Clinical signs generally develop progressively between 4 and 10 weeks post-infection, with severity closely linked to water temperature and parasite load (Clifton-Hadley *et al.*, 1987a,b; Schmidt-Posthaus *et al.*, 2012).

Severity of PKD varies between host species, reflecting differences in susceptibility, parasite development and host–pathogen interactions (Okamura *et al.*, 2011). Obvious clinical signs typically characterize rainbow trout and brown trout (Hedrick *et al.*, 1993), with milder clinical signs or asymptomatic infections observed in other salmonids and close relatives (Bucke *et al.*, 1991; Feist and Bucke, 1993) (Table 7.1).

7.2.2. Gross pathology and histology

The disease process reflects a combination of parasite-induced tissue damage and exuberant host immune activation, culminating in impaired renal and haematopoietic function. The pronounced enlargement of the posterior kidney during PKD is driven by interstitial inflammation due to infiltrating lymphoid tissue (MacConnell *et al.*, 1989) and granulomatous response (Hedrick *et al.*, 1993). In severe infections, splenic lesions may progress to extensive collagen formation, enlargement and discoloration (Clifton-Hadley *et al.*, 1987a). In hosts where clinical signs are weak, gross lesions are subtle or absent.

Histologically, the kidney exhibits severe interstitial lymphocytic hyperplasia and varying degrees of renal atrophy (Hedrick *et al.*, 1993) (Fig. 7.5). Amoeboid and pre-sporogonic parasites are localized within the renal parenchyma, where the associated pathology includes thrombus formation and necrotizing vasculitis, along with marked hyperplastic response. This progresses to extensive proliferative and diffuse granulomatous nephritis, which disrupts the renal architecture and may lead to degeneration of the renal tubuli (Kent and Hedrick, 1985). In other hosts, or less severe infections, histological findings may be limited to mild interstitial lymphoid proliferation and the presence of an inflammatory profile, with only occasional detection of pre-sporogonic parasite stages. In such cases, the parasite development may remain incomplete, suggesting low-competency or incidental host dynamics (Hedrick *et al.*, 1993).

General blood profiles have been described in rainbow trout in the USA (Clifton-Hadley *et al.*, 1987b) and Europe (Palikova *et al.*, 2017), with similar conclusions, despite the difference in co-evolutionary history between rainbow trout and the North American and European strains of the parasite. Skin haemorrhages and the presence of haemorrhagic fluid in the internal cavities indicate pronounced haemorrhagic and haemolytic anaemia (Palikova *et al.*, 2017), with substantial reductions in red blood cell count, haematocrit and haemoglobin concentration, associated with peak gross pathology (Clifton-Hadley *et al.*, 1987b). The pathology in the kidney and spleen coincides with impaired erythropoiesis and morphological alterations of erythrocytes.

A parallel leucocyte shift in the blood profile is observed, with reduced lymphocyte numbers and increased phagocyte counts, particularly macrophages and neutrophils (Palikova *et al.*, 2017). Complement activity and total plasma immunoglobulin (Ig) levels are elevated during early infection, reflecting strong humoral immune activation. Particularly notable is the rise in IgT levels, with IgT^{+} B cells becoming the dominant lymphocyte subset in the kidney as pathology progresses. Intriguingly, red blood cells begin to express surface IgM, with up to 99% of erythrocytes being IgM^{+} in heavily infected individuals, revealing a putative novel immunomodulatory role for nucleated red blood cells during PKD (Chan *et al.*, 2023). Notably, fish that survive PKD and transition

Table 7.1. Fish species susceptible to infection with *Tetracapsuloides bryosalmonae* and examples of outbreaks in cultured and wild populations. (Author's own table.)

Fish host species	Scientific name	*T. bryosalmonae* strain[a]	Affected cultured populations	Affected wild populations	Level of sporogenesis observed
Rainbow trout (landlocked)	*Oncorhynchus mykiss*	NA	Idaho, USA (Smith *et al.*, 1984) California, USA (Foott *et al.*, 2007)	None reported	Mature spores in urine (Hedrick *et al.*, 2004)
Steelhead trout (anadromous)	*O. mykiss*	NA	California, USA (Hedrick *et al.*, 1984) Oregon, USA (A. Reed, Oregon Department of Fish and Wildlife, Fish Health Section, 2020, unpublished results)	Montana, USA (Klontz *et al.*, 1986)	Intraluminal sporogonic stages with polar capsules (Das *et al.*, 2026)
Rainbow trout (landlocked)	*O. mykiss*	EU	Spain (Peribáñez *et al.*, 1997) UK (Ferguson and Ball, 1979) Switzerland (Wahli *et al.*, 2002) Czech Republic (Palikova *et al.*, 2017)	UK (Bucke *et al.*, 1991) Germany (Hoffman and Dangschat, 1981)	Pre-sporogonic stages in interstitium
Brown trout	*Salmo trutta*	EU	Spain (Peribáñez *et al.*, 1997) Austria (Gorgoglione *et al.*, 2016) UK (Ellis *et al.*, 1982)	Austria (Waldner *et al.*, 2020) Germany (Arndt *et al.*, 2019) Switzerland (Wahli *et al.*, 2002)	Intraluminal sporogonic stages with polar capsules
Brook trout	*Salvelinus fontinalis*	EU	None reported	None reported	Intraluminal sporogonic stages
Cutthroat trout	*Oncorhynchus clarkii*	NA	None reported	Montana, USA (MacConnell and Peterson, 1992)	Intraluminal sporogonic stages
Chinook salmon	*Oncorhynchus tshawytscha*	NA	California, USA (Hedrick *et al.*, 1984) Oregon, USA (A. Reed, Oregon Department of Fish and Wildlife, Fish Health Section, 2020, personal communication) British Columbia, Canada (Kent *et al.*, 1995)	None reported	Intraluminal sporogonic stages with polar capsules
Coho salmon	*Oncorhynchus kisutch*	NA	California, USA (Hedrick *et al.*, 1984)	None reported	Intraluminal sporogonic stages with polar capsules
Kokanee salmon (landlocked)	*Oncorhynchus nerka*	NA	None reported	None reported	Intraluminal sporogonic stages with polar capsules (Kent *et al.*, 1995)
Sockeye salmon (anadromous)	*O. nerka*	NA	None reported	Alaska, USA (Gorgoglione *et al.*, 2020)	Intraluminal sporogonic stages

Chum salmon	*Oncorhynchus keta*	NA	None reported	None reported	Intraluminal sporogonic stages (Gorgoglione *et al*., 2020)
Arctic charr	*Salvelinus alpinus*	NA	Newfoundland, Canada (Brown *et al*., 1991)	None reported	Intraluminal sporogonic stages with polar capsules
Arctic charr	*S. alpinus*	EU	None reported	None reported	Intraluminal sporogonic stages with polar capsules (Mo and Jørgensen, 2017)
Pink salmon	*Oncorhynchus gorbuscha*	NA	None reported	None reported	Intraluminal sporogonic stages (Braden *et al*., 2010)
Mountain whitefish	*Prosopium williamsoni*	NA	None reported	Montana, USA (Hutchins *et al*., 2021)	Not reported
European whitefish	*Coregonus lavaretus*	EU	None reported	None reported	Not reported (Sobociński *et al*., 2018)
Whitefish	*Coregonus albula*	EU	None reported	None reported	Intraluminal sporogonic stages (Naldoni *et al*., 2019)
Grayling	*Thymallus thymallus*	EU	None reported	None reported	Intraluminal sporogonic stages with polar capsules (Bucke *et al*., 1991)
Atlantic salmon	*Salmo salar*	EU	Scotland (Ellis *et al*., 1982)	Norway (Sterud *et al*., 2007)	Intraluminal sporogonic stages with polar capsules
Marble trout	*Salmo trutta marmoratus*	EU	Italy (Beraldo *et al*., 2006)	None reported	Mature spores in renal tubules
Golden trout	*Oncorhynchus aguabonita*	EU	UK (Morris *et al*., 2003)	None reported	Intraluminal sporogonic stages
Northern pike	*Esox lucius*	NA	None reported	None reported	Not reported (Bucke *et al*., 1991)

[a]NA, North American strain; EU, European strain.

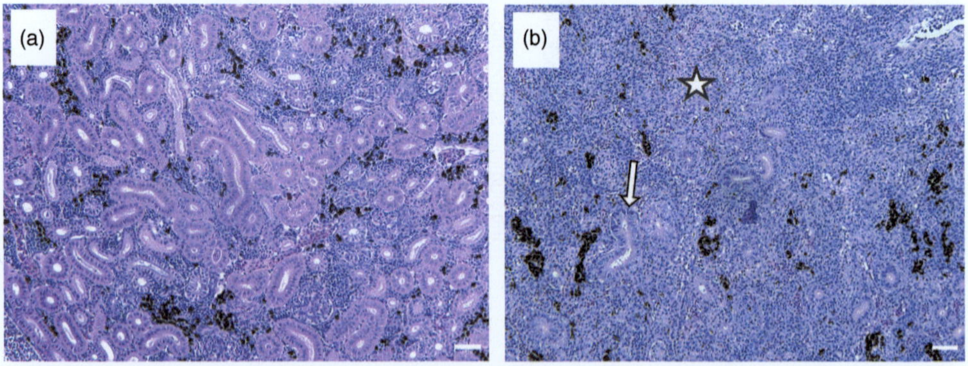

Fig. 7.5. Histology of the posterior kidney in (a) healthy and (b) *Tetracapsuloides bryosalmonae*-infected *Oncorhynchus mykiss*. (b) Characteristic pathology of PKD can be observed, including hyperplasia of the interstitium (star) and a reduction in the number of renal tubules (arrow). Haematoxylin and eosin stain; bar = 100 μm. (Author's own image.)

into recovery undergo full haematological rehabilitation (Palikova *et al.*, 2017).

7.2.3. Diagnosis

The standard protocol for diagnosing PKD involves a combination of gross examination, histopathology and molecular techniques, as external and behavioural signals are not specific to PKD alone. Necropsy focuses on the posterior kidney, and most commonly, the degree of kidney swelling is assessed on a scale from 0 to 4 (Clifton-Hadley *et al.*, 1987a). Visual and tactile criteria include the degree of enlargement, extent of pallor or mottling, firmness or friability of the tissue, and distortion of the kidney's normal shape. A score of 0 indicates a normal kidney, while scores of 1 and 2 reflect mild to moderate swelling, and scores of 3 or 4 indicate severe enlargement and severe clinical disease. The scale also includes the score H, which is used to indicate a kidney with an advanced sign of healing. This scoring scale provides a standardized, semi-quantitative measure of PKD progression, allowing comparison across time points, populations or treatment groups. Figure 7.6 and Table 7.2 provide an expanded scoring guide for PKD based on the original framework developed by Clifton-Hadley *et al.* (1987a), with additional criteria to enhance clarity and consistency in the field and laboratory (L. King Wolf, Nottingham, 2025, unpublished results).

Three other measures of swelling are also used. The Kidney Somatic Index (KSI) represents a ratio of the kidney weight to the fish weight and thus requires the isolation and weighing of the kidney. KSI correlates well with parasite intensity and histopathological grade, and standardizes for fish size (Bailey *et al.*, 2021). The Posterior Kidney Somatic Index (PKSI) is very similar to KSI but only utilizes the posterior kidney instead of the entire organ. The third measure is the kidney to body ratio (K/B), calculated as the ratio of the kidney thickness to body thickness. The measurements are obtained from a transverse cross-section made through the mid region of the posterior kidney, usually at a standardized anatomical point such as the midpoint between the head and tail. The cut is made perpendicular to the fish's longitudinal axis to produce a clean cross-sectional view that exposes the internal kidney structure for imaging and analysis (Bruneaux *et al.*, 2017). It is important to note the method used, as they are not comparable, despite kidney swelling index (Fig. 7.6) being often referred to as KSI.

For histological analysis tissue samples from the kidney should be fixed in 10% v/v neutral buffered formalin before being embedded into paraffin. Paraffin embedded sections are stained with haematoxylin and eosin to identify characteristic lesions, such as interstitial lymphoid hyperplasia and the presence of *T. bryosalmonae* stages within the renal parenchyma (Klontz and Chacko, 1983; Hedrick *et al.*, 1992; Rubin *et al.*, 2019). Immunohistochemistry using anti-*T. bryosalmonae* antibodies can enhance diagnostic specificity by precisely localizing parasite stages within host tissue sections, particularly within the renal interstitium (Longshaw *et al.*, 1999; Schmidt-Posthaus *et al.* 2012;

Grade 0

Grade 1

Grade 2

Grade 3

Grade 4

Grade H

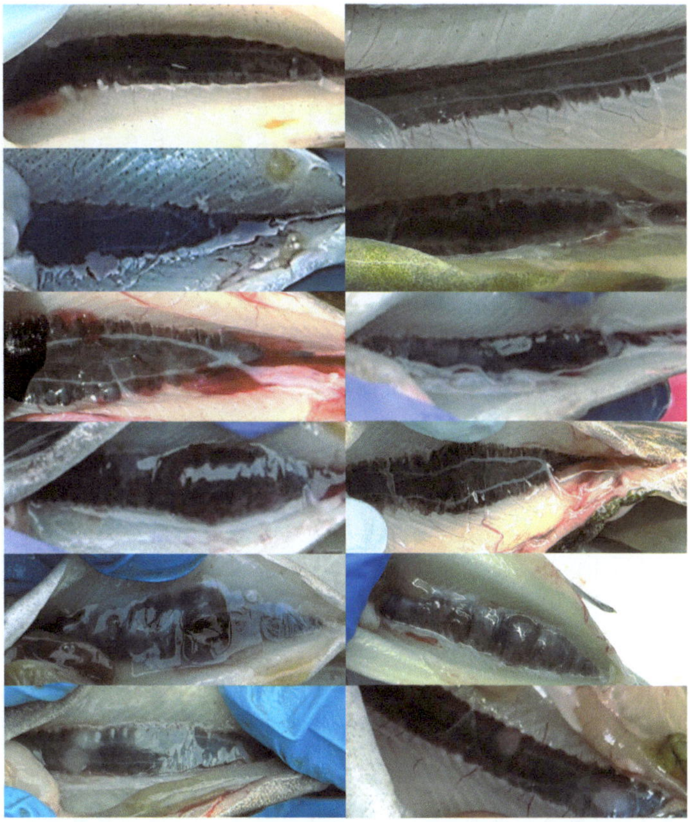

Fig. 7.6. Different grades of kidney swelling caused by PKD. Grade 0 = normal kidney, 1 = mild swelling, 2 = mild to moderate swelling, 3 = moderate swelling, 4 = severe swelling and H = kidney with advanced stages of healing. (Author's own image.) Refer to Table 7.2 for more information.

Kumar *et al.*, 2013). Lectin histochemistry has also been applied to demonstrate carbohydrate-binding patterns of *T. bryosalmonae* stages within renal tissue (Castagnaro *et al.*, 1991; Hedrick *et al.*, 1992; Skovgaard and Buchmann, 2012).

For definitive confirmation, molecular diagnostics such as PCR or quantitative PCR (qPCR) targeting parasite-specific DNA (e.g. 18S rRNA or ITS regions) can be performed on fresh or ethanol-preserved kidney tissue (Kent *et al.*, 1998; Bettge *et al.*, 2009; Hutchins *et al.*, 2018) (Table 7.3). The 18S primers have been shown to perform particularly well, with highest sensitivity attributed to the primer/probe combination published by Bettge *et al.* (2009) (Stelzer *et al.*, 2024). qPCR has also been used to detect active shedding of *T. bryosalmonae* non-invasively from a small volume of water in which the target host has been incubated (Duval *et al.*, 2021).

Environmental DNA (eDNA) detection has become an important diagnostic tool for *T. bryosalmonae* in both wild and farmed fish environments (Fontes *et al.*, 2017; Sieber *et al.*, 2020). Parasite DNA (from fragments to whole malacospores), shed by infected fish through urine and by bryozoan hosts, is captured by filtration, the DNA is extracted from the membrane and the parasite presence detected via PCR/qPCR with *T. bryosalmonae*-specific primers. eDNA allows for early, non-invasive detection of the parasite, without the need to capture or euthanize fish (Bass *et al.*, 2023). eDNA is especially valuable for temporal evaluation of the dynamics of parasite pressure in farm inlets and for monitoring wild fish populations. Monitoring the proliferation and occurrence of bryozoans hosts contributes by predicting seasonal PKD outbreaks in natural habitats and helping in management of stocking.

Table 7.2. Scoring scale for grading the severity of PKD. Refer to Fig. 7.6 for accompanying images. (Author's own table.)

Grade	Kidney swelling	Kidney tissue coloration	Kidney visual appearance	Kidney tissue texture	Swelling location	Fish appearance
0	Concave	Uniform dark red	Smooth with smooth edges	Smooth and uniform	No general or localized visible swelling	Healthy
1	Flat	Uniform dark red	Swollen with smooth edges	Smooth and uniform	Entire kidney appearing flat, no localized swelling	Healthy
2	Slightly enlarged and convex	Slightly mottled red with a grey sheen	Renal tissue swollen with serrated (sawtooth) edges	Uniform with slight grey granules	Posterior	Minor abdominal swelling
3	Clearly enlarged and swollen	Formed renal compartments exhibit a matted red appearance with a grey-blue surface sheen	Corrugated renal tissue with sawtooth edges and early formation of tissue compartments	Tougher, less uniform and grainy. Still bloody when sampled	Mainly posterior moving towards anterior	Mild abdominal swelling, pale gills and reduced blood pigmentation
4	Extremely enlarged and clearly swollen	Matted grey/blue with clear liquid between 'compartments'	Marked bulging and corrugation of renal tissue, forming distinct compartments of swollen tissue	Grainy and tough with little to no blood surrounding formed renal tissue compartments	Entire kidney	Abdominal swelling, gill pallor and reduced blood pigmentation
H	Flat and moving towards concave	Red kidney tissue with nodules that are lighter	Kidney appears uniform except for discrete white/light red nodular lesions	Nodules are firm, kidney texture is smooth and uniform	Pale nodules can be found along the kidney	No external abnormalities. Spleen exhibits irregular texture

Table 7.3. PCR and qPCR primers used for diagnosis of *Tetracapsuloides bryosalmonae* in tissue and eDNA samples. (Author's own table.)

Forward (5′–3′)	Reverse (5′–3′)	TaqMan probe	Amplicon length	Target region[a]	Method	Reference
CCTATTCAATTGAGTAGGAGA	GGACCTTACTCGTTCCGACC	Not applicable	435	18S	PCR	Kent *et al.* (1998)
GCGAGATTTGTTGCATTTAAAAAG	GCACATGCAGTGTCCAATCG	CAAAATTGTGGAACCGTCC GACTACGA	73	18S	PCR qPCR	Bettge *et al.* (2009)
CAGGTCCATTCGTGAGTAACAA	TGCCTCCTTAGTTAGGTAGACAAA	Not applicable	182	18S	PCR qPCR	Fontes *et al.* (2017)
CGAACGAGACTTCTTCCTT	CTTCCTACGCTTTTAAATAGCG	CCCTTCAATTAGTTGATCTAAA CCCCAATT	90	18S	PCR qPCR	Hutchins *et al.* (2017)
GGTTGTTTAGTTTGGGCTCACC	TCCCTGTAGGGACAGCTATTG	CAAGATCTTATTTTAT GGCTGCCAC	103	COI	PCR qPCR	Carraro *et al.* (2018)
TCATGATACGGTGAAAGGTG	CTTCCTACGCTTTTAAATAGCG	Not applicable	170	18S	PCR	Hutchins *et al.* (2018)

[a]18S, 18S ribosomal RNA; COI, cytochrome oxidase subunit 1.

7.2.4. Pathophysiology

Parasite development within the renal interstitium triggers intense lymphoid hyperplasia and inflammation, compressing functional nephrons, which impairs critical kidney functions such as osmoregulation, ion balance and nitrogenous waste excretion (Schmidt-Posthaus *et al.*, 2012; Bailey *et al.*, 2020). Compromised kidney function leads to physiological stress that affects metabolic efficiency (Hedrick *et al.*, 1993), overall fish fitness (Ellis *et al.*, 1982), blood chemistry and homeostasis (Palikova *et al.*, 2017), making the fish more vulnerable to secondary infections (Feist and Bucke, 1993) and environmental stressors.

7.2.5. Immune response

The pathophysiological responses are a product of parasite activity and host immune response to the presence of the parasite. The posterior kidney, which is the primary proliferation site of *T. bryosalmonae*, has both renal and important immunological functions as it is a prime location for activated B cells and Toll-like receptors (TLRs) (reviewed by Bailey *et al.*, 2020). In both brown and rainbow trout, the immune response to *T. bryosalmonae* is characterized by B-cell activity and T-helper-like cells with lymphocyte-like functions (Holland *et al.*, 2003; Bailey *et al.*, 2017b). Additionally, in brown trout, TLRs are suggested to be key components in the activation of the innate immune system, with receptors such as TLR1 being upregulated during the early stages of infection (Sudhagar *et al.*, 2020). Macrophages also play a vital role during infection by infiltrating the renal interstitium and contributing to parasite clearance through phagocytosis and the secretion of reactive oxygen and nitrogen species, which damage and kill the parasite (Gorgoglione *et al.*, 2013; Bailey *et al.*, 2017b).

Recognition of conserved pathogen-associated molecular patterns (PAMPs) on *T. bryosalmonae* triggers signalling cascades that activate the inflammatory responses within the innate immune response (Sudhagar *et al.*, 2020). Prolonged or excessive activation of these responses can facilitate parasite persistence and contribute to the lymphoid hyperplasia and tissue remodelling that is the signature of *T. bryosalmonae* infection (Chilmonczyk *et al.*, 2002; Bailey *et al.*, 2020).

The adaptive immune response also includes a strong humoral component. Parasite-specific antibodies help neutralize extracellular stages of *T. bryosalmonae* and limit its spread within the host, while T-cell responses are involved in controlling intracellular stages and modulating inflammation (Yamaguchi and Dijkstra, 2019; Shivam *et al.*, 2021). However, due to the putative immune evasion strategies of *T. bryosalmonae*, these adaptive responses are often delayed or suboptimal, contributing to chronic infection and progressive kidney damage (Bailey *et al.*, 2020).

7.2.6. Recovery

Recovery from PKD has been documented in most host species and characterized in greatest detail in rainbow (Hedrick *et al.*, 1993) and brown trout (Abd-Elfattah *et al.*, 2014b; Rubin *et al.*, 2019) infected by the European strains of *T. bryosalmonae*. In the kidney, recovery is characterized by reduction in swelling, return of normal coloration, but occasionally with presence of white or pale nodules along the tissue (Clifton-Hadley *et al.*, 1987a) (Fig. 7.6, Stage H). Recovery from infection can begin as early as 4 weeks post-exposure, but depending on species can be delayed until approximately 14 weeks, reflecting variability in host response and disease progression (Bailey *et al.*, 2020; Shivam *et al.*, 2021).

Recovery is temperature dependent; rainbow trout held at 15°C recovered and completely cleared the parasite (Bailey *et al.*, 2020), whereas in fish held at 18°C, recovery was observed in only ~90% of fish, 9 months after infection (Morris *et al.*, 2005). In brown trout, recovery follows a similar timeline (Strepparava *et al.*, 2018); however, the parasite is not cleared and recovered individuals become chronically infected hosts, capable of passing the parasite to bryozoans (Abd-Elfattah *et al.*, 2014b).

The mechanisms underlying recovery are not well understood, however it is clear that reduction of inflammation and repair processes work in tandem to induce restoration of the kidney tissue (Schmidt-Posthaus *et al.*, 2012; Bailey *et al.*, 2020). During recovery, as parasite loads decline, innate immune activity subsides, and regulatory tissue recovery pathways, such as interleukin-10 (IL-10) and transforming growth factor-β1 (TGF-β1), become activated to promote the resolution of inflammation and support kidney tissue repair. Anti-inflammatory cytokines and regulatory immune cells help prevent further tissue damage caused by prolonged immune activation (Gorgoglione *et al.*, 2013; Abos *et al.*, 2018). Restoration of homeostasis involves clearing cellular debris and repairing damaged nephrons, processes supported by macrophages with tissue remodelling functions (Gorgoglione *et al.*, 2013; Bailey *et al.*, 2020). Notably, fish that recovered from a prior clinical PKD infection exhibit increased numbers of IgM^+ B cells in circulation compared to naïve fish, highlighting the importance of the B-cell activation to develop immunity against the parasite (Bailey *et al.*, 2017b). Transcriptomic analyses during this recovery stage have revealed a distinct expression profile, including continued upregulation of immunoglobulin genes (IgM, IgT), expression of anti-inflammatory mediators (IL-10), and the emergence of gene expression associated with tissue repair and immune regulation, indicating a shift from immune pathology to adaptive immune resolution and renal restoration (Bailey *et al.*, 2020).

Histologically, the recovery phase in the kidney is marked by decreased lymphoid hyperplasia and fibrosis, accompanied by regeneration of nephrons (Schmidt-Posthaus *et al.*, 2012). In the spleen, a key lymphoid organ involved in immune responses, recovery is evidenced by normalization of splenic size and cellular composition (Bailey *et al.*, 2020; Shivam *et al.*, 2021). Splenic tissue analyses have recorded nodular splenomegaly with surface irregularities in specimens sampled during the late recovery phase of PKD, coinciding with kidney swelling index H classification (L. King Wolf, Nottingham, 2025, unpublished results) (Fig. 7.7).

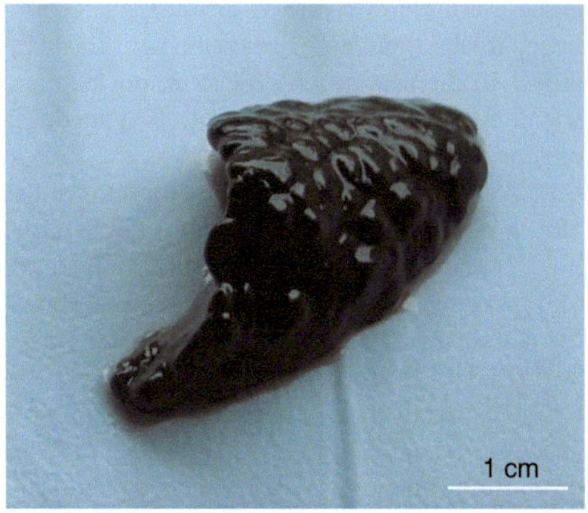

Fig. 7.7. Spleen during the recovery stage of PKD in rainbow trout (*Oncorhynchus mykiss*). Nodular splenomegaly with surface irregularities is visible. (Author's own image.)

7.2.7. Disease drivers

The most significant driver of PKD is temperature, as both within-host infection dynamics and host ecology are temperature dependent (Bettge *et al.*, 2009; Tops *et al.*, 2009; Schmidt-Posthaus *et al.*, 2012). Water temperature of 15°C has emerged as a threshold above which clinical PKD and mortality develop in most hosts (Schmidt-Posthaus and Wahli, 2015), and above these temperatures, recovery is impaired (Morris *et al.*, 2003). The effect of temperature was first suggested by comprehensive field surveys in Switzerland, which found PKD presence typically below 800 m above sea level (Wahli *et al.*, 2008), and further field surveys confirm that mean temperature in June and number of days with mean temperature >15°C correlate strongly with parasite prevalence and intensity (Rubin *et al.* 2019). Despite the clear relationship of PKD and temperature, the within-host mechanisms of increased mortality are not fully understood (Schmidt-Posthaus and Wahli, 2015). Severity of histological lesions does not appear to respond to increasing temperature beyond 15°C (Schmidt-Posthaus *et al.*, 2012); however, rate of lesion development and parasite numbers in kidney correlate positively with increasing temperature (Bettge *et al.*, 2009).

Higher spore doses and continuous infection are promoted by warmer water temperatures, as they accelerate parasite development in the bryozoan hosts, provoke overt infection development (Tops *et al.*, 2006), and lead to earlier and more intense release of infective spores (Tops *et al.*, 2006). Temporal parasite-density-dependent effects may modulate and drive disease, although infection by a single *T. bryosalmonae* malacospore has been shown to elicit clinical disease (McGurk *et al.*, 2006). Regardless, parasite spore dose does seem to drive an increase in the rate at which lesions develop and shorten the time post-infection to first shedding of spores (Strepparava *et al.*, 2020).

Water quality and nutrient dynamics also play a role, and experimental and field studies have observed an increase in PKD prevalence and severity when exposed to treated wastewater (El-Matbouli and Hoffmann, 2002; Bailey *et al.*, 2018). However, it is unclear whether this is due to direct effects of the water quality on the fish, or indirectly by increasing spore dose by promoting infected bryozoan growth. Nutrient loading can enhance infected bryozoan densities and colony size (Hartikainen *et al.*, 2009), which reflects spatial patterns of PKD risk (Carraro *et al.*, 2017). Therefore, habitat structure and hydrological variability also influence PKD transmission, although few measurements of spore dispersal and flow dynamics exist. Changes in flow regime, whether from natural drought, damming or channel modification, can alter these dynamics (Sterud *et al.*, 2007).

7.3. Protective/Control Strategies

Recovery from PKD and subsequent resistance to reinfection by *T. bryosalmonae* point towards control strategies via immunization. While the precise mechanisms underlying protective immunity remain incompletely understood, evidence from aquaculture indicates that induction of *T. bryosalmonae*-specific immunity will significantly reduce the severity of reinfection, prevent epidemics and enhance survival.

7.3.1. Aquaculture

The development of a vaccine to mitigate PKD is of central importance, and the early stages of development efforts have shown some promise. The first trials have established the potential to induce specific antibody production by targeting key parasite antigens prior to environmental exposure to *T. bryosalmonae* (Faber *et al.*, 2019). However, significant challenges are presented by the complex life cycle and immune evasion strategies of *T. bryosalmonae* and a key knowledge gap needs to be closed in the host–parasite molecular interactions before robust vaccine targets and optimized immunization protocols are viable. Most fish vaccines are utilizing whole cultured and purified pathogens, which is problematic when dealing with pathogens that are difficult to culture, such as parasites (Pollard and Bijker, 2020). Therefore, vaccine control of PKD will likely be reliant on the development of a recombinant subunit vaccine, which requires an in-depth knowledge of the functional genomics of *T. bryosalmonae*.

A widely applied method to mitigate PKD is by controlled pre-exposure to *T. bryosalmonae*, which was developed as a strategy by the trout industry in the UK as a response to the increasing PKD mortalities since the 1980s (O. Robinson, UK, 2021, personal communication) (Fig. 7.8). This method exploits the partial immunity that develops during recovery from PKD (Bailey *et al.*, 2017a). Clinical PKD is not a requirement for development of protective immunity during pre-exposure in rainbow trout (L. King Wolf, Nottingham, 2025, unpublished results).

Controlled pre-exposure involves exposing fish to the parasite under conditions that allow parasite development but also promote recovery. In practice this is realized by stocking fish into a PKD-endemic farm during late summer, which results in infection and upregulation of the innate and adaptive immune systems to elicit a response. The method then relies on predictably cooler autumn water temperatures to avoid the development of overwhelming clinical pathology. This immune priming is effective in protecting the fish in the following summer when temperatures again become permissive for clinical PKD and infectious spore loads in water increase.

Establishing successful pre-exposures takes repeated trial and error and has to be optimized separately to each fish-farming location (O. Robinson, UK, 2021, personal communication). Despite reduction in mortality and improvement in welfare, pre-exposures remain economically costly. This is because of the logistical complexities involved in stocking raceways only in certain periods of the year, the resulting complications in the production cycle, and due to the uncertainty associated with natural pre-exposure, which still remains liable to failure due to e.g. anomalous weather conditions (British Trout Association, UK, 2021, personal communication).

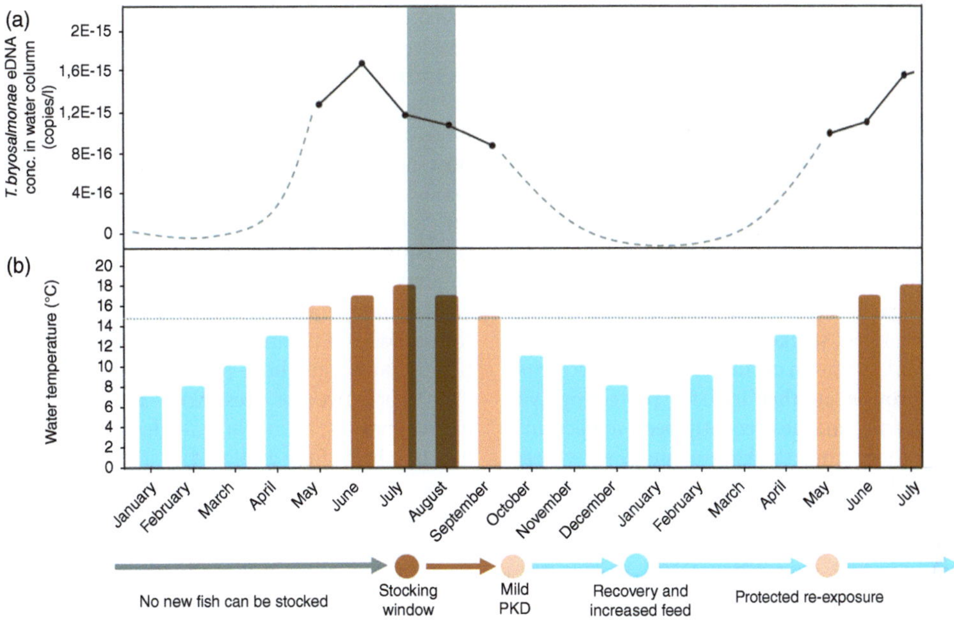

Fig. 7.8. Conceptual illustration of the pre-exposure principle. (a) Proposed seasonal dynamics of *Tetracapsuloides bryosalmonae* DNA concentrations in the water column, with spore release initiated upon water temperatures exceeding a 15°C threshold (dotted black line). (b) Seasonal temperature profile, with light red bars indicating temperatures approaching 15°C and dark red bars representing periods exceeding this threshold. The grey shaded area highlights the pre-exposure window, where parasite presence coincides with declining water temperatures, representing a potential opportunity for controlled, low-intensity exposure that may confer disease protection upon future exposure. (Author's own image.)

Selective breeding for resistance to PKD has been investigated, with some supportive evidence for genetic variation in susceptibility in rainbow trout (Butterfield, 2008), brown trout (Debes *et al.*, 2017) and Atlantic salmon (Cauwelier *et al.*, 2010). Comparative phenotypic studies of different rainbow trout lineages have revealed variation in kidney swelling scores, parasite burdens and survivorship among species and lineages (Grabner and El-Matbouli, 2009; Syrová *et al.*, 2020). Brown trout exhibit significantly milder kidney pathology than rainbow trout strains tested simultaneously (Grabner and El-Matbouli, 2009). Among the rainbow trout, the Hofer strain consistently demonstrated reduced kidney swelling scores and parasite burdens, with approximately 20–30% higher survival rates compared to more susceptible strains, indicating enhanced resistance (Grabner and El-Matbouli, 2009). Despite these results, the selective breeding approaches have not yet broadly translated into applied tools for the aquaculture industry.

7.3.2. Wild populations

Controlling PKD in wild fish populations is challenging due to the complex life cycle. The key strategy is habitat management aimed at improving conditions for trout in general (reviewed in Borsuk *et al.*, 2006; Ros *et al.*, 2022), which may also indirectly reduce bryozoan population density. Enhancing the thermal regulation of water bodies may aid PKD control in the wild but is difficult to achieve. Suggested approaches include preserving or restoring riparian vegetation to provide shade that can help moderate water temperatures, and evidence for the active use of thermal refugia by infected trout is emerging (Ros *et al.*, 2023; Ros and Brinker, 2024). Strategic management of dam releases has been employed to control other myxozoan diseases (e.g. see Bartholomew *et al.*, 2023), although this is not possible in many smaller riverine habitats and it is not known how effective increased flow rates could be in reducing infected bryozoan densities.

Biological monitoring and surveillance remain essential components of PKD management in wild fish populations. Regular assessment of parasite prevalence using eDNA is now well established (Carraro *et al.*, 2017; Stelzer *et al.*, 2024) and enables early detection of emerging parasite hot spots. This information supports adaptive management strategies, and may include actions such as restricting fish translocations, minimizing disturbance to vulnerable populations during peak transmission periods and guiding conservation stocking practices (Ros *et al.*, 2022). Application of the pre-exposure principle may provide another tool for protecting wild populations and has recently been applied in a wild brown trout stocking context, where pre-exposed fish experienced lower parasite loads and reduced kidney pathology compared to naïve controls released directly into the wild (Ros *et al.*, 2022). While no single control method is sufficient in isolation, integrated, ecosystem-based management approaches offer the most promising pathway to mitigating PKD impacts on wild fish populations.

7.4. Conclusions and Suggestions for Future Studies

The severity and geographic range of PKD are closely linked to water temperature, which influences all stages and phases of the parasite's complex life cycle. With climate change, there is an urgent need for vaccine-based control strategies and early, rapid diagnostic tools in aquaculture. River-basin-level improvement of water and habitat quality, perhaps through rewilding, is crucial to ensure PKD-resilient future freshwater ecosystems.

Future studies should focus on fully resolving the functional basis of immunity, resistance and recovery in the fish hosts in natural and farm conditions. Drivers of mortality in fish hosts, and the immune evasion strategies of the parasite, present promising avenues for future studies relevant for vaccine development and other control strategies. Investigations into the genetic diversity of *T. bryosalmonae* will reveal its evolutionary history and speciation patterns, while adaptive responses of both the parasite and the hosts can be used to inform on how shifting thermal conditions will modulate PKD. For example, while *T. bryosalmonae* may exhibit increased replication and transmission efficiency at higher temperatures, long-term selection pressures could drive changes in virulence or host specificity. Similarly, host populations might exhibit plastic or evolutionary responses, including enhanced immune tolerance. Insight into such questions require longitudinal field studies combined with experimental infections under varying temperature regimes to determine the thresholds and tipping points that govern infection dynamics and host–pathogen co-evolution.

Alternative or reservoir hosts among non-salmonids, as subclinical infection carriers, has not been fully explored. Targeted surveillance and molecular screening of diverse non-salmonid species across PKD-endemic and -emerging regions could clarify their role in transmission networks and inform risk assessments under changing ecological conditions. Studying the effects of environmental change on the thresholds that promote bryozoan survival, their reproductive and dispersal dynamics and their susceptibility to infection will be important for integrating ecology into disease modelling.

Proactive management strategies will require predictive tools capable of incorporating complex interactions between environmental variables, host physiology and pathogen biology. Mechanistic models that couple hydrological, thermal and disease dynamics could help forecast future PKD outbreaks and guide mitigation efforts. These models should be grounded in robust empirical data from field observations, experimental studies and molecular diagnostics, including eDNA-based detection of parasite and bryozoan presence in rivers and reservoirs.

Key priorities for future research include:

- defining environmental thresholds for transmission and parasite development (e.g. water velocity and effective transmission to either host);
- understanding the physiological and genetic basis of host resistance and recovery;
- developing climate-informed models to predict outbreak risk in salmonids;
- producing a viable control method for farms (e.g. a vaccine);

- characterizing strain variation among *T. bryosalmonae*;
- understanding closely related malacosporeans and speciation;
- describing immune responses and mode of virulence in different salmonid species;
- determining mitigation in wild thermal refugia and rewilding;
- understanding bases of local host–parasite adaptation, and scope for future climate adaptations in the hosts and the parasite; and
- investigating the impacts of stocking on PKD and host–parasite co-evolution.

Acknowledgements

Florian Melzer (University of Nottingham) kindly created the *T. bryosalmonae* transmission diagram (Fig. 7.2). Oliver Robinson and the British Trout Association provided data on PKD impacts in the UK trout sector and their use of pre-exposure programmes. Drs Aimee Reed and Sarah Bjork (Oregon Department of Fish and Wildlife, Fish Health Section) provided the Oregon hatchery data. Ashley Hatleberg (Oregon Department of Fish and Wildlife, Leaburg Hatchery) provided the steelhead for the North American *T. bryosalmonae* transmission trial. The Oregon Veterinary Diagnostic Laboratory processed (cut and stained) the histological samples. Dr Michael Kent (Oregon State University) provided guidance with histopathology. H.H. and L.K.W. were supported by NC3Rs grant NC/W001942/1. S.L.H. and N.D. were supported in part by the Oregon State University College of Agricultural Sciences–US Department of Agriculture Animal Health Disease Research programme.

References

Abd-Elfattah, A., Fontes, I., Kumar, G., Soliman, H., Hartikainen, H. *et al.* (2014a) Vertical transmission of *Tetracapsuloides bryosalmonae* (Myxozoa), the causative agent of salmonid proliferative kidney disease. *Parasitology* 141, 482–490. DOI: 10.1017/S0031182013001650.

Abd-Elfattah, A., Kumar, G., Soliman, H. and El-Matbouli, M. (2014b) Persistence of *Tetracapsuloides bryosalmonae* (Myxozoa) in chronically infected brown trout *Salmo trutta*. *Diseases of Aquatic Organisms* 111, 41–49. DOI: 10.3354/DAO02768.

Abos, B., Estensoro, I., Perdiguero, P., Faber, M., Hu, Y. *et al.* (2018) Dysregulation of B cell activity during proliferative kidney disease in rainbow trout. *Frontiers in Immunology* 9, 1203. DOI: 10.3389/FIMMU.2018.01203.

Anderson, C.L., Canning, E.U. and Okamura, B. (1999) Molecular data implicate bryozoans as hosts for PKX (phylum Myxozoa) and identify a clade of bryozoan parasites within the Myxozoa. *Parasitology* 119, 555–561. DOI: 10.1017/S003118209900520X.

Arkush, K.D. and Hedrick, R.P. (1990) Experimental transmission of PKX, the causative agent of proliferative kidney disease, to three species of Pacific salmon. *Journal of Applied Ichthyology* 6, 237–243. DOI: 10.1111/j.1439-0426.1990.tb00584.x.

Arndt, D., Fux, R., Blutke, A., Schwaiger, J., El-Matbouli, M. *et al.* (2019) Proliferative kidney disease and proliferative darkening syndrome are linked with brown trout (*Salmo trutta fario*) mortalities in the pre-alpine Isar river. *Pathogens* 8, 177. DOI: 10.3390/pathogens8040177.

Bailey, C., Segner, H. and Wahli, T. (2017a) What goes around comes around: an investigation of resistance to proliferative kidney disease in rainbow trout *Oncorhynchus mykiss* (Walbaum) following experimental re-exposure. *Journal of Fish Diseases* 40, 1599–1612. DOI: 10.1111/jfd.12628.

Bailey, C., Segner, H., Casanova-Nakayama, A. and Wahli, T. (2017b) Who needs the hotspot? The effect of temperature on the fish host immune response to *Tetracapsuloides bryosalmonae* the causative agent of proliferative kidney disease. *Fish and Shellfish Immunology* 63, 424–437. DOI: 10.1016/j.fsi.2017.02.039.

Bailey, C., Rubin, A., Strepparava, N., Segner, H., Rubin, J.F. and Wahli, T. (2018) Do fish get wasted? Assessing the influence of effluents on parasitic infection of wild fish. *PeerJ* 6, e5956. DOI: 10.7717/peerj.5956.

Bailey, C., Segner, H., Wahli, T. and Tafalla, C. (2020) Back from the brink: alterations in B and T cell responses modulate recovery of rainbow trout from chronic immunopathological *Tetracapsuloides bryosalmonae* infection. *Frontiers in Immunology* 11, 1093. DOI: 10.3389/fimmu.2020.01093.

Bailey, C., Strepparava, N., Ros, A., Wahli, T., Schmidt-Posthaus, H. *et al.* (2021) It's a hard knock life for some: heterogeneity in infection life history of salmonids influences parasite disease outcomes. *Journal of Animal Ecology* 90, 2573–2593. DOI: 10.1111/1365-2656.13562.

Bartholomew, J.L., Alexander, J.D., Alvarez, J., Atkinson, S.D., Belchik, M. *et al.* (2023) Deconstructing dams and disease: predictions for salmon disease risk following Klamath River dam removals. *Frontiers in Ecology and Evolution* 11, 1245967. DOI: 10.3389/fevo.2023.1245967.

Bass, D., Christison, K.W., Stentiford, G.D., Cook, L.S.J. and Hartikainen, H. (2023) Environmental DNA/RNA for pathogen and parasite detection, surveillance, and ecology. *Trends in Parasitology* 39, 285–304. DOI: 10.1016/j.pt.2022.12.010.

Beraldo, P., Berton, D., Giavenni, R. and Galeotti, M. (2006) First report on proliferative kidney disease (PKD) in marble trout (*Salmo trutta marmoratus*, Cuvier 1817). *Bulletin of the European Association of Fish Pathologists* 26, 143–150.

Bettge, K., Wahli, T., Segner, H. and Schmidt-Posthaus, H. (2009) Proliferative kidney disease in rainbow trout: time- and temperature-related renal pathology and parasite distribution. *Diseases of Aquatic Organisms* 83, 67–76. DOI: 10.3354/dao01989.

Borgwardt, F., Unfer, G., Auer, S., Waldner, K., El-Matbouli, M. and Bechter, T. (2020) Direct and indirect climate change impacts on brown trout in central Europe: how thermal regimes reinforce physiological stress and support the emergence of diseases. *Frontiers in Environmental Science* 8, 59. DOI: 10.3389/fenvs.2020.00059.

Borsuk, M.E., Reichert, P., Peter, A., Schager, E. and Burkhardt-Holm, P. (2006) Assessing the decline of brown trout (*Salmo trutta*) in Swiss rivers using a Bayesian probability network. *Ecological Modelling* 192, 224–244. DOI: 10.1016/j.ecolmodel.2005.07.006.

Braden, L.M., Prosperi-Porta, G., Kim, E. and Jones, S.R.M. (2010) *Tetracapsuloides bryosalmonae* in spawning pink salmon, *Oncorhynchus gorbuscha* (Walbaum), in the Quinsam River, British Columbia, Canada. *Journal of Fish Diseases* 33, 617–621. DOI: 10.1111/j.1365-2761.2010.01145.

Brown, J.A., Thonney, J.P., Holwell, D. and Wilson, W.R. (1991) A comparison of the susceptibility of *Salvelinus alpinus* and *Salmo salar ouananiche* to proliferative kidney disease. *Aquaculture* 96, 1–6. DOI: 10.1016/0044-8486(91)90134-S.

Bruneaux, M., Visse, M., Gross, R., Pukk, L., Saks, L. and Vasemägi, A. (2017) Parasite infection and decreased thermal tolerance: impact of proliferative kidney disease on a wild salmonid fish in the context of climate change. *Functional Ecology* 31, 216–226. DOI: 10.1111/1365-2435.12701.

Bucke, D., Feist, S.W. and Clifton-Hadley, R.S. (1991) The occurrence of proliferative kidney disease (PKD) in cultured and wild fish: further investigations. *Journal of Fish Diseases* 14, 583–588. DOI: 10.1111/j.1365-2761.1991.tb00614.x.

Butterfield, G.M. (2008) Genetic variation for disease resistance in rainbow trout (*Oncorhynchus mykiss*). PhD thesis, University of Stirling, Stirling, UK.

Canning, E.U., Curry, A., Feist, S.W., Longshaw, M. and Okamura, B. (2000) A new class and order of myxozoans to accommodate parasites of bryozoans with ultrastructural observations on *Tetracapsula bryosalmonae* (PKX organism). *Journal of Eukaryotic Microbiology* 47, 456–468. DOI: 10.1111/j.1550-7408.2000.tb00075.x.

Canning, E.U., Curry, A. and Okamura, B. (2008) Early development of the myxozoan *Buddenbrockia plumatellae* in the bryozoans *Hyalinella punctata* and *Plumatella fungosa*, with comments on taxonomy and systematics of the Myxozoa. *Folia Parasitologica* 55(4), 241–255. DOI: 10.14411/fp.2008.032.

Carraro, L., Bertuzzo, E., Mari, L., Fontes, I., Hartikainen, H. *et al.* (2017) Integrated field, laboratory, and theoretical study of PKD spread in a Swiss prealpine river. *Proceedings of the National Academy of Sciences USA* 114, 11992–11997. DOI: 10.1073/pnas.1713691114.

Carraro, L., Hartikainen, H., Jokela, J., Bertuzzo, E. and Rinaldo, A. (2018) Estimating species distribution and abundance in river networks using environmental DNA. *Proceedings of the National Academy of Sciences USA* 115, 11724–11729. DOI: 10.1073/pnas.1813843115.

Castagnaro, M., Marin, M., Ghittino, C. and Hedrick, R.P. (1991) Lectin histochemistry and ultrastructure of rainbow trout *Oncorhynchus mykiss* kidneys affected by proliferative kidney. *Diseases of Aquatic Organisms* 10, 173–183. DOI: 10.3354/dao010173.

Cauwelier, E., Gilbey, J., Jones, C.S., Noble, L.R. and Verspoor, E. (2010) Genotypic and phenotypic correlates with proliferative kidney disease-induced mortality in Atlantic salmon. *Diseases of Aquatic Organisms* 89, 125–135. DOI: 10.3354/dao02191.

Chan, J.T.H., Picard-Sánchez, A., Majstorović, J., Rebl, A., Koczan, D. *et al.* (2023) Red blood cells in proliferative kidney disease – rainbow trout (*Oncorhynchus mykiss*) infected by *Tetracapsuloides bryosalmonae harbor* IgM^{+} red blood cells. *Frontiers in Immunology* 14, 1041325. DOI: 10.3389/fimmu.2023.1041325.

Chilmonczyk, S., Monge, D. and de Kinkelin, P. (2002) Proliferative kidney disease: cellular aspects of the rainbow trout, *Oncorhynchus mykiss* (Walbaum), response to parasitic infection. *Journal of Fish Diseases* 25, 217–226. DOI: 10.1046/j.1365-2761.2002.00362.x.

Clifton-Hadley, R.S. and Bucke, D. (1986) Economic importance of proliferative kidney disease of salmonid fish in England and Wales. *Veterinary Record* 12, 305–306.

Clifton-Hadley, R.S., Bucke, D. and Richards, R.H. (1987a) A study of the sequential clinical and pathological changes during proliferative kidney disease in rainbow trout, *Salmo gairdneri* Richardson. *Journal of Fish Diseases* 10, 335–352. DOI: 10.1111/j.1365-2761.1987.tb01081.x.

Clifton-Hadley, R.S., Richards, R.H. and Bucke, D. (1987b) Further consideration of the haematology of proliferative kidney disease (PKD) in rainbow trout, *Salmo gairdneri* Richardson. *Journal of Fish Diseases* 10, 435–444. DOI: 10.1111/j.1365-2761.1987.tb01094.x.

Das, N., Atkinson, S.D. and Hallett, S.L. (2026) The salmonid *Oncorhynchus mykiss* and bryozoan *Fredericella borealis* serve as active hosts for the North American strain of *Tetracapsuloides bryosalmonae*, the cause of proliferative kidney disease. *Journal of Parasitology* 112 (2), DOI: 10.1645/25-47.

De Kinkelin, P., Gay, M. and Forman, S. (2002) The persistence of infectivity of *Tetracapsula bryosalmonae*, infected water for rainbow trout, *Oncorhynchus mykiss* (Walbaum). *Journal of Fish Diseases* 25, 477–482. DOI: 10.1046/j.1365-2761.2002.00382.x.

Debes, P.V., Gross, R. and Vasemägi, A. (2017) Quantitative genetic variation in, and environmental effects on, pathogen resistance and temperature-dependent disease severity in a wild trout. *The American Naturalist* 190, 244–265. DOI: 10.1086/692536.

Duval, E., Blanchet, S., Quéméré, E., Jacquin, L., Veyssière, C. *et al.* (2021) Urine DNA (uDNA) as a non-lethal method for endoparasite biomonitoring: development and validation. *Environmental DNA* 3, 1035–1045. DOI: 10.1002/edn3.228.

Ellis, A.E., McVicar, A.H. and Munro, A.L.S. (1982) A preliminary report on the epidemiology of proliferative kidney disease in brown trout (*Salmo trutta*) and Atlantic salmon parr (*S. salar*) in Scotland. *Bulletin of the European Association of Fish Pathologists* 2, 13–15.

El-Matbouli, M. and Hoffmann, R.W. (1994) Proliferative kidney disease (PKD) as an important myxosporean infection in salmonid fish. In: Pike, A.W. and Lewis, J.W. (eds) *Parasitic Diseases of Fish*. Samara Publishing Ltd, Tresaith, UK, pp. 3–15.

El-Matbouli, M. and Hoffmann, R.W. (2002) Influence of water quality on the outbreak of proliferative kidney disease – field studies and exposure experiments. *Journal of Fish* Diseases 25, 459–467. DOI: 10.1046/j.1365-2761.2002.00393.

Faber, M.N., Holland, J.W. and Secombes, C.J. (2019) Vaccination strategies and IgM responses against PKD in rainbow trout. *Fish and Shellfish Immunology* 91, 423. DOI: 10.1016/j.fsi.2019.04.159.

Feist, S.W. and Bucke, D. (1993) Proliferative kidney disease in wild salmonids. *Fisheries Research* 17, 51–58. DOI: 10.1016/0165-7836(93)90006-S.

Feist, S.W., Longshaw, M., Canning, E.U. and Okamura, B. (2001) Induction of proliferative kidney disease (PKD) in rainbow trout *Oncorhynchus mykiss* via the bryozoan *Fredericella sultana* infected with *Tetracapsula bryosalmonae. Diseases of Aquatic Organisms* 45, 61–68. DOI: 10.3354/dao045061.

Feist, S.W., Morris, D.J., Alama-Bermejo, G. and Holzer, A.S. (2015) Cellular processes in myxozoans. In: Okamura, B., Gruhl, A. and Bartholomew, J.L. (eds) *Myxozoan Evolution, Ecology and Development*. Springer, Cham, Switzerland, pp. 139–154. DOI: 10.1007/978-3-319-14753-6_8.

Ferguson, H.W. and Ball, H.J. (1979) Epidemiological aspects of proliferative kidney disease amongst rainbow trout *Salmo gairdneri* Richardson in Northern Ireland. *Journal of Fish Diseases* 2, 219–225. DOI: 10.1111/j.1365-2761.1979.tb00161.x.

Fontes, I., Hartikainen, H., Holland, J.W., Secombes, C.J. and Okamura, B. (2017) *Tetracapsuloides bryosalmonae* abundance in river water. *Diseases of Aquatic Organisms* 124, 145–157. DOI: 10.3354/dao03116.

Foott, J., Stone, R. and Nichols, K. (2007) Proliferative kidney disease (*Tetracapsuloides bryosalmonae*) in Merced River Hatchery juvenile Chinook salmon: mortality and performance impairment in 2005 smolts. *California Fish and Game* 93, 57–76.

Fusianto, C.K., Meuninck, D., Ingersoll, A., Leachman, K. and Gorgoglione, B. (2024) The first detection of *Tetracapsuloides bryosalmonae* in trout from Indiana and Ohio. Presented at: *American Fisheries Society, Fish Health Section Annual Meeting*, Boise, Idaho. Available at: https://event.fourwaves.com/wfdw64/abstracts/ca28e6b6-6e25-423a-9c8d-a2e624dd5abb (accessed 15 November 2025).

Gorgoglione, B., Wang, T., Secombes, C.J. and Holland, J.W. (2013) Immune gene expression profiling of proliferative kidney disease in rainbow trout *Oncorhynchus mykiss* reveals a dominance of anti-inflammatory, antibody and T helper cell-like activities. *Veterinary Research* 44, 55. DOI: 10.1186/1297-9716-44-55.

Gorgoglione, B., Kotob, M.H., Unfer, G. and El-Matbouli, M. (2016) First proliferative kidney disease outbreak in Austria, linking to the aetiology of black trout syndrome threatening autochthonous trout populations. *Diseases of Aquatic Organisms* 119, 117–128. DOI: 10.3354/dao02993.

Gorgoglione, B., Bailey, C. and Ferguson, J.A. (2020) Proliferative kidney disease in Alaskan salmonids with evidence that pathogenic myxozoans may be emerging north. *International Journal for Parasitology* 50, 797–807. DOI: 10.1016/j.ijpara.2020.03.010.

Grabner, D.S. and El-Matbouli, M. (2008) Transmission of *Tetracapsuloides bryosalmonae* (Myxozoa: Malacosporea) to *Fredericella sultana* (Bryozoa: Phylactolaemata) by various fish species. *Diseases of Aquatic Organisms* 79, 133–139. DOI: 10.3354/dao01894.

Grabner, D.S. and El-Matbouli, M. (2009) Comparison of the susceptibility of brown trout (*Salmo trutta*) and four rainbow trout (*Oncorhynchus mykiss*) strains to the myxozoan *Tetracapsuloides bryosalmonae*, the causative agent of proliferative kidney disease (PKD). *Veterinary Parasitology* 165, 200–206. DOI: 10.1016/j.vetpar.2009.07.028.

Gruhl, A. and Okamura, B. (2015) Tissue characteristics and development in Myxozoa. In: Okamura, B., Gruhl, A. and Bartholomew, J.L. (eds) *Myxozoan Evolution, Ecology and Development*. Springer, Cham, Switzerland, pp. 155–174. DOI: 10.1007/978-3-319-14753-6_9.

Hartikainen, H. and Okamura, B. (2015) Ecology and evolution of malacosporean-bryozoan interactions. In: Okamura, B., Gruhl, A. and Bartholomew, J.L. (eds) *Myxozoan Evolution, Ecology and Development*. Springer, Cham, Switzerland, pp. 201–216. DOI: 10.1007/978-3-319-14753-6_11.

Hartikainen, H., Johnes, P., Moncrieff, C. and Okamura, B. (2009) Bryozoan populations reflect nutrient enrichment and productivity gradients in rivers. *Freshwater Biology* 54, 2320–2334. DOI: 10.1111/j.1365-2427.2009.02262.x.

Hartikainen, H., Fontes, I. and Okamura, B. (2013) Parasitism and phenotypic change in colonial hosts. *Parasitology* 140, 1403–1412. DOI: 10.1017/S0031182013000899.

Hedrick, R.P., Kent, M.L., Rosemark, R. and Manzer, D. (1984) Proliferative kidney disease (PKD) in Pacific salmon and steelhead trout. *Journal of the World Mariculture Society* 15, 318–325. DOI: 10.1111/j.1749-7345.1984.tb00166.x.

Hedrick, R.P., Marin, M., Castagnaro, M., Monge, D. and de Kinkelin, P. (1992) Rapid lectin-based staining procedure for the detection of the myxosporean causing proliferative kidney disease in salmonid fish. *Diseases of Aquatic Organisms* 13, 129–132. DOI: 10.3354/dao013129.

Hedrick, R.P., MacConnell, E. and de Kinkelin, P. (1993) Proliferative kidney disease of salmonid fish. *Annual Review of Fish Diseases* 3, 277–290. DOI: 10.1016/0959-8030(93)90039-E.

Hedrick, R.P., Baxa, D.V., de Kinkelin, P. and Okamura, B. (2004) Malacosporean-like spores in urine of rainbow trout react with antibody and DNA probes to Tetracapsuloides *bryosalmonae*. *Parasitology Research* 92, 81–88. DOI: 10.1007/S00436-003-0986-3.

Henderson, M. and Okamura, B. (2004) The phylogeography of salmonid proliferative kidney disease in Europe and North America. *Proceedings of the Royal Society B: Biological Sciences* 271, 1729–1736. DOI: 10.1098/RSPB.2004.2677.

Hoffman, R. and Dangschat, H. (1981) A note on the occurrence of proliferative kidney disease in Germany. *Bulletin of the European Association of Fish Pathologists* 1, 33.

Holland, J.W., Gould, C.R.W., Jones, C.S., Noble, L.R. and Secombes, C.J. (2003) The expression of immune-regulatory genes in rainbow trout, *Oncorhynchus mykiss,* during a natural outbreak of proliferative kidney disease (PKD). *Parasitology* 126, S95–S102. DOI: 10.1017/S0031182003003767.

Hutchins, P.R., Sepulveda, A.J., Martin, R.M. and Hopper, L.R. (2018) A probe-based quantitative PCR assay for detecting *Tetracapsuloides bryosalmonae* in fish tissue and environmental DNA water samples. *Conservation Genetics Resources* 10, 317–319. DOI: 10.1007/S12686-017-0812-3.

Hutchins, P.R., Sepulveda, A.J., Hartikainen, H., Staigmiller, K.D., Opitz, S.T. *et al.* (2021) Exploration of the 2016 Yellowstone River fish kill and proliferative kidney disease in wild fish populations. *Ecosphere* 12, e03436. DOI: 10.1002/ecs2.3436.

Kent, M. (2014) Proliferative kidney disease. In: AFS-FHS (ed.) *FHS Blue Book: Suggested Procedures for the Detection and Identification of Certain Finfish and Shellfish Pathogens*. American Fisheries Society – Fish Health Section, Bethesda, Maryland, p. VIII 3.2.7. Available at: https://units.fisheries.org/fhs/wp-content/uploads/sites/30/2017/08/3.2.7-PKD-2014.pdf (accessed 20 November 2025).

Kent, M.L. and Hedrick, R.P. (1985) PKX, the causative agent of Proliferative Kidney Disease (PKD) in Pacific salmonid fishes and its affinities with the Myxozoa. *The Journal of Protozoology* 32, 254–260. DOI: 10.1111/J.1550-7408.1985.TB03047.X.

Kent, M.L., Higgins, M., Whitaker, D.J. and Yokoyama, H. (1995) Proliferate kidney disease and *Sphaerospora oncorhynchi* in wild-caught salmonids from the Puntledge River system, Vancouver Island, British Columbia. *Canadian Journal of Fisheries and Aquatic Sciences* 52, 13–17. DOI: 10.1139/F95-503.

Kent, M.L., Khattra, J., Hervio, D.M.L. and Devlin, R.H. (1998) Ribosomal DNA sequence analysis of isolates of the PKX myxosporean and their relationship to members of the genus Sphaerospora. *Journal of Aquatic Animal Health* 10, 12–21. DOI: 10.1577/1548-8667 (1998)010<0012:RDSAOI>2.0.CO;2.

Kent, M.L., Khattra, J., Hedrick, R.P. and Devlin, R.H. (2000) *Tetracapsula renicola* n. sp. (Myxozoa: Saccosporidae); the PKX myxozoan—the cause of proliferative disease of salmonid fishes. *Journal of Parasitology* 86, 103–111. DOI: 10.1645/0022-3395(2000)086[0103:TRNSMS]2.0.CO;2.

Klontz, G.W. and Chacko, A.J. (1983) Methods to detect the organism causing proliferative kidney disease in salmonids. *Bulletin of the European Association of Fish Pathologists* 3, 33–36.

Klontz, G.W., Rourke, A.W. and Eckblad, W. (1986) The immune response during proliferative kidney disease in rainbow trout: a case history. *Veterinary Immunology and Immunopathology* 12, 387–393. DOI: 10.1016/0165-2427(86)90145-5.

Kristmundsson, Á., Rut Svavarsdóttir, F., Árnason, F., Antonsson, Þ., Guðbergsson, G. *et al.* (2023) *Tetracapsuloides bryosalmonae* and proliferative kidney disease in Icelandic salmonids – comparative data from two different time periods. *International Journal for Parasitology* 53, 207–220. DOI: 10.1016/j.ijpara.2022.11.011.

Kumar, G., Abd-Elfattah, A., Saleh, M. and El-Matbouli, M. (2013) Fate of *Tetracapsuloides bryosalmonae* (Myxozoa) after infection of brown trout *Salmo trutta* and rainbow trout *Oncorhynchus mykiss. Diseases of Aquatic Organisms* 107, 9–18. DOI: 10.3354/dao02665.

Lauringson, M., Nousiainen, I., Kahar, S., Burimski, O., Gross, R. *et al.* (2021) Climate change-driven disease in sympatric hosts: temporal dynamics of parasite burden and proliferative kidney disease in wild brown trout and Atlantic salmon. *Journal of Fish Diseases* 44, 689–699. DOI: 10.1111/jfd.13330.

Longshaw, M., Feist, S., Canning, E.U. and Okamura, B. (1999) First identification of PKX in bryozoans from the United Kingdom – molecular evidence. *Bulletin of the European Association of Fish Pathologists* 4, 146–148.

MacConnell, E. and Peterson, J.E. (1992) Proliferative kidney disease in feral cutthroat trout from a remote Montana reservoir: a first case. *Journal of Aquatic Animal Health* 4, 182–187. DOI: 10.1577/1548-8667 (1992)004<0182:PKDIFC>2.3.CO;2.

MacConnell, E., Smith, C.E., Hedrick, R.P. and Speer, C.A. (1989) Cellular inflammatory response of rainbow trout to the protozoan parasite that causes proliferative kidney disease. *Journal of Aquatic Animal Health* 1, 108–118. DOI: 10.1577/1548-8667(1989)001<0108:CIRORT>2.3.CO;2.

McGurk, C., Morris, D.J., Bron, J.E. and Adams, A. (2005) The morphology of *Tetracapsuloides bryosalmonae* (Myxozoa: Malacosporea) spores released from *Fredericella sultana* (Bryozoa: Phylactolaemata). *Journal of Fish Diseases* 28, 307–312. DOI: 10.1111/j.1365-2761.2005.00627.x.

McGurk, C., Morris, D.J., Auchinachie, N.A. and Adams, A. (2006) Development of T*etracapsuloides bryosalmonae* (Myxozoa: Malacosporea) in bryozoan hosts (as examined by light microscopy) and quantitation of infective dose to rainbow trout (*Oncorhynchus mykiss*). *Veterinary Parasitology* 135, 249–257. DOI: 10.1016/j.vetpar.2005.07.022.

Mo, T.A., and Jørgensen, A. (2017) A survey of the distribution of the PKD-parasite *Tetracapsuloides bryosalmonae* (Cnidaria: Myxozoa: Malacosporea) in salmonids in Norwegian rivers – additional information gleaned from formerly collected fish. *Journal of Fish Diseases* 40, 621–627. DOI: 10.1111/jfd.12542.

Morris, D.J. and Adams, A. (2006) Proliferative, presaccular stages of *Tetracapsuloides bryosalmonae* (Myxozoa: Malacosporea) within the invertebrate host *Fredericella sultana* (Bryozoa: Phylactolaemata). *Journal of Parasitology* 92, 984–989. DOI: 10.1645/GE-868R.1.

Morris, D.J. and Adams, A. (2007) Sacculogenesis and sporogony of *Tetracapsuloides bryosalmonae* (Myxozoa: Malacosporea) within the bryozoan host *Fredericella sultana* (Bryozoa: Phylactolaemata). *Parasitology Research* 100, 983–992. DOI: 10.1007/S00436-006-0371-0.

Morris, D.J., Adams, A. and Richards, R.H. (2000) *In situ* hybridisation identifies the gill as a portal of entry for PKX (phylum Myxozoa), the causative agent of proliferative kidney disease in salmonids. *Parasitology Research* 86, 950–956. DOI: 10.1007/pl00008525.

Morris, D.J., Longshaw, M. and Adams, A. (2003) California golden trout *Oncorhynchus mykiss aguabonita* are susceptible to proliferative kidney disease. *Journal of Aquatic Animal Health* 15, 184–187. DOI: 10.1577/H03-003.

Morris, D.J., Ferguson, H.W. and Adams, A. (2005) Severe, chronic proliferative kidney disease (PKD) induced in rainbow trout *Oncorhynchus mykiss* held at a constant 18°C. *Diseases of Aquatic Organisms* 66, 221–226. DOI: 10.3354/dao066221.

Naldoni, J., Adriano, E.A., Hartigan, A., Sayer, C. and Okamura, B. (2019) Malacosporean myxozoans exploit a diversity of fish hosts. *Parasitology* 146, 968–978. DOI: 10.1017/S0031182019000246.

Okamura, B., Anderson, C.L., Longshaw, M., Feist, S.W. and Canning, E.U. (2001) Patterns of occurrence and 18S rDNA sequence variation of PKX (*Tetracapsula bryosalmonae*), the causative agent of salmonid proliferative kidney disease. *Journal of Parasitology* 87, 379–385. DOI: 10.1645/0022-3395(2001)087[0379:POOARS]2.0.CO;2.

Okamura, B., Hartikainen, H., Schmidt-Posthaus, H. and Wahli, T. (2011) Life cycle complexity, environmental change and the emerging status of salmonid proliferative kidney disease. *Freshwater Biology* 56, 735–753. DOI: 10.1111/j.1365-2427.2010.02465.x.

Palikova, M., Papezikova, I., Markova, Z., Navratil, S., Mares, J. *et al.* (2017a) Proliferative kidney disease in rainbow trout (*Oncorhynchus mykiss*) under intensive breeding conditions: pathogenesis and haematological and immune parameters. *Veterinary Parasitology* 238, 5–16. DOI: 10.1016/j.vetpar.2017.03.003.

Peribáñez, M.A., Luco, D.F., García, L. and Castillo, J.A. (1997) The prevalence of proliferative kidney disease from the kidney and muscle of rainbow and brown trout in Aragón (Spain). *Preventive Veterinary Medicine* 32, 287–297. DOI: 10.1016/S0167-5877(97)00032-9.

Pollard, A.J. and Bijker, E.M. (2020) A guide to vaccinology: from basic principles to new developments. *Nature Reviews Immunology* 21(2), 83–100. DOI: 10.1038/s41577-020-00479-7.

Ros, A. and Brinker, A. (2024) Thermotactic behaviour in lacustrine and riverine forms of Salmo trutta and its relevance to an emerging parasitic disease (PKD) in the wake of climate change. *Scientific Reports* 14, 13539. DOI: 10.1038/s41598-024-64137-x.

Ros, A., Baer, J., Basen, T., Chucholl, C., Schneider, E. *et al.* (2021) Current and projected impacts of the parasite *Tetracapsuloides bryosalmonae* (causative to proliferative kidney disease) on Central European salmonid populations under predicted climate change. *Freshwater Biology* 66, 1182–1199. DOI: 10.1111/fwb.13709.

Ros, A., Schmidt-Posthaus, H. and Brinker, A. (2022) Mitigating human impacts including climate change on proliferative kidney disease in salmonids of running waters. *Journal of Fish Diseases* 45, 497–521. DOI: 10.1111/jfd.13585.

Ros, A., Baer, J. and Brinker, A. (2023) Does treatment of brown trout with the parasite causing PKD increase stocking success and boost resilience against the disease? *Fisheries Management and Ecology* 30, 333–337. DOI: 10.1111/fme.12626.

Rubin, A., de Coulon, P., Bailey, C., Segner, H., Wahli, T. and Rubin, J.F. (2019) Keeping an eye on wild brown trout (*Salmo trutta*) populations: correlation between temperature, environmental parameters, and proliferative kidney disease. *Frontiers in Veterinary Science* 6, 281. DOI: 10.3389/fvets.2019.00281.

Schager, E., Peter, A. and Burkhardt-Holm, P. (2007) Status of young-of-the-year brown trout (*Salmo trutta fario*) in Swiss streams: factors influencing YOY trout recruitment. *Aquatic Sciences* 69, 41–50. DOI: 10.1007/s00027-007-0845-x.

Schmidt-Posthaus, H. and Wahli, T. (2015) Host and environmental influences on development of disease. In: Okamura, B., Gruhl, A. and Bartholomew, J.L. (eds) *Myxozoan Evolution, Ecology and Development*. Springer, Cham, Switzerland, pp. 281–293. DOI: 10.1007/978-3-319-14753-6_15.

Schmidt-Posthaus, H., Bettge, K., Forster, U., Segner, H. and Wahli, T. (2012) Kidney pathology and parasite intensity in rainbow trout *Oncorhynchus mykiss* surviving proliferative kidney disease: time course and influence of temperature. *Diseases of Aquatic Organisms* 97, 207–218. DOI: 10.3354/dao02417.

Schwaha, T., Hirose, M. and Wanninger, A. (2016) The life of the freshwater bryozoan *Stephanella hina* (Bryozoa, Phylactolaemata) – a crucial key to elucidating bryozoan evolution. *Zoological Letters* 2, 25. DOI: 10.1186/S40851-016-0060-5.

Seagrave, C.P., Bucke, D., Hudson, E.B. and McGregor, D. (1981) A survey of the prevalence and distribution of proliferative kidney disease (PKD) in England and Wales. *Journal of Fish Diseases* 4, 437–439. DOI: 10.1111/j.1365-2761.1981.tb01155.x.

Shivam, S., El-Matbouli, M. and Kumar, G. (2021) Kinetics of parasite-specific antibody and B-cell-associated gene expression in brown trout, *Salmo trutta* during proliferative kidney disease. *Biology* 10, 1244. DOI: 10.3390/biology10121244.

Sieber, N., Hartikainen, H. and Vorburger, C. (2020) Validation of an eDNA-based method for the detection of wildlife pathogens in water. *Diseases of Aquatic Organisms* 141, 171–184. DOI: 10.3354/dao03524.

Skovgaard, A. and Buchmann, K. (2012) *Tetracapsuloides bryosalmonae* and PKD in juvenile wild salmonids in Denmark. *Diseases of Aquatic Organisms* 101, 33–42. DOI: 10.3354/dao02502.

Smith, C.E., Morrison, J.K., Ramsey, H.W. and Ferguson, H.W. (1984) Proliferative kidney disease: first reported outbreak in North America. *Journal of Fish Diseases* 7, 207–216. DOI: 10.1111/j.1365-2761.1984.tb00925.x.

Sobociński, B., Huusko, A. and Vasemägi, A. (2018) First record of *Tetracapsuloides bryosalmonae* (Myxozoa; Malacosporea) in European whitefish (*Coregonus lavaretus*). *Bulletin of the European Association of Fish Pathologists* 38, 115–120.

Soliman, H., Kumar, G. and El-Matbouli, M. (2018) *Tetracapsuloides bryosalmonae* persists in brown trout *Salmo trutta* for five years post exposure. *Diseases of Aquatic Organisms* 127, 151–156. DOI: 10.3354/dao03200.

Stelzer, M., Ord, J., Neyrinck, S., Steiner, J., Hartikainen, H. *et al.* (2024) Optimal detection protocol of *Tetracapsuloides bryosalmonae* by environmental DNA: a comparison of qPCR and ddPCR approaches. *Environmental DNA* 6, e501. DOI: 10.1002/edn3.501.

Sterud, E., Forseth, T., Ugedal, O., Poppe, T.T., Jørgensen, A. *et al.* (2007) Severe mortality in wild Atlantic salmon *Salmo salar* due to proliferative kidney disease (PKD) caused by *Tetracapsuloides bryosalmonae* (Myxozoa). *Diseases of Aquatic Organisms* 77, 191–198. DOI: 10.3354/dao01846.

Strepparava, N., Segner, H., Ros, A., Hartikainen, H., Schmidt-Posthaus, H. and Wahli, T. (2018) Temperature-related parasite infection dynamics: the case of proliferative kidney disease of brown trout. *Parasitology* 145, 281–291. DOI: 10.1017/S0031182017001482.

Strepparava, N., Ros, A., Hartikainen, H., Schmidt-Posthaus, H., Wahli, T. *et al.* (2020) Effects of parasite concentrations on infection dynamics and proliferative kidney disease pathogenesis in brown trout (*Salmo trutta*). *Transboundary and Emerging Diseases* 67, 2642–2652. DOI: 10.1111/tbed.13615.

Sudhagar, A., El-Matbouli, M. and Kumar, G. (2020) Identification and expression profiling of Toll-like receptors of brown trout (*Salmo trutta*) during proliferative kidney disease. *International Journal of Molecular Sciences* 21, 3755. DOI: 10.3390/ijms21113755.

Syrová, E., Palíková, M., Mendel, J., Seidlová, V., Papežíková, I. *et al.* (2020) Field study indicating susceptibility differences between salmonid species and their lineages to proliferative kidney disease. *Journal of Fish Diseases* 43, 1201–1211. DOI: 10.1111/jfd.13221.

Tops, S., Lockwood, W. and Okamura, B. (2006) Temperature-driven proliferation of *Tetracapsuloides bryosalmonae* in bryozoan hosts portends salmonid declines. *Diseases of Aquatic Organisms* 70, 227–236. DOI: 10.3354/dao070227.

Tops, S., Hartikainen, H.L. and Okamura, B. (2009) The effects of infection by *Tetracapsuloides bryosalmonae* (Myxozoa) and temperature on *Fredericella sultana* (Bryozoa). *International Journal for Parasitology* 39, 1003–1010. DOI: 10.1016/j.ijpara.2009.01.007.

Vasemägi, A., Nousiainen, I., Saura, A., Vähä, J.P., Valius, J. and Huusko, A. (2017) First record of proliferative kidney disease agent *Tetracapsuloides bryosalmonae* in wild brown trout and European grayling in Finland. *Diseases of Aquatic Organisms* 125, 73–78. DOI: 10.3354/dao03126.

Wahli, T., Knuesel, R., Bernet, D., Segner, H., Pugovkin, D. *et al.* (2002) Proliferative kidney disease in Switzerland: current state of knowledge. *Journal of Fish Diseases* 25, 491–500. DOI: 10.1046/j.1365-2761.2002.00401.x.

Wahli, T., Bernet, D., Segner, H. and Schmidt-Posthaus, H. (2008) Role of altitude and water temperature as regulating factors for the geographical distribution of *Tetracapsuloides bryosalmonae* infected fishes in Switzerland. *Journal of Fish Biology* 73, 2184–2197. DOI: 10.1111/j.1095-8649.2008.02054.x.

Waldner, K., Bechter, T., Auer, S., Borgwardt, F., El-Matbouli, M. and Unfer, G. (2020) A brown trout (*Salmo trutta*) population faces devastating consequences due to proliferative kidney disease and temperature increase: a case study from Austria. *Ecology of Freshwater Fish* 29, 465–476. DOI: 10.1111/eff.12528.

Wood, T.S. (2022) Phylactolaemate bryozoans at the Zoological Survey of India and a taxonomic key to Indian Phylactolaemata. *Zootaxa* 5200, 401–435. DOI: 10.11646/zootaxa.5200.5.1.

Wood, T.S. and Marsh, T.G. (1999) Biofouling of wastewater treatment plants by the freshwater bryozoan, *Plumatella vaihiriae* (Hastings, 1929). *Water Research* 33, 609–614. DOI: 10.1016/S0043-1354(98)00274-7.

Yamaguchi, T. and Dijkstra, J.M. (2019) Major histocompatibility complex (MHC) genes and disease resistance in fish. *Cells* 8, 378. DOI: 10.3390/cells8040378.

8 *Myxobolus cerebralis* and *Ceratonova shasta*

Sascha L. Hallett*, Julie D. Alexander and Stephen D. Atkinson
Department of Microbiology, Oregon State University, USA

Abstract

Like all >3000 members of the cnidarian subphylum Myxozoa Grasse, 1970, *Myxobolus cerebralis* and *Ceratonova shasta* are microscopic, spore-forming parasites. They have indirect, freshwater life cycles with two spore stages that develop alternately in fish and annelids. *M. cerebralis* originated in Europe and has spread across the world through anthropogenic activities, whereas *C. shasta* remains restricted to its native range in North America. Both pathogens were described following disease outbreaks in hatchery rainbow trout (*Oncorhynchus mykiss*) and are problematic in North America where they have ecological and economic impacts on juvenile salmonids.

8.1. *Myxobolus cerebralis*

8.1.1. Introduction

8.1.1.1. Description

Myxobolus cerebralis has been called one of the most notorious myxosporean species (Lom and Hoffman, 1971). This tiny, metazoan endoparasite was first reported in Germany in 1893. The parasite targets cartilage and infection can manifest in whirling disease (Drehkrankheit). Cultured rainbow trout (*Oncorhynchus mykiss*) and brook trout (*Salvelinus fontinalis*) became infected in Europe, after being imported as specific pathogen-free eggs from the USA (Hofer, 1903). The disease continues to plague fish hatcheries and wild salmonid populations in North America. The organism underwent several name changes (e.g. *Myxosoma cerebralis*) in the years that followed its discovery but eventually reverted back to the original binomen (Lom and Noble, 1984). *M. cerebralis* is probably the most well-known and certainly the most thoroughly scrutinized member of the Myxozoa.

M. cerebralis spores have two morphologically distinct infective phenotypes: (i) a triactinomyxon-type actinospore; and (ii) a myxobolus-type myxospore (Figs 8.1 and 8.2, Table 8.1). The myxospores are broadly oval in frontal view, broadly lenticular in side view with length 8.7 µm, width 8.2 µm and thickness 6.3 µm (Lom and Hoffman, 1971). Two hard valve cells encapsulate a binucleate sporoplasm and two polar capsules which each house a coiled (five to six loops), solid, extrudable polar tubule. The actinospore has a tri-radially symmetric anchor shape. Three valve cells form an axis (~150 µm) with three caudal processes (each ~194 µm) (El-Matbouli and Hoffmann, 1998). Within the

*E-mail: sascha.hallett@oregonstate.edu

(eds P.T.K. Woo and K. Buchmann)
DOI: 10.1079/9781800628748.0008

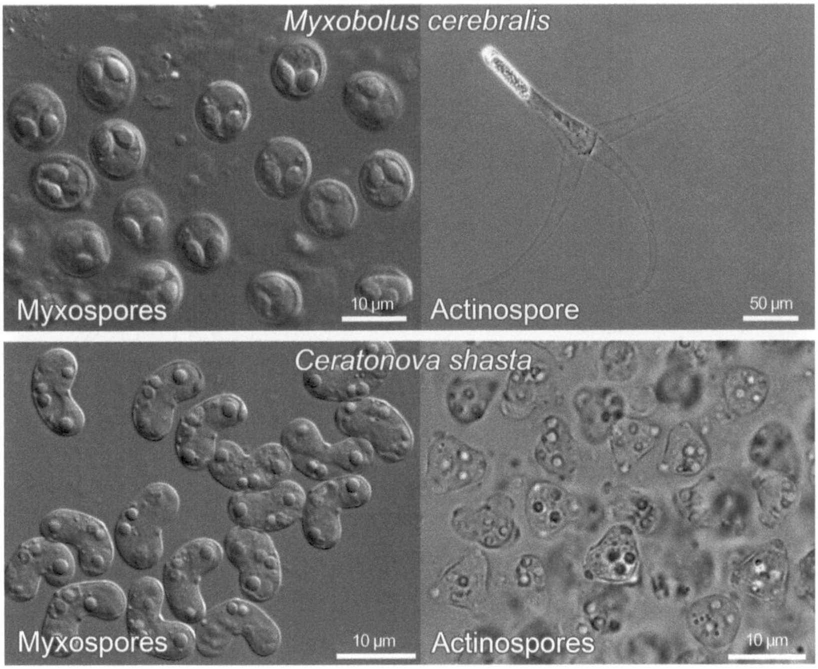

Fig. 8.1. Life-cycle counterparts of *Myxobolus cerebralis* (Mc) and *Ceratonova shasta* (Cs). Myxospores are from infected rainbow trout and actinospores are from infected annelid hosts, *Tubifex tubifex* (Mc) and *Manayunkia occidentalis* (Cs). Myxospores, Nomarski phase contrast; Mc actinospore, phase contrast; Cs actinospore, bright field; all freshly isolated and unstained. (Author's own image.)

apex of the axis are three polar capsules (nematocysts) that each contain a coiled polar tubule (five loops), and below the capsules is a sporoplasm that contains 64 germ cells.

Contemporary descriptions of myxozoans typically include both morphological and molecular (DNA sequence data) details. *M. cerebralis* was one of the first myxozoans to have its small-subunit ribosomal RNA gene (ssrRNA) sequenced (Andree *et al.*, 1997). Other genes that have been used to characterize this species are listed in Table 8.1. Genetic information has proven indispensable in separating closely related and morphologically similar (cryptic) species. It has also permitted development of sensitive and specific diagnostic assays, and investigation of myxozoan dispersal and distribution.

8.1.1.2. Transmission

The life cycle of *M. cerebralis* was the first elucidated for a myxozoan and this momentous discovery revolutionized our understanding not only of a species but of the entire 'Phylum Myxozoa'. In 1983, Markiw and Wolf found that a tubificid oligochaete was required for the development of the infective stage for fish (Markiw and Wolf, 1983), and the following year they described the complete sequence of steps (Wolf and Markiw, 1984), which involves two immotile water-borne stages and various developmental stages within each obligate host (Fig. 8.2). The two spore phenotypes were later confirmed as the same genotype (Andree *et al.*, 1997). As a consequence, the class Actinosporea was suppressed (Kent *et al.*, 1994). The parasite is propagated by only one invertebrate species (actually a species assemblage), *Tubifex tubifex* Muller, 1774 (Wolf *et al.*, 1986), and only fishes of the family Salmonidae (Hedrick and El-Matbouli, 2002). However, compatibility and susceptibility within each host group vary widely (MacConnell and Vincent, 2002; Hallett *et al.*, 2009; Steinbach *et al.*, 2009).

The triactinomyxon actinospore, released from the invertebrate host, is the infective stage for fish. Chemical signals in the aquatic environment (fish mucous-derived; primarily nucleosides) and mechanical stimulation by close proximity to a

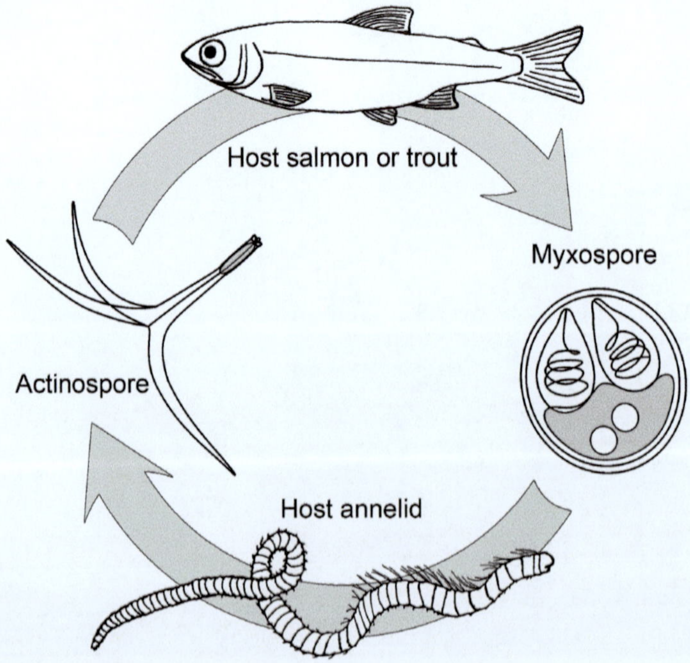

Fig. 8.2. Life cycle of *Mxyobolus cerebralis*. Actinospores released into fresh water from infected *Tubifex tubifex* oligochaetes develop into myxospores in the cartilage of salmonid fishes, which are released into the environment, to be consumed by oligochaetes. (Author's own image.)

Table 8.1. Characteristics of two ecologically and economically significant freshwater myxozoan parasites. (Author's own table.)

Parasite species	*Myxobolus cerebralis*	*Ceratonova shasta*
Disease	Whirling disease	Enteronecrosis
Vertebrate host (intermediate)	Salmonid fish	Salmonid fish
Invertebrate host (definitive)	Oligochaete (*Tubifex tubifex*)	Annelid (*Manayunkia occidentalis*)
Actinospore morphotype	Triactinomyxon	Tetractinomyxon
Point of entry	Epidermis	Gills
Migration route	Nervous system	Circulatory system
Target organ	Cartilage	Intestine
Development time in fish	Months	Weeks
Origin/current distribution	Europe/worldwide	Pacific Northwest of North America
Sequence data available	rRNA[a] plus many other protein-coding genes; partial genome and transcriptome from actinospores	rRNA, plus many other protein-coding genes; genome and transcriptomes from infected fish and isolated myxospores

[a]rRNA, ribosomal RNA gene array comprising small subunit, internal transcribed spacer region 1, internal transcribed spacer region 2 and large subunit.

fish trigger the discharge of the polar tubules (Kallert *et al.*, 2005, 2011), which anchor the parasite to a fish (Fig. 8.3). Within a few minutes of attachment, the amoeboid sporoplasm emerges from between the valve cells and enters the fish epidermis through the secretion opening of a mucous cell (Fig. 8.3; El-Matbouli *et al.*, 1999a). Epithelial damage caused by this initial attachment of high

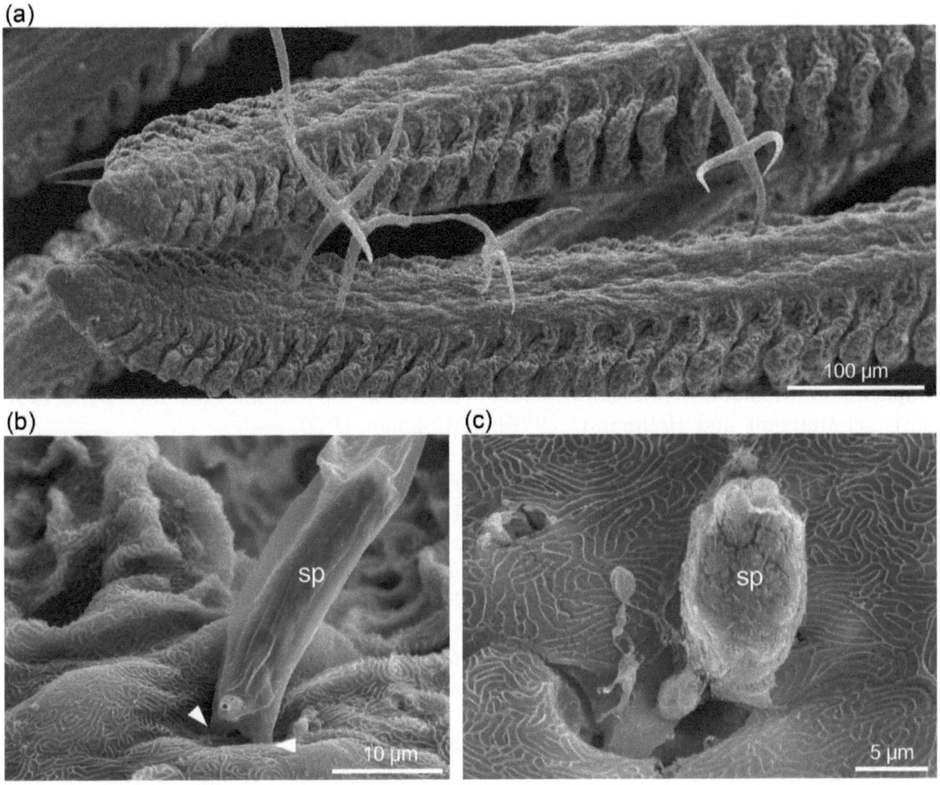

Fig. 8.3. Scanning electron microscope images of *Myxobolus cerebralis* triactinomyxon stages attaching to the gill of rainbow trout: (a) multiple actinospores attached to gill epithelium; (b) higher magnification showing spore attached at two points (arrowheads) by discharged polar tubules (not visible) and sporoplasm (sp) not yet emerged; (c) emergent sporoplasm (sp) after detachment of the now-empty spore shell. (Author's own image.)

numbers of triactinomyxon spores can cause mortality in some fish, but its contribution to overall mortality due to the parasite is not known (Americus *et al.*, 2021b). Particular parasite genes are involved in the invasion process of fish (Eszterbauer *et al.*, 2009). The initial steps of the invasion process – tubule attachment and sporoplasm emergence – can occur also upon contact with non-salmonids (Kallert *et al.*, 2009; Eszterbauer *et al.*, 2019), but the sporoplasm can only successfully penetrate and infect salmonids (El-Matbouli *et al.*, 1999a). Actinospores more frequently attach to the fins in comparison to the gills or skin (Eszterbauer *et al.*, 2019).

After penetration, the parasite multiplies mitotically as it migrates through the epidermis, peripheral nerves, blood and central nervous system to reach cartilage (El-Matbouli *et al.*, 1995, 1999a; Sipos *et al.*, 2018). The host immune response can be effective in eliminating the parasite, but varies widely among salmonids (MacConnell and Vincent, 2002; Akram *et al.*, 2023). Early in the infection, parasites that do not reach the nerves are eliminated by host cellular and/or humoral responses (Hedrick *et al.*, 1998). Suppression of pro-inflammatory and anti-inflammatory cytokines and stimulation of T helper 17 cell (Th17)-mediated immunity occur in resistant fish (Saleh *et al.*, 2020). Once within the nerves, developmental stages are sheltered from the host response until they reach the cartilage, where the parasite trophozoites elicit an inflammatory response as they consume host chondrocytes during myxospore formation (Hedrick *et al.*, 1998; MacConnell and Vincent, 2002).

There is some evidence that mature parasite spores are released while the fish host is alive (Taylor and Haber, 1974; Nehring *et al.*, 2002). However, most tissue-trapped myxospores are probably liberated into sediments when the fish dies (Hedrick *et al.*, 1998) then are dispersed passively by water currents (Kerans and Zale, 2002). As *T. tubifex* forage, they ingest myxospores; polar filaments discharge and attach to the gut epithelium, shell valves open and the sporoplasm penetrates between the cells of the intestinal epithelium. Here ensues an asynchronous developmental series of multiplication, including both mitosis and meiosis (El-Matbouli and Hoffmann, 1998). Ultimately, sporulation creates pansporocysts that contain eight, folded, triactinomyxon-type actinospores. Mature actinospores exit their host via the intestinal tract, inflate upon contact with water, then passively float until they contact a fish, or disintegrate. Infected annelids can each harbour thousands of spores (Gilbert and Granath, 2001; Hallett *et al.*, 2009), which are released as early as 74 days post-infection at 15°C (Gilbert and Granath, 2001). The water-borne triactinomyxons are viable for 6–15 days at 7–15°C (Markiw, 1992b; El-Matbouli *et al.*, 1999b). Two to ten actinospores are sufficient to infect susceptible fish (Hallett and Bartholomew, 2008) and cause disease (Markiw, 1992a). An infected fish may harbour several million myxospores 52–120 days post-exposure at 7–17°C (Halliday, 1973). The parasite is only transmitted via alternating spore stages; there is no horizontal or vertical transmission within fish or worm populations.

M. cerebralis is dispersed primarily via infected fish (Steinbach *et al.*, 2009) but, as discussed earlier, must metamorphose in a worm to reinfect fish. Intra- and inter-basin transfers can occur naturally when infected anadromous fish stray during migration (Engelking, 2002; Zielinski *et al.*, 2010) or via piscivorous fish and birds (Taylor and Lott, 1978; El-Matbouli and Hoffmann, 1991; Arsan and Bartholomew, 2008; Koel *et al.*, 2010). Dissemination may also occur through anthropogenic activities, primarily commercial transfer and stocking of infected fishes, but also during recreational pursuits. Fish eggs do not become infected but associated water may contain spores.

8.1.1.3. Geographic distribution

M. cerebralis originated in Europe but is now exotic in four continents (Asia, Africa, North America and Oceania). Establishment outside its native range was possible because of: (i) the wide distribution of the invertebrate host; (ii) spatial/temporal overlap of these worms with infected fish; and (iii) a combination of environmental factors conducive to parasite persistence. The route of dissemination followed the transfer of live rainbow trout, although imported frozen fish were also implicated as a possible additional source of entry to the USA during the 1950s (Hoffman, 1970).

Whirling disease was first described in rainbow trout that were imported from the USA into Germany. *M. cerebralis* existed in that region in wild brown trout (*Salmo trutta*), which exhibit some resistance to the disease, but the introduced rainbow trout were naïve to the parasite and were decimated by the infection. In the early 1900s, the pathogen spread throughout trout-rearing facilities in Germany and was detected in Denmark and Finland. Translocated infected rainbow trout may have introduced the parasite, or uninfected fish may have provided a susceptible population in areas where the parasite was enzootic (Hoffman, 1970).

Spread and detection of *M. cerebralis* accelerated post-World War II. Between 1952 and 1975, the parasite was detected in 18 more European countries (France, Italy, Czech Republic, Poland, Bulgaria, Yugoslavia, Sweden, Scotland, Norway, Austria, Belgium, Hungary, England, Ireland, Liechtenstein, Luxemburg, the Netherlands and Spain) and in the USSR, Lebanon, South Africa, Morocco, New Zealand, the USA and Canada. *M. cerebralis* has been detected in 27 states in the USA, most recently in North Carolina and Tennessee, and in two provinces in Canada (Alberta Environment and Parks, 2017; Ruiz *et al.*, 2017; Ksepka *et al.*, 2020; Barry *et al.*, 2021; CFIA, 2024). Its global dissemination has been reviewed earlier (Bartholomew and Reno, 2002).

Dissemination of the parasite to new locations is largely attributable to anthropogenic activities. This is supported by the low intraspecific variation of ssrRNA (<1%) and internal transcribed spacer region 1 (1.7%) DNA sequences between European and North American isolates of *M. cerebralis* (Whipps *et al.*, 2004; Arsan *et al.*, 2007a).

8.1.1.4. Impact

Whirling disease was initially only a problem for fish culture operations. These facilities raised trout for food, recreation, restoration and conservation. They sustained large economic losses from the reduced quality and quantity of fish and increased costs from the implementation of treatment and control measures. In some cases, destruction of infected fish or closure of the facility was necessary to curtail contamination of neighbouring waterways (Bartholomew and Reno, 2002; Bartholomew *et al.*, 2007).

In Europe, wild trout populations had presumably evolved resistance to the parasite and were not impacted by the disease (Christensen, 1972). In stark contrast, following its introduction to the USA, the parasite had devastating effects on wild rainbow trout and cutthroat trout (*Oncorhynchus clarkii*) populations, particularly in the Intermountain West (e.g. about 90% reduction of some stocks; Vincent, 1996; Nehring *et al.*, 1998). Whirling disease continues to be a significant fish health issue in the USA (CFIA, 2024; Gilbert and Granath, 2003; Krueger *et al.*, 2006). The malady has changed fish community structure, as vulnerable species are replaced by more resistant species such as brown trout (Baldwin *et al.*, 1998; Granath *et al.*, 2007). Losses have persisted in some areas, while elsewhere populations are recovering (Steinbach *et al.*, 2009). Despite focal points of decimation, there has been no obvious long-term economic harm to recreational fishing in the USA because of a shift to fishing more resistant species (Steinbach *et al.*, 2009).

A range of variables (water flow rates, temperature, sediment, host life histories) governs the impact of *M. cerebralis* on wild fish. Populations may be affected severely in some locations (Vincent, 1996; Nehring *et al.*, 1998), yet persist alongside the parasite elsewhere (see Modin, 1998; Kaeser *et al.*, 2006). Water temperature appears to be the most influential factor, with the critical window being 10–15°C. Temperature affects: (i) parasite development time; (ii) level and duration of spore release from the worm host (El-Matbouli *et al.*, 1999b; Kerans and Zale, 2002; Blazer *et al.*, 2003; Kerans *et al.*, 2005); and (iii) prevalence and severity of infection in the fish host (Baldwin *et al.*, 2000; Schisler *et al.*, 2000; Hiner and Moffitt, 2002; Vincent, 2002; Krueger *et al.*, 2006). Differences in impact have also been associated with the presence of susceptible *T. tubifex* (Beauchamp *et al.*, 2005; Krueger *et al.*, 2006) – a hardy annelid with broad distribution from pristine to polluted sediments (Kathman and Brinkhurst, 1998; Granath and Gilbert, 2002; Shirakashi and El-Matbouli, 2010).

8.1.2. Pathobiology

8.1.2.1. Diagnosis of infection

Efficient detection in the vertebrate host is critical, as there is no effective treatment for *M. cerebralis* or whirling disease (Andree *et al.*, 2002). Some infected fish may be carriers of viable stages and do not display clinical signs. Detection methods: (i) permit documentation of parasite distribution; (ii) identify localities with high parasite abundance; (iii) monitor spread; and (iv) determine prevalence and severity of infection in hosts. Accurate detection and diagnosis measure the success of management procedures (Andree *et al.*, 2002).

Myxozoans are identified primarily on the morphological and morphometrical characteristics of the myxospore in the vertebrate host (Atkinson *et al.*, 2015). Host species and tissue tropism are also considered, and contemporary novel descriptions are expected to be augmented with molecular (DNA sequence) data.

Diagnosis of whirling disease requires multiple steps. Characteristic gross clinical signs are not unique to the disease and must be observed in combination with the identification of *M. cerebralis* myxospores in cartilage (Andree *et al.*, 2002). Myxozoan species cannot readily be distinguished based on developmental stages, and formation of mature myxospores takes several months. The genus *Myxobolus* Bütschli, 1882 contains over 970 described species (Eiras *et al.*, 2021). Several species resemble *M. cerebralis* morphologically and six inhabit the cranial tissues of salmonids (Markiw, 1992c; Hogge *et al.*, 2008). *M. cerebralis* is found in cartilage or bone, while *Myxobolus neurobius* (Schuberg and Schroder,

1905), *Myxobolus kisutchi* (Yasutake and Wood, 1957), *Myxobolus arcticus* (Pugachev and Khokhlov, 1979) and *Myxobolus farionis* (Gonzalez-Lanza and Alvarez-Pellitero, 1984) have been described in nerve tissue and *Myxobolus neurotropus* from brain and spinal cord (Hogge *et al.*, 2008). Another commonly encountered myxobolid of salmonids, *Myxobolus squamalis*, is similar in size to *M. cerebralis* but has two distinctive ridges on either side of the suture and is found in scale pockets (Hoffman, 1999; Polley *et al.*, 2013). Histopathology can resolve fine tissue tropic differences and discriminate between co-occurring cranial myxobolids whose close proximity would lead to co-purification using other methods. DNA-based methods provide unambiguous identification of *M. cerebralis* (Hogge et al., 2008).

Diagnostic methods for *M. cerebralis* (reviewed by Andree *et al.*, 2002; Steinbach *et al.*, 2009; Sarker *et al.*, 2015) range in complexity and vary in sensitivity and specificity. The chosen technique depends on the intended purpose (research, monitoring, diagnostics or fish health inspection), and on the source of the sample (fish, annelid, water or sediment). There are strict guidelines for inspection purposes in the USA (American Fisheries Society-Fish Health Section, 2020).

Most procedures are lethal and, for non-DNA based methods, the infection must be sufficiently advanced. Sporogenesis of the parasite is temperature dependent and takes 90 days at 12–13°C or 11 months at 0–7°C (Hedrick and El-Matbouli, 2002). In young fish, spore production peaks 5 months after exposure (>10°C). The general approach is to isolate and/or concentrate spores and then identify these through microscopy (location, spore morphology) or molecular methods. Entire heads or bodies of young fish can be processed, whereas larger fish may need to be subsampled by taking a core through the head or halving the head down the midline sagittal plane.

The most common approach for diagnosis is isolation of spores using pepsin–trypsin digest (PTD) and presumptive identification of myxospores, followed by confirmation based on histology (spores of the correct dimensions located in appropriate tissues) or PCR amplification of parasite DNA. PTD uses enzymes and centrifugation to digest and concentrate spores from cartilage, which can then be quantified using a haemocytometer (Markiw and Wolf, 1974; Lorz and Amandi, 1994). Microscopic examination of stained histological sections reveals all stages of development and allows scoring of disease severity (Lorz and Amandi, 1994; Baldwin *et al.*, 2000). The MacConnell–Baldwin numerical scale goes from grade 0 (no abnormalities visible and *M. cerebralis* is not detected) to grade 5 (multifocal to coalescing areas of cartilage necrosis visible with loss of normal architecture). Lack of parasite detection using PTD does not confirm absence, given the high detection threshold, hence PTD can be followed by PCR.

PCR-based detection methods include: (i) single-round (Schisler *et al.*, 2001; Baldwin and Myklebust, 2002); (ii) nested (Andree *et al.*, 1998); and (iii) quantitative PCR (qPCR) (Cavender *et al.*, 2004; Kelley *et al.*, 2004). A multi-laboratory comparison of these molecular assays determined that the Kelley *et al.* (2004) qPCR was robust and supported its inclusion as a gold standard in the American Fisheries Society-Fish Health Section Blue Book (Cavender *et al.*, 2024). The sensitivity and specificity of PCR/qPCR allow detection of any life-cycle stage. PCR/qPCR also permits detection of early or light infections and can distinguish between phenotypically similar species. Nested PCR of non-lethal caudal fin clips appears effective for detection of early parasite stages but becomes less accurate as the infection progresses (Skirpstunas *et al.*, 2006; Chiaramonte *et al.*, 2018). To ensure meaningful results, appropriate negative and positive controls as well as relevant reference or calibration standards should be included (Hallett and Bartholomew, 2008). It is important to remember, when using sensitive methods (such as PCR) that do not include direct observation of the parasite, that detection of pathogen DNA does not imply disease.

Other detection methods include: (i) plankton centrifugation to concentrate spores (O'Grodnick, 1975; Lemmon and Kerans, 2001); (ii) molecular based *in situ* hybridization (Antonio *et al.*, 1998); and (iii) loop-mediated isothermal amplification (LAMP) (El-Matbouli and Soliman, 2005).

8.1.2.2. Clinical signs

Whirling disease was unknown until rainbow trout were introduced to Europe, where native brown trout are disease-resistant hosts of *M. cerebralis*. Clinical signs include whirling behaviour, blacktail, skeletal deformities, stunted growth and death (Fig. 8.4). Abnormal behaviour and a blackened tail may not be evident in fish with chronic infections, and both disappear from dead fish.

Parasite development in the fish causes granulomatous inflammation that constricts the spinal cord and compresses the brain stem. This constriction appears responsible for the abnormal swimming behaviour in infected fish (Rose *et al.*, 2000). 'Whirling disease' is named for the repeated episodes of tail-chasing – rapid circular swimming – followed by a series of anterior body contractions (Hofer, 1903; Rose *et al.*, 2000). Additionally, fish may adopt an elevated tail posture when not swimming and, less often, brain-stem compression may cause fish to abruptly cease all movement, except opercular movements, and sink (Rose *et al.*, 2000). Swimming performance generally decreases with increased parasite burden (Ryce *et al.*, 2001, 2005; DuBey *et al.*, 2007).

Blacktail is a consequence of infection of the posterior spinal cartilage (Fig. 8.4); inflammation exerts pressure on root ganglia that control skin melanocytes in the caudal area (Halliday, 1976; Schäperclaus, 1991; El-Matbouli *et al.*, 1995). Skeletal deformities result from disrupted osteogenesis following cartilage damage and associated inflammation, and may include a shortened operculum, indented skull, reduced nose, misaligned jaws and a crooked spine (Fig. 8.4; Andree *et al.*, 2002; MacConnell and Vincent, 2002). Growth may be reduced during the active phase of infection in severely infected fish but resume thereafter except in crippled fish (Hedrick *et al.*, 2001; MacConnell and Vincent, 2002). Mortality may occur either directly through internal physical damage, or indirectly from an inability to feed or evade predators (Hedrick *et al.*, 1998; Steinbach *et al.*, 2009).

Clinical signs may appear 3–8 weeks post-exposure to *M. cerebralis* actinospores (MacConnell and Vincent, 2002). Development and severity of clinical signs depend on: (i) exposure dose and duration; and (ii) the age, size and strain/species/genus of the salmonid host (Table 8.2; Markiw, 1991, 1992a; MacConnell and Vincent, 2002; Bartholomew *et al.*, 2003; Ryce *et al.*, 2004, 2005). Salmonids can become infected at any age from 2 days post-hatch (Markiw, 1991), but younger fish are most vulnerable to infection

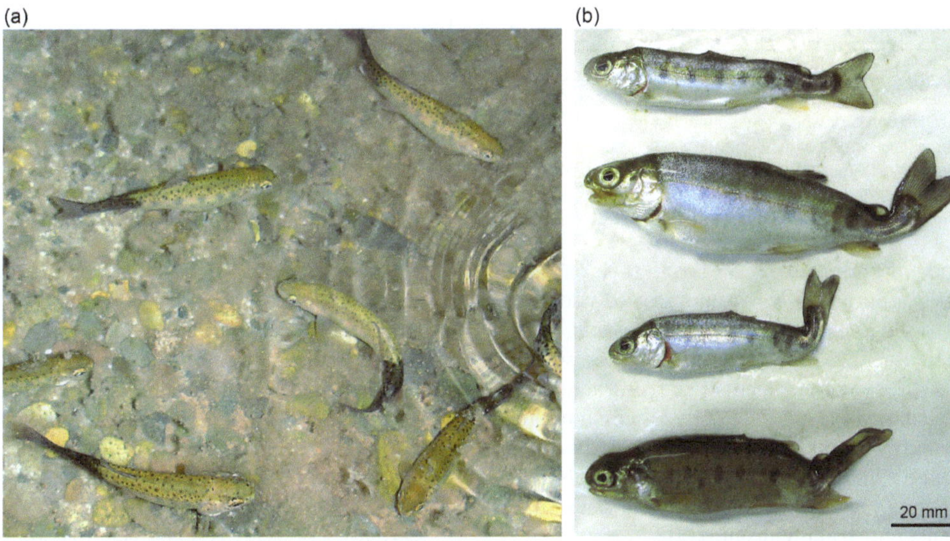

Fig. 8.4. Clinical signs of whirling disease in rainbow trout. Fish were infected with *Myxobolus cerebralis* as fry in the laboratory through cohabitation with infected *Tubifex tubifex*. (a) Live fish have distinct black tails and exhibit whirling behaviour when disturbed; (b) skeletal deformities in fish cohabited with infected annelids for 6 weeks post-hatch, then held on well water for 5 months and euthanized (Hallett and Bartholomew, 2008). (Author's own image).

Table 8.2. Susceptibility to whirling disease among species of salmonids following laboratory or natural exposure to *Myxobolus cerebralis* at a vulnerable life stage. (From: MacConnell and Vincent, 2002; Sollid *et al.*, 2002, 2004; Vincent, 2002; Wagner *et al.*, 2006; Steinbach *et al.*, 2009; Thompson *et al.*, 2010; Americus *et al.*, 2021b.)

Genus	Species/subspecies	Common name	Susceptibility[a]
Oncorhynchus	*mykiss*	Rainbow trout	S–hS
	mykiss	Steelhead trout	S–hS
	clarkii	Cutthroat trout	S–hS
	clarkii bouvieri	Yellowstone cutthroat	S–hS
	clarkii lewisi	Westslope cutthroat	S
	clarkii pleuriticus	Colorado River cutthroat	S
	clarkii virginalis	Rio Grande cutthroat	S
	clarkii stomias	Greenback cutthroat	S
	tshawytscha	Chinook salmon	S
	nerka	Sockeye salmon	hS
	keta	Chum salmon	pR, U
	gorbuscha	Pink salmon	pR, U
	masu	Cherry salmon	pR, U
	kisutch	Coho salmon	pR
	gilae	Gila	hS[b]
	gilae apache	Apache	hS[b]
Salvelinus	*fontinalis*	Brook trout	S
	malma	Dolly varden	pR, U
	confluentus	Bull trout	pR
	namaycush	Lake trout	R
Salmo	*salar*	Atlantic salmon	S, U
	trutta	Brown trout	pR
Prosopium	*williamsoni*	Mountain whitefish	S[b]
Thymallus	*thymallus*	European grayling	S, U
	arcticus	Arctic grayling	R–pR
Hucho	*hucho*	Danube salmon	hS

[a]hS, Highly susceptible, clinical disease common; pR, partially resistant, clinical disease rare and develops only when exposed to very high parasite doses; R, resistant, no spores develop; S, susceptible, clinical disease common at high parasite doses or when very young, but greater resistance to disease at low doses; U, susceptibility is unclear (conflicting reports or insufficient data).
[b]Rapid mortality has been observed in juvenile trout and mountain whitefish exposed to high doses of actinospores in laboratory exposures.

and most prone to disease before their cartilage ossifies. Surprisingly, resistance is not associated with the level of skeletal ossification but rather with other age- and size-related factors, such as the stage of development of the central nervous system (Ryce *et al.*, 2005). Myxospore burden is not proportional to disease severity, and both decrease with host age. Survivors of long-term infections may only exhibit skeletal deformities (MacConnell and Vincent, 2002).

8.1.2.3. Lesions

A successful *M. cerebralis* infection culminates in internal, microscopic lesions filled with myxospores (Fig. 8.5). Lesions can form in the peripheral nerves and epineurium during parasite migration but are predominant in cartilage (Baldwin *et al.*, 2000). Parasite trophozoites digest cartilage as they multiply and mature. Lesions only develop if fish are exposed to a sufficiently high parasite dose (Hedrick *et al.*, 1999a) and only fish that develop lesions have active acquired immunity (MacConnell and Vincent, 2002).

Cartilage lesions are best characterized from rainbow trout, but progress similarly for other species (Hedrick *et al.*, 1999b; Baldwin *et al.*, 2000). Initially, they are small, discrete foci of trophozoites and cartilage degeneration with minimal associated tissue damage and no inflammation

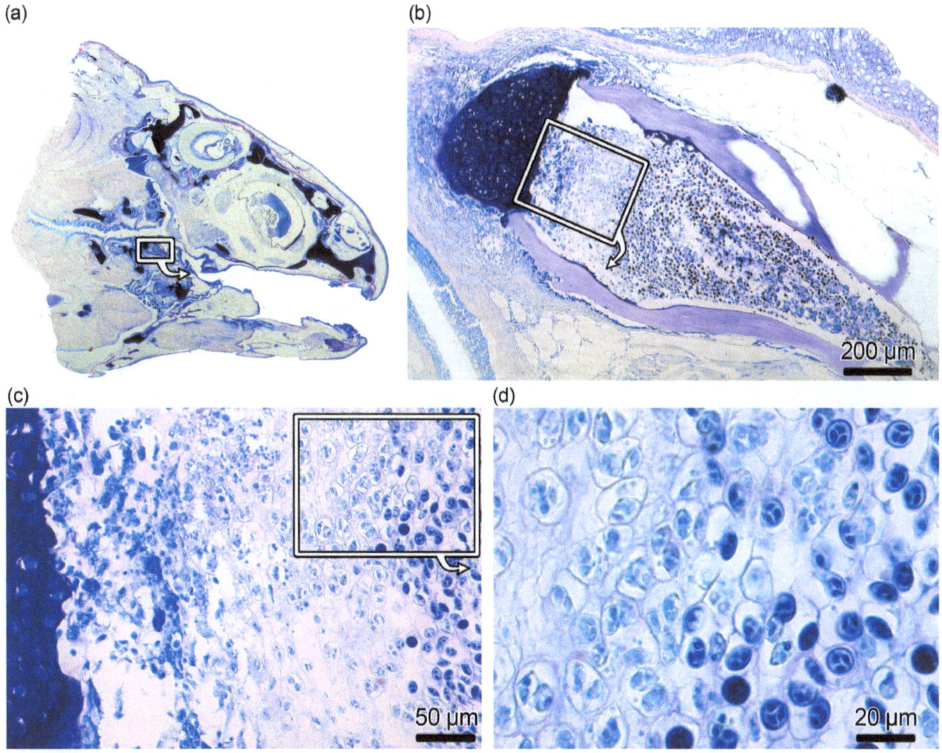

Fig. 8.5. Histological sections of rainbow trout cranial tissues 3 months post-exposure to *Myxobolus cerebralis* showing cartilage damage. (a) Cross-section through head showing location of subsequent images (box); (b) lesion showing succession of cartilage degradation and progression of parasite front; (c) higher magnification of coalescing regions; (d) developmental stages – mature myxospores with dark-staining polar capsules and sporoplasm are conspicuous. Giemsa stain. (Author's own image.)

(Baldwin *et al.*, 2000; MacConnell and Vincent, 2002). These early lesions progress to extensive cartilage necrosis and degeneration with numerous parasite stages. Older stages are centrally located in necrotic foci with younger stages at the leading edges (Baldwin *et al.*, 2000). Surrounding tissues become involved and granulomatous inflammation is evident (MacConnell and Vincent, 2002). Closely associated with infected cartilage in adjacent soft tissues are mononuclear leucocytes. These and multinuclear leucocytes border and/or infiltrate advanced lesions (Baldwin *et al.*, 2000). As the disease advances, large granulomatous lesions may have necrotic centres that contain spores (Plehn, 1905; Hedrick *et al.*, 1998). Coalescing areas of granulomatous inflammation may become so extensive that the normal structural framework of the cartilage is destroyed (Hedrick *et al.*, 1998; MacConnell and Vincent, 2002). Myxospores can become encased in bone as remaining cartilage ossifies.

Lesions in more resistant brown trout: (i) are smaller than those in highly susceptible rainbow trout; (ii) contain fewer parasite stages; and (iii) have fewer associated leucocytes but more multinucleated giant cells (Baldwin *et al.*, 2000). Any cartilage (cranium, spine, fins, vertebrae, ribs and operculum) can be infected (Antonio *et al.*, 1998) and the principal location of parasite lesions varies among salmonid species. In highly susceptible fish, such as rainbow trout, lesions are found throughout the body but consistently in cranial regions, primarily the ventral calvarium then gill arches (Baldwin *et al.*, 2000). In Yellowstone cutthroat trout, lesions are most prevalent in the lower jaw cartilage (Murcia *et al.*, 2011). In brown trout, lesions are most common in the gill arches and rarely in the calvarial or other cartilages (Hedrick *et al.*, 1999a; Baldwin *et al.*, 2000). In bull trout (*Salvelinus confluentus*) and mountain whitefish (*Prosopium williamsoni*), lesions may be found in the cranium but are often limited to the axial skeleton (MacConnell and Vincent, 2002).

8.1.2.4. Pathophysiology

In contrast to the profound physical effects *M. cerebralis* has on fish there are only a few described pathophysiological effects. These include chronic inflammation, disrupted osteogenesis and suppressed growth.

Whirling disease is a chronic cartilaginous inflammatory malady of salmonid fish. The early developmental stages of *M. cerebralis* do not cause cellular reaction of the epidermal or nervous tissues, despite the parasite commencing replication soon after entering the fish host and occupying the central nervous system for several weeks. However, passage through the nerves may affect key neurological responses (Hedrick and El-Matbouli, 2002).

Once in the cartilage, maturing developmental stages lyse and digest chondrocytes. As the infection becomes widespread, trophozoites elicit an intense inflammatory response in most susceptible fish species (MacConnell and Vincent, 2002). Following cartilage degeneration, lesions form, which contain granulomatous inflammation. Inflamed regions may coalesce, and the normal structure disappears. Granulomatous inflammation can extend into the perineural space and produce ring-like constrictions of the upper spinal cord, sometimes compressing and deforming the lower brain stem (Rose *et al.*, 2000). Pathways that connect the medulla with the spinal cord may also degenerate.

The inflammatory response to the trophozoite stage can disrupt osteogenesis (El-Matbouli *et al.*, 1995; MacConnell and Vincent, 2002). Phagocytosis of chondrocytes destroys the structural framework required for healthy osteocyte formation (Schäperclaus, 1991; MacConnell and Vincent, 2002), which results in irregular bone formation and permanent skeletal deformities.

In severely infected fish, growth rates may be reduced during the active phase of infection, but resume thereafter, except in disabled fish (Hedrick *et al.*, 2001; MacConnell and Vincent, 2002; Fetherman *et al.*, 2011). The physiological parameters associated with these outcomes are unknown. Bioenergetic costs of the disease have not been fully evaluated.

8.1.3. Protective/control strategies

Any management or control programme for *M. cerebralis* necessarily requires a holistic approach that incorporates an understanding of environmental factors of the particular locality (Alexander *et al.*, 2011; Murcia *et al.*, 2011) and surveys and monitoring programmes of water, fish and annelids (Bartholomew *et al.*, 2007). Numerous control strategies for the parasite have been tested experimentally but few of these have been implemented on a large scale. Current and possible control measures are covered in detail by Wagner (2002) and Ramazi *et al.* (2022). The present discussion is an update on successful and novel approaches.

Evaluations of chemical and physical stressors on spore viability show the actinospore is the more fragile of the two spore stages of *M. cerebralis*. Viability staining indicates that actinospores are killed by: (i) freezing (–20°C); (ii) drying for 1 h; (iii) chlorine concentrations of 130 ppm for 1 min or longer; (iv) hydrogen peroxide concentrations of greater than 10% w/v; and (v) temperatures above 75°C for at least 5 min (Wagner *et al.*, 2003). These approaches are applicable to disinfection of equipment rather than water supply. Water treatment approaches for inactivation or impairment of triactinomyxons include sand filtration (Arndt and Wagner, 2003; Arndt, 2005), ozonation, chlorination and/or ultraviolet (UV) light (20–80 mJ/cm^2) (Markiw, 1992c; Hedrick *et al.*, 2000, 2007, 2012). Research has recently focused on triactinomyxon deactivation via fish host mucus-derived nucleosides (Kallert *et al.*, 2014) and cations (Americus *et al.*, 2020).

More recent assessments of myxospore viability have involved exposure experiments rather than vital staining (which tends to overestimate live spores) and demonstrated that the myxospore stage is rather less hardy than previously described (Hedrick *et al.*, 2008; Nehring *et al.*, 2015). Infectivity is eliminated by: (i) freezing (–20°C) for 7 days; (ii) heating to 20°C for 2 months; (iii) drying; and (iv) treating with alkyl dimethyl benzyl ammonium chloride at 1500 mg/l for 10 min. A UV dose of 40–480 mJ/cm^2 and chlorine bleach at 500 mg/l for 15 min are largely effective at inactivating myxospores.

Drug efficacy varies widely among myxozoan species and genera (Feist and Longshaw, 2006). No drug or therapeutant treatment exists for *M. cerebralis*. Eleven drugs have been assessed (acetarsone, amprolium, benomyl, clamoxyquin, fumagillin and its analogue TNP-470, furazolidone/Furoxone®, nicarbazin, oxytetracycline, proguanil and sulfamerazine) but none progressed past the testing phase (Wagner, 2002). Several drugs (e.g. furazolidone, proguanil, benomyl) reduced infection and suppressed disease (inhibited spore formation and/or deformed spores), but none prevented or eliminated infection and some had side effects including toxicity (TNP-470) and reduced growth (furazolidone) (Hoffman *et al.*, 1962; Taylor *et al.*, 1973; O'Grodnick and Gustafson, 1974; Alderman, 1986; El-Matbouli and Hoffmann, 1991; Staton *et al.*, 2002). Efficacy may depend on the timing of application, relative to parasite development, in particular whether treatment occurred before or after sporulation. Drug development is further impeded by the regulatory environment (at least in the USA) and issues of drug application to wild fish (Wagner, 2002; Steinbach *et al.*, 2009).

An alternative being explored are salt treatments. Actinospore nematocysts are affected by endogenous cations that may offer an effective therapeutant in hatcheries when salmonids are young and most vulnerable (Americus *et al.*, 2020).

Direct sampling and quantification of parasite stages or parasite DNA in water or sediment through qPCR offers a means to identify areas and times of high parasite abundance and avoids sampling fishes (Richey *et al.*, 2018; Barry *et al.*, 2021). Coupled with sentinel fish exposures, thresholds for infection and disease in the salmonid host can be determined. If parasite density can be measured in near real-time, the data can inform and assess management actions.

8.1.3.1. Fish culture facilities

Hatcheries and ponds offer greater possibilities for control measures than natural settings. Effective strategies include:

- Conversion of earth-bottom ponds and raceways to concrete, and the regular removal of accumulated organics to eliminate *T. tubifex* habitat.
- Use of a pathogen-free water supply (usually converting from surface water to groundwater supply) and a strong water flow (Hoffman, 1990; Hallett and Bartholomew, 2008), at least while fish are young and most vulnerable to disease.
- Treatment of incoming water to kill incoming actinospores using ozonation, chlorination and/or UV light (40 mJ/cm^2) (Markiw, 1992c; Hedrick *et al.*, 1998, 2000, 2007, 2012) rather than copper (Fetherman *et al.*, 2019) or filtration (sand–charcoal rather than membrane) (Hoffman, 1962, 1974; Wagner, 2002; Arndt and Wagner, 2003; Arndt, 2005) to remove actinospores.
- Disinfection of ponds with calcium cyanide, calcium cyanamide or chlorine to render both spore stages non-viable and to kill the invertebrate host.
- Regular fish health inspections to detect *M. cerebralis* and careful tracking of fish transfers and stocking.
- Regular water sampling to enumerate water-borne parasite stages.

8.1.3.2. Natural settings

Once *M. cerebralis* is established, few options exist for its eradication; the goals are to reduce disease severity and mitigate effects on salmonid populations. Risk assessment models and analyses can identify locations at high risk of parasite introduction and establishment, as well as highlight the most important variable(s) (Bartholomew *et al.*, 2005; Kaeser *et al.*, 2006; Krueger *et al.*, 2006; Arsan and Bartholomew, 2008, 2009; Turner *et al.*, 2014; Ramazi *et al.*, 2022).

In rivers where the fishery is managed for recreational purposes, one of the most simple and effective management strategies is to stock larger fish (Steinbach *et al.*, 2009). Although these fish can still become infected they are less susceptible and produce fewer spores (Ryce *et al.*, 2004). Another effective approach is to selectively stock species or strains of salmonids that are naturally resistant to disease, or whose life histories limit the overlap of fry with seasonal peaks of water-borne actinospores. Two other strategies are being explored: (i) foster the breeding of wild fish populations with high genetic diversity (Miller and Vincent, 2008; Steinbach *et al.*, 2009); and (ii) selective breeding whereby vulnerable native populations are crossed with *M. cerebralis*-resistant fish, such as the domesticated German Hofer strain (Schisler *et al.*, 2006; Fetherman *et al.*, 2014; Avila *et al.*, 2018, 2022). The aim is to produce progeny with resistance to whirling disease while retaining genetic traits important for survival in the wild.

Comparison of resistant and susceptible fish strains indicates whirling disease severity has a genetic component (Schisler *et al.*, 2006; Fetherman *et al.*, 2012). A major effect quantitative trait locus (*WDRES9*) region for disease resistance has been identified on chromosome Omy9 of *O. mykiss* (Baerwald *et al.*, 2011). This locus controls a large percentage (50–86%) of phenotypic variation that contributes to whirling disease resistance.

Non-salmonids have been proposed as interceptor fish to lower infection intensity in trout (Kallert *et al.*, 2009). Under laboratory conditions, *M. cerebralis* actinospores attach indiscriminately to fish of any species and more actinospores attach to carp, for example, than to trout (Kallert *et al.*, 2009; Eszterbauer *et al.*, 2019).

The invertebrate host, *T. tubifex*, is small and often inconspicuous. Significantly, different populations of *T. tubifex* can vary considerably in prevalence of infection and level of actinospore production, or amplification (Beauchamp *et al.*, 2002; Kerans *et al.*, 2004; Rassumssen *et al.*, 2008). This provides one explanation for the patchy geographic distribution of infection and severity (Beauchamp *et al.*, 2005; Hallett *et al.*, 2009; Alexander *et al.*, 2011; Lodh *et al.*, 2011; Fytilis *et al.*, 2013) and suggests surveying *T. tubifex* lineages in a stream offers a tool for risk assessment. Variation in the ability to propagate the parasite have been correlated with host mitochondrial 16S rDNA 'lineage': at the extremes, lineage III is described as the most susceptible (Beauchamp *et al.*, 2002; Rasmussen *et al.*, 2008; Hallett *et al.*, 2009; Zielinski *et al.*, 2011), lineage I as compatible (Rassmussen *et al.*, 2008; Lodh *et al.*, 2011), and lineages IV and V as non-compatible (DuBey *et al.*, 2005; Arsan *et al.*, 2007b; Baxa and Nehring, 2022). However, in Alberta, *cox1* (cytochrome c oxidase subunit 1) was observed to be more reliable than 16S rDNA for assessing *M. cerebralis* propagation by *T. tubifex* populations (Barry *et al.*, 2021). Our understanding of compatibility and susceptibility remains somewhat unresolved in the annelid host. The increased availability and use of high-throughput molecular tools (e.g. barcoding) suggest a wider invertebrate host base may exist than was previously described (North Carolina, Ksepka *et al.*, 2021; Alberta, Turnbull, 2024). However, as with molecular detection of *M. cerebralis* in fish hosts from new geographic regions, positive results must be validated through demonstrated propagation of mature parasite spores – in this case, triactinomyxons.

Resistant *T. tubifex* outcompete susceptible strains in exposure experiments conducted under laboratory conditions (Beauchamp *et al.*, 2006; Nehring *et al.*, 2013) and triactinomyxon production per individual infected worm was reduced in populations dominated by refractory annelid species/strains (Kerans *et al.*, 2004; Hallett *et al.*, 2009; Nehring *et al.*, 2013). Myxospore deactivation has also been demonstrated by refractory annelids (Nehring *et al.*, 2016). Exploiting these interactions may offer alternative approaches for the control of whirling disease in streams; however they are most applicable to contained water bodies, such as private ponds. The density of infected *T. tubifex* is positively correlated with whirling disease risk and is associated with fine sediments and lower water temperatures (Krueger *et al.*, 2006). The association between *T. tubifex* populations and point sources of organic enrichment can explain occurrence of the parasite in some systems (Kaeser *et al.*, 2006). Several environmental engineering approaches are being evaluated for their ability to decrease parasite abundance, primarily through reduction of *T. tubifex* populations. Sediment removal reduces favourable *T. tubifex* habitat and can be achieved through direct excavation or by flushing flows in regulated rivers (Hallett and Bartholomew, 2008). Construction of permeable berms has been used in an attempt to filter and isolate areas of high parasite abundance. Stream restoration efforts include exclusion of grazing livestock along waterways to increase riparian vegetation for shade that lowers stream temperatures. Livestock also contribute significant quantities of nutrients and generate fine sediment (Steinbach *et al.*, 2009; Granath, 2014).

Public education is also paramount to restricting inadvertent dissemination of *M. cerebralis* through aquatic recreational activities. Pertinent, practical information is provided to the public via websites, brochures and signage. Recommended precautions include: (i) no transportation of fish between water bodies; (ii) rinsing all mud and aquatic plants from vehicles, boats, trailers, anchors, axles, waders, boots and fishing equipment with clean water; (iii) draining all water from boats; (iv) allowing boats and gear to dry between trips; and (v) disposing of fish away from waterways, preferably in compost or garbage rather than kitchen disposal (Steinbach *et al.*, 2009). Private fish-pond owners and home aquarists also have a responsibility: individuals should be aware of fish health regulations and appreciate that live invertebrate fish food and associated water can harbour myxozoan infective stages (Lowers and Bartholomew, 2003; Hallett *et al.*, 2005, 2006).

8.2. *Ceratonova shasta*

8.2.1. Introduction

8.2.1.1. Description

Ceratonova shasta (Noble, 1950) has been labelled 'a dangerous pathogen of North American salmonids' (Lom and Dyková, 2006). It was first reported in 1948 as the cause of an epizootic among rainbow trout reared at a hatchery in Shasta County, California, USA. The disease, enteronecrosis (originally ceratomyxosis), was described as unusual in the number of tissues and organs affected (Wales and Wolf, 1955); however, the parasite has a tropism for the intestine. Originally assigned as a *Ceratomyxa*, the species was long recognized as being atypical for the genus – most *Ceratomyxa* species are coelozoic parasites of marine fishes – and these distinctions were recognized formally in Atkinson *et al.* (2014).

C. shasta has two morphologically distinct spore stages (Fig. 8.1): (i) a ceratomyxa/ceratonova-type myxospore; and (ii) a tetractinomyxon-type actinospore. Myxospores measure 14–17 μm thick and 6–8 μm long at the suture line (Yamanoto and Sanders, 1979). Characteristic of the genus, the two spore valves are smooth, elongated and crescent shaped (hence the description as a kidney bean-shaped spore), and the suture line is distinct. Two subspherical polar capsules, each containing a coiled polar tubule, are located mid-spore near the suture line. Mature actinospores are smaller (10 μm × 8 μm). They have three valve cells that encapsulate three polar capsules and one binucleate sporoplasm (Fig. 8.1; Bartholomew *et al.*, 1997).

C. shasta has multiple strains (internal transcribed spacer region 1 (ITS1) genotypes) that differ in their host affinity (Atkinson and Bartholomew, 2010a,b; Atkinson *et al.*, 2018). Generally, the parasite genotypes are host-species specific. An exception is host *O. mykiss*, in which the two different life history forms, steelhead and rainbow trout, are differentially infected.

8.2.1.2. Transmission

The *C. shasta* life cycle involves two hosts. The actinospore stage develops in a freshwater annelid, *Manayunkia occidentalis* (formerly misidentified as *Manayunkia speciosa*; Atkinson *et al.*, 2020), and the myxospore stage develops in a salmonid fish (Fig. 8.6; Bartholomew *et al.*, 1997). The life-cycle counterparts of *C. shasta* were determined through laboratory experiments and, for the first time, supported concurrently by DNA (rRNA) sequence data. The parasite requires both hosts to complete its life cycle: there is no horizontal or vertical transmission between fish or between annelids.

Myxospores ingested by the filter-feeding annelid release their sporoplasms in the gut, which then penetrate between the epithelial cells (Meaders and Hendrickson, 2009). The parasite multiplies and migrates through the nervous system to the epidermal layer of the integument where most development occurs (Bartholomew *et al.*, 1997; Meaders and Hendrickson, 2009) and parallels that described for *M. cerebralis* (El-Matbouli and Hoffmann, 1998). Development to mature actinospores occurs in approximately 7 weeks at water temperatures averaging 17°C (Meaders and Hendrickson, 2009). Pansporocysts are released through secretory pores in the annelid epidermis and rupture, each releasing eight actinospores (Bartholomew *et al.*, 1997; Bjork, 2010), but unlike *M. cerebralis* they do not inflate or change morphologically upon contact with water. Asynchronous development permits prolonged spore release and host survival.

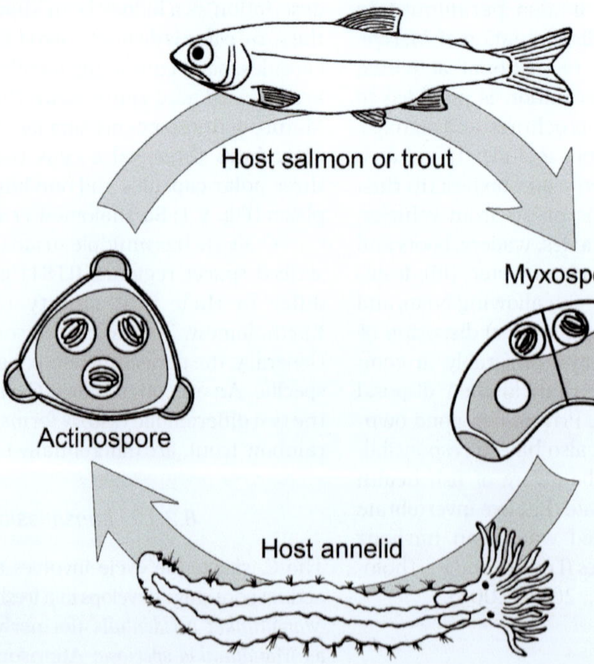

Fig. 8.6. Life cycle of *Ceratonova shasta*. Actinospores released into fresh water from infected *Manayunkia occidentalis* annelids develop into myxospores in the intestine of salmonid fishes and are released subsequently into the environment where they are consumed by naïve annelids. (Author's own image.)

Several hundred actinospores may be released in a single day from an infected annelid (Bartholomew *et al.*, 2004; Meaders and Hendrickson, 2009). Viability of the actinospores decreases with increasing temperature. Actinospores are viable for up to 13 days at 11°C (Ratliff, 1983) and 3–7 days at 18°C (Foott *et al.*, 2007) under field conditions. In the laboratory actinospores are physically intact for up to 18 days at 4°C and 15 days at 12°C, but for only 6 days at 20°C (Bjork, 2010). Enteronecrosis occurs seasonally, with release of actinospores in the spring as temperatures rise above 8°C (Bartholomew *et al.*, 2022), although infection can occur at lower temperatures (e.g. 7°C; Ratliff, 1983). Infection by a single actinospore is sufficient to result in death of highly susceptible strains of salmon and trout (Ratliff, 1983; Bjork and Bartholomew, 2009).

Actinospores attach to the fish gill, and their sporoplasm penetrates the epithelium (Bjork and Bartholomew, 2010). The parasite migrates to the blood vessels of the gill arch where it replicates in the vessel endothelium, then is delivered to the intestine and other organs via the circulatory system (Bjork and Bartholomew, 2010). Here it develops in small disporic pseudoplasmodia (Yamanoto and Sanders, 1979), which culminate in the myxospore stage at 2 weeks post-exposure at 18°C (Ray *et al.*, 2010). In semelparous fishes such as Chinook salmon (*Oncorhynchus tshawytscha*) and coho salmon (*Oncorhynchus kisutch*), myxospores are released upon maturation in juvenile fish, but not until post-mortem in adult fish; adult salmon that die on spawning grounds release millions of spores (Foott *et al.*, 2016), thus returning the parasite to the upper portions of watersheds. In iteroparous fish (such as steelhead trout), mature parasites are observed in the intestinal lumen and faecal casts of infected fish throughout their lifespan.

8.2.1.3. Geographic distribution

C. shasta occurs in salmonids in freshwater environments of the Pacific Northwest region of North America. Unlike the widely dispersed

M. cerebralis, *C. shasta* remains restricted to the Pacific Northwest's larger river systems. The distribution of the parasite requires both salmonid and annelid hosts, and it does not encompass the geographic distribution of either. *C. shasta* is not established in many rivers in the Pacific Northwest where infected salmon migrate. Although Pacific salmon have been introduced to the eastern USA, the parasite has not become established. This is likely because *M. occidentalis* appears absent from this region (a closely related annelid, *M. speciosa*, is present but is not known to host *C. shasta*). The distribution of *C. shasta* in the Pacific Northwest has been mapped using sentinel fishes and water sampling (Hallett and Bartholomew, 2006; Stinson *et al.*, 2018). Naïve fish held in cages detect the fragile actinospore stage released from annelid hosts which indicates parasite establishment. First identified from the Pit River drainage (Schafer, 1968), California, *C. shasta* is now considered endemic in most major Pacific Northwest river drainages, including the San Joaquin, Sacramento, Pit, Klamath, Rogue, Columbia, Fraser and Deschutes Rivers, plus several smaller rivers (e.g. Nehalem, Alsea and Chehalis) and Lake Washington (Sanders *et al.*, 1970; Ratliff, 1983; Ching and Munday, 1984a; Hoffmaster *et al.*, 1988; Hendrickson *et al.*, 1989; Stocking *et al.*, 2006, 2007; Stinson *et al.*, 2018). In Alaska, distribution has been inferred from detection of *C. shasta* in adult salmon, indicating that the parasite is present in several south-central and interior drainages, including the Yukon (Meyers *et al.*, 2008).

8.2.1.4. Host distribution

The resulting mosaic distribution of the parasite is reflected in patterns of resistance among salmon and trout, with relative resistance to infection and disease occurring in fish populations that have evolved in waters where *C. shasta* is endemic. Thus, strains of salmonids within the same species may show different susceptibilities to *C. shasta* (Zinn *et al.*, 1977; Buchanan and Sanders, 1983; Ching and Munday 1984b; and reviewed in Bartholomew, 1998; Alama-Bermejo *et al.*, 2020). These variations in susceptibility of populations of salmon and trout to infection and disease are one of the best-documented examples of heritable resistance in fishes (Ibarra *et al.*, 1992; Bartholomew, 1998; Bartholomew *et al.*, 2001; Nichols *et al.*, 2003).

C. shasta has been regarded as a single species throughout both its geographic and its host ranges based on: (i) similarities in the site of infection in fish; (ii) disease manifestations; and (iii) morphology of the myxospore. This conclusion was largely supported by genetic studies, as the rRNA sequences of isolates from different geographic locations and from different species were homogeneous (Atkinson and Bartholomew, 2010a). However, studies on *C. shasta* in the Klamath River system documented the presence of multiple parasite strains based on differences in the ITS1 (Atkinson and Bartholomew, 2010a,b; Breyta *et al.*, 2020). In rivers with mixed salmonid species, parasite genotypes occur in sympatry yet show marked differences in infection success in different hosts, indicating evolution of host-specific parasite genotypes. Similar to the distribution of their anadromous hosts, some of these parasite strains have been extirpated from portions of rivers with the construction of dams that have blocked fish passage (Atkinson and Bartholomew, 2010a).

8.2.1.5. Impact

C. shasta enteronecrosis is considered one of the most virulent myxozoan diseases, in part as a result of early epizootics in hatcheries where susceptible strains of salmon and trout were reared on surface waters containing the parasite. Hatcheries where outbreaks occurred were forced to change water sources, treat the water supply or rear more resistant strains of fish. While these practices have decreased epizootics in hatcheries, outbreaks still occur when treatment systems fail, environmental conditions change to favour the parasite, or when susceptible strains of fish are brought on to these facilities. Even when protected from infection in the hatchery, these juvenile fish will be exposed to *C. shasta* following release into rivers where parasite levels are high. Naturally reared fish are similarly at risk of disease, and in some cases this risk may be even higher because of the longer period these fish are exposed to the parasite.

In contrast to whirling disease, size and age of the fish have little effect on the severity of enteronecrosis (Bjork and Bartholomew, 2009). Estimates of infection and mortality in natural populations of juvenile salmonids and among hatchery fish following release are difficult to determine and vary widely (Ratliff, 1981; Bartholomew *et al.*, 1992; Margolis *et al.*, 1992; Foott *et al.*, 2004). Information can be deduced from sentinel fish exposures, water sampling and fish trapping (e.g. Foott *et al.*, 2004; Hallett and Bartholomew, 2006; Stocking *et al.*, 2006). It is generally acknowledged that the parasite may significantly affect juvenile survival during years when water flows are low and water temperatures high; however, the consistent high mortality of juvenile salmon that occurs in certain rivers may be indicative of an imbalance in the host–parasite relationship. In the Klamath River (which rises in Oregon and flows through northern California, USA), *C. shasta* infections have caused significant mortality of migrating juvenile salmon (Foott *et al.*, 2004; Stocking *et al.*, 2006), with consequences for commercial fisherfolk and Native Americans who rely on these fish for their livelihood and culture. Elsewhere in the Pacific Northwest, *C. shasta* is an important contributor to pre-spawn mortality of infected adult fish (Sanders *et al.*, 1970; Chapman, 1986; Bartholomew *et al.*, 1992).

8.2.2. Pathobiology

8.2.2.1. Diagnosis of infection

As with other myxozoan infections, visual diagnosis is complicated by the long period required for development of mature myxospores in the fish and by the pleomorphic appearance of the pre-sporogonic stages. However, in contrast to *M. cerebralis*, the location of the parasite in the intestine provides an accessible tissue to sample. Spore maturation is often simultaneous with death of the fish host and the process is temperature dependent: for example, the mean time from infection to death for rainbow trout held at 12°C is 55 days; this decreases to 19 days at 20.5°C (Udey *et al.*, 1975). Presumptive diagnosis of *C. shasta* is confirmed by the identification of myxospores with the appropriate morphology or by specific amplification of DNA of pre-sporogonic life stages (Bartholomew, 2012). While other myxozoans such as *Myxidium minteri*, *Chloromyxum* spp. and *Myxobolus* spp. may co-occur with *C. shasta* infections, the ceratomyxid is distinct in its bean-like morphology. Of almost 340 species of morphologically similar *Ceratomyxa* Thélohan, 1892, and *Ceratonova* Atkinson, Foott & Bartholomew, 2014, only some 20 are known from fresh water, and only *C. shasta* infects salmonid fishes and intestinal tissue (Lom and Dyková, 2006; Whipps *et al.*, 2025).

PRESUMPTIVE DIAGNOSIS. Wet mounts prepared from the wall of the posterior intestine or from ascites are examined for spores. Lesions in any tissue should also be examined. An anal swab permits non-lethal sampling of larger fish. Wet mounts can be scanned in a systematic manner under phase contrast or brightfield microscopy at 200–400× magnification. Presumptive diagnosis is based on identification of multicellular myxosporean pre-sporogonic stages (trophozoites; Fig. 8.7a) (Bartholomew, 2012). Infected salmonids may not show signs of enteronecrosis. An alternative to wet mounts is tissue imprints or histological sections of intestinal or other grossly infected tissues. These may be stained with either Giemsa or haematoxylin and eosin stain. In Giemsa-stained sections, multicellular trophozoites appear light blue with the nuclei containing a dark-staining karyosome surrounded by a clear halo (Fig. 8.7d).

CONFIRMATORY DIAGNOSIS. Visual confirmation of *C. shasta* infection is by identification of the characteristic kidney bean-shaped myxospores in wet mounts or histological sections (Fig. 8.7b). Spores are most often detected in the posterior intestine, but may be found in other tissues, particularly the kidney, liver, gall bladder and pyloric caeca. Confirmation using molecular diagnosis is standard, and *C. shasta*-specific PCR primers have been developed (Palenzuela *et al.*, 1999; Palenzuela and Bartholomew, 2002; Bartholomew, 2012).

Non-lethal sampling techniques for adult salmon include intestinal lavage, which uses a syringe and flexible tubing to flush the posterior intestine with saline (Coley *et al.*, 1983). Although that study used visual examination to detect spores, molecular methods could also have been employed. Fox *et al.* (2000) modified this technique for juvenile fish and used a swab for collection of intestinal contents combined with PCR for detection. Although this test was

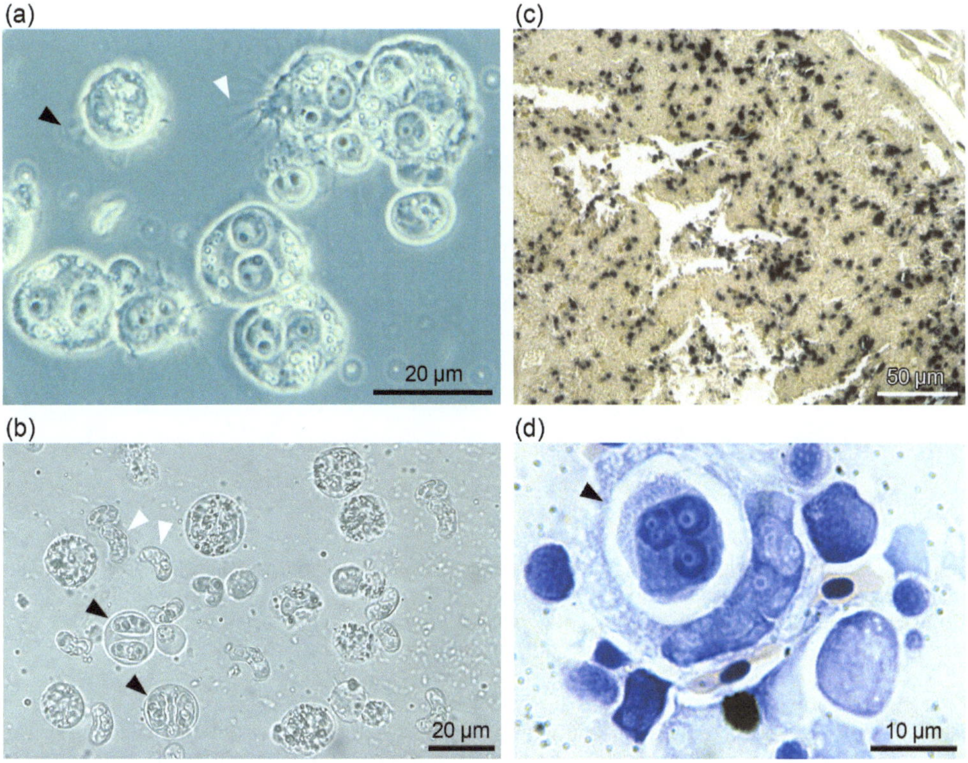

Fig. 8.7. Diagnosis of *Ceratonova shasta* infections. (a) Pre-sporogonic (= trophozoite) stages of the parasite in fresh ascites showing filopodia (white arrowhead) and blebbing (black arrowhead); (b) sporogonic (= disporoblast) stages (black arrowheads) and mature myxospores (white arrowheads) in ascites from a more advanced infection; (c) *in situ* hybridization staining of posterior intestine of a heavily infected rainbow trout, labelled parasites stain dark brown; (d) pre-sporogonic stage (arrowhead) in kidney imprint, stained with Giemsa. (Author's own image.)

not as sensitive as the lethal PCR assay, the parasite could be detected as early as 13 days post-exposure. PCR primers have also been adapted for *in situ* hybridization on histological sections (Fig. 8.7c), although this remains primarily a research tool (Palenzuela and Bartholomew, 2002; Bjork and Bartholomew, 2010). qPCR allows estimation of parasite density in a sample and, when combined with water filtration, has been used to monitor for water-borne spores in rivers and to predict mortality in migrating juvenile fish (Hallett and Bartholomew, 2006).

8.2.2.2. Clinical signs

Clinical signs of enteronecrosis vary with level of infection, fish species and fish age. Infected juvenile salmon typically become anorexic, lethargic and darken in colour (especially rainbow trout/steelhead). The anus becomes swollen and haemorrhaged, and the abdomen may be distended with ascites (Fig. 8.8a). Exophthalmia is common in fish with ascites. Acutely infected fish may die before clinical signs develop.

8.2.2.3. Lesions

MACROSCOPIC. The most common external lesion is a haemorrhagic anus that results from severe intestinal lesions. Internally, macroscopic and microscopic lesions are common in *C. shasta*-infected fish and are not restricted to the primary site of infection. In susceptible fish, *C. shasta* invades all intestinal tissue layers and causes necrosis and haemorrhaging, resulting in mortality approaching 100%. Internally, the digestive tract may be grossly swollen, necrotic and haemorrhagic with mucoid contents (Fig. 8.8b and c).

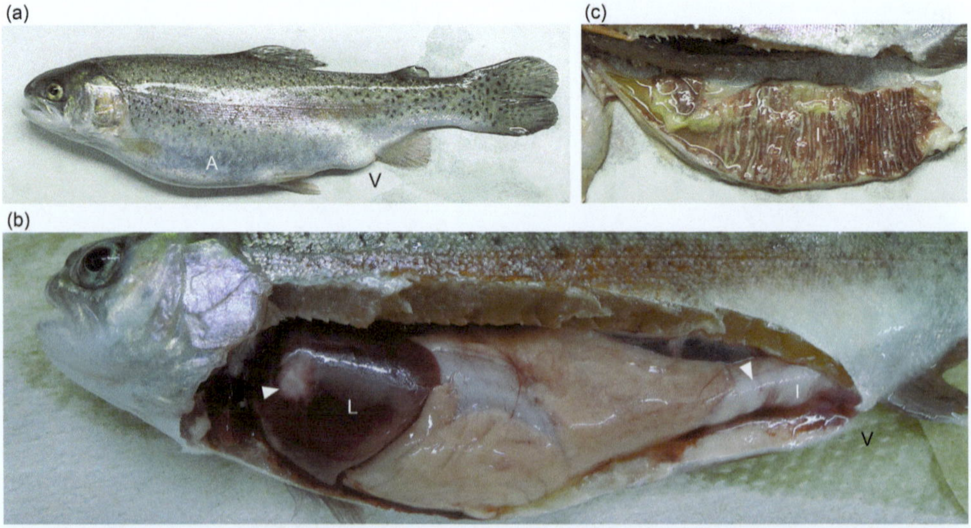

Fig. 8.8. External and internal gross signs of *Ceratonova shasta* infection. (a) Clinical enteronecrosis in an allopatric rainbow trout showing swollen vent (V) and abdomen (A) distended with ascites; (b) dissected rainbow trout with swollen, pale intestine (I: arrow head) and lesions on the liver (L: arrow head); (c) opened intestine showing haemorrhaging. (Author's own image.)

The intestine and pyloric caeca may also be lined with caseous material. Additional characteristics may include ascites, lesions in the kidney or liver (fluid filled blebs/pustules to firm creamy white nodules) and haemorrhaging and (or) necrosis of liver, gallbladder, spleen, gonads, kidney, heart, gills and skeletal musculature.

In adult salmonids, the walls of the intestine and pyloric caeca may be thickened and haemorrhagic. Nodular lesions may develop in the intestinal wall and perforate the intestine. Gross lesions (which may abscess) can occur in liver, kidney, spleen or musculature (Fig. 8.8b; Conrad and Decew, 1966; Schafer, 1968; Bartholomew *et al.*, 1989).

MICROSCOPIC. In the intestine, the parasite triggers an acute inflammatory reaction involving polymorphonuclear leucocytes (PMNLs), fibroblasts and macrophages. In severe infections, the epithelial lining necrotizes, fragments and ultimately sloughs, and is replaced by fibrous connective tissue that contains host cells and parasite stages (Bartholomew *et al.*, 2004). The intestinal lumen may contain epithelial cells, epithelial cell fragments, PMNLs, fibroblasts and different parasite stages (Bartholomew *et al.*, 1989; Bjork and Bartholomew, 2010). As the trophozoite stages of *C. shasta* proliferate in the intestine and blood vessels, the infection spreads to other organs (Fig. 8.9). Parasites may be detected subsequently in the pyloric caeca, kidney (Fig. 8.9e) and liver, and finally in the capsule of the spleen. Parasites may also congregate in the eye (Fig. 8.9f) causing opaqueness and vision loss; it is unclear whether this tissue is directly infected or is part of a systemic infection.

In resistant hosts the parasite can successfully invade the gills and establish in the blood vessels (Bjork, 2010); however, it is cleared from the bloodstream within 2 weeks. Two defence strategies have been observed histologically: (i) parasites are isolated in granulomatous lesions and eliminated; and (ii) parasites migrate through the intestinal layers to the lumen without evidence of host tissue reactions (Bartholomew *et al.*, 1989, 2004; Ibarra *et al.*, 1991; Foott *et al.*, 2007; Bjork, 2010). The latter response may indicate immunological tolerance.

8.2.2.4. Pathophysiology

Despite our understanding of the pathological effects, the physiological aspects of the disease are largely unknown. Afflicted fish may be immunocompromised and have hampered nutrient uptake and transportation, resulting in reduced

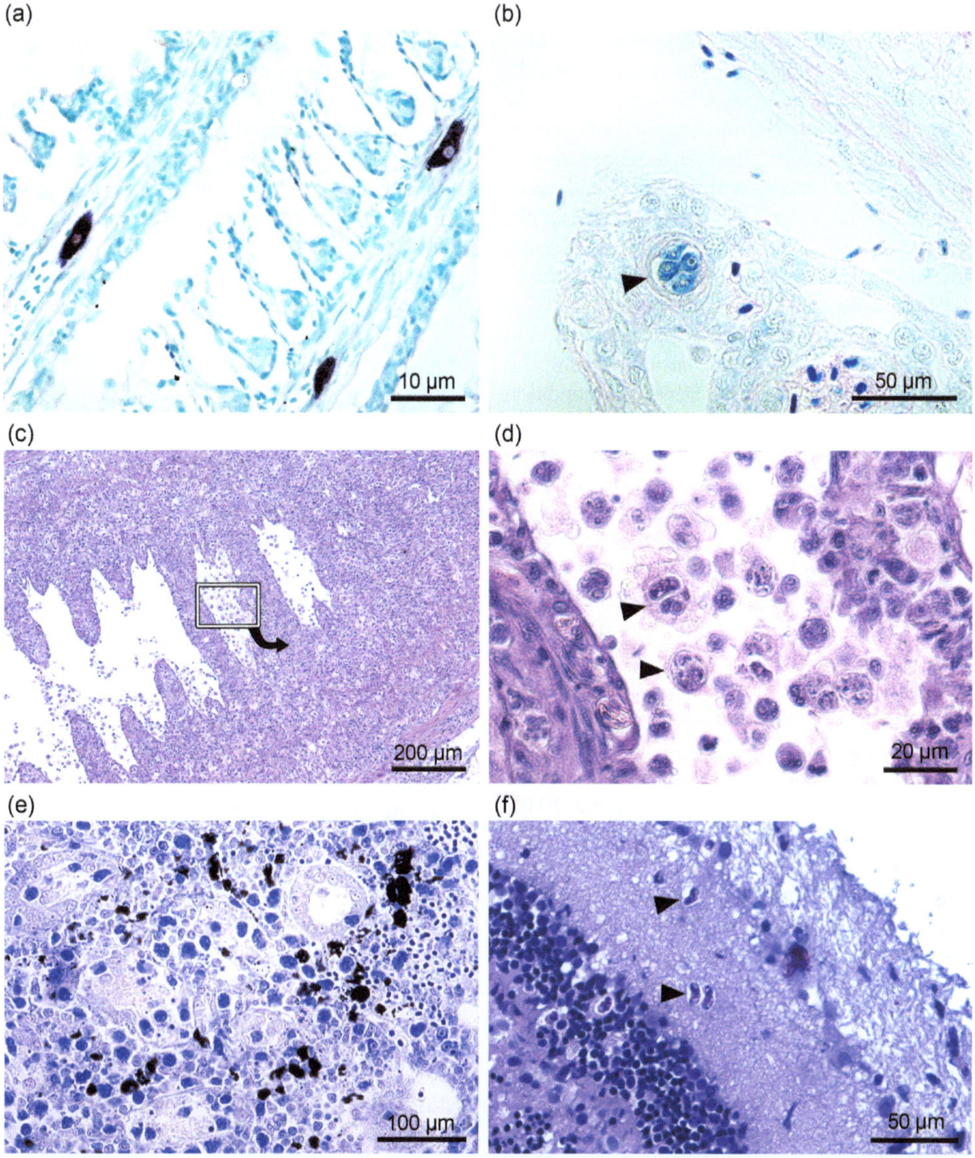

Fig. 8.9. Histological sections of salmonids at different times post-infection, in chronological order. (a) Parasites (dark staining) in gill arch blood vessels; (b) parasite (arrowhead) in blood vessel supplying the intestine; (c) longitudinal section of the posterior intestine late in the infection showing destruction of intestinal epithelium and proliferation of parasites and host immune cells; (d) higher magnification of (c), showing a variety of parasite stages, including disporoblasts (arrowheads); (e) kidney with parasite stages proliferating throughout; (f) section through eye showing mature spores (arrowheads) in multiple tissue layers. (Image in (a) provided by Sarah Bjork, Oregon State University; (b–f) author's own image.)

growth (Barker *et al.*, 1993). Disease severity is related to: (i) the parasite dose; (ii) the inherent resistance of the fish strain; and (iii) water temperature.

For fish that succumb to infection, death may be a direct result of damage to the intestine or may result from secondary invasion in the damaged tissue by bacterial pathogens. Although empirical observations indicate that parasitized fish are more prone to secondary infection by other pathogens, this has rarely been experimentally demonstrated. In some cases, co-infections may be a result of a lowered immune capacity as a result of myxozoan infection. However, the coincidence of infections of *C. shasta* with bacterial pathogens of low virulence, such as *Aeromonas hydrophila*, suggests that the lesions that result from *C. shasta* infection allow the environmental bacterium to invade and become a primary pathogen.

The severe granulomatous enteritis that develops in response to *C. shasta* infection also appears to contribute to diminished body condition (Bartholomew *et al.*, 2004), possibly by disturbance of adsorption and transport functions in the intestine (Barker *et al.*, 1993). Protein-losing enteropathy, wasting and ascites are commonly associated with these lesions and negatively impact growth of infected fish. Survivors of infections in hatcheries are undersized (Tipping, 1988) and it has been suggested that *C. shasta* probably affects post-release survival during migration and seawater acclimatization either indirectly by decreasing fitness or directly as the disease progresses.

Despite the presence of this parasite in the gills both early (Bjork and Bartholomew, 2010) and late (Bartholomew *et al.*, 1989) in the infection, there is no direct evidence that the parasite interferes with osmoregulatory functions. This should be examined more thoroughly, particularly during the process of smoltification and seawater transition of anadromous fishes.

Advances in sequencing techniques and the ability to maintain annelid hosts and thereby culture pure *C. shasta* genotypes in the laboratory have enabled identification of candidate genes related to virulence, parasite motility, venoms and proteases (Alama-Bermejo *et al.*, 2020, 2022; Americus *et al.*, 2021a). Insights into these factors, molecules and mechanisms indicate that they are differentially associated with different genotypes (Bartholomew *et al.*, 2022). Proteases and their inhibitors are important in host–parasite interactions and infection outcomes. Four proteases of different catalytic types, namely cathepsin D (aspartic), cathepsin L and Z-like (cysteine), aminopeptidase-N (metallo) and a stefin (cysteine protease inhibitor), have been identified for *C. shasta* and their expression during infection and parasite development appears genotype dependent (Alama-Bermejo *et al.*, 2022). Additionally, venom-like compounds have been identified and their expression varied considerably during infection, with expression at early infection time points being associated with parasite invasion and proliferation (Americus *et al.*, 2021a). Ongoing genomic and transcriptomic investigations will further inform our understanding of the complex host–parasite interactions among *C. shasta* genotypes and their respective hosts, both allopatric and sympatric.

8.2.3. Protective/control strategies

8.2.3.1. Hatcheries

Because *C. shasta* infections are not transmitted directly between fish, outbreaks in hatcheries occur only by introduction of actinospores through the water supply. The invertebrate host for *C. shasta* has different habitat preferences to the host of *M. cerebralis* and is less likely to accumulate in a hatchery environment. Thus the most effective means of disease prevention in a hatchery is by use of uncontaminated water or by rearing *C. shasta*-resistant strains of salmon and trout. In hatcheries where parasite-free water supplies are unavailable, UV irradiation or chlorination of water supplies can reduce or eliminate the infective actinospore (Bedell, 1971). Sand filtration in combination with either of these methods is more effective in reducing incidence of disease (Sanders *et al.*, 1972; Bower and Margolis, 1985) and ozone treatment of water reduces mortality from *C. shasta* and also increases fish growth (Tipping, 1988). There has been limited testing of therapeutants for controlling enteronecrosis. Two studies investigated the efficacy of fumagillin and its analogue TNP-470 and found no substantial protection when administered either prophylactically or for 53 days post-infection (Ibarra *et al.*, 1990; Whipple *et al.*, 2002). Similarly, glucans fed prophylactically did not provide protection to subsequent parasite exposure (Whipple *et al.*, 2002).

8.2.3.2. Wild

This parasite has not been as broadly disseminated as other fish pathogens because *C. shasta* is not transmitted horizontally or vertically and the annelid host apparently has a restricted range. However, in natural waters where it is present, it continues to cause severe disease as control options are limited. The most widely applied management tool for maintaining sports fisheries in endemic waters has been the stocking of resistant salmonids (Buchanan and Sanders, 1983). Interestingly, a corollary to this practice is based on concerns about hatchery fish interbreeding with native fish. Because of this, highly susceptible strains of fish from non-endemic waters have been used to stock certain watersheds, with the knowledge that these fish would not survive infection to interbreed. While this has been an effective management tool, it elevated parasite levels in some waters to very high levels that could potentially affect natural fish populations (Hurst *et al.*, 2012). Another strategy for minimizing infection of hatchery fish is to time release to occur during periods when parasite abundance is low; this approach also avoids amplification of the parasite by the released fish (Bartholomew *et al.*, 2022).

In many rivers, construction of dams, diversion of water and destruction of riparian habitat have stabilized water flows, raised water temperatures and reduced sediment transport (Bartholomew *et al.*, 2023). These changes may increase habitat for the annelid host (Alexander *et al.*, 2015, 2016), promote the overlap of hosts and parasite stages, and increase transmission efficiency. In these systems, the need to develop predictive tools for parasite effects has led to the development of water-sampling methods that both quantify the parasite and distinguish between parasite genotypes (Hallett and Bartholomew, 2006; Atkinson and Bartholomew, 2010a,b). Data from parasite density and fish infection severity studies conducted concurrently has enabled the determination of species-specific mortality thresholds (e.g. 10 spores of *C. shasta* genotype I per litre is associated with 40% mortality in Chinook salmon; Hallett *et al.*, 2012) that trigger adaptive management responses. These advances in molecular techniques allow predictions of which fish species are likely to become infected and what level of mortality may be expected so that managers can make real-time decisions about water allocation and timing of fish release from hatcheries. These tools also allow better resolution of where focal points for infection occur, which can be targeted for habitat restoration (Hallett *et al.*, 2012; Homel and Alexander, 2022; Foott *et al.*, 2023).

In regulated river systems, infection prevalence and severity in free-ranging fishes can be reduced through prescribed flow events (water released from reservoirs behind dams). Higher flows can reduce parasite concentration through dilution, flush the water-borne stages downstream, reduce transmission efficiency, affect movement of salmonids, and disturb the annelid habitat (Alexander *et al.*, 2016; Bartholomew *et al.*, 2022, 2023). The impact depends on the timing, magnitude and duration of the event. For example, in the Klamath River in North America, three types of flow have been identified and implemented to achieve these outcomes: (i) a deep flushing flow; (ii) a surface flushing flow; and (iii) an emergency flow (Hillemeier *et al.*, 2017; Bartholomew *et al.*, 2023). Return to natural flow regimes, present before host–parasite dynamics became unbalanced with large-scale anthropogenic habitat modifications, should help mitigate disease.

Removal of adult salmon carcasses from spawning grounds was proposed as a management action to reduce myxospore input into the Klamath River system, but the approach was deemed impractical. Although many fish (up to 87%) were infected, myxospores were not always observed. Only a few fish (<10%) contributed high numbers of spores (>half a million) back into the system (Foott *et al.*, 2016) and the effect of carcass removal efforts could not easily be measured.

Natural strategies salmonids adopt to decrease infection and its severity include heritable/evolution of disease resistance (Bartholomew *et al.*, 2001), altering migration timing to reduce encounters, and use of tributaries and refugia characterized by cooler water and lower parasite abundance (Chiaramonte *et al.*, 2016).

An epizootiological model, a theoretical predictive tool, was developed to identify parameters important for parasite transmission and persistence (Ray *et al.*, 2010). Continued refinement and validation of the model as quantitative data fills data gaps (e.g. transmission efficiency) allow the model to be used to identify links in the cycle where management actions can be leveraged to achieve the best outcomes for managing disease in wild and stocked fish populations. Other modelling approaches have also been developed to investigate mechanisms driving infection and disease risk (e.g. Robinson *et al.*, 2022) and the effects of management actions (Alexander *et al.*, 2016).

8.3. Conclusions and Suggestions for Future Studies

Few other pathogens in North America have received as much attention or raised as much public awareness on the importance of healthy fisheries as *M. cerebralis* (Bartholomew and Wilson, 2002). In response to the impact of the parasite on wild fish populations in the USA, a cooperative research effort was developed between private individuals, federal and state governments and the scientific community (Bartholomew and Wilson, 2002). This was a unique endeavour that endured more than a decade. Research was funded to combat the disease from a number of approaches and resulted in a tremendous increase in our knowledge of this parasite. *M. cerebralis* now serves as a model for studies on other myxozoans, and progress in our understanding of this organism has radically altered our view of the entire subphylum Myxozoa and impelled myxozoan research.

Identification of the causative agent for whirling disease and its source permitted more extensive and better controlled studies, as evidenced by the explosion of scientific literature in the 1990s (see Hedrick *et al.*, 1998; Bartholomew and Wilson, 2002). Outbreaks of whirling disease in wild trout populations in the US Intermountain West (Nehring and Walker, 1996; Vincent, 1996) further spurred research. Similarly, identification of the infectious stage for enteronecrosis, identification of its invertebrate host and discovery of its host-specific genotypes permitted new avenues of experimentation. Continued episodic disease outbreaks in hatcheries and imperilled wild salmonid stocks have funnelled state and federal finances to *C. shasta* research. Of note is the unique long-term, extensive collaboration among state and federal agencies, tribes and universities to monitor *C. shasta* in the Klamath River, USA, where it is responsible for declines in native salmonid populations (Bartholomew *et al.*, 2023). The multi-pronged approaches developed and applied in that system enable adaptive management and the development of models to guide disease mitigation, which are used as an example to direct efforts in other systems (e.g. Lehman *et al.*, 2020).

Despite advances in our knowledge of both *M. cerebralis* and *C. shasta*, we have numerous questions because of the impediments and limitations to working with organisms that cannot be directly cultured, and that require two different hosts to complete their life cycles. In contrast to *M. cerebralis*, *C. shasta* remains a problematic parasite to study under laboratory conditions. A parasite-free stock of annelids is difficult to obtain and maintain. This host is sensitive to handling (it dwells in a self-made tube), is almost microscopic and is fastidious. A high actinospore dose is required for infection of some fish strains, yet annelids have a low infection prevalence and actinospore development is asynchronous. Improvements in annelid culture and laboratory challenge models have been made, but working with the parasite remains a challenging venture.

The lack of an adequate test for spore viability has hampered assessments of physical and chemical stressors on spore longevity, particularly for *C. shasta*. Vital stains such as methylene blue, fluorescein diacetate (FDA) and propidium iodide (PI) (Hoffman and Markiw, 1977; Markiw, 1992b; Yokoyama *et al.*, 1997; Wagner *et al.*, 2003) have been used to indicate viability of myxozoans, but produce variable results, and infectivity studies have demonstrated that vital staining underestimates the inactivation of *M. cerebralis* actinospores (Hedrick *et al.*, 2007; Kallert and El-Matbouli, 2008). Thus, the ability to infect the next host remains the best metric for evaluating spore viability (Hedrick *et al.*, 2008) but a simpler, faster method that circumvents such infection experiments would be beneficial.

Less is known about *C. shasta* than *M. cerebralis*. But for both parasites, it is still unclear why they have failed to establish in certain regions and why disease effects differ among regions where they are established. Preliminary investigations of the annelid host of *C. shasta* indicate that there are multiple strains (cytochrome oxidase subunit 1 genotypes) of *M. occidentalis* in the Pacific Northwest. In contrast to the oligochaete host of *M. cerebralis*, there is no evidence to suggest that susceptibility of annelids to *C. shasta* varies with host genotype or that there is a correlation between host genotype and parasite strain. Additional research should reveal whether there are genetic differences among the annelid host populations and how these differences map across different river basins and relate to *C. shasta* genotype abundances.

The discovery that *C. shasta* comprises multiple, host-specific genotypes has led to re-evaluation of previous conclusions regarding susceptibilities of different salmonid species and strains, as initial testing may have been done using inappropriate parasite genotypes. Determining the specific genotype–specific dose thresholds for each salmonid species (infection and clearing an infection versus succumbing) presents opportunities for management, as severe infection in one salmonid species does not necessarily mean all species are at risk. Furthermore, Chinook salmon are able to clear infection of type I if the dose and river temperature are not too high; however, whether this applies to coho salmon and its type II is unknown, as is whether any *C. shasta* genotypes persist in anadromous fish after entering the ocean. Thus, we need further refinement of genotyping tools to allow better predictive ability for effects and examination of other salmonid species across the parasite range to determine how they are affected by different genotypes at different phases of their life histories.

The development of methods for quantification of parasites in environmental samples leads to opportunities for close to real-time monitoring of parasite levels that can be used to predict disease mortality and facilitate rapid management responses. Establishment of monitoring programmes on key river systems has provided information for epizootic models and should allow examination of how anthropogenic factors and climate change affect parasite and host distribution. Of particular interest is the unique, large-scale natural experiment with the reconnection of waterways following dam removal and habitat restoration in the Klamath River, USA.

A great deal of progress has been made in understanding host responses to parasite invasion for both species, and this research avenue should be pursued with the aim of determining protective host responses. We are still developing our understanding of genes that are upregulated during parasite invasion (Severin and El-Matbouli, 2007; Bjork, 2010; Zhang *et al.*, 2010; Baerwald, 2013; Alama-Bermejo *et al.*, 2020), and investigations should continue into corollary functional studies to determine how these molecules interact with the parasites. Questions persist on: (i) factors related to parasite virulence; (ii) the mechanisms they use to invade and proliferate in their hosts; and (iii) their migration to very specific tissues. Understanding these mechanisms could provide clues to what treatments might be efficacious in culture and particularly indicate those that might provide protection after fish are released into endemic waters. However, because the regulatory environment will probably continue to limit chemical therapeutic options in aquaculture, research should proceed down other avenues such as marker-assisted selection for disease resistance traits in captive populations and risk assessments to identify means to minimize disease outbreaks for natural populations.

Acknowledgements

Sam Onjukka (Oregon Department of Fish and Wildlife) and George Schisler (Colorado Parks and Wildlife) kindly provided fish infected with *M. cerebralis*. Harriet Lorz and Laila Brubaker (Oregon State University) isolated the *M. cerebralis* myxospores and actinospores. Rich Holt (Oregon State University) sampled the *C. shasta*-infected eye. Jerri Bartholomew (Oregon State University) contributed to the original version of this chapter.

References

Akram, N., El-Matbouli, M. and Saleh, M. (2023) The immune response to the myxozoan parasite *Myxobolus cerebralis* in salmonids: a review on whirling disease. *International Journal of Molecular Sciences* 24, 17392.

Alama-Bermejo, G., Meyer, E., Atkinson, S.D., Holzer, A.S., Wiśniewska, M.M. *et al.* (2020) Transcriptome-wide comparisons and virulence gene polymorphisms of host-associated genotypes of the cnidarian parasite *Ceratonova shasta* in salmonids. *Genome Biology and Evolution* 12, 1258–1276.

Alama-Bermejo, G., Bartošová-Sojková, P., Atkinson, S.D., Holzer, A.S. and Bartholomew, J.L. (2022) Proteases as therapeutic targets against the parasitic cnidarian *Ceratonova shasta*: characterization of molecules key to parasite virulence in salmonid hosts. *Frontiers in Cellular and Infection Microbiology* 11, 804864.

Alberta Environment and Parks (2017) Whirling disease in Bow River watershed. Edmonton, Alberta. Available at: https://www.alberta.ca/release.cfm?xID=46262A00CB125-CCE0-5AC7-9815E058B20176B3 (accessed 17 November 2025).

Alderman, D.J. (1986) Whirling disease chemotherapy. *Bulletin of the European Association of Fish Pathologists* 6, 38–40.

Alexander, J.D., Kerans, B.L., Koel, T.M. and Rasmussen, C. (2011) Context-specific parasitism in *Tubifex tubifex* in geothermally influenced stream reaches in Yellowstone National Park. *Journal of the North American Benthological Society* 30, 853–867.

Alexander, J.D., Kerans, B.L., El-Matbouli, M., Hallett, S.L. and Stevens, S.L. (2015) Annelid–myxosporean interactions. In: Okamura, B., Gruhl, A. and Bartholomew, J.L. (eds) *Myxozoan Evolution, Ecology and Development*. Springer, Cham, Switzerland, pp. 217–234.

Alexander, J.D., Bartholomew, J.L. Wright, K.A. Som, N.A. and Hetrick, N.J. (2016) Integrating models to predict distribution of the invertebrate host of myxosporean parasites. *Freshwater Science* 35, 1263–1275.

American Fisheries Society-Fish Health Section (2020) *Suggested Procedures for the Detection and Identification of Certain Finfish and Shellfish Pathogens, Blue Book*, 2020 edn. Fish Health Section, American Fisheries Society, Bethesda, Maryland.

Americus, B., Austin, B.M., Lotan, T., Bartholomew, J.L. and Atkinson, S.D. (2020) *In vitro* and *in vivo* assays reveal that cations affect nematocyst discharge in *Myxobolus cerebralis* (Cnidaria: Myxozoa). *Parasitology* 147, 1352–1358.

Americus, B., Hams, N., Klompen, A.M.L., Alama-Bermejo, G., Lotan, T. *et al.* (2021a) The cnidarian parasite *Ceratonova shasta* utilizes inherited and recruited venom-like compounds during infection. *PeerJ* 9, e12606.

Americus, B., Schisler, G.J., Bartholomew, J.L. and Atkinson, S.D. (2021b) *Myxobolus cerebralis* causes presporogonic mortality in juvenile mountain whitefish. *Journal of Aquatic Animal Health* 33, 116–122.

Andree, K.B., Gresoviac, S.J. and Hedrick, R.P. (1997) Small subunit ribosomal RNA sequences unite alternate actinosporean and myxosporean stages of *Myxobolus cerebralis* the causative agent of whirling disease in salmonid fish. *Journal of Eukaryotic Microbiology* 44, 208–215.

Andree, K.B., MacConnell, E. and Hedrick, R.P. (1998) A nested polymerase chain reaction for the detection of genomic DNA of *Myxobolus cerebralis* in rainbow trout *Oncorhynchus mykiss*. *Diseases of Aquatic Organisms* 34, 145–154.

Andree, K.B., Hedrick, R.P. and MacConnell, E. (2002) A review of the approaches to detect *Myxobolus cerebralis*, the cause of salmonid whirling disease. In: Bartholomew J.L. and Wilson J.C. (eds) *Whirling Disease: Reviews and Current Topics.* Symposium 29. American Fisheries Society, Bethesda, Maryland, pp. 197–212.

Antonio, D.B., Andree, K.B., McDowell, T.S. and Hedrick, R.P. (1998) Detection of *Myxobolus cerebralis* in rainbow trout and oligochaete tissues by using a non-radioactive *in situ* hybridization (ISH) protocol. *Journal of Aquatic Animal Health* 10, 338–347.

Arndt, R. (2005) Pilot project at Midway Hatchery to evaluate several whirling disease filtration techniques. *Utah Division of Wildlife Resources Fisheries Experiment Station Ichthyogram* 16, 1–3.

Arndt, R.E. and Wagner, E.J. (2003) Filtering *Myxobolus cerebralis* triactinomyxons from contaminated water using rapid sand filtration. *Aquacultural Engineering* 29, 77–91.

Arsan, E.L. and Bartholomew, J.L. (2008) Potential for dissemination of the non-native salmonid parasite *Myxobolus cerebralis* in Alaska. *Journal of Aquatic Animal Health* 20, 136–149.

Arsan, E.L. and Bartholomew, J.L. (2009) Potential dispersal of the non-native parasite *Myxobolus cerebralis* in the Willamette River Basin, Oregon: a qualitative analysis of risk. *Reviews in Fisheries Science* 17, 360–372.

Arsan, E.L., Atkinson, S.D., Hallett, S.L., Meyers, T. and Bartholomew, J.L. (2007a) Expanded geographical distribution of *Myxobolus cerebralis*: first detections from Alaska. *Journal of Fish Diseases* 30, 483–491.

Arsan, E.L., Hallett, S.L. and Bartholomew, J.L. (2007b) *Tubifex tubifex* from Alaska: distribution and susceptibility to *Myxobolus cerebralis*. *Journal of Parasitology* 93, 1332–1342.

Atkinson, S.D. and Bartholomew, J.L. (2010a) Disparate infection patterns of *Ceratomyxa shasta* (Myxozoa) in rainbow trout *Oncorhynchus mykiss* and Chinook salmon *Oncorhynchus tshawytscha* correlate with ITS-1 sequence variation in the parasite. *International Journal for Parasitology* 40, 599–604.

Atkinson, S.D. and Bartholomew, J.L. (2010b) Spatial, temporal and host factors structure the *Ceratomyxa shasta* (Myxozoa) population in the Klamath River basin. *Infection, Genetics and Evolution* 10, 1019–1026.

Atkinson, S.D., Foott, J.S. and Bartholomew, J.L. (2014) Erection of *Ceratonova* n. gen. (Myxosporea: Ceratomyxidae) to encompass freshwater species *C. gasterostea* n. sp. from threespine stickleback (*Gasterosteus aculeatus*) and *C. shasta* n. comb. from salmonid fishes. *Journal of Parasitology* 100, 640–645.

Atkinson, S.D., Bartošová-Sojková, P., Whipps, C.M. and Bartholomew, J.L. (2015) Approaches for characterising myxozoan species. In: Okamura, B., Gruhl, A. and Bartholomew, J.L. (eds) *Myxozoan Evolution, Ecology and Development.* Springer, Cham, Switzerland, pp. 111–123.

Atkinson, S.D., Hallett, S.L. and Bartholomew, J.L. (2018) Genotyping of individual *Ceratonova shasta* (Cnidaria: Myxosporea) myxospores reveals intra-spore ITS-1 variation and invalidates the distinction of genotypes II and III. *Parasitology* 145, 1588–1593.

Atkinson, S.D., Bartholomew, J.L. and Rouse, G.W. (2020) The invertebrate host of salmonid fish parasites *Ceratonova shasta* and *Parvicapsula minibicornis* (Cnidaria: Myxozoa), is a novel fabriciid annelid, *Manayunkia occidentalis* sp. nov. (Sabellida: Fabriciidae). *Zootaxa* 4751, 320.

Avila, B.W., Winkelman, D.L. and Fetherman, E.R. (2018) Survival of whirling-disease-resistant rainbow trout fry in the wild: a comparison of two strains. *Journal of Aquatic Animal Health* 30, 280–290.

Avila, B.W., Winkelman, D.L. and Fetherman, E.R. (2022) Dual resistance to *Flavobacterium psychrophilum* and *Myxobolus cerebralis* in rainbow trout (*Oncorhynchus mykiss*, Walbaum). *Journal of Fish Diseases* 45, 801–813.

Baerwald, M.R. (2013) Temporal expression patterns of rainbow trout immune-related genes in response to *Myxobolus cerebralis* exposure. *Fish and Shellfish Immunology* 35, 965–971.

Baerwald, M.R., Petersen, J.P., Hedrick, R.P., Schisler, G.J. and May, B. (2011) A major effect quantitative trait locus for whirling disease resistance identified in rainbow trout (*Oncorhynchus mykiss*). *Heredity* 106, 920–926.

Baldwin, T.J. and Myklebust, K.A. (2002) Validation of a single-round polymerase chain reaction assay for identification of *Myxobolus cerebralis* myxospores. *Diseases of Aquatic Organisms* 49, 185–190.

Baldwin, T.J., Peterson, J.E., McGhee, G.C., Staigmiller, K.D., Motteram, E.S. *et al.* (1998) Distribution of *Myxobolus cerebralis* in salmonid fishes in Montana. *Journal of Aquatic Animal Health* 10, 361–371.

Baldwin, T.J., Vincent, E.R., Silflow, R.M. and Stanek D. (2000) *Myxobolus cerebralis* infection in rainbow trout (*Oncorhynchus mykiss*) and brown trout (*Salmo trutta*) exposed under natural stream conditions. *Journal of Veterinary Diagnostic Investigation* 12, 312–321.

Barker, I.K., Van Dreumel, A.A. and Palmer, N. (1993) The alimentary system: chronic inflammatory disease. In: Jubb, K.V.F., Kennedy, P.C. and Palmer, N. (eds) *Pathology of Domestic Animals*, Vol. 2, 4th edn. Academic Press, New York, pp. 120–124.

Bartholomew, J.L. (1998) Host resistance to infection by the myxosporean parasite *Ceratomyxa shasta*: a review. *Journal of Aquatic Animal Health* 10, 112–120.

Bartholomew, J.L. (2012) Salmonid ceratomyxosis. In: AFS-FHS (American Fisheries Society-Fish Health Section) (ed.) *FHS Blue Book: Suggested Procedures for the Detection and Identification of Certain Finfish and Shellfish Pathogens*, 2020 edn. Available at: https://units.fisheries.org/fhs/fish-health-section-blue-book-2020/ (accessed 17 November 2025).

Bartholomew, J.L. and Reno, P.W. (2002) The history and dissemination of whirling disease. In: Bartholomew, J.L. and Wilson, J.C. (eds) *Whirling Disease: Reviews and Current Topics*. Symposium 29. American Fisheries Society, Bethesda, Maryland, pp. 3–24.

Bartholomew, J.L. and Wilson, J.C. (eds) (2002) *Whirling Disease: Reviews and Current Topics*. Symposium 29. American Fisheries Society, Bethesda, Maryland.

Bartholomew, J.L., Smith, C.E., Rohovec, J.S. and Fryer, J.L. (1989) Characterization of the host response to the myxosporean parasite, *Ceratomyxa shasta* (Noble), by histology, scanning electron microscopy, and immunological techniques. *Journal of Fish Diseases* 12, 509–522.

Bartholomew, J.L., Fryer, J.L. and Rohovec, J.S. (1992) Impact of the myxosporean parasite, *Ceratomyxa shasta*, on survival of migrating Columbia River basin salmonids. In: Svrjcek, R.S. (ed.) *Proceedings of the 19th US Japan Meeting on Aquaculture*, Ise, Mie Prefecture, Japan, 29–30 October 1990.

Bartholomew, J.L., Whipple, M.J., Stevens, D.G. and Fryer, J.L. (1997) The life cycle of *Ceratomyxa shasta*, a myxosporean parasite of salmonids, requires a freshwater polychaete as an alternate host. *American Journal of Parasitology* 83, 859–868.

Bartholomew, J.L., Whipple, M.J. and Campton, D. (2001) Inheritance of resistance to *Ceratomyxa shasta* in progeny from crosses between high- and low-susceptibility strains of rainbow trout (*Oncorhynchus mykiss*). *Bulletin of the National Research Institute of Aquaculture* (Suppl. 5), 71–75.

Bartholomew, J.L., Lorz, H.V., Sollid, S.A. and Stevens, D.G. (2003) Susceptibility of juvenile and yearling bull trout to *Myxobolus cerebralis*, and effects of sustained parasite challenges. *Journal of Aquatic Animal Health* 15, 248–255.

Bartholomew, J.L., Ray, E., Torell, B., Whipple, M.J. and Heidel, J.R. (2004) Monitoring *Ceratomyxa shasta* infection during a hatchery rearing cycle: comparison of molecular, serological and histological methods. *Diseases of Aquatic Organisms* 62, 85–92.

Bartholomew, J.L., Kerans, B.L., Hedrick, R.P., MacDiarmid, S.C. and Winton, J.R. (2005) A risk assessment based approach for the management of whirling disease. *Reviews in Fisheries Science* 13, 205–230.

Bartholomew, J.B., Lorz, H.V., Atkinson, S.D., Hallett, S.L., Stevens, D.G. *et al.* (2007) Evaluation of a management strategy to control the spread of *Myxobolus cerebralis* in a lower Columbia River tributary. *North American Journal of Fisheries Management* 27, 542–550.

Bartholomew, J.L., Alexander, J.D., Hallett, S.L., Alama-Bermejo, G. and Atkinson, S.D. (2022) *Ceratonova shasta*: a cnidarian parasite of annelids and salmonids. *Parasitology* 149, 1862–1875.

Bartholomew, J.L., Alexander, J.D., Alvarez, J., Atkinson, S.D., Belchik, M. *et al.* (2023) Deconstructing dams and disease: predictions for salmon disease risk following Klamath River dam removals. *Frontiers in Ecology and Evolution* 11, 1245967.

Barry, D.E., Veillard, M., James, C.T., Brummelhuis, L., Pila, E.A. *et al.* (2021) qPCR-based environmental monitoring of *Myxobolus cerebralis* and phylogenetic analysis of its tubificid hosts in Alberta, Canada. *Diseases of Aquatic Organisms* 145, 119–137.

Baxa, D.V. and Nehring, R.B. (2022) Effect of substrate on the proliferation of *Myxobolus cerebralis* in the mitochondrial lineages of the *Tubifex tubifex* host. *Parasitology Research* 121, 2503–2516.

Beauchamp, K.A., Gay, M., Kelley, G.O., El-Matbouli, M., Kathman, R.D. *et al.* (2002) Prevalence and susceptibility of infection to *Myxobolus cerebralis*, and genetic differences among populations of *Tubifex tubifex*. *Diseases of Aquatic Organisms* 51, 113–121.

Beauchamp, K.A., Kelley, G.O., Nehring, R.B. and Hedrick, R.P. (2005) The severity of whirling disease among wild trout corresponds to the differences in genetic composition of *Tubifex tubifex* populations in central Colorado. *Journal of Parasitology* 91, 53–60.

Beauchamp, K.A., El-Matbouli, M., Gay, M., Georgiadis, M.P., Nehring, R.B. and Hedrick, R.P. (2006) The effect of cohabitation of *Tubifex tubifex* (Oligochaeta: Tubificidae) populations on infections to *Myxobolus cerebralis* (Myxozoa: Myxobolidae). *Journal of Invertebrate Pathology* 91, 1–8.

Bedell, G.W. (1971) Eradicating *Ceratomyxa shasta* from infected water by chlorination and ultraviolet irradiation. *The Progressive Fish-Culturist* 33, 51–54.

Bjork, S.J. (2010) Factors affecting the *Ceratomyxa shasta* infectious cycle and transmission between polychaete and salmonid hosts. PhD thesis, Oregon State University, Corvallis, Oregon, 207 pp.

Bjork, S.J. and Bartholomew, J.L. (2009) Effects of *Ceratomyxa shasta* dose on a susceptible strain of rainbow trout and comparatively resistant Chinook and coho salmon. *Diseases of Aquatic Organisms* 86, 29–37.

Bjork, S.J. and Bartholomew, J.L. (2010) Invasion of *Ceratomyxa shasta* (Myxozoa) and comparison of migration to the intestine between susceptible and resistant fish hosts. *International Journal for Parasitology* 40, 1087–1095.

Blazer, V.S., Waldrop, T.B., Schill, W.B., Densmore, C.L. and Smith, D. (2003) Effects of water temperature and substrate type on spore production and release in eastern *Tubifex tubifex* worms infected with *Myxobolus cerebralis*. *Journal of Parasitology* 89, 21–26.

Bower, S.M. and Margolis, L. (1985) Microfiltration and ultraviolet irradiation to eliminate *Ceratomyxa shasta* (Myxozoa: Myxosporea), a salmonid pathogen, from Fraser River water, British Columbia. *Canadian Technical Report of Fisheries and Aquatic Sciences* 1364, 11.

Breyta, R., Atkinson, S.D. and Bartholomew, J.L. (2020) Evolutionary dynamics of *Ceratonova* species (Cnidaria: Myxozoa) reveal different host adaptation strategies. *Infection, Genetics and Evolution* 78, 104081.

Buchanan, D.V. and Sanders, J.E. (1983) Relative susceptibility of four strains of summer steelhead to infection by *Ceratomyxa shasta*. *Transactions of the American Fisheries Society* 14, 541–543.

CFIA (Canadian Food Inspection Agency) (2024) Notice to Industry – Update on Zoning for Whirling Disease – British Columbia and Columbia River Watershed. Available at: https://inspection.canada.ca/en/animal-health/aquatic-animals/diseases/reportable-diseases/whirling-disease/update-zoning-whirling-disease (accessed 4 December 2025).

Cavender, W.P., Wood, J.S., Powell, M.S., Overturf, K.E. and Cain, K.D. (2004) Real-time quantitative polymerase chain reaction (qPCR) to identify *Myxobolus cerebralis* in rainbow trout *Oncorhynchus mykiss*. *Diseases of Aquatic Organisms* 60, 205–213.

Cavender, W., Swan, C., Wolf, S., Van Vliet, D., Johnson, A.A. *et al.* (2024) Comparative evaluation of three real-time polymerase chain reaction assays to detect *Myxobolus cerebralis*. *Journal of Aquatic Animal Health* 36, 250–264.

Chapman, P.F. (1986) Occurrence of the non-infective stage of *Ceratomyxa shasta* in mature summer chinook salmon in the South fork Salmon River, Idaho. *The Progressive Fish-Culturist* 48, 304–306.

Chiaramonte, L.V., Ray, R.A., Corum, R.A., Soto, T., Hallett, S.L. and Bartholomew, J.L. (2016) Klamath River thermal refuge provides juvenile salmon reduced exposure to the parasite *Ceratonova shasta*. *Transactions of the American Fisheries Society* 145, 810–820.

Chiaramonte, L.V., Burbank, D., Scott, R. and Trushenski, J.T. (2018) Comparison of sampling and detection methods for chinook salmon and steelhead naturally infected with *Myxobolus cerebralis*. *Journal of Aquatic Animal Health* 30, 57–64.

Ching, H.L. and Munday, D.R. (1984a) Geographic and seasonal distribution of the infectious stage of *Ceratomyxa shasta* Noble, 1950, a myxozoan salmonid pathogen in the Fraser River system. *Canadian Journal of Zoology* 62, 1075–1080.

Ching, H.L. and Munday, D.R. (1984b) Susceptibility of six Fraser chinook salmon stocks to *Ceratomyxa shasta* and the effects of salinity on ceratomyxosis. *Canadian Journal of Zoology* 62, 1081–1083.

Christensen, N.O. (1972) Panel review on myxosomiasis (whirling disease in salmonid fishes). *FI:EIFAC 72/ SC II-Symposium* 8, 6.

Coley, T.C., Chacko, A.J. and Klontz, G.W. (1983) Development of a lavage technique for sampling *Ceratomyxa shasta* in adult salmonids. *Journal of Fish Diseases* 6, 317–319.

Conrad, J.F. and Decew, M. (1966) First report of *Ceratomyxa* in juvenile salmonids in Oregon. *The Progressive Fish-Culturist* 28, 238.

DuBey, R., Caldwell, C. and Gould, W.R. (2005) Effects of temperature, photoperiod, and *Myxobolus cerebralis* infection on growth, reproduction, and survival of *Tubifex tubifex* lineages. *Journal of Aquatic Animal Health* 17(4), 338–344. DOI: 10.1577/H04-061.1.

DuBey, R.J., Caldwell, C.A. and Gould, W.R. (2007) Relative susceptibility and effects on performance of Rio Grande cutthroat trout and rainbow trout challenged with *Myxobolus cerebralis*. *Transactions of the American Fisheries Society* 136, 1406–1414.

Eiras, J.C., Cruz, C.F., Saraiva, A. and Adriano, E.A. (2021) Synopsis of the species of *Myxobolus* (Cnidaria, Myxozoa, Myxosporea) described between 2014 and 2020. *Folia Parasitologica* 68, 012.

El-Matbouli, M. and Hoffmann, R.W. (1991) Effects of freezing, aging, and passage through the alimentary canal of predatory animals on the viability of *Myxobolus cerebralis* spores. *Journal of Aquatic Animal Health* 3, 260–262.

El-Matbouli, M. and Hoffmann, R.W. (1998) Light and electron microscopic studies on the chronological development of *Myxobolus cerebralis* to the actinosporean stage in *Tubifex tubifex*. *International Journal for Parasitology* 28, 195–217.

El-Matbouli, M. and Soliman, H. (2005) Development of a rapid assay for the diagnosis of *Myxobolus cerebralis* in fish and oligochaetes using loop-mediated isothermal amplification. *Journal of Fish Diseases* 28, 549–557.

El-Matbouli, M., Hoffmann, R.W. and Mandok, C. (1995) Light and electron microscopic observations on the route of the triactinomyxon-sporoplasm of *Myxobolus cerebralis* from epidermis into rainbow trout cartilage. *Journal of Fish Biology* 46, 919–935.

El-Matbouli, M., Hoffmann, R.W., Shoel H., McDowell, T.S. and Hedrick, R.P. (1999a) Whirling disease: host specificity and interaction between the actinosporean stage of *Myxobolus cerebralis* and rainbow trout (*Oncorhynchus mykiss*) cartilage. *Diseases of Aquatic Organisms* 35, 1–12.

El-Matbouli, M., McDowell, T.S., Antonio, D.B., Andree, K.B. and Hedrick, R.P. (1999b) Effect of water temperature on the development, release and survival of the triactinomyxon stage of *Myxobolus cerebralis* in its oligochaete host. *International Journal for Parasitology* 29, 627–641.

Engelking, H.M. (2002) Potential for introduction of *Myxobolus cerebralis* into the Deschutes River watershed in central Oregon from adult anadromous salmonids. In: Bartholomew, J.L. and Wilson, J.C. (eds) *Whirling Disease: Reviews and Current Topics*. Symposium 29. American Fisheries Society, Bethesda, Maryland, pp. 25–31.

Eszterbauer, E., Kallert, D.M., Grabner, D. and El-Matbouli, M. (2009) Differentially expressed parasite genes involved in host recognition and invasion of the triactinomyxon stage of *Myxobolus cerebralis* (Myxozoa). *Parasitology* 136, 367–377.

Eszterbauer, E., Sipos, D., Szakály, Á. and Herczeg, D. (2019) Distinctive site preference of the fish parasite *Myxobolus cerebralis* (Cnidaria, Myxozoa) during host invasion. *Acta Veterinaria Hungarica* 67, 212–223.

Feist, S.W. and Longshaw, M. (2006) Phylum Myxozoa. In: Woo, P.T.K. (ed.) *Fish Diseases and Disorders, Volume 1: Protozoan and Metazoan Infections*, 2nd edn. CAB International, Wallingford, UK, pp. 230–296.

Fetherman, E.R., Winkelman, D.L., Schisler, G.J. and Myrick, C.A. (2011) The effects of *Myxobolus cerebralis* on the physiological performance of whirling disease resistant and susceptible strains of rainbow trout. *Journal of Aquatic Animal Health* 23, 169–177.

Fetherman, E.R., Winkelman, D.L., Schisler, G.J. and Antolin, M.F. (2012) Genetic basis of differences in myxospore count between whirling disease-resistant and susceptible strains of rainbow trout. *Diseases of Aquatic Organisms* 102, 97–106.

Fetherman, E.R., Winkelman, D.L., Baerwald, M.R. and Schisler G.J. (2014) Survival and reproduction of *Myxobolus cerebralis*-resistant rainbow trout introduced to the Colorado river and increased resistance of age-0 progeny. *PLoS One* 9, e96954.

Fetherman, E.R., Cadmus, P., Jefferson, A.L. and Hura, M.K. (2019) Increasing copper concentrations do not affect *Myxobolus cerebralis* triactinomyxon viability. *Journal of Fish Diseases* 42, 1327–1331.

Foott, J.S., Harman, R. and Stone, R. (2004) Effect of water temperature on non-specific immune function and ceratomyxosis in juvenile Chinook salmon and steelhead from the Klamath River. *California Fish and Game* 90, 71–84.

Foott, J.S., Stone, R., Wiseman, E., True, K. and Nichols, K. (2007) Longevity of *Ceratomyxa shasta* and *Parvicapsula minibicornis* actinospore infectivity in the Klamath River. *Journal of Aquatic Animal Health* 19, 77–83.

Foott, J.S., Stone, R., Fogerty, R., True, K., Bolick, A. *et al.* (2016) Production of *Ceratonova shasta* myxospores from salmon carcasses: carcass removal is not a viable management option. *Journal of Aquatic Animal Health* 28, 75–84.

Foott, J.S., Kindopp, J., Gordon, K., Imrie, A. and Hikey, K. (2023) *Ceratonova shasta* infection in lower Feather River Chinook juveniles and trends in water-borne spore stages. *California Fish and Wildlife Journal* 109, e9.

Fox, M.D., Palenzuela, O. and Bartholomew, J.L. (2000) Strategies for diagnosis of *Ceratomyxa shasta* using the PCR: comparison of lethal and non-lethal sampling with microscopic examination. *Journal of Aquatic Animal Health* 12, 100–106.

Fytilis, N., Rizzo, D.M., Lamb, R.D., Kerans, B.L. and Stevens, L. (2013) Using real-time PCR and Bayesian analysis to distinguish susceptible tubificid taxa important in the transmission of *Myxobolus cerebralis*, the cause of salmonid whirling disease. *International Journal for Parasitology* 43, 493–501.

Gilbert, M.A. and Granath, W.O. Jr (2001) Persistent infection of *Myxobolus cerebralis*, the causative agent of salmonid whirling disease, in *Tubifex tubifex*. *Journal of Parasitology* 87, 101–107.

Gilbert, M.A. and Granath, W.O. Jr (2003) Whirling disease of salmonid fish: life cycle, biology, and disease. *Journal of Parasitology* 89, 658–667.

Gonzalez-Lanza, M. and Alvarez-Pellitero, M.P. (1984) *Myxobolus farionis* n.sp and *M. ibericus* n.sp. of *Salmo trutta* f. *fario* from the Duero basin (NW Spain). Description and population dynamics. *Angewandte Parasitologie* 25, 181–189.

Granath, W.O. Jr (2014) Effects of habitat alteration on the epizootiology of *Myxobolus cerebralis*, the causative agent of salmonid whirling disease. *Journal of Parasitology* 100, 157–165.

Granath, W.O. Jr and Gilbert, M.A. (2002) The role of *Tubifex tubifex* (Annelida: Oligochaeta: Tubificidae) in the transmission of *Myxobolus cerebralis* (Myxozoa: Myxosporea: Myxobolidae). In: Bartholomew, J.L. and Wilson, J.C. (eds) *Whirling Disease: Reviews and Current Topics*. Symposium 29. American Fisheries Society, Bethesda, Maryland, pp. 79–85.

Granath, W.O. Jr, Gilbert, M.A., Wyatt-Pescador, E.J. and Vincent, E.R. (2007) Epizootiology of *Myxobolus cerebralis*, the causative agent of salmonid whirling disease in the Rock Creek drainage of west-central Montana. *Journal of Parasitology* 93, 104–119.

Hallett, S.L. and Bartholomew, J.L. (2006) Application of a real-time PCR assay to detect and quantify the myxozoan parasite *Ceratomyxa shasta* in water samples. *Diseases of Aquatic Organisms* 71, 109–118.

Hallett, S.L. and Bartholomew, J.L. (2008) Effects of water flow on the infection dynamics of *Myxobolus cerebralis*. *Parasitology* 135, 371–684.

Hallett, S.L., Atkinson, S.D., Erséus, C. and El-Matbouli, M. (2005) Dissemination of triactinomyxons (Myxozoa) via oligochaetes used as live food for aquarium fishes. *Diseases of Aquatic Organisms* 65, 137–152.

Hallett, S.L., Atkinson, S.D., Erséus, C. and El-Matbouli, M. (2006) Myxozoan parasites disseminated via oligochaete worms as live food for aquarium fishes: descriptions of aurantiactinomyxon and raabeia actinospore types. *Diseases of Aquatic Organisms* 69, 213–225.

Hallett, S.L., Lorz, H.V., Atkinson, S.D., Rasmussen, C., Xue, L. and Bartholomew, J.L. (2009) Propagation of the myxozoan parasite *Myxobolus cerebralis* by different geographic and genetic populations of *Tubifex tubifex*: an Oregon perspective. *Journal of Invertebrate Pathology* 102, 57–68.

Hallett, S.L., Ray, R.A., Hurst, C.N., Holt, R.A., Buckles, G.R. *et al.* (2012) Density of the waterborne parasite *Ceratomyxa shasta* and its biological effects on salmon. *Applied and Environmental Microbiology* 78, 3724–3731.

Halliday, M.M. (1973) Studies on *Myxosoma cerebralis*, a parasite of salmonids. II. Development and pathology of *Myxosoma cerebralis* in experimentally infected rainbow trout (*Salmo gairdneri*) fry reared at different water temperatures. *Nordisk Veterinaermedicin* 25, 349–358.

Halliday, M.M. (1976) The biology of *Myxosoma cerebralis*: the causative organism of whirling disease of salmonids. *Journal of Fish Biology* 9, 339–357.

Hedrick, R.P. and El-Matbouli, M. (2002) Recent advances with taxonomy, life cycle, and development of *Myxobolus cerebralis* in the fish and oligochaete hosts. In: Bartholomew, J.L. and Wilson, J.C. (eds) *Whirling Disease: Reviews and Current Topics*. Symposium 29. American Fisheries Society, Bethesda, Maryland, pp. 45–53.

Hedrick, R.P., El-Matbouli, M., Adkison, M.A. and MacConnell, E. (1998) Whirling disease: re-emergence among wild trout. *Immunological Reviews* 166, 365–376.

Hedrick, R.P., McDowell, T.S., Gay, M., Marty, G.D., Georgiadis, M.P. and MacConnell, E. (1999a) Comparative susceptibility of rainbow trout *Oncorhynchus mykiss* and brown trout *Salmo trutta* to *Myxobolus cerebralis*, the cause of salmonid whirling disease. *Diseases of Aquatic Organisms* 37, 173–183.

Hedrick, R.P., McDowell, T.S., Mukkatira, K., Georgiadis, M.P. and MacConnell, E. (1999b) Susceptibility of selected inland salmonids to experimentally induced infections with *Myxobolus cerebralis*, the causative agent of whirling disease. *Journal of Aquatic Animal Health* 11, 330–339.

Hedrick, R.P., McDowell, T.S., Marty, G.D., Mukkatira, K., Antonio, K. *et al.* (2000) Ultraviolet irradiation inactivates the waterborne infective stages of *Myxobolus cerebralis*: a treatment for hatchery water supplies. *Diseases of Aquatic Organisms* 42, 53–59.

Hedrick, R.P., McDowell, T.S., Mukkatira, K., Georgiadis, M.P. and MacConnell, E. (2001) Salmonids resistant to *Ceratomyxa shasta* are susceptible to experimentally induced infections with *Myxobolus cerebralis*. *Journal of Aquatic Animal Health* 13, 35–42.

Hedrick, R.P., Petri, B., McDowell, T.S., Mukkatira, K. and Sealey, L.J. (2007) Evaluation of a range of doses of ultraviolet irradiation to inactivate waterborne actinospore stages of *Myxobolus cerebralis*. *Diseases of Aquatic Organisms* 74, 113–118.

Hedrick, R.P., McDowell, T.S., Mukkatira, K., MacConnell, E. and Petri, B. (2008) The effects of freezing, drying, ultraviolet irradiation, chlorine and quaternary ammonium treatments in the infectivity of myxospores of *Myxobolus cerebralis* for *Tubifex tubifex*. *Journal of Aquatic Animal Health* 20, 116–125.

Hedrick, R.P., McDowell, T.S., Adkison, M.A., Myklebust, K.A., Mardones, F.O. and Petri, B. (2012) Invasion and initial replication of ultraviolet irradiated waterborne infective stages of *Myxobolus cerebralis* results in immunity to whirling disease in rainbow trout. *International Journal for Parasitology* 42, 657–666.

Hendrickson, G.L., Carlton, A. and Manzer, D. (1989) Geographic and seasonal distribution of the infective stage of *Ceratomyxa shasta* (Myxozoa) in northern California. *Diseases of Aquatic Organisms* 7, 165–169.

Hillemeier, D., Belchik, M., Soto, T., Tucker, S.C. and Ledwin, S. (2017) Measures to reduce *Ceratonova shasta* infection of Klamath River salmonids: a guidance document. Available at: https://www.waterboards.ca.gov/waterrights/water_issues/programs/bay_delta/california_waterfix/exhibits/docs/PCFFA&IGFR/part2/pcffa_154.pdf (accessed 26 November 2025).

Hiner, M. and Moffitt, C.M. (2002) Modeling *Myxobolus cerebralis* infections in trout: associations with habitat variables. In: Bartholomew, J.L. and Wilson, J.C. (eds) *Whirling Disease: Reviews and Current Topics*. Symposium 29. American Fisheries Society, Bethesda, Maryland, pp. 167–179.

Höfer, B. (1903) Ueber die Drehkrankheit der Regenbogenforelle. *Allgemeine Fischerei Zeitung* 28, 7–8.

Hoffman, G.L. (1962) *Whirling Disease of Trout*. Fishery Leaflet 508. US Department of the Interior, Fish and Wildlife Service, Washington, DC.

Hoffman, G.L. (1970) Intercontinental and transcontinental dissemination and transfaunation of fish parasites with emphasis on whirling disease. In: Snieszko, S.F. (ed.) *Symposium on Diseases of Fishes and Shellfishes*. American Fisheries Society, Bethesda, Maryland, pp. 69–81.

Hoffman, G.L. (1974) Disinfection of contaminated water by ultraviolet irradiation, with emphasis on whirling disease (*Myxosoma cerebralis*) and its effect on fish. *Transactions of the American Fisheries Society* 103, 541–550.

Hoffman, G.L. (1990) *Myxobolus cerebralis*, a worldwide cause of salmonid whirling disease. *Journal of Aquatic Animal Health* 2, 30–37.

Hoffman, G.L. (1999) *Parasites of North American Freshwater Fishes*, 2nd edn. Cornell University Press, Ithaca, New York, p. 71.

Hoffman, G.L. and Markiw, M.E. (1977) Control of whirling disease (*Myxosoma cerebralis*). Use of methylene blue staining as a possible indicator of effect of heat on spores. *Journal of Fish Biology* 10, 181–183.

Hoffman, G.L., Dunbar, C.E. and Bradford, A. (1962) *Whirling Disease of Trouts Caused by Myxosoma cerebralis in the United States*. US Fish and Wildlife Service, Special Scientific Report Fishery Leaflet 427. US Department of the Interior, Fish and Wildlife Service, Washington, DC.

Hoffmaster, J.L., Sanders, J.E., Rohovec, J.S., Fryer, J.L. and Stevens, D.G. (1988) Geographic distribution of the myxosporean parasite, *Ceratomyxa shasta* Noble, 1950, in the Columbia River basin. *Journal of Fish Diseases* 11, 97–100.

Hogge, C.I., Campbell, M.R. and Johnson, K.A. (2008) A new species of myxozoan (Myxosporea) from the brain and spinal cord of rainbow trout (*Oncorhynchus mykiss*) from Idaho. *Journal of Parasitology* 94, 218–222.

Homel, K. and Alexander, J.D. (2022) Spatiotemporal distribution of *Ceratonova shasta* in the lower Columbia River Basin and effects of exposure on survival of juvenile chum salmon *Oncorhynchus keta*. *PLoS One* 17, e0273438.

Hurst, C.N., Holt, R.A. and Bartholomew, J.L. (2012) Dam removal and implications for fish health: *Ceratomyxa shasta* in the Williamson River, Oregon, USA. *Journal of North American Fisheries Management* 32, 14–23.

Ibarra, A.M., Gall, G.A.E. and Hedrick, R.P. (1990) Trials with fumagillin DCH and malachite green to control ceratomyxosis in rainbow trout (*Oncorhynchus mykiss*). *Fish Pathology* 25, 217–223.

Ibarra, A.M., Gall, G.A.E. and Hedrick, R.P. (1991) Susceptibility of two strains of rainbow trout *Oncorhynchus mykiss* to experimentally induced infections with the myxosporean *Ceratomyxa shasta*. *Diseases of Aquatic Organisms* 10, 191–194.

Ibarra, A.M., Hedrick, R.P. and Gall, G.A.E. (1992) Inheritance of susceptibility to *Ceratomyxa shasta* (Myxozoa) in rainbow trout and the effect of length of exposure on the liability to develop ceratomyxosis. *Aquaculture* 104, 219–229.

Kaeser, A.J., Rasmussen, C. and Sharpe, W.E. (2006) An examination of environmental factors associated with *Myxobolus cerebralis* infection of wild trout in Pennsylvania. *Journal of Aquatic Animal Health* 18, 90–100.

Kallert, D.M. and El-Matbouli, M. (2008) Differences in viability and reactivity of actinospores of three myxozoan species upon ageing. *Folia Parasitologica* 55, 105–110.

Kallert, D.M., El-Matbouli, M. and Haas, W. (2005) Polar filament discharge of *Myxobolus cerebralis* actinospores is triggered by combined non-specific mechanical and chemical cues. *Parasitology* 131, 609–616.

Kallert, D.M., Eszterbauer, E., Grabner, D. and El-Matbouli, M. (2009) *In vivo* exposure of susceptible and non-susceptible fish species to *Myxobolus cerebralis* actinospores reveals nonspecific invasion behaviour. *Diseases of Aquatic Organisms* 84, 123–130.

Kallert, D.M., Bauer, W., Haas, W. and El-Matbouli, M. (2011) No shot in the dark: myxozoans chemically detect fresh fish. *International Journal for Parasitology* 41, 271–276.

Kallert, D.M., Forró B. and Eszterbauer, E. (2014) Inosine-arginine salt as a promising agent for *in vitro* activation of waterborne fish-pathogenic myxozoan actinospores. *Diseases of Aquatic Organisms* 109, 149–154.

Kathman, R.D. and Brinkhurst, R.O. (1998) *Guide to Freshwater Oligochaetes in North America*. Aquatic Resources Center, College Grove, Tennessee.

Kelley, G.O., Zagmutt-Vergara, F.J., Leutenegger, C.M., Myklebust, K.A., Adkison, M.A. *et al.* (2004) Evaluation of five diagnostic methods of the detection and quantification of *Myxobolus cerebralis*. *Journal of Veterinary Diagnostic Investigation* 16, 202–211.

Kent, M.L., Margolis, L. and Corliss, J.O. (1994) The demise of a class of protists: taxonomic and nomenclatural revisions proposed for the protist phylum Myxozoa Grasse, 1970. *Canadian Journal of Zoology* 72, 932–937.

Kerans, B.L. and Zale, A.V. (2002) The ecology of *Myxobolus cerebralis*. In: Bartholomew, J.L. and Wilson, J.C. (eds) *Whirling Disease: Reviews and Current Topics*. Symposium 29. American Fisheries Society, Bethesda, Maryland, pp. 145–166.

Kerans, B.L., Rasmussen, C., Stevens, R., Colwell, A.E.L. and Winton, J.R. (2004) Differential propagation of the metazoan parasite *Myxobolus cerebralis* by *Limnodrilus hoffmeisteri*, *Ilyodrilus templetoni*, and genetically distinct strains of *Tubifex tubifex*. *Journal of Parasitology* 90, 1366–1373.

Kerans, B.L., Stevens, R.I. and Lemmon, J.C. (2005) Water temperature affects a host–parasite interaction: *Tubifex tubifex* and *Myxobolus cerebralis*. *Journal of Aquatic Animal Health* 17, 216–221.

Koel, T.M., Kerans, B.L., Barras, S.C., Hanson, K.C. and Wood, J.S. (2010) Avian piscivores as vectors for *Myxobolus cerebralis* in the greater Yellowstone ecosystem. *Transactions of the American Fisheries Society* 139, 976–988.

Krueger, R.C., Kerans, B.L., Vincent, E.R. and Rasmussen, C. (2006) Risk of *Myxobolus cerebralis* infection to rainbow trout in the Madison River, Montana, USA. *Ecological Applications* 16, 770–783.

Ksepka, S.P., Rash, J.M., Simcox, B.L., Besler, D.A., Dutton, H.R. *et al.* (2020) An updated geographic distribution of *Myxobolus cerebralis* (Hofer, 1903) (Bivalvulida: Myxobolidae) and the first diagnosed case of whirling disease in wild-caught trout in the south-eastern United States. *Journal of Fish Diseases* 43, 813–820.

Ksepka, S.P., Rash, J.M., Cai, W. and Bullard, S.A. (2021) Detection of *Myxobolus cerebralis* (Bivalvulida: Myxobolidae) in two non-*Tubifex tubifex* oligochaetes in the southeastern USA. *Diseases of Aquatic Organisms* 143, 51–56.

Lehman, B.M., Johnson, R.C., Adkison, M., Burgess, O.T., Connon, R.E. *et al.* (2020) Disease in Central Valley salmon: status and lessons from other systems. *San Francisco Estuary and Watershed Science* 18, 1–31.

Lemmon, J.C. and Kerans, B.L. (2001) Extraction of whirling disease myxospores from sediments using the plankton centrifuge and sodium hexametaphosphate. *Intermountain Journal of Sciences* 7, 57–62.

Lodh, N., Stevens, L. and Kerans, B. (2011) Prevalence of *Myxobolus cerebralis* infections among genetic lineages of *Tubifex tubifex* at three locations in the Madison River, Montana. *Journal of Parasitology* 97, 531–534.

Lom, J. and Dyková, I. (2006) Myxozoan genera: definition and notes on taxonomy, life-cycle terminology and pathogenic species. *Folia Parasitologia* 53, 1–36.

Lom, J. and Hoffman, G.L. (1971) Morphology of the spores of *Myxosoma cerebralis* (Höfer, 1903) and *M. cartilaginis* (Hoffman, Putz, and Dunbar, 1965). *Journal of Parasitology* 56, 1302–1308.

Lom, J. and Noble, E.R. (1984) Revised classification of the *myxosporea Bütschli*, 1881. *Folia Parasitologica* 31, 193–205.

Lorz, H.V. and Amandi, A. (1994) VI. Whirling disease of salmonids. In: Thoesen, J.C. (ed.) *Blue Book Version 1 Suggested Procedures for the Detection and Identification of Certain Finfish and Shellfish Pathogens*. Fish Health Section, American Fisheries Society, Bethesda, Maryland, pp. 1–7. Available at: https://units.fisheries.org/fhs/wp-content/uploads/sites/30/2025/03/1994-Blue-Book.pdf (accessed 4 December 2025).

Lowers, J.M. and Bartholomew, J.L. (2003) Detection of myxozoan parasites in oligochaetes imported as food for ornamental fish. *Journal of Parasitology* 89, 84–91.

MacConnell, E. and Vincent, E.R. (2002) The effects of *Myxobolus cerebralis* on the salmonid host. In: Bartholomew, J.L. and Wilson, J.C. (eds) *Whirling Disease: Reviews and Current Topics*. Symposium 29. American Fisheries Society, Bethesda, Maryland, pp. 95–107.

Margolis, L., McDonald, T.E. and Whitaker, D.J. (1992) Assessment of the impact of the myxosporean parasite *Ceratomyxa shasta* on survival of seaward migrating juvenile chinook salmon, *Oncorhynchus tshawytscha*, from the Fraser River, British Columbia. *Canadian Journal of Fisheries and Aquatic Sciences* 49(9), 1883–1889.

Markiw, M.E. (1991) Whirling disease: earliest susceptible age of rainbow trout to the triactinomyxid of *Myxobolus cerebralis*. *Aquaculture* 92, 1–6.

Markiw, M.E. (1992a) Experimentally induced whirling disease. I. Dose response of fry and adults of rainbow trout exposed to the triactinomyxon stage of *Myxobolus cerebralis*. *Journal of Aquatic Animal Health* 4, 40–43.

Markiw, M.E. (1992b) Experimentally induced whirling disease. II. Determination of longevity of the infective triactinomyxon stage of *Myxobolus cerebralis* by vital staining. *Journal of Aquatic Animal Health* 4, 44–47.

Markiw, M.E. (1992c) *Salmonid Whirling Disease*. Leaflet 17. US Fish and Wildlife Service, Washington, DC.

Markiw, M.E. and Wolf, K. (1974) *Myxosoma cerebralis*: isolation and concentration from fish skeletal elements – sequential enzymatic digestions and purification by differential centrifugation. *Journal of the Fisheries Research Board of Canada* 31, 15–20.

Markiw, M.E. and Wolf, K. (1983) *Myxosoma cerebralis* (Myxozoa: Myxosporea) etiologic agent of salmonid whirling disease requires tubificid worm (Annelida: Oligochaeta) in its life cycle. *Journal of Protozoology* 30, 561–564.

Meaders, M. and Hendrickson, G. (2009) Chronological development of *Ceratomyxa shasta* in the polychaete host, *Manayunkia speciosa*. *Journal of Parasitology* 95, 1397–1407.

Meyers, T.R., Burton, T., Bentz, C. and Starkey, N. (2008) *Common Diseases of Wild and Cultured Fishes in Alaska*. Alaska Department of Fish and Game, Commercial Fisheries Division, Juneau, Anchorage, Alaska, 105 pp.

Miller, M.P. and Vincent, R.E. (2008) Rapid natural selection for resistance to an introduced parasite of rainbow trout. *Evolutionary Applications* 1, 336–341.

Modin, J. (1998) Whirling disease in California: a review of its history, distribution, and impacts, 1965–1997. *Journal of Aquatic Animal Health* 10, 132–142.

Murcia, S., Kerans, B.L., MacConnell, E. and Koel, T.M. (2011) Correlation of environmental attributes with histopathology of native Yellowstone cutthroat trout naturally infected with *Myxobolus cerebralis*. *Diseases of Aquatic Organisms* 93, 225–234.

Nehring, R.B. and Walker, P.G. (1996) Whirling disease in the wild: the new reality in the intermountain west. *Fisheries* 21, 28–30.

Nehring, R.B., Thompson, K.G. and Hebein, S. (1998) Impacts of whirling disease on wild trout populations in Colorado. In: Wadsworth, K.G. (ed.) *Transactions of the 63rd North American Wildlife and Natural Resources Conference*. Wildlife Management Institute, Washington, DC, pp. 82–94.

Nehring, R.B., Thompson, K.G., Taurman, K.A. and Shuler, D.L. (2002) Laboratory studies indicating that living brown trout *Salmo trutta* expel viable *Myxobolus cerebralis* myxospores. In: Bartholomew, J.L. and Wilson, J.C. (eds) *Whirling Disease: Reviews and Current Topics*. Symposium 29. American Fisheries Society, Bethesda, Maryland, pp. 125–134.

Nehring, R.B., Hancock, B., Catanese, M., Stinson, M.E., Winkelman, D. *et al.* (2013) Reduced *Myxobolus cerebralis* actinospore production in a Colorado reservoir may be linked to changes in *Tubifex tubifex* population structure. *Journal of Aquatic Animal Health* 25, 205–220.

Nehring, B., Schisler, G., Chiaramonte, L., Horton, A. and Poole, B. (2015) Assessment of the long-term viability of the myxospores of *Myxobolus cerebralis* as determined by production of the actinospores by *Tubifex tubifex*. *Journal of Aquatic Animal Health* 27, 50–56.

Nehring, R.B., Schisler, G.J., Chiaramonte, L., Horton, A. and Poole B. (2016) Accelerated deactivation of *Myxobolus cerebralis* myxospores by susceptible and non-susceptible *Tubifex tubifex*. *Diseases of Aquatic Organisms* 121, 37–47.

Nichols, K.M., Bartholomew, J.L. and Thorgaard, G.H. (2003) Mapping multiple genetic loci associated with *Ceratomyxa shasta* resistance in *Oncorhynchus mykiss*. *Diseases of Aquatic Organisms* 56, 145–154.

Noble, E.R. (1950) On a myxosporidian (protozoan) parasite of California trout. *Journal of Parasitology* 36, 457–460.

O'Grodnick, J.J. (1975) Whirling disease *Myxosoma cerebralis* spore concentration using the continuous plankton centrifuge. *Journal of Wildlife Diseases* 11, 54–57.

O'Grodnick, J.J. and Gustafson, C.C. (1974) *A Study of the Transmission, Life History, and Control of Whirling Disease of Trout*. Federal Aid to Fish Restoration Progress Report F-35-R-6. US Fish and Wildlife Service, Washington, DC.

Palenzuela, O. and Bartholomew, J.L. (2002) Molecular tools for the diagnosis of *Ceratomyxa shasta* (Myxozoa). In: Cunningham, C. (ed.) *Molecular Diagnosis of Fish Diseases*. Springer, Dordrecht, The Netherlands, pp. 285–298.

Palenzuela, O., Trobridge, G. and Bartholomew, J.L. (1999) Development of a polymerase chain reaction diagnostic assay for *Ceratomyxa shasta*, a myxosporean parasite of salmonid fish. *Diseases of Aquatic Organisms* 36, 45–51.

Plehn, M. (1905) Uber die drehkrankheit der salmoniden [(*Lentospora cerebralis*) (Höfer) Plehn]. *Archiv für Protistenkunde* 5, 145–166.

Polley, T.M., Atkinson, S.D., Jones, G.R. and Bartholomew, J.L. (2013) Supplemental description of *Myxobolus squamalis* (Myxozoa). *Journal of Parasitology* 99, 725–728.

Pugachev, O.N. and Khokhlov, P.P. (1979) Myxosporean parasites of genus *Myxobolus* – parasites of the salmonids head and spinal brain. In: *Sistematika i ekologiya ryb kontinental'nykh vodoemov Dal'nego*

Vostoka (Systematics and Ecology of Fish of Continental Water Bodies of the Russian Far East). Dal'nevost, Vladivostok, Russia, pp. 137–139.

Ramazi, P., Fischer, S., Alexander, J. James, C., Paul, A. *et al.* (2022) *Myxobolus cerebralis* establishment and spread: a graphical synthesis. *Canadian Journal of Fisheries and Aquatic Sciences* 79, 677–691.

Rasmussen, C., Zickovich, J., Winton, J.R. and Kerans, B.L. (2008) Variability in triactinomyxon production in *Tubifex tubifex* populations from the same mitochondrial linage infected with *Myxobolus cerebralis*, the causative agent of whirling disease in salmonids. *Journal of Parasitology* 94, 700–708.

Ratliff, D.E. (1981) *Ceratomyxa shasta*: epizootiology in chinook salmon of central Oregon. *Transactions of the American Fisheries Society* 110, 507–513.

Ratliff, D.E. (1983) *Ceratomyxa shasta*: longevity, distribution, timing and abundance of the infective stage in central Oregon. *Canadian Journal of Fisheries and Aquatic Sciences* 40, 1622–1632.

Ray, R.A., Rossignol, P.A. and Bartholomew, J.L. (2010) Mortality threshold for Chinook salmon (*Oncorhynchus tshawytscha*) in an epidemiological model of *Ceratomyxa shasta*. *Diseases of Aquatic Organisms* 93, 63–70.

Richey, C.A., Kenelty, K.V., Van Stone, H.K., Stevens, B.N., Martínez-López, B. *et al.* (2018) Distribution and prevalence of *Myxobolus cerebralis* in postfire areas of Plumas National Forest: utility of environmental DNA sampling. *Journal of Aquatic Animal Health* 30, 130–143.

Robinson, H.E., Alexander, J.D., Bartholomew, J.L., Hallett, S.L., Hetrick, N.J. *et al.* (2022) Using a mechanistic framework to model the density of an aquatic parasite *Ceratonova shasta*. *PeerJ* 10, e13183. DOI: 10.7717/peerj.13183.

Rose, J.D., Marrs, G.S., Lewis, C. and Schisler, G. (2000) Whirling disease behavior and its relation to pathology of brain stem and spinal cord in rainbow trout. *Journal of Aquatic Animal Health* 12, 107–118.

Ruiz, F., Rash, J.M., Arias, C.R., Besler, D.A., Orélis-Ribeiro, R. *et al.* (2017) Morphological and molecular confirmation of *Myxobolus cerebralis myxospores* infecting wild caught and cultured trout in North Carolina (SE USA). *Diseases of Aquatic Organisms* 126, 185–198.

Ryce, E.K.N., Zale, A.V. and Nehring, R.B. (2001) Lack of selection for resistance to whirling disease among progeny of Colorado River rainbow trout. *Journal of Aquatic Animal Health* 13, 63–68.

Ryce, E.K.N., Zale, A.V. and MacConnell, E. (2004) Effects of fish age and parasite dose on the development of whirling disease in rainbow trout. *Diseases of Aquatic Organisms* 59, 225–233.

Ryce, E.K.N., Zale, A.V., MacConnell, E. and Nelson, M. (2005) Effects of fish age versus size on the development of whirling disease in rainbow trout. *Diseases of Aquatic Organisms* 63, 69–76.

Saleh, M., Friedl, A., Srivastava, M., Secombes, C.J. and El-Matbouli, M. (2020) Modulation of local and systemic immune responses in brown trout (*Salmo trutta*) following exposure to *Myxobolus cerebralis*. *Fish and Shellfish Immunology* 106, 844–851.

Sanders, J.E., Fryer, J.L. and Gould, R.W. (1970) Occurrence of the myxosporidian parasite *Ceratomyxa shasta*, in salmonid fish from the Columbia River basin and Oregon coastal streams. In: Snieszko, S.F. (ed.) *A Symposium on Diseases of Fishes and Shellfishes*. American Fisheries Society Special Publication 5. American Fisheries Society, Bethesda, Maryland, pp. 133–144.

Sanders, J.E., Fryer, J.L., Leith, D.A. and Moore, K.D. (1972) Control of the infectious protozoan *Ceratomyxa shasta* by treating hatchery water supplies. *The Progressive Fish-Culturist* 34, 13–17.

Sarker, S., Kallert, D.M., Hedrick, R.P. and El-Matbouli, M. (2015) Whirling disease revisited: pathogenesis, parasite biology and disease intervention. *Diseases of Aquatic Organisms* 114, 155–175.

Schafer, W.E. (1968) Studies on the epizootiology of the myxosporidian *Ceratomyxa shasta* Noble. *California Fish and Game* 54, 90–99.

Schäperclaus, W. (1991) *Fish Diseases*, Vol. 2, 5th edn (translated from German). Akademie-Verlag, Berlin.

Schisler, G.J., Bergersen, E.P. and Walker, P.G. (2000) Effects of multiple stressors on morbidity and mortality of fingerling rainbow trout infected with *Myxobolus cerebralis*. *Transactions of the American Fisheries Society* 129, 859–865.

Schisler, G.J., Bergersen, E.P., Walker, P.G., Wood, J. and Epp, J.K. (2001) Comparison of single-round polymerase chain reaction (PCR) and pepsin–trypsin digest (PTD) methods for detection of *Myxobolus cerebralis*. *Diseases of Aquatic Organisms* 45, 109–114.

Schisler, G.L., Myklebust, K.A. and Hedrick, R.P. (2006) Inheritance of *Myxobolus cerebralis* resistance among F_1-generation crosses of whirling disease resistant and susceptible rainbow trout strains. *Journal of Aquatic Animal Health* 18, 109–115.

Schuberg, A. and Schröder, O. (1905) Myxosporidien aus dem nervensystem und der haut der bachforelle. *Archiv für Protistenkunde* 6, 46–60.

Shirakashi, S. and El-Matbouli M. (2010) Effect of cadmium on the susceptibility of *Tubifex tubifex* to *Myxobolus cerebralis* (Myxozoa), the causative agent of whirling disease. *Diseases of Aquatic Organisms* 89, 63–70.

Severin, V.I. and El-Matbouli, M. (2007) Relative quantification of immune-regulatory genes in two rainbow trout strains, *Oncorhynchus mykiss*, after exposure to *Myxobolus cerebralis*, the causative agent of whirling disease. *Parasitology Research* 101, 1019–1027.

Sipos, D., Ursu, K., Dán, Á., Herczeg, D. and Eszterbauer, E. (2018) Susceptibility-related differences in the quantity of developmental stages of *Myxobolus* spp. (Myxozoa) in fish blood. *PLoS One* 13, e0204437.

Skirpstunas, R.T., Hergert, J.M. and Baldwin, T.J. (2006) Detection of early stages of *Myxobolus cerebralis* in fin clips from rainbow trout (*Onchorynchus* (sic) *mykiss*). *Journal of Veterinary Diagnostic Investigation* 18, 274–277.

Sollid, S.A., Lorz, H.V., Stevens, D.G. and Bartholomew. J.L. (2002) Relative susceptibility of selected Deschutes River, Oregon, salmonid species to experimentally induced infection by *Myxobolus cerebralis*. In: Bartholomew, J.L. and Wilson, J.C. (eds) *Whirling Disease: Reviews and Current Topics*. Symposium 29. American Fisheries Society, Bethesda, Maryland, pp. 117–124.

Sollid, S.A., Lorz, H.V., Stevens, D.G., Reno, P.W. and Bartholomew, J.L. (2004) Prevalence of *Myxobolus cerebralis* at juvenile salmonid acclimation sites in northeastern Oregon. *North American Journal of Fisheries Management* 24, 146–153.

Staton, L., Erdahl, D. and El-Matbouli, M. (2002) Efficacy of fumagillin and TNP-470 to prevent experimentally induced whirling disease in rainbow trout *Oncorhynchus mykiss*. In: Bartholomew, J.L. and Wilson, J.C. (eds) *Whirling Disease: Reviews and Current Topics*. Symposium 29. American Fisheries Society, Bethesda, Maryland, pp. 239–247.

Stinson, M.E.T., Atkinson, S.D. and Bartholomew, J.L. (2018) Widespread distribution of *Ceratonova shasta* (Cnidaria: Myxosporea) genotypes indicates evolutionary adaptation to its salmonid fish hosts. *Journal of Parasitology* 104, 645–650.

Steinbach, E.L.C., Stromberg, K.E., Ryce, E.K.N. and Bartholomew, J.L. (2009) *Whirling Disease in the United States. A Summary of Progress in Research and Management 2009*. Trout Unlimited Whirling Disease Foundation, Bozeman, Montana, 61 pp.

Stocking, R.W., Holt, R.A., Foott, J.S. and Bartholomew, J.L. (2006) Spatial and temporal occurrence of the salmonid parasite *Ceratomyxa shasta* (Myxozoa) in the Oregon–California Klamath River Basin. *Journal of Aquatic Animal Health* 18, 194–202.

Stocking, R.W., Lorz, H.L., Holt, R.A. and Bartholomew, J.L. (2007) Surveillance for *Ceratomyxa shasta* in the Puget Sound watershed, WA, USA. *Journal of Aquatic Animal Health* 19, 116–120.

Taylor, R.E.L. and Haber, M.H. (1974) Opercular cyst formation in trout infected with *Myxosoma cerebralis*. *Journal of Wildlife Diseases* 10, 347–351.

Taylor, R.L. and Lott, M. (1978) Transmission of salmonid whirling disease by birds fed trout infected with *Myxosoma cerebralis*. *Journal of Protozoology* 25, 105–106.

Taylor, R.E.L., Coli, S.J. and Junell, D.R. (1973) Attempts to control whirling disease by continuous drug feeding. *Journal of Wildlife Diseases* 9, 302–305.

Thompson, J.B., Snekvik, K.R. and Vincent, E.R. (2010) The effects of *Myxobolus cerebralis* on Apache and Gila trout in laboratory exposures. *Journal of Aquatic Animal Health* 22, 87–91.

Tipping, J.M. (1988) Ozone control of ceratomyxosis: survival and growth benefits to steelhead and cutthroat trout. *The Progressive Fish-Culturist* 50, 202–210.

Turnbull, A. (2024) Molecular characterization of *Tubifex* populations in Alberta, Canada, and their role in the spread of whirling disease. MSc thesis, University of Alberta, Edmonton, Alberta, Canada, p. 55.

Turner, K.G, Smith, M.J. and Ridenhour, B.J. (2014) Whirling disease dynamics: an analysis of intervention strategies. *Preventive Veterinary Medicine* 113, 457–468.

Udey, L.R., Fryer, J.L. and Pilcher, K.S. (1975) Relation of water temperature to ceratomyxosis in rainbow trout (*Salmo gairdneri*) and coho salmon (*Oncorhynchus kisutch*). *Journal of the Fisheries Research Board of Canada* 32, 1545–1551.

Vincent, E.R. (1996) Whirling disease and wild trout: the Montana experience. *Fisheries* 21, 32–33.

Vincent, E.R. (2002) Relative susceptibility of various salmonids to whirling disease with emphasis on rainbow and cutthroat trout. In: Bartholomew, J.L. and Wilson, J.C. (eds) *Whirling Disease: Reviews and Current Topics*. Symposium 29. American Fisheries Society, Bethesda, Maryland, pp. 109–115.

Wagner, E. (2002) Whirling disease prevention, control, and management: a review. In: Bartholomew, J.L. and Wilson, J.C. (eds) *Whirling Disease: Reviews and Current Topics*. Symposium 29. American Fisheries Society, Bethesda, Maryland, pp. 217–225.

Wagner, E.J., Smith, M., Arndt, R. and Roberts, D.W. (2003) Physical and chemical effects on viability of the *Myxobolus cerebralis* triactinomyxon. *Diseases of Aquatic Organisms* 53, 133–142.

Wagner, E.J., Wilson, C., Arndt, R., Goddard, P., Miller, M. *et al.* (2006) Evaluation of disease resistance of the Fish Lake–DeSmet, Wounded Man, and Harrison Lake strains of rainbow trout exposed to *Myxobolus cerebralis*. *Journal of Aquatic Animal Health* 18, 128–135.

Wales, J.H. and Wolf, H. (1955) Three protozoan diseases of trout in California. *California Fish and Game* 41, 183–187.

Whipple, M.J., Gannam, A.L. and Bartholomew, J.L. (2002) Lack of a prophylactic effect of orally administered glucan and fumagillin on naturally acquired infection with *Ceratomyxa shasta* in juvenile rainbow and steelhead trout (*Oncorhynchus mykiss*). *North American Journal of Aquaculture* 64, 1–9.

Whipps, C.M., El-Matbouli, M., Hedrick, R.P., Blazer, V. and Kent, M.L. (2004) *Myxobolus cerebralis* internal transcribed spacer 1 (ITS-1) sequences support recent spread of the parasite to North America and within Europe. *Diseases of Aquatic Organisms* 60, 105–108.

Whipps, C.M., Atkinson, S.D. and Hoeksema, B.W. (2025) World List of Myxozoa. Available at: https://www.marinespecies.org/myxozoa (accessed 26 November 2025).

Wolf, K. and Markiw, M.E. (1984) Biology contravenes taxonomy in the Myxozoa: new discoveries show alternation of invertebrate and vertebrate hosts. *Science* 225, 1449–1452.

Wolf, K., Markiw, M.E. and Hiltunen, J.K. (1986) Salmonid whirling disease: *Tubifex tubifex* (Müller) identified as the essential oligochaete in the protozoan life cycle. *Journal of Fish Diseases* 9, 83–85.

Yamanoto, T. and Sanders, J.E. (1979) Light and electron microscopic observations of sporogenesis in the myxosporida, *Ceratomyxa shasta* (Noble, 1950). *Journal of Fish Diseases* 2, 411–428.

Yasutake, W.T. and Wood, E.M. (1957) Some myxosporidia found in Pacific Northwest salmonids. *Journal of Parasitology* 43, 633–642.

Yokoyama, H., Danjo, T., Ogawa, K. and Wakabayashi, H. (1997) A vital staining technique with fluorescein diacetate (FDA) and propidium iodide (PI) for the determination of viability of myxosporean and actinosporean spores. *Journal of Fish Diseases* 20, 281–286.

Zhang, Y.A., Salinas, I., Li, J., Parra, D., Bjork, S. *et al.* (2010) IgT, a primitive immunoglobulin class specialized in mucosal immunity. *Nature Immunology* 11, 827–835.

Zielinski, C.M., Lorz, H.V. and Bartholomew, J.L. (2010) Detection of *Myxobolus cerebralis* in the lower Deschutes River basin, Oregon, USA. *North American Journal of Fishery Management* 30, 1032–1040.

Zielinski, C.M., Lorz, H.V., Hallett, S.L., Xue, L. and Bartholomew, J.L. (2011) Comparative susceptibility of Deschutes River, Oregon, *Tubifex tubifex* populations to *Myxobolus cerebralis*. *Journal of Aquatic Animal Health* 23, 1–8.

Zinn, J.L., Johnson, K.A., Sanders, J.E. and Fryer, J.L. (1977) Susceptibility of salmonid species and hatchery strains of chinook salmon (*Oncorhynchus tshawytscha*) to infections by *Ceratomyxa shasta*. *Journal of the Fisheries Research Board of Canada* 34, 933–936.

9 *Enteromyxum* Species

Ariadna Sitjà-Bobadilla*, Itziar Estensoro, M. Carla Piazzon and Oswaldo Palenzuela
Instituto de Acuicultura Torre de la Sal, CSIC, Castellón, Spain

Abstract

Enteromyxum includes four myxozoan species that primarily infect the gastrointestinal tract of marine fish, causing enteritis and severe emaciation. These microscopic parasites pose significant challenges to wild, aquarium and farmed populations worldwide due to difficulties in diagnosis, treatment and limited understanding of host–parasite interactions. This chapter reviews recent advances in transmission, pathophysiology, invasion strategies and disease management. Molecular tools have enabled the discovery of new species, revealed genetic diversity, and improved diagnostic speed and accuracy. Nevertheless, critical aspects including host–parasite dynamics and environmental drivers of transmission – remain unclear. The pathobiology of enteromyxosis reveals complex host–parasite interactions involving immune evasion, epithelial barrier disruption and nutrient malabsorption. These mechanisms can affect different hosts in markedly different ways, underscoring a clear immunopathological component in disease progression and outcome. The severity of clinical manifestations highlights the need for early detection and targeted intervention. Although no effective treatments currently exist, protective strategies such as selective breeding, improved biosecurity, environmental monitoring and vaccine development show promise. Multidisciplinary research is essential to develop effective control measures and reduce the impact of *Enteromyxum* on aquaculture and wild stocks, aligning with broader goals of sustainable disease management in aquatic systems.

9.1. Introduction

9.1.1. Taxonomic remarks

Myxozoans (phylum Cnidaria) are microscopic metazoan parasites with a debated phylogeny. Over the past decades, genetic evidence revealed myxozoans as highly evolved cnidarians, possessing cnidarian-specific genes such as minicollagens and nematogalectins (Feng *et al.*, 2014; Foox *et al.*, 2015). Phylogenomic analyses suggest that within Cnidaria, Myxozoa forms a sister clade to Medusozoa (Feng *et al.*, 2014; Chang *et al.*, 2015). However, more recent evidence, specifically the discovery of circular mitochondrial chromosomes in *Kudoa* and *Enteromyxum*, supports an alternative positioning outside Medusozoa (Yahalomi *et al.*, 2017). Myxozoa comprises two classes, Myxosporea and Malacosporea. The genus *Enteromyxum* (Palenzuela *et al.*, 2002) belongs to the former, a class that includes primarily parasites of fish and only rarely of other vertebrates. This genus comprises four gastrointestinal species. *Enteromyxum leei*,

*Email: ariadna.sitja@csic.es

DOI: 10.1079/9781800628748.0009

described as *Myxidium leei* (Diamant *et al.*, 1994), was first reported in cultured gilthead seabream (GSB) (*Sparus aurata*) from southern Cyprus. Susceptible hosts include >70 wild and farmed marine fishes, with a global distribution across the Mediterranean, Atlantic and Pacific Oceans (Tables 9.1 and 9.2). The parasite has been experimentally transmitted to freshwater fishes (Diamant *et al.*, 2006b).

However, *Enteromyxum scophthalmi* (Palenzuela *et al.*, 2002) has only been reported in cultured turbot (*Psetta maxima*) and Senegalese sole (*Solea senegalensis*) (Palenzuela *et al.*, 2007). *Enteromyxum fugu* (Yanagida *et al.*, 2004), originally described as *Myxidium fugu* (Tun *et al.*, 2000), occurs exclusively in cultured tiger puffer (*Takifugu rubripes*) in Japan, but has been experimentally transmitted to red seabream (*Pagrus major*) (Table 9.2). The most recently described species, *Enteromyxum caesio* (Freeman *et al.*, 2020), was found in the stomach of a wild redbelly yellowtail fusilier (*Caesio cuning*) from Malaysia. The genus is now placed in the newly established Enteromyxidae family, within suborder Variisporina Lom et Noble, 1984, to separate it from the Myxidiidae *sensu stricto*. The Enteromyxidae are phylogenetically related to other histozoic myxosporeans from the marine environment, but remain a discrete group. Within this family there is a significant genetic range with respect to small-subunit ribosomal DNA (SSU rDNA) data, and likely other species are yet to be discovered (Freeman *et al.*, 2020).

9.1.2. Impact

Most myxosporea are not highly pathogenic to fish, but some are responsible for severe economic losses in aquaculture (Kent *et al.*, 2001; Feist and Longshaw, 2006; Lom and Dyková, 2006). The impact of *Enteromyxum* species is not only limited to direct mortality but also to weight loss, poor feed conversions, delayed growth and reduced marketability of infected fish. *E. leei* is one of the most devastating parasites in warm-water marine cultures in the Mediterranean Sea and in Japanese and Korean waters (Palenzuela, 2006; Rigos and Katharios, 2010; Sekiya *et al.*, 2016; Golomazou *et al.*, 2017; Yanagida, 2017). The severity of *E. leei* infections largely depends on the susceptibility of the host, the aquaculture model and environmental conditions (Table 9.1B). Among aquacultured species, sharpsnout seabream (*Diplodus puntazzo*) is probably the most susceptible species, to the extent that its cultivation is considered doomed in specific enzootic locations (Rigos and Katharios, 2010). It develops as a subacute syndrome in juvenile fish (<50 g), a few weeks after introduction into netpens, with heavy mortality, while larger fish may remain relatively unaffected. Culture of other sparids such as red porgy (*Pagrus pagrus*) is also hampered by enteromyxosis (Fioravanti *et al.*, 2020). In contrast, *E. leei* usually causes a milder, subchronic disease in GSB, ranging from undetected in sea cages to conspicuous or even severe in some facilities. Tiger puffer and olive flounder (*Paralichthys olivaceus*) are also highly susceptible hosts and their aquaculture has been severely affected in Japanese waters since the mid-1990s (Tun *et al.*, 2000; Yasuda *et al.*, 2005). Major *E. leei* outbreaks have also been reported in Japan affecting other species such as red seabream or spotted knifejaw (*Oplegnathus punctatus*) (Yanagida *et al.*, 2008) and malabar grouper (*Epinephelus malabaricus*) (China *et al.*, 2013). In Korea, where olive flounder is a major aquacultured fish, emaciation disease was first noticed in 2007, but not clearly associated to *E. leei* until more recently (Kim *et al.*, 2015), and the disease has generated great concern to the local aquaculture industry because of the devastating effects. *E. leei* infections can also have a severe impact in exhibition aquarium facilities (Table 9.1A), affecting temperate and tropical fish species. Multi-species outbreaks can cause significant disturbance and affect very valuable and long-lived specimens such as sunfish (*Mola mola*) and the humphead wrasse (*Cheilinus undulatus*) (Padrós *et al.*, 2001; Katharios *et al.*, 2011).

E. scophthalmi is very pathogenic to cultured turbot causing serious disease with 100% mortality in some fish stocks (Branson *et al.*, 1999) and forcing production breaks and even cease of operations in several farms since the late 1990s (O. Palenzuela, M.J. Redondo and P. Álvarez-Pellitero, 2001, unpublished results). This species is not as cosmopolitan as *E. leei*, and besides turbot it has only been reported in sole (Palenzuela *et al.*, 2007). *E. fugu*, the least pathogenic species, causes minor impact in tiger puffer cultures. Experimentally infected fish show no

Table 9.1A. List of wild and aquarium-reared marine fish species reported to be infected by *Enteromyxum leei*. Details on the cases are included as available in the original reports; when not available appear as –. (*) Presumably ascribed to *E. leei* by spore morphology and clinical signs. (Author's own table.)

Fish order/family	Fish species	Location	Type of facility, water conditions	Prevalence (%)	Mortality detected, clinical signs	Reference
Acanthuriformes						
Acanthuridae	*Acanthurus leucosternon*	New Jersey, USA (Asian/African origin)	Aquarium	18.1	Yes, outbreak, emaciation	Hyatt *et al.* (2018)
	Acanthurus nigrofuscus	Israel	Wild captured	–		Diamant *et al.* (2004)
	Zebrasoma flavescens(*)	Florida, USA	Aquarium	–	Yes, emaciation	Hyatt (2009)
Lutjanidae	*Lutjanus kasmira*	New Jersey, USA (Asian/African origin)	Aquarium	4.3	Yes, outbreak, emaciation	Hyatt *et al.* (2018)
Pomacanthidae	*Pomacanthus imperator*	New Jersey, USA (Asian/African origin)	Aquarium	33.3	Yes, outbreak, emaciation	Hyatt *et al.* (2018)
	Centropyge acanthops	Barcelona, Spain	Aquarium (tropical)	–	Yes, mortality	C. Hispano, F. Padrós and O. Palenzuela (2025, unpublished results)
Batrachoidiformes						
Batrachoididae	*Halobatrachus didactylus*	Barcelona, Spain	Aquarium	100	Yes, outbreak	Padrós *et al.* (2001)
Perciformes						
Blenniidae	*Blennius* sp. *Parablennius* sp. *Scartella* sp.	Barcelona, Spain	Aquarium	81.2	Yes, outbreak	Padrós *et al.* (2001)
	Cirripectes filamentosus	Northern Red Sea, Israel	Wild captured	–	–	Diamant *et al.* (2004)
	Lipophrys pavo	Barcelona, Spain	Aquarium	100	Yes, outbreak	Padrós *et al.* (2001)
Carangidae	*Decapterus russelli*	Northern Gulf of Eilat, Red Sea, Israel	Wild captured	33.3	–	Álvarez-Pellitero *et al.* (2005)
	Trachurus indicus	Ashdod Harbour, Mediterranean, Israel	Wild captured	33.3	–	Álvarez-Pellitero *et al.* (2005)
		Northern Gulf of Eilat, Red Sea, Israel	Wild captured	20–50	–	Álvarez-Pellitero *et al.* (2005)
	Trachurus mediterraneus	Mediterranean coast, Gandía, Spain	Wild intruders in sea cages of *Diplodus puntazzo* infected	100	–	Montero *et al.* (2007)

Gobiidae	*Gobius niger*	Barcelona, Spain	Aquarium	33.3	Yes, outbreak	Padrós *et al.* (2001)
Labridae	*Cheilinus undulatus*	Crete, Greece	Aquarium	1 unique case	No clinical signs, but severe enteritis, mortality, chronic inflammation	Katharios *et al.* (2011)
	Clepticus parrae	Mississippi, USA	Aquarium	3 cases	–	Woodyard *et al.* (2024)
	Coris aygula	New Jersey, USA (Asian/African origin)	Aquarium	60	Yes, outbreak, emaciation	Hyatt *et al.* (2018)
	Coris julis	Barcelona, Spain	Aquarium	9.4	Yes, outbreak	Padrós *et al.* (2001)
	Labrus viridis	Barcelona, Spain	Aquarium	16.7	Yes, outbreak	Padrós *et al.* (2001)
	Labrus bergylta	Barcelona, Spain	Aquarium	100	Yes, outbreak	Padrós *et al.* (2001)
	Labrus merula	Barcelona, Spain	Aquarium	100	Yes, outbreak	Padrós *et al.* (2001)
	Symphodus cinereus	Barcelona, Spain	Aquarium	100	Yes, outbreak	Padrós *et al.* (2001)
	Symphodus mediterraneus	Barcelona, Spain	Aquarium	40	Yes, outbreak	Padrós *et al.* (2001)
	Symphodus melops	Barcelona, Spain	Aquarium	100	Yes, outbreak	Padrós *et al.* (2001)
	Symphodus ocellatus	Barcelona, Spain	Aquarium	100	Yes, outbreak	Padrós *et al.* (2001)
	Symphodus roissali	Barcelona, Spain	Aquarium	20	Yes, outbreak	Padrós *et al.* (2001)
	Symphodus rostratus	Barcelona, Spain	Aquarium	15.4	Yes, outbreak	Padrós *et al.* (2001)
	Symphodus tinca	Barcelona, Spain	Aquarium	39.1	Yes, outbreak	Padrós *et al.* (2001)
	Thalassoma pavo	Barcelona, Spain	Aquarium	37.5	Yes, outbreak	Padrós *et al.* (2001)
	Xyrichtys novacula	Barcelona, Spain	Aquarium	50	Yes, outbreak	Padrós *et al.* (2001)
Lethrinidae	*Lethrinus variegatus*	Red Sea, Eilat, Israel	Wild captured	100	–	Álvarez-Pellitero *et al.* (2005)
Mugilidae	*Chelon labrosus*	Mediterranean coast, Israel	Wild fish in brackish channels and coastline adjacent to mariculture	25–40	–	Diamant (1998)
	Liza aurata	Mediterranean coast, Israel	Wild fish in brackish channels and coastline adjacent to mariculture	25–40	–	Diamant (1998)

Continued

Table 9.1A. Continued.

Fish order/family	Fish species	Location	Type of facility, water conditions	Prevalence (%)	Mortality detected, clinical signs	Reference
		Mediterranean coast, Spain	Intruders in sea cages of *D. puntazzo* infected	100	–	Montero *et al.* (2007)
	Liza ramada	Mediterranean coast, Israel	Wild fish in brackish channels and coastline adjacent to mariculture	40	–	Diamant (1998); Álvarez-Pellitero *et al.* (2005)
	Mugil cephalus	Western Orbetello Lagoon, Italy	Wild captured	8.1	–	Álvarez-Pellitero *et al.* (2005)
	Mugil saliens	Mediterranean coast, Israel	Wild fish in brackish channels and coastline adjacent to mariculture	25–40	–	Diamant (1998)
Mullidae	*Mullus surmuletus*	Barcelona, Spain	Aquarium	4.8	Yes, outbreak	Padrós *et al.* (2001)
	Mulloidichthys vanicolensis	Israel	Wild captured	–	–	Diamant *et al.* (2004)
Nemipteridae	*Scolopsis ghanam*	Israel	Wild captured	–	–	Diamant *et al.* (2004)
Pomacentridae	*Chromis chromis*	Black Sea coast, Turkey	Wild	8	–	Özer *et al.* (2014)
		Barcelona, Spain	Aquarium	33.3	Yes, outbreak	Padrós *et al.* (2001)
	Chromis viridis	Barcelona, Spain	Aquarium (tropical)	–	Yes, mortality	C. Hispano, F. Padrós and O. Palenzuela (2025, unpublished results)
	Abudelduf saxatilis	Barcelona, Spain	Aquarium (Tropical)	–	Yes, mortality	C. Hispano, F. Padrós and O. Palenzuela (2025, unpublished results)
	Neopomacentrus miryae	Northern Gulf of Eilat, Red Sea, Israel	Wild captured	25	–	Diamant *et al.* (2004); Álvarez-Pellitero *et al.* (2005)
	Teixeirichthys jordani	Red Sea, Eilat, Israel	Wild captured	6.25	–	Álvarez-Pellitero *et al.* (2005)

Scaridae	*Sparisoma cretense*	Crete, Greece	Aquarium, quarantine facilities. Borehole water	–	Emaciation and bilateral body depression rare, most fish no external clinical signs. 60% mortality over 3.5 months	Katharios *et al.* (2014)
Siganidae	*Siganus luridus*	Northern Gulf of Eilat, Red Sea, Israel	Wild captured	11.4–100	–	Álvarez-Pellitero *et al.* (2005)
	Siganus rivulatus	Northern Gulf of Eilat, Red Sea, Israel	Wild captured	23.1	–	Álvarez-Pellitero *et al.* (2005)
		Ashdod Harbour, Mediterranean, Israel	Wild captured	10	–	Álvarez-Pellitero *et al.* (2005)
Sparidae	*Boops boops*	Greece	Wild captured	–	–	Álvarez-Pellitero *et al.* (2005)
	Diplodus noct	Red Sea, Eilat, Israel	Wild captured	11.1	–	Diamant *et al.* (2004); Álvarez-Pellitero *et al.* (2005)
	Diplodus sargus	Barcelona, Spain	Aquarium	33.3	Yes, outbreak	Padrós *et al.* (2001)
	Diplodus vulgaris	Barcelona, Spain	Aquarium	100	Yes, outbreak	Padrós *et al.* (2001)
	Sparus aurata	Barcelona, Spain	Aquarium	12.5	Yes, outbreak	Padrós *et al.* (2001)
		Western Mediterranean, France	Wild captured	11.1	–	Álvarez-Pellitero *et al.* (2005)
	Spicara maena	Barcelona, Spain	Aquarium	3.4	Yes, outbreak	Padrós *et al.* (2001)
Scorpaeniformes						
Scorpaenidae	*Scorpaena porcus*	Barcelona, Spain	Aquarium	14.3	Yes, outbreak	Padrós *et al.* (2001)
Tetraodontiformes						
Molidae	*Mola mola*	Barcelona, Spain	Aquarium	100	Yes, outbreak	Padrós *et al.* (2001)

Table 9.1B. List of farmed marine fish species reported to be infected by *Enteromyxum leei.* Details on the location and culture conditions are included as available in the original report; when not available appear as –. (Author's own table.)

Fish order/family	Fish species	Location	Type of facility, water conditions	Prevalence (%)	Mortality detected, clinical signs	Reference
Carangiformes						
Paralichthyidae	*Paralichthys olivaceus*	Miyazaki, Japan	Land-based farm: concrete tanks, Vicinity of infected puffer fish farm. Open flow	–	Yes, outbreak, emaciation	Yasuda *et al.* (2005))
		Jeju Island, South Korea	–	–	–	Kim *et al.* (2015)
		Wando, South Korea	–	–	–	Lee *et al.* (2024b)
	Platichthys stellatus	Jeju Island, South Korea	–	50–100	Decreased condition factor	Shin and Lee (2023)
	Paralichthys adspersus	Eastern Pacific, Peru	Earth ponds	–	Yes, emaciation and mortality	J.M. Leiro and O. Palenzuela (2014, unpublished results)
	Solea senegalensis	Western Mediterranean	Concrete raceways	–	Yes, emaciation and mortality	F. Padrós and O. Palenzuela (2002, unpublished results)
Scophthalmidae	*Scophthalmus maximus*	Jeju Island, South Korea	Flow-through system of land-based facilities	Isolated case	Emaciation	Sekiya *et al.* (2016)
Perciformes						
Moronidae	*Dicentrarchus labrax*	France	Vicinity of infected *S. aurata*	–	–	Renaud *et al.* (2004)
		Italy	Inland: concrete tanks	1.2–15	–	Fioravanti *et al.* (2006)
		Greece	Commercial farms	–	–	Varvarigos (2003)
Oplegnathidae	*Oplegnathus punctatus*	Kagoshima Prefecture, Japan	Commercial farms	–	Emaciation	Yanagida *et al.* (2008)
Sciaenidae	*Argyrosomus regius*	Mediterranean, Spain	Sea cages	–	Emaciation	O. Palenzuela and A. Girons, 2024 (unpublished results)
Serranidae	*Epinephelus malabaricus*	Okinawa Prefecture, Japan	Tanks	0–100	Severe emaciation, 20–50% mortality	China *et al.* (2013)
Sparidae	*Dentex dentex*	Greece	–	–	–	Rigos *et al.* (1997)
	Diplodus puntazzo	Sicily and Sardinia, Italy	Inland farm: tanks	100	Yes, enteritis	Caffara *et al.* (1999)
		North and South Italy	Sea cages	80–100	36–100% mortality	Beraldo *et al.* (2011)
		Western Greece	Growing unit, sea cages		Yes, 33% outbreak, emaciation	Le Breton and Marques (1995)

		Greece	Sea cages	80	Yes, 80% mortality, emaciation	Athanassopoulou *et al.* (1999)
		Greece	Sea cages	5–45	Yes, associated to peak of prevalence and temperature	Golomazou *et al.* (2014)
		Mediterranean, Spain	Sea cages	75–100	–	Montero *et al.* (2007)
	Diplodus sargus	Mediterranean, Greece	Sea cages	0–40	–	Golomazou *et al.* (2006c)
	Pagrus major	Western Greece	Sea cages	90	Yes	Le Breton and Marques (1995)
		Mie and Kagoshima Prefectures, Japan	Commercial farms	0–35	9.1–9.7% mortality	Yanagida *et al.* (2008)
	Pagrus pagrus	Mediterranean	–	–	–	Diamant (1995)
	Pagellus bogavareo	Mediterranean, Italy	Research experimental facilities	–	Yes, anorexia, lethargy	Marino *et al.* (2004)
	Sparus aurata	South Cyprus	Grow-out tanks	–	Yes, emaciation	Diamant (1992)
		Canary Islands, Spain	Land-based farm: concrete tanks	8.3	–	Diamant *et al.* (2006)
		North Atlantic, France	Land-based farm, powerplant water, concrete tanks	0–100	Yes	Diamant *et al.* (2006)
		Eastern Orbetello Lagoon, Italy	Land-based farm: PVC tanks and earth ponds	36.6–58	–	Diamant *et al.* (2006)
		Piombino, Italy	Land-based farm	86.6	–	Diamant *et al.* (2006)
		Mediterranean, Spain	Sea cages	36.6	–	Diamant *et al.* (2006)
		Mediterranean, France	Sea cages	5	–	Diamant *et al.* (2006)
		Ionian Sea, Greece	Sea cages	3.3–10	–	Diamant *et al.* (2006)
		Red Sea, Israel	Sea cages	9.2–60	–	Diamant *et al.* (2006)
		Italy	Sea cages: offshore	43–71	–	Fioravanti *et al.* (2006)
			Inland: concrete tanks	11.6–20		
Tetraodontiformes						
Tetraodontidae	*Takifugu rubripes*	Western Japan	Sea cages	–	Severe emaciation	Ogawa and Yokoyama (2001)

Table 9.2. List of experimental infections achieved for *Enteromyxum leei* by feeding (F) or intubating orally (O) or anally (A) with infected gut scrapings, by cohabitation (C), or by contact with effluent (E) water from infected donor tanks. (Author's own table.)

Route	Donor species	Recipient species	Days pe	Prevalence (%)[a]	Reference
F, O	*Sparus aurata*	*S. aurata*	35	13	Diamant (1997)
			28–29	–	Diamant and Wajsbrot (1997)
				0–93.3	Sitjà-Bobadilla *et al.* (2007a)
		Puntius tetrazona[b,c]	35	80	Diamant *et al.* (2006)
		Oreochromis mossambicus[b,c]	43	90	Diamant *et al.* (2006)
		Astronotus ocellatus[b,c]	35	85	Diamant *et al.* (2006)
		Danio rerio[b,c]	40	53	Diamant *et al.* (2006)
F	*Takifugu rubripes*	*T. rubripes*	42	100	Yasuda *et al.* (2002); Yanagida *et al.* (2006)
		Pagrus major	42	57.1	Yanagida *et al.* (2004)
	Paralichthys olivaceus	*P. olivaceus*	32	100	Yasuda *et al.* (2005)
			63	73.3–93.3	Shin *et al.* (2022)
		T. rubripes	23	40	Yasuda *et al.* (2005)
		Takifugu niphobles[b]	–	–	Yokoyama and Shirakashi (2007)
		Amphiprion clarkii[b]	28	50	Yokoyama and Shirakashi (2007)
		Amphiprion ocellaris[b]	28	67	Yokoyama and Shirakashi (2007)
		P. major	70	28.6	Cho *et al.* (2024)
	Epinephelus malabaricus	*E. malabaricus*	33	80	China *et al.* (2013)
A	*S. aurata*	*S. aurata*	60–216	46.1–100	Estensoro *et al.* (2010b)
	P. olivaceus	*P. olivaceus*	63	46.7–93.3	Shin *et al.* (2022)
C	*S. aurata*	*S. aurata*	63	31.6	Diamant (1997)
			56	50	Diamant and Wajsbrot (1997)
			71–113	10–92	Sitjà-Bobadilla *et al.* (2007a)
		Sciaenops ocellatum	43	45.8	Diamant (1998)
		D. puntazzo	10	100	Álvarez-Pellitero *et al.* (2008)
	Diplodus puntazzo	*D. puntazzo*	19	100	Golomazou *et al.* (2006a)
			19	100	Muñoz *et al.* (2007)
			28	77	Henry *et al.* (2020)
	T. rubripes	*T. rubripes*	128	28.5	Yasuda *et al.* (2002)
		P. major	70	42.8	Yanagida *et al.* (2008)
	E. malabaricus	*E. malabaricus*	33	100	China *et al.* (2013)

E	*S. aurata*	*S. aurata*	63	33.3	Diamant (1997)
			56	40	Diamant and Wajsbrot (1997)
			77–84	2.4–78	Sitjà-Bobadilla *et al.* (2007a)
		Sciaenops ocellatus	43	35	Diamant (1998)
		Dicentrarchus labrax	139	53.3	Sitjà-Bobadilla *et al.* (2007)
	T. rubripes	*T. rubripes*	41	40	Yasuda *et al.* (2002)
		P. major	70	25	Yanagida *et al.* (2008)

[a]Highest value achieved, when different sampling times post-exposure (pe) were reported from a single experiment. A minimum–maximum range is provided when different experiments, or different infection doses, applied.

[b]Indicates this infection has not been detected naturally, or no data is available under farming conditions.

[c]Freshwater species. The remaining ones are marine fish.

significant intestinal pathology or disease signs despite high infection prevalence and rapid intestinal colonization (Yanagida *et al.*, 2006). There is no data on the impact of *E. caesio*, which has been reported only once from a Malaysian wild catch (Freeman *et al.*, 2020).

9.1.3. Transmission

Life cycles of myxozoans are generally heteroxenous, involving a fish and an invertebrate host. The known invertebrates are bryozoans in Malacosporea and annelids in Myxosporea, and these are, *sensu stricto*, the primary hosts (i.e. where sexual conjugation occurs). In the typical myxosporean cycle, spores released from fish (myxospores) are ingested by annelids, in which the sporoplasm infects the gut epithelium or the epidermis and finally develops into actinospores, infective for fish (Eszterbauer *et al.*, 2015). It is quite possible, but not proved, that members of *Enteromyxum* also have similar cycles involving invertebrate hosts in the wild. Some of the closest known relatives of *Enteromyxum*, based on phylogenetic analyses, have life cycles that involve polychaete hosts. For example, *Ceratonova shasta* and *Parvicapsula minibicornis* develop in the polychaete *Manayunkia occidentalis* (Atkinson *et al.*, 2020), while stages of *Ellipsomyxa* have been identified in *Nereis* spp. (Køie *et al.*, 2013). Rangel *et al.* (2011) described a new type of myxozoan actinospore, termed unicapsulactinomyxon, from the polychaete *Diopatra neapolitana*, with 81–84% similarity in SSU rDNA sequences to *Enteromyxum* genotypes. While this level of similarity is probably too low to suggest the two are congeneric, *Enteromyxum* spp. remain the closest known matches. The most exceptional characteristic of *Enteromyxum* is that three of the four known species can be directly transmitted (fish-to-fish) without the involvement of invertebrate hosts. The infective stages are either developmental stages or even cells present in the developing sporoblasts, but not the myxospores (see Fig. 9.3a and d, below). These stages are shed in epithelium remnants and faeces, often within mucous casts that preserve parasite viability for up to 24 h in sea water (Redondo *et al.*, 2004). Infection occurs through grazing or pecking at rectal prolapses which can develop in some infected species. Direct horizontal transmission greatly facilitates the spread of enteromyxosis across populations and stocks, with major implications for the parasites' pathobiology. Experimental transmission of *E. scophthalmi* has been achieved within the same host species using three methods: (i) exposure to water from tanks containing infected fish (effluent transmission); (ii) cohabitation with infected individuals; and (iii) oral intubation with infected intestinal scrapings (Redondo *et al.*, 2004). In the case of *E. leei*, these same methods have successfully enabled both intraspecific and interspecific transmission. Additionally, the anal intubation method is effective for this species (Table 9.2). For *E. fugu*, *per os* transmission is also effective (Yanagida *et al.*, 2006). Detailed protocols for experimental transmission of *E. leei* to GSB and *E. scophthalmi* to turbot can be found in the book *Fish Parasites: A Handbook of Protocols for their Isolation, Culture and Transmission* (Palenzuela *et al.*, 2021b; Sitjà-Bobadilla *et al.*, 2021).

9.1.4. Infection dynamics and epidemiology

The infection dynamics of *Enteromyxum* spp. largely depend on host susceptibility and culture system. *E. leei* has been described in all types of farming facilities (concrete/PVC tanks, earth ponds and sea cages, see Table 9.1B). Although *E. scophthalmi* infections have been observed in experimental sea cages located in drowned estuaries and in small-scale intertidal raceways (O. Palenzuela, 2006, unpublished results), most outbreaks occur in land-based, pump-ashore farms. In intensive farming set-ups, the first cases of enteromyxosis typically appear in the larger (older) size classes during the grow-out phase. As clinical signs become more evident in some of these older fish, the infection progressively spreads to additional culture units, eventually reaching younger age classes, where mortality is often highest. Since there is a variable but considerable pre-patent period (i.e. several weeks), by the time the outbreak is diagnosed, the number of parasites released in the system has multiplied exponentially and likely contaminated the entire facility.

The dynamics of the infections by *E. leei* in sea cages are more unpredictable, particularly in GSB, due to the relative resistance of this species and the diversity of environmental and management-related factors. In a wide-scale horizontal cross-sectional study of 40 Mediterranean farms (Palenzuela *et al.*, 2021a), the parasite was found to be widely distributed, even in sites where farmers did not notice disease signs. This survey revealed that farms removing mortalities more frequently, and those with better water exchange, had lower prevalence of infection. The number of hatcheries sourcing juveniles to the farm and the size of fish at harvest showed the strongest positive association with infection prevalence. Farms with more cages, larger cage sizes and higher annual production tended to have higher prevalence. Fish which had been exposed to higher minimum temperature during the grow-out phase, and those introduced to the cages with larger size, presented higher prevalence, whereas shorter times on the farm and higher specific growth rates (SGRs) were associated with lower infection prevalence. For GSB facilities, several risk or aggravating factors have been highlighted: (i) poor water exchange and/or re-intake of contaminated effluent water; (ii) recirculation systems; (iii) prolonged culture periods for production of large fish (Jublanc *et al.*, 2005; Diamant *et al.*, 2006a); and (iv) age/size of fish at entering sea cages (Golomazou *et al.*, 2014).

Enteromyxosis may be associated with overfeeding of high fat content diets (Rigos *et al.*, 1999). Indeed, a worse disease outcome was reported in experimentally infected GSB fed a diet containing vegetable oils as the major source of lipids (Estensoro *et al.*, 2011). This has also been reported in aquarium-reared parrotfish (*Sparisoma cretense*), in which clinical signs appeared after switching from herbivorous to carnivorous diet (Katharios *et al.*, 2014). Other triggering or aggravating factors are related to the infective pressure, namely duration of exposure time and fish density, as demonstrated for *E. leei* in GSB experimental infections (Sitjà-Bobadilla *et al.*, 2007a; Picard-Sánchez *et al.*, 2020b) and for *E. scophthalmi* in farm infections (Quiroga *et al.*, 2006). The existence of genetically based differences in parasite virulence has not been analysed for *Enteromyxum* spp., but it cannot be disregarded.

9.1.5. Water temperature

A clear relationship between infection and water temperature has been demonstrated for three species (Redondo *et al.*, 2002; Yanagida *et al.*, 2006; Estensoro *et al.*, 2010b; Shin *et al.*, 2018). Under culture conditions, GSB develops enteromyxosis clinical signs above 18–22°C (Le Breton and Marques, 1995; Rigos *et al.*, 1999; Fleurance *et al.*, 2008). Infection prevalence in olive flounder farmed in Korea has increased in recent years with rising water temperatures (Lee *et al.*, 2024b). Disease onset is largely delayed or suppressed at low temperatures, and in temperate regions, winter infective doses appear too low to establish the infection (Golomazou *et al.*, 2014). However, the infection can persist latently during cooler periods and re-emerge as temperatures rise (Yanagida *et al.*, 2006; Estensoro *et al.*, 2010b). This has key epizootiological implications, as fish testing negative in winter may act as reservoirs once conditions become favourable. However, high water temperature seems to prevent or eliminate the infections in some fish species (China *et al.*, 2014; Piazzon *et al.*, 2022; Toxqui-Rodríguez *et al.*, 2025). This effect could be partly due to a better immune performance of these hosts at higher temperature (Picard-Sánchez *et al.*, 2020b).

In turbot, clinical infections by *E. scophthalmi* are seldom noticed below 12°C, but become devastating above 18°C (Redondo *et al.*, 2002; Quiroga *et al.*, 2006). At 18°C, the pre-patent period can last up to 6 weeks post-exposure (pe), with mortality reaching 100% between 12 and 15 weeks pe. Empirical and experimental data indicates that parasite development is arrested below 11–12°C, and epizootics are uncommon at these temperatures unless parasite loads are exceptionally high. Nevertheless, *E. scophthalmi* may persist and transmit at low levels during colder months, with outbreaks often emerging after spring temperature increases.

9.2. Clinical Signs (Microscopic and Macroscopic Lesions)

Common field observations include loss of appetite (anorexia), poor food conversion rates and difficulties to reach commercial size in the final months of production. Clinical signs of enteromyxosis usually consist of a severe emaciation with epaxial muscle atrophy (Fig. 9.1). This emaciation can be noticed externally as a knife or razor-like aspect typical of compressiform species (e.g. Sparidae) (Fig. 9.1a, b and d), or as conspicuous head bony ridges and 'sunken head syndrome' in depressiform species (e.g. turbot, sole, olive flounder) (Fig. 9.1e–g). The emaciation is best noticed in subchronic infections at mild temperatures, with dead fish usually appearing wasted, and it can be imperceptible in very susceptible species and/or at high temperatures (e.g. sharpsnout seabream infections with *E. leei*) because fish die before reaching a cachectic condition. The weight loss is clearly reflected in

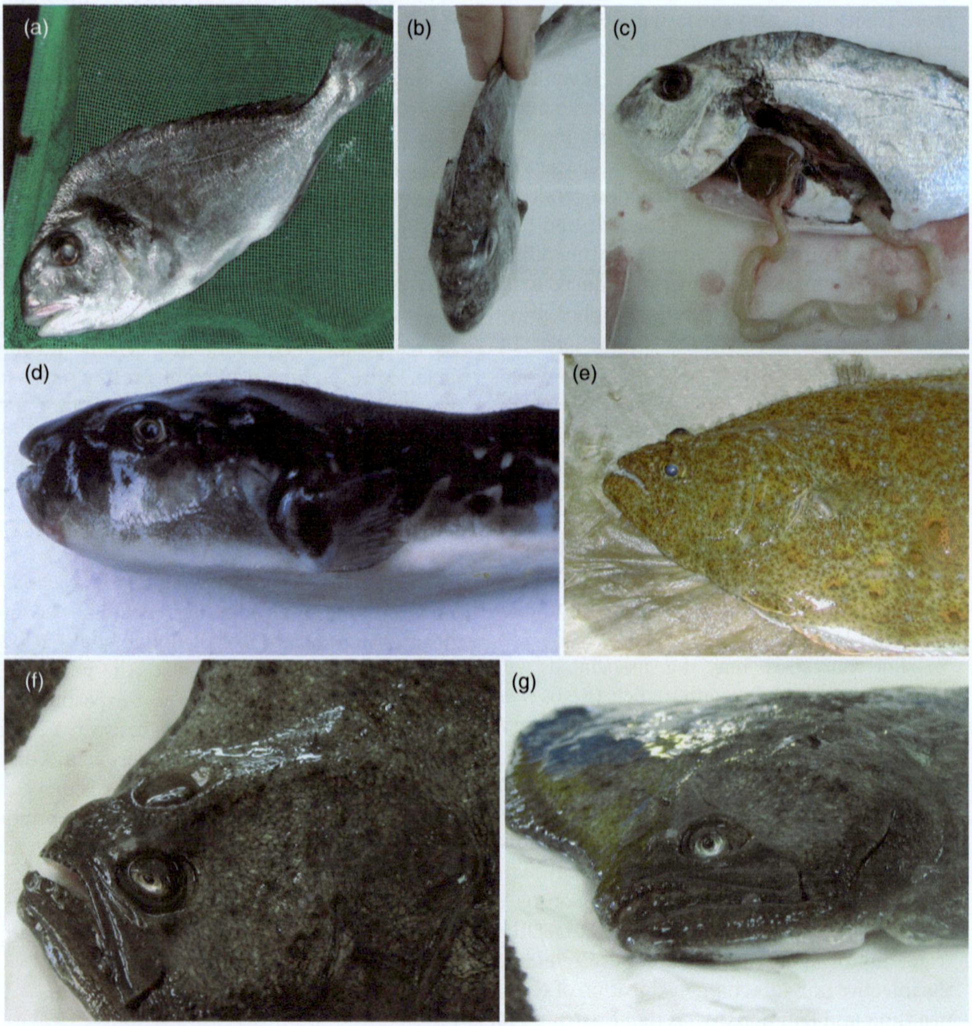

Fig. 9.1. Macroscopic clinical signs of enteromyxosis. *Enteromyxum* produces atrophy of epaxial muscle, with a razor-like aspect typically in *Enteromyxum leei*-infected gilthead seabream (a, b) and tigger puffer (d). Abnormal liver coloration, empty and semi-translucid digestive track filled with liquid, and absence of visceral fat are common in *E. leei*-infected gilthead seabream (c). Conspicuous cranial bony ridges and 'sunken head' are visible in *E. leei*-infected olive flounder (e) and *Enteromyxum scophthalmi*-infected turbot (f, g). (All figures are original from the authors, except (d) is courtesy of Dr Hiroshi Yokoyama (Okayama University of Science, Japan) and (b, c, f, g) are courtesy of Carlos Zarza (Skretting, Spain).)

the worsening of the relative condition factor (CF) (Estensoro *et al.*, 2011; Shin *et al.*, 2022; Cho *et al.*, 2024). A clear negative relationship between *E. leei* burden and CF was found in olive flounder and starry flounder (*Platichthys stellatus*) (Shin *et al.*, 2019; Shin and Lee, 2023). In GSB, the intensity of infection and the spreading of *E. leei* in the intestine were negatively correlated with the host CF and SGR (Picard-Sánchez *et al.*, 2020b). Ascites, distended abdomen and/or rectal prolapse occur in olive flounder and tiger puffer infected by *E. leei* or in turbot infected by *E. scophthalmi*. Discoloration and scale loss are less frequent (Athanassopoulou *et al.*, 1999).

Internal macroscopical signs in clinically infected fish are typically confined to the intestine, which often shows focal congestion, haemorrhages, fragility, semi-transparent appearance, and can be completely empty or containing seromucous fluid (Fig. 9.1c). Affected fish commonly exhibit reduced perivisceral fat and pale organs. The liver may appear greenish, occasionally atrophied or darkened (Hyatt *et al.*, 2018). Enlarged or discolored gallbladders are common in some hosts (e.g. sharpsnout seabream).

The histopathological analysis of intestine sections infected by *E. scophthalmi* and *E. leei* reveals different degrees of desquamative enteritis and myxozoan stages between enterocytes, or free in the lumen in severe infections (Fig. 9.2). Ribbons of epithelium containing parasite stages are sloughed to the lumen, and the lamina propria-submucosae often appear detached from the epithelial layer or hypertrophied and infiltrated by immune cells (Fig. 9.2a, c and d). Stages of *E. scophthalmi* often reach beyond the intestinal epithelium and can be found within the connective tissue of the lamina propria-submucosa and in blood vessels (Redondo *et al.*, 2002). Oedema is common in infected turbot. In turbot and olive flounder, the intestinal villi often lack epithelial lining (Sekiya *et al.*, 2016). The nature and intensity of the inflammatory response (Fig. 9.2b) vary by host–parasite model. Generally, more susceptible species exhibit stronger inflammation and earlier epithelial detachment, whereas more resistant hosts may harbour high parasite loads with minimal inflammation. Re-epithelization is frequent, though newly formed epithelia can be recolonized. Detailed histopathological studies are available elsewhere (Tun *et al.*, 2002; Golomazou *et al.*, 2006c; Álvarez-Pellitero *et al.*, 2008; Fleurance *et al.*, 2008; Bermúdez *et al.*, 2010; Sekiya *et al.*, 2016; Estensoro *et al.*, 2018; Ronza *et al.*, 2019).

Parasite distribution is limited to the digestive system, mainly the intestine. However, *E. leei* is often reported in the gallbladder lumen of some hosts, such as sharpsnout seabream or white seabream (*Diplodus sargus*) (Athanassopoulou *et al.*, 1999; Golomazou *et al.*, 2006c), but rarely in the gallbladder and intrahepatic biliary ducts of GSB (Le Breton and Marques, 1995; Fleurance *et al.*, 2008). Spores have been reported in the gastric lumen of heavily infected GSB although parasites were rare in the gastric mucosa (Le Breton and Marques, 1995; Fleurance *et al.*, 2008). Stages of *E. leei* have also been reported in the gastric mucosa and urinary bladder of olive flounder (Sekiya *et al.*, 2016; Shin *et al.*, 2018). *E. scophthalmi* stages are also detected occasionally in the stomach and oesophagus, haematopoietic organs, skeletal muscle, pancreatic tissue, heart, gills, skin and peripheral blood (Redondo *et al.*, 2002, 2004). These locations, however, are neither primary nor consistent. Scattered parasite foci at early stages of infection spread to the remaining intestine following different directional patterns depending on the host–parasite model. In turbot, *E. scophthalmi* stages are initially detected in the mucosa of the pyloric coeca and anterior intestine (Redondo *et al.*, 2004; Álvarez-Pellitero *et al.*, 2008), whereas *E. leei* stages are first found in the rectum and distal intestine in GSB, then spread/extend to the anterior intestine and later on to the middle intestinal region (Fleurance *et al.*, 2008; Cuadrado, 2009; Estensoro *et al.*, 2010b, 2011, 2014, 2018).

E. caesio has only been reported in the stomach (glandular tissue and lumen), but other possible locations cannot be disregarded (Freeman *et al.*, 2020). *E. fugu* is the only species which does not exhibit histozoic trophozoite proliferation in the paracellular space between enterocytes, making it the least pathogenic species. It has been observed only at epicellular sites on the intestinal mucosa of tiger puffer, attached by pseudopodia to brush-border microvilli. Sporogenesis of this species remains undocumented (Yanagida *et al.*, 2006; Freeman *et al.*, 2020). The parasite detaches easily and spreads along

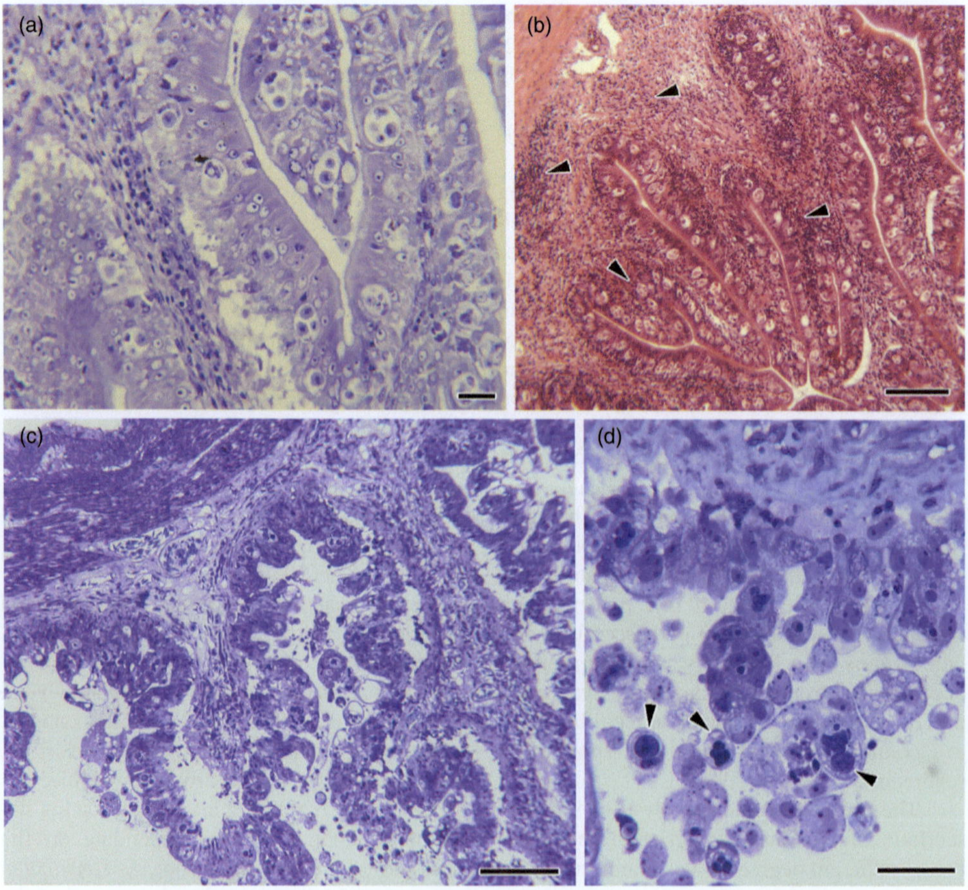

Fig. 9.2. Histopathological effects of *Enteromyxum leei* (a, b) and *Enteromyxum scophthalmi* (c, d). Note the detachment of the epithelium from the lamina propria (a, c) and the disintegration of the epithelial layer (b, c). (b) Lymphocyte infiltration is visible at the epithelial base and in the lamina propria-submucosae (arrowheads). (d) Parasite stages (arrowheads) and cell debris are released to the intestinal lumen. Stainings: Giemsa (a), haematoxylin and eosin (b), toluidine blue (c, d). Bars = 20 μm (a), 100 μm (b, c), 10 μm (d). (Author's own image.)

the intestine, facilitating rapid progression from anterior to posterior sections.

9.3. Diagnosis

Diagnosis of enteromyxosis based solely on gross clinical signs is unreliable due to variability across host species. However, clinical infection should be suspected in susceptible cultured marine fish during the grow-out phase when signs such as severe cachexia, enteritis, emaciation and/or dehydration are observed. Field confirmatory diagnosis typically relies on detecting *Enteromyxum* spores in intestinal mucosa smears, either fresh or stained (e.g. Diff-Quick or May–Grünwald Giemsa) (Fig. 9.3c, e and h). However, *E. leei* spores may be unevenly distributed along the intestine or accumulate in the gallbladder (Breton and Marques, 1995; Katharios *et al.*, 2014; Özer *et al.*, 2014). Spores are often scarce or absent in *E. scophthalmi*-infected turbot (Palenzuela *et al.*, 2021b) and may be undetectable in *E. leei* infections in some hosts or under certain conditions (Yanagida *et al.*, 2006; O. Palenzuela and A. Sitjà-Bobadilla, 2012, unpublished results). Identification of pre-sporogonic developmental stages in fresh smears requires considerable

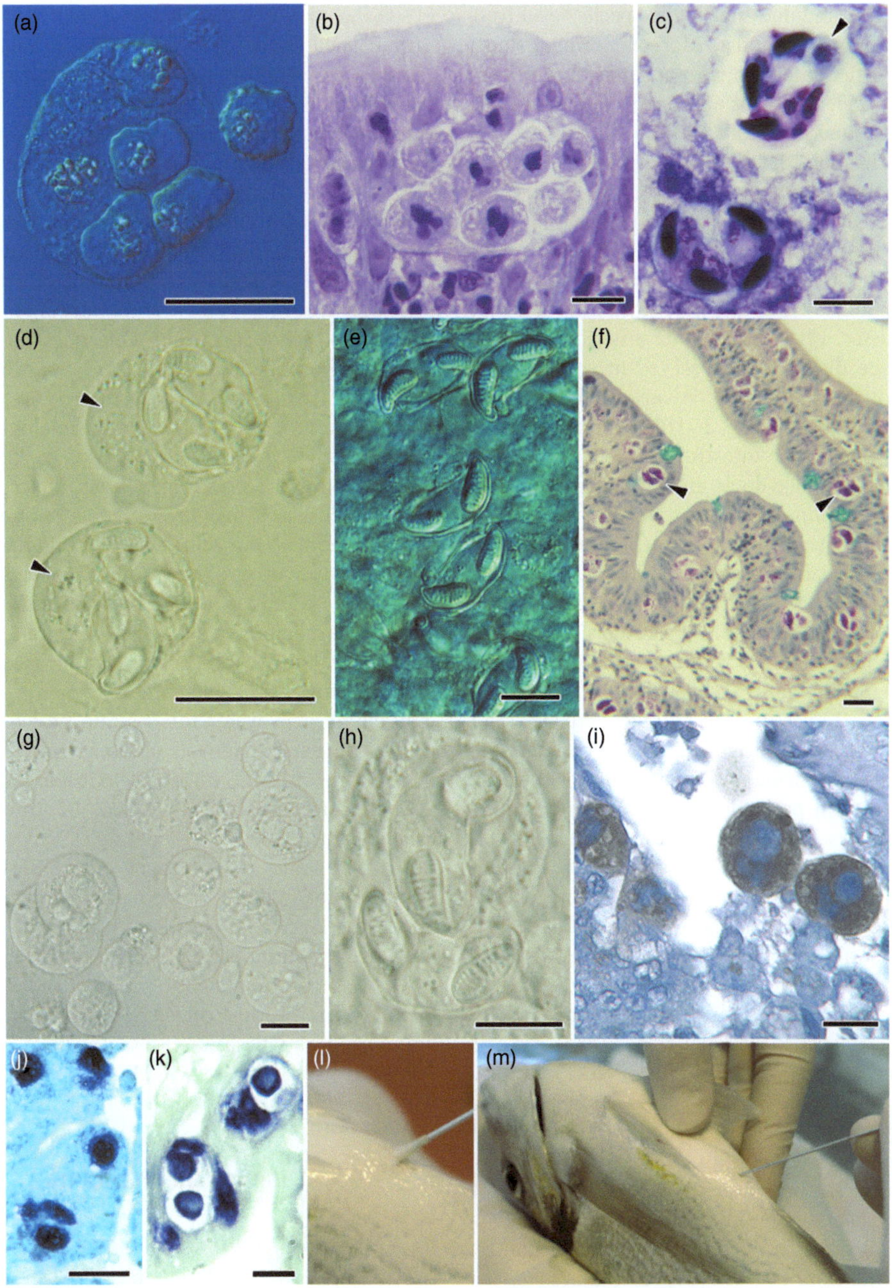

Fig. 9.3. Microscopic detection of *Enteromyxum leei* (a–f, k) and *Enteromyxum scophthalmi* (g–j) stages in fresh intestinal scrapings (a, d, e, g, h), May–Grünwald-stained smear (c), Alcian blue–PAS-stained histological section (f), lectin-stained histological section (soybean agglutinin from *Glycine max*) (i) and by ISH (j, k). Note the presence of developmental stages with the cell-in-a-cell pattern (a, b, g, k), the labelling of the primary cells (i), the disporoblasts with accompanying cells (arrowheads) (c, d) and the mature spores with dark-stained polar capsules (c). Parasite stages are fuchsine-stained (arrowheads) in (f). Coiled polar filaments are more visible with Nomarski microscopy (e). Rectal probing for non-lethal sampling diagnostic of *E. leei* by PCR (l, m). Bars = 20 μm (a, d, f, j), 10 μm (b, c, e, g, h, i, k). (All figures are original from the authors except (j) which is courtesy of Dr M.J. Redondo (Instituto de Acuicultura Torre de la Sal, CSIC, Spain); (i) was taken from Redondo *et al*., 2008, with permission from the publisher).

expertise and does not allow species-level resolution (Fig. 9.3a and g). Moreover, similar stages from other enteric myxozoans may compromise the specificity of this approach (Yanagida *et al.*, 2004; Cuadrado *et al.*, 2007).

Histological examination of target tissues is the reference procedure. Periodic acid–Schiff (PAS) (Fig. 9.3f), Giemsa and toluidine blue (Fig. 9.3b) stainings, or some lectins (Fig. 9.3i), can aid parasite visualization. However, infections with low parasite loads and patchy distribution may be missed. Given the distinct anterior–posterior parasite distribution observed in several hosts (Redondo *et al.*, 2004; Álvarez-Pellitero *et al.*, 2008; Estensoro *et al.*, 2010b), sampling should include multiple intestinal regions, as well as intrahepatic bile ducts and gallbladder in some species, to improve diagnostic sensitivity.

Since gene data on *Enteromyxum* spp. is available (Palenzuela *et al.*, 2002), oligonucleotide probes have been used for the diagnosis of enteromyxosis using PCR (Palenzuela *et al.*, 2004; Yanagida *et al.*, 2005) and *in situ* hybridization (ISH) (Fig. 9.3j and k) (Redondo, 2005; Cuadrado *et al.*, 2007). In general, *Enteromyxum* rDNA genes present sufficient variability compared to the closest marine myxozoan lineages to facilitate efficient probe designs for molecular diagnostic tests. These have evolved from the earliest end-point PCR tests to more advanced quantitative PCR (qPCR) tests using DNA-binding dyes or fluorescent hydrolysis probes in absolute or relative quantification assays for *E. leei*, *E. fugu* and *E. scophthalmi* (Table 9.3). Single-tube colorimetric, loop-mediated isothermal amplification (LAMP) assays have also been developed for *E. leei* and *E. scophthalmi* (Torres-Bocero, 2013; Katata and Okuyama, 2017). However, comprehensive analytical and clinical validation of several of these assays remains quite limited. In addition, as for any other clinical testing, the choice of methods of sample collection and DNA extraction impact largely on the assay performance. The intestinal mucosal niche of *Enteromyxum* spp. allows non-lethal sampling via rectal swabs. This technique, first developed for *C. shasta* infections in trout (Fox *et al.*, 2000), was later adapted to *Enteromyxum* infections in our laboratory (Fig. 9.3l and m). For *E. leei*, rectal swabbing was validated against whole-digestive tract histology by three independent laboratories, showing high sensitivity (0.96) and specificity (1) (O. Palenzuela and P. Álvarez-Pellitero, 2005, unpublished results). In turbot, the non-lethal rectal swab method also shows excellent diagnostic performance, despite the anterior-to-posterior intestine infection progression and typically lower parasite load at the posterior end (Redondo *et al.*, 2004). Many farms routinely use non-lethal PCR (NL-PCR) for *Enteromyxum* detection due to its convenience and heightened sensitivity, enabling early diagnosis. This approach is also preferred in our laboratory for monitoring infections in experimental trials (Palenzuela *et al.*, 2021b; Sitjà-Bobadilla *et al.*, 2021). However, enhanced sensitivity can be obtained by sampling tissues from portions with the highest parasite load for each species, or by using homogenates of larger intestinal sections. Molecular methods, besides being powerful tools for disease monitoring and surveillance, are invaluable for studying parasite entry routes, subclinical infections, potential invertebrate hosts and co-infections, among others. Environmental DNA (eDNA) methods have been successfully used to monitor presence of *Enteromyxum* spp. DNA in land-based farm water intakes and outlets, as well as for early diagnosis of tanks or culture units prior to the onset of clinical signs (O. Palenzuela and C. Díez-Vives, 2009, unpublished results). However, validating eDNA detection for reliable prediction of enteromyxosis remains challenging – particularly in netpens – due to the large volumes of sea water involved and the discontinuous concentration of parasite DNA (of uncertain viability) shed in fish faeces. Broader limitations of eDNA methods for diagnosing aquatic animal diseases have been discussed elsewhere (WOAH, 2022).

9.4. Disease Mechanisms

9.4.1. Pathophysiology

Enteromyxum triggers a cascade of physiological and metabolic events leading to cachexia, characterized by reduced haematological parameters (haematocrit, haemoglobin) and impaired growth performance (weight, length, CF, SGR). Cachexia primarily results from reduced food intake, caused not only by damaged intestinal epithelium impairing absorption but also by anorexia,

Table 9.3. Details of the molecular tools available for the diagnostic of *Enteromyxum* species. (Author's own table.)

Test	Species	Probe name	Sequence (5′ → 3′)[a]	Type[b]	Notes (target, applications)[c]	Reference
qPCR (SYBR)	*Enteromyxum leei*	EL-qF	ACT CGG CTA TGT GGG CAG TG	Primer (F)	LSU rDNA	Sohn *et al.* (2021)
		EL-qR	ATT GTT AAT TGC TAG TCG TAA AGA GCA AG	Primer (R)		
qPCR (SYBR)	*E. leei*	EL1F	ACC AAG TCT TCG GGC TCT G	Primer (F)	SSU rDNA	Golomazou *et al.* (2014)
		EL1R	TCT GTCA TTC TGT CAA TCC TAT CG	Primer (R)		
PCR and qPCR (SYBR)	*E. leei*	ELNMF	CGG TGA CGC CAA TCC GTG	Primer (F)	SSU rDNA; end point multiplex to discriminate from other species; reused for qPCR	Shin *et al.* (2018, 2019)
		MyNMR	GAC GGT ATC TGA TCG TCT TCG A	Primer (R)		
PCR	*E. leei*	EL-F	GGA TAT TGT CAG AGT ATG TT	Primer (F)	SSU rDNA; end point (species identification)	Yanagida *et al.* (2005)
		EL-R	AGA AGC CAA CGT ATA TGA TT(T)* A	Primer (R)		
	Enteromyxum fugu	EF-F	GGA GCA GTT CCA ATG GGA TT	Primer (F)	SSU rDNA	
		EF-R	AGA ACC TAC AAT TGG TCT GT	Primer (R)		
		EF-1F	TAT CGT AGG CGG AAG CCT GG	Primer (F)	SSU rDNA; end point multiplex for *E. fugu*/*E. leei*; combined with EF-R and EF-F for end-point species discrimination (one-round, and nested PCR)	Lee *et al.* (2024)
		EF-2R	CGG TGA GAC TAA CAT GTA TC	Primer (R)		
qPCR (SYBR)	*E. fugu*	REF-R	ATA CCA CAA TAG CTT CAA CT	Primer (R)	SSU rDNA; combined with EF-F for qPCR	
PCR	*E. leei*	EL-1F	CTA TTC GAT GGT ATA CAT AG	Primer (F)	SSU rDNA; end point species discrimination (one-round, and nested PCR)	
		EL-1R	GTC TAC TCT TTC GAG CAA AC	Primer (R)		
		EL-2F	ACT AGC TAG AAA CCA ACA AG	Primer (F)		
		El-2R	AAC ACG GAT TGG CGT CAC CG	Primer (R)	EL-2F and EL-1R for end point multiplex for *E. leei*/*E. fugu*	
qPCR (Nuclease assay)	*Enteromyxum scophthalmi*	ENTEROMYX F	GGC TTA ATT TGA CTC AAC A	Primer (F)	SSU rDNA	Alonso *et al.* (2015)
		ENTEROMYX R	CTC CAC CAA CTA AGA ACG	Primer (R)		
		ENTEROMYX PROBE	(6-FAM)-CCA TGC ACC ACC AAT CAT TGT ATC AT-(BHQ1)	Hydrolysis probe		
ISH	*E. leei*	EMXL ISH763U20	GAA TAT CGG TGA CGC CAA TC-(DIG)	ISH probes	SSU rDNA	Cuadrado *et al.* (2007)
		EMXL ISH1029L18	CCG GAG AAG CCA ACG TAT-(DIG)		SSU rDNA and rRNA	
	E. scophthalmi	EMXS ISH1344U22	GAG TTG AAC TCA GTA GTC TCT C-(DIG)		SSU rDNA	Redondo (2005)
		EMXS ISH637L20	CGT AAG ATA CTG ACA CAT CAC-(DIG)		SSU rDNA and rRNA	

Continued

Table 9.3. Continued.

Test	Species	Probe name	Sequence (5′ → 3′)[a]	Type[b]	Notes (target, applications)[c]	Reference
qPCR (SYBR)	*E. scophthalmi*	EMXS_626F	CAG TAT CTT ACG CAA GTG AG	Primer (F)	SSU rDNA; author's laboratory (routine diagnostics)	O. Palenzuela (2009, unpublished results)
		EMXS_719R	CAC AAG TGA CCA TCT ACA AA	Primer (R)		
qPCR (SYBR)	*E. leei*	EMXL_1374U20	TGA TGC CCT TCG ATG TTC TG	Primer (F)		
		EMXL_1451L29	AGT CTA CTC TTT CGA GCA AAC AAC TAT TT	Primer (R)		
LAMP	*E. leei*	EMXL-LAMP1_FIP	ACA CCA ATC CAA AAC CAA CAC G -TTTT- CGC TCG AAT GTA GTA GC	Looping inner FIP	SSU rDNA	Torres-Bocero (2013)
		EMXL-LAMP1_BIP	AAG GGA CAT TTT GAG GGC GTT -TTTT- TTG GTG GGT CTA AAG AAT TTC AC	Looping inner BIP		
		EMXL-LAMP1_F3	AAA GTG CTC AAT ACA AAG CG	Outer F3		
		EMXL-LAMP1_B3	GCT TTC GCA TTA GTG AGT CT	Outer B3		
LAMP	*E. scophthalmi*	EMXS-LAMP2_FIP	CCT GTT ATT GCC ACA CTT CCC-TTTT-GTT GTA ACT GAT CTT AGA GAG ACT	Looping inner FIP		
		EMXS-LAMP2_BIP	TGA TGC CCT TCG ATG TTC TG-TTTT-CGA CTC TCT CAA GTT AGG TAC	Looping inner BIP		
		EMXS-LAMP2_F3	CCA CAA TCT CTA ATT CAT TAC AGT	Outer F3		
		EMXS-LAMP2_B3	ATG ACA GCA ATT GCA AGT T	Outer B3		
LAMP	*E. leei*	EL-F3	AAA GTG CTC AAT ACA AGC G	Outer F3		Katata and Okuyama (2017)
		EL-B3	GCT TTC GCA TTA GTG AGT CT	Outer B3		
		EL-FIP	ACC AAT CCA AAA CCA ACA CGG ACC GCT CGA ATG TAG TAG C	Looping inner FIP		
		EL-BIP	AAG GGA CAT TTG AGG GCG TTT TGG TGG GTC TAA GAA TTT CAC	Looping inner BIP		

[a]6-FAM, 6-carboxyfluorescein; BHQ1, black hole quencher 1; DIG, digoxigenin; *, indicates EL-R modified by Sekiya *et al.* (2016) as mEL-R by removing (T) at 3′.
[b]F, forward; R, reverse; FIP, forward inner primer; BIP, backward inner primer.
[c]SSU, small subunit; LSU, large subunit.

which in GSB can reduce feeding by up to 45% compared to controls. However, anorexia accounts only for about half of the weight loss (Estensoro *et al.*, 2011). Weight loss may also stem from osmoregulatory failure, as shown in *E. leei*-infected tiger puffer (Ishimatsu *et al.*, 2007). Molecular analyses in turbot infected with *E. scophthalmi* revealed downregulation of genes related to structural proteins and digestive metabolism, underlying cachexia's causes and effects (Robledo *et al.*, 2014). *E. leei* disrupts intestinal water uptake, evidenced by a negative correlation between plasma chloride and CF, and elevated plasma osmolarity and intestinal fluid ion concentration in infected fish. Hepatic function was also impaired (Ishimatsu *et al.*, 2007), and a significant decrease of the lipid depots in hepatocytes was reported from *E. leei*-infected GSB (Picard-Sánchez *et al.*, 2020a). Additionally, respiratory frequency significantly declines in experimentally infected GSB, as measured by opercular accelerometers (Rosell-Moll *et al.*, 2021).

These pathophysiological effects of *Enteromyxum* arise from disruption of tight junctions and the associated electrolyte balance, compromising the epithelial barrier. Electrophysiology revealed decreased transepithelial resistance and a diarrhoeic profile in infected GSB (Sitjà-Bobadilla *et al.*, 2019). Intestinal barrier integrity may also be impaired by enterocyte apoptosis and necrosis (Bermúdez *et al.*, 2010), although it remains unclear whether apoptosis is a host defence limiting parasite spread or a parasite-facilitated mechanism enhancing survival by releasing partially protected, parasite-bearing enterocytes into the lumen (Redondo *et al.*, 2003a). Alterations in tight junction-associated proteins have also been documented. In turbot, E-cadherin immunostaining patterns shifted from regular to irregular at the host–parasite interface, although gene expression remained unchanged. Conversely, in GSB, no changes in E-cadherin protein distribution were observed, but gene expression was significantly downregulated in advanced infection (Ronza *et al.*, 2020). Similarly, immunodetection of tight junction proteins Tjp1 and Cldn3 was significantly reduced in parasitized GSB, while E-cadherin levels remained largely unaffected (Sitjà-Bobadilla *et al.*, 2019).

Parasite exposure stimulates intestinal epithelial cell turnover, increasing the proliferative rate of enterocytes and immune cells across all intestinal segments in GSB as a host response to counteract enterocyte damage (Estensoro *et al.*, 2018). The thickened lamina propria-submucosa, along with neovascularization and fibrosis patterns, further indicate ongoing tissue repair (Fleurance *et al.*, 2008). Apoptosis of enterocytes in *E. scophthalmi* and *E. leei* infections has been demonstrated by caspase-3 quantification, with increased cell death closely linked to epithelial desquamation and infection severity (Estensoro *et al.*, 2009; Losada *et al.*, 2014b). Enterocyte damage may result from direct parasite compression, epithelial detachment or parasite excretory/secretory products, especially when apoptotic cells are not in direct parasite contact.

The host immune response imposes metabolic costs and adverse effects on growth and feed intake involving anorexigenic factors, including gastrointestinal neuropeptides or growth factors. Exposed GSB showed fewer enteroendocrine cells positive for neuropeptide Y and substance P (Estensoro *et al.*, 2009). In *E. scophthalmi*-infected turbot, numbers of epithelial cells positive for cholecystokinin-8 and serotonin increase, while vasoactive intestinal polypeptide (VIP)-immunoreactive endocrine cells and nerve structures decrease (Bermúdez *et al.*, 2007). Immunohistochemistry revealed reduced anorexigenic peptides bombesin and glucagon in infected turbot, which might normally increase food intake, but gastrointestinal lesions likely impair nutrient absorption (Losada *et al.*, 2014a).

Upregulation of reactive oxygen or nitrogen species production systems and downregulation of antioxidant defence systems upon enteromyxosis are found in turbot and GSB (Sitjà-Bobadilla *et al.*, 2008; Losada *et al.*, 2012). In GSB, it was also demonstrated that these responses can be differentially modulated depending on the dietary background (Estensoro *et al.*, 2011). Thus, infected fish may experience oxidative stress, heightening their susceptibility to lipid peroxidation and oxidative damage.

Blood transcriptomics and metabolomics provide valuable insights into the pathophysiological consequences of enteromyxosis. Serum metabolomics identified 20 compounds that significantly differentiated controls from *E. leei*-infected GSB. Among these, inosine (decreased) and creatine (increased) emerged as potential non-lethal biomarkers of infection and disease progression (Sitjà-Bobadilla *et al.*, 2019). In *E. scophthalmi*-infected turbot, transcriptomic profiling revealed that moderately infected individuals exhibited downregulation of numerous genes involved in innate and adaptive immune responses. These included genes within chemokine signalling, B- and T-cell signalling, and focal adhesion pathways, suggesting an immunosuppressive or immune evasion effect exerted by the parasite during early or moderate stages of disease. In contrast, severely infected turbot displayed an upregulation of genes associated with innate immunity, including the complement cascade and pro-inflammatory mediators. However, components of adaptive immunity, especially genes related to B-cell receptor signalling and antigen processing and presentation, were downregulated (Ronza *et al.*, 2021). These findings are consistent with earlier studies and support the notion of a dysregulated immune response – characterized by excessive inflammation without effective adaptive immunity – which contributes to disease progression and host inability to clear the parasite.

Parasite-induced intestinal disruption also alters the gut microbiota of infected GSB. Notably, there is an over-representation of Proteobacteria and a concurrent decline in Firmicutes and Actinobacteria. These microbial shifts correlate with changes in host gene expression, suggesting that the transcriptomic alterations observed during enteromyxosis may arise directly from parasite activity and indirectly through microbiota dysbiosis (Toxqui-Rodríguez *et al.*, 2025). Maintaining a balanced gut microbiota appears to enhance resistance or resilience to infection. GSB families selected for fast growth harboured more metabolically adaptable and taxonomically stable microbiota, and displayed reduced clinical signs and lower parasite burden, than families with less stable microbial communities (Piazzon *et al.*, 2020). Furthermore, dietary supplementation with sodium butyrate improved gut microbiota stability and structure, significantly attenuating clinical manifestations of enteromyxosis (Piazzon *et al.*, 2017). Figures 9.4 and 9.5 integrate all these cascades of events for *E. leei* and *E. scophthalmi*, respectively.

9.4.2. Pathogenicity and invasion mechanisms

The pathogenic mechanisms of *Enteromyxum* spp. and the processes by which these parasites invade their hosts are not well understood. Proteases are known to contribute to the proliferation of several myxosporeans, but data for *Enteromyxum* is limited. Immunohistochemical detection of caspase-3-like activity in proliferative stages of *E. leei* (Estensoro *et al.*, 2009) suggests the involvement of cysteine proteases, which in mammalian cells are linked to cytoskeletal remodelling and cell proliferation. Moreover, functional gelatinolytic proteases spanning a broad molecular-weight range (49–245 kDa) have been detected in *E. leei* extracts from infected GSB intestines (Estensoro *et al.*, 2013a). In response, infected hosts show elevated levels of serum total antiproteases and α_2-macroglobulin (α_2M), both in sharpsnout seabream (Muñoz *et al.*, 2007) and turbot (Sitjà-Bobadilla *et al.*, 2006). This counteraction is further supported by the upregulation of α_2M gene expression in the intestine of infected GSB (Sitjà-Bobadilla *et al.*, 2008).

We are just starting to decipher the host–parasite interactions at the intestinal epithelium that allow trophozoites to penetrate between enterocytes and dwell in the paracellular space. Receptors in the intestinal mucin layer can act as binding sites for parasites, and lectin–carbohydrate interactions are frequently involved in the adhesion and penetration of parasites. Carbohydrate residues of *E. leei* (Redondo and Álvarez-Pellitero, 2010a; Estensoro *et al.*, 2013a) and *E. scophthalmi* (Redondo *et al.*, 2008) (Fig. 9.3i) and of their host digestive tract (Redondo and Álvarez-Pellitero, 2010a; Estensoro *et al.*, 2012) have been detected with lectin histochemistry and lectin blotting. Mannose and/or glucose and fucose residues are most abundant in membranes of myxosporeans and at the host–parasite interfaces. In the host intestine, terminal mannose and/or glucose, fucose and *N*-acetylglucosamine residues decreased upon enteromyxosis. A dramatic reduction of sialic acid occurred only in *E. leei*-infected GSB, especially at the posterior intestinal segment (Redondo and Álvarez-Pellitero, 2010a; Estensoro *et al.*, 2012). The intestinal mucus layer, primarily composed of *O*-glycosylated mucins secreted by goblet cells, serves as the first line of innate defence by mediating microbial and parasite interactions. Acidic mucins and sialic acid play critical roles in mucosal protection and pathogen recognition. Evidence suggests that GSB would lose the protective sialic acid during enteomyxosis, whereas its absence in

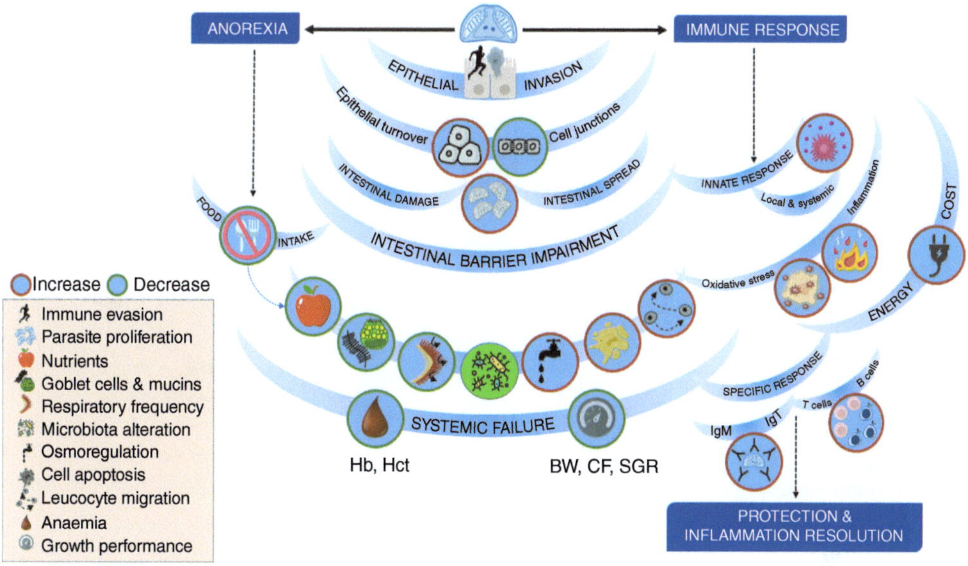

Fig. 9.4. Proposed integrative model of the pathophysiology of *Enteromyxum leei* in gilthead seabream. The parasite invades the intestinal epithelium, in part due to immune evasion, and induces anorexia, immune responses and changes in intestinal integrity. Parasite proliferation and spreading increases host epithelial turnover and changes in cell junctions, resulting in intestinal damage, and intestinal barrier impairment. Intestinal integrity is also affected by vitamin depletion, oxidative stress and inflammation. These changes are translated into gut permeability dysfunction, which, together with decreased food intake, produce nutrient depletion and osmotic intestinal failure. Other changes include decrease of goblet cells and mucins, decrease of respiratory frequency, alteration of the microbiota, and increased cell apoptosis and leucocyte migration. All this, together with the energy cost of mounting an immune response, leads to systemic failure and death. However, if the innate immune response prevents parasite spreading, and the specific immune response is strong enough, inflammation is resolved and fish recover. Typical disease indicators are related to growth retardation (body weight (BW), condition factor (CF) and specific growth rate (SGR)) and anaemia (low haemoglobin (Hb) and haematocrit (Hct)). (Modified from Sitjà-Bobadilla *et al.*, 2019. Created with Biorender and Pixabay icons and illustrations.)

healthy turbot intestines would render the higher disease severity (Redondo and Álvarez-Pellitero, 2010a; Estensoro *et al.*, 2012). Furthermore, a clear reduction in the number of intestinal goblet cells during enteromyxosis was noted (Fleurance *et al.*, 2008). Subsequent studies indicated this cell type was reduced in number and size in parasitized fish, regardless of their mucin content (Redondo *et al.*, 2008; Estensoro *et al.*, 2012). In GSB, the strongest effect on goblet cell depletion was caused by the parasite infection, but also plant-based diets contributed to goblet cell depletion (Estensoro *et al.*, 2012). An intestinal mucin exclusively expressed in the posterior intestinal segment of GSB was highly regulated by the diet and by enteromyxosis (Pérez-Sánchez *et al.*, 2013). In addition, mucins secreted in the intestinal mucus of *E. leei*-infected GSB exhibit altered glycoprotein composition and glycosylation resulting in a terminal glycosylation pattern characteristic of immature mucins, which has been associated with reduced bacterial adhesion (Estensoro *et al.*, 2013b). A glycomic approach in GSB showed a significant shift of the *O*-glycosylation structures with a notable decrease in core 4 structures (J. Benktander, I. Estensoro, A. Sitjà-Bobadilla, M.C. Piazzon and S. Lindén, 2025, unpublished results).

Ultrastructural studies of *E. scophthalmi* indicated that, during the initial phase of infection, unicellular trophozoites occupy an apparently intracellular position within host enterocytes, potentially facilitating early immune evasion (Redondo *et al.*, 2003a,b). As the parasite develops into a multinucleated plasmodium, it transitions to a paracellular location, nestled between adjacent

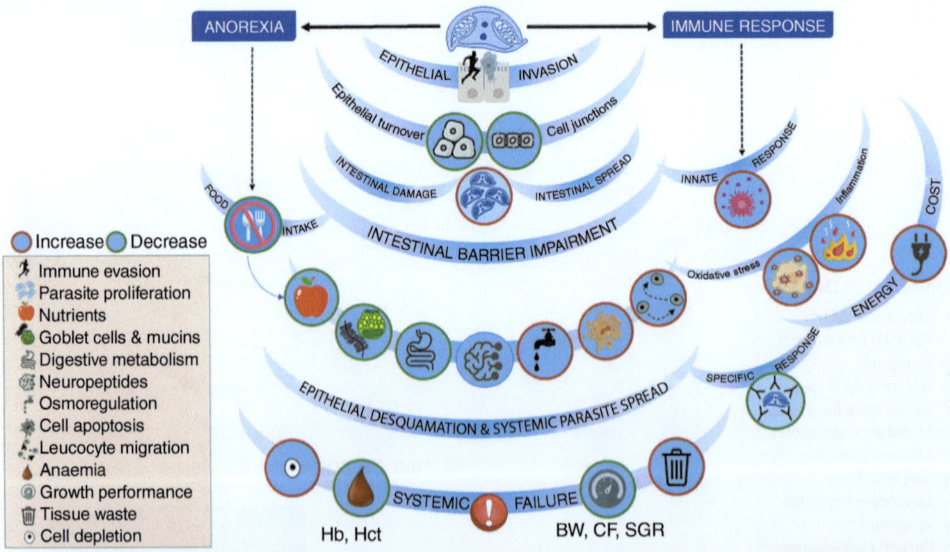

Fig. 9.5. Proposed integrative model of the pathophysiology of *Enteromyxum scophthalmi* in turbot. The parasite invades the intestinal epithelium, in part due to immune evasion, and induces anorexia, immune responses and changes in intestinal integrity. Parasite proliferation and spreading decreases host epithelial turnover and changes in cell junctions, resulting in intestinal damage, and intestinal barrier impairment. Intestinal integrity is also affected by oxidative stress and inflammation. These changes are translated into gut permeability dysfunction and decreased food intake, that produce nutrient depletion and osmotic intestinal failure. Other changes include decrease of digestion metabolism, goblet cells and mucins, modulation of neuropeptides, and increased cell apoptosis and leucocyte migration. In spite of the energy cost of mounting an immune response, this is unable to prevent the infection, leading to systemic failure and death. Typical disease indicators are related to growth retardation (body weight (BW), condition factor (CF) and specific growth rate (SGR)), waste, cell depletion and anaemia (low haemoglobin (Hb) and haematocrit (Hct)). (Based on Ronza *et al.*, 2019). Created with Biorender and Pixabay icons and illustrations.)

enterocytes. At this stage, *Enteromyxum* stages develop numerous convoluted cytoplasmic projections that establish direct contact with host cell membranes – some resembling gap junctions (Redondo *et al.*, 2003b; Cuadrado *et al.*, 2008). These structures are presumed to facilitate both attachment and communication with host cells, while also increasing the parasite's absorptive surface area to optimize nutrient uptake. This ability to integrate into and mimic the host epithelial environment likely contributes to immune evasion during the initial phases of infection, allowing rapid parasite expansion. Consequently, host recognition of the parasite and subsequent antigen presentation by cellular and humoral immune effectors may be delayed, hindering the timely production of specific antibodies and compromising the host's capacity to control the infection (see Section 9.5.3).

9.5. Protective/Control Strategies

Once *Enteromyxum* is established in an aquaculture facility, it can have devastating consequences and eradication typically requires aggressive measures. These may include production breaks and thorough sanitation of facilities. In many cases, significant modifications to the infrastructure and/or a shift towards farming less susceptible species are necessary. Prevention and continuous monitoring remain the cornerstones of effective management. In the following sections, we outline the main strategies available for the control of these infections.

9.5.1. Environmental-management measures

Usually, myxosporean infections of fish are first acquired from actinospores developed in annelids.

This exposure can be continuous or, more likely, in waves responding to the annelid cycles and environmental conditions (Eszterbauer *et al.*, 2015). In *Enteromyxum* spp., these cycles possibly occur in the wild – which would explain index cases in new outbreaks at isolated facilities. However, these cycles have not been confirmed for *Enteromyxum* spp. and for disease management, outbreaks in farmed conditions are triggered by the spreading of parasite stages from other infected fish. The geographical extension of the parasite, combined with its exceptionally broad host range and variable pathogeny, facilitates its persistence in the wild, particularly in regions where warmwater aquaculture is practised.

Avoiding *Enteromyxum* infections in marine aquaculture is challenging and management strategies depend on the type of facility. Epidemiological data from outbreaks in north-western Spain, Portugal and Japan (2000–2015) indicates that land-based, flow-through systems are particularly susceptible to massive infections by *E. scophthalmi* and *E. leei* in numerous fish species. These outbreaks usually occur in estuaries, enclosed bays or harbours, where suboptimal positioning of water inlets and outlets – combined with tidal forces, water currents or other environmental factors – allow plant effluent water to re-enter the system. Large-scale water recirculation promotes exponential amplification of the parasite, often resulting in the collapse of aquaculture operations. Some parasite-free facilities on open oceanic shores with well-designed water inlet and outlet systems have experienced catastrophic *E. scophthalmi* outbreaks when technical failures in water supply forced sustained water reuse (R. Romero, J. Fernández-Casal, A. Ruiz-Cruz and O. Palenzuela, 2013, unpublished results).

Temperature modulates the development of enteromyxosis, providing a potential intervention point for managing infections. Parasite development and proliferation decrease or cease at the lower end of the temperature range specific for each *Enteromyxum* species: <11°C for *E. scophthalmi* and <15°C for *E. leei* and *E. fugu* (Yanagida *et al.*, 2006). Conversely, evidence from malabar grouper and anemonefish (*Amphiprion ocellaris*) has shown that some diseased fish recovered and cleared *E. leei* infections when water temperature increased to 27–30°C (China *et al.*, 2014). Our own infection trials in GSB also indicate that *E. leei* is inhibited at sustained temperatures above 28°C (Piazzon *et al.*, 2022; Toxqui-Rodríguez *et al.*, 2025). This approach was recently applied in an exhibition aquarium, in combination with chemotherapy (Farmer *et al.*, 2025). The upper thermal limit for *E. scophthalmi* remains unknown. However, infections become particularly severe at the highest temperatures tolerated by turbot aquaculture, ~22–23°C. Hyposalinity (<8 ppt) has also been shown effective for the control of *E. leei* infection (Yokoyama and Shirakashi, 2007).

The management of *Enteromyxum* infections through environmental control is limited to set-ups where it is technically and economically viable, and within tolerable ranges for the fish. However, data on the practical effectivity of these approaches in aquaculture settings is missing. In sea cages rearing GSB and other sparids, the options are limited. For prevention, it is essential to avoid risk or aggravating factors: (i) sustainedly elevated water temperatures such as those using heated water (e.g. effluents from powerplants, springs or lagoons in geothermal areas); (ii) poor water exchange and accumulation of contaminated water, commonly found in enclosed bays or lagoons; and (iii) prolonged culture periods necessary for production of large-size fish (Jublanc *et al.*, 2005; Diamant *et al.*, 2006a). Daily removal of carcasses reduced the impact of *E. leei* infections in cage-based GSB farms (A. Diamant, National Centre for Mariculture, Israel Oceanographic and Limnological Research, 2010, personal communication).

All turbot kept in mechanically filtered water (i.e. using self-cleaning drum filters with 50 μm nominal mesh size) in pump-ashore, flow-through farms remained uninfected by *E. scophthalmi* (Quiroga *et al.*, 2006). However, the use of such filtration in turbot farms as a routine prophylaxis is not always affordable due to the large volume of water needed, and it is only used during the early grow-out phases. In addition, these systems cannot completely shield farms, particularly in high-risk environments. Some facilities located in enzootic waters have managed to overcome the infections by treating incoming water (e.g. with ozone, utltraviolet light and/or filtration) and effluent treatment with ozone, in addition to rigorous disease surveillance and early culling of infected stocks.

However, no data on the relative efficacy of these measures or recommended dosages is available.

Periodic surveys are always suggested for early detection. Immediate culling of affected stocks is, most often, the wisest measure to avoid exponential concentration of infective material and dispersion of the disease through contagion or transportation of stocks to disease-free facilities. Marine exhibition aquaria are especially vulnerable to *E. leei* outbreaks due to the wide host range of this species, as evidenced by outbreaks across Europe and the USA (Padrós *et al.*, 2001; Katharios *et al.*, 2011, 2014; Hyatt *et al.*, 2018; Woodyard *et al.*, 2024). Quarantine protocols with NL-PCR testing are recommended when introducing new imported or wild-captured fish.

9.5.2. Chemotherapeutic approaches

There are no specific antiparasitic drugs against myxosporeans, and those tested experimentally have mixed results. Oral treatment with toltrazuril did not ameliorate the clinical progress of the disease in *E. scophthtalmi*-infected turbot, though the drug induced some cytological alterations on the parasite (Bermúdez *et al.*, 2006a). This drug has been evaluated *in vivo* and *in vitro* against *E. leei* infection in olive flounder (Lee *et al.*, 2025). The combination of salinomycin and amprolium significantly reduced prevalence, intensity and mortality in *E. leei*-infected sharpsnout seabream, without apparent toxic effects (Golomazou *et al.*, 2006b). It also increased survival rates of turbot infected with *E. scophthalmi* (Palenzuela *et al.*, 2009). More recently, it was found effective to cease mortalities and reduced clinical signs in a multi-species aquarium outbreak (Hyatt *et al.*, 2018). However, mass mortality of false pilchards (*Harengula clupeola*) and scad (*Decapterus macarellus*) followed application of these chemicals, along with prolonged temperature increase, to address an *E. leei* outbreak at a recreational aquarium (Farmer *et al.*, 2025). Toxic effects have also been reported with other drugs, such as fumagillin (Golomazou *et al.*, 2006b) or the combination of narasin and nicarbazin (Palenzuela *et al.*, 2009). Other chemotherapeutic combinations like robenidine plus sulfamides, or diets supplemented with proprietary phytogenic natural extracts, temporarily improve survival rate of infected turbot and the lower mortality seemed to be due to reduced parasite loads, more restricted intestinal invasion, and a more equilibrated rate of infected epithelium desquamation and re-epithelization (Palenzuela *et al.*, 2009). However, none of the treatments stopped the infection (100% final prevalence). In addition, regulatory restrictions prevent use of most of these chemicals at farm level.

Some *in vitro* studies have explored the parasiticidal effect of phytogenic compounds against freshly isolated *E. leei* stages, and citral at 100–250 μg/ml was the most effective (Kim *et al.*, 2025). However, large-scale investigations and studies on the mechanisms of action of these compounds are hampered by the low *in vitro* survival of isolated *Enteromyxum* cells and the lack of a longer-term *in vitro* maintenance model (Redondo *et al.*, 2003a). Additional *in vitro* studies using intestinal turbot explants have shown that some parasite carbohydrates are involved in parasite entry, since the addition of the corresponding blocking lectin can inhibit *E. scopththalmi* penetration in the tissues (Redondo and Álvarez-Pellitero, 2010b). This may open a new set of therapeutic targets that need further robust studies.

The activity of natural extracts and phytobiotics warrants further investigation, as their use in aquaculture is subject to fewer regulatory restrictions than conventional chemotherapeutics. Several phytogenic ingredients are available as proprietary in-feed additives formulated to combine microbiocidal and immune-boosting effects, and some of these products reduced the prevalence and intensity of infections and mitigated clinical signs of enteromyxosis in experimentally infected GSB (Palenzuela *et al.*, 2020). However, the same formula failed to mitigate the infection in sharpsnout seabream under high temperature and parasite pressure (Henry *et al.*, 2020). Other commercial in-feed additives containing phytobiotics have been tested for protection against *E. scophthalmi* in turbot and *E. leei* in GSB, but no significant protective effects were demonstrated (O. Palenzuela and A. Sitjà-Bobadilla, 2012, unpublished results). In general, the direct microbiocidal effect on the parasites is unclear and their benefits, if any, are probably related to immune boosting in the host (see Section 9.5.3).

Although the above information suggests some potential for combined therapies in enteromyxosis, the high susceptibility of some hosts, especially under high water temperatures, does not allow complete clearance of the parasite. In addition, the lack of efficacious antiparasitic products licensed for aquaculture further restricts the options, particularly in warmwater Mediterranean aquaculture (Rigos *et al.*, 2024).

9.5.3. Strategies based on exploitation of the host immune system

Understanding the host immune response to *Enteromyxum* and how the parasite evades or modulates this defence is essential for developing future vaccines, preventive measures, and selecting resistant fish strains. Key aspects of the immune response to *E. scophthalmi* and *E. leei* have been studied (Sitjà-Bobadilla, 2008; Holzer *et al.*, 2021) and are summarized here.

Parasite invasion of the enteric paracellular space triggers a local cellular immune response, initially activating leucopoiesis, followed by leucocyte depletion in lymphohaematopoietic organs. Consequently, granulocytes (Álvarez-Pellitero *et al.*, 2008) and Ig^+ (immunoglobulin-positive) cell numbers (Bermúdez *et al.*, 2006b) increase at the intestine but decrease in the head kidney and spleen of *Enteromyxum*-infected fish (Cuesta *et al.*, 2006b; Sitjà-Bobadilla *et al.*, 2006; Álvarez-Pellitero *et al.*, 2008; Bermúdez *et al.*, 2010). In GSB, transcriptional and immunohistochemical studies revealed an increase in $Zap70^+$ (ζ-chain-associated protein kinase 70-positive) cells in the intestines, coinciding with a decrease in lymphohaematopoietic tissues. Proliferation assays supported the migration of these cells from central immune organs (Piazzon *et al.*, 2018). In turbot, immune cell recruitment was also inferred, as elevated counts of $Tnf\text{-}\alpha^+$ (tumour necrosis factor-α-positive) cells did not correlate with increased gene expression, suggesting mobilization of cells harbouring preformed intracellular cytokine pools (Ronza *et al.*, 2015). Enteromyxosis also induces increased respiratory burst activity in circulating phagocytes (Sitjà-Bobadilla *et al.*, 2008), elevated serum nitric oxide levels (Golomazou *et al.*, 2006a) and enhanced cell-mediated cytotoxicity (Cuesta *et al.*, 2006b). Despite this cellular activation, the parasite continues to develop and ultimately colonizes the entire intestinal tract in susceptible species.

Humoral innate factors such as peroxidases, lysozyme and complement are altered during enteromyxosis, though no single molecule appears critical for parasite clearance. Lysozyme levels decrease in exposed turbot and GSB (Sitjà-Bobadilla *et al.*, 2006, 2008), whereas in sharpsnout seabream, lysozyme is undetectable in both infected and healthy fish (Golomazou *et al.*, 2006b; Sitjà-Bobadilla *et al.*, 2007c), suggesting its absence may contribute to higher pathogenicity in this host (Álvarez-Pellitero *et al.*, 2008). The alternative complement pathway eventually becomes exhausted during infection (Cuesta *et al.*, 2006a; Sitjà-Bobadilla *et al.*, 2006, 2007c). Whether strategies aimed at enhancing basal levels of these factors could mitigate disease remains unclear.

Both turbot and GSB can mount a specific humoral immune response against *Enteromyxum* spp. (Sitjà-Bobadilla *et al.*, 2004; Estensoro *et al.*, 2010a), but antibody production is relatively slow. In turbot challenged with *E. scophthalmi*, specific antibodies were detected at 48 days pe in previously exposed fish (Sitjà-Bobadilla *et al.*, 2007b), while naïve fish developed disease and died without producing antibodies between 40 and 49 days pe (Redondo *et al.*, 2002; Sitjà-Bobadilla *et al.*, 2006). In GSB, enteromyxosis increases serum IgM and IgT titres, upregulates transcription of both isotypes (Piazzon *et al.*, 2016), and raises IgM^+ and plasma cell numbers in the gut (Estensoro *et al.*, 2014). Passive immunization showed that parasite-specific Igs are essential for overcoming infection. Although the parasite disrupts Ig expression as an evasion strategy, some fish mount a protective response, mainly via IgT (Picard-Sánchez *et al.*, 2020a). The importance of a proper IgT response was further supported by diet trials, where plant-based feeds suppressed intestinal soluble IgT and worsened disease outcomes (Piazzon *et al.*, 2016).

Although some information is available on parasite antigenic molecules (Sitjà-Bobadilla *et al.*, 2004; Estensoro *et al.*, 2010a), the specific antigens triggering this response remain unknown. A polyclonal antibody against *E. leei* detected several proteins in parasite extracts, highlighting two glycoproteins that cross-reacted with an antibody against *Myxobolus pendula* polar filament.

The identity of these antigens is still unknown (Estensoro *et al.*, 2013a). Tandem mass spectrometry (MS/MS) sequencing of *E. leei* proteins recognized by IgM from naturally immunized GSB revealed 12 candidate antigenic proteins, some of which are promising vaccine targets due to their secreted or transmembrane nature (Picard-Sánchez, 2021). The improvement of the quality of *Enteromyxum* genomes, along with further characterization of these antigens, are essential.

T-cell responses, Zap70$^+$ and Tbet$^+$ (T-box transcription factor 21-positive) cells increased significantly in the intestine of *E. leei*-infected GSB. Gene expression analyses showed a concurrent rise in cytotoxic T lymphocyte and Th1 (type 1 helper T cell) markers, indicating local T-cell activation modulated by the simultaneous upregulation of regulatory cytokines (Pérez-Cordón *et al.*, 2014, Piazzon *et al.*, 2018). *E. scophthalmi* also induced upregulation of type I response markers in the intestine and systemic tissues of turbot during early infection (Ronza *et al.*, 2016). However, at advanced stages, lymphocyte depletion, downregulation of T-cell markers, thymic atrophy and general suppression of the adaptive immune response were associated with greater susceptibility and pathology in this species (Bermúdez *et al.*, 2006b, 2010; Ronza *et al.*, 2020, 2021).

Genetically based intraspecific differences in host susceptibility have seldom been studied. The difference in the brood stock origin could contribute to differences in prevalence of different stocks during an observational study at an enzootic turbot farm (Quiroga *et al.*, 2006). However, experimental infections of selected turbot cohorts with *E. scophthalmi* did not reveal important differences in disease outcome (O. Palenzuela, A. Riaza, M.J. Redondo and P. Álvarez-Pellitero, 2005, unpublished results). Field and experimental data suggests that some GSB stocks are partially resistant to *E. leei* (Jublanc *et al.*, 2006; Sitjà-Bobadilla *et al.*, 2007a; Fleurance *et al.*, 2008). However, the influence of environmental conditions under natural conditions and the difficulty of applying homogeneous infective pressures in experimental infections hinder definitive conclusions. In any case, genetic selection, based on innate resistance, has not been exploited. None the less, heritability for innate resistance to these parasites and genetic correlations with other traits are not known. Therefore, estimating these parameters for enteromyxosis should be a priority to decide the best strategy for genetic breeding programmes. Some turbot companies have started selective breeding programmes, which may be a promising future strategy.

Acquired resistance to certain enteromyxoses offers a promising avenue for future vaccine development. Red seabream, sharpsnout seabream, GSB and turbot that had recovered from infection were refractory to reinfection and exhibited earlier and higher specific antibody titres (Golomazou *et al.*, 2006a; Sitjà-Bobadilla *et al.*, 2007b; Yanagida *et al.*, 2008; Picard-Sánchez *et al.*, 2019). In GSB, re-exposed individuals displayed a post-inflammatory phenotype characteristic of inflammation resolution Moreover, GSB injected with parasite-specific antibodies became infected but showed reduced disease signs and infection intensity (Picard-Sánchez *et al.*, 2020a). These findings underscore the crucial role of specific antibody responses and lay the groundwork for effective treatments or prophylactic strategies.

Different commercial aquafeeds include immunostimulant compounds, or nutraceuticals, which are presumed to enhance the fish immune system, mucosal barriers and overall potential against pathogens. In GSB, diets supplemented with Sanacore®GM mitigated the anorexia and growth arrestment and fish showed lower prevalence of infection and parasite load (Palenzuela *et al.*, 2020). Also in GSB, a diet supplemented with sodium butyrate avoided growth retardation in parasitized fish (Piazzon *et al.*, 2017), most likely due to a more efficient repair and improvement of the intestinal integrity and function (Estensoro *et al.*, 2016).

9.6. Conclusions and Suggestions for Future Studies

Over the past two decades, intensive research on *Enteromyxum* species has significantly advanced our understanding of their biology and host–pathogen interactions. However, key gaps remain, such as identifying the invertebrate host and developing *in vitro* culture or cryopreservation methods – crucial for producing consistent parasite sources for vaccine and drug screening. There is also a need for rapid, point-of-care diagnostic tools and environmental risk assessment methods. Exploring global genetic diversity, including intraspecific variation in *E. leei* and the discovery of new species, may reveal important insights into the evolution, virulence and control of the genus. Comprehensive characterization at structural, genetic, transcriptomic, proteomic and antigenic levels is essential to better understand host–parasite dynamics and identify therapeutic targets. Emerging technologies, such as specific cell markers, immune cell isolation and single-cell transcriptomics, will be instrumental in uncovering immune mechanisms and resistance genes, ultimately clarifying the basis of host susceptibility and guiding disease control strategies.

Acknowledgements

The authors thank Dr Hiroshi Yokoyama (Okayama University of Science, Japan) and Carlos Zarza (Skretting, Spain) for providing updated information on disease status in aquaculture and diseased fish images. We would also like to show our recognition to Prof. Pilar Álvarez-Pellitero, who pioneered research on these parasites in the late 1990s at the Instituto de Acuicultura Torre de la Sal, CSIC Fish Pathology Group. Part of the information gathered in this chapter was obtained through different research projects: (i) *MucosalFrontier* (PID2020-115070RA-I00) funded by Spanish MCIN/AEI/10.13039/501100011033; (ii) the Generalitat Valenciana through the *ThinkInAzul* programme, supported by MICIU (Spanish Ministry of Science, Innovation and Universities) with funding from European Union NextGenerationEU (PRTR-C17.I1) and by Generalitat Valenciana (GVA-THINKINAZUL/2021/22), and CIAICO/2022/144 to Consolidated Groups; and (iii) the European Union, through the Horizon2020 research and innovation programme grant agreement 634429 (*ParaFishControl*). This publication reflects only the authors' view, and the European Union cannot be held responsible for any use that may be made of the information contained herein.

References

Alonso, M., Lago, F.C., Gómez-Reino, M., Fernández Casal, J., Martín Varela, I. *et al.* (2015) Non-invasive fast real-time PCR assay for detection of the enteric parasite *Enteromyxum scophthalmi* in cultured turbot (*Scophthalmus maximus* L.). *Aquaculture Research* 46(9), 2104–2115. DOI: 10.1111/are.12366.

Álvarez-Pellitero, P., Crespo, S., Marques, A., Athanassopoulou, F., Ghittino, C. and Diamant, A. (2005) MyxFishControl European Project (QLK2-CT-2001-00722) Internal Report. Available at: https://cordis.europa.eu/project/id/QLK2-CT-2002-00722/results (accessed 3 December 2025).

Álvarez-Pellitero, P., Palenzuela, O. and Sitjà-Bobadilla, A. (2008) Histopathology and cellular response in *Enteromyxum leei* (Myxozoa) infections of *Diplodus puntazzo* (Teleostei). *Parasitology International* 57(2), 110–120. DOI: 10.1016/j.parint.2007.09.004.

Athanassopoulou, F., Prapas, T. and Rodger, H. (1999) Diseases of *Puntazzo puntazzo* Cuvier in marine aquaculture systems in Greece. *Journal of Fish Diseases* 22(3), 215–218. DOI: 10.1046/j.1365-2761.1999.00151.x.

Atkinson, S.D., Bartholomew, J.L. and Rouse, G.W. (2020) The invertebrate host of salmonid fish parasites *Ceratonova shasta* and *Parvicapsula minibicornis* (Cnidaria: Myxozoa), is a novel fabriciid annelid, *Manayunkia occidentalis* sp. nov. (Sabellida: Fabriciidae). *Zootaxa* 4751(2), 310–320–310–320. DOI: 10.11646/zootaxa.4751.2.6.

Beraldo, P., Volpatti, D., Bulfon, C., Fioravanti, M.L. and Galeotti, M. (2011) Histopathological surveys during spontaneous *Enteromyxum leei* infection in sharpsnout seabream (*Diplodus puntazzo*, Cetti 1777). *Ittiopatologia* 8(1–3), 63–78.

Bermúdez, R., Aleman, N., Vigliano, F., Vázquez, S., Quiroga, M.I. and Nieto, J.M. (2006a) Effects of symmetric triazinone (toltrazuril) on developmental stages of *Enteromyxum scophthalmi* parasitizing turbot (*Scophthalmus maximus* L.): a light and electron microscopic study. *Aquaculture* 254(1–4), 65–71. DOI: 10.1016/j.aquaculture.2005.10.042.

Bermúdez, R., Vigliano, F., Marcaccini, A., Sitjà-Bobadilla, A., Quiroga, M.I. and Nieto, J.M. (2006b) Response of Ig-positive cells to *Enteromyxum scophthalmi* (Myxozoa) experimental infection in turbot, *Scophthalmus maximus* (L.): a histopathological and immunohistochemical study. *Fish and Shellfish Immunology* 21(5), 501–512. DOI: 10.1016/j.fsi.2006.02.006.

Bermúdez, R., Vigliano, F., Quiroga, M.I., Nieto, J.M., Bosi, G. and Domeneghini, C. (2007) Immunohistochemical study on the neuroendocrine system of the digestive tract of turbot, *Scophthalmus maximus* (L.), infected by *Enteromyxum scophthalmi* (Myxozoa). *Fish and Shellfish Immunology* 22(3), 252–263.

Bermúdez, R., Losada, A.P., Vazquez, S., Redondo, M.J., Álvarez-Pellitero, P. and Quiroga, M.I. (2010) Light and electron microscopic studies on turbot *Psetta maxima* infected with *Enteromyxum scophthalmi*: histopathology of turbot enteromyxosis. *Diseases of Aquatic Organisms* 89(3), 209–221. DOI: 10.3354/dao02202.

Branson, E., Riaza, A. and Álvarez-Pellitero, P. (1999) Myxosporean infection causing intestinal disease in farmed turbot, *Scophthalmus maximus* (L.), (Teleostei: Scophthalmidae). *Journal of Fish Diseases* 22(5), 395–399. DOI: 10.1046/j.1365-2761.1999.00193.x.

Caffara, M., Delgado, M., Fioravanti, M., Quaglio, F. and Restani, R. (1999) *Myxidium leei* (Myxozoa, Myxosporea) in sparidi (*Sparus aurata* e *Diplodus puntazzo*) allevati in Italia. *Bollettino Società Italiana Patologia Ittica* 27, 10–17. Available at: https://hdl.handle.net/11577/2517783 (accessed 20 November 2025).

Chang, E.S., Neuhof, M., Rubinstein, N.D., Diamant, A., Philippe, H. *et al.* (2015) Genomic insights into the evolutionary origin of Myxozoa within Cnidaria. *Proceedings of the National Academy of Sciences USA* 112(48), 14912–14917. DOI: 10.1073/pnas.1511468112.

China, M., Nakamura, H., Hamakawa, K., Tamaki, E., Miwa, S. *et al.* (2013) Occurrence of the myxosporean emaciation disease caused by *Enteromyxum leei* in cultured Malabar grouper *Epinephelus malabaricus*. *Fish Pathology* 48(3), 88–96. DOI: 10.3147/jsfp.48.88.

China, M., Nakamura, H., Hamakawa, K., Tamaki, E., Yokoyama, H. *et al.* (2014) Efficacy of high water temperature treatment of myxosporean emaciation disease caused by *Enteromyxum leei* (Myxozoa). *Fish Pathology* 49(3), 137–140. DOI: 10.3147/jsfp.49.137.

Cho, Y.-G., Hur, S.-P. and Shin, S.P. (2024) Experimental infection of *Enteromyxum leei* to red seabream *Pagrus major*. *Journal of Fish Pathology* 37(2), 269–275. DOI: 10.7847/jfp.2024.37.2.269.

Cuadrado, M. (2009) Enteromixosi produïda per *Enteromyxum leei* (Diamant, Lom i Dyková, 1994) en espàrids d'interès comercial del Mediterrani. PhD thesis, Universitat Autònoma de Barcelona, Barcelona, Spain.

Cuadrado, M., Albinyana, G., Padrós, F., Redondo, M.J., Sitjà-Bobadilla, A. *et al.* (2007) An unidentified epi-epithelial myxosporean in the intestine of gilthead sea bream *Sparus aurata* L. *Parasitology Research* 101(2), 403–411.

Cuadrado, M., Marques, A., Diamant, A., Sitjà-Bobadilla, A., Palenzuela, O. *et al* (2008) Ultrastructure of *Enteromyxum leei* (Diamant, Lom, & Dykova, 1994) (Myxozoa), an enteric parasite infecting gilthead sea bream (*Sparus aurata*) and sharpsnout sea bream (*Diplodus puntazzo*). *Journal of Eukaryotic Microbiology* 55(3), 178–184. DOI: 10.1111/j.1550-7408.2008.00325.x.

Cuesta, A., Muñoz, P., Rodríguez, A., Salinas, I., Sitjà-Bobadilla, A. *et al.* (2006a) Gilthead seabream (*Sparus aurata* L.) innate defence against the parasite *Enteromyxum leei* (Myxozoa). *Parasitology* 132(1), 95–104. DOI: 10.1017/S0031182005008759.

Cuesta, A., Salinas, I., Rodríguez, A., Muñoz, P., Sitjà-Bobadilla, A. *et al.* (2006b) Cell-mediated cytotoxicity is the main innate immune mechanism involved in the cellular defence of gilthead seabream (Teleostei: Sparidae) against *Enteromyxum leei* (Myxozoa). *Parasite Immunology* 28(12), 657–665. DOI: 10.1111/j.1365-3024.2006.00905.x.

Diamant, A. (1992) A new pathogenic histozoic *Myxidium* (Myxosporea) in cultured gilthead sea bream *Sparus aurata* L. *Bulletin of the European Association of Fish Pathologists* 12(2), 64–66.

Diamant, A. (1995) *Myxidium leei* (Myxosporea) infections in sharpsnout sea bream *Diplodus puntazzo* (Cetti) and common sea bream *Pagrus pagrus* (L.) (Sparidae). In: *Program and Book of Abstracts, IV International Symposium of Fish Parasitology*, Munich, Germany, 3–7 October 1995, Abstract #8.

Diamant, A. (1997) Fish-to-fish transmission of a marine myxosporean. *Diseases of Aquatic Organisms* 30(2), 99–105.

Diamant, A. (1998) Red drum *Sciaenops ocellatus* (Sciaenidae), a recent introduction to Mediterranean mariculture, is susceptible to *Myxidium leei* (Myxosporea). *Aquaculture* 162(1–2), 33–39. DOI: 10.1016/S0044-8486(97)00307-4.

Diamant, A. and Wajsbrot, N. (1997) Experimental transmision of *Myxidium leei* in gilthead sea bream *Sparus aurata*. *Bulletin of the European Association of Fish Pathologists* 17(3–4), 99–103.

Diamant, A., Lom, J. and Dyková, I. (1994) *Myxidium leei* n. sp., a pathogenic myxosporean of cultured sea bream *Sparus aurata*. *Diseases of Aquatic Organisms* 20(2), 137–141. DOI: 10.3354/dao020137.

Diamant, A., Colorni A and Ucko, M. (2004) *Monitoring program of mortality and disease in wild fish populations in the Gulf of Eilat, northern Red Sea*. Israeli Ministry of Environmental Protection, International Expert

Team Project No. 22. Available at: https://www.gov.il/en/pages/studies_and_surveys_in_the_gulf_of_eilat (accessed 20 November 2020).

Diamant, A., Palenzuela, O., Álvarez-Pellitero, P., Athanassopoulou, F., Golomazou, E. (2006a) Epizootiology of *Enteromyxum leei* (Myxozoa: Myxosporea) in Mediterranean mariculture systems. In: *5th International Symposium on Aquatic Animal Health Proceedings*, San Francisco, California, 2–6 September 2006.

Diamant, A., Ram, S. and Paperna, I. (2006b) Experimental transmission of *Enteromyxum leei* to freshwater fish. *Diseases of Aquatic Organisms* 72(2), 171–178.

Estensoro, I., Bermúdez, R., Losada, A.P., Quiroga, M.I., Álvarez-Pellitero, P. and Sitjà-Bobadilla, A. (2009) Effect of *Enteromyxum leei* (Myxozoa) on gastrointestinal neuromodulators and cell apoptosis of gilthead sea bream (*Sparus aurata*). In: *Abstract Book, 14th International Conference of the European Association of Fish Pathologists (EAFP) on Diseases of Fish and Shellfish*, Prague, 14–19 September 2007. European Association of Fish Pathologists, Prague, pp. 142–143. Available at: https://digital.csic.es/handle/10261/255106 (accessed 20 November 2025).

Estensoro, I., Redondo, M.J., Álvarez-Pellitero, P. and Sitjà-Bobadilla, A. (2010a) Detection of specific antibodies against *Enteromyxum leei* (Myxozoa: Myxosporea) in gilthead sea bream (*Sparus aurata*) by ELISA and immunohistochemistry. In: *Abstract Book, 1st Symposium of the European Organisation of Fish Immunology*, Viterbo, Italy, p. 44.

Estensoro, I., Redondo, M.J., Álvarez-Pellitero, P. and Sitjà-Bobadilla, A. (2010b) Novel horizontal transmission route for *Enteromyxum leei* (Myxozoa) by anal intubation of gilthead sea bream *Sparus aurata*. *Diseases of Aquatic Organisms* 92(1), 51–58.

Estensoro, I., Benedito-Palos, L., Palenzuela, O., Kaushik, S., Sitjà-Bobadilla, A. and Pérez-Sánchez, J. (2011) The nutritional background of the host alters the disease course in a fish-myxosporean system. *Veterinary Parasitology* 175(1–2), 141–150. DOI: 10.1016/j.vetpar.2010.09.015.

Estensoro, I., Redondo, M.J., Salesa, B., Kaushik, S., Pérez-Sánchez, J. and Sitjà-Bobadilla, A. (2012) Effect of nutrition and *Enteromyxum leei* infection on gilthead sea bream Sparus aurata intestinal carbohydrate distribution. *Diseases of Aquatic Organisms* 100(1), 29–42. DOI: 10.3354/dao02486.

Estensoro, I., Álvarez-Pellitero, P. and Sitjà-Bobadilla, A. (2013a) Antigenic characterization of *Enteromyxum leei* (Myxozoa: Myxosporea). *Diseases of Aquatic Organisms* 106(2), 149–162. DOI: 10.3354/dao02651.

Estensoro, I., Jung-Schroers, V., Álvarez-Pellitero, P., Steinhagen, D. and Sitjà-Bobadilla, A. (2013b) Effects of *Enteromyxum leei* (Myxozoa) infection on gilthead sea bream (*Sparus aurata*) (Teleostei) intestinal mucus: glycoprotein profile and bacterial adhesion. *Parasitology Research* 112(2), 567–576. DOI: 10.1007/s00436-012-3168-3.

Estensoro, I., Mulero, I., Redondo, M.J., Álvarez-Pellitero, P., Mulero, V. and Sitjà-Bobadilla, A. (2014) Modulation of leukocytic populations of gilthead sea bream (*Sparus aurata*) by the intestinal parasite *Enteromyxum leei* (Myxozoa: Myxosporea). *Parasitology* 141(3), 425–440. DOI: 10.1017/S0031182013001789.

Estensoro, I., Ballester-Lozano, G., Benedito-Palos, L., Grammes, F., Martos-Sitcha, J.A. *et al.* (2016) Dietary butyrate helps to restore the intestinal status of a marine teleost (*Sparus aurata*) fed extreme diets low in fish meal and fish oil. *PLoS One* 11(11), e0166564. DOI: 10.1371/journal.pone.0166564.

Estensoro, I., Pérez-Cordón, G., Sitjà-Bobadilla, A. and Piazzon, M.C. (2018) Bromodeoxyuridine DNA labelling reveals host and parasite proliferation in a fish-myxozoan model. *Journal of Fish Diseases* 41(4), 651–662. DOI: 10.1111/jfd.12765.

Eszterbauer, E., Atkinson, S., Diamant, A., Morris, D., El-Matbouli Mansour, M. and Hartikainen, H. (2015) Myxozoan life cycles: practical approaches and insights. In: Okamura, B., Gruhl, A. and Bartholomew, J. (eds) *Myxozoan Evolution, Ecology and Development*. Springer, Cham, Switzerland, pp. 175–198. DOI: 10.1007/978-3-319-14753-6_10.

Farmer, K., Perry, S.M., Meredith, A., Woodyard, E.T., Rosser, T.G. *et al.* (2025) Acute mortality event in false pilchards *Harengula clupeola* after salinomycin and amprolium treatment for myxozoan (*Enteromyxum leei*) infection. *Diseases of Aquatic Organisms* 161, 23–28. DOI: 10.3354/dao03835.

Feist, S.W. and Longshaw, M. (2006) Phylum myxozoa. In: Woo, P.T.K. (ed.) *Fish Diseases and Disorders, Volume 1: Protozoan and Metazoan Infections*. CAB International, Wallingford, UK, pp. 230–296.

Feng, J.M., Xiong, J., Zhang, J.Y., Yang, Y.L., Yao, B. *et al.* (2014) New phylogenomic and comparative analyses provide corroborating evidence that Myxozoa is Cnidaria. *Molecular Phylogenetics and Evolution* 81, 10–18. DOI: 10.1016/j.ympev.2014.08.016.

Fioravanti, M.L., Caffara, M., Florio, D., Gustinelli, A. and Marcer, F. (2006) A parasitological survey of European sea bass (*Dicentrarchus labrax*) and gilthead sea bream (*Sparus aurata*) cultured in Italy. *Veterinary Research Communications* 30(2), 249–252. DOI: 10.1007/s11259-006-9021-3.

Fioravanti, M., Mladineo, I., Palenzuela, O., Beraldo, P., Massimo, M. *et al.* (2020) *Fish Farmer's Guide to Combating Parasitic Infections in European Sea Bass and Gilthead Sea Bream Aquaculture.*

A Series of Para Fish Control Guides to Combating Fish Parasite Infections in Aquaculture. Publicaciones CSIC, Madrid. e-NIPO:833-20-104-5.

Fleurance, R., Sauvegrain, C., Marques, A., Le Breton, A., Guereaud, C. *et al.* (2008) Histopathological changes caused by *Enteromyxum leei* infection in farmed sea bream *Sparus aurata*. *Diseases of Aquatic Organisms* 79(3), 219–228.

Foox, J., Ringuette, M., Desser, S.S. and Siddall, M.E. (2015) *In silico* hybridization enables transcriptomic illumination of the nature and evolution of Myxozoa. *BMC Genomics* 16(1), 840. DOI: 10.1186/s12864-015-2039-6.

Fox, M.D., Bartholomew, J.L. and Palenzuela, O. (2000) Strategies for the diagnosis of *Ceratomyxa shasta* using the polymerase chain reaction: comparison of lethal and nonlethal sampling with microscopic examination. *Journal of Aquatic Animal Health* 12(2), 100–106. DOI: 10.1577/1548-8667(200006)012<0100:SFTDOC>2.0.CO;2.

Freeman, M.A., Yanagida, T. and Kristmundsson, À. (2020) A novel histozoic myxosporean, *Enteromyxum caesio* n. sp., infecting the redbelly yellowtail fusilier, *Caesio cuning*, with the creation of the Enteromyxidae n. fam., to formally accommodate this commercially important genus. *PeerJ* 2020(7), e9529. DOI: 10.7717/peerj.9529.

Golomazou, E., Athanassopoulou, F., Karagouni, E., Tsagozis, P., Tsantilas, H. and Vagianou, S. (2006a) Experimental transmission of *Enteromyxum leei* Diamant, Lom and Dykova, 1994 in sharpsnout sea bream, *Diplodus puntazzo* C. and the effect on some innate immune parameters. *Aquaculture* 260(1–4), 44–53.

Golomazou, E., Athanassopoulou, F., Karagouni, E., Vagianou, S., Tsantilas, H. and Karamanis, D. (2006b) Efficacy and toxicity of orally administrated anti-coccidial drug treatment on *Enteromyxum leei* infections in sharpsnout seabream (*Diplodus puntazzo* C.). *Israeli Journal of Aquaculture – Bamidgeh* 58(3), 157–169. DOI: 10.46989/001C.20444.

Golomazou, E., Athanassopoulou, F., Vagianou, S., Sabatakou, O., Tsantilas, H. *et al.* (2006c) Diseases of white sea bream (*Diplodus sargus* L.) reared in experimental and commercial conditions in Greece. *Turkish Journal of Veterinary and Animal Sciences* 30(4), 389–396.

Golomazou, E., Exadactylos, A., Malandrakis, E.E., Karatzinos, T., Gkafas, G. *et al.* (2014) Early diagnosis of enteromyxosis in intensively reared sharpsnout seabream, *Diplodus Puntazzo*. *Aquatic Living Resources* 27(2), 99–106. DOI: 10.1051/alr/2014010.

Golomazou, E., Karagouni, E. and Athanassopoulou, F. (2017) The most important Myxosparean parasite species affecting cultured Mediterranean fish. *Journal of the Hellenic Veterinary Medical Society* 55(4), 342–352. DOI: 10.12681/jhvms.15145.

Henry, M.A., Kokou, F., Palenzuela, O., Pyrenis, G. and Rigos, G. (2020) Experimental infection model with the bivalvulid *Enteromyxum leei* (Myxidiidae) in the sharpsnout seabream, *Diplodus puntazzo* (Sparidae), and evaluation of the antiparasitic efficacy of a functional diet. *Folia Parasitologica* 67, 024. DOI: 10.14411/fp.2020.024.

Holzer, A.S., Piazzon, M.C., Barrett, D., Bartholomew, J.L. and Sitjà-Bobadilla, A. (2021) To react or not to react: the dilemma of fish immune systems facing myxozoan infections. *Frontiers in Immunology* 12, 734238. DOI: 10.3389/fimmu.2021.734238.

Hyatt, M.W. (2009) Successful treatment on enteric myxosporiosis in a collection of yellow tangs *Zebrasoma flavescens* at a public aquarium. *Florida Aqua News* 4, 1–6.

Hyatt, M.W., Waltzek, T.B., Kieran, E.A., Frasca, S. and Lovy, J. (2018) Diagnosis and treatment of multi-species fish mortality attributed to *Enteromyxum leei* while in quarantine at a US aquarium. *Diseases of Aquatic Organisms* 132(1), 37–48. DOI: 10.3354/dao03303.

Ishimatsu, A., Hayashi, M., Nakane, M. and Sameshima, M. (2007) Pathophysiology of cultured tiger puffer *Takifugu rubripes* suffering from the myxosporean emaciation disease. *Fish Pathology* 42(4), 12.

Jublanc, E., Elkiric, N., Toubiana, M., Widada, J.S., Le Breton, A. *et al.* (2005). Observation on a *Enteromyxum leei* (Myxozoa Myxosporea) parasitosis on farming sea bream *Sparus aurata*. *Journal of Eukaryotic Microbiology* 52(2), 28S–34S. DOI: 10.1111/j.1550-7408.2005.05202003_3_19.x.

Jublanc, E., Toubiana, M., Sri Widada, J., Le Breton, A., LeFebvre, G. *et al.* (2006) Observation of a survival case following infestation by *Enteromyxum leei* (Myxozoa Myxosporea), a pathogenic myxosporidian of the digestive duct of the gilthead sea bream (*Sparus aurata*) in pisciculture. *Journal of Eukaryotic Microbiology* 53, 20S.

Katata, M. and Okuyama, Y. (2017) Development of loop-mediated isothermal amplification methods for detection of the enteric myxosporeans causing myxosporean emaciation disease. *Fish Pathology* 52(2), 1–16. DOI: 10.3147/jsfp.52.104.

Katharios, P., Rigos, G. and Divanach, P. (2011) *Enteromyxum leei* (Myxozoa), a lethal intruder of tropical pet fish: first case in humphead wrasse, *Cheilinus undulatus* (Rüppell, 1835). *Journal of Exotic Pet Medicine* 20(2), 138–143. DOI: 10.1053/j.jepm.2011.02.009.

Katharios, P., Kokkari, C., Sterioti, A., Smyrli, M. and Kalatzis, P.G. (2014) *Enteromyxum leei* infection in parrotfish, *Sparisoma cretense*: histopathological, morphological and molecular study. *Veterinary Parasitology* 199(3–4), 136–143. DOI: 10.1016/j.vetpar.2013.10.011.

Kent, M.L., Andree, K.B., Bartholomew, J.L., El-Matbouli, M., Desser, S.S. *et al.* (2001) Recent advances in our knowledge of the Myxozoa. *Journal of Eukaryotic Microbiology* 48(4), 395–413. DOI: 10.1111/j.1550-7408.2001.tb00173.x.

Kim, J., Yoon, S., Mansoor, S., Jung, C.Y., Kim, C.S. and Boo, K.H. (2025) Parasiticidal activity of citral against *Enteromyxum leei* (myxozoa: Myxosporea) in olive flounder (*Paralichthys olivaceus*). *Acta Parasitologica* 70(2), 74. DOI: 10.1007/S11686-025-01011-4.

Kim, S.M., Jun, L.J., Park, M.A., Jeong, H.D. and Jeong, J.B. (2015) Characterization of the myxosporean parasite isolated from emaciated olive flounders *Paralichthys olivaceus* on Jeju Island. *Korean Journal of Fisheries and Aquatic Sciences* 48(3), 337–345. DOI: 10.5657/kfas.2015.0337.

Køie, M., Whipps, C.M. and Kent, M.L. (2013) *Ellipsomyxa gobii* (Myxozoa: Ceratomyxidae) in the common goby *Pomatoschistus microps* (Teleostei: Gobiidae) uses *Nereis* spp. (Annelida: Polychaeta) as invertebrate hosts. *Folia Parasitologica* 51(1), 14–18. DOI: 10.14411/FP.2004.002.

Le Breton, A. and Marques, A. (1995) Occurrence of an histozoic *Myxidium* infection in two marine cultured species: *Puntazzo puntazzo* C. and *Pagrus major*. *Bulletin of the European Association of Fish Pathologists* 15(6), 210–212.

Lee, Y.J., Jun, L.J., Kim, Y.J., Han, J.E., Ko, Y.J. *et al.* (2024a) Comparison of specificity and sensitivity of diagnostic methods for *Enteromyxum leei* and *Enteromyxum fugu* detected from cultured tiger puffer, *Takifugu rubripes* in Korea. *Journal of Fish Diseases* 47(1), e13865. DOI: 10.1111/jfd.13865.

Lee, Y.J, Jun, L.J, Oh, Y.E, Lee, E.J. and Jeong, J.B. (2024b) Case report of *Enteromyxum leei*, the causative agent of emaciation disease in olive flounder (*Paralichthys olivaceus*) farm in Wando. *Journal of Fish Pathology* 37(2), 277–283. DOI: 10.7847/JFP.2024.37.2.277.

Lee, Y.J., Oh, Y.E., Lee, E.J., Jun, L.J. and Jeong, J.B. (2025) Evaluation of cytotoxicity and antiparasitic effects of toltrazuril against *Enteromyxum leei* in olive flounders: *in vitro* and *in vivo* studies. *Journal of Fish Diseases* 48(11), e14125. DOI: 10.1111/jfd.14125.

Lom, J. and Dyková, I. (2006) Myxozoan genera: definition and notes on taxonomy, life-cycle terminology and pathogenic species. *Folia Parasitologica* 53(1), 1–36. DOI: 10.14411/fp.2006.001.

Losada, A.P., Bermúdez, R., Faílde, L.D. and Quiroga, M.I. (2012) Quantitative and qualitative evaluation of iNOS expression in turbot (*Psetta maxima*) infected with *Enteromyxum scophthalmi*. *Fish and Shellfish Immunology* 32(2), 243–248. DOI: 10.1016/j.fsi.2011.11.007.

Losada, A.P., Bermúdez, R., Faílde, L.D., Di Giancamillo, A., Domeneghini, C. and Quiroga, M.I. (2014a) Effects of *Enteromyxum scophthalmi* experimental infection on the neuroendocrine system of turbot, *Scophthalmus maximus* (L.). *Fish and Shellfish Immunology* 40(2), 577–583. DOI: 10.1016/j.fsi.2014.08.011.

Losada, A.P., Bermúdez, R., Faílde, L.D., de Ocenda, M.V.R. and Quiroga, M.I. (2014b) Study of the distribution of active caspase-3-positive cells in turbot, *Scophthalmus maximus* (L.), enteromyxosis. *Journal of Fish Diseases* 37(1), 21–32. DOI: 10.1111/jfd.12029.

Marino, F., Macri, D., Paruta, S., Busalacchi, B., Genovese, L. and De Vico, G. (2004) Black spot seabream (*Pagellus bogaraveo*), a new susceptible host for *Myxidium leei*. In: Adams, S. and Olafsen, J.A. (eds) *Extended Abstracts and Short Communications Booklet*. European Aquaculture Society Special Publication No. 34. European Aquaculture Society, Barcelona, Spain, pp. 524–525.

Montero, F.E., Cuadrado, M., Padrós, F., Crespo, S. and Raga, J.A. (2007) *Cryptocaryon irritans* and *Enteromyxum leei*, two threats for the culture of *Diplodus puntazzo* in the Mediterranean. *Bulletin of the European Association of Fish Pathologists* 27(6), 242–249.

Muñoz, P., Cuesta, A., Athanassopoulou, F., Golomazou, H., Crespo, S. *et al.* (2007) Sharpsnout sea bream (*Diplodus puntazzo*) humoral immune response against the parasite *Enteromyxum leei* (Myxozoa). *Fish and Shellfish Immunology* 23(3), 636–645. DOI: 10.1016/j.fsi.2007.01.014.

Ogawa, K. and Yokoyama, H. (2001) Emaciation disease of cultured tiger puffer *Takifugu rubripes*. *Bulletin of the National Research Institute of Aquaculture* 5S, 210–212.

Özer, A., Öztürk, T., Özkan, H. and Çam, A. (2014) First report of *Enteromyxum leei* (Myxozoa) in the Black Sea in a potential reservoir host *Chromis chromis*. *Fish Pathology* 49(2), 57–60. Available at: https://www.jstage.jst.go.jp/article/jsfp/49/2/49_57/_pdf (accessed 20 November 2025).

Padrós, F., Palenzuela, O., Hispano, C., Tosas, O., Zarza, C. *et al.* (2001) *Myxidium leei* (Myxozoa) infections in aquarium-reared Mediterranean fish species. *Diseases of Aquatic Organisms* 47(1), 57–62. DOI: 10.3354/dao047057.

Palenzuela, O. (2006) Myxozoan infections in Mediterranean mariculture. *Parassitologia* 48(1–2), 27–29. Available at: http://www.ncbi.nlm.nih.gov/entrez/query.fcgi?cmd=Retrieve&db=PubMed&dopt=Citation&list_uids=16881390 (accessed 20 November 2025).

Palenzuela, O., Redondo, M.J. and Álvarez-Pellitero, P. (2002) Description of *Enteromyxum scophthalmi* gen. nov., sp. nov. (Myxozoa), an intestinal parasite of turbot (*Scophthalmus maximus* L.) using morphological and ribosomal RNA sequence data. *Parasitology* 124(4), 369–379. DOI: 10.1017/S0031182001001354.

Palenzuela, O., Agnetti, F.G.A., Álvarez-Pellitero, P.F.A., Crespo, S., Diamant, A. and Ghittino, C. (2004) Applicability of PCR screening for the monitoring of *Enteromyxum leei* (Myxozoa) infection in Mediterranean aquaculture: an epidemiological survey in sparid facilities. In: Adams, S. and Olafsen, J.A. (eds) *Extended Abstracts and Short Communications Booklet*. European Aquaculture Society Special Publication No. 34. European Aquaculture Society, Barcelona, Spain, pp. 639–640.

Palenzuela, O., Redondo, M.J., López-Grandal, E. and Álvarez-Pellitero, M. del P. (2007) Cultured sole, *Solea senegalensis* is susceptible to *Enteromyxum scophthalmi*, the myxozoan parasite causing turbot emaciative enteritis. In: Matiucci, S., Damiano, S. and Paoletti (eds) *7th International Symposium on Fish Parasites Abstract Book. Parassitologia* 49(), 73.

Palenzuela, O., López-Grandal, E., Zarza, C. and Álvarez-Pellitero, M. del P. (2009) Treatment of turbot enteromyxosis with antiparasitic drugs and bioactive natural extracts-suplemented feeds. In: *Abstract Book, 14th International Conference of the European Association of Fish Pathologists (EAFP) on Diseases of Fish and Shellfish*, Prague, 14–19 September 2007. European Association of Fish Pathologists, Prague, pp. 142–143. Available at: https://digital.csic.es/handle/10261/255112 (accessed 20 November 2025).

Palenzuela, O., Del Pozo, R., Piazzon, M.C., Isern-Subich, M.M., Ceulemans, S. *et al.* (2020) Effect of a functional feed additive on mitigation of experimentally induced gilthead sea bream *Sparus aurata* enteromyxosis. *Diseases of Aquatic Organisms* 138, 111–120. DOI: 10.3354/dao03453.

Palenzuela, O., Cook, A., Del Pozo, R., Mladineo, I., Hrabar, J. *et al.* (2021a) *Enteromyxum leei* in Mediterranean gilthead sea bream farms: how much is out there? In: *Abstract Book, Aquaculture Europe 21 'Oceans of Opportunity'*, Funchal, Madeira, Portugal, 4–7 October 2021, pp. 925–926. Available at: https://digital.csic.es/handle/10261/267363 (accessed 20 November 2025).

Palenzuela, O., Piazzon, M.C. and Sitjà-Bobadilla, A. (2021b) *Enteromyxum scophthalmi*. In: Sitjà-Bobadilla, A., Bron, J., Wiegertjes, G. and Piazzon, M.C. (eds) *Fish Parasites: A Handbook of Protocols for their Isolation, Culture and Transmission*. European Association of Fish Pathologists (EAFP)/5m Books Series. CAB International, Wallingford, UK, pp. 143–156. DOI: 10.1079/9781800629127.0010.

Pérez-Cordón, G., Estensoro, I., Benedito-Palos, L., Calduch-Giner, J.A., Sitjà-Bobadilla, A. and Pérez-Sánchez, J. (2014) Interleukin gene expression is strongly modulated at the local level in a fish-parasite model. *Fish and Shellfish Immunology* 37(2), 201–208. DOI: 10.1016/j.fsi.2014.01.022.

Pérez-Sánchez, J., Estensoro, I., Redondo, M.J., Calduch-Giner, J.A., Kaushik, S. and Sitjà-Bobadilla, A. (2013) Mucins as diagnostic and prognostic biomarkers in a fish–parasite model: transcriptional and functional analysis. *PLoS One* 8(6), e65457. DOI: 10.1371/journal.pone.0065457.

Piazzon, M.C., Galindo-Villegas, J., Pereiro, P., Estensoro, I., Calduch-Giner, J.A. *et al.* (2016) Differential modulation of IgT and IgM upon parasitic, bacterial, viral, and dietary challenges in a perciform fish. *Frontiers in Immunology* 7, 637. DOI: 10.3389/fimmu.2016.00637.

Piazzon, M.C., Calduch-Giner, J.A., Fouz, B., Estensoro, I., Simó-Mirabet, P. *et al.* (2017) Under control: how a dietary additive can restore the gut microbiome and proteomic profile, and improve disease resilience in a marine teleostean fish fed vegetable diets. *Microbiome* 5(1), 164. DOI: 10.1186/S40168-017-0390-3.

Piazzon, M.C., Estensoro, I., Calduch-Giner, J.A., Pozo, R. Del, Picard-Sánchez, A. *et al.* (2018) Hints on T cell responses in a fish–parasite model: *Enteromyxum leei* induces differential expression of T cell signature molecules depending on the organ and the infection status. *Parasites and Vectors* 11(1), 443. DOI: 10.1186/s13071-018-3007-1.

Piazzon, M.C., Naya-Català, F., Perera, E., Palenzuela, O., Sitjà-Bobadilla, A. and Pérez-Sánchez, J. (2020) Genetic selection for growth drives differences in intestinal microbiota composition and parasite disease resistance in gilthead sea bream. *Microbiome* 8(1), 168. DOI: 10.1186/s40168-020-00922-w.

Piazzon, M.C., Naya-Català, F., Pereira, G.V., Estensoro, I., Del Pozo, R. *et al.* (2022) A novel fish meal-free diet formulation supports proper growth and does not impair intestinal parasite susceptibility in gilthead sea bream (*Sparus aurata*) with a reshape of gut microbiota and tissue-specific gene expression patterns. *Aquaculture* 558, 738362. DOI: 10.1016/j.aquaculture.2022.738362.

Picard-Sánchez, M.A. (2021) Control of enteric parasitic diseases of farmed gilthead sea bream: new insights into *Enteromyxum leei* (Myxozoa) and *Enterospora nucleophila* (Microsporidia) infections. [PhD Thesis] Universitat Politècnica de Valencia, Valencia, Spain. DOI: 10.4995/Thesis/10251/167035.

Picard-Sánchez, A., Estensoro, I., del Pozo, R., Piazzon, M.C., Palenzuela, O. and Sitjà-Bobadilla, A. (2019) Acquired protective immune response in a fish–myxozoan model encompasses specific antibodies and inflammation resolution. *Fish and Shellfish Immunology* 90(April), 349–362. DOI: 10.1016/j.fsi.2019.04.300.

Picard-Sánchez, A., Estensoro, I., Perdiguero, P., del Pozo, R., Tafalla, C. *et al.* (2020a) Passive immunization delays disease outcome in gilthead sea bream infected with *Enteromyxum leei* (Myxozoa), despite the moderate changes in IgM and IgT repertoire. *Frontiers in Immunology* 11, 581361. DOI: 10.3389/fimmu.2020.581361.

Picard-Sánchez, A., Estensoro, I., Pozo, R. Del, Palenzuela, O.R., Piazzon, M.C. and Sitjà-Bobadilla, A. (2020b) Water temperature, time of exposure and population density are key parameters in *Enteromyxum leei* fish-to-fish experimental transmission. *Journal of Fish Diseases* 43(4), 491–502. DOI: 10.1111/jfd.13147.

Quiroga, M.I., Redondo, M.J., Sitjà-Bobadilla, A., Palenzuela, O., Riaza, A. *et al.* (2006) Risk factors associated with *Enteromyxum scophthalmi* (Myxozoa) infection in cultured turbot, *Scophthalmus maximus* (L.). *Parasitology* 133(4), 433–442. DOI: 10.1017/S0031182006000515.

Rangel, L.F., Cech, G., Székely, C. and Santos, M.J. (2011) A new actinospore type Unicapsulactinomyxon (Myxozoa), infecting the marine polychaete, *Diopatra neapolitana* (Polychaeta: Onuphidae) in the Aveiro Estuary (Portugal). *Parasitology* 138(6), 698–712. DOI: 10.1017/S0031182011000163.

Redondo, M.J. (2005) Estudios sobre el ciclo vital y transmisión de *Enteromyxum scophthalmi* (Myxozoa), parásito entérico del rodaballo. PhD thesis, Universidad de Valencia, Valencia, Spain. Available at: http://hdl.handle.net/10261/253671 (accessed 20 November 2025).

Redondo, M.J. and Álvarez-Pellitero, P. (2010a) Carbohydrate patterns in the digestive tract of *Sparus aurata* L. and *Psetta maxima* (L.) (Teleostei) parasitized by *Enteromyxum leei* and *E. scophthalmi* (Myxozoa). *Parasitology International* 59(3), 445–453. DOI: 10.1016/j.parint.2010.06.005.

Redondo, M.J. and Álvarez-Pellitero, P. (2010b) The effect of lectins on the attachment and invasion of *Enteromyxum scophthalmi* (Myxozoa) in turbot (*Psetta maxima* L.) intestinal epithelium *in vitro*. *Experimental Parasitology* 126(4), 577–581. DOI: 10.1016/j.exppara.2010.06.008.

Redondo, M.J., Palenzuela, O., Riaza, A., Macías, A. and Álvarez-Pellitero, P. (2002) Experimental transmission of *Enteromyxum scophthalmi* (Myxozoa), an enteric parasite of turbot *Scophthalmus maximus*. *Journal of Parasitology* 88(3), 482–488. DOI: 10.2307/3285435.

Redondo, M.J., Palenzuela, O. and Álvarez-Pellitero, P. (2003a) *In vitro* studies on viability and proliferation of *Enteromyxum scophthalmi* (Myxozoa), an enteric parasite of cultured turbot *Scophthalmus maximus*. *Diseases of Aquatic Organisms* 55(2), 133–144. DOI: 10.3354/dao055133.

Redondo, M.J., Quiroga, M.I., Palenzuela, O., Nieto, J.M. and Álvarez-Pellitero, P. (2003b) Ultrastructural studies on the development of *Enteromyxum scophthalmi* (Myxozoa), an enteric parasite of turbot (*Scophthalmus maximus* L.). *Parasitology Research* 90(3), 192–202. DOI: 10.1007/S00436-002-0810-5.

Redondo, M.J., Palenzuela, O. and Álvarez-Pellitero, P. (2004) Studies on transmission and life cycle of *Enteromyxum scophthalmi* (Myxozoa), an enteric parasite of turbot *Scophthalmus maximus*. *Folia Parasitologica* 51(2–3), 188–198. DOI: 10.14411/fp.2004.022.

Redondo, M.J., Cortadellas, N., Palenzuela, O. and Álvarez-Pellitero, P. (2008) Detection of carbohydrate terminals in the enteric parasite *Enteromyxum scophthalmi* (Myxozoa) and possible interactions with its fish host *Psetta maxima*. *Parasitology Research* 102(6), 1257–1267. DOI: 10.1007/s00436-008-0903-x.

Renaud, F., Manet, D., Toubiana, M., Siau, Y., Le Breton, A. *et al.* (2004) *Enteromyxum leei* infection in sea bass, *Dicentrarchus labrax*, reared with infested sea bream, *Sparus aurata*. *Journal of Eukaryotic Microbiology* 51(2), 27A.

Rigos, G. and Katharios, P. (2010) Pathological obstacles of newly-introduced fish species in Mediterranean mariculture: a review. *Reviews in Fish Biology and Fisheries* 20(1), 47–70. DOI: 10.1007/s11160-009-9120-7.

Rigos, G., Grigorakis, L, Christophilogannis, P., Nengas, I. and Alexis, M. (1997) *Ceratomyxa* spp. (Myxosporea) infection in cultured common dentex from Greece. *Bulletin of the European Association of Fish Pathologists* 17(5), 174–176.

Rigos, G., Christophilogiannis, P., Yiagnisi, M., Andriopoulou, A., Koutsodimou, M. *et al.* (1999) Myxosporean infections in Greek mariculture. *Aquaculture International* 7(5), 361–364. DOI: 10.1023/a:1009200732200.

Rigos, G., Padrós, F., Golomazou, E. and Zarza, C. (2024) Antiparasitic approaches and strategies in European aquaculture, with emphasis on Mediterranean marine finfish farming: present scenarios and future visions. *Reviews in Aquaculture* 16(2), 622–643. DOI: 10.1111/RAQ.12857.

Robledo, D., Ronza, P., Harrison, P.W., Losada, A.P., Bermúdez, R. *et al.* (2014) RNA-seq analysis reveals significant transcriptome changes in turbot (*Scophthalmus maximus*) suffering severe enteromyxosis. *BMC Genomics* 15(1), 1149. DOI: 10.1186/1471-2164-15-1149.

Ronza, P., Bermúdez, R., Losada, A.P., Sitjà-Bobadilla, A., Pardo, B.G. and Quiroga, M.I. (2015) Immunohistochemical detection and gene expression of TNFα in turbot (*Scophthalmus maximus*) enteromyxosis. *Fish and Shellfish Immunology* 47(1), 368–376. DOI: 10.1016/j.fsi.2015.09.032.

Ronza, P., Robledo, D., Bermúdez, R., Losada, A.P., Pardo, B.G. *et al.* (2016) RNA-seq analysis of early enteromyxosis in turbot (*Scophthalmus maximus*): new insights into parasite invasion and immune evasion strategies. *International Journal for Parasitology* 46(8), 507–517. DOI: 10.1016/j.ijpara.2016.03.007.

Ronza, P., Robledo, D., Bermúdez, R., Losada, A.P., Pardo, B.G. *et al.* (2019) Integrating genomic and morphological approaches in fish pathology research: The case of turbot (*Scophthalmus maximus*) enteromyxosis. *Frontiers in Genetics* 10, 26. DOI: 10.3389/fgene.2019.00026.

Ronza, P., Estensoro, I., Bermúdez, R., Losada, A.P., Pérez-Cordón, G. *et al.* (2020) Effects of *Enteromyxum* spp. (Myxozoa) infection in the regulation of intestinal E-cadherin: turbot against gilthead sea bream. *Journal of Fish Diseases* 43(3), 337–346. DOI: 10.1111/jfd.13130.

Ronza, P., Álvarez-Dios, J.A., Robledo, D., Losada, A.P., Romero, R. *et al.* (2021) Blood transcriptomics of turbot *Scophthalmus maximus*: a tool for health monitoring and disease studies. *Animals* 11(5), 1296. DOI: 10.3390/ani11051296.

Rosell-Moll, E., Piazzon, M.C., Sosa, J., Ferrer, M., Cabruja, E. *et al.* (2021) Use of accelerometer technology for individual tracking of activity patterns, metabolic rates and welfare in farmed gilthead sea bream (*Sparus aurata*) facing a wide range of stressors. *Aquaculture* 539, 736609. DOI: 10.1016/j.aquaculture.2021.736609.

Sekiya, M., Setsuda, A., Sato, H., Song, K., Han, J.K. *et al.* (2016) *Enteromyxum leei* (Myxosporea: Bivalvulida) as the cause of myxosporean emaciation disease of farmed olive flounders (*Paralichthys olivaceus*) and a turbot (*Scophthalmus maximus*) on Jeju Island, Korea. *Parasitology Research* 115(11), 4229–4237. DOI: 10.1007/s00436-016-5200-5.

Shin, S.P. and Lee, J. (2023) Infection of *Enteromyxum leei* in cultured starry flounder *Platichthys stellatus*. *Fisheries and Aquatic Sciences* 26(3), 234–240. DOI: 10.47853/fas.2023.e20.

Shin, S.P., Sohn, H.C., Jin, C.N., Kang, B.J. and Lee, J. (2018) Molecular diagnostics for verifying an etiological agent of emaciation disease in cultured olive flounder *Paralichthys olivaceus* in Korea. *Aquaculture* 493, 18–25. DOI: 10.1016/j.aquaculture.2018.04.041.

Shin, S.P., Sohn, H.C., Jin, C.N., Kang, B.J. and Lee, J. (2019) Quantitative investigation of *Enteromyxum leei* (Myxozoa: Myxosporea) infection and relative condition factor in cultured olive flounder *Paralichthys olivaceus* (Temminck and Schlegel). *Journal of Fish Diseases* 42(2), 159–165. DOI: 10.1111/jfd.12912.

Shin, S.P., Jin, C.N., Sohn, H. and Lee, J. (2022) Comparison of oral and anal inoculation of *Enteromyxum leei* into olive flounder *Paralichthys olivaceus*. *Aquaculture* 561, 738641. DOI: 10.1016/j.aquaculture.2022.738641.

Sitjà-Bobadilla, A. (2008) Fish immune response to Myxozoan parasites. *Parasite* 15(3), 420–425. DOI: 10.1051/parasite/2008153420.

Sitjà-Bobadilla, A., Redondo, M.J., Macias, M.A., Ferreiro, I., Riaza, A. and Álvarez-Pellitero, P. (2004) Development of immunohistochemistry and enzyme-linked immunosorbent assays for the detection of circulating antibodies against *Enteromyxum scophthalmi* (Myxozoa) in turbot (*Scophthalmus maximus* L.). *Fish and Shellfish Immunology* 17(4), 335–345. DOI: 10.1016/j.fsi.2004.04.007.

Sitjà-Bobadilla, A., Redondo, M.J., Bermúdez, R., Palenzuela, O., Ferreiro, I. *et al.* (2006) Innate and adaptive immune responses of turbot, *Scophthalmus maximus* (L.), following experimental infection with *Enteromyxum scophthalmi* (Myxosporea: Myxozoa). *Fish and Shellfish Immunology* 21(5), 485–500. DOI: 10.1016/j.fsi.2006.02.004.

Sitjà-Bobadilla, A., Diamant, A., Palenzuela, O. and Álvarez-Pellitero, P. (2007a) Effect of host factors and experimental conditions on the horizontal transmission of *Enteromyxum leei* (Myxozoa) to gilthead sea bream, *Sparus aurata* L., and European sea bass, *Dicentrarchus labrax* (L.). *Journal of Fish Diseases* 30(4), 243–250. DOI: 10.1111/j.1365-2761.2007.00804.x.

Sitjà-Bobadilla, A., Palenzuela, O., Riaza, A., Macías, M.A. and Álvarez-Pellitero, P. (2007b) Protective acquired immunity to *Enteromyxum scophthalmi* (Myxozoa) is related to specific antibodies in *Psetta maxima* (L.) (Teleostei). *Scandinavian Journal of Immunology* 66(1), 26–34. DOI: 10.1111/j.1365-3083.2007.01942.x.

Sitjà-Bobadilla, A., Palenzuela, O. and Álvarez-Pellitero, P. (2007c) The innate immune response of sharpsnout sea bream (*Diplodus puntazzo*) in relation to enteromyxosis progression. *Parassitologia* 49, 77.

Sitjà-Bobadilla, A., Calduch-Giner, J., Saera-Vila, A., Palenzuela, O., Álvarez-Pellitero, P. and Pérez-Sánchez, J. (2008) Chronic exposure to the parasite *Enteromyxum leei* (Myxozoa: Myxosporea) modulates the immune response and the expression of growth, redox and immune relevant genes in gilthead sea bream, *Sparus aurata* L. *Fish and Shellfish Immunology* 24(5), 610–619. DOI: 10.1016/j.fsi.2008.01.014.

Sitjà-Bobadilla, A., Gil-Solsona, R., Estensoro, I., Piazzon, M.C., Martos-Sitcha, J.A. *et al.* (2019) Disruption of gut integrity and permeability contributes to enteritis in a fish–parasite model: a story told from serum metabolomics. *Parasites and Vectors* 12(1), 486. DOI: 10.1186/S13071-019-3746-7.

Sitjà-Bobadilla, A., Estensoro, I. and Palenzuela, O. (2021) *Enteromyxum leei*. In: Sitjà-Bobadilla, A., Bron, J., Wiegertjes, G. and Piazzon, M.C. (eds). *Fish Parasites: A Handbook of Protocols for their Isolation, Culture and Transmission*. European Association of Fish Pathologists (EAFP)/5m Books Series. CAB International, Wallingford, UK, pp. 127–142. DOI: 10.1079/9781800629127.0009.

Sohn, H., Jin, C.N., Kang, B.J., Shin, S.P. and Lee, J. (2021) Infection dynamics of *Enteromyxum leei* (Myxozoa, Myxosporea) in culture water and its effects on cultured olive flounder, *Paralichthys olivaceus* (Temminck & Schlegel). *Journal of Fish Diseases* 44(9), 1475–1479. DOI: 10.1111/jfd.13449.

Torres-Bocero, I.F. (2013) Diagnóstico de *Enteromyxum* spp. mediante la técnica LAMP (loop-mediated isothermal amplification). MSc thesis, Universitat Jaume I, Castelló de la Plana, Spain.

Toxqui-Rodríguez, S., Estensoro, I., Domingo-Bretón, R., Del Pozo, R., Pérez-Sánchez, J. *et al.* (2025) Interactions between gilthead seabream intestinal transcriptome and microbiota upon *Enteromyxum leei* infection: a multi–omic approach. *Animal Microbiome* 7(1), 22. DOI: 10.1186/s42523-025-00388-x.

Tun, T., Yokoyama, H., Ogawa, K. and Wakabayashi, H. (2000) Myxosporeans and their hyperparasitic microsporeans in the intestine of emaciated tiger puffer. *Fish Pathology* 35(3), 145–156. DOI: 10.3147/jsfp.35.145.

Tun, T., Ogawa, K. and Wakabayashi, H. (2002) Pathological changes induced by three myxosporeans in the intestine of cultured tiger puffer, *Takifugu rubripes* (Temminck and Schlegel). *Journal of Fish Diseases* 25(2), 63–72. DOI: 10.1046/j.1365-2761.2002.00333.x.

Varvarigos, P. (2003) Health status and the most economically important pathologies of the marine fish cultured in Greece and the Eastern Aegean Sea. In: *Treatment and Prevention. X Convegno Nazionale Societa Italiana Patologia Ittica, Tavola Rotonda: Principali patologie nella maricoltura Mediterranea*, Terano, Italy, pp. 70–72. Available at: https://www.sipi-online.it/convegni/2003/atti2003.pdf (accessed 3 December 2025).

WOAH (2022) The Use of Environmental DNA Methods for Detection of WOAH Listed Aquatic Animal Diseases. Available at: https://www.woah.org/app/uploads/2022/07/edna-final-ang.pdf (accessed 21 November 2025).

Woodyard, E., Stilwell, J., Perry, S., Delaune, A., Stilwell, N. *et al.* (2024) *Enteromyxum leei* from Creole wrasse *Clepticus parrae*. In: *Fish Health Section Annual Meeting and 63rd Western Fish Disease Workshop (American Fisheries Society FHS/WFDW)*, Boise, Idaho, p. 53. Available at: https://event.fourwaves.com/wfdw63/abstracts/814b231f-93ed-4410-a40a-c273c8391cef (accessed 20 November 2025).

Yahalomi, D., Haddas-Sasson, M., Rubinstein, N.D., Feldstein, T., Diamant, A. and Huchon, D. (2017) The multipartite mitochondrial genome of *Enteromyxum leei* (Myxozoa): Eight fast-evolving megacircles. *Molecular Biology and Evolution* 34(7), 1551–1556. DOI: 10.1093/molbev/msx072.

Yanagida, T. (2017) Myxosporean emaciation disease. *Fish Pathology* 52(2), 63–67. DOI: 10.3147/jsfp.52.63.

Yanagida, T., Nomura, Y., Kimura, T., Fukuda, Y., Yokoyama, H. and Ogawa, K. (2004) Molecular and morphological redescriptions of enteric myxozoans, *Enteromyxum leei* (formerly *Myxidium* sp. TFI) and *Enteromyxum fugu* comb. n. (syn. *Myxidium fugu*) from cultured tiger puffer. *Fish Pathology* 39(3), 137–143. DOI: 10.3147/jsfp.39.137.

Yanagida, T., Freeman, M.A., Nomura, Y., Takami, I., Sugihara, Y. *et al.* (2005) Development of a PCR-based method for the detection of enteric myxozoans causing the emaciation disease of cultured tiger puffer. *Fish Pathology* 40(1), 23–28. DOI: 10.3147/jsfp.40.23.

Yanagida, T., Sameshima, M., Nasu, H., Yokoyama, H. and Ogawa, K. (2006) Temperature effects on the development of *Enteromyxum* spp. (Myxozoa) in experimentally infected tiger puffer, *Takifugu rubripes* (Temminck & Schlegel). *Journal of Fish Diseases* 29(9), 561–567. DOI: 10.1111/j.1365-2761.2006.00752.x.

Yanagida, T., Palenzuela, O., Hirae, T., Tanaka, S., Yokoyama, H. and Ogawa, K. (2008) Myxosporean emaciation disease of cultured red sea bream *Pagrus major* and spotted knifejaw *Oplegnathus punctatus*. *Fish Pathology* 43(1), 45–48. DOI: 10.3147/jsfp.43.45.

Yasuda, H., Ooyama, T., Iwata, K., Tun, T., Yokoyama, H. and Ogawa, K. (2002) Fish-to-fish transmission of *Myxidium* spp. (Myxozoa) in cultured tiger puffer suffering from emaciation disease. *Fish Pathology* 37(1), 29–33.

Yasuda, H., Ooyama, T., Nakamura, A., Iwata, K., Palenzuela, O. and Yokoyama, H. (2005) Occurrence of the myxosporean emsaciation disease caused by *Enteromyxum leei* in cultured Japanese flounder *Paralichthys olivaceus*. *Fish Pathology* 40(4), 175–180.

Yokoyama, H. and Shirakashi, S. (2007) Evaluation of hyposalinity treatment on infection with *Enteromyxum leei* (Myxozoa) using anemonefish *Amphiprion* spp. as experimental host. *Bulletin of the European Association of Fish Pathologists* 27(2), 74–78.

10 *Henneguya ictaluri*

Matt J. Griffin[1,3], T. Graham Rosser[2], Justin M. Stilwell[3] and Lester H. Khoo[1,3]*
[1]*Thad Cochran National Warmwater Aquaculture Center, Mississippi State University, Stoneville, Mississippi, USA;* [2]*Department of Comparative Biomedical Sciences, Mississippi State University, Mississippi State, Mississippi, USA;* [3]*Department of Pathobiology and Population Medicine, Mississippi State University, Mississippi State, Mississippi, USA*

Abstract

Proliferative gill disease (PGD), caused by the myxozoan *Henneguya ictaluri*, is a major impediment to catfish aquaculture in the USA. The two-host life cycle involves a myxospore stage in the gills of channel catfish (*Ictalurus punctatus*) and an actinospore stage released by the benthic oligochaete *Dero digitata*. Continuous exposure of channel catfish and channel catfish × blue catfish hybrids to water-borne actinospores leads to destructive branchitis, characterized by epithelial hyperplasia, lamellar fusion and chondrolysis of the filament cartilage, which compromise gill integrity and impair respiratory function. This disease is most common in fingerlings stocked into grow-out ponds in the spring, outbreaks can affect catfish of all sizes and occur year-round however, causing significant economic losses through direct mortality, reduced feeding activity and disruption of production cycles. This chapter provides a comprehensive overview on PGD pathogenesis and epidemiology with highlights on recent advances in pond-level surveillance, risk assessment tools and control strategies.

10.1. Introduction

The commercial production of channel catfish (*Ictalurus punctatus*) is the largest warmwater aquaculture sector in the USA. As of 2024, the total production area encompassed approximately 53,545 water acres (21,668 ha), with 93.6% of operations concentrated in Alabama, Arkansas, Mississippi and Texas (USDA–NASS, 2024). The estimated inventory of market-size catfish in 2024 was approximately 139 million fish. Based on the 2018 Census of Aquaculture, 489 farms were engaged in catfish production nationwide (USDA–NASS, 2019).

Commercial channel catfish (*I. punctatus*) and channel catfish (*I. punctatus*) × blue catfish (*Ictalurus furcatus*) hybrids are intensively cultured in open earthen ponds ranging from 8 to 20 acres (3.2–8.1 ha), although recent industry trends favour ponds at the lower end of that range. Stocking rates vary widely, ranging from 1293 to 24,710 fish/ha (USDA, 1997; Avery and Steeby, 2004; Boyd, 2004). Pond design and industry management practices have created an environment conducive for the introduction and maintenance of numerous fish parasites. Hegde *et al.* (2022) also reported the adoption of new technologies, including split-pond systems, intensive aeration, hybrid catfish and automatic oxygen monitoring, which support higher stocking rates, may further support parasite persistence. Several factors contribute to the difficulty

*Email: khoo@cvm.msstate.edu

(eds P.T.K. Woo and K. Buchmann)
DOI: 10.1079/9781800628748.0010

of controlling and eradicating parasitic agents from these systems: (i) multiple age classes of fish are often raised together; (ii) ponds are rarely drained; and (iii) diverse wildlife species live in or around the ponds year-round.

One parasite that has plagued this industry since its commercialization in the early 1980s is the myxozoan *Henneguya ictaluri*, the causative agent of proliferative gill disease (PGD) in channel and hybrid catfish. Outbreaks of this disease have devastating effects on the industry, with mortality rates often exceeding 50% in affected ponds. While early diagnostic reports and case studies implicated *Henneguya* spp. were associated with this disease (Bowser and Conroy, 1985; Bowser *et al.*, 1985; MacMillan *et al.*, 1989), it was not until the late 1990s and early 2000s that PGD was linked to the myxozoan *H. ictaluri* (Burtle *et al.*, 1991; Pote *et al.*, 2000).

Currently, 12 *Henneguya* spp. (*Henneguya adiposa*, *Henneguya angingensis*, *Henneguya bulbosus*, *Henneguya diversis*, *Henneguya exilis*, *Henneguya extensa*, *Henneguya longicauda*, *Henneguya limatula*, *Henneguya mississippiensis*, *Henneguya postexilis*, *Henneguya sutherlandi* and *H. ictaluri*) have been described from channel catfish. Species identifications are based on cyst and myxospore morphology, as well as location in the catfish host (Kudo, 1929; Minchew, 1977; Lin *et al.*, 1999; Pote *et al.*, 2000; Griffin *et al.*, 2008b, 2009b; Rosser *et al.*, 2014, 2015; Woodyard *et al.*, 2022; Zhang *et al.*, 2023). The 18S small-subunit ribosomal RNA (SSU rDNA) has been sequenced for *H. adiposa*, *H. exilis*, *H. extensa*, *H. ictaluri*, *H. missisippiensis*, *H. postexilis* and *H. sutherlandi*.

The life cycles of several ictalurid-associated *Henneguya* spp. have also been confirmed using molecular techniques, wherein the actinospore stages of *H. ictaluri*, *H. mississippiensis* and *H. exilis* have been definitively linked to their corresponding myxospore stages in the fish. Ten of these species were originally described in the USA, with two recently described from channel catfish introduced in China. *H. extensa*, originally described from China (Zhang *et al.*, 2023), was molecularly identical to what Stilwell *et al.* (2022) described as Unclassified Myxozoan 11, identified during a targeted metagenomic sequencing assessment of clinical PGD cases in the USA. *H. postexilis*, originally reported from farm-raised catfish in Mississippi, USA (Woodyard *et al.*, 2022), has additionally been reported in channel catfish from Japan (Nitta and Ishikawa, 2024). Several of the ictalurid-associated *Henneguya* spp. (*H. bulbosus*, *H. exilis*, *H. extensa*, *H. longicauda*, *H. mississippiensis*, *H. postexilis* and *H. ictaluri*) exhibit plasmodia and myxospore development within the gills of the catfish host. Additionally, *H. adiposa* may infect and complete an initial series of pre-sporogonic replication within the gills before proceeding to the adipose fin for plasmodia formation and myxospore development (Stilwell *et al.*, 2019b, 2022, 2023b).

Molecular and morphological studies have confirmed that *H. ictaluri* follows a typical myxozoan life cycle (Wolf and Markiw, 1984) with the myxospore stage in the catfish host *I. punctatus* (Fig. 10.1a) and the actinospore stage (formerly *Aurantiactinomyxon ictaluri*) (Fig. 10.1b) in the aquatic oligochaete host *Dero digitata* (Fig. 10.1c) (Styer *et al.*, 1991; Pote *et al.*, 2000).

The only oligochaete identified as a suitable invertebrate host for *H. ictaluri* is *D. digitata*, which has been confirmed experimentally and molecularly (Styer *et al.*, 1991; Pote *et al.*, 2000). Comparably, other aquatic oligochaetes and invertebrates in North American catfish ponds have not been observed shedding *H. ictaluri*, even during active PGD outbreaks (Bellerud *et al.*, 1995).

D. digitata is a ubiquitous freshwater oligochaete, found in natural and man-made freshwater systems throughout North America. It is present throughout the year in the benthic sediment of commercial catfish ponds, with population estimates ranging from 1400 to 20,000 oligochaetes/m^2 (Bellerud, 1993; Bellerud *et al.*, 1995). Although *D. digitata* is present year-round, population levels peak in the spring, with a smaller secondary peak in the autumn, corresponding to pond-water temperatures between 19 and 24°C (Wax *et al.*, 1987; Mischke *et al.*, 2016). This seasonal pattern aligns with the occurrence of PGD, which is most prevalent in the spring (March–May) and less common in the autumn (September–October) (Bellerud, 1993; Bellerud *et al.*, 1995; Wise *et al.*, 2004).

H. ictaluri-infected *D. digitata* maintained in the laboratory can remain infected for several weeks. These oligochaetes reproduce asexually (Pote *et al.*, 1994), and the progeny of an infected worm also retain the infection. Actinospores

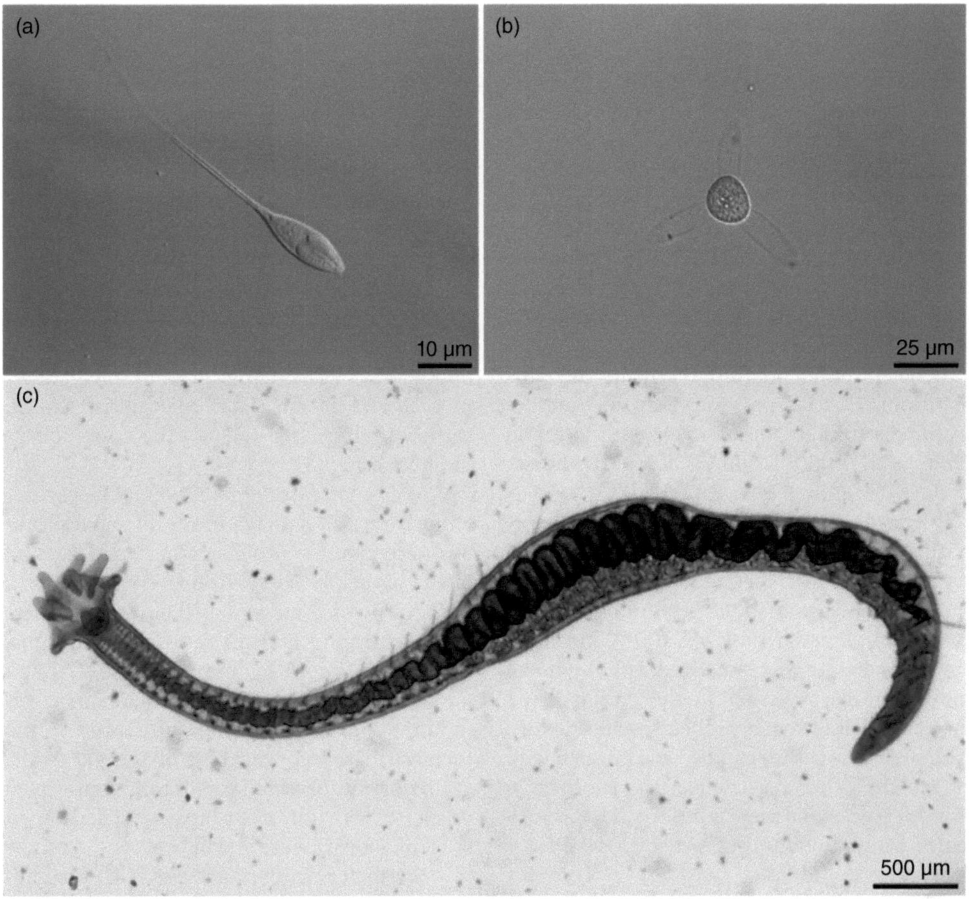

Fig. 10.1. Spore stages of *Henneguya* spp. in US catfish aquaculture systems. (a) Typical *Henneguya* spp. myxospore isolated from the gills of channel catfish; (b) *Henneguya ictaluri* actinospore; (c) the oligochaete host *Dero digitata* involved in the life cycle of *H. ictaluri*. (Author's own image.)

develop within the gastrointestinal tract for release with the faeces. During asexual reproduction, the gastrointestinal tract is divided between progeny, resulting in vertical transmission of the infection to both oligochaetes, effectively doubling the prevalence of infected invertebrate hosts with each reproductive cycle. This contributes to the rapid amplification of infected *D. digitata* populations and the sudden onset of PGD outbreaks in the field. While the prevalence and number of *D. digitata* infected with *H. ictaluri* are higher in ponds experiencing PGD outbreaks, even ponds considered PGD-negative or with low disease activity harbour infected *D. digitata*, maintaining a constant reservoir for the parasite (Bellerud, 1993; Bellerud *et al.*, 1995).

H. ictaluri actinospores released by infected *D. digitata* remain infective for at least 24 h, with infectivity decreasing rapidly over time (Wise *et al.*, 2008). Belem and Pote (2001) demonstrated the route of infection for the *H. ictaluri* actinospore into the catfish host occurs through the skin, gills or orally. *In vitro* studies demonstrated that exposure of *H. ictaluri* actinospores to channel catfish blood, mucus and gill tissues resulted in the discharge of a pseudopodia-like motile stage, which indicates this may be one of the cues for host penetration (Pote and Waterstrat, 1993; Richardson *et al.*, 2022). Research on other myxozoans indicates that non-specific mechanical and chemical cues can initiate similar responses (Kallert *et al.*, 2005; Richardson *et al.*, 2022). Notably, mucus from non-ictalurid fish species can also activate the motile stage of *H. ictaluri*, a phenomenon observed in other myxozoans (Kallert *et al.*, 2015; Richardson *et al.*, 2022). However, the specific factors mediating *H. ictaluri* actinospore interactions with catfish hosts remain poorly understood.

Once the actinospore infects the catfish, the parasite stage can be found in the blood within 24 h post-infection (Belem and Pote, 2001; Griffin *et al.*, 2010). Pre-sporogonic stages of *H. ictaluri* can be observed histologically in the gills beginning 3 days post-infection and mature plasmodia from 18 to 24 weeks post-infection (Pote *et al.*, 2000; Griffin *et al.*, 2010; Rosser *et al.*, 2019; Stilwell *et al.*, 2023b).

The channel catfish appears to be the only natural host for *H. ictaluri*. There have been reports of PGD in wild-caught channel catfish in the USA (Thiyagarajah, 1993) and in channel catfish in Italy (Marcer *et al.*, 2004), but in all cases this disease was associated with unknown myxozoan-like parasites in the gills with no molecular data to confirm their specific identity. Although blue catfish can become infected with *H. ictaluri*, it does not complete its life cycle in this fish species and there is little pathology associated with infection (Griffin *et al.*, 2010; Rosser *et al.*, 2019).

Interestingly, hybrid catfish (*I. punctatus* × *I. furcatus*) are susceptible to the acute stages of *H. ictaluri* infection and exhibit pathology comparable to those in channel catfish, including similar early lesions and subsequent resolution and healing (Griffin *et al.*, 2010; Rosser *et al.*, 2019; Stilwell *et al.*, 2023b). However, efforts to complete the *H. ictaluri* life cycle in hybrid catfish, including the development of myxospores, have been unsuccessful. In controlled laboratory exposures using pond water from active PGD outbreaks, hybrid catfish failed to develop *H. ictaluri* myxospores, while concurrently exposed channel catfish produced myxospores between 12 and 20 weeks post-challenge. These findings suggest, at a minimum, reduced transmission and proliferation of *H. ictaluri* in hybrid catfish compared to channel catfish, indicating less efficient parasite development and possible inadequate adaptation of *H. ictaluri* to the hybrid host (Griffin *et al.*, 2010; Rosser *et al.*, 2019; Stilwell *et al.*, 2023b).

10.2. Diagnosis of Infection

Presumptive diagnosis of the disease is based on clinical signs, gross lesions and microscopic examination of wet mounts from gill biopsies. Because acute infections impair respiratory function, affected fish often show signs of hypoxia and are typically observed piping at the water surface or swimming listlessly near the pond margins or behind aerators, even when dissolved oxygen levels are adequate. Affected gills are swollen and fragile, with a mottled appearance resembling ground meat. This mottled and haemorrhagic appearance has led catfish producers to refer to the condition as 'hamburger gill'.

Microscopic examination of gill biopsy wet mounts reveals damage to the filament cartilage, accompanied by haemorrhage and swelling of the branchial tissue. In fingerling-sized fish, the severity of these lesions typically correlates with infection intensity and clinical signs. However, in larger, food-size fish (0.7–0.9 kg), far fewer gill filaments can be examined on wet mounts compared to fingerlings due to the increased size and thickness of the gill tissue. Consequently, observed cartilage fractures may be sparse, with only a few breaks visible, even in cases of active disease and mortality.

Mortality rates during severe PGD outbreaks can exceed 50% of the affected fish population, with the most significant losses typically occurring in the spring and to a lesser extent in the autumn, when pond-water temperatures range from 15 to 20°C in the south-eastern USA (Wise *et al.*, 2004). Although PGD is most prevalent in the spring, sporadic outbreaks can occur year-round. Additionally, lesions in the filament cartilage may heal more slowly at cooler temperatures, so gill damage observed in clinical cases submitted during the winter may reflect delayed healing from a previous infection rather than an active outbreak.

A definitive diagnosis can be made by histological examination of fixed and stained tissues, identifying the characteristic changes together with the presence of the pre-sporogonic vegetative stage. Confirmation can also be made using species-specific PCR or quantitative PCR (qPCR) (Whitaker *et al.*, 2001; Pote *et al.*, 2003; Griffin *et al.*, 2008a) or species-specific *in situ* hybridization (ISH) (Stilwell *et al.*, 2023b). Histological identification of the infective organism may require examination of multiple gill sections as the organisms may not be present in all planes of a tissue section. Also, the characteristic pre-sporogonic stages are usually only present during the acute stages of infection and in controlled experimental infections, are not readily evident after 14 days post-infection. However, clinical cases generally represent more continuous, prolonged exposure and organisms present within gill tissue sections represent multiple stages of development.

While the vast majority of lesions are caused by *H. ictaluri*, pre-sporogonic stages of other catfish-infecting *Henneguya* spp. may resemble those of *H. ictaluri* and can induce similar lesions (Stilwell *et al.*, 2023b). These pre-sporogonic stages can only be differentiated in histological sections using *Henneguya* species-specific ISH techniques as morphological characters are not present at this stage of development. Additionally, plasmodia of other myxozoans may be present due to mixed species presence in pond water (Stilwell *et al.*, 2023a,b). In clinical cases where lesions are suggestive of PGD but organisms are not readily evident, *H. ictaluri* infection can be confirmed using PCR or ISH, which can detect early stages of infection that cannot be discerned by routine haematoxylin and eosin (H&E) staining and microscopy (Whitaker *et al.*, 2001; Pote *et al.*, 2003, Stilwell *et al.*, 2023b). Building on the assay developed by Whitaker *et al.* (2001), a quantitative real-time PCR (qPCR) assay was developed, providing a means to not only detect low numbers of these organisms in the tissue but also quantify the amount of parasite DNA present (Griffin *et al.*, 2008a). Molecular techniques, however, have the disadvantage that they cannot discriminate between acute infection (when mortalities are often occurring) and more chronic subclinical cases. Thus, an accurate diagnosis requires the use of confirmatory tests in conjunction with information from the presumptive diagnosis.

In addition, both molecular assays have been modified to detect *H. ictaluri* actinospores in pond water (Whitaker *et al.*, 2005; Griffin *et al.*, 2009a); consequently, they can be used to identify ponds with *H. ictaluri* actinospores in the water, even in the absence of clinical disease in the resident fish population. For reasons that are currently unclear, resident fish in a pond have varying degrees of susceptibility to PGD (Wise *et al.*, 2004; Griffin *et al.*, 2009a; Richardson *et al.*, 2025).

10.3. External/Internal Lesions

10.3.1. Gross

Gills of catfish fingerlings with moderate to severe PGD often have a red and white mottled appearance, are swollen, fragile and bleed easily (Fig. 10.2a). These gills are often shortened or truncated with portions of the filament tips missing. In larger food-size fish, the affected gills may only show multiple foci of haemorrhage rather than the 'meaty' appearance seen in fingerlings and the gill filaments are usually not truncated.

10.3.2. Microscopic

Presumptive diagnosis of this disease is based on microscopic examination of gill biopsies, with particular attention on defects in the filament cartilage, typically appearing as semicircular gaps or fractures (Fig. 10.2b and c). Acute infections often have multifocal haemorrhage and swelling of the branchial tissue, along with loss of secondary lamellar detail. However, in food-size fish, the severity of microscopic lesions may not correspond with the clinical severity of disease. One limitation in these larger fish is that the size and thickness of the gill filaments restrict the number that can be placed on a glass slide for wet mount examination, reducing the likelihood of detecting representative lesions and complicating diagnosis.

Histologically, PGD lesions in experimentally infected fish are dependent on the severity and the chronicity of the disease. At 1 day post-exposure (pe) in sublethal experimental infections, where naïve channel catfish fingerlings are exposed to pond water from a confirmed PGD outbreak, lesions are often relatively non-specific. These may include: (i) multifocal areas of inflammation with haemorrhage; (ii) epithelial hyperplasia; and (iii) mucus cell hyperplasia, which partially fills or completely obliterates the lamellar troughs (Fig. 10.3a).

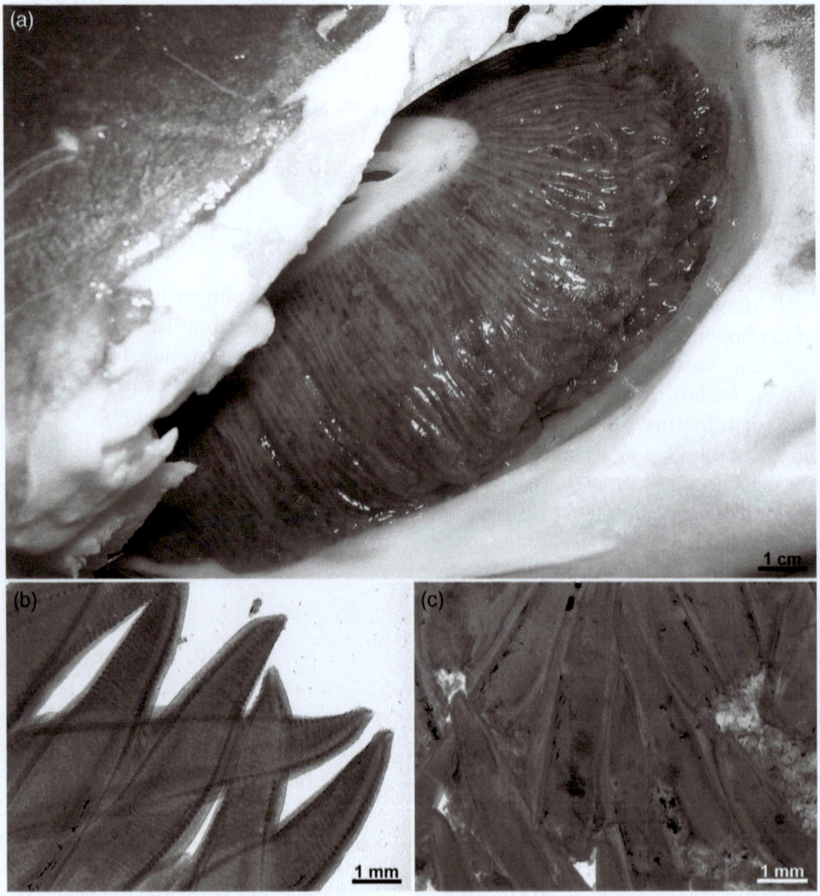

Fig. 10.2. Mottled appearance of gills (a) of a channel catfish fingerling affected by PGD or 'hamburger gill'. The operculum has been removed. Wet mount of gill clip from a normal (b) and a PGD-affected (c) channel catfish. Note the defects in the cartilage and swelling and haemorrhage of the branchial tissue in the affected fish (c). (Author's own image.)

By 7 days pe, the inflammatory response is granulomatous and is more intense and expansile. The infiltrate of mononuclear inflammatory cells fills and expands the central portion of the gill filament separating the two ends of the cartilage (Fig. 10.3b). Often, though not always, one or more granular structures (~20–40 µm in diameter) containing basophilic clusters of the developing pre-sporogenic vegetative stage (as seen in H&E-stained sections) are associated with these foci of intense inflammation. These pre-sporogenic structures are typically surrounded by a distinct ring of large, palisading mononuclear inflammatory cells, presumed to be epithelioid macrophages. They are consistent with descriptions by Bowser and Conroy (1985) and Duhamel *et al.* (1986) who initially ascribed the lesions to *H. exilis* based upon the concurrent presence of mature *H. exilis* plasmodia and myxospores. These descriptions occurred prior to the identification and molecular characterization of *H. ictaluri* by Pote *et al.* (2000) and disease associated with *H. exilis* in catfish has since been shown to represent a separate condition from PGD (Stilwell *et al.*, 2019a, 2024).

By 14 days pe, there is partial resolution of the inflammatory response, with evidence of ongoing healing marked by bridging of cartilaginous defects and early callus formation (Fig. 10.3c). This regenerative tissue is characterized by disorganized, dyschondroplastic growth composed of large, pale, basophilic chondrocytes.

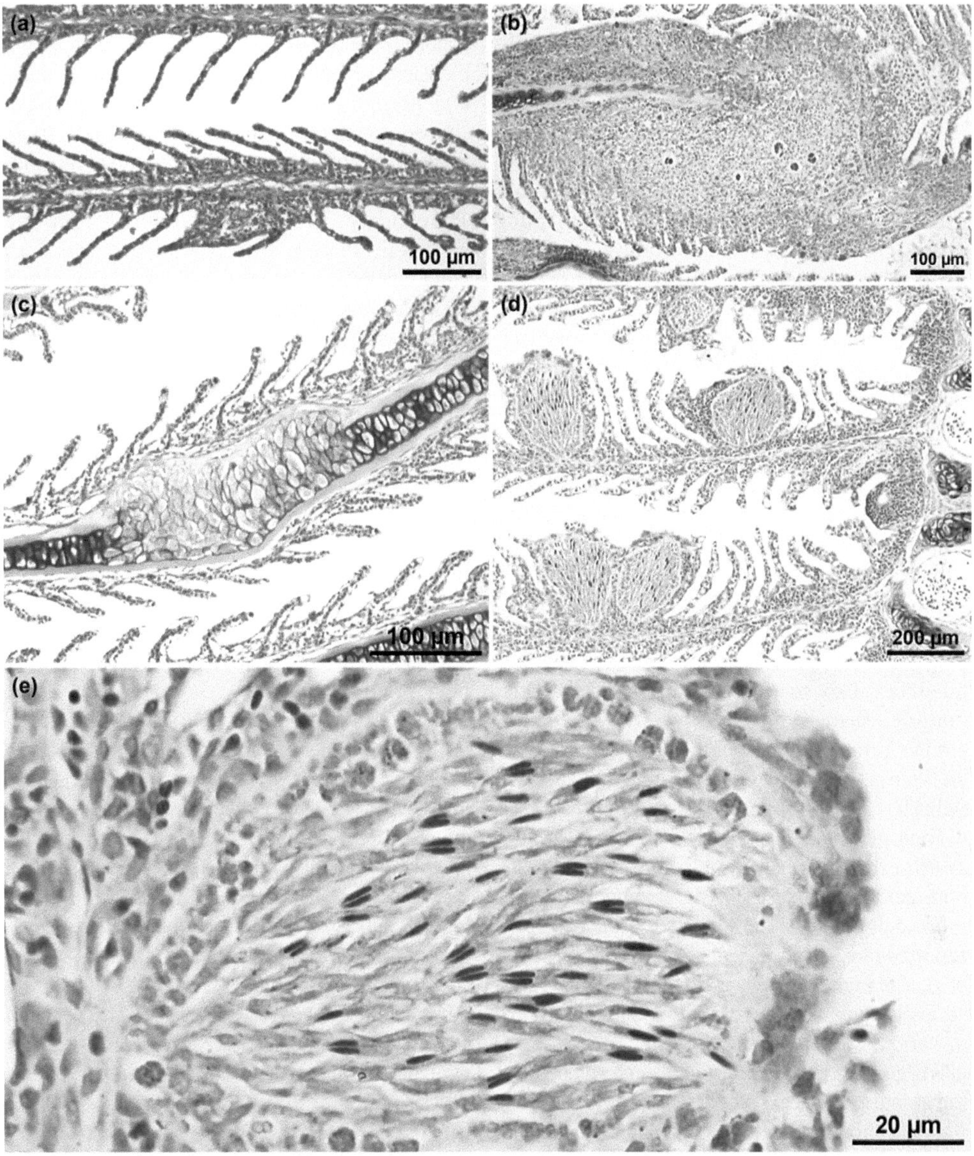

Fig. 10.3. Gills from a channel catfish experimentally infected with PGD. (a) At 1 day pe, the inflammation and epithelial proliferation partially fill the lamellar troughs and lamellar synechia, bridging the troughs. H&E stain. (b) At 7 days pe, the central portion of the gill is markedly expanded by the influx of inflammatory cells. At least five pre-vegetative spore stages of *Henneguya ictaluri* can be seen surrounded by macrophages. Giemsa stain. (c) At 14 days pe, the break in the cartilage has been bridged by cartilaginous hyperplasia. There is still an inflammatory component present; however, pre-vegetative spore stages are no longer readily evident. Giemsa stain. (d) At 70 days pe, note the distention due to numerous pseudocysts containing mature and developing myxospores and the lack of an inflammatory component. Giemsa stain. (e) Higher magnification of a pseudocyst containing mature and developing myxospores. Giemsa stain. (Author's own image.)

Interestingly, by this stage, the infectious agent is no longer readily apparent under light microscopy. The only remaining indication of the parasite is a ring of epithelioid macrophages encircling faint eosinophilic fibrillar material in H&E-stained sections.

By 21 days pe, the inflammation continues to subside, and early remodelling of the cartilaginous callus becomes apparent, including partial calcification along the peripheral margins. At this point, developing sporozoites are generally absent, even in regions where cartilage repair is actively underway. *H. ictaluri* may exhibit extrasporogenic development similar to that described for other myxozoans such as *Sphaerospora* spp., in which parasite replication occurs in tissues separate from the site of sporulation (Kent *et al.*, 2001). However, no pathological findings have been attributed to *H. ictaluri* in non-branchial tissues, and potential alternative sites of development remain unconfirmed.

By 28 days pe, continued remodelling of the cartilaginous callus is accompanied by multifocal infiltrates of mononuclear inflammatory cells, which are often not directly associated with the callus itself. At this stage, developing sporozoites remain inconspicuous. No significant histological changes are noted between 28 and 35 days pe.

After 35 and 70 days pe, non-epithelium-lined cyst-like structures have characteristic mature *Henneguya* spores each with two prominent pyriform polar capsules that stained dark blue on Giemsa sections (Fig. 10.3d) (Pote *et al.*, 2000). Stilwell *et al.* (2023b) used *H. ictaluri*-specific ISH to confirm the developmental timeline of *H. ictaluri* in fish exposed to pond water from natural PGD outbreaks, revealing similar development but on a more delayed timeline. Stilwell *et al.* (2023b) reported rare, mononuclear pre-sporogonic stages of *H. ictaluri* in channel catfish gill tissues at 7 and 12 weeks pe, with sporogonic plasmodia of *H. ictaluri* in various stages of maturity in channel catfish gills beginning 14 weeks post-challenge and persisting as late as 20 weeks pe.

Plasmodia may not be at or adjacent to the nodular remnant of the callus. The plasmodia of this histozoic myxosporean is often intralamellar (Molnár, 2002), arising just beneath the lamellar epithelium and often balloons out to fill the lamellar trough. The plasmodia may exceed the dimensions of the lamellar trough and distort the adjacent branchial architecture. The myxozoan spores are separated from the branchial tissue by a thin (~1–2 μm), pale eosinophilic hyaline (on H&E-stained sections) parasitic wall and there is usually no inflammatory component associated with the intact plasmodia. With additional time, the cyst-like structures enlarge and through asynchronous development, are filled with mature myxospores. Mature myxospores released from these plasmodia when gill biopsies are examined have the typical *Henneguya* morphology (Pote *et al.*, 2000) (i.e. spindle-shaped spores with an oval-to-pyriform spore body containing two pyriform polar capsules and a bifurcated caudal process or appendage). The caudal process is split the entire length, and each is the continuation of the one valve. Both polar capsules are usually the same size and width and are dark blue in Giemsa-stained histological sections (Fig 10.3e).

10.4. Pathophysiology

Belem and Pote (2001) demonstrated that *H. ictaluri* appears to enter channel catfish primarily through the stomach but can also enter through the buccal cavity, gills and skin. After entry the developing sporozoites move or are transported via the blood, appearing in the heart and hepatic vessels and are disseminated to the spleen, kidneys, liver and gills.

Besides respiration, the other major functions of the gills are ion regulation, acid–base balance and excretion (Evans *et al.*, 1999; Speare and Ferguson, 2006), all of which are adversely affected in fish with PGD. There is a dearth of literature concerning the pathophysiology of PGD. Beecham *et al.* (2010) documented the physiological effects of PGD in sublethally infected channel catfish and channel catfish × blue catfish hybrids at 24, 96 and 168 h pe to the parasite. Besides respiratory distress, there was a significant reduction in pO_2 and an increase in pCO_2 at 96 h. There also was a decrease in haematocrit values at 96 h pe, which corresponds to the haemorrhage seen grossly and microscopically in the gills, that they concluded could also contribute to the changes in pO_2 and pCO_2. Blue catfish concurrently exposed in the same study did not exhibit pathology or any physiological changes. In their study, Beecham *et al.* (2010) did not see changes in blood-plasma calcium concentration, concluding the negative effects of PGD on gaseous exchange were more significant than on osmoregulation.

In other gill diseases, such as bacterial gill disease (BGD) caused by *Flavobacterium branchiophilum*, physiological changes beyond hypoxemia have been observed. For instance, affected brook trout (*Salvelinus fontinalis*) exhibited hyponatraemia, hypochloraemia, hypoosmolality, hypoproteinaemia and increased haematocrit, the latter considered a compensatory response to hypoxemia (Byrne *et al.*, 1991). Similar changes, along with hypercapnia and elevated blood ammonia, were noted in rainbow trout (*Oncorhynchus mykiss*), though less pronounced in unfed fish (Byrne *et al.*, 1995). In contrast, rainbow trout infected with *Loma salmonae* had only slight increases in hypernatraemia and hyperchloraemia, with no significant changes in plasma K^+ (Powell *et al.*, 2006). In respiratory henneguyosis of African sharptooth catfish (*Clarias gariepinus*), a closely related disease, Sabri *et al.* (2009) observed decreases in serum proteins, albumin and Na^+/K^+-ATPase activity, and an increase in globulin levels. Viral diseases that affect gills are known to negatively impact not only respiration, osmoregulatory functions and nitrogenous waste excretion but also energy metabolism. The effects of the latter increase the stress response and immunosuppression, increasing the possibility of secondary infections (Zawisza *et al.*, 2024). Given the severity of inflammation and gill damage in PGD, similar physiological changes could be expected, though studies confirming these alterations are scarce.

Targeted metagenomic sequencing of gill tissues from natural PGD outbreaks revealed a wider diversity of previously known and unknown myxozoan taxa infecting catfish (Stilwell *et al.*, 2022). Several of these myxozoans were found within PGD lesions forming secondary pathology including inflammation, epithelial hyperplasia, haemorrhage, and space-occupying lesions such as interlamellar plasmodia (Stilwell *et al.*, 2023b). As such, other myxozoans appear to exacerbate the pathology of PGD and the subsequent respiratory distress and compromise, though *H. ictaluri* induces the most significant damage (Stilwell *et al.*, 2023b). Furthermore, other agents including *Edwardsiella* spp. and *Flavobacterium covae* may secondarily colonize PGD lesions.

10.5. Protective/Control Strategies

10.5.1. Chemical treatments

Several drugs have been experimented with for the control of myxosporidian infections in fish. Fumagillin dicyclohexylamine has been used for the treatment of *Myxobolus cerebralis* infections but with mixed results (Wagner, 2002). This same drug was successful in treating *Thelohanellus hovorkai* in koi carp (*Cyprinus rubrofuscus*) and *Sphaerospora renicola* in common carp (*Cyprinus carpio*), but the drug was unsuccessful for treating *Myxobolus cyprini* and *Thelohanellus nikolskii*. Wagner (2002) concluded there was different susceptibility of the various myxozoans to the drug. However, Buchmann *et al.* (1993) found that the time for drug application is very important. If the drug is distributed in the fish tissue before sporogony it will be effective. In contrast, if the drug is administered following sporogony it is not efficacious against spores that are encapsulated and protected in the tissue. Furazolidone, acetarsone, amprolium, nicarbazin, as well as oxytetracycline and sulfamerazine have also been used for treating *M. cerebralis* infections but with mixed results (Wagner, 2002). The anticoccidials amprolium and salinomycin have also been demonstrated to be effective against myxozoan infections in other fish species (Athanassopoulou *et al.*, 2004). However, at present, none of these drugs have been shown to be efficacious against *H. ictaluri*.

Mischke *et al.* (2001) investigated several potential chemical therapeutics to eradicate the oligochaete host (*D. digitata*) without negatively affecting the pond ecosystem and adversely affecting the resident fish populations. Formalin, chloramine-T, sodium chloride (NaCl), potassium permanganate ($KMnO_4$), copper sulfate ($CuSO_4$), hydrogen peroxide (H_2O_2), rotenone ($C_{23}H_{22}O_5$, 5% solution; Prentiss, Inc., Sandersville, Georgia, USA) and Bayluscide® (niclosamide, 70% wettable powder; Bayer Chemical Co., Kansas City, Missouri, USA) were all tested for their ability to eliminate *D. digitata*. Unfortunately, doses required for these agents were cost prohibitive, and required multiple treatments, thus making them an impractical treatment option. Although these chemical agents can be useful tools after an outbreak has occurred and the pond has been drained, they have limited utility while fish are present. The benthic substrate and organic matter in these ponds also inhibit the efficacy of chemical treatments, requiring higher doses to achieve an LC_{50} (lethal concentration for 50% of the population) for *D. digitata*, resulting in doses that are also lethal to catfish (Mischke *et al.*, 2001). One study investigated the potential for potassium permanganate to eradicate *D. digitata* from commercial catfish ponds, revealing doses as high as 20 mg/l did not successfully eradicate *D. digitata* populations from the pond (Mischke *et al.*, 2014). At present, no pond treatments have been identified to successfully remove *D. digitata* from catfish pond muds.

10.5.2. Biological control

Biological control of PGD has also been explored. This includes polyculture with common carp that initially reduced the numbers of *D. digitata* in ponds but changed their feeding preference as they grew and no longer preferred oligochaetes. Thus, repeated stocking with an appropriate-size crop is required and this is not practical in commercial settings (Burtle and Styer, 1996). Fathead minnows (*Pimephales promelas*) that also feed on benthic organisms and algae were tried as well but these fish can also serve as dietary supplement for catfish. It has proven to be difficult to maintain adequate densities of fathead minnows in catfish ponds to be an effective biological control (Burtle, 1998). Finally, smallmouth buffalo (*Ictiobus bubalus*) were also co-cultured and as with common carp, early results were promising when the fish were small; however, as the smallmouth buffalo grew, their effectiveness declined. In experimental settings, they showed no measurable impact on reducing *D. digitata* abundance in ponds or lesion development in sentinel fish exposures (Mischke *et al.*, 2016).

10.5.3. Supplemental treatments

Palliative therapies for PGD involve restricted feeding to reduce the oxygen demand of the fish, and increased aeration and pond salinity to ameliorate the respiratory insult and help the fish deal with osmoregulatory stress, respectively (Mitchell *et al.*, 1998; Wise *et al.*, 2004). Chloride levels in the pond should also be monitored closely to prevent the onset of nitrite-induced methaemoglobinaemia, which decreases the oxygen-carrying capacity of the blood, potentially exacerbating losses to PGD (Huey *et al.*, 1980; Bowser *et al.*, 1985). Since it is often difficult or almost impossible to remove all of the dead fish, this often leads to an increase in ammonia in the water that is converted to nitrites. Adding salt reduces the deleterious effects of nitrite toxicity because there is competitive uptake of chloride ions and nitrite ions by the chloride cells in the gills.

In addition to managing water chemistry, maintaining adequate oxygen levels is critical during a PGD outbreak. Supplemental aeration is the most effective strategy for reducing losses during PGD outbreaks. Although benthic oligochaetes are unevenly distributed in ponds (Bellerud *et al.*, 1995), the infective actinospore stage is dispersed uniformly throughout the water column (Griffin *et al.*, 2009a). While mechanical aerators might seem likely to further spread actinospores, they contribute no more to their distribution than natural physical processes. In salmonid aquaculture, myxozoan life cycles can be disrupted by rearing fish in concrete raceways or other systems that exclude the oligochaete host by eliminating the required earthen substrate (Wagner, 2002). However, such infrastructure-based solutions are not economically viable for catfish farming.

Another option during a PGD outbreak is to move the fish to a pond free of *H. ictaluri*. If done early in the outbreak, relocating the fish to a clean, well-oxygenated environment reduces mortality and morbidity. However, this approach comes with significant costs in both labour and time, and transport-induced stress can lead to additional losses, especially among clinically and subclinically infected fish. The decision to relocate fish should be based on the expected losses if they remain in the current pond and the number of fish likely to survive transport (Wise *et al.*, 2004). There is also the risk of introducing the disease to a previously uninfected pond. However, research suggests that *H. ictaluri* is endemic on most catfish farms, meaning it is likely already present in many commercial ponds (Bellerud *et al.*, 1995; Wise *et al.*, 2004, 2008).

10.5.4. Pond monitoring

The most effective way of reducing losses with PGD is an efficient management strategy. In short, naïve fish should not be stocked into ponds with high concentrations of *H. ictaluri* actinospores or active PGD outbreaks; and, if possible, in the incident of a severe outbreak, fish should be moved to an environment where *H. ictaluri* actinospores are absent or at significantly lower levels. Monitoring and surveillance for *H. ictaluri* abundance within a pond using qPCR to detect environmental DNA (eDNA) in water and/or naïve sentinel fish in cages allows producers to determine whether a pond is predisposed to developing or actively experiencing a PGD epizootic. This is not only important when identifying ponds for the relocation of fish, but also in determining when a pond is safe to restock following a severe PGD outbreak.

Fingerlings stocked into food-fish production ponds are at the greatest risk of developing PGD, especially in the spring or following a severe PGD outbreak. For reasons that are currently unclear, resident populations within a pond have varying degrees of susceptibility to PGD. The multi-batch system of stocking used in most commercial catfish ponds means that at any given time there are several populations of fish within a pond. Often, younger fish that have most recently been added to the pond will suffer significant mortalities during an epizootic, while older fish that have been in the pond for a longer period demonstrate little or no clinical signs of the disease. Whether this has to do with an acquired immunity or it simply takes a much higher challenge dose to result in the same level of damage in older, larger fish remains unclear. As such, the resident population of fish does not always provide an accurate assessment of the concentration of *H. ictaluri* actinospores present within the pond. This has necessitated the development of an assessment strategy to determine the risk of losing fish to PGD in newly stocked catfish ponds.

There is a strong correlation between the percentage of damaged or affected gill filaments in sentinel fish and mortality rates in newly introduced fish (Wise *et al.*, 2008). To assess PGD severity in ponds, the Fish Health Management Program at the Thad Cochran National Warmwater Aquaculture Center (Mississippi State University, Stoneville, Mississippi, USA) developed a lesion scoring system (Wise *et al.*, 2004). Using parasite-free sentinel fish, the levels of *H. ictaluri* actinospores in the pond can be indirectly estimated, allowing prediction of infection severity. Naive fish are held in netpens or cages that allow free water exchange for 7 days. Afterwards, gill biopsy wet mounts (~40–80 filaments) are examined microscopically for chondrolytic lesions. Infection severity is quantified by calculating the percentage of primary gill lamellae with at least one lytic lesion in the cartilage. If moderate to severe infection is present, the sampling protocol is repeated.

Based on examination of 40–80 gill filaments, a mild infection, which is defined as 1–5% of filaments exhibiting chondrolytic lesions, has little to no impact on fish health. Moderate infections, which do not cause direct mortality, typically involve 6–15% of filaments with chondrocytic lysis. Severe infections, resulting in mortality within 1–2 weeks, involve lesions in more than 15% of the examined filaments. If the percentage of filaments with chondrolysis drops below 5% between sampling periods and no mortality occurs in sentinel fish, the pond can be stocked with minimal risk of loss in newly introduced fish.

However, in ponds with high levels of infective actinospores, severe gill damage and mortality can occur in caged fish within 7 days, necessitating repeated sampling and delaying infection assessment (Wise *et al.*, 2004, 2008). The sentinel fish approach is also resource-intensive, requiring a supply of naive fish, transport tanks and equipment. Additionally, if sentinel fish die before sampling, determining the cause of death can be challenging. Improper acclimatization to ambient pond-water temperatures, especially in early spring, can lead to mortality or increased susceptibility to other diseases such as saprolegniasis and columnaris, which may be misattributed to PGD. During summer months, oxygen depletion from algal blooms or restricted water flow due to heavy algal growth on netpens can also result in mortality. To prevent oxygen depletion, netpens are often placed near mechanical aerators, but strong currents can exhaust fish and lead to death. Consequently, post-mortem autolysis can introduce sampling bias, preventing accurate evaluation of gill damage and reducing the number of fish available for analysis.

Alternatively, a qPCR assay was developed to directly quantify the number of *H. ictaluri* actinospores within the pond (Griffin *et al.*, 2009a). This has eliminated the need for sentinel fish since the PGD status of a pond can be determined using qPCR analysis of water samples.

This has drastically reduced the amount of labour associated with pond monitoring and provided more rapid results. Water samples collected on two separate days, preferably 6–10 days apart, can measure the level of *H. ictaluri* actinospores in the water and determine whether the actinospore level is increasing, decreasing or remaining stable. With levels ranging between 10 and 25 actinospores/l, there is a moderate risk of losing fish, especially if water quality parameters are suboptimal. At actinospore concentrations ≥ 25/l, stocking fish would not be recommended. Alternatively, research has shown that with actinospore concentrations ≤ 10 actinospores/l, and a marked decrease from the first to last sampling, producers can stock fish with relatively low risk of losing them to PGD (Griffin *et al.*, 2009a; Richardson *et al.*, 2025).

10.5.5. Alternative catfish species

Another potential control measure is to culture a catfish species less susceptible to PGD, or at least occasionally rotate between channel catfish and a less susceptible catfish species, periodically breaking the life cycle in the ponds. Blue catfish possess several attributes that make them desirable for aquaculture. They have a higher dress-out percentage than channel catfish, are relatively easy to seine, have high individual weight gains in temperate regions and are more resistant to several diseases (such as enteric septicaemia and channel catfish virus) that affect channel catfish (Graham, 1999; Hargreaves and Tucker, 2004). Also *H. ictaluri* rarely infects blue catfish (Bosworth *et al.*, 2003) and when infection does occur, it may be rapidly cleared by host defences (Griffin *et al.*, 2010; Rosser *et al.* 2019). However, blue catfish grow more slowly than channel catfish in the first 2 years of life under culture conditions and are less tolerant to poor water quality. Current processing techniques would also have to be modified due to slight differences in body conformation.

Similarly, blue catfish × channel catfish hybrids have increased in popularity in recent years. Their superior growth and relative disease resistance compared to channel catfish also make them desirable to catfish producers. In controlled studies, channel catfish and hybrid catfish suffer similar levels of gill damage and mortality when concurrently exposed to water from ponds with active PGD outbreaks (Bosworth *et al.*, 2003; Griffin *et al.*, 2010; Rosser *et al.*, 2019; Stilwell *et al.*, 2023b). However, the route of infection does not appear to be the same in the two fish, evident by significantly reduced levels of parasite DNA in hybrid catfish blood and tissues compared to channel catfish (Griffin *et al.*, 2010; Rosser *et al.*, 2019). Similarly, *H. ictaluri* abundance is reduced in ponds dedicated to continuous monoculture of hybrid catfish compared to channel catfish (Griffin *et al.*, 2020; Stilwell *et al.*, 2023a). This suggests that *H. ictaluri* may not be able to complete its life cycle in hybrid catfish as efficiently as it does in channel catfish. To date, *H. ictaluri* plasmodia and myxospores have not been isolated from hybrid catfish following laboratory exposures to *H. ictaluri* actinospores (Griffin *et al.*, 2010; Rosser *et al.*, 2019; Stilwell *et al.*, 2023b). This may offer an explanation as to why severe PGD outbreaks do not seem to occur in hybrid catfish ponds as frequently as in channel catfish ponds. If the parasite is unable to complete its life cycle in hybrid catfish, or does so only rarely, ponds used regularly for production of hybrid catfish may not provide the opportunity for the parasite to accumulate within the system to levels that result in catastrophic fish kills.

10.5.6. Single-batch versus multi-batch culture

Because hybrid catfish do not grade as readily as channel catfish, rotating production between the two would require producers to abandon the multi-batch production system currently used by most channel catfish operations. In a multi-batch system, fingerlings are continuously stocked into food-fish grow-out ponds to replace market-size fish that are regularly harvested, ensuring a steady supply of fish ready for market. As a consequence of this strategy, ponds on a given operation have fish at various ages and sizes throughout the year allowing producers to capitalize on demand during favourable periods. Furthermore, in instances where fish from a specific pond are temporarily rendered unmarketable due to the development of off-flavours, the presence of market-size fish across multiple ponds allows producers to maintain harvest schedules by selecting unaffected ponds. Despite this operational advantage, the multi-batch production system, when used in conjunction with conventional earthen-bottom ponds, creates optimal conditions for the establishment and perpetuation of myxozoan life cycles. Continuous stocking and harvesting, without seasonal production breaks, ensures a steady introduction of susceptible fish hosts. In addition, because most ponds remain in uninterrupted production for several years before draining for levee maintenance and sediment removal, there is no disruption to the parasitic cycle. The absence of pond drying further enables the persistence of benthic oligochaete populations, which serve as obligate intermediate hosts, thereby supporting ongoing transmission dynamics.

Alternatively, a single-batch system, where ponds are stocked only once at the beginning of the production cycle without replacing harvested fish, would provide an opportunity at the end of the production cycle, once all fish have been harvested, to drain and dry the pond prior to the next production cycle. This, in theory, could reduce the number of oligochaete hosts within the system, reducing the level of *H. ictaluri* within the pond, and indirectly preventing the parasite from reaching levels that can result in mortality and lost production. If fingerlings are confirmed to be parasite-free prior to stocking, there is less chance for the parasite to be introduced into the system. A potential drawback to instituting the single-batch culture, at least in terms of PGD, is that each time a pond is dried and drained it essentially becomes a new pond, which could theoretically increase the incidence of PGD rather than decrease it. For reasons that are poorly understood, the most severe outbreaks are often observed in new or recently reworked catfish ponds. This is thought to be the consequence of an ecological shift in the oligochaete host populations, favouring the establishment of *D. digitata*, which is considered an intermediate colonizing organism (Soster and McCall, 1990). In the first several months following new pond construction, or reworking of the pond sediment, *D. digitata* can be one of the predominant oligochaete species within the pond, providing more opportunities for *H. ictaluri* to complete its life cycle.

Admittedly, single-batch culture does not mitigate the potential for exogenous introduction of *H. ictaluri* via avian or other mechanical vectors. Although the specific role of such vectors in the dissemination of *H. ictaluri* has not been empirically demonstrated, their involvement cannot be discounted. Notably, Koel *et al.* (2010) showed that the closely related myxozoan *M. cerebralis*, the causative agent of whirling disease in salmonids, remained viable after passage through the gastrointestinal tract of great blue herons. Faecal material from herons fed infected fish subsequently infected oligochaete worms in laboratory cultures, confirming the potential for avian-mediated dissemination and life-cycle perpetuation. The continued occurrence of PGD in hybrid catfish production ponds, despite multiple studies suggesting that *H. ictaluri* cannot complete its life cycle in hybrid hosts, may therefore be partially explained by mechanical introduction of the parasite. Further research is needed to evaluate the extent to which single-batch systems may reduce PGD incidence, as well as to clarify the role of piscivorous birds and other potential vectors in maintaining and spreading *H. ictaluri* within and between commercial catfish operations.

10.6. Conclusions and Suggestions for Future Studies

Although *H. ictaluri* remains a persistent challenge for the commercial catfish industry, several emerging strategies offer promise for improved control and long-term management of this parasite. qPCR assays targeting *H. ictaluri* are increasingly being used not only to assess pond status following PGD outbreaks but also as a proactive management tool. In particular, several producers in the Mississippi Delta now use qPCR-based surveillance data to guide springtime stocking schedules, thereby reducing the risk of introducing naïve fingerlings into ponds harbouring lethal levels of *H. ictaluri* actinospores (Richardson *et al.*, 2025). Longitudinal monitoring of historically affected ponds is also being used to inform predictive models of PGD risk based on environmental and temporal parameters. In parallel, host susceptibility studies have shown that blue catfish exhibit reduced susceptibility to *H. ictaluri*, prompting ongoing efforts to elucidate the genetic and immunological determinants of resistance. These findings support the feasibility of selective breeding programmes aimed at developing *H. ictaluri*-resistant catfish strains, which may complement improved diagnostic and management strategies in mitigating the impact of PGD.

While raising catfish in closed recirculating aquaculture systems would in theory eliminate the occurrence of PGD, the associated production costs make this approach economically unfeasible for producers (Losordo *et al.*, 2004). Although the life cycle of *H. ictaluri* and its causal role in PGD have been established, substantial gaps remain in our understanding of the parasite's biology and host–parasite interactions. To date, the complete life cycle has not been successfully propagated under laboratory conditions, which continues to limit experimental investigations to periods of natural outbreak. The development of an *in vitro* or *in vivo* laboratory propagation system would represent a critical advancement, enabling controlled studies on the transmission dynamics, virulence mechanisms and environmental persistence of the parasite. Foundational research is also needed to elucidate: (i) the immune response of catfish species to *H. ictaluri* infection; (ii) the pathogenesis of this myxozoan in both the fish and oligochaete hosts; and (iii) the biochemical and molecular interactions that facilitate host invasion and establishment. Comparative studies examining host susceptibility between channel and blue catfish could uncover genetic or immunological correlates of resistance, potentially leading to the identification of potential markers that could aid in selective breeding programmes targeting PGD-resistant strains of channel and hybrid catfish. Furthermore, better characterization of the population dynamics, spatial distribution and ecological factors influencing *D. digitata* in production ponds will be essential to understanding transmission risk and designing targeted interventions. Importantly, these insights will inform the development of novel control strategies, including the application of targeted antiparasitic compounds capable of disrupting the *H. ictaluri* life cycle in either or both hosts. The integration of chemotherapeutic agents with selective breeding, pond management and predictive diagnostic tools may ultimately provide a multifaceted approach to reducing the incidence and severity of PGD in commercial catfish aquaculture.

References

Athanassopoulou, F., Karagouni, E., Dotsika, E., Ragias, V., Tavla, J. *et al.* (2004) Efficacy and toxicity of orally administrated anti-coccidial drugs for innovative treatments of *Myxobolus* sp. infection in *Puntazzo puntazzo*. *Diseases of Aquatic Organisms* 62, 217–226.

Avery, J.L. and Steeby, J.A. (2004) Hatchery management. In: Tucker, C.S. and Hargreaves, J.A. (eds) *Biology and Culture of the Channel Catfish*, 1st edn. Elsevier BV, Amsterdam, pp. 145–165.

Beecham, R.V., Griffin, M.J., LaBarre, S.B., Wise, D., Mauel, M. *et al.* (2010) The effects of proliferative gill disease on the blood physiology of channel catfish, blue catfish and channel catfish × blue catfish hybrid fingerlings. *North American Journal of Aquaculture* 72, 213–218.

Belem, A.M. and Pote, L.M. (2001) Portals of entry and systemic localization of proliferative gill disease organisms in channel catfish *Ictalurus punctatus*. *Diseases of Aquatic Organisms* 48, 37–42.

Bellerud, B.L. (1993) Etiological and epidemiological factors effecting outbreaks of proliferative gill disease on Mississippi channel catfish farms. PhD thesis, Mississippi State University, Stoneville, Mississippi.

Bellerud, B.L., Pote, L.M., Lin, T.L., Johnson, M.J. and Boyle, C.R. (1995) Etiological and epizootological factors associated with outbreaks of proliferative gill disease in channel catfish. *Journal of Aquatic Animal Health* 7, 124–131.

Bosworth, B.G., Wise, D.J., Terhune, J.S. and Wolters, W.R. (2003) Family and genetic group effects for resistance to proliferative gill disease in channel catfish, blue catfish and channel catfish × blue catfish backcross hybrids. *Aquaculture Research* 34, 569–573.

Bowser, P.R. and Conroy, J.D. (1985) Histopathology of gill lesions in channel catfish associated with *Henneguya*. *Journal of Wildlife Diseases* 21, 177–179.

Bowser, P.R., Munson, A.D., Jarboe, H.H. and Stiles, F.N. (1985) Transmission trials of proliferative gill disease in channel catfish (*Ictalurus punctatus*). *Mississippi Agricultural and Forestry Experiment Station Research Report*, Vol. 10(8). Mississippi State University, Stoneville, Mississippi.

Boyd, C.E. (2004) Pond hydrology. In: Tucker, C.S. and Hargreaves, J.A. (eds) *Biology and Culture of the Channel Catfish*, 1st edn. Elsevier BV, Amsterdam, pp. 196–214.

Buchmann, K., Slotved, H.-C. and Dana, D. (1993) Epidemiology of gill parasites from carp (*Cyprinus carpio*) in Indonesia and possible control methods. *Aquaculture* 118, 9–21.

Burtle, G.J. (1998) Control of the oligochaete vector of proliferative gill disease in catfish. In: *1998 Annual Report of the Department of Animal and Dairy Science*. The University of Georgia, College of Agricultural and Environmental Sciences, Athens, Georgia, pp. 22–25.

Burtle, G.J. and Styer, E.L. (1996) Biological control of proliferative gill disease of channel catfish: fish as predators. In: *1996 Annual Report of the Department of Animal and Dairy Science*. The University of Georgia, College of Agricultural and Environmental Sciences, Athens, Georgia, pp. 1–5.

Burtle, G.J., Harrison, L.R. and Styer, E.L. (1991) Detection of a triactinomyxid myxozoan in an oligochaete from ponds with proliferative gill disease in channel catfish. *Journal of Aquatic Animal Health* 3, 281–287.

Byrne, P.J., Ferguson, H.W., Lumsden, J.S. and Ostland, V.E. (1991) Blood chemistry of bacterial disease in brook trout *Salvelinus fontinalis*. *Diseases of Aquatic Organisms* 10, 1–6.

Byrne, P.J., Ostland, V.E., Lumsden, J.S., MacPhee, D.D. and Ferguson, H.W. (1995) Blood chemistry and acid–base balance in rainbow trout *Oncorhynchus mykiss* with experimentally induced acute bacterial gill disease. *Fish Physiology and Biochemistry* 14(6), 509–518.

Duhamel, G.E., Kent, M.L., Dybdal, N.O. and Hedrick, R.P. (1986) *Henneguya exilis* Kudo associated with granulomatous branchitis of channel catfish *Ictalurus punctatus*. *Veterinary Pathology* 23, 354–361.

Evans, D.H., Piermarini, D.R. and Potts, W.T.W. (1999) Ionic transport in fish gill epithelium. *Journal of Experimental Zoology* 282, 641–652.

Graham, K. (1999) A review of the biology and management of blue catfish. *American Fisheries Society Symposium* 24, 37–49.

Griffin, M.J., Wise, D.J., Camus, A.C., Mauel, M.J., Greenway, T.E. and Pote, L.M. (2008a) A real-time polymerase chain reaction assay for the detection of the myxozoan parasite *Henneguya ictaluri* in channel catfish. *Journal of Veterinary Diagnostic Investigation* 20(5), 559–566.

Griffin, M.J., Wise, D.J., Camus, A.C., Mauel, M.J., Greenway, T.E. and Pote, L.M. (2008b) A novel *Henneguya* sp. from channel catfish (*Ictalurus punctatus*) described by morphological, histological and molecular characterization. *Journal of Aquatic Animal Health* 20(3), 127–135.

Griffin, M.J., Pote, L.M., Camus, A.C., Mauel, M.J., Greenway, T.E. and Wise, D.J. (2009a) Application of a real-time PCR assay for the detection of *Henneguya ictaluri* in channel catfish ponds. *Diseases of Aquatic Organisms* 86, 223–233.

Griffin, M.J., Wise, D.J. and Pote, L.M. (2009b) Morphology and small-subunit ribosomal DNA sequence of *Henneguya adiposa* (Myxosporea) from *Ictalurus punctatus* (Siluriformes). *Journal of Parasitology* 95, 1076–1085.

Griffin, M.J., Wise, D.J., Camus, A.C., Greenway, T.E., Mauel, M.J. and Pote, L.M. (2010) Variation in susceptibility to *Henneguya ictaluri* infection by two species of catfish and their hybrid cross. *Journal of Aquatic Animal Health* 22, 21–35.

Griffin, M.J., Ware, C., Rosser, T.G., Woodyard, E.T., Mischke, C.C. *et al.* (2020) Monoculture of ♀ channel (*Ictalurus punctatus*) × ♂ blue (*I. furcatus*) hybrid catfish mitigates proliferative gill disease caused by *Henneguya ictaluri* (Cnidaria: Myxobolidae) in catfish aquaculture ponds. *Journal of the World Aquaculture Society* 51(3), 729–739

Hargreaves, J.A. and Tucker, C.S. (2004) Industry development. In: Tucker, C.S. and Hargreaves, J.A. (eds) *Biology and Culture of the Channel Catfish*, 1st edn. Elsevier BV, Amsterdam, pp. 1–14.

Hegde, S., Kumar, G., Engle, C., Hanson, T., Roy, L.A. *et al.* (2022) Technological progress in the US catfish industry. *Journal of the World Aquaculture Society* 53(2), 367–383.

Huey, D.W., Simco, B.A. and Criswell, D.W. (1980) Nitrite-induced methemoglobin formation in channel catfish. *Transactions of the American Fisheries Society* 109, 558–562.

Kallert, D.M., El-Matbouli, M. and Haas, W. (2005) Polar filament discharge of *Myxobolus cerebralis* actinospores is triggered by combined non-specific mechanical and chemical cues. *Parasitology* 131, 1–8.

Kallert, D.M., Grabner, D.S., Yokoyama, H., El-Matbouli, M. and Eszterbauer, E. (2015) Transmission of myxozoans to vertebrate hosts. In: Okamura, B., Gruhl, A. and Bartholomew, J.L. (eds) *Myxozoan Evolution, Ecology and Development*. Springer, Cham, Switzerland, pp. 235–251.

Kent, M.L., Andree, K.B., Bartholomew, J.L., El-Matbouli, M., Desser, S.S. *et al.* (2001) Recent advances in our knowledge of the myxozoa. *Journal of Eukaryotic Microbiology* 48(4), 395–413.

Koel, T.M., Kerans, B.L., Barras, S.C., Hanson, K.C. and Wood, J.S. (2010) Avian piscivores as vectors for *Myxobolus cerebralis* in the Greater Yellowstone ecosystem. *Transactions of the American Fisheries Society* 139(4), 976–988.

Kudo, R.R. (1929) Histozoic myxosporidia found in freshwater fishes in Illinois, USA. *Archiv für Protistenkunde* 65, 364–378.

Lin, D., Hanson, L.A. and Pote, L.M. (1999) Small subunit ribosomal RNA sequence of *Henneguya exilis* (class Myxosporea) identifies the actinosporean stage from an oligochaete host. *Journal of Eukaryotic Microbiology* 46, 66–68.

Losordo, T.M., Ray, L.E. and Delong, D.P. (2004) Flow-through and recirculating systems. In: Tucker, C.S. and Hargreaves, J.A. (eds) *Biology and Culture of the Channel Catfish*, 1st edn. Elsevier BV, Amsterdam, pp. 545–560.

MacMillan, J.R., Wilson, C. and Thiyagarajah, A. (1989) Experimental induction of proliferative gill disease in specific-pathogen-free channel catfish. *Journal of Aquatic Animal Health* 1, 245–254.

Marcer, F., Quaglio, F., Caffara, M., Ferraresi, M. and Floravanti, M. (2004) Proliferative gill disease in channel catfish farmed in Italy. *Ittopatologia* 1, 120–126.

Minchew, C.D. (1977) Five new species of *Henneguya* (Protozoa: Myxosporidia) from ictalurid fishes. *Journal of Protozoology* 24, 213–220.

Mischke, C.C., Terhune, J.S. and Wise, D.J. (2001) Acute toxicity of several chemicals to the oligochaete *Dero digitata*. *Journal of the World Aquaculture Society* 32, 184–188.

Mischke, C.C., Griffin, M.J., Wise, D.J. and Greenway, T.E. (2014) Potassium permanganate is not an effective pond disinfectant to control *Dero digitata*. *Journal of the World Aquaculture Society* 45(3), 350–353.

Mischke, C.C., Griffin, M.J., Wise, D.J. and Greenway, T.E. (2016) Effects of co-stocking smallmouth buffalo, *Ictiobus bubalus*, with channel catfish, *Ictalurus punctatus*. *Journal of the World Aquaculture Society* 47(2), 212–219

Mitchell, A.J., Durborow, R.M. and Crosby, M.D. (1998) *Proliferative Gill Disease*. Southeastern Regional Aquaculture Center (SRAC) Publication No. 475. US Department of Agriculture Cooperative State Research, Education, and Extension Service, Stoneville, Mississippi.

Molnár, K. (2002) Site preference of fish myxosporeans in the gill. *Diseases of Aquatic Organisms* 48, 197–207.

Nitta, M. and Ishikawa, T. (2024) New Japanese record of *Henneguya postexilis* (Cnidaria: Myxobolidae) from gills of alien channel catfish *Ictalurus punctatus* (Siluriformes: Ictaluridae) in Japan. *Species Diversity* 29(1), 23–30.

Pote, L.M. and Waterstrat, P. (1993) Motile stage of *Aurantiactinomyxon* sp. (Actinosporea: Actinomyxia: Triactinomyxidae) isolated from *Dero digitata* found in channel catfish ponds. *Journal of Aquatic Animal Health* 5, 213–218.

Pote, L.M., Bellerud, B.L., Lin, D.L. and Chenney, E.F. (1994) The isolation and propagation of *Dero digitata* infected with *Aurantiactinomyxon* sp. *Journal of the World Aquaculture Society* 25, 303–307.

Pote, L.M., Hanson, L.A. and Shivaji, R. (2000) Small subunit ribosomal RNA sequences link the cause of proliferative gill disease in channel catfish to *Henneguya* n. sp. (Myxozoa: Myxosporea). *Journal of Aquatic Animal Health* 12, 230–240.

Pote, L.M., Hanson, L.A. and Khoo, L. (2003) Proliferative gill disease. In: *Suggested Procedures for the Detection and Identification of Certain Finfish and Shellfish Pathogens, Blue Book*, 2010 edn. Fish Health Section, American Fisheries Society, Bethesda, Maryland.

Powell, M.D., Speare, D.J. and Becker, J.A. (2006) Whole body net ion fluxes, plasma electrolyte concentrations and haematology during a *Loma salmonae* infection of juvenile rainbow trout, *Oncorhynchus mykiss* (Walbaum). *Journal of Fish Diseases* 29, 727–735.

Richardson, B.M., Mischke, C.C., Rosser, T.G., Woodyard, E.T., Ware, C. *et al.* (2022) Activation of *Henneguya ictaluri* actinospores by nonictalurid fish species, with implications for management of proliferative gill disease in catfish aquaculture. *North American Journal of Aquaculture* 84(3), 313–324.

Richardson, B.M., Noor Ul-Huda, Ware, C., Camus, A.C., Older, C.E. *et al.* (2025) Fingerling stocking size has no influence on proliferative gill disease severity in farm-raised channel catfish. *Journal of Aquatic Animal Health* 37(1), 1–10.

Rosser, T.G., Griffin, M.J., Quiniou, S.M.A., Khoo, L.H. and Pote, L.M. (2014) 18S rRNA gene sequencing identifies a novel species of *Henneguya* parasitizing the gills of the channel catfish (Ictaluridae). *Parasitology Research* 113, 4651–4658.

Rosser, T.G., Griffin, M.J., Quiniou, S.M.A., Khoo, L.H., Greenway, T.E. *et al.* (2015) Small subunit ribosomal RNA sequence links the myxospore stage of *Henneguya mississippiensis* n. sp. from channel catfish *Ictalurus punctatus* to an actinospore released by the benthic oligochaete *Dero digitata*. *Parasitology Research* 114, 1595–1602.

Rosser, T.G., Khoo, L.H., Wise, D.J., Mischke, C.C., Greenway, T.E. *et al.* (2019) Arrested development of *Henneguya ictaluri* (Cnidaria: Myxobolidae) in ♀ channel catfish × ♂ blue catfish hybrids. *Journal of Aquatic Animal Health* 31, 201–213.

Sabri, D.M., Danasoury, M.A., Eissa, I.A.M. and Khouraiba, H.M. (2009) Alterations in serum protein fractions and Na^+K^+ATPase activity in *Clarias gariepinus* infested with henneguyosis in Ismailia, Egypt. *African Journal of Aquatic Science* 34(1), 103–107.

Soster, F.M. and McCall, P.L. (1990) Benthos response to disturbance in western Lake Erie: field experiments. *Canadian Journal of Aquatic Animal Science* 47(10), 1970–1985.

Speare, D.J. and Ferguson, H.W. (2006) Gills and pseudobranchs. In: Ferguson H.W. (ed.) *Systemic Pathology of Fish*. Scotian Press, London, pp. 24–63.

Stilwell, J.M., Camus, A.C., Leary, J.H., Khoo, L.H. and Griffin, M.J. (2019a) Pathologic changes associated with respiratory compromise and morbidity due to massive interlamellar *Henneguya exilis* infection in channel × blue catfish. *Journal of Parasitology* 105(5), 686–692.

Stilwell, J.M., Camus, A.C., Leary, J.H., Mohammed, H.H. and Griffin, M.J. (2019b) Molecular confirmation of Henneguya adiposa (Cnidaria: Myxozoa) and associated histologic changes in adipose fins of channel catfish, Ictalurus punctatus (Teleost). Parasitology Research 118(5), 1639–1645. DOI: 0.1007/s00436-019-06295-w.

Stilwell, J.M., Griffin, M.J., Waldbieser, G.C., Stanton, J.B., Leary, J.H. *et al.* (2022) Myxozoan community composition and diversity in clinical cases of proliferative gill disease in Mississippi catfish aquaculture. *Journal of Parasitology* 108, 132–140.

Stilwell, J.M., Camus, A.C., Ware, C., Walker, C.M., Stanton, J.B. *et al.* (2023a) Influence of channel catfish and channel × blue catfish hybrids on myxozoan community composition in catfish aquaculture ponds. *North American Journal of Aquaculture,* 85(3), 241–251.

Stilwell, J.M., Camus, A.C., Woodyard, E.T., Ware, C., Rosser, T.G. *et al.* (2023b) Species-specific *in situ* hybridization confirms arrested development of *Henneguya ictaluri* in hybrid catfish (channel catfish × blue catfish) under experimental conditions, with notes on mixed-species infections in clinical cases of proliferative gill disease from Mississippi catfish aquaculture. *Journal of Aquatic Animal Health* 35, 223–237.

Stilwell, J.M., Griffin, M.J., Leary, J.H., Khoo, L.H. and Camus, A.C. (2024) Massive branchial-henneguyosis of catfish: a distinct, myxozoan-induced disease caused by severe interlamellar *Henneguya exilis* infection in catfish aquaculture. *Veterinary Pathology* 61, 965–972.

Styer, E.L., Harrison, L.R. and Burtle, G.J. (1991) Experimental production of proliferative gill disease in channel catfish exposed to myxozoan-infected oligochaete, *Dero digitata*. *Journal of Aquatic Animal Health* 3, 288–291.

Thiyagarajah, A. (1993) Proliferative gill disease from the Tennessee–Tombigbee Waterway. *Journal of Aquatic Animal Health* 5, 219–222.

USDA (1997) *Catfish Epidemiology and Animal Health*. US Department of Agriculture, Animal and Plant Health Inspection Service, Fort Collins, Colorado.

USDA–NASS (2019) *2018 Census of Aquaculture, AC-17-SS-2*. US Department of Agriculture, National Agricultural Statistics Service, Washington, DC.

USDA–NASS (2024) *2023 Census of Aquaculture, AC-22-SS-2*. US Department of Agriculture, National Agricultural Statistics Service, Washington, DC.

Wagner, E.J. (2002) Whirling disease, prevention, control, and management: a review. *American Fisheries Society Symposium* 29, 217–225.

Wax, C.L., Pote, J.W. and Deliman, N.C. (1987) *A climatology of pond temperatures for aquaculture in Mississippi*. Mississippi Agricultural and Forestry Experiment Station Bulletin No. 149. Mississippi State University, Stoneville, Mississippi.

Whitaker, J.W., Pote, L.M., Khoo, L., Shivaji, R. and Hanson, L.A. (2001) The use of polymerase chain reaction assay to diagnose proliferative gill disease in channel catfish (*Ictalurus punctatus*). *Journal of Veterinary Diagnostic Investigation* 13, 394–398.

Whitaker, J.W., Pote, L.M. and Hanson, L.A. (2005) Assay to detect the actinospore and myxospore stages of proliferative gill disease in oligochaetes and pond water. *North American Journal of Aquaculture* 67, 133–137.

Wise, D.J., Camus, A., Schwedler, T. and Terhune, J. (2004) Health management. In: Tucker, C.S. and Hargreaves, J.A. (eds) *Biology and Culture of the Channel Catfish*, 1st edn. Elsevier BV, Amsterdam, pp. 482–488.

Wise, D.J., Griffin, M.J., Terhune, J.S., Pote, L.M. and Khoo, L. (2008) Induction and evaluation of proliferative gill disease in channel catfish fingerlings. *Journal of Aquatic Animal Health* 20(4), 236–244.

Wolf, K. and Markiw, M.E. (1984) Biology contravenes taxonomy in the Myxozoa: new discoveries show alternation of invertebrate and vertebrate hosts. *Science* 255, 1449–1452.

Woodyard, E.T., Rosser, T.G., Stilwell, J.M., Camus, A.C., Khoo, L.H. *et al.* (2022) New data on *Henneguya postexilis* Minchew, 1977, a parasite of channel catfish *Ictalurus punctatus*, with notes on resolution of molecular markers for myxozoan phylogeny. *Systematic Parasitology* 99, 41–62.

Zawisza, M., Chadzinska, M., Steinhagen, D., Rakus, K. and Adamek, M. (2024) Gill disorders in fish: lessons from poxvirus infections. *Reviews in Aquaculture* 16(1), 234–253.

Zhang, B., Tu, X. and Gu, Z. (2023) Henneguyosis: a novel threat to the exotic channel catfish *Ictalurus punctatus* cultivated in China. *Aquaculture* 576, 739831.

11 *Gyrodactylus salaris* and *Gyrodactylus derjavinoides*

Kurt Buchmann*
Department of Veterinary and Animal Sciences, Faculty of Health and Medical Sciences, University of Copenhagen, Denmark

Abstract

Gyrodactylus salaris and *Gyrodactylus derjavinoides* are monogenean parasites on fins and skin of certain salmonid species. They are hermaphroditic, viviparous and readily spread in vulnerable host populations. *G. salaris* was introduced to Norway in the 1970s and subsequently spread to 53 rivers with Atlantic salmon (*Salmo salar*). Most Baltic salmon strains have high natural resistance, but East Atlantic salmon strains are very susceptible to infection, which leads to severe stock depletion. Continuous monitoring of parasite occurrence is recommended. Control strategies are needed to eradicate these parasites, but some chemical methods have had ecological impacts. *G. derjavinoides* targets brown trout (*Salmo trutta*) in natural streams and rivers and rainbow trout (*Oncorhynchus mykiss*) in farms, which may call for control measures. However, the two host species are also able to mount protective mucosal responses on fins and skin to prevent epidemic outbreaks.

11.1. Introduction

Monogenean flatworms of the genus *Gyrodactylus* occur on a wide array of fishes, possess a high degree of host specificity and it has been estimated that the number of species may exceed 20,000 (Bakke *et al.*, 2002), with a few of these parasites infecting salmonids worldwide (Malmberg, 1993). In Europe the Atlantic salmon (*Salmo salar*), brown trout (*Salmo trutta*) and rainbow trout (*Oncorhynchus mykiss*) are hosts to several important species of which *Gyrodactylus salaris* and *Gyrodactylus derjavinoides* are considered the most pathogenic. The biological characteristics of *G. salaris* and *G. derjavinoides*, which are both freshwater parasites, have been studied in detail and these species will be discussed here.

G. salaris Malmberg, 1957 (Fig. 11.1) was first described from Baltic salmon sampled at a freshwater hatchery in the Swedish Hölle Laboratory, where the infection had caused problems in the early 1950s (Malmberg, 2004). The parasite probably originated in rivers draining into the Baltic Sea, which is populated by a Baltic strain of the Atlantic salmon. This fish stock comprises numerous subpopulations homing to rivers in Sweden, Finland, Russia, Latvia, Lithuania, Estonia, Poland and Germany draining into the Baltic Sea (Nilsson *et al.*, 2001; Ozerov *et al.*, 2010). The stock has been isolated from other races of Atlantic salmon for thousands of years following the end of the last glacial period. Norwegian salmon populating rivers draining into the Atlantic had probably always been free

*Email: kub@sund.ku.dk

 Fish Parasites: Pathobiology and Protection, 2nd Edition
(eds P.T.K. Woo and K. Buchmann)
DOI: 10.1079/9781800628748.0011

of *G. salaris* but anthropogenic transfer of infected salmon from Sweden into Norway occurred in the 1970s on several occasions. This was based on a high demand for salmon for stocking and experimental purposes (Johnsen and Jensen, 1991; Malmberg, 1993; Mo, 1994; Bakke *et al.*, 2007). The parasite was new to Norwegian stocks of wild salmon, but these fish showed up to be extremely susceptible to the worm which subsequently spread to at least 53 rivers in Norway resulting in severe ecological and economic problems (Mo, 2024). It is commonly called the 'the Norwegian salmon killer' (Malmberg, 1993; Bakke *et al.*, 2007). Economic losses are related to: (i) diminished fish stocks; (ii) loss of angler tourism; and (iii) parasitological surveys and control measures that have been estimated to cost more than 1.5 billion Norwegian Kroner (NOK) in the last decades (Mo, 2024). Other types of East Atlantic salmon (such as Scottish and Danish strains) are also very susceptible to the parasite and show no effective host response, whereas Baltic strains activate a clear protective response a few weeks after infection (Bakke *et al.*, 1990; Bakke and MacKenzie, 1993; Dalgaard *et al.*, 2003; Lindenstrøm *et al.*, 2006; Heinecke *et al.*, 2007; Kania *et al.*, 2007a, 2010). Several different fish species including stickleback (*Gasterosteus aculeatus*) and flounder (*Platichthys flesus*) have transient and non-lasting infections (Bakke *et al.*, 2007), whereas others such as Arctic charr (*Salvelinus alpinus*) allow significant persistence and propagation of the parasite (Winger *et al.*, 2008). The introduced and domesticated rainbow trout *O. mykiss* is susceptible to *G. salaris* and transfers of infected fish between farms spread the disease (Ieshko *et al.*, 2016; Hansen *et al.*, 2022). Recent studies have shown that some strains are pathogenic while others are non-pathogenic to East Atlantic salmon (Lindenstrøm *et al.*, 2003b; Jørgensen *et al.*, 2007; Robertsen *et al.*, 2007).

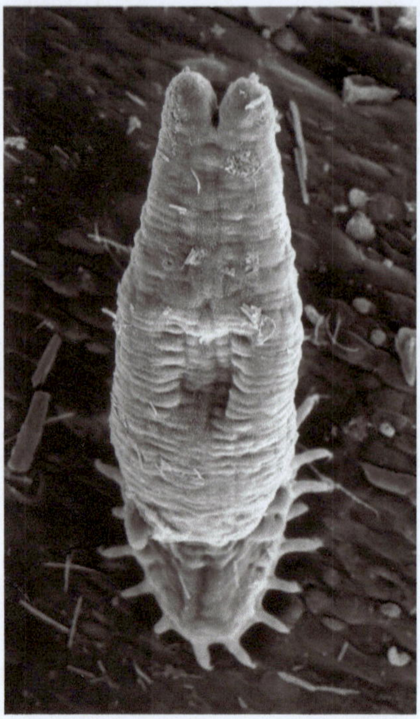

Fig. 11.1. *Gyrodactylus salaris*, *in toto*, on the fin of a Scottish River Conon salmon, dorsal view. Total length of the parasite = 800 μm. (Scanning electron microscopy (SEM) image by K. Buchmann and J. Bresciani.)

The parasite *G. derjavinoides* (Fig. 11.2) has been studied extensively (under the name *Gyrodactylus derjavini*) in European trout populations (Malmberg and Malmberg, 1993; Mo, 1993, 1997; Buchmann *et al.*, 2000). *G. derjavini* was originally recovered from the Caspian trout (*Salmo trutta caspius*) and described by Mikailov (1975). However, recent studies of *Gyrodactylus* from Iranian trout (*S. trutta caspius*) have suggested that the European parasite (up until then referred to as *G. derjavini*) differs from the parasite originally described by Mikailov (1975). Consequently the parasite in European trout was renamed *G. derjavinoides* by Malmberg *et al.* (2007). This parasite has probably been endemic in Eurasian populations of brown trout (*S. trutta*)

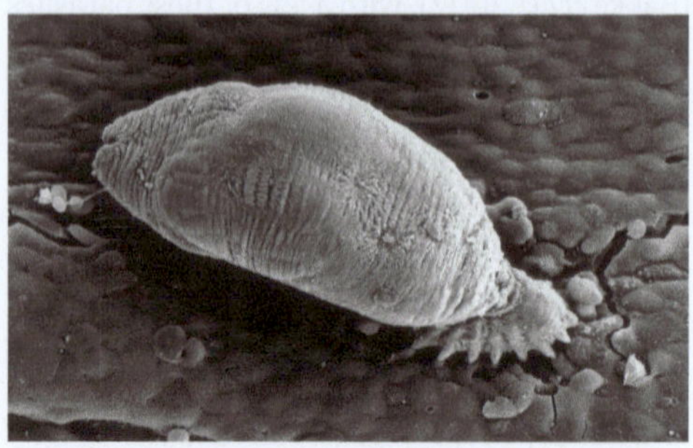

Fig. 11.2. *Gyrodactylus derjavinoides*, *in toto*, on the fin of a rainbow trout, dorsolateral view. Total length of the parasite = 800 μm. (SEM image by K. Buchmann and J. Bresciani.)

and rarely causes epidemics in natural water bodies although heavy parasite burdens in wild fish have been noted (Ergens, 1983; Buchmann *et al.*, 2000). However, the introduced domesticated *O. mykiss* is a susceptible and vulnerable host to this parasite, which may call for treatment (Buchmann and Bresciani, 1997; Buchmann and Uldal, 1997). Atlantic salmon may host the parasite but rarely allow a significant parasite population increase (Mo, 1993, 1997; Buchmann and Uldal, 1997; Olafsdottir *et al.*, 2003; Jørgensen *et al.*, 2008, 2009).

11.1.1. Description of the parasites

Both species are ectoparasitic flatworms with a length of less than 1 mm and a body width of around 0.1 mm. However, the soft body parts of gyrodactylids are affected by compression during slide preparation and their dimensions should not be used for diagnosis. In contrast, hard parts are of taxonomic importance. The ventrally directed opisthaptor is equipped with two large hamuli and 16 marginal hooklets (Figs 11.3 and 11.4). Shapes and dimensions of these sclerotized parts are used for diagnosis (see Mo, 1991, 1993; Malmberg, 1993). The dimensions of the hard structures are negatively correlated to temperature; consequently if parasites are propagated at low temperatures the anchors increase in size (Mo, 1991, 1993). The anterior part of the body is equipped with cephalic glands and ducts producing secretions. These structures and secretions are for attachment to the host surfaces and are used during migration of the worm from one host to the other or to objects in the aquatic environment (stones, gravel). Using light microscopy the intestinal caeca, pharynx and the cirrus are clearly visible. The most prominent character is the uterus in which the embryo develops. The parasite is viviparous and gives birth to a live young (which may already have an embryo in its uterus). The newborn is about the same size as the mother, and this spectacular organization with three generations in one parasite specimen has inspired parasitologists to call the system a Russian doll arrangement (Bakke *et al.*, 2007). Sequencing of genes encoding ribosomal DNA (the internal transcribed spacer (ITS) and intergenic spacer (IGS) regions) and mitochondrial enzymes have

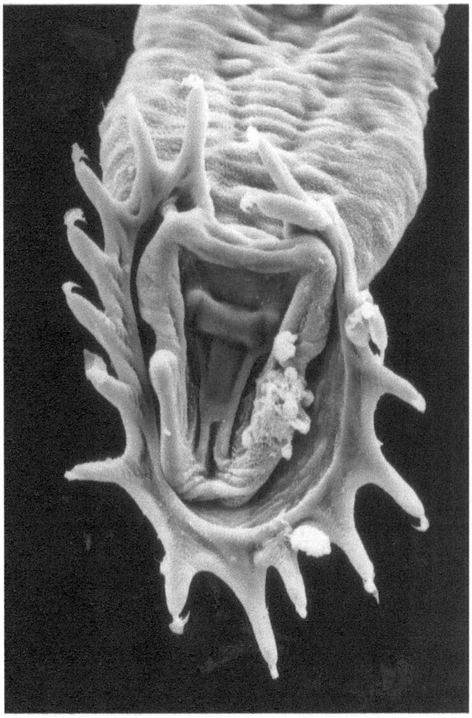

Fig. 11.3. Opisthaptor of *Gyrodactylus salaris*, ventral view showing hamuli and marginal hooklets. (SEM image by K. Buchmann and J. Bresciani.)

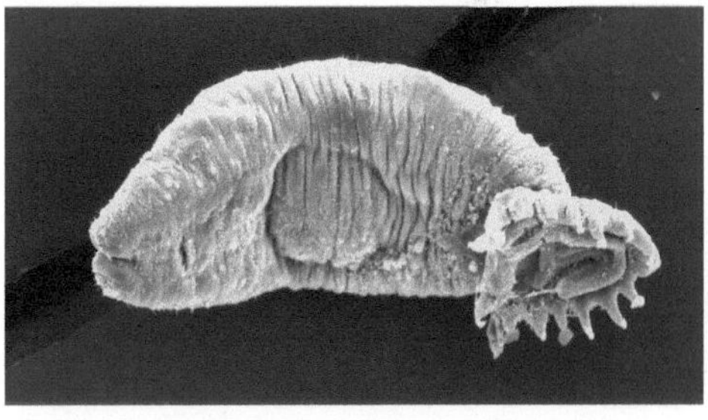

Fig. 11.4. *Gyrodactylus derjavinoides*, *in toto*, lateroventral view showing ventrally directed hamuli and marginal hooklets. (SEM image by K. Buchmann and J. Bresciani.)

proved to be excellent tools for species and strain discrimination (Cunningham *et al.*, 1995, 2003; Cunningham, 1997; Meinilä *et al.*, 2002; Hansen *et al.*, 2003; Huyse *et al.*, 2007, 2008; Collins *et al.*, 2010; Zietara *et al.*, 2010). These molecular tools have also improved detection sensitivity, which is the basis for the development of an alternative monitoring approach using environmental DNA (eDNA) to identify infected water bodies (Rusch *et al.*, 2018).

11.1.2. Location on the host

Both *G. derjavinoides* and *G. salaris* infect preferentially the fins of the fish but may also be found on the body proper and the head (including nostrils, mouth cavity and cornea). The gills are only rarely infected. However, the location on the host is influenced by: (i) the host strain; (ii) the parasite load; and (iii) the duration of the infection. During its initial colonization *G. salaris* selects preferentially fins and especially the pectoral fins (Fig. 11.5) of East Atlantic salmon. During an 8-week infection course the relative occurrence on pectoral fins decreases whereas a larger part of the parasite population can be found on the caudal fin. In contrast, the parasites will be found at higher frequency at the caudal fin of Baltic salmon at the initial stage of infection (Heinecke *et al.*, 2007). Heavily parasitized salmon will harbour parasites all over the body, including skin, fins and corneal surfaces. Moderately infected wild Norwegian salmon harbour the main part of the parasite population on the dorsal, anal and pectoral fins. Heavily infected salmon have parasites at all body sites (Jensen and Johnsen, 1992).

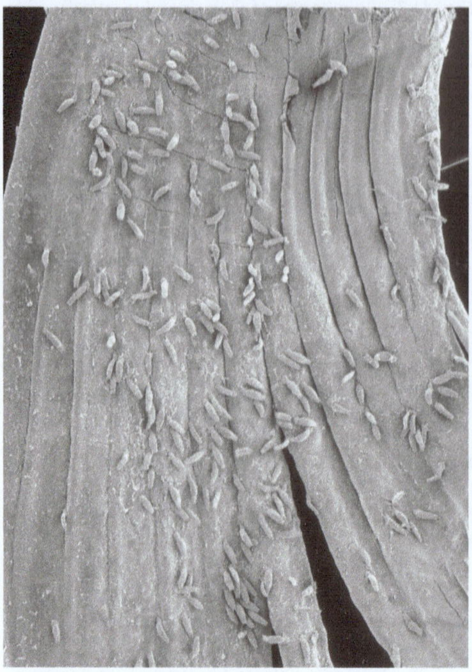

Fig. 11.5. *Gyrodactylus salaris* colonizing a salmon fin. (SEM image by K. Buchmann and J. Bresciani.)

The *G. derjavinoides* population is on the pectoral and pelvic fins on rainbow and brown trout shortly after the initial colonization. During a 6-week infection course the host mounts a mucosal response in the skin and the relative distribution on the fins and the body changes. The initial colonization sites become partly abandoned whereas previously less colonized sites such as the corneal surface and the tail fin become increasingly populated (Buchmann and Uldal, 1997; Buchmann and Bresciani, 1998). East Atlantic salmon and Baltic salmon obtain merely a weak infection by *G. derjavinoides* and then the parasites are found mostly on the tail fin, the pectoral, pelvic and anal fins, and the corneal surface of the host (Buchmann and Uldal, 1997).

11.1.3. Transmission

Both parasite species are able to spread from one host to another by direct contact between hosts or between hosts and detached parasites occurring on the substrate (stones or gravel or fish-tank walls) or floating in the water column. Both parasite species can detach from the host and move (using leech-like movements) in the fish tank (bottom, walls) or on stones, gravel, plant materials or alternative hosts in their natural aquatic habitat (river, lake). Also direct parasite transmission from dead hosts to live hosts is considered significant (Olstad *et al.*, 2006). The lifespan at the detached stage is temperature dependent but may for *G. derjavinoides* last for up to 5 days (Buchmann and Bresciani, 1999) and at least 25 h and probably several days for *G. salaris* (Larsen and Buchmann, 2006). Spreading of the parasite between different rivers and water bodies is mostly observed in connection with translocation of fish (transport and restocking). Fishing tackle which has not been disinfected may allow live parasites to be translocated from one river to another with anglers moving between fishing sites. *G. salaris* is not able to survive in high-salinity sea water but may persist for 240 h in 10 ppt and for 42 h in 20 ppt (Soleng and Bakke, 1997). Therefore, migration of infected salmon from infected rivers through low-salinity fjords may explain some cases of parasite introduction to previously uninfected rivers (Soleng and Bakke, 1997). *G. derjavinoides* may survive in water with 7 ppt sodium chloride and will also be able to spread between rivers in low-salinity waters but may not survive on trout migrating in high-salinity marine waters (Buchmann, 1997). A series of alternative hosts, especially Arctic charr, may represent an important reservoir for parasites which can infect salmon in previously uninfected sites or following chemical treatment of rivers (Winger *et al.*, 2008).

11.1.4. Geographical distribution

The pathogenic form of *G. salaris* is found in Norway where a series of subpopulations have been recognized (Hansen *et al.*, 2003). Probably the *G. salaris* in Sweden (Malmberg, 1993; Malmberg and Malmberg, 1993), Finland (Rintamäki-Kinnunen and Valtonen, 1996), Russia (Cunningham *et al.*, 2003; Zietara *et al.*, 2008; Kalinina and Kravets, 2020; Hansen *et al.*, 2022), Latvia (Hansen *et al.*, 2003) and Poland (Rokicka *et al.*, 2007) may be virulent to East Atlantic salmon. Recent reports from Northern Russia, where the parasite seems to spread along with rainbow trout transportation, indicate that the local parasite strain may have a potential to spread in rivers of the White Sea drainage system (Hansen *et al.*, 2022). In Denmark a confirmed non-pathogenic form of *G. salaris* has been isolated from rainbow trout in farms. It shows a predilection towards rainbow trout whereas Atlantic salmon (both East Atlantic and Baltic strains) are not able to sustain the parasite population (Jørgensen *et al.*, 2007). A similar *G. salaris* has been reported from Germany (Cunningham *et al.*, 2003) and Italy (Paladini *et al.*, 2009) as well. However, experimental studies on host preference and pathogenicity towards various salmonid species and strains of salmon have not yet been performed for German and Italian isolates. Due to the documented history of frequent rainbow trout transportations from Denmark to Germany and Italy, it is likely that at least some of the *G. salaris* from these countries belong to the same non-pathogenic type as reported by Lindenstrøm *et al.* (2003b) and Jørgensen *et al.* (2007). Thus, the *G. salaris* form pathogenic to East Atlantic salmon does not exist in Denmark (Jørgensen *et al.*, 2008) and it can be questioned if the *G. salaris* forms in Italy and Germany are pathogenic to salmon.

11.1.5. Diagnosis

The common approach to investigate if a stream, river or lake is populated by *Gyrodactylus*-infected fish is to sample fish and subsequently conserve fins and/or body in ethanol (70 or 96% v/v). Parasites can then be isolated in the laboratory from the preserved material and be subjected to morphometric and molecular analysis. An alternative parasite collection method was presented by Thrush *et al.* (2019) to allow survival of fish, reduce labour during the sampling process, reduce time for sampling and can sample a higher number of fish. By exposing the fish shortly after sampling to a low concentration of hydrogen peroxide these authors found that the majority of *G. derjavinoides* and *Gyrodactylus truttae* were removed from fins and skin in brown trout. Parasites could then be recovered from the water by filtration for diagnostic studies. Rusch *et al.* (2018) showed that a water sample taken for eDNA analysis is sufficient to detect infection in water using molecular techniques.

The classical diagnostic technique is based on morphometric analysis of the opisthaptoral hard parts including anchors and marginal hooklets (Mo, 1991, 1993; Malmberg, 1993; Shinn *et al.*, 1995). Also the location and arrangement of protonephridia can be used for diagnostic purposes (Malmberg, 1970) and the distribution of argentophilic structures on the parasite surface may aid differentiation of species (Shinn *et al.*, 1998). The morphometric method is valuable but the existence of parasite variants possessing different virulence has made it necessary to supplement with alternative methods. Cunningham *et al.* (1995) showed that small-subunit (18S) ribosomal RNA (rRNA) gene sequences could be used to differentiate some species (*G. salaris*, *G. derjavinoides* and *G. truttae*). *In situ* hybridization methods using specific probes binding to immobilized parasite DNA on various membrane types were applied with some success (Cunningham *et al.*, 1995). The ITS gene spanning from 18S over ITS1, 5.8S, ITS2 to 28S was different between *G. salaris*, *G. derjavinoides* and *G. truttae* and several restriction fragment length polymorphism (RFLP) methods could be used for fast identification (Cunningham, 1997). This method was later used to study a congeneric species *Gyrodactylus teuchis* (Cunningham *et al.*, 2001). Direct sequencing of DNA following PCR and subsequent comparison is time-consuming and therefore RFLP based on PCR, restriction enzyme incubation and finally agarose gel electrophoresis in ethidium bromide is used. Kania *et al.* (2007b) showed that non-pathogenic *G. salaris* could be differentiated from the pathogenic strain using an RFLP technique based on a single base substitution in the ITS region. Using a TaqMan probe real-time multiplex PCR assay, Collins *et al.* (2010) could reduce the time needed for a valid diagnosis based on ITS sequences even further. The rRNA genes are tandemly repeated and separated by gene regions called the IGS. The sequence variability within the IGS regions is very high and cannot easily be used for species identification (Cunningham *et al.*, 2003). Mitochondrial gene sequences encoding various enzymes within both *G. salaris* and *G. derjavinoides* can be used not only for strain identification but also for species identification (Meinila *et al.*, 2002; Hansen *et al.*, 2003; Huyse *et al.*, 2007, 2008; Zietara *et al.*, 2010). Different diagnostic techniques were evaluated by Shinn *et al.* (2010) in a multi-centre study which concluded that combining morphometric and molecular methods provides the most accurate diagnosis.

11.2. Pathobiology

Infection of salmonid fish with gyrodactylids has been the focus for numerous studies due to the obvious pathogenic effect of infection on the commercially important fish species. The rapid spread and impact on wild Atlantic salmon in Norwegian rivers since the 1970s accelerated the research efforts significantly. Effects are seen on the overall fish production and the behaviour and clinical signs of infected fish, which primarily are caused by the pathophysiological impact.

11.2.1. Impact of the disease on fish production

Susceptible Atlantic salmon can have extremely heavy *G. salaris* infections. Several thousand parasites per fish can be on Norwegian, Scottish and Danish salmon if fish are not treated. Farmed and wild fish start dying within 3–5 weeks of infection. At the population level, the impact of infection in wild fish becomes obvious after 1–2 years when the fish density has decreased. *G. derjavinoides* infections elicit morbidity and mortality of rainbow trout and brown trout (Ergens, 1983; Buchmann and Uldal, 1997) and call for frequent use of auxiliary substances in trout farms (Malmberg, 1993; Buchmann and Bresciani, 1997). However, the impact is highly dependent on the intensity of infection. Thus, young fry of brown trout may suffer seriously (30% mortality) already at a parasite load of five to ten parasites per trout. Further, the infection may predispose fish to subsequent bacterial pathogens such as *Flavobacterium psychrophilum* (Busch *et al.*, 2003).

11.2.2. Clinical signs

Heavy mortalities may be the first obvious sign of a *G. salaris* epidemic. Behavioural changes of infected fish may be restricted to lethargy, anorexia and seeking sheltered habitats. External macroscopic lesions and change of appearance may be darkening of the skin and emaciated fins (Fig. 11.5). The microscopic lesions responsible for the disease are visible using scanning electron microscopy (SEM). The worm attaches to the fin or skin surface of the host by inserting 16 marginal hooklets into the epidermis. This action is clearly associated with injuries to the epithelial cells (Fig. 11.6). Also feeding activities of the worm impose epithelium damage. The stimulation of the epidermis elicits an inflammatory reaction which can be seen as a slightly elevated epithelial surface around the

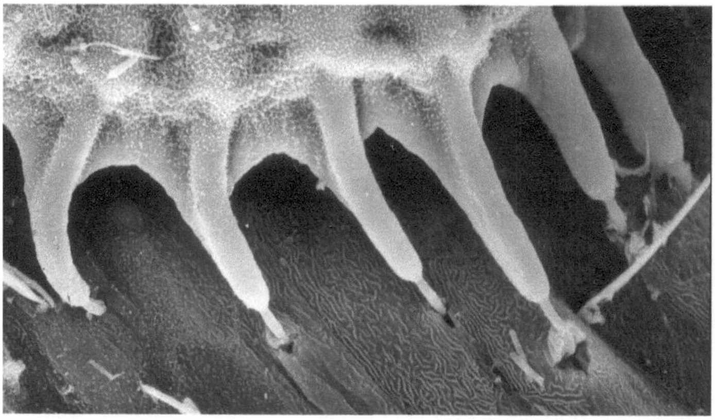

Fig. 11.6. *Gyrodactylus salaris*, marginal hooklets penetrating epithelial cells of the fin of a River Conon salmon. (SEM image by K. Buchmann and J. Bresciani.)

parasite's attachment site and feeding area (Fig. 11.7). In heavy infections the injuries are directly correlated to the number of worms on a given surface area of the fish skin, and the pathological disturbances induced by the individual worms may not be discernible in the totally emaciated skin. Also in *G. derjavinoides* infections the insertion of hooklets (Fig. 11.8) and feeding on epithelium produce openings and lesions (Buchmann and Bresciani, 1997).

11.2.3. Pathophysiology of the disease

The extensive emaciation of host epithelia following heavy gyrodactylid infections is likely to challenge the osmoregulatory system of the fish. Significant changes of the body fluid composition were measured in *G. salaris*-infected Atlantic salmon (Pettersen *et al.*, 2013), and it may be argued that the direct effect of the perforation of epidermal cells may cause problems for the fish when coping with the external ion concentrations. The infection may affect the host indirectly as well. Stimulation of trout skin by *G. derjavinoides* infection elicits a stress response with the release of cortisol in the host. Fish with even low infections have elevated cortisol levels in body fluids (Stoltze and Buchmann, 2001). Due to the immunosuppressive action of cortisol this stress reaction may leave the host more vulnerable to bacterial and fungal pathogens in the environment. Also the physical disturbance of the skin epidermis may give these pathogens an easy access to subepidermal compartments in the host and further aggravate the disease.

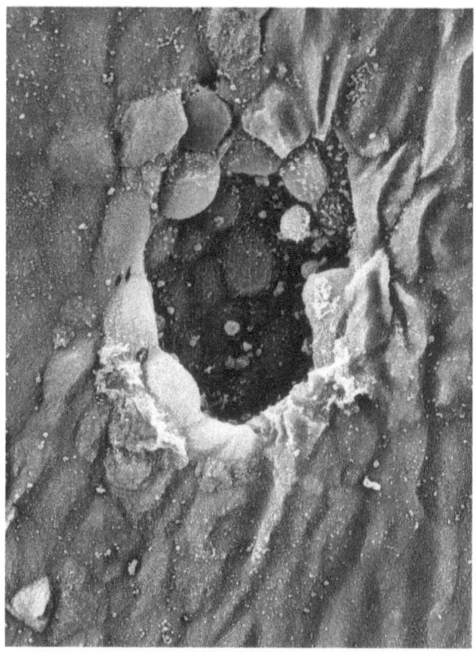

Fig. 11.7. Epithelial damage of salmon fin epidermis following *Gyrodactylus salaris* attachment and feeding. The wound is healing following escape of the worm. (SEM image by K. Buchmann and J. Bresciani.)

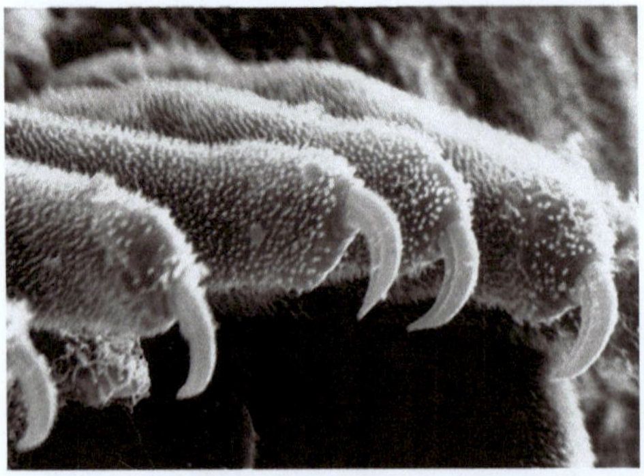

Fig. 11.8. *Gyrodactylus derjavinoides* marginal hooklets. (SEM image by K. Buchmann and J. Bresciani.)

11.3. Protective and Control Strategies

11.3.1. Immunity

The host immune responses against *G. salaris* and *G. derjavinoides* reflect intricate interactions between host specificity mechanisms and immunological factors (Buchmann, 1999; Bakke *et al.*, 2002). Host specificity may be influenced by immunological factors comprising both innate and adaptive immune factors. Antimicrobial peptides and complement factors may play a role but it is possible that other receptor/ligand interactions such as carbohydrate/lectin binding may be involved (Buchmann, 2001; Jørndrup and Buchmann, 2005). However, despite the presence of a host response against *G. derjavinoides* (Lindenstrøm and Buchmann, 2000) in rainbow trout and against *G. salaris* in Baltic salmon (Bakke *et al.*, 1990; Dalgaard *et al.*, 2003), no vaccines are available.

11.3.1.1. Gyrodactylus salaris

The Norwegian, Scottish and Danish strains of the East Atlantic salmon are not able to activate immune factors which confer protection to the host against the Norwegian *G. salaris*. In contrast, some subpopulations of the Baltic salmon strain will, with a few exceptions (Bakke *et al.*, 2004), clearly mount a host response following an infection (Bakke *et al.*, 1990; Bakke and MacKenzie, 1993; Dalgaard *et al.*, 2003; Lindenstrøm *et al.*, 2006; Kania *et al.*, 2007a, 2010). The mechanisms behind the response were elucidated by Harris *et al.* (1998), Buchmann *et al.* (2004), Lindenstrøm *et al.* (2006) and Kania *et al.* (2007a, 2010). Complement-like activity in serum and mucus of the host has an adverse effect on *G. salaris in vitro* (Harris *et al.*, 1998). However, this factor from both susceptible and resistant fish did not show differential activity and their involvement *in situ* is still to be described. The skin mucous cells of salmon are clearly part of the interactions between the host and *G. salaris* (Sterud *et al.*, 1998) and the content of immunologically active substances in these cells is likely to play a role (Buchmann, 1999). Using Western blotting, Buchmann *et al.* (2004) demonstrated that plasma antibodies (both from susceptible and resistant salmon exposed for more than 6 weeks) did not bind to *G. salaris* antigens. This suggests that host antibodies are not part of the response. Gene-expression studies have shown that the susceptible salmon elicits a fast cytokine response (interleukin-1β (IL-1β)) and a more extensive epithelial reaction whereas the less susceptible salmon are non-responsive (Lindenstrøm *et al.*, 2006; Kania *et al.*, 2007a, 2010) in the initial phase of the infection. The factor associated with resistance/low susceptibility in the response phase of Baltic salmon increased expression of: (i) the gene encoding serum amyloid protein A (SAA), which binds to pathogens; and (ii) interferon-γ (IFN-γ), which indicates lymphocyte involvement. Expression of major histocompatibility complex class II (MHC-II) (indicating macrophage activity) and of the regulating cytokine IL-10 is also part of the armament activated in responding salmon. It was hypothesized that a fast but non-specific epithelial skin reaction may benefit propagation of the parasites due to their feeding preference for epithelial cells and mucus. In contrast, resistant salmon restrict proliferation of epithelial cells and thereby limit nutritional uptake by the parasites which eventually are affected by SAA and other effector molecules and cells in the skin (Kania *et al.*, 2010). This corresponds well with the finding that susceptible salmon exhibit a higher mucous cell density in fins compared to resistant fish and that corticosteroid-treated susceptible salmon have an even higher infection concomitant with an increased mucous cell proliferation (Dalgaard *et al.*, 2003).

11.3.1.2. Gyrodactylus derjavinoides

It is well documented that brown trout and rainbow trout develop a temperature-dependent skin response against *G. derjavinoides* (Buchmann and Uldal, 1997; Buchmann and Bresciani, 1998; Andersen and Buchmann, 1998; Lindenstrøm and Buchmann, 2000). Following infection the parasite propagates on fins and skin but within 4–6 weeks the parasite population decreases markedly. The mechanisms involved in the antiparasitic response are corticosteroid labile (Lindenstrøm and Buchmann, 1998), which may indicate that the skin factors affecting the parasite adversely are immunological elements. Epidermal mucous cells are affected by *G. derjavinoides* (Buchmann and Bresciani, 1998; Lindenstrøm and Buchmann, 2000) and a series of mucous factors may affect the worms adversely (Buchmann, 1999). During an infection, specific antibodies binding to the parasite are not detected (Buchmann, 1998); this corresponds to the fact that adoptive transfer of serum from immune individuals does not confer protection to naïve fish (Lindenstrøm and Buchmann, 2000). Complement may be involved as judged from immediate killing following exposure to functional complement (Fig. 11.9). At least complement factor C3 has been shown to bind to epitopes of *G. derjavinoides* at the tegument, the opisthaptor and the cephalic gland ducts (Buchmann, 1998). Also leucocyte products and activity have adverse effects on this parasite (Buchmann and Bresciani, 1999). Molecular studies demonstrated that the reaction is initiated by the production of pro-inflammatory cytokines such IL-1β and tumour necrosis factor-α (TNF-α), events which are followed by expression of the gene encoding nitric oxide synthase (iNOS) (Lindenstrøm *et al.*, 2003a, 2004). Atlantic salmon can obtain an infection with *G. derjavinoides* but will not experience a build-up of infection unless treated with corticosteroids (Olafsdottir *et al.*, 2003). This suggests that host specificity mechanisms, at least partly, are dependent on corticosteroid-labile factors, such as immune factors.

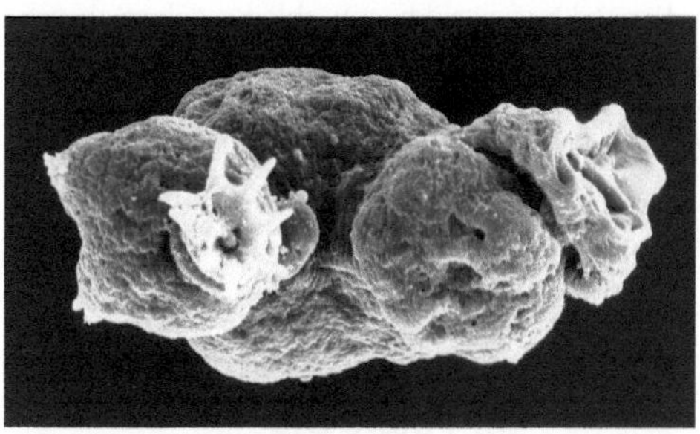

Fig. 11.9. *Gyrodactylus derjavinoides* after immediate killing due to exposure to complement-containing plasma from rainbow trout. (SEM image by K. Buchmann and J. Bresciani.)

11.3.2. Chemotherapy

The treatment strategies are dependent on whether the infection affects wild salmonids in natural rivers and lakes or occurs in confined environments (fish tanks). Application of rotenone for eliminating host fishes with *G. salaris* in natural river systems has been used for decades in Norwegian rivers (see Section 11.3.3) with some success (Mo, 2024). *Gyrodactylus* infections in aquaculture facilities are treated using various anthelmintics and auxiliary substances. Formaldehyde has been applied in traditional fish farming for treatment, but the substance must be avoided due to its carcinogenicity, mutagenicity and allergenic properties (Liu *et al.*, 2006; Nielsen and Wolkoff, 2010). Bath treatments (24 h) using mebendazole (1–5 mg/l) and praziquantel (5 mg/l) will eradicate *G. derjavinoides*. Raising temperature from 11–12 to 18–20°C during exposure augments the efficacy (Lindenstrøm and Buchmann, 1999). Also auxiliary substances and disinfectants such as sodium percarbonate (Buchmann and Kristensson, 2003) and hydrogen peroxide (10 mg/l) eliminate *G. derjavinoides* from the trout skin (Lindenstrøm and Buchmann, 1999). *G. salaris* may be similarly vulnerable to these treatments which mainly can be applied under fish-farm conditions, and the disinfectant Virkon® S (an oxidizing agent) applied in a concentration of 1% (v/v) for 15 min killed *G. salaris* (Koski *et al.*, 2016). Infections of wild fish in natural habitats pose a special challenge. None the less, chemotherapeutical strategies have been applied against *G. salaris* in wild salmon in Norway. Soleng *et al.* (1999) discovered that low pH and aluminium hydroxide are lethal to this parasite. Based on these observations field trials to eradicate *G. salaris* were performed in a series of Norwegian river systems in which aluminium sulfate was dosed continuously. The infection level in fish fell significantly when using aluminium in concentrations of 100–600 μg/l but success was dependent on temperature and buffer capacity of the water. Many river systems are not suitable for this practice and may need fish fences and rotenone treatment for a satisfactory control of the infection (Poleo *et al.*, 2004). Addition of sodium hypochlorite to water has parasiticidal effect on *G. salaris* without seriously affecting the host (Hagen *et al.*, 2014) and this chemotherapeutical approach may be used in future attempts to clear natural water bodies of this invasive parasite species (Mo, 2024). Effects of these compounds on the environment and other aquatic organisms should be investigated.

11.3.3. Zoosanitary measures and hygiene

Eradication of infections at farm level is most efficiently achieved through stamping out (euthanizing and removal of all fish), fallowing, disinfection and drying of ponds and tanks. Subsequently stocking parasite-free fish will secure a healthy fish population. Due to the high pathogenicity of *G. salaris* this approach has been taken with good success in Norwegian fish farms. When the *G. salaris* infection has reached an entire river ecosystem, more drastic measures are needed. Norwegian authorities treat entire river systems with the poison rotenone in order to eradicate the infected salmon population, whereby the parasite is eliminated as well because it cannot survive without its host (Guttvik *et al.*, 2004; Sandodden *et al.*, 2018). Subsequent stocking with non-infected salmon may secure repopulation of the river. These non-infected salmon are obtained from disease-free live genebank hatcheries. This strategy has been used in most infected Norwegian rivers, which may be declared parasite-free after 2 years of monitoring. Additional measures combined with rotenone treatments have been used. Thus, establishing fish fences at river outlets has proved effective in prevention of upward migration of infected fish. Some rivers have been reinfected following rotenone treatment (Guttvik *et al.*, 2004), but the parasite has been eradicated from at least 43 rivers by using this approach (Mo, 2024). As mentioned above, additional trials have involved continuous dosing of aluminium sulfate into rivers. This method could keep the infection level at a satisfactory level but was not able to eradicate the parasite population. During the latest years the use of chlorine compounds, poured directly into rivers, has shown parasiticidal effects on *G. salaris* under field conditions without harming the Atlantic salmon (Hagen *et al.*, 2014). The promising effects call for its use in various river systems in the future (Mo, 2024).

11.3.4. Biotic and abiotic manipulation to interrupt transmission

From a theoretical point of view, it would be worth considering the introduction of genes from less susceptible or resistant salmon into salmon with confirmed vulnerability and susceptibility to *G. salaris*. In line with this approach, Baltic salmon stocks could be used for stocking in infected areas in order to elevate survival and increase the stock. However, due to conservation issues and a general aim of protecting the original gene pool and diversity of the Norwegian salmon populations, this approach is at present unacceptable. Selection of parasite-resistant Norwegian salmon following experimental exposure to *G. salaris* and subsequent use of these fish in a breeding programme was suggested by Salte and Bentsen (2004). Extensive breeding studies using quantitative trait loci (QTLs) in Atlantic salmon populations pointed to at least ten genomic regions associated with resistance to *G. salaris* (Gilbey *et al.*, 2006). The authors concluded that resistance traits were polygenic inherited but could be suitable for selection programmes. However, Norwegian authorities are reluctant to use this breeding approach because it would change the original Norwegian salmon genome just to eradicate/control this parasite (Mo, 2024).

11.4. Conclusions with Suggestions for Future Studies

The *G. salaris* story from Norway emphasizes that anthropogenic transfer of fish to new areas with no history of previous occurrence can be catastrophic. The subsequent spread among vulnerable subpopulations has caused serious ecological and economic problems. This should serve as a lesson for fish transporters and authorities. At the least, stringent quarantine precautions should be taken in all cases involving similar transports. *G. derjavinoides* has not been shown to elicit similar problems among infected host populations in natural water bodies. However, it cannot be excluded that trout populations exist with a similar high susceptibility to infection. Accidental infection through similar fish movements and concomitant parasite transfer would prove harmful in such cases. Introduction of genes encoding resistance against parasites from foreign host populations, or alternatively establishment of breeding programmes based on Norwegian salmon, would be a theoretical possibility. However, such an approach would also be considered to be genetic interference of a salmon population which conservationists wish to keep intact. Constant dosing of substances into natural waters in order to kill parasites without harming the host fishes may be questioned from an environmental point of view. In addition, the use of rotenone for killing off infected hosts for eradication purposes may be discussed from both ethical and environmental points of view. Alternative measures call for basic research into the physiology of the parasite and especially of host–parasite interactions.

References

Andersen, P.S. and Buchmann, K. (1998) Temperature dependent population growth of *Gyrodactylus derjavini* on rainbow trout, *Oncorhynchus mykiss*. *Journal of Helminthology* 72, 9–14.

Bakke, T.A. and MacKenzie, K. (1993) Comparative susceptibility of native Scottish and Norwegian stocks of Atlantic salmon, *Salmo salar*, to *Gyrodactylus salaris* Malmberg: laboratory experiments. *Fisheries Research* 17, 69–85.

Bakke, T.A., Jansen, P.A. and Hansen, L.P. (1990) Differences in host resistance of Atlantic salmon, *Salmo salar* L., stocks to the monogenean *Gyrodactylus salaris* Malmberg, 1957. *Journal of Fish Biology* 37, 577–587.

Bakke, T.A., Harris, P.D. and Cable, J. (2002) Host specificity dynamics: observations on gyrodactylid monogeneans. *International Journal for Parasitology* 32, 281–308.

Bakke, T.A., Harris, P.D., Hansen, H., Cable, J. and Hansen, L.P. (2004) Susceptibility of Baltic and East Atlantic salmon *Salmo salar* stocks to *Gyrodactylus salaris* (Monogenea). *Diseases of Aquatic Organisms* 58, 171–177.

Bakke, T.A., Cable, J. and Harris, P.D. (2007) The biology of gyrodactylid monogeneans: the 'Russian-doll killers'. *Advances in Parasitology* 64, 161–376.

Buchmann, K. (1997) Salinity tolerance of *Gyrodactylus derjavini* from rainbow trout *Oncorhynchus mykiss*. *Bulletin of the European Association of Fish Pathologists* 17, 123–125.

Buchmann, K. (1998) Binding and lethal effect of complement from *Oncorhynchus mykiss* on *Gyrodactylus derjavini* (Platyhelminthes: Monogenea). *Diseases of Aquatic Organisms* 32, 195–200.

Buchmann, K. (1999) Immune mechanisms in fish skin against monogenean infections – a model. *Folia Parasitologica* 46, 1–9.

Buchmann, K. (2001) Lectins in fish skin: do they play a role in host–monogenean interactions? *Journal of Helminthology* 75, 227–231.

Buchmann, K. and Bresciani, J. (1997) Parasitic infections in pond-reared rainbow trout *Oncorhynchus mykiss* in Denmark. *Diseases of Aquatic Organisms* 28, 125–138.

Buchmann, K. and Bresciani, J. (1998) Microenvironment of *Gyrodactylus derjavini*: association between mucous cell density and microhabitat selection. *Parasitology Research* 84, 17–24.

Buchmann, K. and Bresciani, J. (1999) Rainbow trout leucocyte activity: influence on the ectoparasitic monogenean *Gyrodactylus derjavini*. *Diseases of Aquatic Organisms* 35, 13–22.

Buchmann, K. and Kristensson, R.T. (2003) Efficacy of sodium percarbonate and formaldehyde bath treatments against *Gyrodactylus derjavini*. *North American Journal of Aquaculture* 65, 25–27.

Buchmann, K. and Uldal, A. (1997) *Gyrodactylus derjavini* infections in four salmonids: comparative host susceptibility and site selection of parasites. *Diseases of Aquatic Organisms* 28, 201–209.

Buchmann, K., Lindenstrøm, T., Nielsen, M.E. and Bresciani, J. (2000) Diagnosis and occurrence of ectoparasite infections (*Gyrodactylus* spp.) in Danish salmonids. *Dansk Veterinaertidsskrift (Danish Veterinary Journal)* 83, 15–19.

Buchmann, K., Madsen, K.K. and Dalgaard, M.B. (2004) Homing of *Gyrodactylus salaris* and *G. derjavini* (Monogenea) on different hosts and response post-attachment. *Folia Parasitologica* 51, 263–267.

Busch, S., Dalsgaard, I. and Buchmann, K. (2003) Concomitant exposure of rainbow trout fry to *Gyrodactylus derjavini* and *Flavobacterium psychrophilum*: effects on infection and mortality of host. *Veterinary Parasitology* 117, 117–122.

Collins, C.M., Kerr, R., McIntosh, R. and Snow, M. (2010) Development of a real-time PCR assay for the identification of *Gyrodactylus* parasites infecting salmonids in northern Europe. *Diseases of Aquatic Organisms* 90, 135–142.

Cunningham, C.O. (1997) Species variation within the internal transcribed spacer (ITS) region of *Gyrodactylus* (Monogenea: Gyrodactylidae) ribosomal RNA genes. *Journal of Parasitology* 83, 215–219.

Cunningham, C.O., McGillivray, D.M., MacKenzie, K. and Melvin, W.T. (1995) Discrimination between *Gyrodactylus salaris*, *G. derjavini* and *G. truttae* (Platyhelminthes: Monogenea) using restriction fragment length polymorphisms and an oligonucleotide probe within small subunit ribosomal RNA gene. *Parasitology* 111, 87–94.

Cunningham, C.O., Mo, T.A., Collins, C.M., Buchmann, K., Thiery, R. *et al.* (2001) Redescription of *Gyrodactylus teuchis* Lautraite, Blanc, Thiery, Daniel and Vigneulle, 1999 (Monogenea: Gyrodactylidae), a species identified by ribosomal RNA sequence. *Systematic Parasitology* 48, 141–150.

Cunningham, C.O., Collins, C.M., Malmberg, G. and Mo, T.A. (2003) Analysis of ribosomal RNA intergenic spacer (IGS) sequences in species and populations of *Gyrodactylus* (Platyhelminthes: Monogenea) from salmonid fish in northern Europe. *Diseases of Aquatic Organisms* 57, 237–246.

Dalgaard, M.B., Nielsen, C.V. and Buchmann, K. (2003) Comparative susceptibility of two races of *Salmo salar* (Baltic Lule river and Atlantic Conon river strains) to infection with *Gyrodactylus salaris*. *Diseases of Aquatic Organisms* 53, 173–176.

Ergens, R. (1983) *Gyrodactylus* from Eurasian freshwater salmonidae and thymallidae. *Folia Parasitologica* 30, 15–26.

Gilbey, J., Verspoor, E., Mo, T.A, Sterud, E., Olstad, K. *et al.* (2006) Identification of genetic markers associated with *Gyrodactylus salaris* resistance in Atlantic salmon *Salmo salar*. *Diseases of Aquatic Organisms* 71, 119–29. DOI: 10.3354/dao071119.

Guttvik, K.T., Moen, A. and Skår, K. (2004) Control of the salmon parasite *Gyrodactylus salaris* by the use of the plant-derived poison rotenone. *Norsk Veterinaertidsskrift* 3, 172–174.

Hagen, A.G., Hytterød, S. and Olstad, K. (2014) Low concentrations of sodium hypochlorite affect population dynamics in *Gyrodactylus salaris* (Malmberg, 1957): practical guidelines for the treatment of the Atlantic salmon, *Salmo salar* L. parasite. *Journal of Fish Diseases* 37, 1003–1011.

Hansen, H., Bachmann, L. and Bakke, T.A. (2003) Mitochondrial DNA variation of *Gyrodactylus* spp. (Monogenea, Gyrodactylidae) populations infecting Atlantic salmon, grayling, and rainbow trout in Norway and Sweden. *International Journal for Parasitology* 33, 1471–1478.

Hansen, H., Ieshko, E., Rusch, J.C., Samokhvalov, I., Melnik, V. *et al.* (2022) *Gyrodactylus salaris* Malmberg, 1957 (Monogenea, Gyrodactylidae) spreads further – a consequence of rainbow trout farming in Northern Russia. *Aquatic Invasions* 17, 224–237.

Harris, P.D., Soleng, A. and Bakke, T.A. (1998) Killing of *Gyrodactylus salaris* (Platyhelminthes, Monogenea) mediated by host complement. *Parasitology* 117, 137–143.

Heinecke, R.D., Martinussen, T. and Buchmann, K. (2007) Microhabitat selection of *Gyrodactylus salaris* Malmberg on different salmonids. *Journal of Fish Diseases* 30, 733–743.

Huyse, T., Plaisance, L., Webster, B.L., Mo, T.A., Bakke, T.A. *et al.* (2007) The mitochondrial genome of *Gyrodactylus salaris* (Platyhelminthes: Monogenea), a pathogen of Atlantic salmon (*Salmo salar*). *Parasitology* 134, 739–747.

Huyse, T., Buchmann, K. and Littlewood, T. (2008) The mitochondrial genome of *Gyrodactylus derjavinoides* (Platyhelminthes: Monogenea) – a mitogenomic approach for *Gyrodactylus* species and strain identification. *Gene* 417, 27–34.

Ieshko, E., Barskaya, Y., Parshukov, A., Lumme, J. and Khlunov, O. (2016) Occurrence and morphogenetic characteristics of *Gyrodactylus* (Monogenea: Gyrodactylidae) from a rainbow trout farm (Lake Ladoga, Russia). *Acta Parasitologia* 61, 151–157.

Jensen, A.J. and Johnsen, B.O. (1992) Site specificity of *Gyrodactylus salaris* Malmberg, 1957 (Monogenea) on Atlantic salmon (*Salmo salar* L.) in the river Lakselva, Northern Norway. *Canadian Journal of Zoology* 70, 264–267.

Johnsen, B.O. and Jensen, A.J. (1991) The *Gyrodactylus* story in Norway. *Aquaculture* 98, 289–302.

Jørgensen, L.V.G., Heinecke, R.D. Kania, P. and Buchmann, K. (2008) Occurrence of gyrodactylids on wild Atlantic salmon, *Salmo salar* L., in Danish rivers. *Journal of Fish Diseases* 31, 127–134.

Jørgensen, T.R., Larsen, T.B., Jørgensen, L.G., Bresciani, J. and Buchmann, K. (2007) Isolation and characterisation of non-pathogenic form of *Gyrodactylus salaris* from rainbow trout. *Diseases of Aquatic Organisms* 73, 235–244.

Jørgensen, T.R., Jørgensen, L.G., Heinecke, R.D., Kania, P.W. and Buchmann, K. (2009) Gyrodactylids on Danish salmonids with emphasis on wild Atlantic salmon *Salmo salar*. *Bulletin of the European Association of Fish Pathologists* 29, 123–130.

Jørndrup, S. and Buchmann, K. (2005) Carbohydrate localization on *Gyrodactylus salaris* Malmberg, 1957 and *G. derjavini* Mikailov, 1975 and corresponding carbohydrate binding capacity of their hosts *Salmo salar* L. and *S. trutta* L. *Journal of Helminthology* 79, 41–46.

Kalinina, N. and Kravets, P. (2020) Activities for prevention of *Gyrodactylus salaris* distribution in the Kola Peninsula rivers. In: *International Applied Research Conference 'Biological Resources Development and Environmental Management'*, KnE Life Sciences, pp. 676–685. DOI: 10.18502/kls.v5i1.6149.

Kania, P.W., Larsen, T.B., Ingerslev, H.C. and Buchmann, K. (2007a) Baltic salmon activates immune relevant genes in fin tissue when responding to *Gyrodactylus salaris* infection. *Diseases of Aquatic Organisms* 76, 81–85.

Kania, P.W., Jørgensen, T.R. and Buchmann, K. (2007b) Differentiation between a pathogenic and a non-pathogenic form of *Gyrodactylus salaris* using PCR-RFLP. *Journal of Fish Diseases* 30, 123–126.

Kania, P.W., Evensen, O., Larsen, T.B. and Buchmann, K. (2010) Molecular and immunohistochemical studies on epidermal responses in Atlantic salmon *Salmo salar* L. induced by *Gyrodactylus salaris* Malmberg, 1957. *Journal of Helminthology* 84, 166–172.

Koski, P., Anttila, P. and Kuusela, J. (2016) Killing of *Gyrodactylus salaris* by heat and chemical disinfection. *Acta Veterinaria Scandinavica* 58, 21. DOI: 10.1186/s13028-016-0202-y.

Larsen, T.B. and Buchmann, K. (2006) Host specific *in vitro* colonisation of fish epithelia by gyrodactylids. *Acta Ichthyologica et Piscatoria* 36, 113–118.

Lindenstrøm, T. and Buchmann, K. (1998) Dexamethasone treatment increases susceptibility of rainbow trout, *Oncorhynchus mykiss* (Walbaum), to infections with *Gyrodactylus derjavini* Mikailov. *Journal of Fish Diseases* 21, 29–38.

Lindenstrøm, T. and Buchmann, K. (1999) Screening chemotherapeutic compounds against gyrodactylid infections in rainbow trout. Paper presented at the *European Association of Fish Pathologists' 9th Conference, Diseases of Fish and Shellfish*, Rhodes, Greece, 19–24 September.

Lindenstrøm, T. and Buchmann, K. (2000) Acquired resistance in rainbow trout against *Gyrodactylus derjavini*. *Journal of Helminthology* 74, 155–160.

Lindenstrøm, T., Buchmann, K. and Secombes, C.J. (2003a) *Gyrodactylus derjavini* infection elicits IL-1 beta expression in rainbow trout skin. *Fish and Shellfish Immunology* 15, 107–115.

Lindenstrøm, T., Collins, C.M., Bresciani, J., Cunningham, C.O. and Buchmann, K. (2003b) Characterization of a *Gyrodactylus salaris* variant: infection biology, morphology and molecular genetics. *Parasitology* 127, 165–177.

Lindenstrøm, T., Secombes, C.J. and Buchmann, K. (2004) Expression of immune response genes in rainbow trout skin induced by *Gyrodactylus derjavini* infections. *Veterinary Immunopathology and Immunology* 97, 137–148.

Lindenstrøm, T., Sigh, J., Dalgaard, M.B. and Buchmann, K. (2006) Skin expression of IL-1beta in East Atlantic salmon, *Salmo salar* L., highly susceptible to *Gyrodactylus salaris* infection is enhanced compared to a low susceptibility Baltic stock. *Journal of Fish Diseases* 29, 123–128.

Liu, Y.S., Li, C.M., Lu, Z.S., Ding, S.M., Yang, X. and Mo, J.W. (2006) Studies on formation and repair of formaldehyde-damaged DNA by detection of DNA-protein crosslinks and DNA breaks. *Frontiers in Bioscience* 11, 991–997.

Malmberg, G. (1970) The excretory systems and the marginal hooks as a basis for the systematics of *Gyrodactylus* (Trematoda, Monogenea). *Arkiv för Zoologi* Serie, Vol. 2. Royal Swedish Academy of Science, Stockholm, p. 23.

Malmberg, G. (1993) Gyrodactylidae and gyrodactylosis of salmonidae. *Bulletin Français de la Pêche et Pisciculture* 328, 5–46.

Malmberg, G. (2004) How the 'salmon killer' *Gyrodactylus salaris* Malmberg, 1957 was discovered and described in Sweden. Report from the front. In: Buchmann, K. (ed.) *Diagnosis and Control of Fish Diseases*. Research School of Sustainable Control of Fish Diseases in Aquaculture (SCOFDA), Royal Veterinary and Agricultural University, Frederiksberg, Denmark, pp. 12–18.

Malmberg, G. and Malmberg, M. (1993) Species of *Gyrodactylus* (Platyhelminthes, Monogenea) on salmonids in Sweden. *Fisheries Research* 17, 59–68.

Malmberg, G., Collins, C.M., Cunningham, C.O. and Jalai, B.J. (2007) *Gyrodactylus derjavinoides* sp. nov. (Monogenea, Platyhelminthes) on *Salmo trutta trutta* L. and *G. derjavini* Mikailov, 1975 on *S.T. caspius* Kessler, two different species of *Gyrodactylus* – combined morphological and molecular investigations. *Acta Parasitologica* 52, 89–103.

Meinilä, M., Kuusela, J., Zietara, M. and Lumme, J. (2002) Primers for amplifying 820 bp of highly polymorphic mitochondrial COI gene of *Gyrodactylus salaris*. *Hereditas* 137, 72–74.

Mikailov, T.K. (1975) Fish parasites of the waterbasins of Azerbaijan. *Institute of Zoology, Academy of Sciences, Azerbaijan SSR. ELM, Baku* 1, 68–69 (in Russian).

Mo, T.A. (1991) Seasonal variations of opisthaptoral hard parts of *Gyrodactylus salaris* Malmberg, 1957 (Monogenea: Gyrodactylidae) on parr of Atlantic salmon *Salmo salar* L. in laboratory experiments. *Systematic Parasitology* 20, 11–20.

Mo, T.A. (1993) Seasonal variations of opisthaptoral hard parts of *Gyrodactylus derjavini* Mikailov, 1975 (Monogenea: Gyrodactylidae) on brown trout *Salmo trutta* L. parr and of Atlantic salmon *Salmo salar* L. parr in the river Sandvikselva, Norway. *Systematic Parasitology* 26, 225–231.

Mo, T.A. (1994) Status of *Gyrodactylus salaris* problems and research in Norway. In: Pike, A.W. and Lewis, J.W. (eds) *Parasitic Diseases of Fish*. Samara Publishing, Dyfed, UK, pp. 43–56.

Mo, T.A. (1997) Seasonal occurrence of *Gyrodactylus derjavini* (Monogenea) on brown trout, *Salmo trutta*, and Atlantic salmon, *S. salar*, in the Sandvikselva river, Norway. *Journal of Parasitology* 83, 1025–1029.

Mo, T.A. (2024) The battle against the introduced pathogenic monogenean *Gyrodactylus salaris* in Norwegian Atlantic salmon rivers and fish farms. *Journal of Fish Diseases* 47, e13981. DOI: 10.1111/jfd.13981.

Nielsen, G.D. and Wolkoff, P. (2010) Cancer effects of formaldehyde: a proposal for an indoor air guideline value. *Archives of Toxicology* 84, 423–446.

Nilsson, J., Gross, R., Asplund, T., Dove, O., Jansson, H. *et al.* (2001) Matrilinear phylogeography of Atlantic salmon (*Salmo salar* L.) in Europe and postglacial colonisation of the Baltic Sea. *Molecular Ecology* 10, 89–102.

Olafsdottir, S.H., Lassen, H.P.Ø. and Buchmann, K. (2003) Labile resistance of Atlantic salmon, *Salmo salar* L., to infections with *Gyrodactylus derjavini* Mikailov, 1975: implications for host specificity. *Journal of Fish Diseases* 26, 51–54.

Olstad, K., Cable, J., Robertsen, G. and Bakke, T.A. (2006) Unpredicted transmission strategy of *Gyrodactylus salaris* (Monogenea: Gyrodactylidae): survival and infectivity of parasites on dead hosts. *Parasitology* 133, 33–41.

Ozerov, M.Y., Veselov, A.J., Lumme, J. and Primmer, C. (2010) Genetic structure of freshwater Atlantic salmon (*Salmo salar* L.) populations from the lakes Onega and Lodoga of Northwest Russia. *Conservation Genetics* 11, 1711–1724.

Paladini, G., Gustinelli, A., Fioravante, M.L., Hansen, H. and Shinn, A.P. (2009) The first report of *Gyrodactylus salaris* Malmberg, 1957 (Platyhelminthes, Monogenea) on Italian cultured stocks of rainbow trout (*Oncorhynchus mykiss* Walbaum). *Veterinary Parasitology* 165, 290–297.

Pettersen, R. Hytterød, S., Vøllestad, L. and Mo, T. (2013) Osmoregulatory disturbances in Atlantic salmon, *Salmo salar* L., caused by the monogenean *Gyrodactylus salaris*. *Journal of Fish Diseases* 36, 67–70. DOI: 10.1111/j.1365-2761.2012.01441.x.

Poleo, A.B.S., Lydersen, E. and Mo, T.A. (2004) Aluminium against the salmon parasite *Gyrodactylus salaris*. *Norsk Veterinaertidsskrift* 3, 176–180.

Rintamäkki-Kinnunen, P. and Valtonen, T.E. (1996) Finnish salmon resistant to *Gyrodactylus salaris*: a long-term study at fish farms. *International Journal for Parasitology* 26, 723–732.

Robertsen, G., Hansen, H., Bachmann, L. and Bakke, T.A. (2007) Arctic charr (*Salvelinus alpinus*) is a suitable host for *Gyrodactylus salaris* (Monogenea, Gyrodactylidae) in Norway. *Parasitology* 134, 257–267.

Rokicka, M., Lumme, J. and Zietara, M.S. (2007) Identification of *Gyrodactylus* ectoparasites in Polish salmonid farms by PCR-RFLP of the nuclear ITS segment of ribosomal DNA (Monogenea, Gyrodactylidae). *Acta Parasitologica* 52, 185–195.

Rusch, J.C., Hansen, H., Strand, D.A., Markussen, T., Hytterød, S. and Vrålstad, T. (2018) Catching the fish with the worm: a case study on eDNA detection of the monogenean parasite *Gyrodactylus salaris* and two of its hosts, Atlantic salmon (*Salmo salar*) and rainbow trout (*Oncorhynchus mykiss*). *Parasites and Vectors* 11, 333. DOI: 10.1186/s13071-018-2916-3.

Salte, R. and Bentsen, H.B. (2004) Breeding for resistance against *Gyrodactylus salaris*. *Norsk Veterinaertidsskrift* 3, 186–189.

Sandodden, R., Brazier, M., Sandvik, M., Moen, A., Wist, A.N. and Adolfsen, P. (2018) Eradication of *Gyrodactylus salaris* infested Atlantic salmon (*Salmo salar*) in the Rauma River, Norway, using rotenone. *Management of Biological Invasions* 9, 67–77.

Shinn, A.P., Sommerville, C. and Gibson, D.I. (1995) Distribution and characterization of species of *Gyrodactylus* Nordmann, 1832 (Monogenea) parasitizing salmonids in the UK, and their discrimination from *G. salaris* Malmberg, 1957. *Journal of Natural History* 29, 1383–1402.

Shinn, A.P., Sommerville, C. and Gibson, D.I. (1998) The application of chaetotaxy in the discrimation of *Gyrodactylus salaris* Malmberg, 1957 (Gyrodactylidae: Monogenea) from species of the genus parasitizing British salmonids. *International Journal for Parasitology* 28, 805–814.

Shinn, A., Collins, C., Garcia-Vasquez, A., Snow, M., Matejusova, I. *et al.* (2010) Multicentre testing and validation of current protocols for the identification of *Gyrodactylus salaris* (Monogenea). *International Journal for Parasitology* 40, 1455–1467.

Soleng, A. and Bakke, T.A. (1997) Salinity tolerance of *Gyrodactylus salaris* (Platyhelminthes, Monogenea): laboratory studies. *Canadian Journal of Fisheries and Aquatic Sciences* 54, 1837–1845.

Soleng, A., Poleo, A.B.S., Alstad, N.E.W. and Bakke, T.A. (1999) Aqueous aluminium eliminates *Gyrodactylus salaris* (Platyhelminthes, Monogenea) infections in Atlantic salmon. *Parasitology* 119, 19–25.

Sterud, E., Harris, P.H. and Bakke, T.A. (1998) The influence of *Gyrodactylus salaris* Malmberg, 1957 (Monogenea) on the epidermis of Atlantic salmon, *Salmo salar* L., and brook trout, *Salvelinus fontinalis* (Mitchill), experimental studies. *Journal of Fish Diseases* 21, 257–263.

Stoltze, K. and Buchmann, K. (2001) Effect of *Gyrodactylus derjavini* infections on cortisol production in rainbow trout fry. *Journal of Helminthology* 75, 291–294.

Thrush, M.A., Hill, T. and Taylor, N.G.H. (2019) Development of a non-lethal hydrogen peroxide treatment for surveillance of *Gyrodactylus salaris* on trout farms and its application to testing wild salmon populations. *Transboundary and Emerging Diseases* 66, 2107–2119.

Winger, A.C., Kanck, M., Kristoffersen, R. and Knudsen, R. (2008) Seasonal dynamics and persistence of *Gyrodactylus salaris* in two riverine anadromous Arctic charr populations. *Environmental Biology of Fishes* 83, 117–123.

Zietara, M.S., Kuusela, J., Veselov, A. and Lumme, J. (2008) Molecular faunistics of accidental infections of *Gyrodactylus* Nordmann, 1832 (Monogenea) parasitic on salmon *Salmo salar* L. and brown trout *Salmo trutta* in NW Russia. *Systematic Parasitology* 69, 123–135.

Zietara, M.S., Rokicka, M., Stojanovski, S. and Lumme, J. (2010) Introgression of distant mitochondria into the genome of *Gyrodactylus salaris*: nuclear and mitochondrial markers are necessary to identify parasite strains. *Acta Parasitologica* 55, 20–28.

12 *Pseudodactylogyrus anguillae* and *Pseudodactylogyrus bini*

Kurt Buchmann*
Department of Veterinary and Animal Sciences, Faculty of Health and Medical Sciences, University of Copenhagen, Denmark

Abstract

Parasitic monogeneans, *Pseudodactylogyrus anguillae* and *Pseudodactylogyrus bini*, cause severe disease in aquaculture of European eel (*Anguilla anguilla*) and Japanese eel (*Anguilla japonica*). It is hypothesized that the two monogeneans have originated from parasites in Pacific eels and spread to Europe via the fish trade. These monogeneans are hermaphroditic and oviparous with a temperature-dependent life cycle comprising eggs, oncomiracidia, juveniles and adults. Mechanical and chemical stimulations of host gills by opisthaptoral hard parts and parasite feeding elicit hyperplasia, lamellar fusion and clubbing of gill filaments, which reduce the respiratory surface and oxygen uptake. Biosecurity measures are necessary to prevent introduction of parasites, but if parasites are in a facility control measures include filtration of water using fine filters to remove eggs and larvae. Bath treatments of infected eels using praziquantel or mebendazole reduce infection level and eel mortality. European eels develop acquired immunity, but no vaccines are available.

12.1. Introduction

Wild and farmed eels (genus *Anguilla*) suffer from a series of diseases which include the infections caused by monogenean gill parasites (genus *Pseudodactylogyrus*). Two species cause severe outbreaks of pseudodactylogyrosis in eel farms. These are *Pseudodactylogyrus bini*, which was first recorded in Japan (Kikuchi, 1929) and *Pseudodactylogyrus anguillae*, first reported in China (Yin and Sproston, 1948) on Japanese eel (*Anguilla japonica*) during the first half of the 20th century. With increased focus on aquaculture of both Japanese eel (*A. japonica*) and European eel (*Anguilla anguilla*) in the 1970s, the disease attracted attention from researchers both in Europe (Molnar, 1983; Lambert *et al*., 1984; Buchmann *et al*., 1987a) and in Asia (Ogawa and Egusa, 1976; Egusa, 1979). This was linked to the intensification of pond culture of Japanese and European eel in Japan (Ogawa and Egusa, 1976; Egusa, 1979), China and Taiwan (Chan and Wu, 1984; Chung *et al*., 1984) and the subsequent development of the water recirculation system in farming of European eel in Europe since the 1980s. *Pseudodactylogyrus* monogeneans are oviparous with a high potential for rapid spread and propagation. The disease exhibits similarities to the conditions caused by *Dactylogyrus vastator* in common carp (*Cyprinus carpio*) aquaculture (Paperna, 1964), by *Dactylogyrus lamellatus* in grass carp (*Ctenopharyngodon idella*)

*Email: kub@sund.ku.dk

(eds P.T.K. Woo and K. Buchmann)
DOI: 10.1079/9781800628748.0012

ponds (Molnar, 1972) and by *Thaparocleidus vistulensis* in European catfish (*Silurus glanis*) farms (Sajiri *et al.*, 2025). It has been suggested that the two species of *Pseudodactylogyrus* were introduced to European waters due to intercontinental transfer of live infected eels (Buchmann *et al.*, 1987a). Later the two congeners were isolated in North America (Cone and Marcogliese, 1995; Hayward *et al.*, 2001; Kania *et al.*, 2010) and when *P. anguillae* was recorded in anguillid eels on the African continent, a similar mode of spread was suspected (Taraschewski, 2006; Parker *et al.*, 2011; Truter *et al.*, 2021). However, others have hypothesized that parasites might have spread with migrations of eel ancestors millions of years ago during continental drift (Cone and Marcogliese, 1995). Anthropogenic transportation of eels confounds the original distribution of these parasites in the different eel species, but these congeners are considered indigenous in *Anguilla marmorata* in Japan (Katahira and Nagasawa, 2014). The European eel is an endangered species (EC, 2007; ICES, 2007) and regardless of their origin, these eel parasites cause serious concerns and measures should be taken to control the disease, both in farms and, where possible, in wild eels.

12.2. Description of the Parasites

Eight species within the genus *Pseudodactylogyrus* have been described. These include *P. bini*, which was described from Japanese eel in Japan (Kikuchi, 1929), and *P. anguillae*, described from Japanese eel in China (Yin and Sproston, 1948). The former was originally described as *Dactylogyrus bini* by Kikuchi (1929) in Japan and the latter as *Neodactylogyrus anguillae* by Yin and Sproston (1948) in China. The type host in both cases was the Japanese eel (*A. japonica*). The genus *Pseudodactylogyrus* was erected by Gussev (1965) studying parasite specimens recovered from Australian eels (*Anguilla reinhardtii*). Later Ogawa (1984) described *Pseudodactylogyrus haze* from a non-anguillid fish species, the Japanese goby (*Acanthogobius flavimanus*). Further studies by Iwashita *et al.* (2002) led to a description of *Pseudodactylogyrus kamegaii* from wild Japanese eel, and Ogawa *et al.* (2015) described *Pseudodactylogyrus gusevi*, *Pseudodactylogyrus rhodei* and *Pseudodactylogyrus mundayi* from Australian eels. The same authors transferred a species previously described as *Dactylogyrus bialatus* (isolated from a gobiid fish) to the genus *Pseudodactylogyrus*. It cannot be excluded that all these species may have potential to elicit pathological reactions in fish kept in aquaculture and in confined environments allowing propagation of parasite populations. However, it can be documented that *P. bini* and *P. anguillae* are pathogenic to anguillid eels. They are small oviparous monopisthocotylean monogeneans with four eye spots and have a maximum body length of 1.96 mm (*P. bini*) and 1.66 mm (*P. anguillae*). These are hermaphroditic, possessing an ovary, vitellaria (glands producing egg materials), a sclerotized vagina (opening on to the lateral body part), a testis, a prostate gland, a cirrus and an accessory cirrus. The anterior part of the worm is equipped with cephalic openings leading into a series of gland structures producing secretions facilitating attachment during movements (Fig. 12.1). The opisthaptor is located in the posterior part of the body and is equipped with two large ventrally directed hamuli (Fig. 12.2) and 14 marginal hooklets (of larval type) that are used for attachment to the host gills. The parasite uses leech-like movements when translocating on host gills or (when dislodged) on objects in the environment. The oral opening is located at the anteroventral part of the worm, and it feeds on gill epithelia and mucus by grasping the tissue with the mouth and a muscular pharynx (Fig. 12.1). The ingested gill material is digested in the two intestinal caeca which contain esterases, aminopeptidases and phosphatases (Buchmann *et al.*, 1987b;

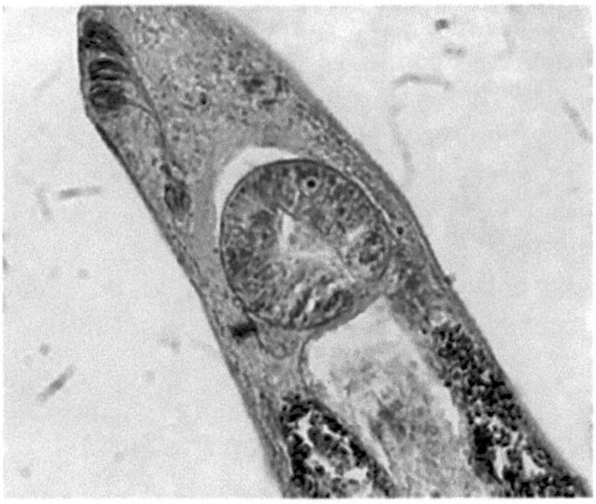

Fig. 12.1. Adult *Pseudodactylogyrus bini*. Histological section (3 μm) showing forepart of worm with cephalic glands and ducts with their openings and a muscular pharynx. (Author's own image.)

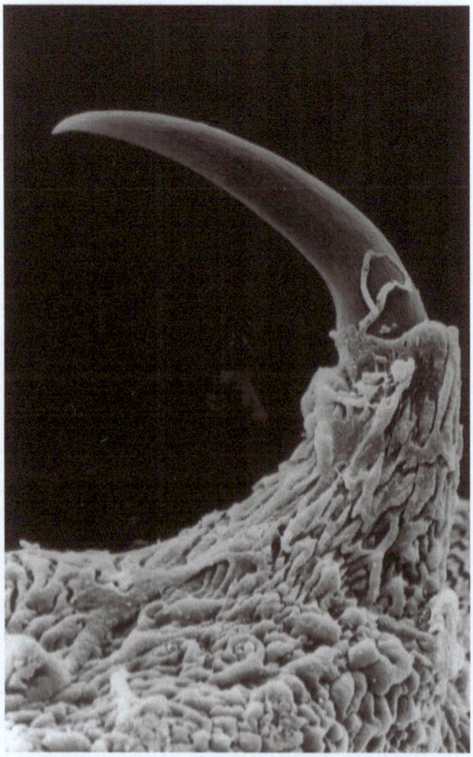

Fig. 12.2. Hamulus tip of *Pseudodactylogyrus anguillae* protruding from the covering tegument of the opisthaptor. Tip length = 25 μm. (Scanning electron microscopy (SEM) image by K. Buchmann and M. Køie).

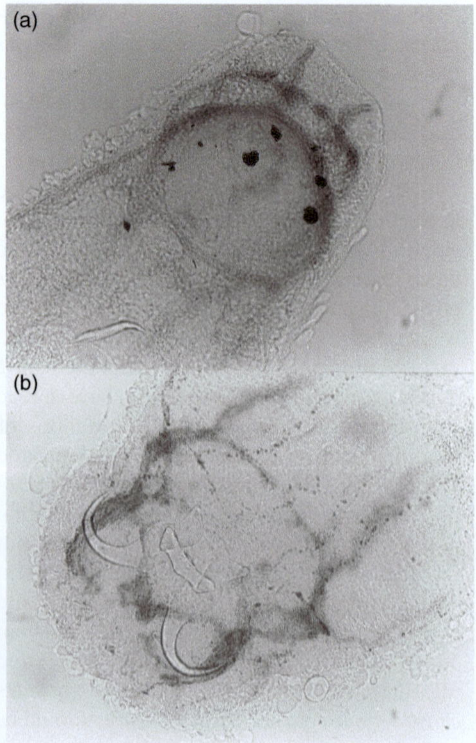

Fig. 12.3. Nervous system of *Pseudodactylogyrus bini* visualized using acetylcholinesterase staining. (a) Front part of worm with four eye spots located over the cerebral ganglia and nerve trunks leading anteriorly and posteriorly. (b) Hind part of worm with opisthaptor possessing hamuli and nerve trunks. Length of entire worm = 1.5 mm. (Author's own image.)

Buchmann, 1988b). The worm has no anus, and undigested material may be regurgitated to the exterior along with enzymes which stimulate the gill epithelium. The excretory system is based on flame cells connected to a system of excretory ducts. The nervous system is composed of a pair of cerebral ganglia connected to ventral and dorsal longitudinal nerves (leading anteriorly and posteriorly) which again are interconnected by transverse commissures (Fig. 12.3). Nervous transmission is based on cholinergic and aminergic elements (Buchmann and Prentø, 1989).

12.3. Location on the Host

Pseudodactylogyrus parasites inhabit fish gills (Fig. 12.4). They attach to the host as larvae (oncomiracidia) by using their larval hooklets. Their primary locations are gill filaments or occasionally head/opercula from where they subsequently migrate to the gill apparatus. Juveniles and adults use their opisthaptors to anchor to the primary gill filaments and their lamellae. The two congeners may be found at all sites in the gill apparatus but studies on smaller eels have shown that these two species have preferred microhabitats. *P. anguillae*, which is more mobile and translocates more easily compared with *P. bini*, selects preferentially the basal and median part of the gill filament on the two posterior gill arches. *P. bini*, in contrast, is more frequently found on the first two gill arches at the median to distal part of the filament (Buchmann, 1989a). Larger eels, possessing a relatively larger gill area, do not show the same parasite distribution (Buchmann, 1989a; Dzika, 1999; Matejusova *et al.*, 2003; Fang *et al.*, 2008). It has been suggested that congeners,

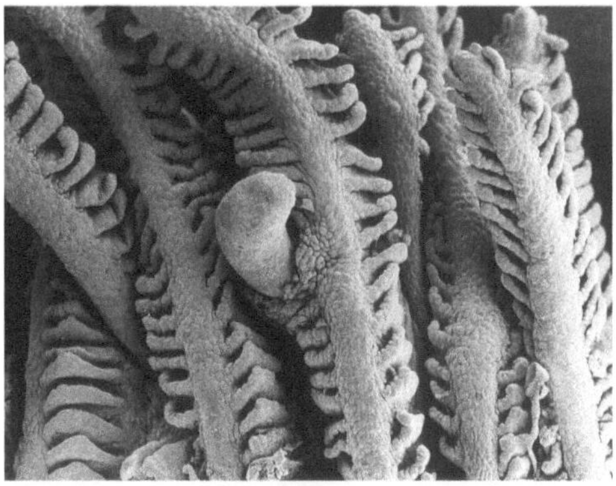

Fig. 12.4. *Pseudodactylogyrus bini* attached to the median part of a primary gill filament of *Anguilla anguilla*. The adult worm, 1.5 mm long, is partly embedded in gill tissue. (SEM image by K. Buchmann and M. Køie.)

due to a selection force through evolution, select different microhabitats to minimize hybridization (Rohde, 1977). The selective force would be that only intraspecific mating leads to fertile offspring. On the other hand, competition could play a role in this segregation. Several competitive mechanisms could be involved. One factor could be based on the fact that *P. bini* elicits severe hyperplasia and epithelial reaction around its attachment site but remains attached despite the host reaction. In contrast, *P. anguillae* may be less able to cope with the distorted gill tissue and escapes from sites with inflammatory reactions in the gill apparatus (Buchmann, 1988c). A similar phenomenon, called competitive exclusion, between *Dactylogyrus* congeners on the gills of carp was described by Paperna (1964).

12.4. Transmission

The life-cycle stages of *Pseudodactylogyrus* parasites (Fig. 12.5) comprise the adult oviparous worm on the gills, the undeveloped egg released (Fig. 12.6), the oncomiracidium developing inside the egg (Fig. 12.7) and the post-larva (Fig. 12.8). Following copulation fertilized eggs are released into the aquatic environment. The oviposition rate is highly dependent on temperature. *P. bini* produces no eggs at temperatures below 10°C. At 15°C, the parasite produces two or three eggs daily; at 20°C, five eggs; at 25°C, 12–13 eggs; and at 30°C, 17 eggs are produced daily. At higher temperatures (e.g. 32 and 34°C) the egg release rate decreases markedly (Buchmann, 1988d). A similar pattern has been observed for *P. anguillae* although the egg production is lower at all temperatures (Buchmann, 1990b). The time from oviposition to hatching is also highly temperature-dependent for both species. Fifty per cent of *P. bini* eggs will hatch after 3 days at 30°C, after 4 days at 25°C, after 6 days at 20°C and at 15°C it takes longer than 11 days (Buchmann, 1988d). *P. anguillae* seems to cope better at lower temperatures. Hatching occurs following 3 days at 30°C, after 3.5 days at 25°C, after 4 days at 20°C, after 18 days at 15°C and after 46 days at 10°C (Buchmann, 1990b).

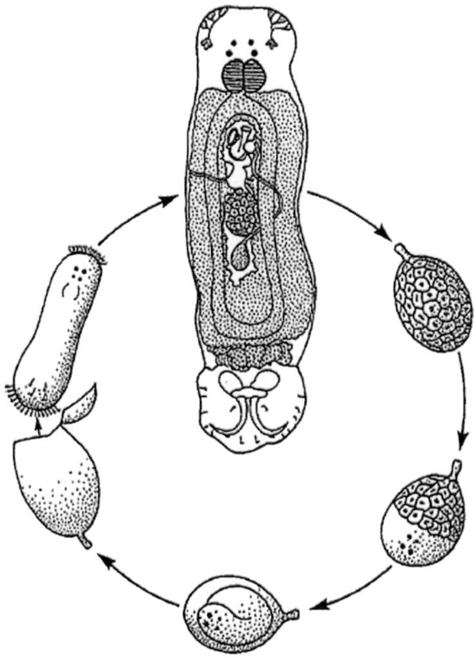

Fig. 12.5. Life cycle of *Pseudodactylogyrus* parasites. The drawing shows a mature hermaphroditic and oviparous worm delivering an egg which embryonates and hatches to a free-swimming ciliated larva (oncomiracidium). This larval stage attaches to the host gill, sheds its ciliated cells and develops through the post-larval stage to the adult egg-producing parasite. (Author's own image.)

The oncomiracidium escaping the shell of the egg is ciliated and equipped with four eye spots, 14 marginal hooklets and two undeveloped

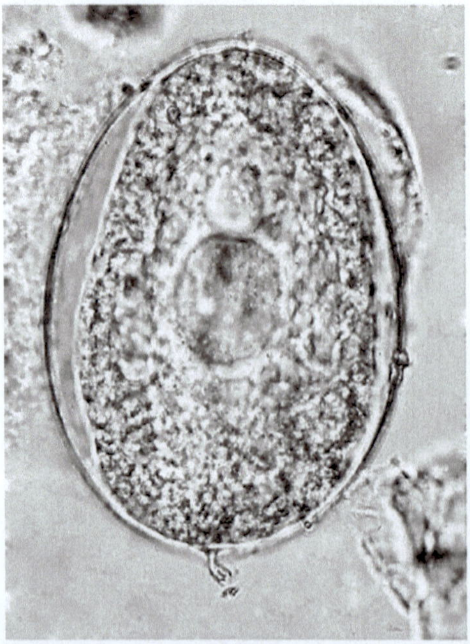

Fig. 12.6. Newly produced and undeveloped egg of *Pseudodactylogyrus anguillae*. Length of egg = 52 µm. (Author's own image.)

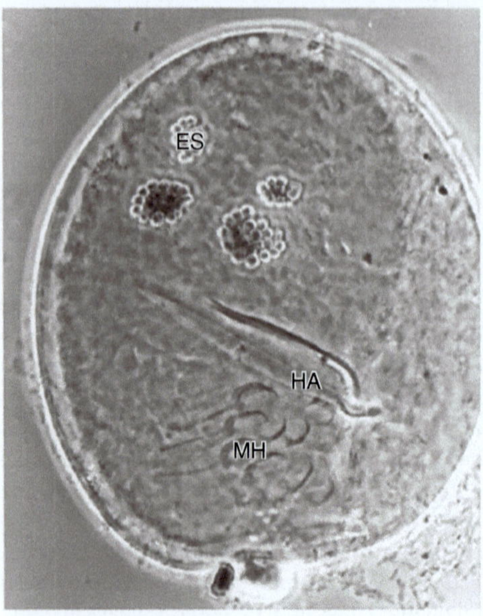

Fig. 12.7. Fully embryonated egg containing an oncomiracidium of *Pseudodactylogyrus anguillae*. The eye spots (ES), hamuli anlagen (HA) and marginal hooklets (MH) are visible in the larva inside the egg's shell. (Author's own image.)

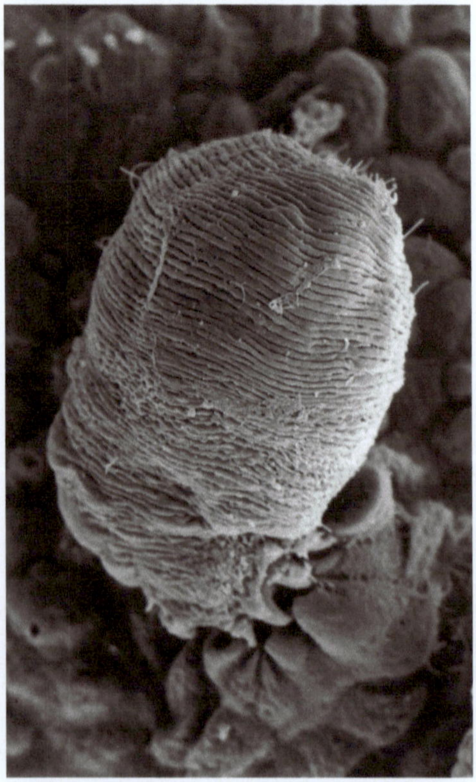

Fig. 12.8. Post-larva of *Pseudodactylogyrus anguillae* attached to a gill filament of *Anguilla anguilla*. Length of post-larva = 200 µm. (SEM image by K. Buchmann and M. Køie.)

hamuli. The oncomiracidium moves in elegant spirals before attaching to the host. This free-living stage is relatively short lived (up to 6 h) (Golovin, 1977; Imada and Muroga, 1978).

Following attachment to the host the oncomiracidium sheds its ciliated cells and starts moving in a leech-like manner to its preferred microhabitat. The time to reach the adult stage is also highly dependent on temperature. At 25–30°C *P. anguillae* produces its first eggs 6–7 days post-infection (Imada and Muroga, 1978; Buchmann, 1990b). This maturation period is 8–9 days for *P. bini* (Buchmann, 1988d).

The lifespan of *P. anguillae* is more than 210 days at 10°C. This is shortened considerably at 20°C (62 days), at 25°C (47 days), at 30°C (30 days) and at 34°C (14 days). The generation time (time from egg deposition to the adult reproducing worm) is around 10 days for *P. anguillae* at

25–30°C and around 11–12 days for *P. bini* (Buchmann, 1988d, 1990b).

12.5. Geographical Distribution

The parasites have been recorded in Japan (Kikuchi, 1929; Ogawa and Egusa, 1976; Fang *et al.*, 2008), China (Yin and Sproston, 1948; Chan and Wu, 1984), Taiwan (Chung *et al.*, 1984), the Indian Ocean (Sasal *et al.*, 2008), Russia (Golovin, 1977), Australia (Gussev, 1965; Hayward *et al.*, 2001), Europe (Molnar, 1983; Lambert *et al.*, 1984; Buchmann *et al.*, 1987a; Køie, 1988; Nie and Kennedy, 1991; Dzika *et al.*, 1995; Saraiva, 1995; Gelnar *et al.*, 1996; Skorikova *et al.*, 1996; Sures *et al.*, 1999; Matejusova *et al.*, 2003; Aguilar *et al.*, 2005; Kania *et al.*, 2010), Africa (Christison and Baker, 2006), North America (Hayward *et al.*, 2001) and Canada (Cone and Marcogliese, 1995; Kania *et al.*, 2010). Due to the initial isolation of the parasites in Japan (Kikuchi, 1929) and China (Yin and Sproston, 1948), it has generally been accepted that their original distribution was the Pacific region. Hence it has been considered an introduced species in Europe, Africa and North America. This is further supported by the finding that the European eel is significantly more susceptible to the parasites when compared with the Japanese eel (Fang *et al.*, 2008). This view has been challenged by Cone and Marcogliese (1995) who suggested the parasites have been associated with both the American eel (*Anguilla rostrata*) and the European eel (*A. anguilla*) since its original ancient spread from the Pacific.

12.6. Disease Impact on Wild and Farmed Fish

Commercial production of European eel (*A. anguilla*) has been severely hampered due to pseudodactylogyrosis both in Europe and Japan (Ogawa and Egusa, 1976; Egusa, 1979). Also farming of Japanese eels is affected (Chan and Wu, 1984; Chung *et al.*, 1984) but generally Japanese eels are less susceptible to the parasite (Fang *et al.*, 2008). In European eel decrease of feed intake and lethargy are some of the first indications of infection. If the parasitosis is left untreated, marked disease signs and high mortality (up to 90%) may subsequently occur. Following introduction of the water recirculation system of eel farming in Europe around 1980, it soon became evident that pseudodactylogyrosis was associated with high mortality and that strict monitoring of parasite occurrence and regular control measures in farms should be implemented to secure stable production (Buchmann *et al.*, 1987a). The impact on wild eels has not been elucidated; however, significant infections of wild European eels have been recorded in some freshwater lakes (Køie, 1988; Nie and Kennedy, 1991; Dzika *et al.*, 1995; Saraiva, 1995; Gelnar *et al.*, 1996; Skorikova *et al.*, 1996; Dzika, 1999; Sures *et al.*, 1999; Matejusova *et al.*, 2003; Aguilar *et al.*, 2005) and it can be assumed that the wild population at certain locations may be affected by this parasitosis. Since Japanese eels appear to be less susceptible to both parasite species (Fang *et al.*, 2008), it may be hypothesized that the wild populations of *A. japonica* are also less affected by these parasites.

12.7. Diagnosis

Correct diagnosis of the infection requires: (i) euthanasia of the host; (ii) dissection of the gill apparatus; (iii) recovery of the gill monogeneans under the dissection microscope; and (iv) subsequent mounting of worms on microscope slides whereby they can be examined at 100–400× magnification for morphometric analysis. Only the hard parts (sclerotized structures) should be used for diagnosis. Soft parts may be stained but due to the distorting effect of compression under slide preparation, these parts should not be used for diagnostic purposes. In order to differentiate between *P. anguillae* and *P. bini* the morphology and size of the hamuli (anchors) and marginal hooklets must be recorded. *P. anguillae* possess long and slender hamuli (Fig. 12.9) whereas *P. bini* anchors are short and stout (Fig. 12.10). The distance between the base of the hamulus curvature and the highest point of the shaft (where it is joining the flexible upper part) is suitable for diagnosis. Thus, this parameter is 53–61 μm in *P. bini* and

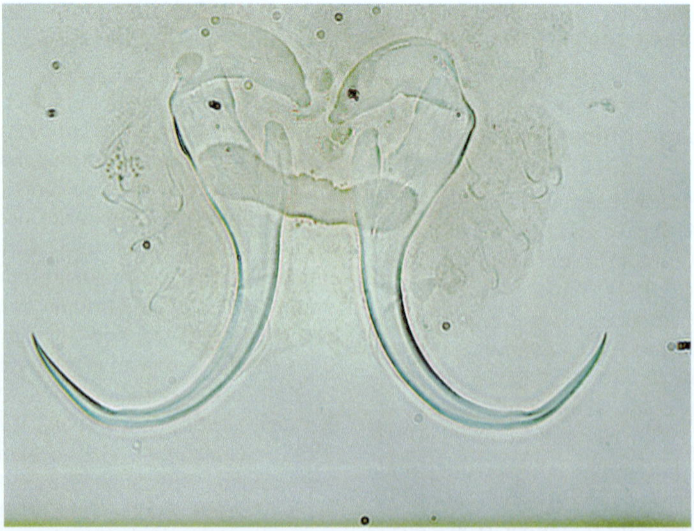

Fig. 12.9. Hamuli from *Pseudodactylogyrus anguillae* showing the long and slender shape to be used for species discrimination (light microscopy). The distance between the hamulus curvature and the upper shaft at the junction with the flexible part is 100 µm. (Author's own image.)

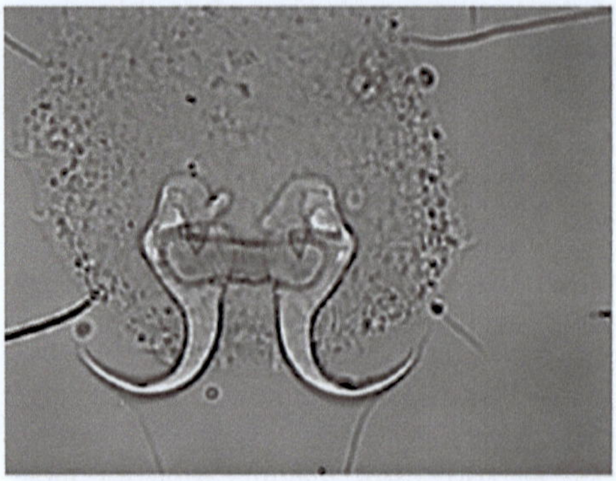

Fig. 12.10. Hamuli from *Pseudodactylogyrus bini* showing the short and stout shape of the anchor (light microscopy). The distance between the hamulus curvature and the upper shaft at the junction with the flexible part is 60 µm. (Author's own image.)

95–114 µm in *P. anguillae*. A key for differentiation of all species within the genus was presented by Ogawa *et al.* (2015).

Molecular techniques may supplement the classical morphometric analysis. The DNA sequence of the genes encoding ribosomal RNA (18S, 28S and the internal transcribed spacer (ITS) region including 5.8S) can be used to differentiate the two species. The methods are dependent on lysis of the parasite (by incubation with proteinase K), subsequent PCR using specific primers and finally sequencing (Hayward *et al.*, 2001; Kania *et al.*, 2010; Ogawa *et al.*, 2015).

A non-lethal and fast diagnostic procedure for clinical use was presented by Buchmann (1990a). This method includes anaesthesia of the host and subsequent insertion of a microendoscope through the opercular opening into the gill chamber of the eel immersed in water. Live parasites present on the gill filaments can be detected and enumerated without killing the host. The parasites will, however, be diagnosed to merely genus level by this technique.

12.8. Clinical Signs and Behavioural Effect of Infection on Eels

Mild infections do not seriously affect the eel. However, if left uncontrolled even weak infections will, due to the short generation time of the parasite, in a few weeks develop into severe infections eliciting serious morbidity and mortality.

The impact of the parasite burden is dependent not on the intensity (number of parasites per fish) but rather on the number of parasites in relation to the size of the eel. The gill surface of fish increases markedly with body length

(Hughes, 1966) and the space available for parasite attachment therefore increases with host size (Buchmann, 1989b). Therefore glass eels and young fingerlings will suffer from even a small number of parasites, which will cause no problems in larger eels. Heavy infections make the eels lethargic and anorectic. The first sign is a decrease of feeding activity, and a second clear sign of gill disease is the fish seeking the water surface (with higher oxygen saturation) due to decreased uptake of oxygen by the affected gills. When reaching a threshold level eels turn upside down and eventually die. In recirculation fish-farming systems (applying a continuous flow of water through tanks and biofilters), the weakened eels are not able to remain at their positions in the fish tank and flow with water currents. This leads eventually to trapping of diseased eels in grids at the outlet.

12.9. Macroscopic and Microscopic Lesions

Severe pathological reaction may be induced by the infection (Egusa, 1979; Buchmann, 1988b,c). The parasite inserts its hamuli and marginal hooklets into gill tissue, which initiates a host inflammatory reaction and cellular response (Fig. 12.11). Hyperplasia of mucous cells is associated with excess production of mucus. Hyperplasia of gill epithelial cells leads to clubbing of primary gill filaments, fusion of gill lamellae and even of adjacent primary filaments (Fig. 12.12). Numerous neutrophilic granulocytes and macrophages are recognized in the gill tissue. These reactions reduce the respiratory gill surface area leading to an impaired gas exchange (release of carbon dioxide from the host and uptake of oxygen). The extensive tissue reaction may lead to partial embedding of *P. bini* (Buchmann, 1988b,c). This parasite species has relatively small hamuli and is less mobile. When the parasite is removed severe malformations of dysfunctional gill tissue can be observed. Haemorrhages due to parasite feeding and insertion of hooks may be evident and telangiectasias are found in heavily infected eels. Further, the injuries produced by the action of attachment hooks and parasite feeding may allow facultative pathogens (bacteria and fungi) to colonize and gain access to the host tissues.

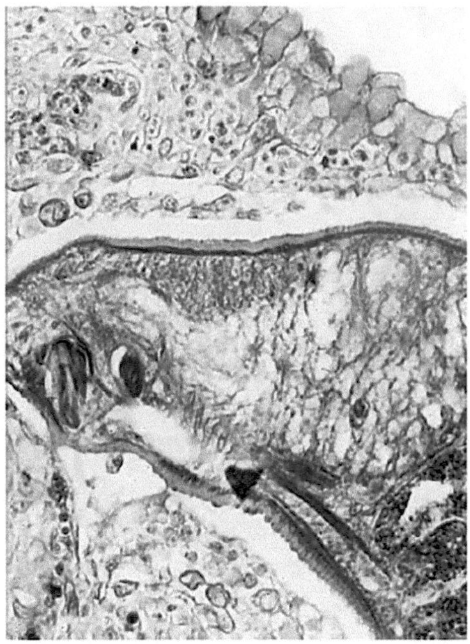

Fig. 12.11. Histological section showing extensive hyperplasia around the opisthaptor of *Pseudodactylogyrus bini* attached to and partly embedded in gill filaments of European eel. (Author's own image.)

12.10. Pathophysiology of the Disease

The effect of the parasites on the host is dependent on the intensity in relation to the host size. Smaller eels (glass eels and fingerlings) suffer from even low infections which cause no or merely a slight problem to larger eels. This is based on the anatomical relationship between host length and gill surface area, which makes the available colonization area of the gills much higher in large eels (Hughes, 1966). Therefore clinical signs in larger eels do normally first occur at relatively high infection intensities. In all cases the surface area of the gill apparatus is markedly reduced due to the severe pathological reactions caused by the infection. This will evidently affect gas exchange and ammonia excretion via gill epithelia. No information from controlled experiments on the effect of *Pseudodactylogyrus* parasites on oxygen uptake and swimming performance of eels is available. However, working with a comparable system

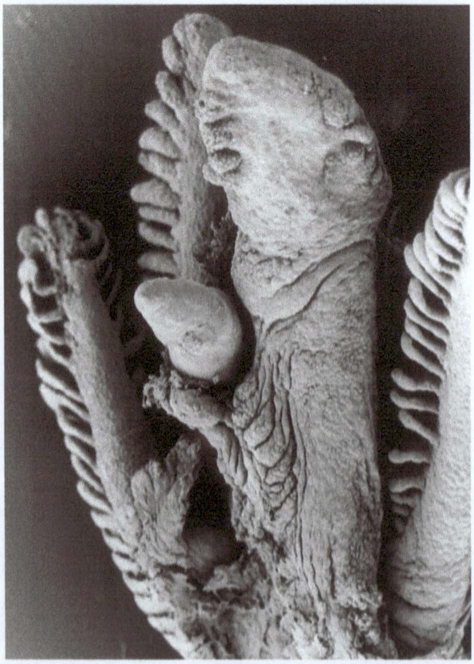

Fig. 12.12. Extensive gill tissue reaction of eel gills with clubbing and fusion of gill filaments due to *Pseudodactylogyrus bini* infection. The adult partly embedded worm is 1.5 mm in length. (SEM image by K. Buchmann and M. Køie.)

(fry of common carp infected with *D. vastator*), Molnar (1994) demonstrated intensity-dependent morbidity of hosts induced by hypoxia. The parasites feed primarily and directly on the gill epithelia and mucus, but in severe cases even blood leaking from haemorrhages may be ingested as well. Since this monopisthocotylean parasite is a surface browser, it normally does not ingest blood; consequently anaemia is not directly linked to pseudodactylogyrosis but may occur as a secondary effect (due to decreased food intake of eels).

12.11. Control Strategies

12.11.1. Immunity

The host reacts strongly to infections by epithelial and mucous cell hyperplasia. The reaction is spectacular in *P. bini* infections where epithelial outgrowth may partly encapsulate and embed the parasite. Also, *P. anguillae* infections are associated with general gill epithelial hyperplasia. An acquired and partly protecting host reaction has been demonstrated in the European eel. Fingerlings of *A. anguilla* were immunized by an experimental primary infection (mixed infection of *P. anguillae* and *P. bini*) which subsequently was eliminated (by bath treatment using the anthelmintic mebendazole). Challenge infections by exposure of eels to infective oncomiracidia at 14 and 33 days post-treatment showed that previously infected eels had a reduced worm burden compared to naïve eels (Slotved and Buchmann, 1993). Although this protective effect on its own is not sufficient for control of the disease under farming conditions, together with additional control measures host immune responses may contribute to acceptable infection levels in farms. The immune reactions mounted in eels comprise both innate and adaptive responses. The cellular elements of the reactions are evident from the histopathological picture discussed earlier, where direct contact between host cells and the tegument of the parasite is noted (Fig. 12.11). The humoral response is represented by a weak, but specific, antibody reactivity in the blood against a few parasite antigens as demonstrated using Western blotting by Buchmann (1993), Mazzanti *et al.* (1999) and Monni and Cognetti-Varriale (2002).

12.11.2. Chemotherapy

Fish farmers have traditionally applied various auxiliary substances such as potassium permanganate, methylene blue, ammonia, formaldehyde, chlorine and sodium chloride in order to control this parasitosis (Chan and Wu, 1984; Buchmann *et al.*, 1987a; Umeda *et al.*, 2006). Formaldehyde has been used frequently (regular bath treatments at 30–90 ppm) with some efficacy. However, the well-defined stress effect of formaldehyde on fish (Jorgensen and Buchmann, 2007) and documented carcinogenic and allergenic properties of this chemical call for alternative measures. Sodium chloride is generally regarded as a relatively environmentally friendly substance for treating ectoparasites. However, it has no effect on adult specimens of *Pseudodactylogyrus*. *P. bini* may be affected by 20 ppt sodium chloride but *P. anguillae* seems to be more salt tolerant and survives this treatment (Buchmann *et al.*, 1992). However, larval stages (oncomiracidia) are sensitive to sodium chloride in high concentrations (25–40 ppt) (Umeda *et al.*, 2006). The organophosphate metrifonate (trichlorphon, Neguvon®) was tested by Chan and Wu (1984) and Umeda *et al.* (2006), who showed efficacy, but due to its high toxicity to eels its use is not recommended. A series of commercially available anthelmintics have been tested. Some anthelmintics were shown to have toxic effects on *A. anguilla* (e.g. niclosamide, ivermectin) and should therefore be avoided (Buchmann *et al.*, 1990a). However, a number of drugs showed high efficacy against the parasites and low toxicity to the host and could be recommended for eel culture. Especially benzimidazoles such as mebendazole, luxabendazole and flubendazole (1 mg/l) were found to have a high parasiticidal effect and low toxicity to the host (Szekely and Molnar, 1987; Buchmann and Bjerregaard, 1990a,b). Also praziquantel (10 mg/l) showed an excellent effect (Buchmann, 1987; Buchmann *et al.*, 1990b). Due to the risk for selection of anthelmintic-resistant parasite populations in frequently treated farms (Waller and Buchmann, 2001), any drug application should be carefully monitored. Alternative herbal extracts, including ginkgolic acids, were suggested as potential parasiticides for European eels by Wang *et al.* (2009).

12.11.3. Zoosanitary measures

Widespread use of mechanical filters in modern fish farming to remove excess organic material from the water has been shown to prevent gill parasite infections as well. Mechanical filters with mesh sizes of 40 μm or less (commonly used in modern fish farms) are able to remove a considerable number of eggs and larvae from the water. The free-living larva may be vulnerable to ultraviolet (UV) irradiation. UV light has been proved to kill infective ciliates with high efficacy (Gratzek *et al.*, 1983) and monogenean larvae are likely to be vulnerable to this energy-rich irradiation. Studies have shown that parasite eggs can be trapped and ingested by elements of the free-living microfauna in recirculation fish-tank systems. Thus, newly produced eggs were ingested and eliminated by turbellarians (*Stenostomum* sp.) and copepods eliminated parasite larvae (Buchmann, 1988a). These organisms may contribute to a reduction of the infection pressure in farms but due to difficulties in controlling the population size of the microfauna, this biocontrol method needs further development before implementation in farms. Disinfection of fish tanks by regular drying of inner fish-tank surfaces (if applicable) may assist killing of parasite eggs and thereby reduce the infection pressure (Umeda *et al.*, 2006).

12.12. Conclusions

The European eel is an endangered species (EC, 2007; ICES, 2007) probably due to deterioration of habitats for juvenile eels in brackish and freshwater locations, but also other species within the genus *Anguilla* are under pressure. Diseases caused by bacterial (Haenen and Davidse, 2001), viral (Haenen *et al.*, 2002) and parasitic organisms (Taraschewski, 2006) may have contributed to the crisis, which may be further aggravated by increasing temperatures in the aquatic environment. These may provide excellent opportunities for the oviparous monopisthocotyleans of the genus *Pseudodactylogyrus* with a proven predilection for higher temperatures. Pseudodactylogyrosis may be controlled in aquaculture enterprises by mechanical and medical measures, but wild eel stocks may be exposed to a less well-defined and uncontrolled infection pressure. Therefore, the disease should be monitored regularly in natural eel populations as part of conservation and management programmes (EC, 2007). The diagnostic methods available are already useful for general purposes but further in-depth research on the genome of the parasites may assist in future high-resolution detection of various strains of parasites.

12.13. Recommendations for Future Studies

Despite clear evidence that the two species of *Pseudodactylogyrus* have been spread through intercontinental transfer of eels, the possibility still exists that a range of parasite species co-evolved with the different anguillid species during colonization (millions of years ago) of new marine habitats arising during periods with continental drift. Development of additional molecular markers, apart from the ITS region (e.g. intergenic spacer (IGS) and mitochondrial genes), may prove to be useful tools in the future for solving these questions. In addition, these tools will still be useful for tracing recent anthropogenic transfer of the two parasites between continents. Sustainable control methods in farms should be further developed. Mechanical filtering and medical methods of control have shown their strength, but alternative methods based on biological control and immune responses of the host may assist this purpose. Immunization may confer a relative protection against reinfection and additional research efforts should be initiated to explore the possibilities for immunoprophylaxis.

References

Aguilar, A., Alvarez, M.F., Leiro, J.M. and Sanmartin, M.L. (2005) Parasite populations of the European eel (*Anguilla anguilla* L.) in the rivers Ulla and Tea (Galicia, northwest Spain). *Aquaculture* 249, 85–94.

Buchmann, K. (1987) The effects of praziquantel on the monogenean gill parasite *Pseudodactylogyrus bini*. *Acta Veterinaria Scandinavica* 28, 447–450.

Buchmann, K. (1988a) Epidemiology of pseudodactylogyrosis in an intensive eel-culture system. *Diseases of Aquatic Organisms* 5, 81–85.

Buchmann, K. (1988b) Feeding of *Pseudodactylogyrus bini* (Monogenea) from *Anguilla anguilla*. *Bulletin of the European Association of Fish Pathologists* 8, 79–81.

Buchmann, K. (1988c) Interactions between the gill-parasitic monogeneans *Pseudodactylogyrus anguillae* and *P. bini* and the fish host *Anguilla anguilla*. *Bulletin of the European Association of Fish Pathologists* 8, 98–100.

Buchmann, K. (1988d) Temperature-dependent reproduction and survival of *Pseudodactylogyrus bini* (Monogenea) on the European eel (*Anguilla anguilla*). *Parasitology Research* 75, 162–164.

Buchmann, K. (1989a) Microhabitats of monogenean gill parasites on European eel (*Anguilla anguilla*). *Folia Parasitologica* 36, 321–329.

Buchmann, K. (1989b) Relations between host-size of *Anguilla anguilla* and the infection level of the monogeneans *Pseudodactylogyrus* spp. *Journal of Fish Biology* 36, 599–601.

Buchmann, K. (1990a) Endoscope-technology for detection of monogenean gill-parasites from eels. *Bulletin of the European Association of Fish Pathologists* 10, 60–61.

Buchmann, K. (1990b) Influence of temperature on reproduction and survival of *Pseudodactylogyrus anguillae* (Monogenea) from the European eel. *Folia Parasitologica* 37, 59–62.

Buchmann, K. (1993) A note on the humoral immune response of infected *Anguilla anguilla* against the gill monogeneans *Pseudodactylogyrus bini*. *Fish and Shellfish Immunology* 3, 397–399.

Buchmann, K. and Bjerregaard, J. (1990a) Comparative efficacies of commercially available benzimidazoles against *Pseudodactylogyrus* infestations in eels. *Diseases of Aquatic Organisms* 9, 117–120.

Buchmann, K. and Bjerregaard, J. (1990b) Mebendazole treatment of pseudodactylogyrosis in intensive eel-culture systems. *Aquaculture* 86, 139–153.

Buchmann, K. and Prentø, P. (1989) Cholinergic and aminergic elements in the nervous system of *Pseudodactylogyrus bini* (Monogenea). *Diseases of Aquatic Organisms* 6, 89–92.

Buchmann, K., Mellergaard, S. and Køie, M. (1987a) *Pseudodactylogyrus* infections in eel: a review. *Diseases of Aquatic Organisms* 3, 51–57.

Buchmann, K., Køie, M. and Prentø, P. (1987b) The nutrition of the gill parasitic monogenean *Pseudodactylogyrus anguillae*. *Parasitology Research* 73, 532–537.

Buchmann, K., Székely, C.S. and Bjerregaard, J. (1990a) Treatment of *Pseudodactylogyrus* infestations of *Anguilla anguilla* I. Trials with niclosamide, toltrazuril, phenolsulfonphthalein and rafoxanide. *Bulletin of the European Association of Fish Pathologists* 10, 14–17.

Buchmann, K., Székely, C.S. and Bjerregaard, J. (1990b) Treatment of *Pseudodactylogyrus* infestations of *Anguilla anguilla* II. Trials with bunamidine, praziquantel and levamisole. *Bulletin of the European Association of Fish Pathologists* 10, 18–20.

Buchmann, K., Felsing, A. and Slotved, H.C. (1992) Effects of metrifonate, sodium chloride and bithionol on an European population of *Pseudodactylogyrus* spp. and the host *Anguilla anguilla*. *Bulletin of the European Association of Fish Pathologists* 12, 57–60.

Chan, B. and Wu, B. (1984) Studies on the pathogenicity, biology, and treatment of *Pseudodactylogyrus* for the eels in fish farms. *Acta Zoologia Sinica* 30, 173–180.

Christison, K.W. and Baker, G.C. (2006) First record of *Pseudodactylogyrus anguillae* (Yin and Sproston, 1948) (Monogenea) from South Africa. *African Zoology* 42, 279–285.

Chung, H.-Y., Lin, I.H. and Kou, G.-H. (1984) Study of the parasites on the gill of cultured eel in Taiwan. *Council of Agriculture Fisheries Series, No. 10, Fish Diseases Research* 4, 24–33.

Cone, D.K. and Marcogliese, D.J. (1995) *Pseudodactylogyrus anguillae* on *Anguilla rostrata* in Nova Scotia – an endemic or an introduction? *Journal of Fish Biology* 47, 177–178.

Dzika, E. (1999) Microhabitats of *Pseudodactylogyrus anguillae* and *P. bini* (Monogenea: Dactylogyridae) on the gills of large-size European eel *Anguilla anguilla* from Lake Gaj, Poland. *Folia Parasitologica* 46, 33–36.

Dzika, E., Wlasow, T. and Gomulka, P. (1995) The first recorded case of the occurrence of two species of the genus *Pseudodactylogyrus* on the eel *Anguilla anguilla* (L.) in Poland. *Acta Parasitologica* 40, 165–167.

Egusa, S. (1979) Notes on culture of the European eel (*Anguilla anguilla* L.) in Japanese eel-farming ponds. *Rapports et Procès-Verbaux des Reunions, Conseil International pour l'Exploration de la Mer* 174, 51–58.

EC (European Community) (2007) Council Regulation (EC) No 1100/2007 of 18 September 2007 establishing measures for the recovery of the stock of European eel. *Official Journal of the European Union* L248/17–L248/23.

Fang, J., Shirakashi, S. and Ogawa, K. (2008) Comparative susceptibility of Japanese and European eels to infections with *Pseudodactylogyrus* spp. (Monogenea). *Fish Pathology* 43, 144–151.

Gelnar, M., Scholz, T., Matejusova, I. and Konecny, R. (1996) Occurrence of *Pseudodactylogyrus anguillae* (Yin and Sproston, 1948) and *P. bini* (Kikuchi, 1929), parasites of eel, *Anguilla anguilla* L., in Austria. *Annalen des Naturhistorischen Museums in Wien* 98B, 1–4.

Golovin, P.P. (1977) Monogeneans of eel during its culture using heated water. *Investigations of Monogeoidea in USSR* (Zoological Institute, USSR, Academy of Sciences, Leningrad) 1, 144–150.

Gratzek, J.B., Gilbert, J.P., Lohr, A.L., Shotts, E.B. and Brown, J. (1983) Ultraviolet light control of *Ichthyophthirius multifiliis* Fouquet in a closed fish culture recirculation system. *Journal of Fish Diseases* 6(2), 145–153.

Gussev, A.V. (1965) A new genus of monogenetic trematodes from the eel, genus *Anguilla*. *Trudy Zoologiya* (Zoological Institute, USSR, Academy of Sciences, Leningrad) 35, 119–125.

Haenen, O.L.M. and Davidse, A. (2001) First isolation and pathogenicity studies with *Pseudomonas anguilliseptica* from diseases European eel *Anguilla anguilla* (L.) in the Netherlands. *Aquaculture* 196(1/2), 27–36.

Haenen, O.L.M., Dijkstra, S.G., van Tulden, P.W., Davidse, A., van Nieuwstadt, A.P. *et al.* (2002) *Herpesvirus anguillae* (HVA) isolations from disease outbreaks in cultured European eel, *Anguilla anguilla*, in the Netherlands since 1996. *Bulletin of the European Association of Fish Pathologists* 22(4), 247–257.

Hayward, C.J., Iwashita, M., Crane, J.S. and Ogawa, K. (2001) First report of the invasive eel pest *Pseudodactylogyrus bini* in North America and in wild American eels. *Diseases of Aquatic Organisms* 44, 53–60.

Hughes, G.M. (1966) The dimensions of fish gills in relation to their function. *Journal of Experimental Biology* 45, 179–195.

Imada, R. and Muroga, K. (1978) *Pseudodactylogyrus microrchis* (Monogenea) on the gills of cultured eels. II. Oviposition, hatching and development on the host. *Bulletin of the Japanese Society for Scientific Fisheries* 44, 571–576.

ICES (International Council for Exploration of the Sea) (2007) European eel. Report of the ICES Advisory Committee on Fishery Management, Advisory Committee on the Marine Environment and Advisory Committee on Ecosystems, 2007. *ICES Advice* 9, 86–92.

Iwashita, M., Hirata, J. and Ogawa, K. (2002) *Pseudodactylogyrus kamegaii* sp. n. (Monogenea: Pseudodactylogyridae) from wild Japanese eel, *Anguilla japonica*. *Parasitology International* 51, 337–342.

Jørgensen, T.R. and Buchmann, K. (2007) Stress response in rainbow trout during infection with *Ichthyophthirius multifiliis* and formalin bath treatment. *Acta Ichthyologica et Piscatoria* 37, 25–28.

Kania, P.W., Taraschewski, H., Han, Y.-S., Cone, D.K. and Buchmann, K. (2010) Divergence between Asian, European and Canadian populations of the monogenean *Pseudodactylogyrus bini* indicated by ribosomal DNA patterns. *Journal of Helminthology* 84, 404–409.

Katahira, H. and Nagasawa, K. (2014) Helminths from the giant mottled eel *Anguilla marmorata* Quoy and Gaimard in Japan, with a description of *Acanthocephalus longiacanthus* n. sp. (Acanthocephala: Echinorhynchidae). *Systematic Parasitology* 88, 91–102.

Kikuchi, H. (1929) Two new species of Japanese trematodes belonging to Gyrodactylidae. *Annotationes Zoologicae Japonenses* 12, 175–186.

Køie, M. (1988) Parasites in European eel *Anguilla anguilla* (L.) from Danish freshwater, brackish and marine localities. *Ophelia* 29, 93–118.

Lambert, A., Le Brun, N. and Pariselle, A. (1984) Presence en France de *Pseudodactylogyrus anguillae* (Yin et Sproston, 1948) Gussev, 1965 (Monogenea, Monopisthocotyles) parasite branchial de l'anguille européenne, *Anguilla anguilla*, en eau douce. *Annales Parasitologie Humaine et Compare* 60, 91–92.

Matejusova, I., Simkova, A., Sasal, P. and Gelnar, M. (2003) Microhabitat distribution of *Pseudodactylogyrus anguillae* and *P. bini* among and within gill arches of the European eel (*Anguilla anguilla* L.). *Parasitology Research* 89, 290–296.

Mazzanti, C., Monni, G. and Varriale, A.M.C. (1999) Observations on antigenic activity of *Pseudodactylogyrus anguillae* (Monogenea) on the European eel (*Anguilla anguilla*). *Bulletin of the European Association of Fish Pathologists* 19, 57–59.

Molnar, K. (1972) Studies on gill parasitosis of the grass carp (*Ctenopharyngodon idella*) caused by *Dactylogyrus lamellatus* Achmerow, 1952. IV. Histopathological changes. *Acta Veterinaria Academiae Scientarum Hungaricae* 22, 9–24.

Molnar, K. (1983) Das Vorkommen von parasitären Hakensaugwürmern bei der Aalaufsucht in Ungarn. *Zeitschrift für Binnenfischerei der DDR* 30, 341–345.

Molnar, K. (1994) Effects of decreased water oxygen content on common carp fry with *Dactylogyrus vastator* (Monogenea) infection of varying severity. *Diseases of Aquatic Organisms* 20, 153–157.

Monni, G. and Cognetti-Varriale, A.M. (2002) Antigenicity of *Pseudodactylogyrus anguillae* and *P. bini* (Monogenea) in the European eel (*Anguillae anguilla*, L.) under different oxygenation conditions. *Fish and Shellfish Immunology* 13, 125–131.

Nie, P. and Kennedy, C.R. (1991) Occurrence and seasonal dynamics of *Pseudodactylogyrus anguillae* (Yin and Sproston) (Monogenea) in eel, *Anguilla anguilla* (L.) in England. *Journal of Fish Biology* 39, 879–900.

Ogawa, K. (1984) *Pseudodactylogyrus haze* sp. n. a gill monogenean from the Japanese goby, *Acanthogobius flavimanus*. *Japanese Journal of Parasitology* 33, 403–405.

Ogawa, K. and Egusa, S. (1976) Studies on eel pseudodactylogyrosis. I. Morphology and classification of three eel dactylogyrids with a proposal of a new species, *Pseudodactylogyrus microorchis*. *Bulletin of the Japanese Society for Scientific Fisheries* 42, 395–404.

Ogawa, K., Iwashita, M., Hayward, C.J. and Kurashima, A. (2015) Three new species of *Pseudodactylogyrus* (Monogenea: Pseudodactylogyridae) from Australian eels. *Folia Parasitologica* 62, 046.

Paperna, I. (1964) Competitive exclusion of *Dactylogyrus extensus* by *D. vastator* (Trematoda, Monogenea) on the gills of reared carp. *Journal of Parasitology* 50, 94–98.

Parker, D., Weyl, O.L.F. and Taraschewski, H. (2011) Invasion of a South African *Anguilla mossambica* (Anguillidae) population by the alien gill worm *Pseudodactylogyrus anguillae* (Monogenea). *African Zoology* 46, 371–377.

Rohde, K. (1977) A non-competitive mechanism responsible for restricting niches. *Zoologischer Anzeiger* 199, 164–172.

Sajiri, W.M.H.W., Szekely, C., Molnar, K., Buchmann, K. and Sellyei, B. (2025) Pathological effects of *Thaparocleidus vistulensis* (Siwak, 1932) infection on the gills of *Silurus glanis* Linnaeus, 1758. *Acta Veterinaria Hungarica* 73, 56–63. DOI: 10.1556/004.2025.01121.

Saraiva, A. (1995) *Pseudodactylogyrus anguillae* (Yin and Sproston, 1948) Gussev, 1965 and *P. bini* (Kikuchi, 1929) Gussev, 1965 (Monogenea:Monopisthocotylea) in Portugal. *Bulletin of the European Association of Fish Pathologists* 15, 81–83.

Sasal, P., Taraschewski, H., Valade, P., Grondin, H., Wielgoss, S. and Moravec, F. (2008) Parasite communities in eels of the Island of Reunion (Indian Ocean): a lesson in parasite introduction. *Parasitology Research* 102, 1343–1350.

Skorikova, B., Scholz, T. and Moravec, F. (1996) Spreading of introduced monogeneans *Pseudodactylogyrus anguillae* and *P. bini* among eel populations in the Czech Republic. *Folia Parasitologica* 43, 155–156.

Slotved, H.-C. and Buchmann, K. (1993) Acquired resistance of *Anguilla anguilla* L. against challenge infections with gill monogeneans. *Journal of Fish Diseases* 16, 585–591.

Sures, B., Knopf, K., Würtz, J. and Hirt, J. (1999) Richness and diversity of parasite communities in European eels *Anguilla anguilla* of the River Rhine, Germany, with special reference to helminth parasites. *Parasitology* 111, 323–330.

Szekely, C.S. and Molnar, K. (1987) Mebendazole is an efficacious drug against pseudodactylogyrosis in the European eel (*Anguilla anguilla*). *Journal of Applied Ichthyology* 3, 183–186.

Taraschewski, H. (2006) Hosts and parasites as aliens. *Journal of Helminthology* 80, 99–128.

Truter, M., Hadfield, K.A., Weyl, O.L.F. and Smit, N.J. (2021) *Pseudodactylogyrus anguillae* (Yin and Sproston, 1948) from the giant mottled eel *Anguilla marmorata* Quoy and Gaimard, 1824, in the Phongolo River, South Africa: an invader on the African continent. *Parasitology Research* 120, 1247–1268.

Umeda, N., Nibe, H., Hara, T. and Hirazawa, N. (2006) Effects of various treatments on hatching of eggs and viability of oncomiracidia of the monogenean *Pseudodactylogyrus anguillae* and *Pseudodactylogyrus bini*. *Aquaculture* 253, 148–153.

Waller, P. and Buchmann, K. (2001) Anthelmintic resistance and parasite control in commercial eel farms: consequences for producers. *The Veterinary Record* 148, 783–784.

Wang, G.X., Jiang, D.X., Zhou, Z., Zhao, Y.K. and Shen, Y.H. (2009) *In vivo* assessment of anthelmintic efficacy of ginkgolic acids (C13:0, C15:1) on removal of *Pseudodactylogyrus* in European eel. *Aquaculture* 297, 38–43.

Yin, W.-Y. and Sproston, N.G. (1948) Studies on the monogenetic trematodes of China, Parts 1–5. *Sinensia* 19, 57–85.

13 *Benedenia seriolae* and *Neobenedenia girellae*

Kate S. Hutson[1,2*] and Ian D. Whittington[†]

[1]Cawthron Institute, Nelson, New Zealand; [2]Centre for Sustainable Tropical Fisheries and Aquaculture, College of Science and Engineering, James Cook University, Townsville, Australia; [†]Deceased, formerly of The South Australian Museum and Australian Centre for Evolutionary Biology and Biodiversity, The University of Adelaide, Australia

Abstract

Ectoparasitic flatworms *Benedenia seriolae* and *Neobenedenia girellae* cause devastating losses of fish in marine aquaculture and marine public aquaria. Strong adhesive and mechanical properties of the parasite's attachment organs, along with feeding on the epidermis, damage fish skin. Individual parasites can produce thousands of eggs which bear a long filament that readily tangles on substrates, so parasite larva hatch near captive fish. New insights into the biology of capsalid monogeneans, enabled through culture techniques, have permitted the development of predictive models with respect to population estimation and spread as well as decision support tools for timed treatments to break parasite life cycles. Recent research effort explores preventive and treatment mechanisms including prolonged hyposalinity in aquaria, antifoulants, novel compounds, breeding for parasite resistance, traps and biocontrols.

13.1. Introduction

Capsalidae are epithelium-feeding platyhelminths (Monopisthocotyla) comprising about 230 known species belonging to ~50 genera (WoRMS Editorial Board, 2025). These ectoparasitic flatworms infect diverse sites on marine teleosts and elasmobranchs (Whittington, 2004). *Benedenia seriolae* (Fig. 13.1, Fig. 13.2a and c) and *Neobenedenia girellae* (Figs 13.2b and d) are capsalids that cause disease, production losses and mortality to teleosts in marine aquaculture and aquaria, threatening profitability and viability (Ogawa, 2005; Whittington, 2005; Whittington and Chisholm, 2008). Estimated production loss in *Seriola* aquaculture can be up to 22% of production costs (see Shinn *et al.*, 2015 for review), while Christie and Foster (2020) describe *Neobenedenia* as a scourge to aquarists maintaining marine fish in public aquaria. The life cycle is direct (Fig. 13.1). Unlike gyrodactylids (see Chapter 11, this volume), capsalids are oviparous and lay tetrahedral eggs singly (Fig. 13.2c and d); and an individual *N. girellae* can produce approximately 3300 eggs in its lifetime (Dinh Hoai and Hutson, 2014). Eggs from parasites on wild hosts drift in sea water where their long filamentous appendage may

*Email: kate.hutson@cawthron.org.nz

 Fish Parasites: Pathobiology and Protection, 2nd Edition (eds P.T.K. Woo and K. Buchmann)
DOI: 10.1079/9781800628748.0013

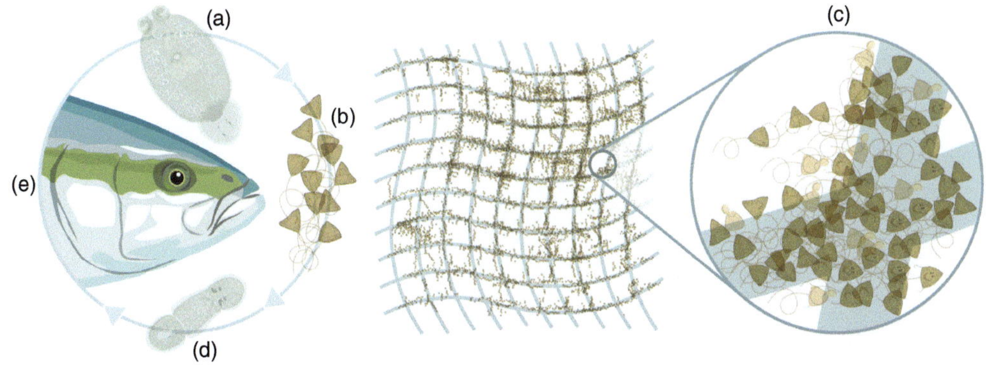

Fig. 13.1. Life cycle of (a) *Benedenia seriolae* infecting skin of *Seriola lalandi* (Carangidae). Eggs (b) typically entangle in large masses on netpens (c). Ciliated larvae (d) hatch, infect a host, and worm populations (e) can grow rapidly on captive fish. (© Eden Cartwright, Bird Circus; used with permission.)

tangle on substrates. After embryonation, an infective larva, the oncomiracidium, hatches (Fig. 13.1d). Eggs from parasites on captive stock may catch on nets, in filters or on other structures (Fig. 13.1c; Ogawa and Yokoyama, 1998) so oncomiracidia hatch close to fish. At 20°C, *B. seriolae* eggs hatch in 10 days and parasites mature in 21 days whereas *N. girellae* eggs hatch in 6 days and mature in 12 days (Hutson *et al.*, 2022). Efficient transmission causes parasite numbers to increase if captive fish densities are high and host immunity is compromised by stress, suboptimal nutrition, water quality and/or other pathogens.

13.2. Taxonomy

13.2.1. Monogenean taxonomy

It has long been considered that there are three major lineages of parasitic flatworms or Neodermata: the trematodes, cestodes and monogeneans. However, recent phylogenies promote two monogenean lineages (the subclasses Monopisthocotylea and Polyopisthocotylea) to class level – Monopisthocotyla and Polyopisthocotyla – and the suppression of the class Monogenea (Brabec *et al.*, 2023). The analysis of these authors showed that non-monophyly of the two monogenean lineages was consistent; however, the Monopisthocotyla were represented by only two *Gyrodactylus* species, and no capsalids were included in the analyses. It appears that monopisthocotyleans are either sister to cestodes or the earliest-diverging lineage of Neodermata. While Brabec *et al.*'s (2023) proposal may represent the evolution of the Neodermata, the current resolution provided for the monogeneans is too low to make definitive conclusions. The current state of flux, the likely suppression of the traditionally recognized class Monogenea and the proposed four major lineages of parasitic flatworms, is duly acknowledged. The term 'monogenean' is used throughout this chapter as a collective to describe members of the family Capsalidae and/or Monopisthocotyla and/or Polyopisthocotyla.

13.2.2. *Benedenia seriolae*

B. seriolae (Yamaguti 1934) Meserve 1938 was first described (as *Epibdella seriolae*) from wild carangids in Japan and became a major pathogen coinciding with the intensification of *Seriola* aquaculture in the 1950s (Egusa, 1983; Whittington *et al.*, 2001a). A supplemental species description was provided by Warren and Bullard (2025) from specimens collected from wild amberjack, *Seriola dumerili*. Sepúlveda and González (2014) proposed that *B. seriolae* is a complex of cryptic species, given morphologically similar but genetically divergent species from at least three geographic localities (Japan, Australia, Chile). This was supported by phylogenetic analysis by Kawato *et al.* (2019), which showed substantial mitogenomic divergence between *B. seriolae* from Australia and Japan. A formal proposal to separate

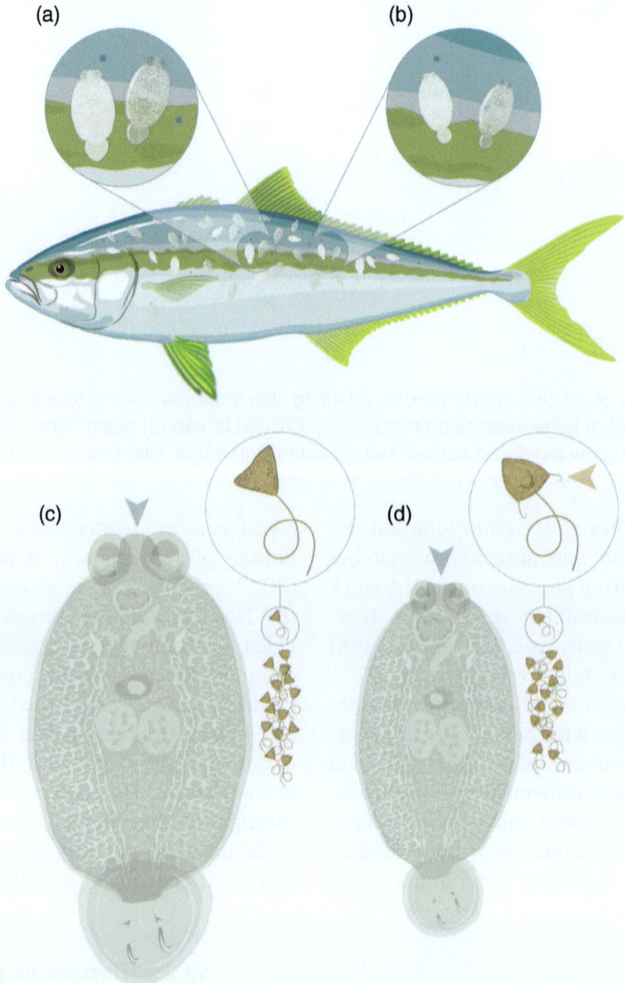

Fig. 13.2. (a) Co-infection of *Benedenia seriolae* and (b) *Neobenedenia girellae* is known to occur on *Seriola dumerili*, *Seriola quinqueradiata* and *Seriola lalandi* (illustrated on the latter species). The body of *B. seriolae* (c) is tapered at the anterior at the level of the attachment organs (grey arrow), while *N. girellae* (d) is broad (grey arrow). The haptor of *B. seriolae* is broadly tapered posteriorly while the *N. girellae* shape is rounder. The eggs of *N. girellae* exhibit short, hooked appendages. (© Eden Cartwright, Bird Circus; used with permission.)

Japanese and Australian *B. seriolae* has not been made to date; however, '*Benedenia seriolae*' infecting wild yellowtail kingfish, *Seriola lalandi*, from Chile was described as a new species, *Benedenia humboldti* Baeza, Sepúlveda, and Gonzalez, 2019. The new species was proposed based on phylogenetic core groups, using the mitochondrial genome and a single morphological difference (shape of the terminal end of the penis; Baeza *et al.*, 2019). This was supported by Warren and Bullard (2025) who suggested additional morphological differences may exist, based on their examination of *B. humboldti* illustrations.

13.2.3. *Seriola* spp. taxonomy

The taxonomy of one of the host species of *B. seriolae*, the yellowtail kingfish, *S. lalandi*, is of considerable scientific interest. It has been suggested that at least three species bear the name '*Seriola lalandi*', with a proposal to reinstate junior synonyms *Seriola aureovittata* Temminck and Schlegel for the north-west Pacific (type locality, Japan), and the north-east Pacific species to *Seriola dorsalis* (type locality, Mexico) and *S. lalandi* Valenciennes, 1833 (type locality, Brazil) to the southern hemisphere (Martinez-Takeshita *et al.*, 2015; Purcell *et al.*, 2015). Others argue that the reinstatement may be premature, and that low genetic divergence supports the more traditional view that *S. lalandi* in the Pacific comprises three distinct populations rather than species (Premachandra *et al.*, 2017). The taxonomy of *Seriola* spp. may be further complicated by the deliberate movement of animals for aquaculture and the potential genetic introgression of aquaculture escapees into wild fish populations (Hutson *et al.*, 2022). Herein, we adopt the conservative approach encouraged by Premachandra *et al.* (2017) but note other authors follow the proposed reinstatement of the species names.

13.2.4. *Neobenedenia girellae*

Neobenedenia are harmful monogenean ectoparasites that infect economically important bony fishes in aquaculture and marine aquaria worldwide. *N. girellae* (Hargis, 1955) Yamaguti, 1963 was originally described infecting opaleye, *Girella nigricans*, Ayres 1860, from California, with a redescription provided by Ogawa *et al.* (1995) from specimens infecting 14 host fish species comprising five families of cultured marine fishes (including *Seriola*) from Japan. The difference between *Neobenedenia melleni* and *N. girellae* was a topic of contention for decades (see Christie and Foster, 2020 for review). Historically, identifications of *Neobenedenia* isolates were overwhelmingly attributed to *N. melleni*; largely the result of a proposal by Whittington and Horton (1996) to synonymize *N. girellae*. However, a global study by Brazenor *et al.* (2018a) – who examined 33 *Neobenedenia* isolates from 22 host species spanning nine countries – confirmed that *N. melleni* and *N. girellae* are separate species, and that *N. girellae* is widespread geographically, able to infest many different host fishes and can be found on wild, farmed and captive fish. This was further supported by Tedesco *et al.* (2021). Importantly, Brazenor *et al.* (2018a) suggested that a large proportion of previous specimens identified as *N. melleni* may be erroneous, and a revision of identifications is needed. Several historical records (as *N. melleni* or *Neobenedenia* sp.) were assigned to *N. girellae* by Brazenor *et al.* (2018a), where specimens were available.

Despite that landmark taxonomic study, many researchers continue to publish studies on '*N. melleni*' in the absence of molecular attribution to this species, compounding continued confusion around delineation of these species. This is particularly fraught because *N. melleni* and *N. girellae* cannot be distinguished through morphology alone. Moreover, Brazenor *et al.* (2018b) highlighted significant intraspecies morphological variation for *N. girellae*, which can exhibit morphological differences between genetically indistinct parasites infesting various host fish species. Seawater temperature also significantly affects body proportions in key taxonomic characters (Brazenor *et al.*, 2018b). For the purposes of this chapter, the evidence that *N. girellae* is the globally cosmopolitan species and likely to be the species most encountered is accepted. The identities from original publications are maintained as presented, except for those assigned to *N. girellae* by Brazenor *et al.* (2018b). Where molecular evidence for species identification of *N. melleni* is not provided by authors, the species is presented in quotation marks (i.e. '*N. melleni*').

13.3. Impacts in Aquaculture and Aquaria

B. seriolae is reported from several wild and farmed *Seriola* species in Japan, Chile, Mexico, Australia and New Zealand (see Table 1 in Warren and Bullard, 2025); but not on *S. dumerili* farmed off the Balearic Islands, western Mediterranean Sea (Grau *et al.*, 1999). A single record from southern bluefin tuna, *Thunnus orientalis*, off Chile is probably erroneous (Baeza and Castro, 1975; Warren and Bullard, 2025). The *Seriola* industry comprises four main species – including Japanese yellowtail, *Seriola quinqueradiata* Temmick

& Schlegel, 1845; *S. lalandi* Valenciennes, 1833; *S. dumerili* (Risso, 1810); and longfin yellowtail or almaco jack, *Seriola rivoliana* Valenciennes, 1833 – which are predominantly farmed in netpens (e.g. Japan, China, USA, Chile and Australia), while production in recirculating aquaculture systems on land is gaining momentum in Europe, South Africa, Chile and New Zealand (see Fig. 2 in Hutson *et al.*, 2022). *S. lalandi* exhibits population subdivisions between some geographic areas (see Section 13.2.3 for discussion on *Seriola* taxonomy). Impacts by *B. seriolae* on cultivated *Seriola* production globally are reported in Japan (e.g. Hoshina, 1968; Egusa, 1983; Ogawa and Yokoyama, 1998; Ogawa, 2005) and Australasia (Whittington *et al.*, 2001c; Ernst *et al.*, 2002; Chambers and Ernst, 2005; Diggles and Hutson, 2005; Hutson *et al.*, 2007) (summarized by Shinn *et al.*, 2015). If unmanaged, infections may kill captive *Seriola* (see Ernst *et al.*, 2002). Production costs in Japan are especially high, reportedly twice those for Atlantic salmon in Norway, and *B. seriolae* may cause 20% mortality with the costs of control around 22% of production expenses (Shinn *et al.*, 2015).

Among the most host specific of all metazoan parasites, commonly a monogenean species may parasitize only one host species (Whittington *et al.*, 2000). *B. seriolae* is specific to host genus so the peculiar ubiquity of *N. girellae* to infect numerous unrelated fish species is extraordinary. Christie and Foster (2020) provided a table of recorded host fishes for '*N. melleni*' and *N. girellae* which now exceeds 52 fish families. An updated list was not attempted given numerous publications on '*N. melleni*' require molecular validation.

Published information about *Neobenedenia* on wild fish is scarce. Brooks and Mayes (1975) reported more than 100 *N. girellae* on the skin of California sheephead, *Pimelometopon pulchrum* (Labridae), and Gaida and Frost (1991) reported up to 42 *N. girellae* on the skin of halfmoon, *Medialuna californiensis* (Kyphosidae), off California. For '*N. melleni*', there are these reports: (i) low mean abundance on skin of red rockfish, *Sebastes capensis* (Sebastidae), off northern Chile (González and Acuña, 1998); (ii) small numbers from the skin of Florida pompano, *Trachinotus carolinus* (Carangidae), in the Gulf of Mexico (Bullard *et al.*, 2003); (iii) low mean abundance on skin of bullseye puffer, *Sphoeroides annulatus* (Tetraodontidae), off Sinaloa, Mexico (Fajer-Ávila *et al.*, 2004); (iv) different infection intensities on skin of three sympatric Caribbean surgeonfish species (Acanthuridae) (see Sikkel *et al.*, 2009); and (v) low infection intensity from skin of largehead hairtail, *Trichiurus lepturus* (Trichiuridae), off Brazil (Carvalho and Luque, 2009). In view of massive infections reported from captive fish, relatively low infection intensities on wild hosts may seem surprising. These, however, probably reflect normal parasitaemia of presumably healthy, wide-ranging hosts at natural population densities in their regular environment.

In contrast, *Neobenedenia* populations on captive fish can be enormous. Jahn and Kuhn (1932) reported more than 2000 adult '*N. melleni*' from a 'Galapagos labroid' in the New York Aquarium and Ogawa *et al.* (1995) observed 2000 *N. girellae* on Japanese flounder, *Paralichthys olivaceus* Temminck and Schlegel (Paralichthyidae), in Japanese sea-cage culture. Pathogenic reports on skin of many teleost species abound globally in public aquaria (Alaska, Australia, Bermuda, Chicago, Las Vegas, Mexico, New York, Philadelphia and Taiwan; Whittington and Chisholm, 2008). In especially heavy aquarium infections, '*N. melleni*' was reported from 'gill and nasal cavities' (Jahn and Kuhn, 1932). In marine aquaculture worldwide, *Neobenedenia* species have caused disease and death to many fish species.

In aquaria, costs to monitor and manage infections and replace fishes killed in outbreaks are incalculable. Impacts in marine aquaculture are huge as demonstrated by several outbreaks, some of which killed stock (Kaneko *et al.*, 1988; Ogawa *et al.*, 1995; Ogawa and Yokoyama, 1998; Deveney *et al.*, 2001; Ogawa *et al.*, 2006). Fifty tonnes of barramundi, *Lates calcarifer*, worth AUS$500,000 died during a 3-week outbreak of *N. girellae* in Australia (Deveney *et al.*, 2001; Brazenor *et al.*, 2018a). There are two characteristics of *Neobenedenia* epizootics in aquaculture: (i) the infection source is often unknown (Kaneko *et al.*, 1988; Deveney *et al.*, 2001; Ogawa *et al.*, 2006); and (ii) fish susceptibility to *Neobenedenia*, and associated inherent difficulties to manage infections, may limit development, progress and expansion of sea-cage culture (e.g. cobia in Taiwan, Liao *et al.*, 2004; and spotted halibut and Japanese flounder in Japan, Hirazawa *et al.*, 2004).

13.4. Diagnosis of the Infection

Both species of ectoparasite are dorsoventrally flattened, generally oval (Fig. 13.2) and infect body surfaces including flanks, head, fins and eyes. Adult worms attach with a large posterior sucker (haptor) and two smaller anterior attachment organs. Live worms can be virtually transparent but are sometimes pigmented (Whittington, 1996). Capsalids feed on epidermis. If skin pigment is ingested, appearance in the branched intestine and worm transparency conceal mild and moderate infections by live parasites. A clinical manifestation of infection may be due to feeding which may 'irritate' fish so that fish rub their body against nearby substrates ('flashing'), presumably trying to dislodge attached, feeding capsalids.

Co-infection of *B. seriolae* and *N. girellae* can occur on a host fish where there is overlap in their distribution and thermal tolerance range (~17–30°C). Co-infections have been reported in Japan from farmed *S. dumerili* and *S. quinqueradiata* (see Kinami *et al.*, 2005; Hirazawa, 2019) and in Western Australia from farmed *S. lalandi* (see Stephens, 2016). It is possible to distinguish adult *B. seriolae* from *N. girellae* on morphology (Ogawa and Shirakashi, 2017; Hutson *et al.*, 2022); however, it is difficult to distinguish immature or poorly preserved specimens and molecular assays may be more appropriate (Kobayashi *et al.*, 2018). Kinami *et al.* (2005) determined distinct shape differences (compare Fig. 13.2c and d) and plotted length of anterior attachment organs against total parasite length to differentiate them. The body of *N. girellae* is broad anteriorly at the level of the attachment organs (Fig. 13.2d), while it is tapered in *B. seriolae* (Fig. 13.2c). The haptor is rounder in *N. girellae*, while broadly tapered posteriorly in *B. seriolae*. Anterior attachment organs and the haptor in *Neobenedenia* species are usually small relative to total parasite size (Fig. 13.1d).

Eggs of both species are laid singly, are straw-coloured and tetrahedral in shape; *N. girellae* eggs have short, hooked appendages on two of the four poles of the tetrahedron, which are absent in *B. seriolae* (Fig. 13.2). *N. girellae* egg size is affected by temperature, with larger eggs laid in cooler sea water (Brazenor *et al.*, 2020); the effect of temperature on egg size has not been investigated for *B. seriolae*. A taxonomically important difference is the presence of a vagina in *Benedenia* species and its absence in *Neobenedenia* species. This however is rarely obvious because it is challenging to detect the narrow vagina in many *Benedenia* species. Insemination behaviour of *B. seriolae* and *N. girellae* was documented by Kearn (1992) and Ogawa *et al.* (2014). Dinh Hoai and Hutson (2014) showed that *N. girellae* successfully reproduced in isolation (i.e. one parasite on a single host fish produced viable offspring) and that multiple generations of isolated individuals remained infective. Egg-laying rhythms have been observed for *N. girellae* with egg production increasing in darkness (64.3%) (Dinh Hoai and Hutson, 2014). Oncomiracidia of both species have light sensory organs, known as eye spots, and are positively phototactic to light (Skilton *et al.*, 2020; Shirakashi *et al.*, 2021).

Molecular characterization of organisms using whole-genome sequencing is becoming increasingly accessible due to its relative affordability. The complete mitochondrial genome is now available for *B. seriolae* (see Kawato *et al.*, 2019) and *B. humboldti* (Baeza *et al.*, 2019), while partial sequence data is available for multiple gene regions for *N. girellae* from published and unpublished sources (see GenBank, National Center for Biotechnology Information: https://www.ncbi.nlm.nih.gov/nuccore/?term=Neobenedenia+girellae, accessed 11 December 2025).

13.4.1. *Benedenia seriolae*

B. seriolae occurs in warm temperate areas, with an assumed thermal tolerance range of 11.5–30°C and optimum of 21.9°C (Hutson *et al.*, 2022). Adults infect skin, sometimes the external surface of the eyes, of *Seriola* species (Fig. 13.2). Adults range from 4 to 12 mm in length, and from 1 to 6 mm in width (Whittington *et al.*, 2001b). Live specimens on hosts may be difficult to detect but a brief dip in dechlorinated tap water highlights infection, turning worms opaque as prominent white, raised, blister-like ovals. This technique rarely detaches parasites from fish. They attach by strong suction maintained even when dead on fish and on smooth inert surfaces like glass and plastic. Attachment is supplemented by proteinaceous sclerites (accessory sclerites, two pairs of hamuli and 14 hooklets at the edge of the posterior attachment organ, the haptor). Tetrahedral eggs (Figs 13.1c and 13.2c; side length = 130–150 µm; Hoshina, 1968) may be detected if infected fish are isolated and tank water is screened (Whittington and Chisholm, 2008) or eggs can be trapped in nylon netting (Kearn *et al.*, 1992). All *Benedenia* species, however, and many monopisthocotyleans including *Neobenedenia* species, lay tetrahedral eggs so their presence does not confirm *B. seriolae* infection. *B. seriolae* lay eggs continuously with no diurnal laying rhythm observed (Mooney *et al.*, 2008).

13.4.2. *Neobenedenia girellae*

N. girellae occur in warm temperate to tropical areas, with an assumed thermal tolerance range of 11.5–30°C and optimum of 21.9°C (Hutson *et al.*, 2022). Adults infect flanks, head, fins and the surface of the eyes, while new recruits may bury beneath the scales of fish (Trujillo-González *et al.*, 2015a). Christie and Foster (2020) describe *Neobenedenia* as a scourge to aquarists maintaining marine fish in marine public aquaria. *Neobenedenia* spp. have been recorded from more than 50 fish families so host taxon provides no diagnostic help (Christie and Foster, 2020). The total length range of adults is 2–7 mm (Whittington and Horton, 1996; Whittington and Chisholm, 2008). Transparency and pigment may hide live worms but bathing in dechlorinated tap water turns specimens *in situ* milky white. Eggs of *Neobenedenia* species bear short, hooked appendages on two of four poles of the tetrahedron plus a long filament (Fig. 13.2d; e.g. MacCallum, 1927; Jahn and Kuhn, 1932; Ogawa and Shirakashi, 2017), which may promote entrapment on substrate (Fig. 13.1c). It is not clear whether hooked appendages are characteristic for all *Neobenedenia* species or only for some species. An egg-laying rhythm was observed in Australia for *N. girellae*, with more eggs laid during darkness (Dinh Hoai and Hutson, 2014). In contrast, *N. girellae* from Japan laid eggs continuously with no obvious diurnal rhythm (Hirano *et al.*, 2015).

13.5. External/Internal Lesions

B. seriolae and *N. girellae* can migrate over the body surface of their host to access selected microhabitats. The strong adhesion of the haptor, mechanical attachment of the hamuli and sclerites as well as the adhesion of the anterior attachment organs when grazing can damage the host's epidermis (Ogawa *et al.*, 2006; Trujillo-González *et al.*, 2015b). There are no studies on feeding by *B. seriolae* or *Neobenedenia* species; however, another well-researched capsalid, *Entobdella soleae*, uses proteolytic secretions from the pharynx to disassociate epithelial cells (Kearn, 1963). Detailed studies on feeding have value. A quantitative assessment of the volume of epidermis ingested per unit time by adult *B. seriolae* and *N. girellae* could inform farm managers about total parasite population trigger levels to alert when stock must be treated to prevent disease and death.

Haptoral sclerites may penetrate host epidermis and injure fish skin (Trujillo-González *et al.*, 2015b) and proliferating parasite numbers can cause lesions. Active feeding by large populations of capsalid monogeneans on mucus and epithelial cells of host fish can cause haemorrhage, inflammation, mucus hyperproduction and epithelial thinning (Paperna, 1991; Hirazawa *et al.*, 2010). Whittington *et al.* (2001c) observed that large capsalid populations grazing on captive fish injured and eroded epithelium faster than it could be replaced. In contrast, wild fish are observed to support smaller capsalid populations and parasite mobility may spread injuries (Whittington, 2005). In farmed fish, lesions may worsen from: (i) epithelial aggravation from flashing; (ii) lack of feeding and associated host health deterioration affecting the immune system; and (iii) secondary infection (bacteria, viruses, fungi) of capsalid-inflicted wounds.

13.5.1. *Benedenia seriolae*

Abrasions and lesions in heavy infections are common (Hoshina, 1968). Feeding erodes epidermis causing attrition and skin haemorrhage (Hoshina, 1968; Ogawa and Shirakashi, 2017), sometimes producing wounds that deeply penetrate the epidermis (Williams *et al.*, 2007). Inflammatory cells and/or secondary infection may also stimulate flashing behaviour. No studies have specifically investigated attachment. Whittington and Chisholm (2008) provided the following observations on infected *S. lalandi* in sea cages in Spencer Gulf, South Australia: (i) flashing behaviour, presumably stimulated by feeding, led to dark epithelial patches; and (ii) lesions worsened by skin damage from flashing. Damage to *Seriola* eyes is not reported.

13.5.2. *Neobenedenia girellae*

The invasion route and site selection of *N. girellae* have been described on Japanese flounder (see Bondad-Reantaso *et al.*, 1995a) and quantified on *S. dumerili* (see Hirayama *et al.*, 2009) and barramundi (see Trujillo-González *et al.*, 2015a). In the two studies, post-larvae were attached to the fins, while older parasites were on the dorsal and ventral body surfaces. These studies used skin scrapings (Bondad-Reantaso *et al.*, 1995a) and stereomicroscopy (Hirayama *et al.*, 2009) to detect live parasites. The infection dynamics and distribution of *N. girellae* throughout its development were examined using fluorescent labelling of oncomiracidia and tracking them from infection to maturity (Trujillo-González *et al.*, 2015a). Oncomiracidia settled opportunistically and then migrated to specific habitats on the fish, notably the head and fins (within 48 h). Aggregations occurred on the eyes, fins and dorsal and ventral extremities of the body, with a marked aggregation on the fins as parasites neared sexual maturity. Trujillo-González *et al.* (2015a) hypothesized these aggregations play a role in mate-finding behaviour. Similarly, Hirayama *et al.* (2009) noted parasite migration as infection progressed, with most adults recovered from the fish belly where haemorrhage was observed at infections of >0.735 ± 0.096 worms/cm^2, but no dermal penetration occurred.

MacCallum (1927) noted pierced and destroyed corneas of several host species in the New York Aquarium within 3 weeks of infection with *N. melleni*. Jahn and Kuhn (1932) confirmed corneal destruction even in mild infections followed by entire damaged eyes, assisted by secondary infections, if parasites were uncontrolled. In heavy outbreaks, body epidermis was severely injured with scale disruption and loss, large areas of connective and muscle tissue exposed, and eventual death. Thoney and Hargis (1991) described open lesions penetrating to the bone in Atlantic spadefish, *Chaetodipterus faber* (Ephippidae), with secondary infection by motile, rod-shaped bacteria. Llewellyn (1957) commented that the eyes of fish are effectively immunologically privileged due to vascular absence and therefore lack blood-borne antibodies. Corneas lack mucous cells (Kearn, 1999) and fish mucus has high immunological activity (Buchmann, 1999). Therefore, *Neobenedenia* epizootics on captive fish may flourish on eyes (Ogawa *et al.*, 2006).

In marine mariculture, '*N. melleni*' infection foci on tilapia, *Oreochromis mossambicus*, in sea cages off Hawaii were in anterodorsal head regions and corneas (Kaneko *et al.*, 1988). Heavily infected fish (>400 '*N. melleni*' per host) had significant mucus secretion, discoloured skin, epithelium and scale loss, and haemorrhagic lesions. Eyes suffered intense pathology with the following chronology: (i) opaque cornea; (ii) corneal ulceration; (iii) eye enlarges; (iv) eye bursts; (v) disintegration of internal eye structure; (vi) scarring; and (vii) blindness (Kaneko *et al.*, 1988). Humpback grouper, *Cromileptes altivelis*, infected by *N. girellae* in Indonesia had eye opacity and excess mucus production and haemorrhagic and abrasive body lesions (Koesharyani *et al.*, 1999). Dusky grouper, *Epinephelus marginatus*, infected by '*N. melleni*' off Brazil showed darkened skin, eye opacity, eye lesions and body haemorrhages (Sanches, 2008).

Ogawa *et al.* (2006) observed *N. girellae* concentrated on the dorsal head region, especially eyes, in cobia, *Rachycentron canadum*, from sea cages in Taiwan. The cornea in uninfected fish comprised several layers of squamous epithelial cells of uniform shape and size but infected eyes were opaque, corneal squamous epithelial cells lost uniformity, became irregularly thickened and were sometimes lost. Below the cornea, upper layers of the collagenous stroma became thickened, oedematous and infiltrated by inflammatory cells; however, no co-infection with other pathogens was apparent. Histological sections of *N. girellae* attached to epithelium surrounding the eye indicated: (i) mucus in the attachment region suggesting a 'strong irritating effect'; (ii) the haptor was applied firmly and closely to epithelium but was lined with cellular debris and mucus; and (iii) the distal tips of the accessory sclerites had penetrated and disrupted epithelial tissue.

Epidermis of fishes experimentally infected by *N. girellae* was thin compared with uninfected fish (Sato *et al.*, 2008; Hirayama *et al.*, 2009;

Hirazawa *et al.*, 2010; Trujillo-González *et al.*, 2015b) suggesting that epithelial cells do comprise the parasites' diet (Sato *et al.*, 2008) or that thinning is a response to infection. Sato *et al.* (2008) also suggested epidermal thinning may lead to increased bruising from flashing behaviour. Mucous cells were seldom observed in epidermis of infected fish compared to uninfected fish, indicating that mucus production at infection sites may be low (Hirazawa *et al.*, 2010; Trujillo-Gonzalez *et al.*, 2015b).

The relative contributions to fish lesions from capsalid infection versus possible secondary pathogen infection are usually unquantified, but Ogawa *et al.* (2006) specifically noted no co-infection by other pathogens in cobia parasitized by *N. girellae*. Lopez *et al.* (2002), however, reported a disease outbreak in caged cobia off Taiwan where vibriosis and photobacteriosis were associated with severe head and eye ulcers and suggested bacteria may gain entry via skin damage from a *Neobenedenia* sp.

13.6. Pathophysiology

At natural population levels, monogeneans typically cause minimal damage with no notable pathogenic response (Whittington, 2005). Epizootics, often due to imbalance(s) in parasite–host–environment interactions, are promoted by unnatural and/or unfavourable conditions. Farmed fish are maintained at one location where parasite eggs, larvae and adults intensify (Fig. 13.1). At high stocking densities, captive fish may become stressed, affecting their ability to manage infections. Captive fish provide a perfect environment for capsalids to reproduce, invade and establish large populations rapidly. Capsalid pathology is inferred but rarely *definitively* credited to a single aetiology and co-infection is seldom discounted. Pathophysiology of monogenean infections (i.e. broad manifestations of parasites and their effects on host organ systems, physiology and metabolism) is totally neglected. It seems logical that epidermal loss, mucus hypersecretion, lesions, appetite loss and emaciation lead to poor nutrition, stress, impaired osmoregulation, growth and immunity, and high incidences of secondary infection that ultimately manifest in fish disease and/or death.

13.6.1. *Benedenia seriolae*

Most research on *B. seriolae* has focused on methods to control infections and not on pathophysiological changes. Hoshina (1968) reported anorexia and growth retardation in infected *S. quinqueradiata*. For infected *S. lalandi*, Whittington and Chisholm (2008) included a time course after appearance of skin lesions: (i) reduced growth and food conversion ratios; (ii) aggravated epithelial lesions; (iii) onset of secondary infections; (iv) appetite loss; and (v) high likelihood for mass stock mortality if parasite and secondary infections are untreated. Miyoshi *et al.* (2019) used challenge trials to evaluate *S. quinqueradiata* susceptibility to *Nocardia seriolae* (Gram-positive bacterium) following mechanical damage and/or *B. seriolae* infestation. The results suggested that *N. seriolae* may have more opportunities to invade fish through skin injuries and that *B. seriolae* contributes to the progression of disease.

13.6.2. *Neobenedenia girellae*

Nigrelli (1932) drew attention to eyes as a preferred site for '*N. melleni*'. In heavy infections, the eye was destroyed and the fish eventually starved to death. Blindness probably occurs at the corneal opacity stage, well before further eye damage. Ogawa *et al.* (2006) speculated that parasitized cobia may be able to suppress *N. girellae* infection via active immune substances in skin mucus (perhaps complement) which may cause parasites to retreat to the eyes.

Heavy parasitaemia is associated with severe body epidermal injuries leading to scale loss, exposure of connective and muscle tissues, and secondary infection by bacteria followed by death within days (Kaneko *et al.*, 1988; Thoney and Hargis, 1991). Robinson *et al.* (2008) reported no significant differences in lymphocytes, plasma cells, neutrophils, monocytes and macrophage counts between uninfected hybrid tilapia, *Oreochromis aureus* × *O. mossambicus*, and those infected by '*N. melleni*' in Jamaica and no evidence of a humoral response. Sato *et al.* (2008) used ^{13}C-labelled fatty acids in supplemented feeding experiments to *S. dumerili* in Japan. No ^{13}C-labelled fatty acids were detected in epidermal mucus suggesting that cell metabolism was fast. Hirayama *et al.* (2009) used the same model system to explore and quantify the effect of different *N. girellae* infection levels on *S. dumerili* growth. At populations >0.285 ± 0.042 worms/cm^2, host growth slowed significantly and the feed conversion ratio was positively correlated with infection size. Lower haematocrit levels when infected by >0.735 ± 0.096 worms/cm^2 were attributed to epidermal haemorrhage. Rare occurrence of epidermal mucous cells was suggested to decrease resistance to bacterial invasion. Ten days after exposure to oncomiracidia, host appetite declined and death occurred after 12 days when infection was 1.393 ± 0.276 worms/cm^2. This study noted that longer infection duration and greater *N. girellae* numbers led to thinner host epidermis. Infected host epidermis was thinner in fish reared at 25 and 30°C but not at 20°C (Hirazawa *et al.*, 2010).

13.7. Management Strategies

Given the broad applicability of prevention and management measures to both *B. seriolae* and *N. girellae* infections, general strategies for both monogenean species are presented together, highlighting specific examples from available studies.

13.7.1. Surveillance

Surveillance involves routine observation of fish for infection and may include visual detection of parasite eggs on structures and parasite counts. Hutson *et al.* (2022) provided guidelines for surveillance of *B. seriolae* and *N. girellae* including visual inspection, sampling fish to attain population estimates, deployment of egg collectors and evaluation of infection status inferred from egg development (also see BeNeZe User Manual; https://beneze.cawthron.org.nz/public/BeNeZe_User_Manual_RAQ_12_21_0320.pdf, accessed 12 December 2025). Visual inspection is recommended daily for behavioural and clinical signs of disease. Evidence of fish rubbing their bodies against sediment, surfaces and each other, as well as scale loss and a grey-black eroded appearance and/or haemorrhage, may indicate infection. Eggs entangle on structures and can be evaluated by placing dedicated egg collectors and monitoring the accumulation of eggs. Eggs collectors can simply comprise a piece of nylon or mesh. Cejas *et al.* (2014) estimated levels of *B. seriolae* infection on *S. dumerili* in rearing tanks based on the number of parasite eggs collected in mesh traps suspended in the tanks. Several factors can influence the number of eggs collected by mesh traps including mesh size, the position of the mesh traps in relation to the water inlets and currents, and the period of suspension. If the infestation level is too high or the mesh traps accumulate excessive amounts of detritus from the tank, observation and egg counts are more challenging, and a single nylon thread may be sufficient.

Chew *et al.* (2024) provided comprehensive suggestions for fish sampling, ectoparasite collection strategies and methods specific to collection of monogeneans. Obtaining accurate representative data of parasite populations in aquaria and marine netpens can be challenging. For example, hook-and-line sampling of farmed *S. lalandi* from netpens introduced selection bias, with the smallest and most heavily parasitized fish captured near the edge of the pen (Fensham *et al.*, 2018). Parasites are difficult to detect with the naked eye due to their transparency, so immersion of fish in fresh water for 3–5 min kills the parasites, making them opaque and thus readily counted. A prototype automated image analysis system for monogenean parasite counts was developed by Whittington *et al.* (2011) and provides a base approach for future artificial intelligence-led parasite counts.

13.7.2. Prevention

Considerable advances have been made in the past two decades, particularly in public aquaria, where hyposalinity has enabled continuous prevention and exclusion.

13.7.2.1. Hyposalinity

Hyposalinity has been used to successfully to eradicate *Neobenedenia* infestations in large public aquaria (Boylan *et al.*, 2021). In the South Carolina Aquarium, a gradual reduction in salinity from an initial 34 ppt to 20 ppt has been maintained for more than a decade, explicitly to control *Neobenedenia*, with no recurrence of monogeneans (Boylan *et al.*, 2021; B.L. Christie, South Carolina Aquarium, 2025, personal communication). The reduced salinity is a barrier to future incursions from the introduction of new fishes, and no negative effects have been noted in the tank's stenohaline and euryhaline fishes. Prolonged hyposalinity as part of parasite prevention and management has been implemented in other large display tanks with similar success (Boylan *et al.*, 2021). The New England Aquarium has a slightly different approach, lowering salinity whenever capsalid eggs appear in screens used for surveillance. However, parasite populations can rebound following low-salinity exposure for long durations and there may be a selection risk for resistance to hyposalinity treatments (B.L. Christie, South Carolina Aquarium, 2025, personal communication).

13.7.2.2. Egg treatments and antifouling

The high occurrence of capsalid monogeneans on fish in netpen aquaculture and commercial aquarium facilities is largely attributed to egg entanglement on infrastructure. *N. girellae* eggs tend to be distributed mainly on shallow areas of netpens, which may be associated with fish feeding near the surface; however, egg accumulation has also been observed at depth (Shirakashi and Hirano, 2015). Eggs can accumulate at astonishing rates – with estimated daily egg accumulation for an entire cage being more than 53 million eggs/day (Shirakashi and Hirano, 2015). As such, any management methods that reduce egg accumulation are highly advantageous. Eggs are largely resistant to disinfection using chemicals due to their proteinaceous shell (Whittington and Chisholm, 2008; Brazenor *et al.*, 2017), thus chemical treatments that may be effective against adult parasites tend to be ineffective on eggs (Sharp *et al.*, 2004).

Ernst *et al.* (2005) studied effects of temperature, salinity, desiccation and chemical treatment on embryonation and hatching success of *B. seriolae* from *S. quinqueradiata* in Japan. Temperature influenced embryonation, with hatching 5 days after laying at 28°C but 16 days at 14°C, and >70% hatching success at each temperature but no hatching at 30°C. The embryonation period increased at low and high salinities: (i) >70% hatched at salinities ranging from 25 to 45 ppt but few or no eggs hatched at 10 and 15 ppt; and (ii) eggs, however, do not hatch if desiccated for 3 min, immersed in water at 50°C for 30 s or treated with 25% w/w ethanol for 3 min. These results are relevant for parasite management in closed or semi-closed systems such as aquaria, nurseries and flow-through hatcheries. Hirazawa (2019) examined the effect of heat, drying, fresh water, benzalkonium chloride and chlorine treatments on eggs of *B. seriolae* and *N. girellae*. They found a heat treatment at ≥50°C for 1 min and drying the eggs for 1 h killed the eggs of both parasite species. Chlorine treatment for 24 h (120 ppm) also killed eggs of both species (see Table 1 in Hirazawa, 2019).

Shirakashi *et al.* (2024) found that copper alloy exhibited notable antifouling efficacy. Antifouling-coated nets reduced the attachment and hatching success of *N. girellae* and *Heteraxine heterocerca*. Monogenean eggs attached to the copper alloy-coated nets showed considerably lower hatching rates, averaging 34.2 ± 3.8%, than those attached to the steel nets (97.3 ± 0.4%).

13.7.3. Protection

13.7.3.1. Farm husbandry

On farms, eggs tangle on net mesh (Fig. 13.1c; Ogawa and Yokoyama, 1998). Regular cleaning or net changes to reduce egg load may have limited efficacy at high summer temperatures when eggs hatch rapidly. In Japan, large cages and steel enclosures cannot be easily changed (Ogawa, 2005). Ernst *et al.* (2002) correlated egg retention on cage material with fouling organisms and noted up to 64,000 eggs/m^2 on nets in Japan which, if distributed evenly over one, 30 m diameter cage, was 165 million eggs! *N. girellae* eggs tend to accumulate near the surface (Shirakashi *et al.*, 2013b), thus 'snorkel' cages used in Norwegian salmon – designed to limit interactions near the surface between salmon and sea lice (Stien *et al.*, 2016) – may have applicability for the management of monogeneans in *Seriola* aquaculture.

Chambers and Ernst (2005) hypothesized that the largest contribution to reinfection of treated stock was from parasites on fish in nearby cages. They assessed infection pressure within and between neighbouring sea-cage leases in South Australia using fish sentinels free of infection. On the same farm, eggs in plankton samples were only found at sites in line with tidal current. Fish sentinels had higher infections when in line with, but not across, tidal current. Infection pressure between farm leases reduced with increased distance from infected stock. For effective parasite management in Spencer Gulf, South Australia, independent management units (i.e. different farm leases) need to be more than 8 km apart due to dispersal of *B. seriolae* eggs. Farms arrange sea cages in line with currents to help maintain cage shape, for functional effectiveness and mooring efficacy. These perceived operational efficiencies may contribute to more efficient monogenean transmission (Chambers and Ernst, 2005). Intensity of sea cages and farms in South Australia is low and independent management units are possible.

13.7.3.2. Acquired immunity

Nigrelli (1932) reported that black triggerfish, *Melichthys bispinosus* = *Melichthys niger* (Balistidae), heavily infected by '*N. melleni*' shed worms and were not reinfected, and that some *Epinephelus* species demonstrated natural immunity throughout epizootics and were not parasitized. Bondad-Reantaso *et al.* (1995b) showed acquired protection by Japanese flounder against larval infection as demonstrated by a reduction in number and size of worms on previously infected fish. No significant difference, however, was found in serum antibody levels between primed and control fish. Experimental inoculation of parasite homogenate indicated that protection from previous infections was not associated with a humoral antibody. In tilapia infected by '*N. melleni*', Robinson *et al.* (2008) showed that mucus of infected fish exhibited maximum parasite killing activity 9 weeks after infection and continued until 15 weeks, which corresponded with a decline in mean infestation intensity, but immunoassays failed to show evidence of a humoral response. Hatanaka *et al.* (2005) identified an antigen expressed on the ciliary surface of larval '*N. girellae*' from spotted halibut, *Verasper variegatus*, which, under *in vitro* conditions, caused agglutination/immobilization of oncomiracidia. Intraperitoneal injection of either sonicated or intact ciliary proteins with adjuvant induced immunoglobulin production that, when injected into Japanese flounder, immobilized parasites *in vitro*. While this discovery may be useful for vaccination, it is unclear whether fish antibodies against this antigen prevent *N. girellae* infection (Hatanaka *et al.*, 2005). Studies have also characterized highly concentrated serum lectins in spotted halibut which bind to the ciliary surface glycoprotein and agglutinate *N. girellae* larvae *in vitro* (Hatanaka *et al.*, 2008).

Experiments by Ohno *et al.* (2008) on susceptibility of different farmed fish species in Japan indicate that *S. dumerili* is more susceptible to *N. girellae* larvae than *S. quinqueradiata* and Japanese flounder. Parasites grow fastest on *S. dumerili*, slowest on Japanese flounder and both species acquired partial protection against reinfection by *N. girellae*. According to Ogawa (2005), Japanese flounder is 'very susceptible' to *N. girellae*. Spotted halibut is thought to be less susceptible to *N. girellae* than other cultured Japanese species and much must be determined about the biological functions of fish lectins including their potential role in pathogen immunity (Hatanaka *et al.*, 2008).

13.7.4. Treatment

13.7.4.1. Fresh water and chemical immersion

An initial step to control infections in hatchery brood stock or aquaria is to quarantine fish before introduction into tanks. Fish are usually given fresh water, hydrogen peroxide or formalin baths before introduction to tanks. Chemical control has been widely studied (Thoney and Hargis, 1991; Whittington and Chisholm, 2008). Nigrelli (1932) dipped tilapia infected by '*N. melleni*' in fresh water, recording death of all parasites and 100% host survival after treatment for 120 and 150 s. By applying 2 min freshwater baths every 2–4 weeks across infected cages on the Hawaiian farm, the '*N. melleni*' population on tilapia declined.

Freshwater bathing is used routinely to control monogeneans on several farmed fish species in South-East Asia (Leong, 1997), *N. girellae* in Japan (Egusa, 1983; Ogawa and Yokoyama, 1998) and '*N. melleni*' off Brazil (Sanches, 2008). In laboratory experiments,

Mueller *et al.* (1992) determined that '*N. melleni*' egg hatching failed from Florida red tilapia, *O. aureus* × *O. mossambicus*, when exposed to fresh water for 72 h or for 96 h. Treatment for 5 days with hyposaline water (15 g/l) prohibited egg hatching and eliminated juveniles and adults from fish (Ellis and Watanabe, 1993). Similar studies at 25°C on *N. girellae* in Japanese experimental culture demonstrated that hyposalinities at 8, 17 and 24 ppt for 5 h reduced egg laying *in vitro*, lowered hatching rates when incubated for 15 days, and the numbers of non-swimming oncomiracidia were higher at 8 and 17 ppt over 5 h (Umeda and Hirazawa, 2004). In tanks in Mexico, a 60 min exposure to fresh water removed 99% of immature and adult *Neobenedenia* sp. from *S. annulatus* (see Fajer-Ávila *et al.*, 2008). Failure to remove all parasites with prolonged freshwater treatment highlights broad variability that is probably dependent on the physiological tolerances of parasites and hosts. A 2 min freshwater bath, however, significantly *increased* susceptibility to reinfection (Ohno *et al.*, 2009). After treatment, a white mucoid material presumed to be host skin mucus was observed in the bath water, and it was suggested loss of this layer probably reduced the resistance of treated *S. dumerili* and *S. quinqueradiata* which led to increased reinfection by *N. girellae*.

In South Australia, freshwater treatment is impractical because cages are some distance offshore and fresh water is scarce. Bathing in 300 ppm hydrogen peroxide is the treatment of choice for *B. seriolae* and *Zeuxapta seriolae* (see Chambers and Ernst, 2005) as it has no food-safety concerns (Mansell *et al.*, 2005); it can, however, be toxic to fish (Treves-Brown, 2000; Hirazawa *et al.*, 2017). Hydrogen peroxide is also an approved treatment in Japan (Ogawa, 2005), eliminates *N. girellae* and *B. seriolae* attached to fish (75 ppm, 30 min; Hirazawa *et al.*, 2016) and has been shown to reduce hatching success of *N. girellae* eggs (Hirazawa *et al.*, 2020). Woolley *et al.* (2022) found that parasite-free *S. lalandi* were relatively tolerant of high concentrations of peroxide with no acute effect on physiological parameters except at very high doses following repeat bathing in warm water.

Caprylic acid, a natural, medium-chain fatty acid in coconut and other edible oils, tested *in vitro* against larvae and adults stopped larval movement immediately, caused lysis within 25 min and death after 2 h, whereas adults contracted in 20 min but remained alive after a 2 h treatment (Hirazawa *et al.*, 2001). Other chemical baths for '*N. melleni*' include: (i) a 14-day treatment using 0.15–0.18 ppm copper sulfate; (ii) a 1 h bath in 250 ppm formalin; (iii) two to three treatments every 2–3 days using 0.5 ppm trichlorfon (Thoney and Hargis, 1991); and (iv) 1:2000 formalin for 10 min (Sanches, 2008).

13.7.4.2. Praziquantel

Praziquantel, an anthelmintic synthesized to treat endoparasitic flatworms of mammals, has been tested against a range of blood- and epidermal-feeding monogeneans from fish as an in-feed treatment (see Nodbury *et al.*, 2022 for review). Praziquantel is the active ingredient of Hadaclean® (Bayer Ltd), Benesaru® (ASKA Animal Health Co., Ltd) and Praziguard flavour for fish® (Riken Vets Pharma, Inc.). However, medicated feed can be unpalatable to fish at high inclusion levels, resulting in feed rejection, regurgitation or reduced feed intake (Williams *et al.*, 2007; Yamamoto *et al.*, 2011), and in many areas fish farmers tend to prefer hydrogen peroxide bathing (Nodbury *et al.*, 2022). Palatability issues may be able to be overcome using particulate praziquantel formulations (beads) incorporated into fish feed (Tang *et al.*, 2022). Nodbury *et al.* (2022; Table 3) summarized praziquantel use against monogeneans, including *B. seriolae* and *N. girellae*, including dose, delivery method and observed efficacy. The maximum efficacy observed for *N. girellae* was >81.4% reduction for chub mackerel, *Scomber japonicus*, in feed (semi-defrosted krill; Yamamoto *et al.*, 2011); and for *B. seriolae*, 100% reduction in *Seriola* spp. in feed (Hirazawa *et al.*, 2013). Hirazawa *et al.* (2013) found that praziquantel was less effective in controlling *N. girellae* compared to *B. seriolae*.

Assessing bioavailability and pharmacokinetics in *S. lalandi*, Tubbs and Tingle (2006a) studied maximum praziquantel concentrations in skin and plasma when administered in solution and in feed. Results suggested oral treatment every 24 h may expose parasites to highly variable praziquantel concentrations. They recommended a dose interval of less than 24 h to potentially alleviate variable, subtherapeutic praziquantel levels in host tissues and ensure it reaches feeding monogeneans. Indeed, higher praziquantel doses are generally required to remove skin-feeding monogeneans compared to blood-feeding monogeneans. Exposure of parasites to sublethal doses could promote the development of drug resistance.

13.8. Predictive Tools, Decision Support Systems and Integrated Parasite Management

Detailed knowledge of monogenean biology, transmission, life cycle, potential biological control and chemical intervention combined into a well-conceived, strategic plan using best-practice husbandry can enable integrated parasite management. Integrated management must account for the influence of environmental parameters (water temperature, salinity) on key life-history stages including: (i) egg size, egg energy reserves and embryonation; (ii) hatching success; (iii) parasite growth; and (iv) development and fecundity (Hoshina and Matsusato, 1967; Ernst *et al.*, 2002, 2005; Tubbs *et al.*, 2005; Lackenby *et al.*, 2007; Mooney *et al.*, 2008; Brazenor *et al.*, 2020). Parasite life-cycle parameter data collected from *in vitro* studies should be interpreted with caution, because live parasite behaviour when attached to hosts is more representative than detached worms in dishes of sea water. Dinh Hoai and Hutson (2014) also advise that monogenean egg production varies with parasite age and time of day, thus average measures from hourly or daily oviposition rates are not readily extrapolated.

An elegant example of how mathematical models can integrate available parasite data to predict growth and spread was provided by Christie and Foster (2020). Using available published data on the lifespan, larval development, adult lifespan, egg incubation, infection rate and fecundity of *Neobenedenia*, they predicted population growth and spread of infection in a closed system. In their estimate, a single infecting founder parasite grew to a total theoretical parasite population of over 2400 parasites by day 25, and to over 96,000 by day 440.

Hutson *et al.* (2022) provided a decision support tool called 'BeNeZe', which corroborates available published data on growth rates and age at sexual maturity for *B. seriolae*, *N. girellae* and *Z. seriolae* to enable strategically timed treatments. Administration of bath or in-feed treatments requires strategically timed dual delivery for optimal results to kill adult parasite populations on fish (first treatment), followed by another delivery (second treatment) to kill immature growing parasites that invaded treated fish as larvae from eggs and oncomiracidia resident in and around the farm (Fig. 13.3). Timing of the second treatment is important because it must kill all new recruits before they become egg layers. Successful treatment timing must use local water temperature and salinity data to predict parasite growth rates.

Available through an open-access app, the BeNeZe tool provides biologically relevant treatment intervals to interrupt the life cycle. The tool was developed from published data and models the effect of temperature on parasite life cycles, enabling determination of treatment intervals for two consecutive medicinal immersion or bathing treatments that kill adult parasites and prevent maturity of subsequent recruits. While readily applied in public aquaria and recirculating aquaculture systems, a logistical constraint

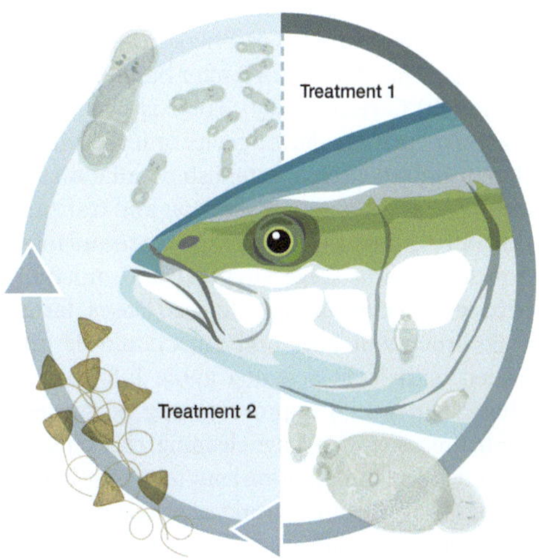

Fig. 13.3. Schematic diagram of *Benedenia seriolae* infecting *Seriola lalandi* showing key parasite life stages and representation of treatment schedules. Treatment 1 kills juvenile and adult stages attached to fish, while the biologically timed Treatment 2 is delivered when all eggs in the environment have hatched and oncomiracidia have infected fish but have not reached sexual maturity. (© Eden Cartwright, Bird Circus; used with permission.)

for application is the recognition of independent management units in marine netpen aquaculture. In many situations, small independent farms (or farm units) operate in a finite area, precluding independent management units and integrated parasite management. Unless netpen and farm density and their arrangement and management can be addressed, prolonged parasite reductions in intense open marine aquaculture remain challenging.

Three-dimensional numerical models have predicted dispersal of sea lice between wild and farmed salmon (Amundrud and Murray, 2009; Murray, 2009). Recent research has provided insights into the dispersal ability of monogeneans. For example, Brazenor *et al.* (2020) showed that *N. girellae* eggs laid under cooler conditions (20 and 25°C) were better provisioned with energetic reserves (compared to those laid at 30°C). They hypothesized this would likely facilitate larval longevity and development success, commensurate with previous observations of parasite epizootics in winter. This was subsequently confirmed by Hirazawa *et al.* (2023), who showed that oncomiracidia remained active and swimming for longer durations at lower seawater temperatures (i.e. oncomiracidia were active for 60, 72 and 108 h after hatching at 30, 25 and 20°C, respectively). There is no information on oncomiracidia longevity or infectivity for *B. seriolae*. Research to establish population size, fecundity, egg viability, dispersion and transmission of eggs, larvae longevity, background infection levels, and stage survival and mortality between infection sources (cages, leases, farms) and throughout bays and gulfs could be integrated with local oceanographic information. These data would improve timing of strategic control measures (e.g. cage cleaning, cage changes and chemical intervention) but may only benefit farms if spatial and temporal coordination of husbandry was viable.

13.9. New Technologies

13.9.1. Chemical treatments, resistance and vaccines

Chemicals applied as baths or in feed, delivered against recommended guidelines (e.g. lower concentrations to cut costs), can lead to subtherapeutic doses, raising the likelihood of the emergence of parasite resistance. Thoney and Hargis (1991) reported acquired resistance to trichlorfon in '*N. melleni*'. Highly variable praziquantel concentrations in *S. lalandi* serum and skin (Tubbs and Tingle, 2006b) suggest its wide use in feed may be ineffective and could lead to resistance. If geographically widespread resistance to hydrogen peroxide and/or praziquantel developed, no effective alternative products are currently available to treat capsalids. Social change has turned against synthetic chemical use in food production. Multidisciplinary approaches incorporating parasitologists, veterinarians, statisticians, chemists, nutritionists, physiologists, ecologists and economists are needed to develop well-designed trials to ensure that environmentally responsible antiparasitic compounds reach parasites at appropriate dose and cost. In-feed immunostimulants to boost the immune system of captive fish is another viable therapy.

Future research will likely lead to development of vaccines. However, there is only one commercially available aquatic parasite vaccine (Providean® AquaTec Sea Lice; Tecnovax), and this is against sea lice (Shivam *et al.*, 2021). Humoral antibody responses and acquired immunity have been observed in fish–monogenean systems (Buchmann, 1999; Kishimori *et al.*, 2021); however, no vaccine candidate antigen has been identified (Ilgová *et al.*, 2021; Kar *et al.*, 2022). Immunoprophylaxis against capsalids requires detailed studies on protection mechanisms to select optimum candidate antigens, adjuvants and formulations for field trials. Benefits of vaccines versus chemicals include specific and sustained action within fish and no/limited environmental impact, withdrawal period or flesh residues. Host responses against many monogeneans are only partially expressed, suggesting the parasites may secrete immune evasion or immunosuppressive substances (Buchmann and Bresciani, 2006), a valuable focus using new technologies.

13.9.2. Advanced sequencing and breeding for parasite resistance

Advanced sequencing enables huge volumes of genetic data to be generated relatively cheaply. Whole genomes are now standard for fish and their parasites. Parasite and fish genomics will provide data which, with appropriate bioinformatics, may help predict and identify new drug targets against reproduction, feeding, metabolism, neurotransmitters and immune evasion. Isolation, characterization and expression of genes and their products will help us to interfere with a parasite's ability to infect, establish, feed and reproduce. RNA interference (RNAi) can produce mutant, deficient and knockdown parasites and hosts to expand knowledge of the parasite–host association (Sitjà-Bobadilla, 2008). Characterization of fish immune mechanisms may help control *B. seriolae* and *N. girellae* infections and several continuous fish cell lines are now available – or being developed – including *S. dumerili* skin cells (Fernandez *et al.*, 1993), enabling studies of their immune systems and *in vitro* parasite cultivation.

Genetic involvement, or breeding for parasite resistance, is a promising approach for the *Seriola* aquaculture industry and has been a focus for 15 years in Japan (Ozaki *et al.*, 2013; Noda *et al.*, 2017; Uchino *et al.*, 2020; Akita *et al.*, 2023). Research efforts have largely focused on *S. quinqueradiata*, which is considered to have a higher inherent resistance to *B. seriolae* compared to *S. lalandi* and *S. dumerili* (see Nagakura *et al.*, 2006, 2010). Nagakura *et al.* (2010) observed some degree of heritable variation in the levels of infestation among individual *S. quinqueradiata*, while Akita *et al.* (2023) examined heritability of resistance over two generations in a long-term field trial using repeated counts – which showed that individual and family performance of resistance was consistent. Ozaki *et al.* (2013) performed quantitative trait locus (QTL) analyses using wild F_1 strains of *S. quinqueradiata* to determine whether there was genetic evidence of resistance to *B. seriolae*. Using a high-density linkage map with microsatellite and single-nucleotide polymorphism (SNP) markers, they identified two major QTL regions contributing to the *Benedenia* disease resistance. This marked the first genetic evidence detailing phenotypic resistance to *B. seriolae* infection. Subsequently, Nakamoto *et al.* (2017) discovered a novel C-type lectin gene for one of the QTL regions, which may control resistance to *B. seriolae*. Concurrently, Noda *et al.* (2017) conducted an epidemiology study to assess changes in *B. seriolae* infection on *S. quinqueradiata* to select *Benedenia*-resistant brood stock candidates. More recently, Uchino *et al.* (2020) conducted a genome scan for QTLs that affect *Benedenia* disease resistance in five full-sib families using SNP markers, finding four significant and five suggestive QTLs. Nguyen and Vu (2022) had less-promising indications for resistance to *B. seriolae* and deformity in *S. lalandi*; their multi-locus linear and threshold mixed-model analyses (for 752 animals) showed that heritabilities for the incidence of skin fluke and deformity were small. They propose future studies could evaluate a larger number of individuals and families to help increase prediction accuracies.

13.9.3. Biological control

Cleaner organisms (fish, shrimp and crabs) live in temperate and tropical waters (Vaughan *et al.*, 2017, 2023) and may be a viable method for reducing capsalid monogenean infestations. Commercial applications have focused on fish as biocontrols for the management of sea lice in salmonid aquaculture, and while biological controls are being increasingly investigated for capsalid monogeneans, they remain largely experimental (Militz and Hutson, 2015; Vaughan *et al.*, 2018a,b; Shirakashi and Takagi, 2020; Martins *et al.*, 2025). Cowell *et al.* (1993) compared the capacity of three tropical cleaner fish species to control parasites and determined that final infections on red tilapia maintained without cleaner fish were significantly greater in two of three experiments. They detected monogeneans in cleaner fish gut contents, found gobies were more effective than a labrid, and suggested cleaning symbionts could provide biological control for '*N. melleni*' in sea-cage tilapia culture. Similarly, Martins *et al.* (2025) evaluated haematological parameters of mullet, *Mugil liza*, parasitized with '*N. melleni*' following cohabitation with cleaner goby, *Elacatinus figaro*, and deduced that cohabitation with cleaners reduced parasite load and host stress.

A field experiment in the Caribbean investigated cleaner shrimps to remove '*N. melleni*' from acanthurids for extended durations open to a constant, natural supply of infective larvae in large enclosures under semi-natural conditions (McCammon *et al.*, 2010). The study allowed shrimps access to natural habitat including alternative food sources, but fish regularly visited shrimps. Pederson shrimp, *Periclimenes pedersoni* (Palaemonidae), significantly reduced the number and size of '*N. melleni*' from the primary host, Atlantic blue tang, *Acanthurus coeruleus* (Acanthuridae) (Sikkel *et al.*, 2009). In Australian-based laboratory experiments, four cleaner shrimp species (*Lysmata amboinensis, Urocaridella antonbruunii, Lysmata vittata* and *Stenopus hispidus*) significantly reduced *N. girellae* infection on grouper (farmed juvenile *Epinephelus coioides*) and reduced *N. girellae* eggs numbers attached to fine mesh (apart from *U. antonbruunii*, which did not reduce egg numbers at all; Vaughan *et al.*, 2018a). In a separate study using simulated recirculating aquaculture conditions, the cleaner shrimp *L. vittata* removed the eggs of *N. girellae* entangled on the mesh of the culture cages and significantly reduced *N. girellae* recruitment to fish by ~87% (Vaughan *et al.*, 2018b).

Cleaner shrimp have been proposed as superior for the treatment of ectoparasitic monogeneans because they are not susceptible to infection by fish ectoparasites and can be reliably bred in captivity (Militz and Hutson, 2015; Vaughan *et al.*, 2018a). Monogenean eggs ingested by shrimp are not viable, while those eaten by fish hatched after excretion (Militz and Hutson, 2015; Shirakashi and Takagi, 2020). Thus, cleaner shrimp can reduce parasite re-infection pressure by consuming parasite life stages that are resistant to chemical therapies. Employing shrimp to reduce parasite life stages in the environment avoids direct contact between shrimp and client fish, and therefore shrimp predation risk can be minimized. Evaluation of the disease risks associated with co-culture (of cleaner fish or shrimp) should be assessed prior to application at commercial scales (e.g. Treasurer and Cox, 1991).

13.9.4. Novel compounds

Social licence to operate, expense of chemical treatments (initial development, then field trials), possible toxicity to fish, barriers to approved use on food fish, deployment and regulation in industry and environmental concerns have stimulated studies seeking alternative treatment methods (Hutson *et al.*, 2012; Militz *et al.*, 2013; Trasviña-Morena *et al.*, 2017; Ingelbrecht *et al.*, 2020). Plant- and seaweed-derived dietary supplements are now commercialized and gaining popularity (Vatsos and Rebours, 2015; Fernández-Montero *et al.*, 2021; Power *et al.*, 2025). Allicin-containing garlic extracts have potential for development as a prophylactic and treatment to manage monogenean infections. Militz *et al.* (2013) found that 30-day dietary supplementation of garlic extracts to barramundi reduced *N. girellae* infection by up to 70% compared to controls. Garlic extracts also significantly inhibited hatching success (5 ± 5%) and oncomiracidia longevity (<2 h) at allicin concentrations of 15.2 μl, while eggs in the seawater control had >95% hatching success and mean oncomiracidia longevity of 37 ± 3 h (Militz *et al.*, 2014). However, juvenile *N. girellae* attached to a host fish are highly resistant to allicin (Militz *et al.*, 2014). Similarly, herbal–seawater solutions containing garlic, rosemary and commercially manufactured herbal products resulted in a significant reduction in the survival of adult *N. girellae* (and *Z. seriolae*) and *N. girellae* oncomiracidia relative to the controls (Ingelbrecht *et al.*, 2020). Aqueous extracts from marine seaweeds, *Asparagopsis taxiformis* and *Ulva* sp., delayed embryonic development and inhibited hatching of *N. girellae* (see Hutson *et al.*, 2012), while in-feed inclusion of the silkworm-derived polysaccharide silkrose reduced *B. seriolae* infection (Miura *et al.*, 2022). Fernandez-Montero *et al.* (2021) compared two commercially available functional dietary additives – one which reduced fish cortisol levels (but not *N. girellae* infection) while another significantly reduced *N. girellae* infection.

13.9.5. Traps

The infective stages of monogeneans exhibit remarkable host-finding strategies which have evolved to maximize survival and infection success. Research into developing traps that attract monogenean oncomiracidia offers considerable promise as a prophylactic measure. The positive phototaxis of *B. seriolae* and *N. girellae* oncomiracidia could help with the development of light traps to guide parasite larvae away from fish stocks and provide an alternative to use of pesticides (Skilton *et al.*, 2020). Indeed, shading can reduce infection intensity under experimental conditions, likely due to accumulation of oncomiracidia into brighter areas, resulting in lowered parasite densities in shaded areas (Ishida *et al.*, 2007; Shirakashi *et al.*, 2013a). LED-based light traps have been used experimentally and in the field to aid sea lice management in salmon farming with promising results for lice larval stages (Flamarique *et al.*, 2009). Skilton *et al.* (2020) proposed synchronously timed deployment of light traps could be used to exploit positive phototaxis and hatching rhythms of *N. girellae* oncomiracidia (Dinh Hoai and Hutson, 2014).

13.9.6. Role of live culture for future technologies

New technologies are likely to emerge from continued fundamental and multidisciplinary approaches to studies of parasite biology, ecology and host–parasite–environment interactions. Parasite cultures permit diverse opportunities to understand these dynamics and are particularly valuable for the identification and production of parasite management strategies, including host species susceptibility trials, vaccine development and efficiency, antigen production for obtaining serological reagents, detection of drug resistance, screening of potential therapeutic agents, treatment strategies and epidemiology (Hutson *et al.*, 2018b). Hutson *et al.* (2018a) reviewed *in vivo* approaches to monogenean cultures including establishment, maintenance, troubleshooting as well as animal ethics and biosecurity considerations. Detailed standard laboratory-based operating procedures for the *in vivo* culture of *N. girellae* are available and can be easily adapted to *B. seriolae* and other capsalid monogeneans (Hutson *et al.*, 2021).

Acknowledgements

Associate Professor Ian D. Whittington (1960–2014) was passionate about monogeneans – he published over 170 articles on their biology and taxonomy – and prepared the first edition of this chapter. For the first edition he acknowledged: Leslie Chisholm, Marty Deveney, Elizabeth Perkins, David Vaughan and Ingo Ernst. For this revised edition: I thank Ingo Ernst and Ian Whittington for enabling my career in marine parasitology. Thank you to all students and colleagues with whom I've had the pleasure to collaborate with on monogeneans. Special thanks to David Vaughan, Central Queensland University, for discussion on monogenean taxonomy; and to Barrett L. Christie, South Carolina Aquarium, who provided valuable commentary on *Neobenedenia* in aquaria. This work was supported by a New Zealand Ministry of Business, Innovation and Employment Endeavour Programme – *Emerging aquatic diseases: A novel diagnostic pipeline and management framework* (CAWX2207).

References

Akita, K. *et al.* (2023) Heritability of resistance to benedeniosis in Japanese yellowtail (*Seriola quinqueradiata*) estimated based on long term repeated measurements in field trials. *Aquaculture* 562, 738856.

Amundrud, T.L. and Murray, A.G. (2009) Modelling sea lice dispersion under varying environmental forcing in a Scottish sea loch. *Journal of Fish Diseases* 32, 27–44.

Baeza, H. and Castro, R. (1975) *Benedenia melleni* (MacCallum, 1927) Ectoparasito en peces de Antofagasta (Platyhelminthes, Monogenea). *Apuntes Oceanológicos* 7, 14–22.

Baeza, J.A. *et al.* (2019) The complete mitochondrial genome and description of a new cryptic species of *Benedenia* Diesing, 1858 (Monogenea: Capsalidae), a major pathogen infecting the yellowtail kingfish *Seriola lalandi* Valenciennes in the South-East Pacific. *Parasites and Vectors* 12, 490.

Bondad-Reantaso, M.G. *et al.* (1995a) Reproduction and growth of Neobenedenia *girellae* (Monogenea: Capsalidae), a skin parasite of cultured marine fishes of Japan. *Fish Pathology* 30, 227–231.

Bondad-Reantaso, M.G. *et al.* (1995b) Acquired protection against *Neobenedenia girellae* in Japanese flounder. *Fish Pathology* 30, 233–238.

Boylan, S.M. *et al.* (2021) Prolonged hypo-salinity to control *Neobenedenia* spp. monogenean infection in large display aquaria. *Zoo Biology* 40, 584–587.

Brabec, J. *et al.* (2023) The evolution of endoparasitism and complex life cycles in parasitic platyhelminths. *Current Biology* 33, 4269–4275.

Brazenor, A.K. *et al.* (2017) Biochemical composition of marine monogenean parasite eggs. *Molecular and Biochemical Parasitology* 218, 1–3.

Brazenor, A.K. *et al.* (2018a) DNA profiling reveals *Neobenedenia girellae* as the primary parasitic monogenean in global fisheries and aquaculture. *Molecular Phylogenetics and Evolution* 129, 130–137.

Brazenor, A.K. *et al.* (2018b) Morphological variation in the cosmopolitan fish parasite *Neobenedenia girellae* (Capsalidae: Monogenea). *International Journal for Parasitology* 48, 125–134.

Brazenor, A.K. *et al.* (2020) Temperature alters reproduction and maternal provisioning in a fish ectoparasite. *International Journal for Parasitology* 50, 839–849.

Brooks, D.R. and Mayes, M.A. (1975) *Phyllodistomum scrippsi* sp. n. (Digenea: Gorgoderidae) and *Neobenedenia girellae* (Hargis, 1955) Yamaguti, 1963 (Monogenea: Capsalidae) from the California sheephead, *Pimelometopon pulchrum* (Ayres) (Pisces: Labridae). *Journal of Parasitology* 61, 407–408.

Buchmann, K. (1999) Immune mechanisms in fish skin against monogeneans – a model. *Folia Parasitologica* 46, 1–9.

Buchmann, K. and Bresciani, J. (2006) Monogenea (phylum Platyhelminthes). In: Woo, P.T.K. (ed.) *Fish Diseases and Disorders, Volume 1: Protozoan and Metazoan Infections*, 2nd edn. CAB International, Wallingford, UK, pp. 297–344.

Bullard, S.A. *et al.* (2003) A new geographic locality and three new host records for *Neobenedenia melleni* (MacCallum) (Monogenea: Capsalidae). *Gulf and Caribbean Research* 15, 1–4.

Carvalho, A.R. and Luque, J.L. (2009) Ocorrência de *Neobenedenia melleni* (Monogenea; Capsalidae) em *Trichiurus lepturus* (Perciformes; Trichiuridae), naturalmente infestados, no litoral do Rio de Janeiro, Brasil. *Revista Brasileira de Parasitologia Veterinaria, Jaboticabal* 18, 74–76.

Cejas, S.J., Doble, A., Almansa, E., Martín, M.V. and Felipe, B.C. (2014) A simple method to monitoring the parasite population of *Benedenia seriolae* in rearing tanks of *Seriola dumerili* J.R. Presented at *IV Simposio Internacional de Ciencias del Mar*, Las Palmas de Gran Canaria, Spain, 11–13 June.

Chambers, C.B. and Ernst, I. (2005) Dispersal of the skin fluke *Benedenia seriolae* (Monogenea: Capsalidae) by tidal currents and implications for sea-cage farming of *Seriola* spp. *Aquaculture* 250, 60–69.

Chew, X.Z. *et al.* (2024) Fish ectoparasite detection, collection and curation. *Advances in Parasitology* 125, 105–157.

Christie, B.L. and Foster, J.W. (2020) A review of the biology of *Neobenedenia melleni* and *Neobenedenia girellae*, and analysis of control strategies in aquaria. *Drum and Croaker* 51, 39–85.

Cowell, L.E. *et al.* (1993) Use of tropical cleaner fish to control the ectoparasite *Neobenedenia melleni* (Monogenea: Capsalidae) on seawater-cultured Florida red tilapia. *Aquaculture* 113, 189–200.

Deveney, M.R., *et al.* (2001) First published record of the pathogenic monogenean parasite *Neobenedenia melleni* (Capsalidae) from Australia. *Diseases of Aquatic Organisms* 46, 79–82.

Diggles, B. and Hutson, K.S. (2005) Diseases of kingfish (*Seriola lalandi*) in Australasia. *Aquaculture Health International* 3, 12–14.

Dinh Hoai, T. and Hutson, K.S. (2014) Reproductive strategies of the insidious fish ectoparasite, *Neobenedenia* sp. (Capsalidae: Monogenea). *PLoS One* 9, e108801.

Egusa, S. (1983) Disease problems in Japanese yellowtail, *Seriola quinqueradiata*, culture: a review. *Rapports et Procès-Verbaux des Réunions, Conseil International pour l'Exploration de la Mer* 182, 10–18.

Ellis, E.P. and Watanabe, W.O. (1993) The effects of hyposalinity on eggs, juveniles and adults of the marine monogenean, *Neobenedenia melleni*: treatment of ecto-parasitosis in seawater-cultured tilapia. *Aquaculture* 117, 15–27.

Ernst, I., *et al.* (2002) Monogenean parasites in sea-cage aquaculture. *Austasia Aquaculture* February/March, 46–48.

Ernst, I. *et al.* (2005) Effects of temperature, salinity, desiccation and chemical treatments on egg embryonation and hatching success of *Benedenia seriolae* (Monogenea: Capsalidae), a parasite of farmed *Seriola* spp. *Journal of Fish Diseases* 28, 157–164.

Fajer-Ávila, E.J. *et al.* (2004) Patterns of occurrence of the platyhelminth parasites of the wild bullseye puffer (*Sphoeroides annulatus*) off Sinaloa, Mexico. *Journal of Parasitology* 90, 415–418.

Fajer-Ávila, E.J. *et al.* (2008) Effectiveness of freshwater treatment against *Lepeophtheirus simplex* (Copepoda: Caligidae) and *Neobenedenia* sp. (Monogenea: Capsalidae), skin parasites of bullseye puffer fish, *Sphoeroides annulatus* reared in tanks. *Aquaculture* 284, 277–280.

Fensham, J.R. *et al.* (2018) Random and systematic sampling error when hooking fish to monitor skin fluke (*Benedenia seriolae*) and gill fluke (*Zeuxapta seriolae*) burden in Australian farmed yellowtail kingfish (*Seriola lalandi*). *Preventive Veterinary Medicine* 153, 7–14.

Fernandez, R.D. *et al.* (1993) Characterization of three continuous cell lines from marine fish. *Journal of Aquatic Animal Health* 5, 127–136.

Fernández-Montero, A. *et al.* (2021) Improving greater amberjack (*Seriola dumerili*) defenses against monogenean parasite *Neobenedenia girellae* infection through functional dietary additives. *Aquaculture* 534, 736317.

Flamarique, I.N. *et al.* (2009) Monitoring and potential control of sea lice using an LED-based light trap. *Canadian Journal of Fisheries and Aquatic Sciences* 66, 1371–1382.

Gaida, I.H. and Frost, P. (1991) Intensity of *Neobenedenia girellae* (Monogenea: Capsalidae) on the halfmoon, *Medialuna californiensis* (Perciformes: Kyphosidae), examined using a new method for detection. *Journal of the Helminthological Society of Washington* 58, 129–130.

González, M.T. and Acuña, E. (1998) Metazoan parasites of the red rockfish *Sebastes capensis* off northern Chile. *Journal of Parasitology* 84, 783–788.

Grau, A. *et al.* (1999) Some protozoan and metazoan parasites of the amberjack from the Balearic Sea (western Mediterranean). *Aquaculture International* 7, 307–317.

Hatanaka, A. *et al.* (2005) A small ciliary surface glycoprotein of the monogenean parasite *Neobenedenia girellae* acts as an agglutination/immobilization antigen and induces an immune response in the Japanese flounder *Paralichthys olivaceus*. *Parasitology* 131, 591–600.

Hatanaka, A. *et al.* (2008) Characterization of highly concentrated serum lectins in spotted halibut *Verasper variegatus*. *Parasitology* 135, 359–369.

Hirano, C. *et al.* (2015) Egg laying and hatching rhythms of the skin fluke *Neobenedenia girellae*. *Fish Pathology* 50, 23–28.

Hirayama T. *et al.* (2009) Effect of *Neobenedenia girellae* (Monogenea) infection on host amberjack *Seriola dumerili* (Carangidae). *Aquaculture* 288, 159–165.

Hirazawa, N. (2019) Killing effects of various treatments on eggs of the skin-parasitic monogeneans *Neobenedenia girellae* and *Benedenia seriolae*. *Aquaculture* 498, 285–288.

Hirazawa, N. *et al.* (2001) *In vitro* assessment of the antiparasitic effect of caprylic acid against several fish parasites. *Aquaculture* 200, 251–258.

Hirazawa, N. *et al.* (2004) Susceptibility of spotted halibut *Verasper variegatus* (Pleuronectidae) to infection by the monogenean *Neobenedenia girellae* (Capsalidae) and oral therapy trials using praziquantel. *Aquaculture* 238, 83–95.

Hirazawa, N. *et al.* (2010) The influence of different water temperatures on *Neobenedenia girellae* (Monogenea) infection, parasite growth, egg production and emerging second generation on amberjack *Seriola dumerili* (Carangidae) and the histopathological effect of this parasite on fish skin. *Aquaculture* 299, 2–7.

Hirazawa, N. *et al.* (2013) Differences in sensitivity to the anthelmintic praziquantel by the skin-parasitic monogeneans *Benedenia seriolae* and *Neobenedenia girellae*. *Aquaculture* 404–405, 59–64.

Hirazawa, N. *et al.* (2016) Anthelmintic effects of 75 ppm hydrogen peroxide treatment on the monogeneans *Benedenia seriolae*, *Neobenedenia girellae*, and *Zeuxapta japonica* infecting the skin and gills of greater amberjack *Seriola dumerili*. *Aquaculture* 450, 244–249.

Hirazawa, N. *et al.* (2017) Investigation of the toxicological and histopathological effects of hydrogen peroxide bath treatments at different concentrations on *Seriola* species and the effectiveness of these treatments on *Neobenedenia girellae* (Monogenea) infestations. *Aquaculture* 479, 217–224.

Hirazawa, N. *et al.* (2020) Effects of hydrogen peroxide on egg laying and hatching of the skin monogenean *Neobenedenia girellae*. *Fish Pathology* 55, 80–83.

Hirazawa, N. *et al.* (2023) Temporal change in the swimming ability and infectivity of the oncomiracidium of a monogenean *Neobenedenia girellae*. *Fish Pathology* 58, 83–90.

Hoshina, T. (1968) On the monogenetic trematode, *Benedenia seriolae*, parasitic on yellowtail, *Seriola quinqueradiata*. *Bulletin de l'Office International des Épizooties* 69, 1179–1191.

Hoshina, T. and Matsusato, T. (1967) *Relation between Egg Hatch of* Benedenia seriolae *and Water Temperature*. Bulletin on Control for the Fish Diseases in 1966, Shizuoka Prefectural Fisheries Experiment Station, Minato City, Japan, pp. 69–71.

Hutson, K.S. *et al.* (2007) Risk assessment for metazoan parasites of yellowtail kingfish *Seriola lalandi* (Perciformes: Carangidae) in South Australian sea-cage aquaculture. *Aquaculture* 271, 85–99.

Hutson, K.S. *et al.* (2012) Seaweed extracts as a natural control against the monogenean ectoparasite, *Neobenedenia* sp., infecting farmed barramundi (*Lates calcarifer*). *International Journal for Parasitology* 42, 1135–1141.

Hutson, K.S. *et al.* (2018a) Monogenean parasite cultures: current techniques and recent advances. *Advances in Parasitology* 99, 61–91.

Hutson, K.S. *et al.* (2018b) Aquatic parasite cultures and their applications. *Trends in Parasitology* 34, 1082–1096.

Hutson, K.S. *et al.* (2021) Chapter 17 – *Neobenedenia girellae*. In: Sitja-Bobadilla, A., Bron, J., Wiegertjes, G. and Piazzon, M.C. (eds) *Fish Parasites: A Handbook of Protocols for their Isolation, Culture and Transmission*. 5m Publishing, Great Easton, UK, pp. 258–271.

Hutson, K.S. *et al.* (2022) A decision support tool for parasite management in fish aquaculture. *Reviews in Aquaculture* 14, 1656–1670.

Ilgová, J. *et al.* (2021) Molecular communication between the monogenea and fish immune system. *Fish and Shellfish Immunology* 112, 179–190.

Ingelbrecht, J. *et al.* (2020) Anthelmintic herbal extracts as potential prophylactics or treatments for monogenean infections in cultured yellowtail kingfish (*Seriola lalandi*). *Aquaculture* 520, 734776.

Ishida, M. *et al.* (2007) Response of *Neobenedenia girellae* (Monogenea) oncomiracidia to brightness and black-and-white contrast. *Parasitology* 134, 1823–1830.

Jahn, T.L. and Kuhn, L.R. (1932) The life history of *Epibdella melleni* MacCallum, 1927, a monogenetic trematode parasitic on marine fishes. *Biological Bulletin (Woods Hole)* 62, 89–111.

Kaneko, J.J. *et al.* (1988) Infection of tilapia, *Oreochromis mossambicus* (Trewavas), by a marine monogenean, *Neobenedenia melleni* (MacCallum, 1927) Yamaguti, 1963 in Kaneohe Bay, Hawaii, USA, and its treatment. *Journal of Fish Diseases* 11, 295–300.

Kar, B. *et al.* (2022) Vaccines for parasitic diseases of fish. In: Makesh M. and Rajendran K.V. (eds) *Fish Immune System and Vaccines*. Springer, Singapore, pp. 125–157.

Kawato, S. *et al.* (2019) Phylogenetic analysis with complete mitochondrial genome sequences of *Benedenia seriolae* specimens derived from Japanese *Seriola* spp. *Fish Pathology* 54, 27–33.

Kearn, G.C. (1963) Feeding in some monogenean skin parasites: *Entobdella soleae* on *Solea solea* and *Acanthocotyle* sp. on *Raia clavata*. *Journal of the Marine Biological Association of the UK* 43, 749–766.

Kearn, G.C. (1992) Mating in the Capsalid Monogenean *Benedenia seriolae*, a skin parasite of the yellowtail, *Seriola quinqueradiata*, in Japan. *Publications of the Seto Marine Biological Laboratory* 35, 273–280.

Kearn, G.C. (1999) The survival of monogenean (platyhelminth) parasites on fish skin. *Parasitology* 119, S57–S88.

Kearn, G.C. *et al.* (1992) Egg production, the oncomiracidium and larval development of *Benedenia seriolae*, a skin parasite of the yellowtail, *Seriola quinqueradiata*, in Japan. *Publications of the Seto Marine Biological Laboratory* 35, 351–362.

Kinami, R. *et al.* (2005) A practical method to distinguish between *Neobenedenia girellae* and *Benedenia seriolae*. *Fish Pathology* 40, 63–66.

Kishimori, J.M. *et al.* (2021) *Neobenedenia melleni*, protection, and mucosal immunity – is it just a fluke? International Association for Aquatic Animal Medicine, Stamford, Connecticut. Available at: https://www.vin.com/apputil/content/defaultadv1.aspx?id=10200673&pid=27093 (accessed 24 November 2025).

Kobayashi, K. *et al.* (2018) Distinction of the skin flukes *Benedenia seriolae* and *Neobenedenia girellae* infecting *Seriola* spp. by PCR-RFLP Assay. *Fish Pathology* 53, 124–127.

Koesharyani, I. *et al.* (1999) Two species of capsalid monogeneans infecting cultured humpback grouper *Cromileptes altivelis* in Indonesia. *Fish Pathology* 34, 165–166.

Lackenby, J.A. *et al.* (2007) Effect of water temperature on reproductive development of *Benedenia seriolae* (Monogenea: Capsalidae) from *Seriola lalandi* in Australia. *Diseases of Aquatic Organisms* 74, 235–242.

Leong, T.S. (1997) Control of parasites in cultured marine finfishes in Southeast Asia – an overview. *International Journal for Parasitology* 27, 1177–1184.

Liao, I.C. *et al.* (2004) Cobia culture in Taiwan: current status and problems. *Aquaculture* 237, 155–165.

Llewellyn, J. (1957) Host-specificity in monogenetic trematodes In: Baer, J.G. (ed.) *First Symposium on Host-Specificity Among Parasites of Invertebrates*. Attinger, Neuchâtel, Switzerland, pp. 199–212.

Lopez, C. *et al.* (2002) Disease outbreak in seafarmed cobia (*Rachycentron canadum*) associated with *Vibrio* spp., *Photobacterium damselae* ssp. *piscicida*, monogenean and myxosporean parasites. *Bulletin of the European Association of Fish Pathologists* 22, 206–211.

MacCallum, G.A., (1927) A new ectoparasitic trematode, *Epibdella melleni*, sp. nov. *Zoopathologica* 291–300.

Mansell, B. *et al.* (2005) Effects of the gill monogenean *Zeuxapta seriolae* (Meserve, 1938) and treatment with hydrogen peroxide on pathophysiology of kingfish, *Seriola lalandi* Valenciennes, 1833. *Journal of Fish Diseases* 28, 253–262.

Martinez-Takeshita, N. *et al.* (2015) A tale of three tails: cryptic speciation in a globally distributed marine fish of the genus *Seriola*. *Copeia* 103, 357–368.

Martins, M.L. *et al.* (2025) The cleaner fish *Elacatinus figaro* can control the monogenean *Neobenedenia melleni*, an ectoparasite of Lebranche mullet *Mugil liza* and does not decrease the hematological response. *Journal of Parasitic Diseases* 49, 472–478.

McCammon, A. *et al.* (2010) Effects of three Caribbean cleaner shrimps on ectoparasitic monogeneans in a semi-natural environment. *Coral Reefs* 29, 419–426.

Militz, T.A. and Hutson, K.S. (2015) Beyond symbiosis: cleaner shrimp clean up in culture. *PLoS One* 10, e0117723.

Militz, T.A. *et al.* (2013) Dietary supplementation of garlic (*Allium sativum*) to prevent monogenean infection in aquaculture. *Aquaculture* 408, 95–99.

Militz, T.A. *et al.* (2014) Efficacy of garlic (*Allium sativum*) extract applied as a therapeutic immersion treatment for *Neobenedenia* sp. management in aquaculture. *Journal of Fish Diseases* 37, 451–461.

Miura, T. *et al.* (2022) The effects of silkworm-derived polysaccharide (silkrose) on ectoparasitic infestations in yellowtail (*Seriola quinqueradiata*) and white trevally (*Pseudocaranx dentex*). *Fishes* 7, 14.

Miyoshi, Y. *et al.* (2019) Skin injuries contribute to nocardiosis in Japanese amberjack *Seriola quinqueradiata*. *Fish Pathology* 54(3), 64–67.

Mooney, A.J. *et al.* (2008) Egg-laying patterns and *in vivo* egg production in the monogenean parasites *Heteraxine heterocerca* and *Benedenia seriolae* from Japanese yellowtail *Seriola quinqueradiata*. *Parasitology* 135, 1295–1302.

Mueller, K.W. *et al.* (1992) Effect of salinity on hatching in *Neobenedenia melleni*, a monogenean ectoparasite of seawater-cultured tilapia. *Journal of the World Aquaculture Society* 23, 199–204.

Murray, A.J. (2009) Using simple models to review the application and implications of different approaches used to simulate transmission of pathogens among aquatic animals. *Preventive Veterinary Medicine* 88, 167–177.

Nagakura, Y. *et al.* (2006) Differences in susceptibility to the monogenean parasite *Benedenia seriolae* among *Seriola quinqueradiata*, *S. lalandi* and their hybrid. *Aquaculture Science* 54, 335–340.

Nagakura, Y. *et al.* (2010) Susceptibility of four families derived from two *Seriola* species to the monogenean parasite (*Benedenia seriolae*) using a new challenge method. *Journal of Fisheries Technology* 3, 21–26.

Nakamoto, M. *et al.* (2017) A novel C-type lectin gene is a strong candidate gene for *Benedenia* disease resistance in Japanese yellowtail, *Seriola quinqueradiata*. *Developmental and Comparative Immunology* 76, 361–369.

Nguyen, N.H. and Vu, N.T. (2022) Threshold models using Gibbs sampling and machine learning genomic predictions for skin fluke disease recorded under field environment in yellowtail kingfish *Seriola lalandi*. *Aquaculture* 547, 737513.

Nigrelli, R.F. (1932) The life history and control of a destructive fish parasite at the New York Aquarium. *Bulletin of the New York Zoological Society* 34, 123–129.

Noda, T. *et al.* (2017) Production of *Benedenia*-resistant yellowtail (*Seriola quinqueradiata*) families – a preliminary approach to the broodstock candidates. *Bulletin of Japan Fisheries Research and Education Agency* 45, 101–105.

Nodbury, L.J. *et al.* (2022) Praziquantel use in aquaculture – current status and emerging issues. *International Journal for Parasitology: Drugs and Drug Resistance* 18, 87–102.

Ogawa, K. (2005) Effects in finfish culture. In: Rohde, K. (ed.) *Marine Parasitology.* CSIRO Publishing, Melbourne, Australia, pp. 378–391.

Ogawa, K. and Shirakashi, S. (2017) Skin fluke infection of cultured marine fish. *Fish Pathology* 52, 186–190.

Ogawa, K. and Yokoyama, H. (1998) Parasitic diseases of cultured marine fish in Japan. *Fish Pathology* 33, 303–309.

Ogawa, K. *et al.* (1995) *Neobenedenia girellae* (Hargis, 1955) Yamaguti, 1963 (Monogenea: Capsalidae) from cultured marine fishes of Japan. *Journal of Parasitology* 81, 223–227.

Ogawa, K. *et al.* (2006) *Neobenedenia girellae* (Monogenea) infection of cultured cobia *Rachycentron canadum* in Taiwan. *Fish Pathology* 41, 51–56.

Ogawa, K. *et al.* (2014) Insemination of the monogenean *Neobenedenia girellae* (Capsalidae, Benedeniinae). *Parasitology International* 63, 473–478.

Ohno, Y. *et al.* (2008) Susceptibility by amberjack (*Seriola dumerili*), yellowtail (*S. quinqueradiata*) and Japanese flounder (*Paralichthys olivaceus*) to *Neobenedenia girellae* (Monogenea) infection and their acquired protection. *Aquaculture* 274, 30–35.

Ohno, Y. *et al.* (2009) The effect of oral antibiotic treatment and freshwater bath treatment on susceptibility to *Neobenedenia girellae* (Monogenea) infection of amberjack (*Seriola dumerili*) and yellowtail (*S. quinqueradiata*) hosts. *Aquaculture* 292, 248–251.

Ozaki, A. *et al.* (2013) Quantitative trait loci (QTL) associated with resistance to a monogenean parasite (*Benedenia seriolae*) in yellowtail (*Seriola quinqueradiata*) through genome wide analysis. *PLoS One* 8, e64987.

Paperna, I. (1991) Diseases caused by parasites in the aquaculture of warm water fish. *Annual Review of Fish Diseases* 1, 155–194.

Power, C. *et al.* (2025) Parasites in aquaculture. In: Smit, N.J. and Sures, B. (eds) *Aquatic Parasitology: Ecological and Environmental Concepts and Implications of Marine and Freshwater Parasites*. Springer, Cham, Switzerland, pp. 595–620.

Premachandra, H.K.A. *et al.* (2017) Genomic DNA variation confirmed *Seriola lalandi* comprises three different populations in the Pacific, but with recent divergence. *Scientific Reports* 7, 9386.

Purcell, C.M. *et al.* (2015) Developing a genetic baseline for the yellowtail amberjack species complex, *Seriola lalandi sensu lato*, to assess and preserve variation in wild populations of these globally important aquaculture species. *Conservation Genetics* 16, 1475–1488.

Robinson, R.D. *et al.* (2008) Interactions between cage-cultured hybrid tilapia and a marine monogenean, *Neobenedenia melleni*, in Jamaica. *North American Journal of Aquaculture* 70, 68–73.

Sanches, E.G. (2008) Controle de *Neobenedenia melleni* (MacCallum, 1927) (Monogenea: Capsalidae) em garoupa-verdadeira, *Epinephelus marginatus* (Lowe, 1834), cultivada em tanques-rede. *Revista Brasileira de Parasitologia Veterinaria* 17, 145–149.

Sato, S. *et al.* (2008) Lipid content and fatty acid composition of the monogenean *Neobenedenia girellae* and comparison between the parasite and host fish species. *Parasitology* 135, 967–975.

Sepúlveda, F.A. and González, M.T. (2014) Molecular and morphological analyses reveal that the pathogen *Benedenia seriolae* (Monogenea: Capsalidae) is a complex species: implications for yellowtail *Seriola* spp. aquaculture. *Aquaculture* 418–419, 94–100.

Sharp, N.J. *et al.* (2004) Efficacy of Aqui-S, formalin and praziquantel against the monogeneans, *Benedenia seriolae* and *Zeuxapta seriolae*, infecting yellowtail kingfish *Seriola lalandi lalandi* in New Zealand. *Aquaculture* 236, 67–83.

Shinn, A. *et al.* (2015) Economic costs of protistan and metazoan parasites to global mariculture. *Parasitology* 142, 196–270.

Shirakashi, S. and Hirano, C. (2015) Accumulation and distribution of skin fluke *Neobenedenia girellae* eggs on a culture cage. *Aquaculture* 443, 1–4.

Shirakashi, S. and Takagi, T. (2020) Consumption of monogenean eggs by crustaceans and fish. *Aquaculture Research* 52, 1915–1924.

Shirakashi, S. *et al.* (2013a) Shading reduced *Neobenedenia girellae* infection on cultured greater amberjack *Seriola dumerili*. *Fish Pathology* 48, 25–28.

Shirakashi, S. *et al.* (2013b) Diurnal pattern of skin fluke infection in cultured amberjack, *Seriola dumerili*, at different water depths. *Aquaculture* 402–403, 19–23.

Shirakashi, S. *et al.* (2021) Phototactic responses in four monogenean oncomiracidia. *Parasitology Research* 120, 3173–3180.

Shirakashi, S. *et al.* (2024) Effects of copper alloy and antifouling-coated nets on the attachment and hatching of monogenean eggs. *Aquaculture* 588, 740954.

Shivam, S. *et al.* (2021) Development of fish parasite vaccines in the omics era: progress and opportunities. *Vaccines* 9, 179.

Sikkel, P.C. *et al.* (2009) Habitat and species differences in prevalence and intensity of *Neobenedenia melleni* (Monogenea: Capsalidae) on sympatric Caribbean surgeonfishes (Acanthuridae). *Journal of Parasitology* 95, 63–68.

Sitjà-Bobadilla, A. (2008) Living off a fish: a trade-off between parasites and the immune system. *Fish and Shellfish Immunology* 25, 358–372.

Skilton, D.C. *et al.* (2020) Parasite attractants: identifying trap baits for parasite management in aquaculture. *Aquaculture* 516, 734557.

Stephens, F.J. (2016) Common pathogens found in yellowtail kingfish *Seriola lalandi* during aquaculture in Australia. *Microbiology Australia* 37, 132–134.

Stien, L.H. *et al.* (2016) 'Snorkel' sea lice barrier technology reduces sea lice loads on harvest-sized Atlantic salmon with minimal welfare impacts. *Aquaculture* 458, 29–37.

Tang, E.K.Y. *et al.* (2022) Effects of formulation on the palatability and efficacy of in-feed praziquantel medications for marine finfish aquaculture. *Marine Drugs* 20, 323.

Tedesco, P. *et al.* (2021) Occurrence of *Neobenedenia girellae* (Monogenea: Capsalidae) in gilthead seabream *Sparus aurata* (Actinopterygii: Sparidae) cultured in Portugal. *Pathogens* 10, 1269.

Thoney, D.A. and Hargis, W.J. (1991) Monogenea (Platyhelminthes) as hazards for fish in confinement. *Annual Review of Fish Diseases* 1, 133–153.

Trasviña-Morena, A.G. *et al.* (2017) Plant extracts as a natural treatment against the fish ectoparasite *Neobenedenia* sp. (Monogenea: Capsalidae). *Journal of Helminthology* 93, 57–65.

Treasurer, J. and Cox, D. (1991) The occurrence of *Aeromonas salmonicida* in wrasse (Labridae) and implications for Atlantic salmon farming. *Bulletin of the European Association of Fish Pathologists* 11, 208–210.

Treves-Brown, K.M. (2000) *Applied Fish Pharmacology*. Kluwer Academic Publishers, Dordrecht, The Netherlands.

Trujillo-González, A. *et al.* (2015a) Tracking transparent monogenean parasites on fish from infection to maturity. *International Journal for Parasitology: Parasites and Wildlife* 4, 316–22.

Trujillo-González, A. *et al.* (2015b) Histopathology associated with haptor attachment of the ectoparasitic monogenean *Neobenedenia* sp. (Capsalidae) to barramundi, *Lates calcarifer* (Bloch). *Journal of Fish Diseases* 38, 1063–1067.

Tubbs, L.A. and Tingle, M.D. (2006a) Bioavailability and pharmacokinetics of a praziquantel bolus in kingfish *Seriola lalandi*. *Diseases of Aquatic Organisms* 69, 233–238.

Tubbs, L.A. and Tingle, M.D. (2006b) Effect of dose escalation on multiple dose pharmacokinetics of orally administered praziquantel in kingfish *Seriola lalandi*. *Aquaculture* 261, 1168–1174.

Tubbs, L.A. *et al.* (2005) Effects of temperature on fecundity *in vitro*, egg hatching and reproductive development of *Benedenia seriolae* and *Zeuxapta seriolae* (Monogenea) parasitic on yellowtail kingfish *Seriola lalandi*. *International Journal for Parasitology* 35, 315–327.

Uchino, T. *et al.* (2020) Novel *Benedenia* disease resistance QTLs in five F1 families of yellowtail (*Seriola quinqueradiata*). *Aquaculture* 529, 735622.

Umeda, N. and Hirazawa, N. (2004) Response of the monogenean *Neobenedenia girellae* to low salinities. *Fish Pathology* 39, 105–107.

Vatsos, I.N. and Rebours, C. (2015) Seaweed extracts as antimicrobial agents in aquaculture. *Journal of Applied Phycology* 27, 2017–2035.

Vaughan, D.B. *et al.* (2017) Cleaner fishes and shrimp diversity and a re-evaluation of cleaning symbioses. *Fish and Fisheries* 18, 698–716.

Vaughan, D.B. *et al.* (2018a) Cleaner shrimp are a sustainable option to treat parasitic disease in farmed fish. *Scientific Reports* 8, 13959.

Vaughan, D.B. *et al.* (2018b) Cleaner shrimp remove parasite eggs on fish cages. *Aquaculture Environment Interactions* 10, 429–436.

Vaughan, D.B. *et al.* (2023) How do fishes manage disease? *Trends in Ecology and Evolution* 38, 396–398.

Warren, M.B. and Bullard, S.A. (2025) Supplemental description of *Benedenia seriolae* (Yamaguti, 1934) Meserve, 1938 (Monogenoidea: Capsalidae) and first record of the parasite infecting a wild greater amberjack, *Seriola dumerili* (Risso, 1810) Hureau and Tortonese, 1973 (Carangiformes: Carangidae) from the northern Gulf of Mexico. *Parasitology International* 104, 102986.

Whittington, I.D. (1996) Benedeniine capsalid monogeneans from Australian fishes: pathogenic species, site-specificity and camouflage. *Journal of Helminthology* 70, 177–184.

Whittington, D.I. (2004) The Capsalidae (Monogenea: Monopisthocotylea): a review of diversity, classification and phylogeny with a note about species complexes. *Folia Parasitologica* 51, 109–122.

Whittington, I.D. (2005) Monogenea Monopisthocotylea (ectoparasitic flukes). In: Rohde, K. (ed.) *Marine Parasitology*. CSIRO Publishing, Melbourne, Australia, pp. 63–72.

Whittington, I.D. and Chisholm, L.A. (2008) Diseases caused by Monogenea. In: Eiras, J.C. *et al.* (eds) *Fish Diseases*, Vol. 2. Science Publishers, Inc., Enfield, New Hampshire, pp. 683–816.

Whittington, I.D. and Horton, M.A. (1996) A revision of *Neobenedenia* Yamaguti, 1963 (Monogenea: Capsalidae) including a redescription of *N. melleni* (MacCallum, 1927) Yamaguti, 1963. *Journal of Natural History* 30, 1113–1156.

Whittington, I.D. *et al.* (2000) Host-specificity of monogenean (platyhelminth) parasites: a role for anterior adhesive areas? *International Journal for Parasitology* 30, 305–320.

Whittington, I.D. *et al.* (2001a) Infections of *Seriola quinqueradiata* Temminck & Schlegel and *S. dumerili* (Risso) in Japan by *Benedenia seriolae* (Monogenea) confirmed by morphology and 28S ribosomal DNA analysis. *Journal of Fish Diseases* 24, 421–425.

Whittington, I.D. *et al.* (2001b) A revision of *Benedenia* Diesling, 1858 including a redescription of *B. sciaenae* (van Beneden, 1856) Odhner, 1905 and recognition of *Menziesia* Gibson, 1976 (Monogenea: Capsalidae). *Journal of Natural History* 35, 663–777.

Whittington, I.D. *et al.* (2001c) Sushi, fish and parasites. *Australasian Science* 2001, 33–36.

Whittington, D.I. *et al.* (2011) *Innovative Solutions for Aquaculture: Assessment of* In Situ *Monitoring Techniques and life History Parameters for Monogenean Skin and Gill Parasites*. Final Report, FRDC Project No. 2003/221. The University of Adelaide, Adelaide, South Australia, p. 43.

Williams, R.E. *et al.* (2007) Efficacy of orally administered praziquantel against *Zeuxapta seriolae* and *Benedenia seriolae* (Monogenea) in yellowtail kingfish *Seriola lalandi*. *Diseases of Aquatic Organisms* 77, 199–205.

Woolley, L.D. *et al.* (2022) The effect of hydrogen peroxide concentration and water temperature on yellowtail kingfish *Seriola lalandi* in a repeated bathing treatment. *Aquaculture* 560, 738545.

WoRMS Editorial Board (2025) *World Register of Marine Species*. Available at: https://www.marinespecies.org at VLIZ (accessed 27 June 2025). DOI: 10.14284/170.

Yamamoto, S. *et al.* (2011) Efficacy of oral praziquantel treatment against the skin fluke infection of cultured chub mackerel, *Scomber japonicus*. *Aquaculture* 319, 53–57.

14 *Heterobothrium okamotoi* and *Neoheterobothrium hirame*

Kazuo Ogawa*
Meguro Parasitological Museum, Tokyo, Japan

Abstract

Heterobothrium okamotoi Ogawa, 1991 and *Neoheterobothrium hirame* Ogawa, 1999 belong to the family Diclidophoridae (Monogenea: Polyopisthocotylea). Infection with the two parasites causes serious disease in their respective host, tiger puffer (*Takifugu rubripes*; Tetraodontidae) and olive flounder or Japanese flounder (*Paralichthys olivaceus*; Paralichthyidae). They share many features concerning biology and pathological effects on their hosts. However, they differ from each other in their origin: *H. okamotoi* is a parasite indigenous to Japan, whereas *N. hirame* is an introduced parasite from the western Atlantic. Besides, *H. okamotoi* infection is a problem in aquaculture, whereas *N. hirame* infection is primarily a problem with wild fish populations.

14.1. *Heterobothrium okamotoi*

14.1.1. Introduction

Monogeneans of the genus *Heterobothrium* infect tetraodontid fishes. Eleven species have been described in Japan, all hosts being members of the genus *Takifugu* (Tetraodontidae) (Ogawa, 1991; Ogawa and Itoh, 2022). The parasites are species specific, and *Heterobothrium okamotoi* is known only from the tiger puffer (*Takifugu rubripes*).

H. okamotoi infection was first reported from tiger puffer cultured in the Inland Sea in western Japan (Okamoto, 1963). Because of its high market value, puffer was cultured in the 1950s–1960s by maintaining fish, caught in the spring and summer, in enclosures until marketed in the winter. Without knowledge of effective control measures, this parasitic disease was a major limiting factor in puffer culture at that time (Okamoto, 1963). Since the 1980s, when artificially produced seedlings were introduced, tiger puffer has been cultured in more locations and on a larger scale in floating net cages. Most typically juvenile puffers are introduced into net cages in the summer and cultured for 1.5 years until the winter of the following year. *H. okamotoi* propagates readily in this culture system, and its infection has since been a recurrent disease problem. This is mainly because of its high fecundity and production of long egg filaments which entangle with the culture nets.

H. okamotoi is a large monogenean, up to 23 mm long, with the body proper attenuated posteriorly in the form of isthmus and haptor bearing four pairs of clamps of typical diclidophorid-type

*Email: ogawak@kiseichu.org

DOI: 10.1079/9781800628748.0014

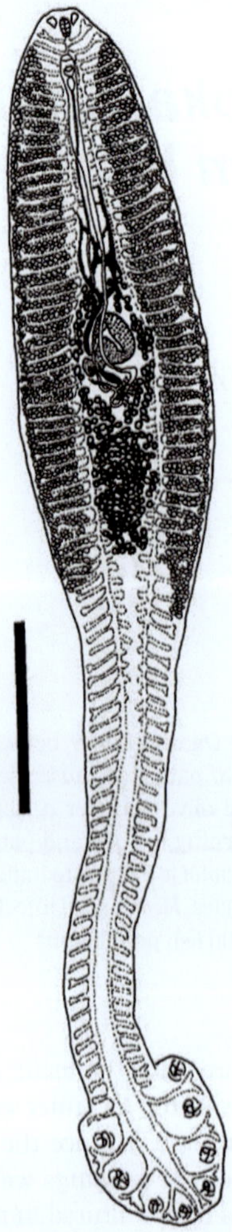

Fig. 14.1. Line drawing of *Heterobothrium okamotoi* Ogawa, 1991. Bar = 3 mm. (From Ogawa, 1991; with permission.)

at its posterior end (Fig. 14.1; Ogawa, 1991). Adult worms infect the branchial cavity wall of the host (Okamoto, 1963; Ogawa and Inouye, 1997a), which is different from typical diclidophorids that infect the gills. In most cases, the site of attachment is on the ventral side of the branchial cavity wall close to the gills. A few to dozens of worms are clustered in heavily infected fish (Fig. 14.2).

Its life cycle is relatively straightforward (Fig. 14.3). Eggs are connected, at both ends, with previous and successive ones through a continuous filament, forming a long egg string (Fig. 14.4; Ogawa, 1997). Eggs hatch and oncomiracidia settle on the gill filaments. Post-larvae are first found on the basal part of the gill filaments; then, with the development of clamps, they gradually move towards the distal part and migrate to the branchial cavity wall, after which they grow on the gills for 1–1.5 months (Ogawa and Inouye, 1997a,b).

There is only one report of *Heterobothrium* infection in wild tiger puffers caught in the Inland Sea (Okamoto and Ogasawara, 1965); only older fish (2+ years) were infected. However, infection among cultured tiger puffer is common. It was detected in all cultured areas in western and southern Japan surrounded by the Pacific, the East China Sea and the Sea of Japan. Tiger puffer cultured in China was also infected with this monogenean (K. Ogawa, 2006, unpublished results). *H. okamotoi* is highly host specific (Ogawa, 1991; Ogawa and Inouye, 1997a; Ohhashi *et al.*, 2007; Hosoya *et al.*, 2013). No similar monogeneans have been recorded from tiger puffer (Ogawa and Yokoyama, 1998).

The oncomiracidium of *H. okamotoi* may recognize its host by detecting the characteristic low body mucus pH of 6.40, compared with the body mucus pH of 7.22–7.30 of four non-host species, for the host-finding (Hirazawa *et al.*, 2003b). Tsutsui *et al.* (2003) identified a novel mannose-specific lectin in the skin mucus of tiger puffer. This lectin is detected in epithelial cells in the skin and gills (Tsutsui *et al.*, 2005) and it binds to *H. okamotoi* under *in vitro* conditions (Tsutsui *et al.*, 2003). Igarashi *et al.* (2017) demonstrated the lectin binding to the D-mannose-specific domain of host immunoglobulin M (IgM), which binds to the ciliated cells of the oncomiracidium, causing shedding of the ciliated cells. Further, Matsui *et al.* (2020) suggested that in addition to the D-mannose-binding ability, the crystallizable fragment domain of IgM plays an important role in host recognition by the oncomiracidia, such as direct binding to the parasites. Fucosylated proteins (FPs), present on the gill surface of non-host *Takifugu* spp. but absent in tiger puffer, might contribute to *H. okamotoi* detachment from the former but not from the latter. From this, Sato *et al.* (2023) suggested that FPs are involved in the host specificity of *H. okamotoi*.

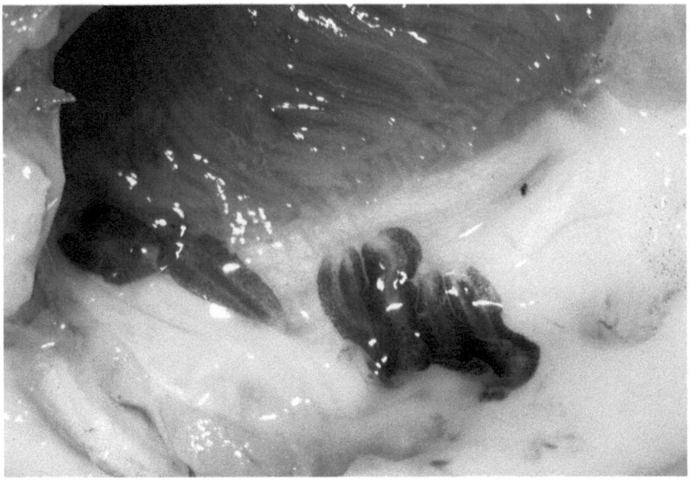

Fig. 14.2. Adults of *Heterobothrium okamotoi* on the branchial cavity wall of tiger puffer (*Takifugu rubripes*). The posterior part of the body is embedded in the host tissue. Note some of them group together to form a cluster. (Photo by M. Nakane; with permission.)

14.1.2. Diagnosis of the infection

The posterior body part (isthmus and haptor) of *H. okamotoi* is embedded within the host tissue and only the body proper appears outside, which is readily observable by the naked eye when the operculum is cut open. Dead worms are sometimes found encapsulated in the host hyperplastic tissue. Worms on the gill filaments are always immature and are up to 6 mm long (Ogawa and Inouye, 1997a).

No signs of external disease are noticed in lightly infected fish. Heavily infected fish are anaemic and lethargic. They tend to swim inactively and leave the school of puffers in the same net cage. Prolonged infection often leads to emaciation and death of the host.

Propagation of *H. okamotoi* is highly temperature dependent. The optimal temperature is approximately 25°C, with the highest mean production rate of 453 eggs/parasite per day (Yamabata *et al.*, 2004). Eggs produced above 26°C are often morphologically abnormal. Eggs laid and kept at 10°C did not hatch, but when transferred to 15°C, they hatched within several days. *Heterobothrium* infections in cultured puffers tend to be milder in the summer than in other seasons (M. Sameshima, Kumamoto Prefectural Fisheries Research Center, 2010, personal communication). Frequency distribution of body length of the parasite collected from a single puffer population indicates that the winter–spring generation mostly disappeared in the summer and it was replaced by an autumn generation (Ogawa and Inouye, 1997a).

The uterus contains a maximum of 1580 eggs, which, when deposited, form an egg string of 2.83 m (Ogawa, 1997). These egg strings entangle with the culture nets, which results in egg accumulation within the culture system. Eggs are easily collected with lines or small pieces of nets hung down from the water surface, and this can be used for monitoring infection.

The oncomiracidium (200–300 μm long; Fig. 14.3) has a lifespan of about 9.1, 7.3 and 4.7 days at 15, 20 and 25°C, respectively (Ogawa, 1998), compared with less than 24 h for oncomiracidia of most monogenean species (Llewellyn, 1963; Buchmann and Bresciani, 2006). Infectivity decreases as the larvae age, but some of the 4-day-old larvae may still be infective (Chigasaki *et al.*, 2000). The oncomiracidium has two types of movements: (i) a swimming phase with strong ciliary beatings; and (ii) a stationary phase with ciliary beatings too weak to generate any directional motion (Shirakashi *et al.*, 2010). It lacks eye spots and hence does not have phototactic reactions. These behavioural characteristics may contribute to its long life at the larval stage.

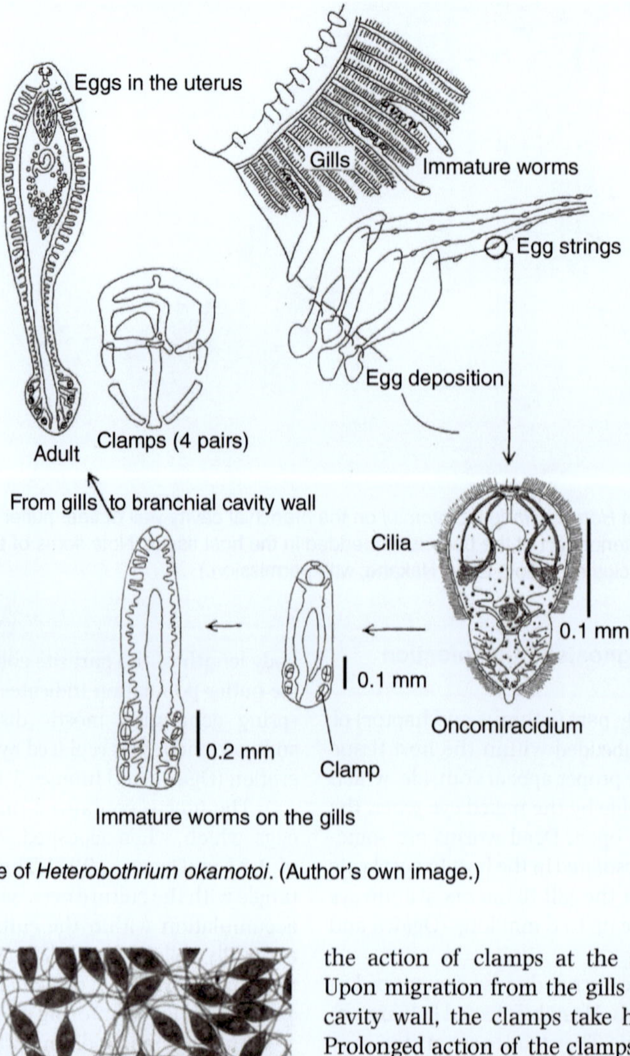

Fig. 14.3. Life cycle of *Heterobothrium okamotoi*. (Author's own image.)

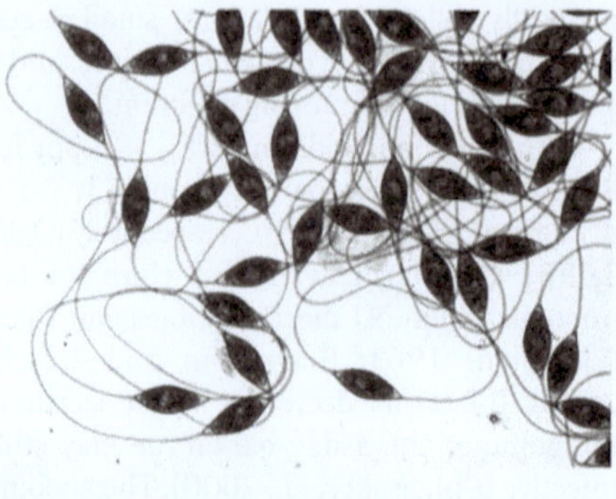

Fig. 14.4. Egg string of *Heterobothrium okamotoi*. (From Ogawa, 2002; with permission from Elsevier.)

14.1.3. External/internal lesions

Infection of immature worms on the gill lamellae induces no apparent responses in the host, whereas adults induce marked inflammation by the action of clamps at the attachment site. Upon migration from the gills to the branchial cavity wall, the clamps take hold of the wall. Prolonged action of the clamps induces disruption of the skin and the haptor reaches the underlining muscle tissue (Fig. 14.5a). The action of clamps also induces host inflammatory responses. Host tissue surrounds the posterior part of the parasite, but as the host encapsulation is incomplete, the surrounding tissue becomes necrotic (Fig. 14.5b) due to invasion of sea water through the eroded tissue (Ogawa and Inouye, 1997a).

14.1.4. Pathophysiology

H. okamotoi is a blood feeder, and heavily infected tiger puffers are anaemic. In an infection experiment, where puffers (205–345 g in body weight) were exposed to an oncomiracidial suspension,

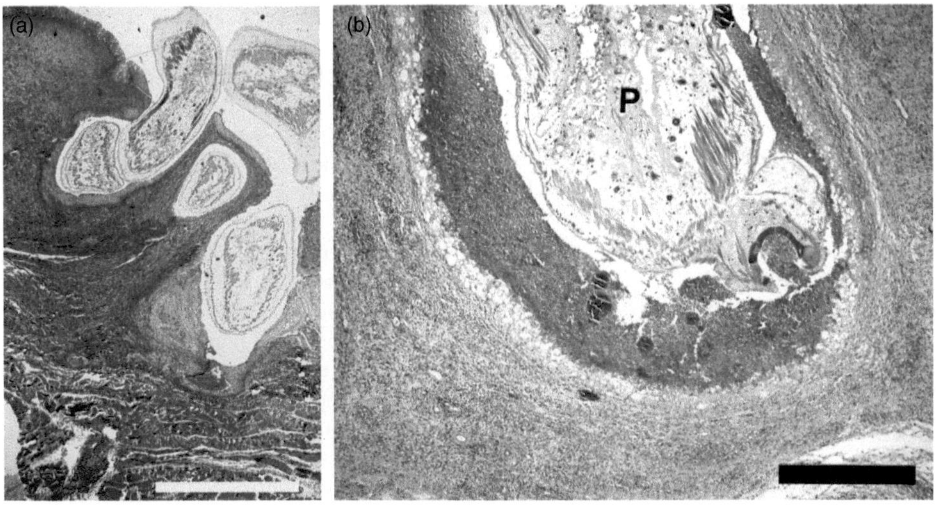

Fig. 14.5. Histological section of an adult *Heterobothrium okamotoi* worm on the branchial cavity wall of tiger puffer (*Takifugu rubripes*). (a) Haptor reaching the underlining muscle tissue of the host. Bar = 2 mm. (b) Host inflammatory responses to the parasite. Note that the host tissue around the parasite (P) is necrotic due to invasion of sea water through the eroded tissue. Bar = 0.5 mm. (From Ogawa, 2002; with permission from Elsevier.)

blood parameters deteriorated as the parasite grew. On 81 days post-exposure (pe) with between two and 38 adults on the branchial cavity, the haemoglobin content was reduced from 6.5 g/100 ml blood to lower than 4.0 g, and the mean haematocrit dropped from 25.1 to 12.8% (Ogawa and Inouye, 1997b).

The number of haematin cells in the gut of the oncomiracidia ranged from 14 in worms at day 7 pe to 114 at day 13 pe and up to 665 at day 19 pe, reflecting a sharp increase in the amount of blood taken by the worms as they grew (Yasuzaki *et al.*, 2004). Ogawa *et al.* (2005) injected fluorescent microspheres (1 μm in diameter) into tiger puffer to estimate the blood taken by a single parasite. In an experimental period of 12 h the volume of blood ingested by a single adult was estimated to be 1.38 μl/day.

14.1.5. Protective/control strategies

14.1.5.1 Host reaction

Nakane *et al.* (2005) showed that persistently infected fish established immunity against *H. okamotoi* infection, though the fish did not completely clear the parasite. When infected fish were cohabited with naïve fish in an aquarium for 70 days, the latter fish obtained a significantly higher parasite load than the former, which showed no change in the infection level. The persistently infected fish had much fewer worms with zero to one pair of clamps on the gills and no new infection on the branchial cavity wall, suggesting that immunity takes effect first when the oncomiracidium settles on the gills, secondly when the parasite develops to one with a pair of clamps, and thirdly when it migrates to the branchial cavity wall (Nakane *et al.*, 2005). These observations suggest that immune-prophylactic measures may have a role in future control programmes.

Naturally infected puffer produced antibody against adult *H. okamotoi* (Wang *et al.*, 1997; Nakane *et al.*, 2005). In contrast, Umeda *et al.* (2007) demonstrated antibody against oncomiracidium and its cilia, but not against immature worms or adults in fish persistently infected for 89 days. Umeda *et al.* (2007) also stated that specific antibodies against adult worms were detected from tiger puffer persistently infected for 2 years, suggesting that tiger puffer would take a considerable period to produce specific antibodies. Puffer intraperitoneally injected with oncomiracidium or its cilia showed no effect on prevention of infection. It is still inconclusive whether antibodies against adult worms play a role in preventing infection.

14.1.5.2. Control measures

In the 1980s–1990s, farmers routinely treated infected fish with diluted formalin, which was subsequently discarded into the sea. For fear of formalin residues in treated fish and pollution of the coastal environment, the use of formalin in aquaculture was banned in 2003. It was replaced with hydrogen peroxide (bath treatment in 0.6 g/l solution for 20–30 min), which is effective to remove immature worms on the gills, but not for adults on the branchial cavity wall (Ogawa and Yokoyama, 1998). In 2004, oral administration of febantel (25 mg/kg fish body weight for five consecutive days), a prodrug of fenbendazole, was approved for commercial use and is now widely used, which is effective both against immature parasites and against adults (Kimura *et al.*, 2006, 2009). Also oral administration of praziquantel (4 g/kg diet) or caprylic acid (2.5 g/kg diet) to tiger puffer was effective to control *Heterobothrium* infection (Hirazawa *et al.*, 2000), but a long-term administration was required (e.g. for 30 consecutive days). These chemicals were used only in experimental studies. Although anthelmintics may show high efficacy, the total eradication of the parasite is not expected using chemotherapy.

Mechanical control and management are also applied. Deposited eggs form long continuous filaments, which easily entangle with the culture nets and constitute a source of reinfection. Thus, at the time of chemical treatment, farmers change the culture nets to remove eggs on the nets (Ogawa and Yokoyama, 1998).

Hatching was completely suppressed when eggs were treated in 40°C sea water or air-dried for 1 h, while freshwater treatment of eggs for 24 h was not effective (Hirazawa *et al.*, 2003a). Heat or air-drying treatment can be used to kill eggs in an aquarium or tanks when they are emptied.

14.1.6. Conclusions and suggestions for future studies

H. okamotoi has been one of the most serious pathogens of cultured tiger puffer, causing severe anaemia (Ogawa and Yokoyama, 1998; Ogawa, 2002). Eradication of the parasite from the culture environments is practically impossible since the infection is maintained between 0-year and 1-year fish at the culture sites. Chemotherapy using hydrogen peroxide and fenbendazole is now widely used for the control of infection. This parasitic disease is now not as serious as it was before chemicals were approved for commercial use. Although no resistance against these anthelmintics has so far been noticed, it should carefully be monitored in puffer farms. Removal of parasite eggs entangled on the culture net is effective to reduce the chances of new infection, but no promising method of egg removal has been developed. It is recommended to use the host immune responses for more effective control, but it remains to be studied in detail. Persistently infected fish produced antibodies against the worm, but it is also not clear how and to what extent the antibodies contribute to protection against infection. Host innate immunity may also be involved, but it needs further careful studies. Tiger puffer is one of the fishes with a completely sequenced genome and the sequences are available, which has opened a way to elucidate how the puffer's defence mechanism works on *H. okamotoi* infection.

The disease problem aside, tiger puffer and *H. okamotoi* provide an ideal model for studies on monogenean infections. Tiger puffer is commercially available and quite easy to maintain in a recirculating water system in a laboratory and *H. okamotoi* is also easily available from puffer culture sites. Tens of thousands of *Heterobothrium* eggs can be collected daily from this laboratory system. Its oncomiracidium has a long lifespan and is easier to handle because it has no phototactic response. For these reasons, experiments using this host–parasite system will contribute to better understanding of monogeneans in general. For example, recent studies on the mechanisms underlining host recognition and host specificity of *H. okamotoi* have made substantial advances at the molecular level.

14.2. *Neoheterobothrium hirame*

14.2.1. Introduction

A disease of wild and, less frequently, cultured olive flounder or Japanese flounder (*P. olivaceus*) with severe anaemia was first confirmed in the

1990s (Michine, 1999; Miwa and Inouye, 1999; Ogawa, 1999; Yoshinaga *et al.*, 2000b). A large-scale epizootiological study conducted of wild flounders showed 31% (130/416) were anaemic, and 90% of the anaemic fish were infected with a monogenean and/or had vestiges of the parasite (Mushiake *et al.*, 2001). Ogawa (1999) described the monogenean as a new diclidophorid species and named it *Neoheterobothrium hirame*.

N. hirame is a slender and large (14–33 mm long) monogenean, with the body proper attenuated posteriorly in the form of isthmus and haptor bearing four pairs of pedunculate clamps (Fig. 14.6). As a member of Diclidophoridae, *N. hirame* has a similar life cycle to that of *H. okamotoi*. Adults attach to the buccal cavity wall. Very young worms attach to the gill filaments with marginal hooks and hamuli and later with clamps. As they grow, they move to the gill arches or rakers, and then to the buccal cavity wall where they mature (Anshary and Ogawa, 2001).

Based on histological observations a viral aetiology was first suspected as the cause of anaemia in olive flounders (Miwa and Inouye, 1999). However, flounders challenged with *N. hirame* and those subjected to repeated bleedings both reproduced the same anaemic condition as found in wild flounder (Yoshinaga *et al.*, 2001b; Nakayasu *et al.*, 2002). Besides, infected flounder recovered from anaemia after the parasite was removed from infected hosts (Yoshinaga *et al.*, 2001c). All these data suggests that the severe anaemia in wild and cultured olive flounders is caused by *N. hirame*.

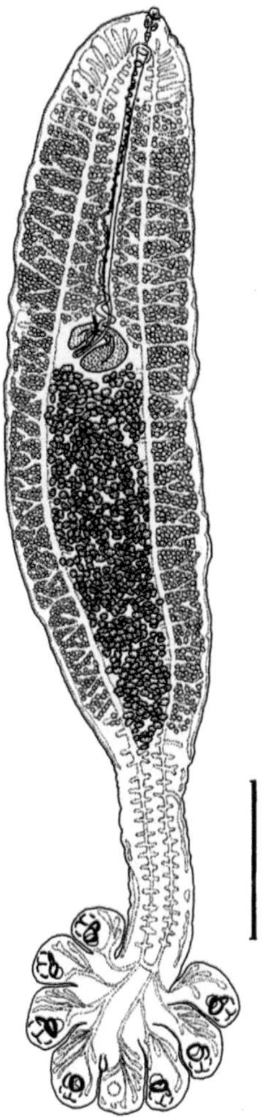

Fig. 14.6. Line drawing of *Neoheterobothrium hirame* Ogawa, 1999. Bar = 3 mm. (From Ogawa, 1999; with permission from The Japanese Society of Fish Pathology.)

N. hirame collected from flounders in different localities from Hokkaido to Kyushu confirmed its existence in the northern Sea of Japan (Anshary *et al.*, 2001) and expanded its distribution to coastal areas of the western Sea of Japan and to the Pacific (Fig. 14.7). Sudden appearance and rapid expansion in the geographical distribution suggest that this monogenean is an introduced parasite.

Hayward (2005), on the other hand, speculated that *N. hirame* naturally spread from the USA through the Bering Sea to Japan; he assumed that *N. hirame* is a synonym of *Neoheterobothrium affine*, a parasite of summer flounders (*Paralichthys dentatus*) in the USA. Yoshinaga *et al.* (2009) morphologically and molecularly compared *N. hirame* from olive flounders with diclidophorids collected from summer flounders and southern flounders (*Paralichthys lethostigma*) from the USA, demonstrating that *N. hirame* is originally a parasite of southern flounders and different from *N. affine* of summer flounders. Also experimental infection demonstrates that southern flounders can serve as the host of *N. hirame* (Yoshinaga *et al.*, 2001a). These findings strongly suggest that *N. hirame* was introduced into Japanese waters with infected southern flounders. Infection was also confirmed on wild olive flounders caught in Korean waters (Hayward *et al.*, 2001).

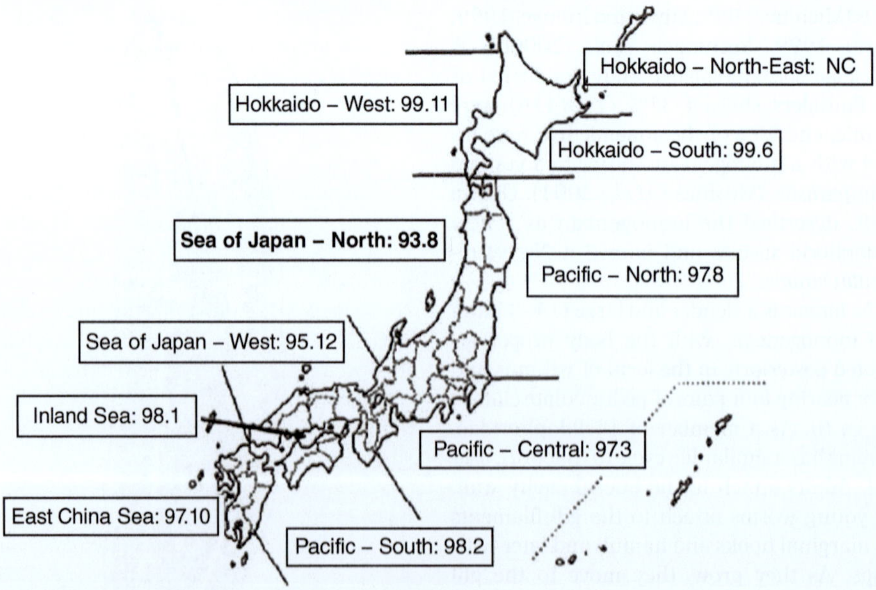

Fig. 14.7. Geographical distribution of *Neoheterobothrium hirame*, with the first record of its occurrence (indicated by the year in 1900s and month) on olive flounder (*Paralichthys olivaceus*) within the ten separated Japanese waters. Earliest specimens were collected from olive flounder caught in the northern Sea of Japan in August 1993, which is surrounded by the box in bold. NC, not collected. (Author's own image.)

Since the mid-1990s, the commercial catch of olive flounders has declined considerably in south-western Japan. In this region, 0-year flounder newly recruited in the spring became infected with *N. hirame* in the summer. Fish density was extremely reduced from late summer to autumn, which was probably caused by the death of heavily infected fish (Anshary *et al.*, 2002). The commercial catch declined by more than 80% which has remained low (Shirakashi *et al.*, 2008). In contrast, no apparent decrease in the commercial catch has been noticed in northern regions of Japan, in spite of high prevalence of infection (Shirakashi *et al.*, 2006; Tomiyama *et al.*, 2009). In the northern Pacific region, where water temperature was below 10°C in the winter, the intensity of infection was about one-third of that in the temperate Sea of Japan area, where the infection level was likely to have no apparent effect on the size of the local host population (Shirakashi *et al.*, 2006).

14.2.2. Diagnosis of the infection

Adult worms can be seen with the naked eye except the posterior part of body (isthmus and haptor) which is embedded within the host tissue. Sometimes worms are clustered at the attachment site. In wild flounders, not only live worms but also vestiges of the posterior part of the parasite are often noticed in hyperplastic tissues of the buccal cavity wall (Mushiake *et al.*, 2001). Worms on the gills are 1.3 ± 0.8 mm long with zero to four pairs of clamps while those on the gill arches or rakers are 5.8 ± 1.9 mm long with four pairs of clamps (Anshary and Ogawa, 2001). Unlike *H. okamotoi*, eggs of *N. hirame* are not connected, and the uterus is narrow and contains only a few eggs (Ogawa, 1999). *N. hirame* has high fecundity, producing 781 eggs daily at 20°C (Tsutsumi *et al.*, 2002). The oncomiracidium are 250–320 μm long (Ogawa, 2000), but their biological characteristics remain to be studied.

Incidence of wild anaemic flounders tends to be low in June–October and high in December–February, and it decreases as fish age: 0-year fish (52.9%), 1-year fish (39.1%) and 2-year fish (28.3%) (Mushiake *et al.*, 2001).

Shirakashi *et al.* (2005) experimentally demonstrated that at 8°C, oncomiracidial attachment and its subsequent development on flounders were negatively affected. A considerable number of worms disappeared from the host before reaching maturation. This suggests that the low temperature is not optimal for the propagation of this parasite.

Infected flounders altered their behaviour in that there is: (i) increased activity level (Fig. 14.8a); (ii) altered diel activity; (iii) poor burrowing performance (Fig. 14.8b); and (iv) lowered swimming endurance (Shirakashi *et al.*, 2008). There is experimental evidence that such infected fish are more susceptible to predation by larger fish. Infected fish also have lowered feeding efficiency, which makes them more vulnerable to predation during feeding (Shirakashi *et al.*, 2009).

14.2.3. External/internal lesions

Infected wild flounder are emaciated, have pale gills (white to pink in colour) and the unpigmented side of the body appears pale blue (Miwa and Inouye, 1999; Mushiake *et al.*, 2001). The heart is enlarged and so is the pale liver (Mushiake *et al.*, 2001).

14.2.4. Pathophysiology

Wild olive flounders had a negative correlation between the number of adult parasites and haemoglobin levels (Mushiake *et al.*, 2001). Haematocrit values of wild anaemic flounders ranged from 1.0 to 12.6% (Miwa and Inouye, 1999). The anaemia is characterized by the appearance of many immature erythrocytes and abnormal staining in the cytoplasm of erythrocytes (Yoshinaga *et al.*, 2000b). As the haemoglobin content lowers, more immature erythrocytes tend to appear in the peripheral blood (Mushiake *et al.*, 2001). In fish with no anaemia (haemoglobin content more than 4 g/100 ml blood), erythrocytes constitute an average of 97.2% mature and 1.7% immature ones, whereas fish with severe anaemia have a haemoglobin content of less than 1 g/100 ml blood and an average of 1.2% mature and 87.9% immature erythrocytes.

14.2.5. Protective/control strategies

14.2.5.1. Host reaction

The host reaction induced by *N. hirame* is similar to that in *H. okamotoi*. The inflammatory response is minimal at the attachment sites on the gill filaments and in the epithelium of the gill arches and rakers, whereas a strong host response including inflammation and hyperplasia and necrosis are associated with the prolonged attachment of adult parasites to the buccal cavity wall (Anshary and Ogawa, 2001). Leucocytes constituting monocytes/macrophages, granulocytes and dense granular cells infiltrate and adhere to adult parasites, with the monocytes/macrophages most often observed. Vacuolation of the parasite tegument (Fig. 14.9) adjacent to the adherent site of the leucocytes is common (Nakayasu *et al.*, 2003). The tegument disrupts partially and is phagocytosed by the infiltrated host cells, which leads to the death and elimination of the parasite (Nakayasu *et al.*, 2005). This host reaction was not observed in infected fish under starvation.

cDNA microarray gene expression patterns of peripheral blood leucocytes were analysed to search for specific molecular biomarkers in response to *N. hirame* (Matsuyama *et al.*, 2007). Some candidate genes were selected, but further analysis is needed to target specific subsets of leucocytes.

In experimentally infected flounders, antibody was detected after the parasite had moved to the buccal cavity wall. Antibody production was enhanced after the death of the parasite induced a host reaction (Tsutsumi *et al.*, 2003).

No investigation has been made as to whether the host inflammatory response and antibody production against *N. hirame* induce immunity to reinfection.

14.2.5.2. Control measures

No chemical has been approved for commercial use to treat *N. hirame*-infected olive flounders. No data is available on the efficacy against *N. hirame* of hydrogen peroxide, febantel or praziquantel, chemicals that are effective to treat *H. okamotoi*-infected tiger puffers. Water temperature, salinity or chlorine treatment of eggs in culture facilities is impractical to prevent infection from *N. hirame* (Yoshinaga *et al.*, 2000a). In culture facilities using running water, eggs released into the water can be flushed out before they hatch (Y. Fukuda, Oita, 2003, personal communication). A treatment of 6% salt water (1 litre sea water supplemented with 30 g NaCl) for 60 min is effective against immature worms on the gills (Yoshinaga *et al.*, 2000c), and 8% salt water (1 litre sea water supplemented with 50 g NaCl) for 5 min is effective against adult worms on the buccal cavity wall (Isshiki *et al.*, 2003).

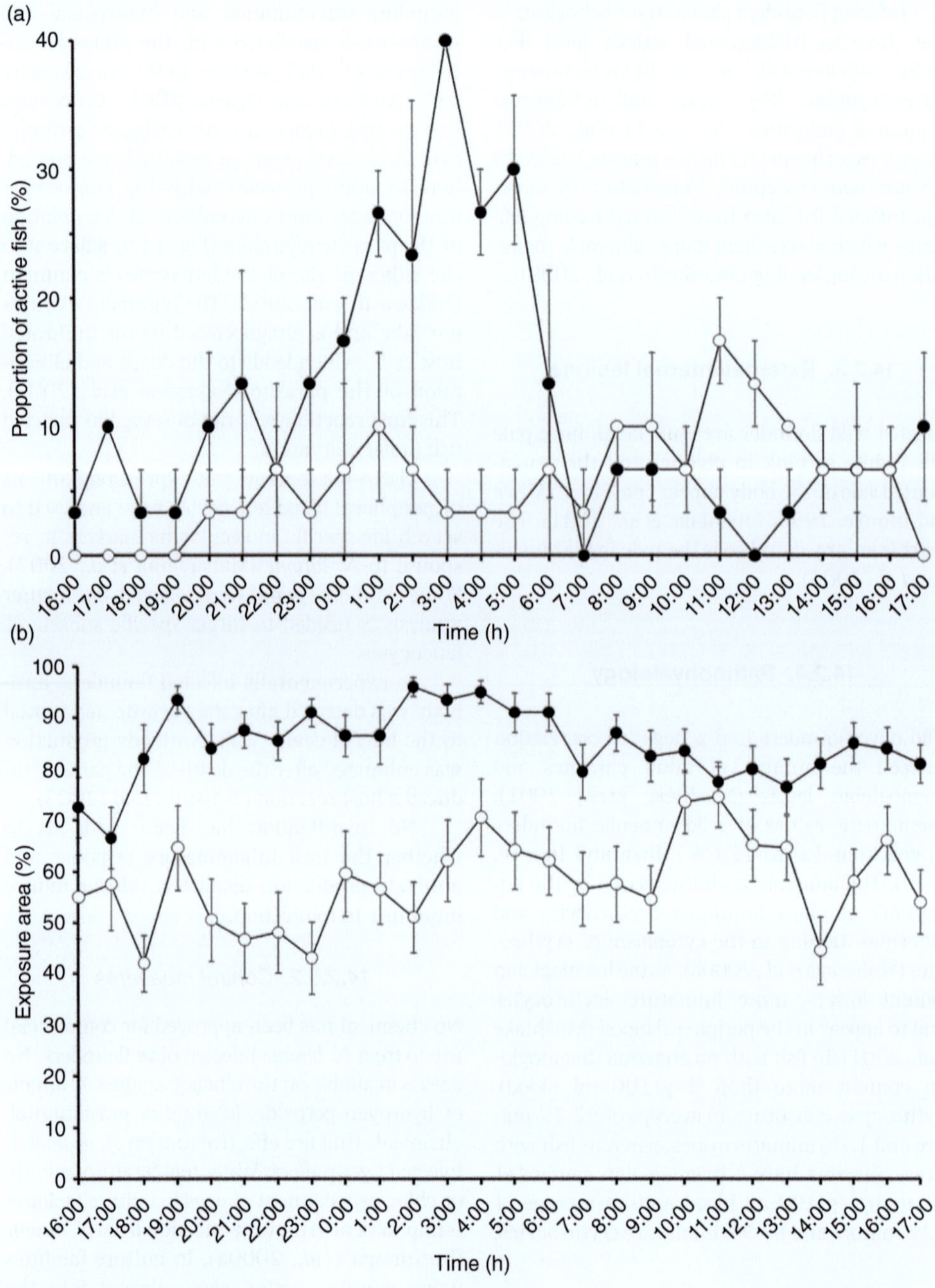

Fig. 14.8. Behavioural changes of olive flounder (*Paralichthys olivaceus*) infected with *Neoheterobothrium hirame*. (a) Temporal change in the proportion of active fish (mean ± SE) during 25 h of monitoring; (b) temporal change in the exposed body area (mean ± SE) during 25 h of monitoring. Light hours were 06:00–18:00. Open circles, uninfected controls; closed circles, infected fish. (From Shirakashi *et al*., 2008; used with permission from Elsevier under the STM Agreement.)

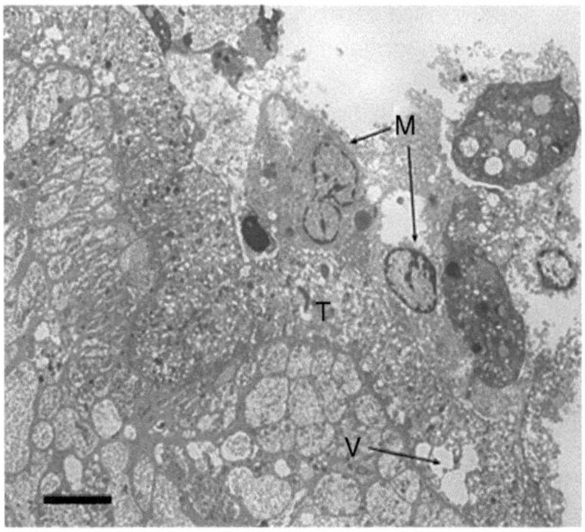

Fig. 14.9. Transmission electron micrograph of olive flounder (*Paralichthys olivaceus*) infected with *Neoheterobothrium hirame*, showing that host leucocytes adhere to the parasite tegument, inducing vacuolation. M, macrophage; T, parasite tegument; V, vacuolation of the tegument. Bar = 4 μm. (Modified from Nakayasu *et al*., 2003; used with permission from The Japanese Society of Fish Pathology.)

The latter treatment can also be used to eliminate parasites from spawner flounders in hatcheries.

14.2.6. Conclusions and suggestions for future studies

N. hirame infection can induce severe anaemia in wild olive flounders and decrease its population considerably in Japan. Severity of infection is dependent on water temperature; in northern Japan, infection is common, but it appears to have no serious effects on flounder populations, whereas in south-western Japan, the intensity of infection is several times higher which results in considerable decline in the flounder catch.

It is still not known how long the high infection levels will continue in the wild flounder populations. *N. hirame* may provide a good example to show how an introduced pathogen can cause serious damage to wild stocks, and such a study requires long-term observations which have been initiated.

References

Anshary, H. and Ogawa, K. (2001) Microhabitats and mode of attachment of *Neoheterobothrium hirame*, a monogenean parasite of Japanese flounder. *Fish Pathology* 36, 21–26.

Anshary, H., Ogawa, K., Higuchi, M. and Fujii, T. (2001) A study of long-term change in summer infection levels of Japanese flounder *Paralichthys olivaceus* with the monogenean *Neoheterobothrium hirame* in the central Sea of Japan, with an application of a new technique for collecting small parasites from the gill filaments. *Fish Pathology* 36, 27–32.

Anshary, H., Yamamoto, E., Miyanaga, T. and Ogawa, K. (2002) Infection dynamics of the monogenean *Neoheterobothrium hirame* infecting Japanese flounder in the western Sea of Japan. *Fish Pathology* 37, 131–140.

Buchmann, K. and Bresciani, J. (2006) Monogenea (phylum Platyhelminthes). In: Woo, P.T.K. (ed.) *Fish Diseases and Disorders, Volume 1: Protozoan and Metazoan Infections*, 2nd edn. CAB International, Wallingford, UK, pp. 297–344.

Chigasaki, M., Ogawa, K. and Wakabayashi, H. (2000) Standardized method for experimental infection of tiger puffer, *Takifugu rubripes* with oncomiracidia of *Heterobothrium okamotoi* (Monogenea: Diclidophoridae) with some data on the oncomiracidial biology. *Fish Pathology* 35, 215–221.

Hayward, C. (2005) Monogenea Polyopisthocotylea (ectoparasitic flukes). In: Rohde, K. (ed.) *Marine Parasitology*. CSIRO Publishing, Melbourne, Australia, pp. 55–63.

Hayward, C.J., Kim, J.H. and Heo, G.J. (2001) Spread of *Neoheterobothrium hirame* (Monogenea), a serious pest of olive flounder *Paralichthys olivaceus*, to Korea. *Diseases of Aquatic Organisms* 45, 209–213.

Hirazawa, N., Ohtaka, T. and Hata, K. (2000) Challenge trials on the anthelmintic effect of drugs and natural agents against the monogenean *Heterobothrium okamotoi* in the tiger puffer *Takifugu rubripes*. *Aquaculture* 188, 1–13.

Hirazawa, N., Goto, T. and Shirasu, K. (2003a) Killing effect of various treatments on the monogenean *Heterobothrium okamotoi* eggs and oncomiracidia and the ciliate *Cryptocaryon irritans* cysts and theronts. *Aquaculture* 223, 1–13.

Hirazawa, N., Oshima, S., Mitsuboshi, T and Yamashita, S. (2003b) Mucus pH of the tiger puffer *Takifugu rubripes* is an important factor for host identification by the monogenean *Heterobothrium okamotoi*. *Parasitology* 127, 225–230.

Hosoya, S., Kido, S., Hirabayashi, Y., Kai, W., Kinami, R. *et al.* (2013) Genomic regions of pufferfishes responsible for host specificity of a monogenean parasite *Heterobothrium okamotoi*. *International Journal for Parasitology* 43, 909–915.

Igarashi, K., Matsunaga, R., Hirakawa, S., Hosoya, S., Suetake, H. *et al.* (2017) Mucosal IgM antibody with D-mannose affinity in fugu *Takifugu rubripes* is utilized by a monogenean parasite *Heterobothrium okamotoi* for host recognition. *Journal of Immunology* 198, 4107–4114.

Isshiki, T., Tochino, M. and Nagano, T. (2003) Treatments of *Neoheterobothrium* infection in Japanese flounder by 8% NaCl-supplemented seawater bathing. *Suisanzoshoku* 51, 363–364.

Kimura, T., Sameshima, M., Nomura, Y., Morita, J., Mizoguchi, H. and Ishihara, M. (2006) Efficacy of orally administered febantel against monogenean *Heterobothrium okamotoi* infection of cultured tiger puffer *Takifugu rubripes*. *Fish Pathology* 41, 147–151.

Kimura, T., Nomura, Y., Kawakami, H., Itano, T., Iwasaki, M. *et al.* (2009) Field trials of febantel against gill fluke disease caused by the monogenean *Heterobothrium okamotoi* in cultured tiger puffer *Takifugu rubripes*. *Fish Pathology* 44, 67–71.

Llewellyn, J. (1963) Larvae and larval development of monogeneans. *Advances in Parasitology* 1, 287–326.

Matsui, S., Goto, T., Tsubouchi, Y., Hirakawa, S., Suetake, H. *et al.* (2020) D-Mannose-specific immunoglobulin M in grass puffer (*Takifugu niphobles*), a nonhost fish of a monogenean ectoparasite *Heterobothrium okamotoi*, can act as a trigger for its parasitism. *Journal of Parasitology* 106, 276–282.

Matsuyama, T., Fujiwara, A., Nakayasu, C., Kamaishi, T., Oseko, N. *et al.* (2007) Microarray analyses of gene expression in Japanese flounder *Paralichthys olivaceus* leucocytes during monogenean parasite *Neoheterobothrium hirame* infection. *Diseases of Aquatic Organisms* 75, 79–83.

Michine, A. (1999) *Neoheterobothrium* sp. found on Japanese flounder cultured commercially or maintained as spawners. *Researches of the Shimane Prefectural Center of Cultural Fisheries* 2, 15–23.

Miwa, S. and Inouye, K. (1999) Histopathological study of the flounder with anemia found in various places in Japanese coastal waters. *Fish Pathology* 34, 113–119.

Mushiake, K., Mori, K. and Arimoto, M. (2001) Epizootiology of anemia in wild Japanese flounder. *Fish Pathology* 36, 125–132.

Nakane, M., Ogawa, K., Fujita, T., Sameshima, M. and. Wakabayashi, H. (2005) Acquired protection of tiger puffer *Takifugu rubripes* against infection with *Heterobothrium okamotoi* (Monogenea: Diclidophoridae). *Fish Pathology* 40, 95–101.

Nakayasu, C., Yoshinaga, T. and Kumagai, A. (2002) Hematology of anemia experimentally induced by repeated bleedings in Japanese flounder with comments on the cause of flounder anemia recently prevailing in Japan. *Fish Pathology* 37, 125–130.

Nakayasu, C., Tsutsumi, N., Yoshitomi, T., Yoshinaga, T. and Kumagai, A. (2003) Identification of Japanese flounder leucocytes involved in the host response to *Neoheterobothrium hirame*. *Fish Pathology* 38, 9–14.

Nakayasu, C., Tsutsumi, N., Oseko, N. and Hasegawa, S. (2005) Role of cellular response in elimination of the monogenean *Neoheterobothrium hirame* in Japanese flounder *Paralichthys olivaceus*. *Diseases of Aquatic Organisms* 64, 127–134.

Ogawa, K. (1991) Redescription of *Heterobothrium tetrodonis* (Monogenea: Diclidophoridae) and other related new species from puffers of the genus *Takifugu* (Teleostei: Tetraodontidae). *Japanese Journal of Parasitology* 40, 388–396.

Ogawa, K. (1997) Copulation and egg production of the monogenean *Heterobothrium okamotoi*, a gill parasite of cultured tiger puffer (*Takifugu rubripes*). *Fish Pathology* 32, 219–223.

Ogawa, K. (1998) Egg hatching of the monogenean *Heterobothrium okamotoi*, a gill parasite of cultured tiger puffer (*Takifugu rubripes*), with a description of its oncomiracidium. *Fish Pathology* 33, 25–30.

Ogawa, K. (1999) *Neoheterobothrium hirame* sp. nov. (Monogenea: Diclidophoridae) from the buccal cavity wall of Japanese flounder *Paralichthys olivaceus*. *Fish Pathology* 34, 195–201.

Ogawa, K. (2000) The oncomiracidium of *Neoheterobothrium hirame*, a monogenean parasite of Japanese flounder *Paralichthys olivaceus*. *Fish Pathology* 35, 229–230.

Ogawa, K. (2002) Impacts of diclidophorid monogenean infections on fisheries in Japan. *International Journal for Parasitology* 32, 373–380.

Ogawa, K. and Inouye, K. (1997a) *Heterobothrium* infection of cultured tiger puffer, *Takifugu rubripes* (Teleostei: Tetraodontidae) – a field study. *Fish Pathology* 32, 15–20.

Ogawa, K. and Inouye, K. (1997b) *Heterobothrium* infection of cultured tiger puffer, *Takifugu rubripes* – experimental infection. *Fish Pathology* 32, 21–27.

Ogawa, K. and Itoh, N. (2022) Five new and two known species of *Heterobothrium* (Monogenea: Diclidophoridae) infecting puffers of the genus *Takifugu* from Japanese waters. *Systematic Parasitology* 99, 317–340.

Ogawa, K. and Yokoyama, H. (1998) Parasitic diseases of cultured marine fish in Japan. *Fish Pathology* 33, 303–309.

Ogawa, K., Yasuzaki, M. and Yoshinaga, T. (2005) Experiments on the evaluation of the blood feeding of *Heterobothrium okamotoi* (Monogenea: Diclidophoridae). *Fish Pathology* 40, 169–174.

Ohhashi, Y., Yoshinaga, T. and Ogawa, K. (2007) Involvement of host recognition and survivability in the host specificity of the monogenean parasite *Heterobothrium okamotoi*. *International Journal for Parasitology* 37, 53–60.

Okamoto, R. (1963) On the problems of a monogenetic trematode infection of tiger puffers from the Inland Sea of Japan. *Suisanzoshoku (Special Issue)* 3, 17–29.

Okamoto, R. and Ogasawara, Y. (1965) Parasite occurrences of tiger puffer in natural waters. *Annual Report of Naikai Regional Fisheries Laboratory, Series A* 2, 42–43.

Sato, Y., Matsunaga, R., Tasumi, S., Mizuno, N., Nakane, M. *et al.* (2003) L-Fucoside localization in the gills of the genus *Takifugu* and its possible implication in the parasitism of *Heterobothrium okamotoi* (Monogenea: Diclidophoridae). *Biochimica et Biophysica Acta – General Subjects* 1867, 130467.

Shirakashi, S., Yoshinaga, T., Oka, M. and Ogawa, K. (2005) Larval attachment and development of the monogenean *Neoheterobothrium hirame* under low temperature. *Fish Pathology* 40, 33–35.

Shirakashi, S., Yamada, T., Yamada, T. and Ogawa, K. (2006) Infection dynamics of *Neoheterobothrium hirame* (Monogenea) on juvenile olive flounder in coastal Japan. *Journal of Fish Diseases* 29, 319–329.

Shirakashi, S., Teruya, K. and Ogawa, K. (2008) Altered behaviour and reduced survival of juvenile olive flounder infected by an invasive monogenean parasite *Neoheterobothrium hirame*. *International Journal for Parasitology* 38, 1513–1522.

Shirakashi, S., Nishioka, N. and Ogawa, K. (2009) *Neoheterobothrium hirame* (Monogenea) alters the feeding behaviour of juvenile olive flounder, *Paralichthys olivaceus*. *Fisheries Science* 75, 121–128.

Shirakashi, S., Nakatsuka, S., Udagawa, A. and Ogawa, K. (2010) Oncomiracidial behavior of *Heterobothrium okamotoi* (Monogenea: Diclidophoridae). *Fish Pathology* 45, 51–57.

Tomiyama, T., Watanabe, M. and Kurita, Y. (2009) Rapid fluctuation in infection levels of *Neoheterobothrium hirame* (Monogenea) in Japanese flounder *Paralichthys olivaceus* in the Joban area, Japan. *Journal of Fish Biology* 75, 172–185.

Tsutsui, S., Tasumi, S., Suetake, H. and Suzuki, Y. (2003) Lectins homologous to those of monocotyledonous plants in the skin mucus and intestine of pufferfish, *Fugu rubripes*. *Journal of Biological Chemistry* 278, 20882–20889.

Tsutsui, S., Tasumi, S., Suetake, H., Kikuchi, K. and Suzuki, Y. (2005) Demonstration of the mucosal lectins in the epithelial cells of internal and external body surface tissues in pufferfish (*Fugu rubripes*). *Developmental and Comparative Immunology* 29, 243–253.

Tsutsumi, N., Mushiake, K., Mori, K., Yoshinaga, T. and Ogawa, K. (2002) Effects of temperature on the egg-laying of the monogenean *Neoheterobothrium hirame*. *Fish Pathology* 37, 41–43.

Tsutsumi, N., Yoshinaga, T., Kamaishi, T., Nakayasu, C. and Ogawa, K. (2003) Effects of temperature on the development and longevity of the monogenean *Neoheterobothrium hirame* on Japanese flounder *Paralichthys olivaceus*. *Fish Pathology* 38, 41–47.

Umeda, N., Hatanaka, A. and Hirazawa, N. (2007) Immobilization antibodies of tiger puffer *Takifugu rubripes* induced by i.p. injection against monogenean *Heterobothrium okamotoi* oncomiracidia do not prevent the infection. *Parasitology* 134, 853–863.

Wang, G., Kim, J.-H., Sameshima, M. and Ogawa, K. (1997) Detection of antibodies against the monogenean *Heterobothrium okamotoi* in tiger puffer by ELISA. *Fish Pathology* 32, 179–180.

Yamabata, N., Yoshinaga, T. and Ogawa, K. (2004) Effects of water temperature on egg production and egg viability of the monogenean *Heterobothrium okamotoi* infecting tiger puffer *Takifugu rubripes*. *Fish Pathology* 39, 215–217.

Yasuzaki, M., Ogawa, K. and Yoshinaga, T. (2004) Early development of the monogenean *Heterobothrium okamotoi* on the gills of tiger puffer *Takifugu rubripes*. *Fish Pathology* 39, 153–158.

Yoshinaga, T., Segawa, I., Kamaishi, T. and Sorimachi, M. (2000a) Effect of temperature, salinity and chlorine treatment on egg hatching of the monogenean *Neoheterobothrium hirame* infecting Japanese flounder. *Fish Pathology* 35, 85–88.

Yoshinaga, T., Kamaishi, T., Segawa, I., Kumagai, A., Nakayasu, C. *et al.* (2000b) Hematology, histopathology and the monogenean *Neoheterobothrium hirame* infection in anemic flounder. *Fish Pathology* 35, 131–136.

Yoshinaga, T., Kamaishi, T., Segawa, I. and Yamamoto, E. (2000c) Effects of NaCl-supplemented seawater on the monogenean, *Neoheterobothrium hirame*, infecting the Japanese flounder. *Fish Pathology* 35, 97–98.

Yoshinaga, T., Tsutsumi, N., Shima, T., Kamaishi, T. and Ogawa, K. (2001a) Experimental infection of the southern flounder *Paralichthys lethostigma* with *Neoheterobothrium hirame* (Monogenea: Diclidophoridae). *Fish Pathology* 36, 237–239.

Yoshinaga, T., Kamaishi, T., Segawa, I., Yamano, K., Ikeda, H. and Sorimachi, M. (2001b) Anemia caused by challenges with the monogenean *Neoheterobothrium hirame* in the Japanese flounder. *Fish Pathology* 36, 13–20.

Yoshinaga, T., Kamaishi, T., Ikeda, H. and Sorimachi, M. (2001c) Experimental recovery from anemia in Japanese flounder challenged with the monogenean *Neoheterobothrium hirame*. *Fish Pathology* 36, 179–182.

Yoshinaga, T., Tsutsumi, N., Hall, K.A. and Ogawa, K. (2009) Origin of the diclidophorid monogenean *Neoheterobothrium hirame* Ogawa, 1999, the causative agent of anemia in olive flounder, *Paralichthys olivaceus*. *Fisheries Science* 75, 1167–1176.

15 *Diplostomum spathaceum* and Related Species

Anssi Karvonen*
Department of Biological and Environmental Science, University of Jyväskylä, Finland

Abstract

Diplostomum eye flukes are among the most common parasites of freshwater fishes. Species infecting the eye lenses (e.g. *Diplostomum spathaceum* and *Diplostomum pseudospathaceum*) cause cataracts in an intensity-dependent manner, which impairs fish vision and results in negative effects like reduced feeding efficiency and growth. The infection also makes the fish more susceptible to predation from avian definitive hosts as well as predatory fish. Infections are also found in aquaculture, where they cause economic losses and necessitate preventive actions such as eradication of the snail intermediate hosts. Recent advances in molecular taxonomy within the *Diplostomum* genus indicate unprecedented species diversity, highlighting the need for further research on life-cycle biology and pathology of individual and co-infecting *Diplostomum* species and genotypes. Research should also investigate genetic variation among host species and populations in defence traits such as parasite avoidance, immunological resistance and tolerance to cataracts.

15.1. Introduction

Trematodes of the genus *Diplostomum* are ubiquitous parasites of freshwater fishes; they infect the eyes of over 100 fish species worldwide (Chappell, 1995). Some of the species are also in other parts of the fish body (Schwelm *et al.*, 2021). *Diplostomum* flukes can be prevalent and also very abundant, with tens or even hundreds of parasites in an individual fish (Chappell, 1969; Wootten, 1974; Valtonen and Gibson, 1997; Valtonen *et al.*, 1997; Francová *et al.*, 2011; Ojaveer *et al.*, 2020). Infections are also found in aquaculture (Stables and Chappell, 1986a; Field and Irwin, 1994; Buchmann and Bresciani, 1997; Karvonen *et al.*, 2006b; Unger *et al.*, 2022), causing significant problems by impairing the fish's vision. This chapter describes the loss of vision in fish (development of parasitic cataracts), explains the effects of the infection (physiology, growth, appearance, behaviour) and discusses control strategies to prevent *Diplostomum* in aquaculture.

Most of the earlier research has focused on *Diplostomum spathaceum sensu lato* (*s.l.*), and more recently on *Diplostomum pseudospathaceum*, as the infection by these species in the eye lenses causes notable deleterious effects in fish of significant economic importance. The taxonomy of *Diplostomum* parasites, however, is very complex and current evidence suggests that the earlier morphology-based species description in this

*Email: anssi.t.karvonen@jyu.fi

DOI: 10.1079/9781800628748.0015

genus was incomplete. Numerous molecular studies have identified new cryptic species of *Diplostomum* in wild fishes (Locke *et al.*, 2010a,b; Georgieva *et al.*, 2013; Blasco-Costa *et al.*, 2014; Faltynková *et al.*, 2014; Kudlai *et al.*, 2017; Hoogendoorn *et al.*, 2020), which has also facilitated research on the spatiotemporal distribution and community organization in *Diplostomum* parasites (Rellstab *et al.*, 2011; Désilets *et al.*, 2013; Locke *et al.*, 2015; Diaz-Suarez *et al.*, 2024). It is clear that the genus *Diplostomum* represents species complexes both in the eye lens and vitreous humour (Georgieva *et al.*, 2013; Blasco-Costa *et al.*, 2014), and that infections of multiple species of *Diplostomum* in fish species and fish individuals are common (Rellstab *et al.*, 2011). However, very little is known about differences between these species regarding their life cycle, transmission and pathology in fish and other hosts. Previously, the species name *D. spathaceum* has been commonly used to collectively describe species found in the lens. For simplicity, the same approach is taken in the present discussion, except when referring to studies in which the species has been reliably identified as other than *D. spathaceum*. Thus, species identity and nomenclature, particularly in earlier literature and in studies based on naturally infected fish, should be interpreted with caution.

15.1.1. Parasite life cycle

The life cycle of *D. spathaceum* is typical for trematodes and includes three host species (Fig. 15.1). Sexual reproduction takes place in the definitive host, which is a fish-eating bird, such as a gull. Adult hermaphroditic worms mate in the intestine and start producing eggs 3–4 days after establishment. An individual bird is typically infected with several hundreds of worms, each of which can release several hundreds of eggs per day (Karvonen *et al.*, 2006a). Eggs are released into the aquatic environment with host faeces, where they hatch to miracidia larvae in 2 weeks in summer temperatures. Miracidia are short lived and actively seek out the first intermediate host, a freshwater snail. Several snail species can act as hosts for *Diplostomum* parasites, but those of the genus *Lymnaea* are the most common. A snail can be infected with one or multiple miracidia and such co-infections tend to be over-represented in a snail population, i.e. parasite genotypes aggregate in certain snail individuals (Louhi *et al.*, 2013).

Within the snail, the parasite reproduces asexually by forming sporocysts, which occupy the reproductive system of the snail leading to castration. Clonal cercariae are formed within the sporocysts and are released into the water in very high numbers (Fig. 15.2). For example, one individual of *Lymnaea stagnalis* can release tens of thousands of cercariae per day for several weeks (Lyholt and Buchmann, 1996; Karvonen *et al.*, 2004b). Cercarial release mainly takes place during the summer months when the water temperature exceeds 10°C (Stables and Chappell, 1986a; Karvonen *et al.*, 2004c). When the snail is infected with more than one miracidium, the cercarial output represents different parasite genotypes, typically in different proportions (Karvonen *et al.*, 2012; Seppälä *et al.*, 2015). These proportions are influenced by the occupancy of sporocysts of different genotypes in snail tissues, which in turn may depend on the order and timing of multiple miracidial infections.

Cercariae are equipped with a bifurcated tail, which is used for short, repeated swimming bursts that maintain the cercariae in the water column. Cercariae rely on finite energy resources, which limits their lifespan to a maximum of 36 h at 20°C, with their ability to infect a fish diminishing already several hours earlier (Karvonen *et al.*, 2003). Upon contact with a fish, cercariae penetrate the epithelium of the gills or skin, drop their tail and enter the host body. Host contact and penetration involve detection of an array of chemical cues by the parasite (Haas *et al.*, 2002). It is not completely understood which routes the cercariae (at this stage called diplostomulae) use in their migration towards the eye, but it is likely to include several tissue types of the host (Ratanarat-Brockelman, 1974). Penetration from the head region and gills of the fish has the highest success (Ratanarat-Brockelman, 1974; Höglund, 1991; Whyte *et al.*, 1991). The key role of the head region in the infection process is also supported by the positive relationship between fish ventilation rate and parasite acquisition (Mikheev *et al.*, 2014).

The tissue migration from host penetration to establishment in the lens is typically completed

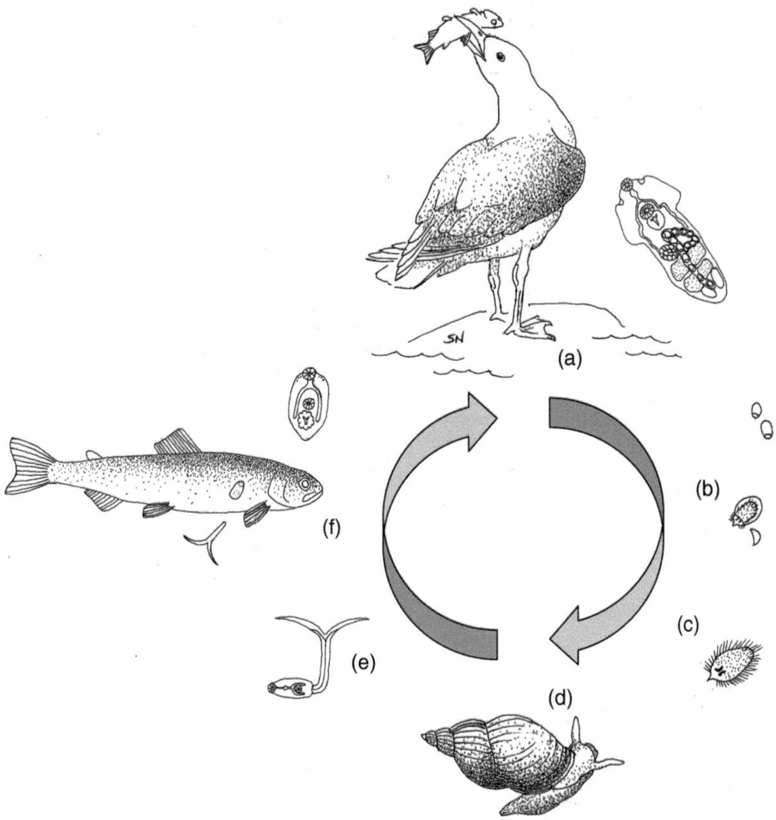

Fig. 15.1. Life cycle of *Diplostomum pseudospathaceum*. Adult worms reproduce in an avian definitive host (a) and produce eggs (b). Eggs hatch in water to miracidia (c), which infect the first intermediate host, an aquatic snail (d). Asexual reproduction in the snail gives rise to thousands of cercariae (e) that penetrate the epithelium of fish (f), the second intermediate host, and settle in the eye lenses as metacercariae (f). The life cycle is completed when an infected fish is eaten by a bird. (Drawing courtesy of Sven Nikander.)

within 24 h (Whyte *et al.*, 1991) but can take longer at low temperatures (Lyholt and Buchmann, 1996). The migration speed and success are also influenced by fish size. In small (and young) fish, most parasites can reach the lens well before the conventional 24 h, even in 10 h or less (Louhi *et al.*, 2015). In larger fish, fewer parasites successfully complete the migration to the eye lenses (Karvonen *et al.*, 2016). This may simply be because larger hosts represent a longer migration distance and time for the parasites, exhausting their limited energy reserves. Another possible reason is that larger (and older) hosts typically have a more developed and/or experienced immune system to fight against the invading parasites. Diplostomulae that fail to reach the eye are cleared by the host immune system.

After reaching the eye lens, diplostomulae develop to metacercariae (Fig. 15.3). They grow considerably in size, first becoming elongated before taking their typical oval or cylindrical shape (Sweeting, 1974). This process is also controlled by the water temperature; development of the metacercariae is completed within a few weeks at 15–20°C but may be halted completely at low temperatures. For example, parasites establishing in fish in late autumn may overwinter as undeveloped metacercariae and continue their development in the following spring (A. Karvonen,

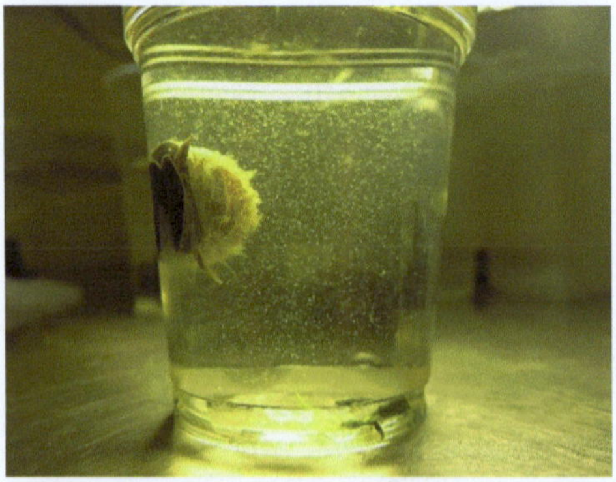

Fig. 15.2. A dense swarm of *Diplostomum pseudospathaceum* cercariae released from an infected *Lymnaea stagnalis* snail, the first intermediate host of the parasite. The cercarial output can include one or several parasite genotypes, depending on the number of miracidial infections in the snail. (Photograph by Anssi Karvonen. Reproduced with permission from Karvonen and Marcogliese, 2020.)

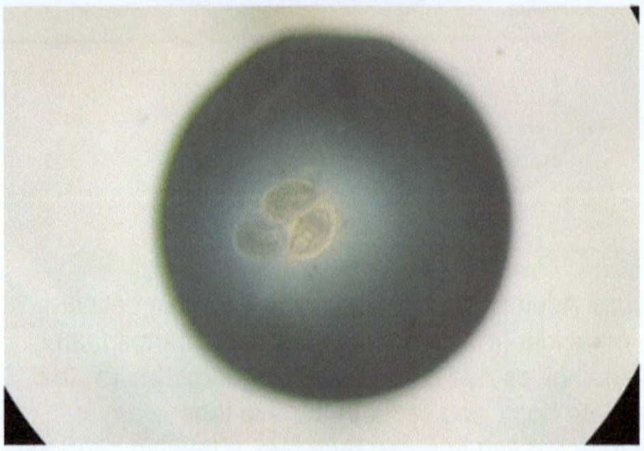

Fig. 15.3. Three metacercariae of *Diplostomum* sp. in an eye lens of Atlantic salmon (*Salmo salar*). (Photograph courtesy of Ines Klemme. Reproduced with permission from Karvonen and Marcogliese, 2020.)

2015, unpublished results). Unlike metacercariae of many other trematode species, metacercariae of *D. spathaceum* and other lens-dwelling species do not form cysts, but move freely in the eye lens, which enables them to cause damage to lens structures. It is generally believed that the metacercariae can survive in fish for years. As such, infections accumulate with time (Marcogliese *et al.*, 2001b). The life cycle of the parasite is completed when an infected fish is eaten by a bird definitive host.

15.2. Pathobiology

15.2.1. Factors influencing *Diplostomum* abundance in fish

As with many macroparasites, the negative effects of *D. spathaceum* infection increase with the intensity of infection, i.e. the number of metacercariae in the lens (see Fig. 15.5 below). Therefore, it is important to consider factors that contribute to parasite numbers and infection success. In nature, the abundance of *D. spathaceum*, as well as other *Diplostomum* species, varies considerably according to geographic location, lake characteristics such as water quality, fish characteristics such as species, age and size, as well as according to composition and abundance of the required host species (McKeown and Irwin, 1997; Valtonen *et al.*, 1997; Marcogliese *et al.*, 2001a,b; Seppälä *et al.*, 2011; Noreikiene *et al.*, 2020). Eye flukes are also aggregated in fish host populations with a small proportion of individuals carrying the highest parasite abundances (Zelmer and Arai, 1998; Karvonen *et al.*, 2004a). Depending on the overall abundance of the infection in a host population, aggregation limits the most severe effects of the infection to the most heavily infected hosts.

The infection process itself is influenced by several parasite- and host-related factors. As cercarial activity functions mainly to maintain the infective stages in the water column, movements of the fish host are decisive for the parasite encounter and infection (Karvonen *et al.*, 2003). Upon contact, parasite numbers in the lens of a fish's eye depend linearly on the dose of the cercarial exposure (Brassard *et al.*, 1982b; Stables and Chappell, 1986c; Whyte *et al.*, 1991; Karvonen *et al.*, 2003). Fish can also be exposed simultaneously to multiple cercarial genotypes of the same *Diplostomum* species, which in species like *D. pseudospathaceum* increases the parasite infection success (Karvonen *et al.*, 2012; Haase *et al.*, 2014; Klemme *et al.*, 2016). Infection success of individual parasite genotypes can also be modified by simultaneous infections of other *Diplostomum* species, either increasing or decreasing their success depending on the specific genotype combination (Seppälä *et al.*, 2009, 2012). Furthermore, infection success of *D. pseudospathaceum* can be altered by co-infection of other helminths, *Schistocephalus solidus* (Piecyk *et al.*, 2019) and *Tylodelphys clavata* (Gopko *et al.*, 2025). Interactions between *Diplostomum* genotypes, as well as those between *Diplostomum* and other parasite species, are likely to be mediated at least partly by the fish immune system, where certain components (such as gene expression of the complement system) can show specificity even to different parasite genotypes (Rauch *et al.*, 2006; Haase *et al.*, 2014, 2016a).

The fish immune system plays a central role in reducing the infection success of *Diplostomum* parasites. Cercarial invasion into an immunologically naïve fish elicits an immune response, which first involves the innate immune system and later also the specific branches of the immune system that work in concert with one another (Chappell *et al.*, 1994; Magnadottir, 2006; Haase *et al.*, 2014, 2016a,b). Specific responses develop within a few weeks from the exposure and significantly reduce the number of parasites establishing in subsequent exposures, but do not provide complete protection (Stables and Chappell, 1986b; Höglund and Thuvander, 1990; Whyte *et al.*, 1990; Karvonen *et al.*, 2005; Rellstab *et al.*, 2013; Haase *et al.*, 2016a). Thus, parasites accumulate with time also in immunologically experienced fish. Immunization, however, changes the parasite infection dynamics. For example, the higher infection success of two simultaneously infecting *D. pseudospathaceum* genotypes is eroded when the target fish has a previous infection from the same parasite species (Klemme *et al.*, 2016). Similarly, previous exposure of the host fish can modify the infection and interspecific interactions between different *Diplostomum* species (Karvonen *et al.*, 2009). Overall, direct and indirect host-mediated interactions between *Diplostomum* species and genotypes can be important not only for the parasite infection success but also for the magnitude of parasite-inflicted damage (eye cataracts).

15.2.2. Parasitic cataracts

The most notable sign of *D. spathaceum* or *D. pseudospathaceum* infection in fish is cataract formation, when the eye lens becomes opaque and grey, and the vision of the fish is impaired (Fig. 15.4). This condition is referred to as diplostomiasis. Quantification of the cataracts is best done with an ophthalmological microscope (Karvonen *et al.*, 2004d). In low-level infections, individual parasites are typically surrounded by small clouds of granules or thread-like formations (Shariff *et al.*, 1980; Karvonen *et al.*, 2004d). In more severe infections, damage caused by individual parasites overlaps resulting in opacity of the lens. Eventually, the eye lens may begin to appear whitish, which is visible just by looking at the fish (Fig. 15.4). This is the chronic stage of the infection. Parasitic cataracts have been described quantitatively both in

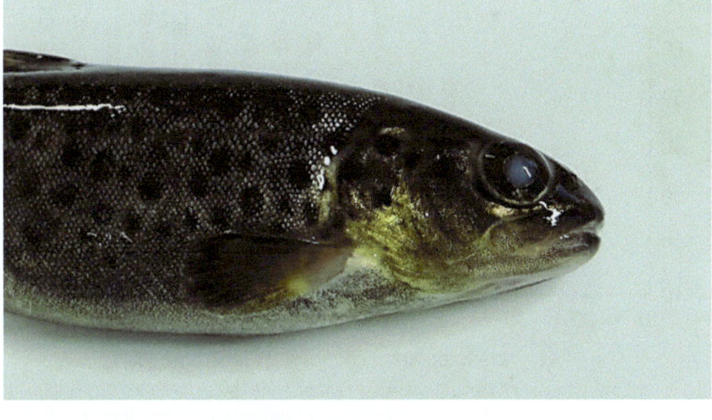

Fig. 15.4. Cataracts caused by *Diplostomum pseudospathaceum* metacercariae in an eye lens of Atlantic salmon (*Salmo salar*) parr. Cataracts intensify with increasing metacercarial abundance so that the lens begins to appear grey and opaque. (Photograph courtesy of Ines Klemme.)

farmed and wild fish species (Marcogliese *et al.*, 2001b; Seppänen *et al.*, 2008; Seppälä *et al.*, 2011; Karvonen and Lindström, 2018; Kuukka-Anttila *et al.*, 2020; Karvonen *et al.*, 2022).

The main factor influencing the severity of cataracts is the number of parasites in the lens (Fig. 15.5). The relationship, however, may be influenced by several factors. For example, cataract coverage typically varies greatly among individual fish so that the same infection intensity does not necessarily cause similar cataracts in all individuals (Fig. 15.5). This can at least partly be explained by metacercarial distribution in the lens; parasites are often found in aggregations resulting in cataracts only in certain parts of the lens. However, in higher infection intensities parasites typically occupy the whole lens area, resulting in cataracts covering the entire lens. In an individual fish, parasites may also be unevenly distributed between the right and left eye. Thus, it is possible that cataracts mainly develop in one eye, while the other remains less affected.

Recently established parasites do not usually cause strong cataracts, but cataracts mainly develop when the metacercariae reach full development (Seppälä *et al.*, 2005a). The rate of metacercarial growth, and consequently their ability to cause damage in the eye lens, may depend on abiotic factors such as temperature (see below) as well as biotic factors such as parasite interactions. For example, *D. pseudospathaceum* genotypes show variation in metacercarial growth rate (Mironova *et al.*, 2025) and ability to cause cataracts (Klemme and Karvonen, 2019), which can also contribute to variation in cataracts between fish individuals. Furthermore, interactions between co-infecting *D. pseudospathaceum* genotypes are known to shape cataract development so that genotypes with a low infectivity and virulence (ability to cause cataracts) in single-genotype infection do better in co-infection, while the pattern is reversed for genotypes with higher performance (Klemme and Karvonen, 2019). As *Diplostomum* genotypes are typically found in co-infections and tend to aggregate in fish (Rauch *et al.*, 2005), genotype interactions are likely to modify cataract development and intensity in most systems.

The rate of metacercarial development and activity is also controlled by water temperature (Chappell *et al.*, 1994). Consequently, temperature also influences cataract formation as parasites become less active in cold water. For example, if fish become infected in late summer or autumn, followed by a decrease in water temperature, development of cataracts may take place in the following spring, several months after the infection (A. Karvonen, 2020, unpublished results). In such cases, it may sometimes be difficult to link the timing of infection and the

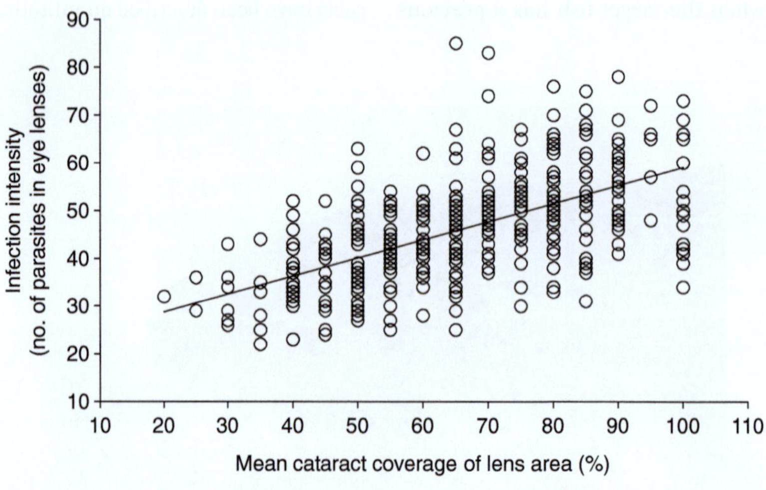

Fig. 15.5. Relationship between intensity of *Diplostomum spathaceum* infection (i.e. the total number of parasites in the lenses of the right and left eye) and mean cataract coverage in the eye lenses of whitefish (*Coregonus lavaretus*) experimentally exposed to the parasite. The fitted line represents linear regression. (Data from Karvonen and Seppälä, 2008a.)

emergence of negative effects in fish. Evidence also suggests that fish can partly recover from cataracts in cold water (Klemme *et al.*, 2021b). This may be because of reduced metacercarial activity, tolerance of the fish host to cataracts (see below), or a combination of both. Regardless of the underlying mechanism, the reduction in cataract intensity in cold water suggests that fish possess means to repair and reduce damage of the infection in the eye lens.

Also other host-related factors, such as fish size, age and species, can result in differences in susceptibility to parasite-inflicted damage. For example, smaller fish may be more susceptible to cataracts as smaller eye lenses may become covered with cataracts even in low infection intensities (Karvonen and Lindström, 2018). This is because the parasite metacercariae reach roughly the same size regardless of the size of their host and cause more damage per capita in a smaller eye lens. Young fish are also often more susceptible to infection before the development of specific immune responses, which may increase parasite abundance and further intensify cataract development. Cataracts may also show differences among fish species, or among populations of one species, because of physiological or genetic predisposition to infection and cataracts (Betterton, 1974; Sweeting, 1974; Rintamäki-Kinnunen *et al.*, 2004; Kuukka-Anttila *et al.*, 2010, 2020; Klemme and Karvonen, 2017; Klemme *et al.*, 2020, 2021a, 2022). For example, salmonid fish populations show genetic variation in different defence traits, avoidance, resistance and tolerance against *D. pseudospathaceum*, as well as trade-offs between the traits (Klemme and Karvonen, 2017; Klemme *et al.*, 2020). This suggests that fish populations invest differently into traits that directly or indirectly influence the degree of parasite-inflicted damage.

15.2.3. Other pathological effects in the eye

A chronic *D. spathaceum* infection may also cause other severe pathological effects in the lens. A fish's eye lens is composed of fibrous cells, which are variably compressed in different parts of the lens. This gives the lens its typical structure with softer outer parts and a very hard nucleus. *Diplostomum* metacercariae commonly occupy the outermost layers of the lens, which may lead to destruction of the crystalline structure of the cells and result in cataract formation (Shariff *et al.*, 1980). In the most severe cases, the lens capsule may rupture releasing materials into the eye and resulting in a significant inflammatory reaction (Shariff *et al.*, 1980). This is often accompanied by retinal detachment and dislocation of the lens to the anterior chamber. At this stage, the vision of the eye is lost completely. Such symptoms, however, are rare and have been reported mainly from aquaculture units in association with very high infection intensities. Their occurrence in wild fish is unknown.

The infection can also result in smaller size of the eye lens, possibly because of leaking of the lens material following the parasite establishment or lower lens growth rate due to parasite development and resource exploitation (Shariff *et al.*, 1980; Karvonen and Seppälä, 2008b). This phenomenon is known in several wild and farmed fish species so that the more heavily infected lens of an individual fish is usually smaller (Karvonen and Seppälä, 2008b). Also, at a population level, more heavily infected fish have smaller eye lenses compared to less infected conspecifics (Karvonen and Seppälä, 2008b). Smaller lens size induced by the infection may lead to increased susceptibility to cataracts, which develop as a function of infection intensity and depend on the lens volume. Also, the ability of fish to focus its vision depends on the lens radius and may therefore be sensitive to changes in lens size. Importantly, the changes in lens size can take place even at low infection intensities (Karvonen and Seppälä, 2008b) and before the development of major pathological changes in the eye. This suggests that focusing and vision ability of the eye could be affected already at lower infection intensities.

15.2.4. Effects of infection on fish

The effects of *Diplostomum* infection can be categorized into two types: (i) acute effects, caused directly by the cercarial invasion; and (ii) chronic effects, induced by metacercariae and cataracts. Several studies have investigated these effects, focusing, for example, on mortality, physiology, feeding, growth and behaviour of infected fish. Most of the research has been conducted using economically important farmed salmonid species, but studies using naturally infected wild fish species also exist.

15.2.4.1. Acute mortality

Penetration by the parasite cercariae and migration of the diplostomulae can be detrimental, especially for young fish. In addition to damage to the epidermis, histological studies have shown that diplostomulae penetrate blood vessels, causing internal haemorrhages and inflammatory responses (Ratanarat-Brockelman, 1974). In a high-level exposure, this can result in acute mortality of fish, the rate of which increases exponentially with the cercarial dose (Brassard *et al.*, 1982b). For example, mortality of small rainbow trout (*Oncorhynchus mykiss*) with a body length of 5–6 cm begins when the fish is simultaneously exposed to 300–600 cercariae and reaches 100% in doses of 1000 cercariae per fish (Larsen *et al.*, 2005). However, larger fish are typically more resistant and rarely experience mortality from the acute infection. Acute mortality of fish from high-level exposure can happen in aquaculture, whereas it is unlikely under natural conditions, where the prevalence of infection in snails is lower and the emerging cercariae are diluted in large water volumes. However, acute infection can also induce indirect mortality by increasing the susceptibility of exposed fish to predation (Brassard *et al.*, 1982a). It is important to note that in this case the increased susceptibility is related to damage or stress caused by the cercarial penetration and not to metacercarial presence and cataracts in the eye lens (see Section 15.2.4.4).

15.2.4.2. Physiology

Acute *Diplostomum* infection typically is a stressor for fish and thus initiates a range of physiological responses. Laitinen *et al.* (1996) showed that an acute exposure to *D. pseudospathaceum* cercariae results in increased heart and ventilation rates in fish. They also observed an increase in swimming activity of fish, which may be related to an attempt to escape the exposure (Karvonen *et al.*, 2004c; Klemme and Karvonen, 2017). Laitinen *et al.* (1996) also demonstrated that fish did not respond to the presence of cercariae of a different parasite species, *Plagiorchis elegans*, which does not infect fish. In other words, the mere presence of cercariae in the water did not elicit the physiological responses; it required the parasites to penetrate host tissues. Some of the observed responses may last for up to 3 days and peak at different stages of parasite establishment (Laitinen *et al.*, 1996), which demonstrates their complexity.

Established *Diplostomum* infection can also have physiological effects in fish. For example, studies have reported increased oxygen consumption among infected Arctic charr (*Salvelinus alpinus*) (Voutilainen *et al.*, 2008) but also decreased standard metabolic rate of the fish (Seppänen *et al.*, 2009). Such effects can be related to increased food intake, as suggested by Voutilainen *et al.* (2008), or reduced efficiency of energy metabolism, as suggested by Seppänen *et al.* (2009). Overall, it is evident that *Diplostomum* infection has metabolic consequences, which again can affect other traits such as growth and fecundity.

15.2.4.3. Feeding and growth

Impaired vision caused by *Diplostomum* parasites may also interfere with fish growth. For example, the infection decreases the weight and condition of rainbow trout in farming conditions (Buchmann and Uldal, 1994), which may be related to reduced feeding efficiency (Crowden and Broom, 1980; Owen *et al.*, 1993). Cataracts play a central role in impairment of vision and typically show high variation among infected individuals (Fig. 15.5). The severity of cataracts is known to correlate negatively with the feeding efficiency of Arctic charr in terms of reaction time to prey and number of prey items caught (Voutilainen *et al.*, 2008). It has also been shown experimentally that growth of whitefish (*Coregonus lavaretus*) is impaired with increasing cataract coverage in aquaculture conditions (Karvonen and Seppälä, 2008a). However, this negative effect is evident only when cataracts cover practically the entire lens area in both eyes (Fig. 15.6). The reason for this may be because fish with poor vision can follow feeding cues (movement to the surface when food is introduced) from less infected conspecifics in a tank using other sensory mechanisms. Conditions in natural systems, however, can be very different and there the negative effects on fish growth may become apparent already at lower cataract

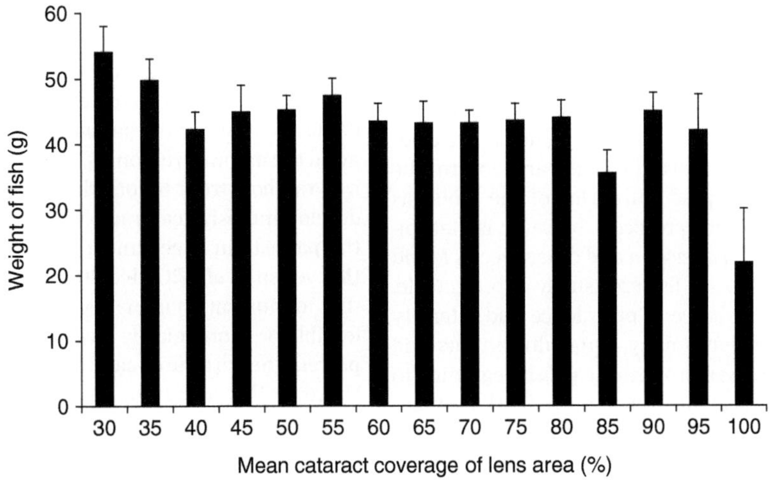

Fig. 15.6. Mean weight (± SE) of whitefish (*Coregonus lavaretus*) in relation to mean cataract coverage in the eye lenses. Fish were experimentally exposed to *Diplostomum spathaceum* and reared thereafter in tanks for 8 weeks. (Data from Karvonen and Seppälä, 2008a.)

intensities. For example, infection of *D. pseudospathaceum* reduces growth of territorial salmonids when the fish rely on natural feed (Klemme *et al.*, 2024) and this effect is correlated with cataract intensity in the range of 10–90% (Karvonen *et al.*, 2023). Overall, these results suggest that the negative effects of the infection on fish growth are likely to be very different in natural and farming conditions.

15.2.4.4. Susceptibility to predation

Predation from the avian definitive hosts is required for the completion of the life cycle of *Diplostomum* parasites. Therefore, parasite-induced phenotypic alterations that increase the susceptibility of the intermediate fish host to predation by suitable next hosts should be beneficial for the parasite. Cryptic coloration is an important mechanism for fish to hide from predators. Coloration of fish is regulated by the amount of light entering the eye; when light intensity increases, fish respond by becoming lighter. However, when the eye lens is infected with *D. spathaceum* metacercariae, observation of light intensity is impaired. This results in infected fish remaining darker and incapable in matching their coloration with a lighter background (Seppälä *et al.*, 2005b). In farming conditions, heavily infected fish are often notably dark and can be separated from less infected individuals.

The lack of cryptic coloration may also be one of the reasons why *D. spathaceum*-infected fish are more vulnerable to predation. Darker fish that cannot properly adjust their colour, or seek shelter from a matching background, are more easily seen by predators (Seppälä *et al.*, 2005b). This is accompanied by their reduced ability to group with conspecifics (Seppälä *et al.*, 2008) or detect approaching avian predators (Seppälä *et al.*, 2004), which is also positively linked with the development and coverage of cataracts (Seppälä *et al.*, 2005a). This increases parasite transmission to final bird hosts. However, the infection and cataracts also make the fish more susceptible to predatory fish (Karvonen *et al.*, 2023; Eronen *et al.*, 2024; Klemme *et al.*, 2024), which are dead-end hosts in terms of parasite life-cycle continuation. Similarly to avian predation (Seppälä *et al.*, 2005a), the increase in susceptibility to predatory fish coincides with the completion of metacercarial development and the timing of cataract formation (Klemme *et al.*, 2024). Overall, these results support cataracts as the definitive mechanism underlying increased predation upon *Diplostomum*-infected fish.

15.3. Protective and Control Strategies

Because of the deleterious effects of *Diplostomum* infection in fish, a range of control strategies have been put forward to limit and control the infections in aquaculture. One of the problems in designing such protocols, however, is that epidemics of *D. spathaceum* and other species found in the eye lenses of fish are usually unpredictable, with high variance in prevalence and intensity of the infection among aquaculture units and years. Moreover, problems (e.g. fish beginning to show cataracts and stopping feeding) often appear with a long time lag after the exposure, when control of the infection is no longer possible. It is to some extent possible to medicate infected fish by chemotherapy (Bylund and Sumari, 1981), but this has not been widely used. Furthermore, the cercariae are released from snails over a period of several months, which makes short-term actions against the cercariae (such as chemical treatments) unfeasible. It is to some extent possible to remove the cercariae from water using mechanical filtering or ultraviolet light (UV), but this is not applicable for large water volumes. However, several strategies against the parasite have been applied, and these can roughly be divided into: (i) those limiting the parasite establishment in fish (immunization); and (ii) those interrupting the parasite life cycle (control strategies against the snail intermediate hosts).

15.3.1. Immunization and other protective mechanisms

D. spathaceum infection evokes innate and specific immune responses in fish, the details of which are fairly well known (see Section 15.2.1). Thus, several researchers have explored the possibility of developing a vaccine against the parasite, for example by using attenuated infective stages (Bortz *et al.*, 1984; Speed and Pauley, 1985; Whyte *et al.*, 1990). Although such protocols decrease subsequent parasite establishment, an effective vaccine against *Diplostomum* has not yet been developed. The effect of the immunization against *D. spathaceum* is also not complete (see Section 15.2.1), meaning that some parasites establish in the lens regardless of acquired immune responses (Karvonen *et al.*, 2005; Rellstab *et al.*, 2013). Considering the efficiency of immunization, it is important to determine the degree of damage caused by the parasites that manage to avoid the immune responses. Previously immunized rainbow trout become heavily infected and develop intensive cataracts when re-exposed to the parasite in cages under natural conditions (Karvonen *et al.*, 2004c, 2010). This suggests that immunization alone is unlikely to provide a feasible or economically sustainable method to prevent the parasite or cataracts in aquaculture. However, this conclusion can depend on the fish species because of their inherent differences in susceptibility to the infection (Betterton, 1974; Klemme *et al.*, 2020).

Fish also use behavioural means in their defence against the parasite and escape the infection (Karvonen *et al.*, 2004c; Klemme *et al.*, 2020), a trait which is effectively eliminated in a limited space such as a tank or cage of a fish farm. The absence of such a defence could very well provide an explanation for the high parasite infection success under those conditions. Tolerance to cataracts (Klemme and Karvonen, 2017; Klemme *et al.*, 2020; Kuukka-Anttila *et al.*, 2020) could also play a role in decreasing the degree of parasite-inflicted damage although it is likely to be most effective at low to moderate infection intensities. Since many of the defence traits against *Diplostomum* have a strong genetic background (Kalbe and Kurtz, 2006; Klemme *et al.*, 2020, 2021a; Kuukka-Anttila *et al.*, 2020), it could also be possible to select for fish populations or hybrids that possess higher resistance or tolerance to the infection and cataracts. However, as none of the defence mechanisms provides a complete protection, their effectiveness in preventing the cataracts is dependent on the overall level of *Diplostomum* exposure.

It also important to note that *Diplostomum* infections are not isolated from other parasitic infections but can interact, probably more commonly than previously acknowledged, with other disease-causing agents. The fish immune system and previous experience of infections can influence such interactions. For example, co-infection of *D. pseudospathaceum* with the pathogenic bacterium, *Flavobacterium columnare*, one of the most harmful fish pathogens in aquaculture, increases the bacterial virulence and changes also the infection success of the flukes (Louhi *et al.*, 2015). These responses are also specific to *D. pseudospathaceum* genotype–*F. columnare* strain combinations. Possible mechanisms of higher bacterial virulence can include co-infection representing a higher challenge for the fish immune system or penetrating flukes opening a route for the bacteria to the fish body, resulting in a faster progression of the disease. These scenarios are supported by the significant increase in fish survival with an interval of 4 h or 5 weeks (fluke first followed by the bacterium) between the two infections (Karvonen *et al.*, 2019). Interactions between *Diplostomum* and bacteria can be shaped further by use of medication such as antibiotics (Sundberg and Karvonen, 2018; Ashrafi *et al.*, 2023). Taken together, these results suggest that infections, as well as prevention, of *Diplostomum* infections can influence the epidemiology of other parasites and diseases as well, supporting the idea that epidemiological patterns in aquaculture should not be considered independently.

15.3.2. Interruption of the parasite life cycle

Perhaps the most efficient strategy to control diplostomiasis in aquaculture is to interrupt the parasite life cycle. In practice, this means eradication of the snail intermediate host since control of the avian definitive host flying over a fish farm is much more challenging. Snails thrive especially in ponds with vegetation and high primary production, and it is common that infection levels differ greatly between individual ponds (Stables and Chappell, 1986a; Field and Irwin, 1994; Karvonen *et al.*, 2006b). Typically, the presence of snail intermediate hosts causes most of the infections within a farm (Stables and Chappell, 1986a), but parasite cercariae can also be brought into a farm by incoming water (Karvonen *et al.*, 2006b). Snails can be removed physically or chemically (Stables and Chappell, 1986a), and this can be ideally done in connection with draining and cleaning of the ponds. Further, establishment of snails can be reduced by removing the vegetation or constructing the ponds in a way that inhibits vegetation growth.

Changes in the infrastructure of a farm can also help in controlling the infections. For example, increasing the water flow rate and turbulence decreases infection intensities in fish (Field and Irwin, 1994). Furthermore, as snails typically inhabit littoral zones of lakes, taking the incoming water from a basin of a lake can decrease the number of cercariae entering the farm. Cercariae can also be filtrated mechanically from the water (Larsen *et al.*, 2005), or killed using chemicals (Larsen *et al.*, 2005) or UV treatment (A. Karvonen, 2025, unpublished results), although these are applicable only with smaller volumes of water. Biological filters, such as filter-feeding mussels, can also reduce *D. pseudospathaceum* cercarial densities and infections in fish (Gopko *et al.*, 2017), but as with other types of filters, the effect is constrained by water volume. Overall, the above actions should be considered complementary to the most important measure of prevention, which is the eradication of snails inside the farm.

15.4. Conclusions and Suggestions for Future Studies

The genus *Diplostomum* is a species complex in which molecular methods have recently enabled significant advances in resolving taxonomy, species identity and diversity, as well as community organization and interspecific interactions. However, details regarding life-cycle biology, host range, migration route in fish, and particularly the pathology of the number of *Diplostomum* species recently discovered around the northern hemisphere are still largely unknown and require further attention. This information is important for evaluating the effects of these parasites on their natural host species, as well as on aquaculture fish. Investigations should also focus on interactions between different *Diplostomum* species and genotypes, which are likely to be common and can contribute significantly to the parasite infection success and virulence. From an applied perspective, interactions between *Diplostomum* species and other aquaculture parasites and pathogens also form an interesting but relatively unexplored research area.

Because of their common occurrence and peculiar site of infection in eye lenses of fish, *D. spathaceum s.l.* continues to cause significant but local problems in aquaculture units using surface water sources. Although a low level of infection may even be beneficial as it evokes immunity against further infections, and heavy infection may be required for the negative effects to emerge in farming conditions, effects of *Diplostomum* infection in fish stocked into more challenging conditions in the wild may become apparent already at low to moderate infection intensities. Stocking protocols are common in many countries to maintain endangered salmonid fish populations. Thus, there is demand for more detailed studies on the effects of these parasites on fish feeding, growth and survival under natural conditions, particularly in relation to different species of *Diplostomum*, intensities of infection and severity of cataracts. Such information would also have a direct applied value when assessing the quality of young fish intended for stocking, as well as evaluating the success of fish stocking protocols in general.

Future studies should also explore the genetic predisposition of different fish species and populations to infection and cataracts. For example, information on less susceptible or more tolerant fish populations or hybrids could be helpful when designing fish breeding protocols which aim to develop fish stocks with better ability to cope with parasite infections. This should be done in parallel with investigations into genetic differences in infectivity and virulence among *Diplostomum* species and genotypes as these are essential in determining damage caused to their hosts. Overall, untangling these interactions requires investigations both from the host's and the parasite's perspective.

Acknowledgements

I thank Ines Klemme for discussions and comments on an earlier draft.

References

Ashrafi, R., Bruneaux, M., Sundberg, L.R., Hoikkala, V. and Karvonen, A. (2023) Multispecies coinfections and presence of antibiotics shape resistance and fitness costs in a pathogenic bacterium. *Molecular Ecology* 32, 4447–4460.

Betterton, C. (1974) Studies on host specificity of eyefluke, *Diplostomum spathaceum*, in brown and rainbow trout. *Parasitology* 69, 11–29.

Blasco-Costa, I., Faltýnková, A., Georgieva, S., Skirnisson, K., Scholz, T. and Kostadinova, A. (2014) Fish pathogens near the Arctic Circle: molecular, morphological and ecological evidence for unexpected diversity of *Diplostomum* (Digenea: Diplostomidae) in Iceland. *International Journal for Parasitology* 44, 703–715.

Bortz, B.M., Kenny, G.E., Pauley, G.B., Garciaortigoza, E. and Anderson, D.P. (1984) The immune response in immunized and naturally infected rainbow trout (*Salmo gairdneri*) to *Diplostomum spathaceum* as detected by enzyme-linked immunosorbent assay (ELISA). *Developmental and Comparative Immunology* 8, 813–822.

Brassard, P., Rau, M.E. and Curtis, M.A. (1982a) Parasite-induced susceptibility to predation in diplostomiasis. *Parasitology* 85, 495–501.

Brassard, P., Rau, M.E. and Curtis, M.A. (1982b) Infection dynamics of *Diplostomum spathaceum* cercariae and parasite-induced mortality of fish hosts. *Parasitology* 85, 489–493.

Buchmann, K. and Bresciani, J. (1997) Parasitic infections in pond-reared rainbow trout *Oncorhynchus mykiss* in Denmark. *Diseases of Aquatic Organisms* 28, 125–138.

Buchmann, K. and Uldal, A. (1994) Effects of eyefluke infections on the growth of rainbow trout (*Oncorhynchus mykiss*) in a mariculture system. *Bulletin of the European Association of Fish Pathologists* 14, 104–107.

Bylund, G. and Sumari, O. (1981) Laboratory tests with Droncit against diplostomiasis in rainbow trout, *Salmo gairdneri* Richardson. *Journal of Fish Diseases* 4, 259–264.

Chappell, L.H. (1969) Parasites of 3-spined stickleback *Gasterosteus aculeatus* L. from a Yorkshire pond. II. Variation of parasite fauna with sex and size of fish. *Journal of Fish Biology* 1, 339–347.

Chappell, L.H. (1995) The biology of diplostomatid eyeflukes of fishes. *Journal of Helminthology* 69, 97–102.

Chappell, L.H., Hardie, L.J. and Secombes, C.J. (1994) Diplostomiasis: the disease and host–parasite interactions. In: Pike, A.W. and Lewis, J.W. (eds) *Parasitic Diseases of Fish.* Samara Publishing Limited, Dyfed, UK, pp. 59–86.

Crowden, A.E. and Broom, D.M. (1980) Effects of the eyefluke, *Diplostomum spathaceum*, on the behavior of dace (*Leuciscus leuciscus*). *Animal Behaviour* 28, 287–294.

Désilets, H.D., Locke, S.A., McLaughlin, J.D. and Marcogliese, D.J. (2013) Community structure of *Diplostomum* spp. (Digenea: Diplostomidae) in eyes of fish: main determinants and potential interspecific interactions. *International Journal for Parasitology* 43, 929–939.

Diaz-Suarez, A., Noreikiene, K., Kahar, S., Ozerov, M.Y., Gross, R. *et al.* (2024) DNA metabarcoding reveals spatial and temporal variation of fish eye fluke communities in lake ecosystems. *International Journal for Parasitology* 54, 33–46.

Eronen, A., Janhunen, M., Hyvärinen, P., Kortet, R. and Karvonen, A. (2024) The effects of hybridization and parasite infection on the survival and behaviour of endangered landlocked salmon subject to predation – implications for genetic rescue. *Evolutionary Applications* 17, e70056.

Faltynková, A., Georgieva, S., Kostadinova, A., Blasco-Costa, I., Scholz, T. and Skírnisson, K. (2014) *Diplostomum* von Nordmann, 1832 (Digenea: Diplostomidae) in the sub-Arctic: descriptions of the larval stages of six species discovered recently in Iceland. *Systematic Parasitology* 89, 195–213.

Field, J.S. and Irwin, S.W.B. (1994) The epidemiology, treatment and control of diplostomiasis on a fish farm in Northern Ireland. In: Pike, A.W. and Lewis, J.W. (eds) *Parasitic Diseases of Fish.* Samara Publishing Limited, Dyfed, UK, pp. 87–100.

Francová, K., Ondračková, M., Polacik, M. and Jurajda, P. (2011) Parasite fauna of native and non-native populations of *Neogobius melanostomus* (Pallas, 1814) (Gobiidae) in the longitudinal profile of the Danube River. *Journal of Applied Ichthyology* 27, 879–886.

Georgieva, S., Soldanova, M., Perez-del-Olmo, A., Dangel, D.R., Sitko, J. *et al.* (2013) Molecular prospecting for European *Diplostomum* (Digenea: Diplostomidae) reveals cryptic diversity. *International Journal for Parasitology* 43, 57–72.

Gopko, M., Mironova, E., Pasternak, A., Mikheev, V. and Taskinen, J. (2017) Freshwater mussels (*Anodonta anatina*) reduce transmission of a common fish trematode (eye fluke, *Diplostomum pseudospathaceum*). *Parasitology* 144, 1971–1979.

Gopko, M., Savina, K., Sotnikov, D. and Mironova, E. (2025) Within-host 'infraecology': asymmetric interactions between two co-infecting eye parasites. *Integrative Zoology* (e-publication ahead of print version). DOI: 10.1111/1749-4877.12991.

Haas, W., Stiegeler, P., Keating, A., Kullmann, B., Rabenau, H. *et al.* (2002) *Diplostomum spathaceum* cercariae respond to a unique profile of cues during recognition of their fish host. *International Journal for Parasitology* 32, 1145–1154.

Haase, D., Rieger, J.K., Witten, A., Stoll, M., Bornberg-Bauer, E. *et al.* (2014) Specific gene expression responses to parasite genotypes reveal redundancy of innate immunity in vertebrates. *PLoS One* 9, e108001.

Haase, D., Rieger, J.K., Witten, A., Stoll, M., Bornberg-Bauer, E. *et al.* (2016a) Immunity comes first: the effect of parasite genotypes on adaptive immunity and immunization in three-spined sticklebacks. *Developmental and Comparative Immunology* 54, 137–144.

Haase, D., Rieger, J.K., Witten, A., Stoll, M., Bornberg-Bauer, E. *et al.* (2016b) Comparative transcriptomics of stickleback immune gene responses upon infection by two helminth parasites, *Diplostomum pseudospathaceum* and *Schistocephalus solidus*. *Zoology* 119, 307–313.

Höglund, J. (1991) Ultrastructural observations and radiometric assay on cercarial penetration and migration of the digenean *Diplostomum spathaceum* in the rainbow trout *Oncorhynchus mykiss*. *Parasitology Research* 77, 283–289.

Höglund, J. and Thuvander, A. (1990) Indications of non-specific protective mechanisms in rainbow trout *Oncorhynchus mykiss* with diplostomosis. *Diseases of Aquatic Organisms* 8, 91–97.

Hoogendoorn, C., Smit, N.J. and Kudlai, O. (2020) Resolution of the identity of three species of *Diplostomum* (Digenea: Diplostomidae) parasitising freshwater fishes in South Africa, combining molecular and morphological evidence. *International Journal for Parasitology: Parasites and Wildlife* 11, 50–61.

Kalbe, M. and Kurtz, J. (2006) Local differences in immunocompetence reflect resistance of sticklebacks against the eye fluke *Diplostomum pseudospathaceum*. *Parasitology* 132, 105–116.

Karvonen, A. and Lindström, K. (2018) Spatiotemporal and gender-specific parasitism in two species of gobiid fish. *Ecology and Evolution* 8, 6114–6123.

Karvonen, A. and Marcogliese, D.J. (2020) Diplostomiasis (*Diplostomum spathaceum* and related species). In: Woo, P.T.K., Leong, J.-A. and Buchmann, K. (eds) *Climate Change and Infectious Fish Diseases.* CAB International, Wallingford, UK, pp. 434–456.

Karvonen, A. and Seppälä, O. (2008a) Effect of eye fluke infection on the growth of whitefish (*Coregonus lavaretus*) – an experimental approach. *Aquaculture* 279, 6–10.

Karvonen, A. and Seppälä, O. (2008b) Eye fluke infection and lens size reduction in fish: a quantitative analysis. *Diseases of Aquatic Organisms* 80, 21–26.

Karvonen, A., Paukku, S., Valtonen, E.T. and Hudson, P.J. (2003) Transmission, infectivity and survival of *Diplostomum spathaceum* cercariae. *Parasitology* 127, 217–224.

Karvonen, A., Hudson, P.J., Seppälä, O. and Valtonen, E.T. (2004a) Transmission dynamics of a trematode parasite: exposure, acquired resistance and parasite aggregation. *Parasitology Research* 92, 183–188.

Karvonen, A., Kirsi, S., Hudson, P.J. and Valtonen, E.T. (2004b) Patterns of cercarial production from *Diplostomum spathaceum*: terminal investment or bet hedging? *Parasitology* 129, 87–92.

Karvonen, A., Seppälä, O. and Valtonen, E.T. (2004c) Parasite resistance and avoidance behaviour in preventing eye fluke infections in fish. *Parasitology* 129, 159–164.

Karvonen, A., Seppälä, O. and Valtonen, E.T. (2004d) Eye fluke-induced cataract formation in fish: quantitative analysis using an ophthalmological microscope. *Parasitology* 129, 473–478.

Karvonen, A., Paukku, S., Seppälä, O. and Valtonen, E.T. (2005) Resistance against eye flukes: naive versus previously infected fish. *Parasitology Research* 95, 55–59.

Karvonen, A., Cheng, G.H., Seppälä, O. and Valtonen, E.T. (2006a) Intestinal distribution and fecundity of two species of *Diplostomum* parasites in definitive hosts. *Parasitology* 132, 357–362.

Karvonen, A., Savolainen, M., Seppälä, O. and Valtonen, E.T. (2006b) Dynamics of *Diplostomum spathaceum* infection in snail hosts at a fish farm. *Parasitology Research* 99, 341–345.

Karvonen, A., Seppälä, O. and Valtonen, E.T. (2009) Host immunization shapes interspecific associations in trematode parasites. *Journal of Animal Ecology* 78, 945–952.

Karvonen, A., Halonen, H. and Seppälä, O. (2010) Priming of host resistance to protect cultured rainbow trout *Oncorhynchus mykiss* against eye flukes and parasite-induced cataracts. *Journal of Fish Biology* 76, 1508–1515.

Karvonen, A., Rellstab, C., Louhi, K.-R. and Jokela, J. (2012) Synchronous attack is advantageous: mixed genotype infections lead to higher infection success in trematode parasites. *Proceedings of the Royal Society B: Biological Sciences* 279, 171–176.

Karvonen, A., Aalto-Araneda, M., Virtala, A.M., Kortet, R., Koski, P. and Hyvärinen, P. (2016) Enriched rearing environment and wild genetic background can enhance survival and disease resistance of salmonid fishes during parasite epidemics. *Journal of Applied Ecology* 53, 213–221.

Karvonen, A., Fenton, A. and Sundberg, L.-R. (2019) Sequential infection can decrease virulence in a fish–bacterium–fluke interaction: implications for aquaculture disease management. *Evolutionary Applications* 12, 1900–1911.

Karvonen, A., Horppila, P., Kuitunen, J., Miettinen, M., Ryynänen, L. and Marjomäki, T.J. (2022) Differences in parasite community composition support ecological differentiation in a freshwater gadoid fish. *Ecology of Freshwater Fish* 31, 693–700.

Karvonen, A., Klemme, I., Räihä, V. and Hyvärinen, P. (2023) Enriched rearing environment enhances fitness-related traits of salmonid fishes facing multiple biological interactions. *Canadian Journal of Fisheries and Aquatic Sciences* 80, 1759–1769.

Klemme, I. and Karvonen, A. (2017) Vertebrate defense against parasites: Interactions between avoidance, resistance, and tolerance. *Ecology and Evolution* 7, 561–571.

Klemme, I. and Karvonen, A. (2019) Within-host interactions shape virulence-related traits of trematode genotypes. *Journal of Evolutionary Biology* 32, 572–579.

Klemme, I., Louhi, K.-R. and Karvonen, A. (2016) Host infection history modifies co-infection success of multiple parasite genotypes. *Journal of Animal Ecology* 85, 591–597.

Klemme, I., Hyvärinen, P. and Karvonen, A. (2020) Negative associations between parasite avoidance, resistance and tolerance predict host health in salmonid fish populations. *Proceedings of the Royal Society B: Biological Sciences* 287, 20200388.

Klemme, I., Hendrikx, L., Ashrafi, R., Sundberg, L.R., Räihä, V. *et al.* (2021a) Opposing health effects of hybridization for conservation. *Conservation Science and Practice* 3, e379.

Klemme, I., Hyvärinen, P. and Karvonen, A. (2021b) Cold water reduces the severity of parasite-inflicted damage: support for wintertime recuperation in aquatic hosts. *Oecologia* 195, 155–161.

Klemme, I., Debes, P.V., Primmer, C.R., Härkönen, L.S., Erkinaro, J. *et al.* (2022) Host developmental stage effects on parasite resistance and tolerance. *American Naturalist* 200, 646–661.

Klemme, I., Pysäys, J., Hyvärinen, P. and Karvonen, A. (2024) Fitness effects of assisted gene flow in an endangered salmonid population. *Conservation Science and Practice* 6, e13058.

Kudlai, O., Oros, M., Kostadinova, A. and Georgieva, S. (2017) Exploring the diversity of *Diplostomum* (Digenea: Diplostomidae) in fishes from the River Danube using mitochondrial DNA barcodes. *Parasites and Vectors* 10, 529.

Kuukka-Anttila, H., Peuhkuri, N., Kolari, I., Paananen, T. and Kause, A. (2010) Quantitative genetic architecture of parasite-induced cataract in rainbow trout, *Oncorhynchus mykiss*. *Heredity* 104, 20–27.

Kuukka-Anttila, H., Peuhkuri, N., Kolari, I. and Kause, A. (2020) Genetically determined resistance and tolerance to *Diplostomum* sp. parasite in farmed rainbow trout. *Aquaculture Research* 51, 4452–4460.

Laitinen, M., Siddall, R. and Valtonen, E.T. (1996) Bioelectronic monitoring of parasite-induced stress in brown trout and roach. *Journal of Fish Biology* 48, 228–241.

Larsen, A.H., Bresciani, J. and Buchmann, K. (2005) Pathogenicity of *Diplostomum* cercariae in rainbow trout, and alternative measures to prevent diplostomosis in fish farms. *Bulletin of the European Association of Fish Pathologists* 25, 20–27.

Locke, S.A., McLaughlin, J.D., Dayanandan, S. and Marcogliese, D.J. (2010a) Diversity and specificity in *Diplostomum* spp. metacercariae in freshwater fishes revealed by cytochrome c oxidase I and internal transcribed spacer sequences. *International Journal for Parasitology* 40, 333–343.

Locke, S.A., McLaughlin, J.D. and Marcogliese, D.J. (2010b) DNA barcodes show cryptic diversity and a potential physiological basis for host specificity among Diplostomoidea (Platyhelminthes: Digenea) parasitizing freshwater fishes in the St. Lawrence River, Canada. *Molecular Ecology* 19, 2813–2827.

Locke, S.A., Al-Nasiri, F.S., Caffara, M., Drago, F., Kalbe, M. *et al.* (2015) Diversity, specificity and speciation in larval Diplostomidae (Platyhelminthes: Digenea) in the eyes of freshwater fish, as revealed by DNA barcodes. *International Journal for Parasitology* 45, 841–855.

Louhi, K.-R., Karvonen, A., Rellstab, C., Louhi, R. and Jokela, J. (2013) Prevalence of infection as a predictor of multiple genotype infection frequency in parasites with multiple-host life cycle. *Journal of Animal Ecology* 82, 191–200.

Louhi, K.-R., Sundberg, L.-R., Jokela, J. and Karvonen, A. (2015) Interactions among bacterial strains and fluke genotypes shape virulence of co-infection. *Proceedings of the Royal Society B: Biological Sciences* 282, 20152097.

Lyholt, H.C.K. and Buchmann, K. (1996) *Diplostomum spathaceum*: effects of temperature and light on cercarial shedding and infection of rainbow trout. *Diseases of Aquatic Organisms* 25, 169–173.

Magnadottir, B. (2006) Innate immunity of fish (overview). *Fish and Shellfish Immunology* 20, 137–151.

Marcogliese, D.J., Compagna, S., Bergeron, E. and McLaughlin, J.D. (2001a) Population biology of eyeflukes in fish from a large fluvial ecosystem: the importance of gulls and habitat characteristics. *Canadian Journal of Zoology* 79, 1102–1113.

Marcogliese, D.J., Dumont, P., Gendron, A.D., Mailhot, Y., Bergeron, E. and McLaughlin, J.D. (2001b) Spatial and temporal variation in abundance of *Diplostomum* spp. in walleye (*Stizostedion vitreum*) and white suckers (*Catostomus commersoni*) from the St. Lawrence River. *Canadian Journal of Zoology* 79, 355–369.

McKeown, C.A. and Irwin, S.W.B. (1997) Accumulation of *Diplostomum* spp. (Digenea: Diplostomatidae) metacercariae in the eyes of 0+ and 1+ roach (*Rutilus rutilus*). *International Journal for Parasitology* 27, 377–380.

Mikheev, V.N., Pasternak, A.F., Valtonen, E.T. and Taskinen, J. (2014) Increased ventilation by fish leads to a higher risk of parasitism. *Parasites and Vectors* 7, 281.

Mironova, E., Spiridonov, S., Sotnikov, D., Shpagina, A., Savina, K. and Gopko, M. (2025) How do trematode clones differ by fitness-related traits and interact within a host? *International Journal for Parasitology* 55, 151–162.

Noreikiene, K., Ozerov, M., Ahmad, F., Koiv, T., Kahar, S. *et al.* (2020) Humic-acid-driven escape from eye parasites revealed by RNA-seq and target-specific metabarcoding. *Parasites and Vectors* 13, 433.

Ojaveer, H., Turovski, A. and Noomaa, K. (2020) Parasite infection of the non-indigenous round goby (*Neogobius melanostomus*) in the Baltic Sea. *Aquatic Invasions* 15, 160–176.

Owen, S.F., Barber, I. and Hart, P.J.B. (1993) Low-level infection by eye fluke, *Diplostomum* spp, affects the vision of 3-spined sticklebacks, *Gasterosteus aculeatus*. *Journal of Fish Biology* 42, 803–806.

Piecyk, A., Ritter, M. and Kalbe, M. (2019) The right response at the right time: exploring helminth immune modulation in sticklebacks by experimental coinfection. *Molecular Ecology* 28, 2668–2680.

Ratanarat-Brockelman, C. (1974) Migration of *Diplostomum spathaceum* (Trematoda) in the fish intermediate host. *Zeitschrift für Parasitenkunde* 43, 123–134.

Rauch, G., Kalbe, M. and Reusch, T.B.H. (2005) How a complex life cycle can improve a parasite's sex life. *Journal of Evolutionary Biology* 18, 1069–1075.

Rauch, G., Kalbe, M. and Reusch, T.B.H. (2006) One day is enough: rapid and specific host–parasite interactions in a stickleback–trematode system. *Biology Letters* 2, 382–384.

Rellstab, C., Louhi, K.R., Karvonen, A. and Jokela, J. (2011) Analysis of trematode parasite communities in fish eye lenses by pyrosequencing of naturally pooled DNA. *Infection, Genetics and Evolution* 11, 1276–1286.

Rellstab, C., Karvonen, A., Louhi, K.-R. and Jokela, J. (2013) Genotype-specific vs. cross-reactive host immunity against a macroparasite. *PLoS One* 8, e78427.

Rintamäki-Kinnunen, P., Karvonen, A., Anttila, P. and Valtonen, E.T. (2004) *Diplostomum spathaceum* metacercarial infection and colour change in salmonid fish. *Parasitology Research* 93, 577–581.

Schwelm, J., Georgieva, S., Grabner, D., Kostadinova, A. and Sures, B. (2021) Molecular and morphological characterisation of *Diplostomum phoxini* (Faust, 1918) with a revised classification and an updated nomenclature of the species-level lineages of *Diplostomum* (Digenea: Diplostomidae) sequenced worldwide. *Parasitology* 148, 1648–1664.

Seppälä, O., Karvonen, A. and Valtonen, E.T. (2004) Parasite-induced change in host behaviour and susceptibility to predation in an eye fluke–fish interaction. *Animal Behaviour* 68, 257–263.

Seppälä, O., Karvonen, A. and Valtonen, E.T. (2005a) Manipulation of fish host by eye flukes in relation to cataract formation and parasite infectivity. *Animal Behaviour* 70, 889–894.

Seppälä, O., Karvonen, A. and Valtonen, E.T. (2005b) Impaired crypsis of fish infected with a trophically transmitted parasite. *Animal Behaviour* 70, 895–900.

Seppälä, O., Karvonen, A. and Valtonen, E.T. (2008) Shoaling behaviour of fish under parasitism and predation risk. *Animal Behaviour* 75, 145–150.

Seppälä, O., Karvonen, A., Valtonen, E.T. and Jokela, J. (2009) Interactions among co-infecting parasite species: a mechanism maintaining genetic variation in parasites? *Proceedings of the Royal Society B: Biological Sciences* 276, 691–697.

Seppälä, O., Karvonen, A. and Valtonen, E.T. (2011) Eye fluke-induced cataracts in natural fish populations: is there potential for host manipulation? *Parasitology* 138, 209–214.

Seppälä, O., Karvonen, A., Rellstab, C., Louhi, K.-R. and Jokela, J. (2012) Reciprocal interaction matrix reveals complex genetic and dose-dependent specificity among coinfecting parasites. *American Naturalist* 180, 306–315.

Seppälä, O., Louhi, K.-R., Karvonen, A., Rellstab, C. and Jokela, J. (2015) Relative reproductive success of co-infecting parasite genotypes under intensified within-host competition. *Infection, Genetics and Evolution* 36, 450–455.

Seppänen, E., Kuukka, H., Huuskonen, H. and Piironen, J. (2008) Relationship between standard metabolic rate and parasite-induced cataract of juveniles in three Atlantic salmon stocks. *Journal of Fish Biology* 72, 1659–1674.

Seppänen, E., Kuukka, H., Voutilainen, A., Huuskonen, H. and Peuhkuri, N. (2009) Metabolic depression and spleen and liver enlargement in juvenile Arctic charr *Salvelinus alpinus* exposed to chronic parasite infection. *Journal of Fish Biology* 74, 553–561.

Shariff, M., Richards, R.H. and Sommerville, C. (1980) The histopathology of acute and chronic infections of rainbow trout *Salmo gairdneri* Richardson with eye flukes, *Diplostomum* spp. *Journal of Fish Diseases* 3, 455–465.

Speed, P. and Pauley, G.B. (1985) Feasibility of protecting rainbow trout, *Salmo gairdneri* Richardson, by immunizing against the eye fluke, *Diplostomum spathaceum*. *Journal of Fish Biology* 26, 739–744.

Stables, J.N. and Chappell, L.H. (1986a) The epidemiology of diplostomiasis in farmed rainbow trout from north-east Scotland. *Parasitology* 92, 699–710.

Stables, J.N. and Chappell, L.H. (1986b) Putative immune response of rainbow trout, *Salmo gairdneri*, to *Diplostomum spathaceum* infections. *Journal of Fish Biology* 29, 115–122.

Stables, J.N. and Chappell, L.H. (1986c) *Diplostomum spathaceum* (Rud 1819) – effects of physical factors on the infection of rainbow trout (*Salmo gairdneri*) by cercariae. *Parasitology* 93, 71–79.

Sundberg, L.-R. and Karvonen, A. (2018) Minor environmental concentrations of antibiotics can modify bacterial virulence in co-infection with a non-targeted parasite. *Biology Letters* 14, 20180663.

Sweeting, R.A. (1974) Investigations into natural and experimental infections of freshwater fish by common eye-fluke *Diplostomum spathaceum* Rud. *Parasitology* 69, 291–300.

Unger, P., Suthar, J., Baustian, F., Neitemeier-Duventester, X., Kleinertz, S. and Palm, H.W. (2022) Seasonality of salmonid parasites from flow-through aquaculture in northern Germany: emphasis on pathogenicity of *Diplostomum* spp. metacercaria. *Aquaculture, Fish and Fisheries* 2, 1–11.

Valtonen, E.T. and Gibson, D.I. (1997) Aspects of the biology of diplostomid metacercarial (Digenea) populations occurring in fishes in different localities of northern Finland. *Annales Zoologici Fennici* 34, 47–59.

Valtonen, E.T., Holmes, J.C. and Koskivaara, M. (1997) Eutrophication, pollution, and fragmentation: effects on parasite communities in roach (*Rutilus rutilus*) and perch (*Perca fluviatilis*) in four lakes in central Finland. *Canadian Journal of Fisheries and Aquatic Sciences* 54, 572–585.

Voutilainen, A., Figueiredo, K. and Huuskonen, H. (2008) Effects of the eye fluke *Diplostomum spathaceum* on the energetics and feeding of Arctic charr *Salvelinus alpinus*. *Journal of Fish Biology* 73, 2228–2237.

Whyte, S.K., Chappell, L.H. and Secombes, C.J. (1990) Protection of rainbow trout, *Oncorhynchus mykiss* (Richardson), against *Diplostomum spathaceum* (Digenea) – the role of specific antibody and activated macrophages. *Journal of Fish Diseases* 13, 281–291.

Whyte, S.K., Secombes, C.J. and Chappell, L.H. (1991) Studies on the infectivity of *Diplostomum spathaceum* in rainbow trout (*Oncorhynchus mykiss*). *Journal of Helminthology* 65, 169–178.

Wootten, R. (1974) Observations on strigeid metacercariae in eyes of fish from Hanningfield Reservoir, Essex, England. *Journal of Helminthology* 48, 73–83.

Zelmer, D.A. and Arai, H.P. (1998) The contributions of host age and size to the aggregated distribution of parasites in yellow perch, *Perca flavescens*, from Garner Lake, Alberta, Canada. *Journal of Parasitology* 84, 24–28.

16 Freshwater Fish Blood Flukes of Sanguinicolidae

Micah B. Warren[1]*, Ruth S. Kirk[2] and Stephen A. Bullard[1,3]

[1]*School of Fisheries, Aquaculture, and Aquatic Sciences, Auburn University, Alabama, USA;* [2]*School of Life Sciences, Pharmacy and Chemistry, Kingston University London, Kingston upon Thames, UK;* [3]*School for Environmental Sciences and Development, North-West University, Potchefstroom, South Africa*

Abstract

This chapter reviews the blood flukes (Sanguinicolidae Poche, 1926), a family of digeneans infecting freshwater ray-finned fishes. Recent revisions based on morphological and nucleotide evidence have redefined this group and its relationship to other fish blood fluke lineages. The life cycle is indirect involving fish definitive hosts and aquatic snail intermediate hosts. Infection causes impairment of respiratory, osmoregulatory and haematopoietic functions, reduced growth and lethargy of young and heavily infected fish. Eggs obstruct gills leading to hyperplasia, ischaemia and necrosis, and haemorrhage when miracidia emigrate from gill tissue. Eggs are sequestered within respiratory and other tissues by granulomatous encapsulation by eosinophils, neutrophils and monocytes/macrophages. Mortalities have been reported from fish farms and hatcheries where infected snails are present, but improvements in husbandry have reduced disease prevalence. Praziquantel is effective in controlling blood fluke infections and is widely used for ornamental fish and under specific veterinary and legislative conditions for food fish.

16.1. Introduction

16.1.1. The parasite

The blood flukes of vertebrates (Schistosomatoidea) have undergone extensive taxonomic and systematic revision (Bullard and Dutton, 2022; Warren and Bullard, 2023). The group comprises a monophyletic group of five families that infect cartilaginous fishes (Chondrichthyes) and ray-finned fishes (Actinopterygii) plus six families that infect marine and freshwater turtles and crocodilians (Bullard *et al.*, 2019; Dutton *et al.*, 2019; Dutton and Bullard, 2020a,b; Bullard and Dutton, 2022). Blood flukes that infect turtles and crocodilians are the sister lineage to the monophyletic bird and mammalian blood flukes (Schistosomatidae), including the causative agents of schistosomiasis. Hence, the study of blood flukes of fishes and turtles could be important in producing novel approaches and perspectives to the study of schistosomiasis. Blood flukes infect all major lineages of jawed vertebrates, and they likely had diversified considerably among aquatic vertebrate hosts (beginning with the most ancient extant gnathostome lineage, the chondrichthyans) long before tetrapods evolved on land.

Fish blood flukes were historically referred to collectively as both 'sanguinicolids' and

*Email: brett.warren@auburn.edu

DOI: 10.1079/9781800628748.0016

'aporocotylids'. Bullard *et al.* (2009) proposed a nomenclatural clarification/solution that was subsequently adopted (considering all fish blood flukes as belonging to Aporocotylidae Odhner, 1912) for several years prior to recent proposed revisions. Subsequent studies on both fish and turtle blood flukes (Bullard *et al.*, 2019; Warren and Bullard, 2019, 2023; Dutton and Bullard, 2020a; Warren *et al.*, 2021, 2023; Bullard and Dutton, 2022), robustly supported by nucleotide-based phylogenetic analyses, recovered clades of genera that can be diagnosed with numerous synapomorphic and autoapomorphic morphological characters. These revisions were conducted within both the fish blood flukes (now including five families) and the turtle blood flukes (now including six families) (Bullard and Dutton, 2022; Warren and Bullard, 2023).

The present chapter is on the Sanguinicolidae. Sanguinicolids (both adults and cercariae) lack the typically large and obvious oral and ventral suckers that many trematodes possess. They also have a pre-oesophageal muscular region resembling a modified sucker (McMichael-Phillips *et al.*, 1994) or pharynx (Poddubnaya *et al.*, 2023) and an uncoiled uterus (Fig. 16.1) (Warren and Bullard, 2023; Warren *et al.*, 2023). The first species of *Sanguinicola* was described as a turbellarian endoparasite of carp (*Cyprinus carpio*) by Plehn (1905) and then as monozoic cestodes (Plehn, 1908) (Table 16.1). However, Odhner (1911) correctly classified them as trematodes. Species-specific life history information is lacking for most species, but several life cycles have been elucidated (Wales, 1958; Erickson and Wallace, 1959; Meade and Pratt, 1965; Schell, 1974; Hoffman *et al.*, 1985; Simon-Martin *et al.*, 1987; Kirk and Lewis, 1993; Warren and Bullard, 2023). Generally, adults in fish blood release eggs that are carried to the gills, where they hatch and release a ciliated, free-swimming miracidium (Kirk and Lewis, 1993; Smith, 1997a; Orélis-Ribeiro *et al.*, 2014; M.B. Warren and S.A. Bullard, 2016, unpublished results).

16.1.2. Taxonomy and systematics

Since the original chapter in the first edition of this volume (Kirk, 2012), several taxonomic revisions and species descriptions have been completed, and many nucleotide sequences have been generated and incorporated into phylogenetic analyses. Orélis-Ribeiro and Bullard (2015) emended *Plehniella* and described two new species (*Plehniella sabajperezi*; *Plehniella armbrusteri*). Continuing this work on catfish infecting blood flukes, Orélis-Ribeiro and Bullard (2016) proposed two new genera (*Kritsky*; *Cladocaecum*) and proposed a new combination and described a new species (*Kritsky platyrhynchi*; *Cladocaecum tomasscholzi*) to accommodate the genera. Truong and Bullard (2013) proposed *Nomasanguinicola* and described *Nomasanguinicola canthoensis* infecting a catfish (Clariidae) from Vietnam. Truong and Bullard (2013) also discussed the morphological similarities (anterior sucker bearing denticles) between *N. canthoensis* and species of *Sanguinicola* and *Plehniella* infecting catfishes (Clariidae: Bagridae) in Israel and Africa (Paperna, 1964; Woodland, 1923; Imam *et al.*, 1984). Shimazu (2013) described a new species of *Sanguinicola* (*Sanguinicola hasegawai*) infecting loach (Nemacheilidae) in Japan. Cutmore *et al.* (2023) examined *Posticobia brazieri* Iredale, 1943 (Tateidae) resulting in five distinct cercarial sequences that nested within the Sanguinicolidae. Warren *et al.* (2023) revised *Sanguinicola*, described a new species (*Sanguinicola plehnae*) infecting pike (Esocidae), provided a supplemental description for *Sanguinicola volgensis*, and reassigned two species to *Nomasanguinicola* (*Nomasanguinicola dentata*; *Nomasanguinicola clarias*). Further, Warren *et al.* (2023) proposed a new genus (*Pseudosanguinicola*) and reassigned a species (*Pseudosanguinicola occidentalis*) to accommodate the genus. Warren and Bullard (2023) and Warren *et al.* (2023) also provided nucleotide sequences for the newly collected species of *Sanguinicola*, *Pseudosanguinicola* and *Nomasanguinicola* as well as including several innominate fish blood fluke sequences for phylogenetic analysis. The revision of *Sanguinicola* and the addition of nucleotide sequences contributed to the revision of the family (Warren and Bullard, 2023). Most recently, Warren *et al.* (2024) collected new specimens of *N. dentata* from sub-Saharan Africa and provided a supplemental description and a nucleotide sequence. Together, these studies underscore the continued refinement of fish blood fluke taxonomy through detailed morphological descriptions and molecular study.

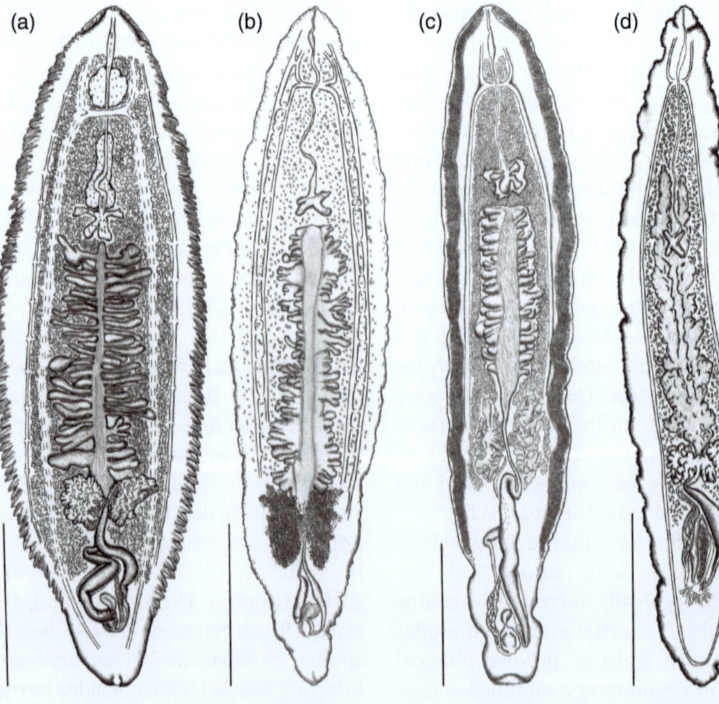

Fig. 16.1. Species of Sanguinicolidae: (a) *Sanguinicola volgensis*. Bar = 250 μm. (b) *Sanguinicola plehnae*. Bar = 500 μm. (c) *Pseudosanguinicola occidentalis*. Bar = 250 μm. (d) *Nomasanguinicola dentata*. Bar = 500 μm. (From Warren *et al*., 2023).

The largest genus, *Sanguinicola*, comprises 26 species that infect a broad range of hosts including carps (Cypriniformes), catfishes (Siluriformes), trout (Salmoniformes), bass (Centrarchiformes) and walleye (Perciformes) across Europe, Asia, Africa, North America, South America and Australia. However, 16 of these 36 species are currently considered *incertae sedis*, *nomen nudum* or *species inquirenda* due to inadequate morphological descriptions and the absence of type specimens, formal diagnoses or illustrations (Warren *et al*., 2023). Species of *Sanguinicola* differ by having lateral tegumental spines that are straight (not recurved) and deeply rooted in the lateral tegument or slightly protruding from it, arranged in a single column, and an intestine comprising four or five radial ceca that collectively appear as an X-shaped structure and terminates in the anterior half of the body.

The monotypic *Parasanguinicola vastispina* infects barramundi (Latidae), while *P. occidentalis* infects walleye (Percidae). *P. vastispina* is reported to have a pre-ovarian female genital pore – an unusual feature within the family that requires confirmation, as no other sanguinicolids are known to possess this character state. *P. occidentalis* is differentiated by the densely compacted transverse rows of lateral tegumental spines and a large seminal vesicle, which may comprise up to one-third of the body length (Warren *et al*., 2023).

All remaining genera within the Sanguinicolidae infect catfishes (Siluriformes). Species of *Nomasanguinicola* (*N. canthoensis*, *N. dentata* and *N. clarias*) are morphologically distinct by having an anterior sucker bearing two rows of denticles flanking the mouth (Paperna, 1964; Imam *et al*., 1984; Truong and Bullard, 2013; Warren *et al*., 2023, 2024; Warren and Bullard, 2023). *N. dentata* and *N. clarias* were recently reassigned and may represent the same species; however, due to the absence of type material, new collections from type localities and type hosts are needed to confirm (Warren *et al*., 2023). Notably, *Sanguinicola chalmersi* was also reported to have two rows

Table 16.1. Species of Sanguinicolidae Poche, 1926.

Species	Type host	Locality	Reference
Cladocaecum tomasscholzi Orélis-Ribeiro and Bullard, 2016	Manduba, *Ageneiosus inermis* Linnaeus, 1766 (Siluriformes: Auchenipteridae)	South America	Orélis-Ribeiro and Bullard (2016)
Kritsky platyrhynchi (Guidelli, Isaac, and Pavanelli, 2002) Orélis-Ribeiro and Bullard, 2016	Porthole shovelnose catfish, *Hemisorubim platyrhynchos* (Valenciennes, 1840) (Siluriformes: Pimelodidae)	South America	Guidelli *et al.* (2002); Orélis-Ribeiro and Bullard (2016)
Nomasanguinicola canthoensis Truong and Bullard, 2013	Bighead catfish, *Clarias macrocephalus* Günther, 1864 (Siluriformes: Clariidae)	South-East Asia	Truong and Bullard (2013)
Nomasanguinicola clarias (Imam, Marzouk, Hassan, and Itman, 1984) Warren and Bullard, 2023	African sharptooth catfish, *Clarias gariepinus* (Burchell, 1822) Teugles, 1982 (Siluriformes: Clariidae)	Northern Africa	Imam *et al.* (1984); Warren *et al.* (2023)
Nomasanguinicola dentata (Paperna, 1964) Warren and Bullard, 2024	African sharptooth catfish, *C. gariepinus* (Burchell, 1822) Teugles, 1982 (Siluriformes: Clariidae)	Israel; southern Africa	Paperna (1964); Warren *et al.* (2024)
Parasanguinicola vastispina Herbert and Shaharom-Harrison, 1995	Barramundi, *Lates calcarifer* (Bloch, 1790) (Carangiformes: Perciformes: Latidae)	South-West Pacific	Herbert and Shaharom-Harrison (1995)
Plehniella armbrusteri Orélis-Ribeiro and Bullard, 2016	Bloch's catfish, *Pimelodus blochii* Valenciennes, 1840 (Siluriformes: Pimelodidae)	South America	Orélis-Ribeiro and Bullard (2015)
Plehniella coelomicola Szidat, 1951	Long whisker catfish, *Iheringichthys labrosus* (Lütken, 1874) (Siluriformes: Pimelodidae)	South America	Szidat (1951)
Plehniella sabajperezi Orélis-Ribeiro and Bullard, 2015	White line catfish, *Pimelodus albofasciatus* Mees, 1974 (Siluriformes: Pimelodidae)	South America	Orélis-Ribeiro and Bullard (2015)
Pseudosanguinicola occidentalis (Van Cleave and Mueller, 1932) Warren and Bullard, 2023	Walleye, *Sander vitreus* (Mitchill, 1818) Bailey *et al.* 2004 (Perciformes: Percidae)	North America	Van Cleave and Mueller (1932); Warren *et al.* (2023)
Sanguinicola alseae (Meade and Pratt, 1965) Holmes, 1971 *incertae sedis*	Cutthroat trout, *Oncorhynchus clarkii* (Richardson, 1836) McAllister, 1990 (Salmoniformes: Salmonidae)	North America	Meade and Pratt (1965)
Sanguinicola argentinensis Szidat, 1951 *incertae sedis*	Streaked prochilod, *Prochilodus lineatus* (Valenciennes, 1837) Malabarba, 1989 (Characiformes: Prochilodontidae) (as *Prochilodus platensis*)	South America	Szidat (1951)
Sanguinicola armata Plehn, 1905 (type species)	Tench, *Tinca tinca* (Linnaeus, 1758) Berg, 1949 (Cypriniformes: Tincidae)	Europe	Plehn (1905)

Continued

Table 16.1. Continued.

Species	Type host	Locality	Reference
Sanguinicola chalmersi Odhner, 1924 *incertae sedis*	Giraffe catfish, *Auchenoglanis occidentalis* (Valenciennes, 1840) Bailey and Stewart, 1984 (Siluriformes: Claroteidae)	Africa	Woodland, (1923); Odhner and Woodland (1924)
Sanguinicola davisi Wales, 1958 *incertae sedis*	Cutthroat trout, *O. clarkii* (Richardson, 1836) McAllister, 1990 (Salmoniformes: Salmonidae)	North America	Wales (1958)
Sanguinicola fontinalis Hoffman, Fried, and Harvey, 1985 *incertae sedis*	Brook trout, *Salvelinus fontinalis* (Mitchill, 1814) Okada, 1961 (Salmoniformes: Salmonidae)	North America	Hoffman *et al.* (1985)
Sanguinicola hasegawai Shimazu, 2013	Loach, *Barbatula toni* (Dybowski, 1869) Okada, 1961 (Cypriniformes: Nemacheilidae)	Japan	Shimazu (2013)
Sanguinicola huronis Fischthal, 1949 *incertae sedis*	Smallmouth bass, *Micropterus dolomieu* Lacepède, 1802 (Centrarchiformes: Centrarchidae)	North America	Fischthal (1949)
Sanguinicola idahoensis Schell, 1974 *incertae sedis*	Rainbow trout, *Oncorhynchus mykiss* (Walbaum, 1792) Tomelleri and Eberle, 1990 (Salmoniformes: Salmonidae)	North America	Schell (1974)
Sanguinicola incognita Akhmerov, 1959 *nomen nudum*	Grass carp, *Ctenopharyngodon idella* (Valenciennes, 1844) (Cypriniformes: Xenocyprididae)	Eastern Europe	Akhmerov (1959)
Sanguinicola inermis Plehn, 1905 *incertae sedis*	Eurasian carp, *Cyprinus carpio* Linnaeus, 1758 (Cypriniformes: Cyprinidae)	Europe	Plehn (1905)
Sanguinicola intermedia Ejsmont, 1926	Crucian carp, *Carassius carassius* (Linnaeus, 1758) Berg, 1949 (Cypriniformes: Cyprinidae)	Eastern Europe	Ejsmont (1926)
Sanguinicola klamathensis Wales, 1958 *incertae sedis*	Cutthroat trout, *O. clarkii* (Richardson, 1836) McAllister, 1990 (Salmoniformes: Salmonidae)	North America	Wales (1958)
Sanguinicola lophophora Erickson and Wallace, 1959	Spottail shiner, *Notropis hudsonius* (Clinton, 1824) Gilbert, 1978 (Cypriniformes: Leuciscidae)	North America	Erickson and Wallace (1959)
Sanguinicola lungensis Tang and Ling, 1975	Goldfish, *Carassius auratus* (Linnaeus, 1758) Berg, 1949 (Cypriniformes: Cyprinidae)	China	Tang and Ling (1975)

Continued

Table 16.1. Continued.

Species	Type host	Locality	Reference
Sanguinicola magnus Hu, Long, and Lee, 1965	Grass carp, *C. idella* (Valenciennes, 1844) (Cypriniformes: Xenocyprididae)	Asia	Hu *et al.* (1965)
Sanguinicola maritimus Nolan and Cribb, 2005 *incertae sedis*	Brownspotted wrasse, *Notolabrus parilus* (Richardson, 1850) Russell, 1988 (Labriformes: Labridae)	South-West Pacific	Nolan and Cribb (2005)
Sanguinicola megalobramae Li, 1980 *nomen nudum*	Wuchang bream, *Megalobrama amblycephala* Yih, 1955 (Cypriniformes: Xenocyprididae)	Asia	Li (1980)
Sanguinicola plehnae Warren, Poddubnaya, Zhokhov, and Bullard, 2022	Northern pike, *Esox lucius* Linnaeus, 1758 (Esociformes: Esocidae)	Russia	Warren *et al.* (2023)
Sanguinicola rhodei Wang, 1983	Giant Chinese bitterling, *Acheilognathus macropterus* (Bleeker, 1871) Chen and Li, 1989 (Cypriniformes: Acheilognathidae) (as *Acanthorhodeus taenianalis*)	Asia	Wang (1983)
Sanguinicola rutili Simón-Martín, Rojo-Vásquez, and Simón-Vicente, 1988	Bermejuela, *Achondrostoma arcasii* (Steindachner, 1866) Robalo *et al.*, 2007 (Cypriniformes: Leuciscidae) (as *Rutilus arcasi*)	Europe	Simon-Martin *et al.* (1987)
Sanguinicola sanliense Wang, 1982 *incertae sedis*	Yellow catfish, presumably *Tachysurus sinensis* Lacepède, 1803 (Siluriformes: Bagridae) (scientific name not included in publication)	Asia	Wang (1982)
Sanguinicola shantsuensis Lung and Chen, 1965 *nomen nudum*	Crucian carp, *C. carassius* (Linnaeus, 1758) Berg, 1949 (Cypriniformes: Cyprinidae)	Asia	Lung and Shen (1965), cited by Li (1980); Tang and Ling (1975); Shimazu (2007)
Sanguinicola skrjabini Akhmerov, 1960	Silver carp, *Hypophthalmichthys molitrix* (Valenciennes, 1844) Berg, 1949 (Cypriniformes: Xenocyprididae)	Eastern Europe	Akhmerov (1960)
Sanguinicola ugui Shimazu, 2007 *incertae sedis*	Big-scaled redfin, *Pseudaspius hakonensis* (Günther, 1877) Dyldin *et al.*, 2020 (Cypriniformes: Leuciscidae) (as *Tribolodon hakonensis*)	Japan	Shimazu (2013)
Sanguinicola volgensis (Rašín, 1929) McIntosh, 1934	Sabrefish, *Pelecus cultratus* (Linnaeus, 1758) Berg, 1949 (Cypriniformes: Leuciscidae)	Russia	Rašín (1929); Warren *et al.* (2023)

of denticles flanking the mouth (Odhner and Woodland, 1924; Imam *et al.*, 1984), but this feature also requires confirmation. Species of *Plehniella* and *Kritsky* infect pimelodid catfishes, whereas *C. tomasscholzi* infects an auchenipterid catfish from South America. All three genera are unique among sanguinicolids because the species infect the body cavity of their fish hosts. Species of *Plehniella* and *K. platyrhynchi* are further distinct by having an intestine composed of six sac-like ceca, while *C. tomasscholzi* has a branched intestine comprising anterior ceca and a single, medial, dendritic posterior cecum (Orélis-Ribeiro and Bullard, 2015, 2016; Warren and Bullard, 2023).

Phylogenetics using nucleotide sequences confirm morphological diagnoses, specifically sequences generated using the large ribosomal subunit (*28S*) gene. While the use of this gene to study fish blood fluke relationships has been incorporated since 2003 (Olson *et al.*, 2003), information regarding the sanguinicolids (as well as several other fish blood fluke families) has been lacking. To highlight this point, no sequence tied to an adult sanguinicolid was available until the most recent revision (Warren *et al.*, 2023). Further, the sequence listed as *Sanguinicola* cf. *inermis* represents cercariae collected from a snail, *Lymnaea stagnalis* (Linnaeus, 1758), in Poland. Presently, three of the seven genera (*Sanguinicola*, *Pseudosanguinicola* and *Nomasanguinicola*) have sequences that are tied to a voucher specimen and are represented in a phylogenetic study (Fig. 16.2) (Warren *et al.*, 2024). Sequences from several innominate species awaiting description from catfishes in Vietnam, centrarchids in North America, and several closely related cercarial sequences from Australia are now available (Cutmore *et al.*, 2023; Warren and Bullard, 2023; Warren *et al.*, 2024). The morphological characters reported from the sanguinicolids infecting catfishes and the phylogenetic placement of several innominate blood fluke sequences highlight the largely undocumented diversity within this group.

16.1.3. Life cycle

The blood flukes of Sanguinicolidae have an indirect life cycle involving fish and aquatic snails.

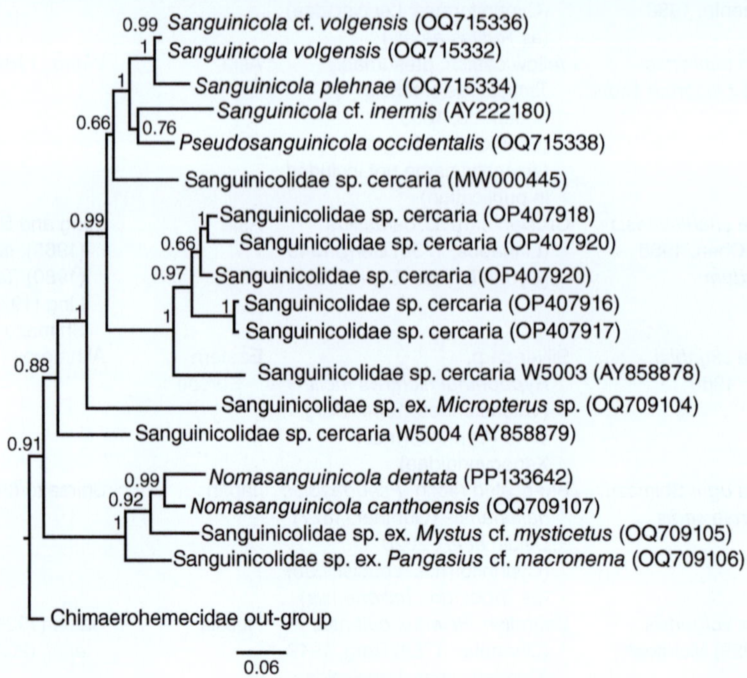

Fig. 16.2. Phylogenetic analysis based on the large ribosomal subunit (*28S*) gene using all available sequences representing species of Sanguinicolidae. Scale bar indicates substitutions per site. (From Warren *et al.*, 2024).

Unlike other digeneans, known life cycles of sanguinicolids involve only a single intermediate host. To date, only gastropods have been confirmed as intermediate hosts – no bivalves or polychaetes, in contrast to other families of fish blood flukes (Warren and Bullard, 2019, 2023). However, the full diversity of intermediate hosts remains to be determined, as only nine life cycles have been elucidated (Warren and Bullard, 2023). Many of the life cycles are associated with cultured fishes (Wales, 1958; Meade and Pratt, 1965; Schell, 1974; Kirk and Lewis, 1993), subsequently limiting our understanding of life cycles in wild definitive and intermediate hosts. Furthermore, several proposed life cycles lack confirmation through experimental infection, underscoring the need for molecular sequencing to verify adult–cercaria relationships, especially since no morphological characters of the cercariae have proven diagnostic for adult identification. Understanding the complete life cycle and the range of intermediate hosts is essential for elucidating the biogeography of sanguinicolid blood flukes. For example, *S. inermis* and likely other congeners have been disseminated between the carp farms and fisheries of Eurasia through anthropogenic movements of carp. By the 1960s, *S. inermis* had become widespread throughout mainland Europe (Bauer, 1962). Establishment of *S. inermis* in new foci has been facilitated by the widespread distribution of the intermediate snail hosts, *Radix auricularia* (Linnaeus, 1758) and *Ampullaceana balthica* (Linnaeus, 1758) (as *Radix*), as well as *L. stagnalis* in cyprinid fisheries (Kirk and Lewis, 1994a).

Fish are infected by the direct penetration of cercariae through the epidermis of the skin, fins, opercular cavity and gill lamellae. Schistosomula migrate through the dermis, connective tissue and muscle to enter the blood vascular system (Schell, 1974; Kirk and Lewis, 1996). The majority of flukes that survive host defences mature in the ventral aorta, afferent branchial arteries, bulbus arteriosus, ventricle and atrium, although flukes can also establish in the dorsal aorta and cephalic, renal and hepatic vessels (Schell, 1974; Kirk and Lewis, 1996). For *S. inermis*, migration to the blood system is completed within 1 month at 20°C (Kirk and Lewis, 1996). Adults cross-fertilize and commence egg development. The maximum lifespan of adults is between 56 and 70 days at 20°C (Meade and Pratt, 1965; Meade, 1967; Schell, 1974; Kirk and Lewis, 1996). The eggs are released from adults while immature and develop further in the blood and tissue of the fish host. Most eggs accumulate in the gills because the majority of adults are present in the ventral blood system as well as branchial arteries (Schell, 1974; Kirk and Lewis, 1993; M.B. Warren and S.A. Bullard, 2016, 2024, unpublished results). They are carried by the ventral blood flow until they lodge in the gill and visceral capillaries. The accumulation of eggs causes the delicate blood vessels to rupture and discharge eggs into adjacent tissue. Miracidia develop inside thin, pliable, non-operculate egg capsules and hatch *in situ* within approximately 7 days (McMichael-Phillips *et al.*, 1992a; Kirk and Lewis, 1996). Those miracidia present in the distal regions of the gills, and some miracidia in the proximal regions, escape into the water using the stylet and rodlet complex of the apical papilla, possibly aided by enzyme secretions from lateral glands (McMichael-Phillips *et al.*, 1992b; Kirk and Lewis, 1996). Ciliated miracidia locate and penetrate snail intermediate hosts. Eggs and miracidia that do not escape from the gills, and those that are sequestered in visceral and connective tissue, become trapped within granulomatous tissue and degrade (Kirk and Lewis, 1996). Within the snail host the miracidium transforms into a mother sporocyst in which daughter sporocysts develop and migrate into the interlobular spaces of the digestive gland. Lophocercous apharyngeate cercariae develop inside daughter sporocysts within 4–5 weeks at 20°C. There is no metacercarial stage. The cercariae emerge from snails in late afternoon to early evening to locate the fish definitive hosts (Kirk and Lewis, 1993).

S. inermis exhibits a well-defined seasonal cycle of development in carp fisheries in temperate regions. Sporocyst infections in snails and miracidial infections in carp overwinter until increasing temperatures in spring facilitate development (Bobiatynska-Ksok, 1964; Lee, 1990). Cercariae emerge from snails in spring/early summer to infect carp, and miracidia migrate from the gill tissue to infect newly hatched snails. Summer adult flukes in carp produce eggs and die by the autumn. Further snails are infected by miracidia. Carp are infected during the second peak of cercarial emergence in the late summer. A second generation of adult flukes develop and produce eggs until declining autumn temperatures inhibit further development. Adults overwintering in the heart of carp hosts reproduce in the spring and then die by early summer (Naumova, 1961; Lee, 1990).

Of the sanguinicolids, life-cycle information is reported only from species of *Sanguinicola* and *Pseudosanguinicola* (Warren and Bullard, 2023). *S. inermis*, *Sanguinicola rutili* and *Sanguinicola lophophora* all infect carps and minnows (Cypriniformes: Cyprinidae and Leuciscidae) and snails from Lymnaeidae, Planorbidae and Valvatidae (Erickson and Wallace, 1959; Simon-Martin *et al.*, 1987; Kirk and Lewis, 1994a). For example, in addition to Eurasian carp (*C. carpio*), *S. inermis* has been reported using bream (*Abramis brama*), crucian carp (*Carassius carassius*), goldfish (*Carassius auratus*), nase (*Chondrostoma nasus*), roach (*Rutilus rutilus*), rudd (*Scardinius erythrophthalmus*), silver bream (*Blicca bjoerkna*) and tench (*Tinca tinca*) as definitive hosts (Smith, 1997b, *Esox lucius* is an error). *Sanguinicola davisi*, *Sanguinicola klamathensis*, *Sanguinicola alseae*, *Sanguinicola idahoensis* and *Sanguinicola fontinalis* all infect trouts (Salmoniformes: Salmonidae) and snails from Hydrobiidae, Semisulcospiridae and Pleuroceridae (Wales, 1958; Meade and Pratt, 1965; Meade, 1967; Schell, 1974; Hoffman *et al.*, 1985; Warren and Bullard, 2023). *P. occidentalis* infects walleye (Perciformes: Percidae) and snails from Viviparidae (Van Cleave and Mueller, 1932; Bacha, 1966; Warren *et al.*, 2023). No life-cycle information regarding species of *Plehniella*, *Cladocaecum*, *Kritsky*, *Nomasanguinicola* and *Parasanguinicola* is currently available but would likely have a significant impact on the group. Further information on intermediate and definitive hosts of sanguinicolids is provided by Smith (1997a,b).

16.1.4. Impact on fish production

Fish mortalities attributed to sanguinicolids have occurred in intensively farmed fish populations. In China, species of *Sanguinicola* have been associated with epizootics of cyprinid fingerlings in pond farms. *Sanguinicola lungensis* caused extensive losses of silver carp (*Hypophthalmichthys molitrix*) and bighead carp (*Hypophthalmichthys nobilis*) in South Fukien (Tang and Ling, 1975). *Sanguinicola megalobramae* killed blunt-snout bream (*Megalobrama amblycephala*) in Hupei Province (Li, 1980). Species of *Sanguinicola* in North America caused mortalities of young salmonids in hatcheries until husbandry was improved to eliminate intermediate hosts from water circulation systems. *S. davisi* was responsible for heavy losses of young rainbow and steelhead trout (*Oncorhynchus mykiss*) and cutthroat trout (*Oncorhynchus clarkii*) in hatcheries in Oregon and California (Wales, 1958; Davis *et al.*, 1961). Wales (1958) also reported mass mortalities of cutthroat trout in an Oregon hatchery attributed to *S. klamathensis*. *S. idahoensis* caused significant disease problems and losses in steelhead trout in a hatchery in Idaho (Schell, 1974). *S. fontinalis* caused severe disease in 400,000 brook trout (*Salvelinus fontinalis*) in a Pennsylvania state hatchery, necessitating a cull of approximately 100,000 of the most severely infected fish (Hoffman *et al.*, 1985). In 1997, a non-peer-reviewed internal report attributed the death of 20,000 brook trout in a North Carolina state hatchery to a blood fluke morphologically similar to *S. fontinalis*. In 2024, we (M.B.W. and S.A.B.) examined dead brook trout infected by *S.* cf. *fontinalis* from the same North Carolina state hatchery where the parasite was previously reported. This ongoing infection, known to cause mortality more than 20 years after its initial report, highlights the need for extensive sampling in wild fish populations for blood fluke infections.

Mortalities attributed to *S. inermis* have occurred in 0–1+-year-old carp in intensively farmed fish populations. The parasite was responsible for serious economic problems on carp farms in mainland Europe and Asia from the 1950s to the 1980s, having caused parasite-induced mortalities and impaired growth of fry and fingerlings (Bauer, 1962; Lucky, 1964; Moravec, 1984). Disease problems were exacerbated by old fish-farming practices of rearing fry with older fish in silted ponds containing high populations of snails (Bobiatynska-Ksok, 1964; Hlond *et al.*, 1977), but improvements in husbandry and use of molluscicides have reduced the prevalence of sanguinicoliasis (Sapozhnikov, 1988). The first epizootic of *S. inermis* in the UK occurred in 1977 resulting in 90% mortality of the year's fry on a Cotswold carp farm in Gloucestershire, England (Sweeting, 1979). The parasite was subsequently reported from numerous sites in southern, eastern and central England translocated by legal and illegal stock movements and caused further mortalities in young carp. Mortalities were lower in extensive fisheries than farms and typically occurred in combination with secondary factors such as post-spawning stress and low dissolved oxygen (Kirk and Lewis, 1994b). Reports of *S. inermis* infections then declined in the UK after the mid-1990s, possibly due to the increasing trend of angling clubs and commercial fisheries to densely populate fishing venues with fish which subsequently predated available aquatic macroinvertebrates, including snail hosts (Brewster, 2000).

16.2. Pathobiology

16.2.1. Diagnosis and clinical signs

Sanguinicolid adult flukes are under-reported from definitive fish hosts because they are small and fragile and will deteriorate within an hour of euthanizing a fish host (Warren *et al.*, 2023). They can be detected by their highly contractile movements when small fish or organs are dissected in water and viewed under a low-power microscope (Kirk and Lewis, 1993). Wet compression mounts of branchial, cardiac, renal, hepatic and cephalic/optic tissue examined by phase contrast microscopy can be used to detect eggs, although egg morphology is not reliable for species discrimination (Fig. 16.3). Previous species identification relied on morphometric analysis but sanguinicolid flukes are difficult to stain, which accounts for the typically poor condition of deposited type and voucher specimens. Molecular diagnostic techniques are in development, particularly use of the *28S* gene. Methods for integrative taxonomic identification are given in Warren *et al.* (2023).

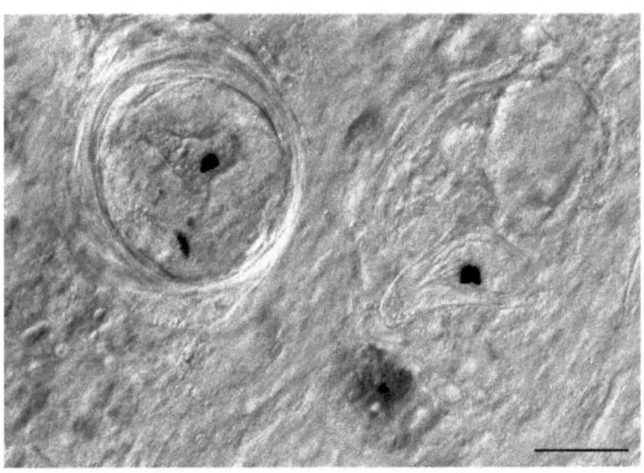

Fig. 16.3. Wet compression mount of kidney tissue from carp showing eggs of *Sanguinicola inermis*. Bar = 25 μm. (Author's own image.)

The diagnoses of the families of fish blood flukes are briefly summarized here (Warren and Bullard, 2023).

- Species of Chimaerohemecidae Yamaguti, 1971 (13 species of 11 genera) infect chimeras, sharks and rays (Chondrichthyes) and have C-shaped lateral tegumental spines and a non-sinusoidal testis or lack spines and have a sinusoidal testis.
- Species of Acipensericolidae Warren and Bullard, 2023 (two species assigned to one genus) infect sturgeons and paddlefish (Acipenseriformes) and have a bowl-shaped, pedunculate anterior sucker, lateral tegumental spines that are spike-like, an inverse U-shaped intestine, six testes, a Laurer's canal, and a dextral common genital pore.
- Species of Sanguinicolidae Poche, 1926 (36 species of seven genera; Table 16.1) infect freshwater ray-finned fishes (Teleostei) and have a diminutive anterior sucker, a medial oesophageal swelling (pouch), short, radial ceca or short anterior ceca plus an elongate, dendritic posterior cecum, testis with appendix-like lateral lobes, and separate or common genital pores.
- Species of Elopicolidae Warren and Bullard, 2023 (four species of two genera) infect ladyfishes, tarpons and catadromous eels (Elopomorpha) and have a bowl-shaped, pedunculate anterior sucker, lateral tegumental spines that are spike-like, short or indistinct anterior ceca, posterior ceca that terminate at level of the testis(es), a single testis or two testes, a Laurer's canal present or absent, and a sinistral common genital pore.
- Species of Aporocotylidae Odhner, 1912 (126 species of 26 genera) primarily infect marine and estuarine ray-finned fishes (Teleostei) and have a spheroid anterior sucker with concentric rows of circumferential spines or the spheroid anterior sucker is lost in adults or adults have a diminutive

> anterior sucker, a sinuous oesophagus lacking a pouch, an X- or H-shaped intestine having four ceca, long anterior ceca (or secondarily lost), posterior ceca that extend posteriad and terminate near the posterior body end, no Laurer's canal, and a sinistral common genital pore or separate genital pores that are sinistral.

The severity of pathological changes is determined by host size and parasite intensity, so young fish and heavily infected fish in hatcheries/intensive fisheries and experimental systems are most likely to exhibit external clinical signs of infection. Anorexia, reduced growth and lethargy of fingerlings with high-intensity infections are typical clinical signs for carp infected with *S. inermis* (Lee, 1990; Kirk and Lewis, 1998) (Fig. 16.4) and cutthroat trout infected with *S. klamathensis* (Evans, 1974a). Respiratory distress due to damage caused by eggs and miracidia accumulating in the gills is exhibited in fingerlings by aggregation at aeration sources (Evans, 1974a; Lee, 1990; Kirk and Lewis, 1998); also observed in brook trout heavily infected with *S. fontinalis* (Hoffman *et al.*, 1985). Not all infected fish show signs of clinical disease. Young carp with low infection intensities and older carp with chronic infections may present with no or few external clinical signs such as reduced growth rate, raised scales, oedema and/or exophthalmia (Sapozhnikov, 1988; Kirk and Lewis, 1994b).

16.2.2. Histopathology

Spines of invading *S. inermis* cercariae form fissures in the epithelial cells of carp and migrating juveniles damage dermal, connective and muscle tissue (Kirk and Lewis, 1998). Adult *S. inermis* flukes perforate the pericardium and blood vessels on entry and then brace against the walls, utilizing club-shaped setae and a lobed tegument to resist the blood flow. Their presence elicits hyperplasia of the endothelial lining and high numbers of aggregated flukes partially occlude blood flow from the heart to the gills (Kirk and Lewis, 1998) (Fig. 16.5). Adult *Sanguinicola armata* flukes dilate the branchial arteries of experimentally infected bighead carp (Shaharom-Harrison *et al.*, 2011). *S. idahoensis* adults show a predilection for the eyes of steelhead trout in addition to the vascular system, damaging the choroid coat and iris stroma. Clusters of flukes near to the optic nerve cause the retina to bulge into the vitreous humour and the vascular stroma is disrupted (Schell, 1974).

Most of the pathology is associated with the presence of eggs in blood vessels and host

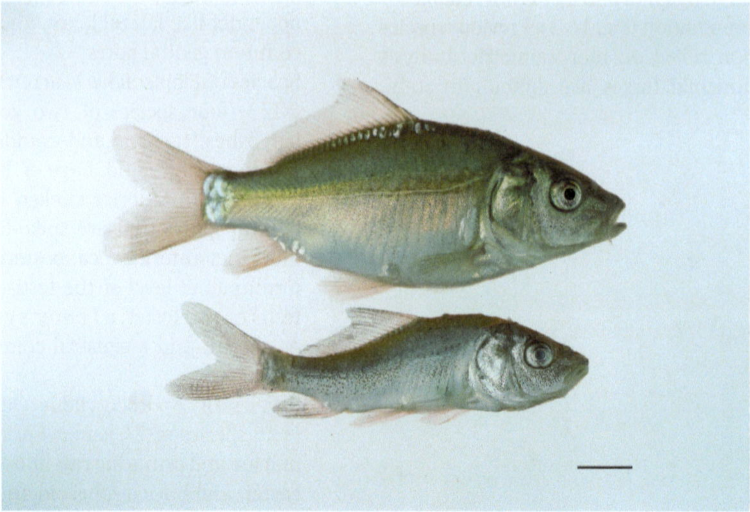

Fig. 16.4. Uninfected 3-month carp fingerling (above) and *Sanguinicola inermis*-infected carp fingerling (below). Bar = 1 cm. (Author's own image.)

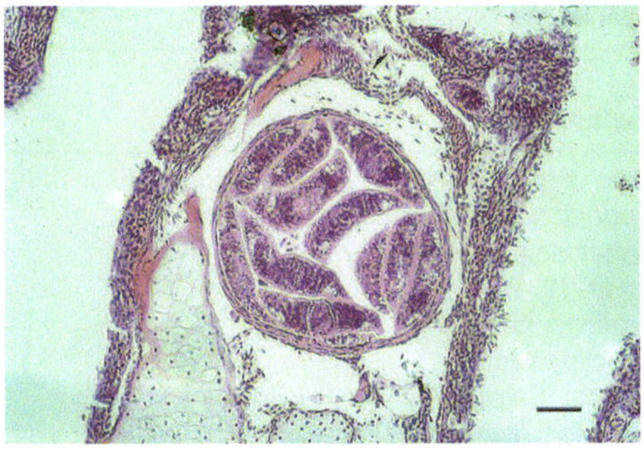

Fig. 16.5. Adult *Sanguinicola inermis* flukes occluding the blood vessel of a carp fingerling. Haematoxylin and eosin section. Bar = 100 μm. (Author's own image.)

tissue and emigration of miracidia from the gills. Egg production of *S. inermis* in experimentally infected carp commences by 28 days post-infection (pi) and peaks at 42 days pi at 20°C, followed by death of adults. Eggs released by adult flukes in the ventral aorta and afferent branchial vessels accumulate in gill vessels (Kirk and Lewis, 1992, 1996). Gill tissue infected by sanguinicolids in wild and laboratory fish exhibits epithelial hyperplasia of primary and secondary lamellae and lamellar fusion, reducing functional respiratory surface. The accumulation of eggs in branchial capillaries ruptures pillar cells and vessel walls, releasing eggs into gill tissue. Eggs elicit eosinophilic infiltration in tissues, and they become surrounded by periovular granulomas (Table 16.2). Vascular embolism by eggs and miracidia and vessel destruction results in ischaemia in the gills, leading to necrosis of gill tissue. The most severe pathology is due to miracidia emigrating from the gills causing mechanical damage, haemorrhage and sometimes death (Fig. 16.6, Table 16.2). Destruction of gill tissue ultimately results in establishment of secondary infections (Kirk and Lewis, 1998). Iqbal and Sommerville (1986) also reported hyperplasia, necrosis and haemorrhage of skin tissue and subsequent osmoregulatory and respiratory failure. Many eggs are sequestered in capillaries in other organs including the renal, hepatic, splenic and cephalic tissue and are eventually degraded within periovular granulomas forming dead-end infections (Table 16.2). Granulomatous inflammation damages eggs, but replaces functional tissue, exacerbating pathophysiological impacts (Kirk and Lewis, 1998).

16.2.3. Pathophysiology

Pathology caused by sanguinicolids results in impairment of respiratory, osmoregulatory and haematopoietic functions, but few studies have been carried out to elucidate and quantify pathophysiological changes. Ivasik and Svirepo (1971) reported that the haemoglobin levels of overwintering carp in the Ukraine, lightly and heavily infected with *S. inermis*, were 20 and 61% lower, respectively, than in uninfected carp. Brook trout with branchial bleeding and high intensities of *S. fontinalis* had significantly reduced haematocrits and plasma osmotic pressure in comparison to uninfected fish (Holliday and Fried, 1986). Cutthroat trout infected with *S. klamathensis* had significantly lower haemoglobin levels and packed cell volume than uninfected fish (Evans, 1974a). When 1–3-year-old bermejuela (*Achondrostoma arcasii*) were experimentally infected with *Sanguinicola* sp. (later identified as *S. rutili*), the haemoglobin concentration of infected fish decreased to a low level in the youngest fish after 3 weeks pi (Gomez-Bautista and Simon-Martin, 1987). Iqbal and Sommerville (1986) measured the growth performance of 14-month-old carp that had been infected with *S. inermis* when 2–3 months old, moved from farm tanks and then maintained in experimental conditions over a 16-week period at 20°C. Carp from the 100% infection prevalence group showed a consistently poor growth performance with a specific growth rate of 1.41%/day compared with logarithmic growth in carp from the 20% prevalence group at 1.62%/day. Food conversion and protein efficiency ratios were reported as below standard in both groups. Daily food intake and daily protein intake were particularly low in the 100% prevalence group (109.17 and 53.49 mg, respectively) compared with the 20% prevalence group (240.83 and 118.01 mg, respectively) due to systemic impairment (Iqbal and Sommerville, 1986). Similarly, cutthroat trout infected with *S. klamathensis* declined in total weight compared to control fish (Evans, 1974a).

Table 16.2. Histopathology caused by freshwater Sanguinicolidae eggs and miracidia.

Location	Histopathological response	Parasite species	Host species	Reference
Gills	Epithelial hyperplasia, lamellar fusion	*Sanguinicola armata* Plehn, 1905	Bighead carp, *Hypophthalmicthys nobilis* (Richardson, 1845) Okada, 1961 (Cypriniformes: Xenocyprididae)	Shaharom-Harrison *et al.* (2011)[a]
		Sanguinicola fontinalis Hoffman, Fried, and Harvey, 1985	Brook trout, *Salvelinus fontinalis* (Mitchill, 1814) Okada, 1961 (Salmoniformes: Salmonidae)	Hoffman *et al.* (1985)[b]
		Sanguinicola idahoensis Schell, 1974	Rainbow trout, *Oncorhynchus mykiss* (Walbaum, 1792) Tomelleri and Eberle, 1990 (Salmoniformes: Salmonidae)	Schell (1974)[a]
		Sanguinicola inermis Plehn, 1905	Eurasian carp, *Cyprinus carpio* Linnaeus, 1758 (Cypriniformes: Cyprinidae)	Hlond *et al.* (1977)[b]; Iqbal and Sommerville (1986)[b]; Lee (1990)[b]; Kirk and Lewis (1998)[a]
		Sanguinicola klamathensis Wales, 1958	Cutthroat trout, *Oncorhynchus clarkii* (Richardson, 1836) McAllister, 1990 (Salmoniformes: Salmonidae)	Evans (1974b)[a]
		Sanguinicola lungensis Tang and Ling, 1975	Bighead carp, *H. nobilis* (Richardson, 1845) Okada, 1961 (Cypriniformes: Xenocyprididae); silver carp, *Hypophthalmichthys molitrix* (Valenciennes, 1844) Berg, 1949 (Cypriniformes: Xenocyprididae)	Tang and Ling (1975)[b]
	Granulomas around eggs	*S. armata* Plehn, 1905	Bighead carp, *H. nobilis* (Richardson, 1845) Okada, 1961 (Cypriniformes: Xenocyprididae)	Shaharom-Harrison *et al.* (2011)[a]
		S. inermis Plehn, 1905	Eurasian carp, *C. carpio* Linnaeus, 1758 (Cypriniformes: Cyprinidae)	Iqbal and Sommerville (1986)[b]; Lee (1990)[b]; Kirk and Lewis (1998)[a]
	Haemorrhage	*S. fontinalis* Hoffman, Fried, and Harvey, 1985	Brook trout, *Salv. fontinalis* (Mitchill, 1814) Okada, 1961 (Salmoniformes: Salmonidae)	Hoffman *et al.* (1985)[b]; Holliday and Fried (1986)[b]

Continued

Table 16.2. Continued.

Location	Histopathological response	Parasite species	Host species	Reference
		S. idahoensis Schell, 1974	Rainbow trout, *O. mykiss* (Walbaum, 1792) Tomelleri and Eberle, 1990 (Salmoniformes: Salmonidae)	Schell (1974)[a]
		S. inermis Plehn, 1905	Eurasion carp, *C. carpio* Linnaeus, 1758 (Cypriniformes: Cyprinidae)	Hlond *et al.* (1977)[b]; Iqbal and Sommerville (1986)[b]; Lee (1990)[b]; Kirk and Lewis (1998)[a]
		S. klamathensis Wales, 1958	Cutthroat trout, *Oncorhynchus clarkii* (Richardson, 1836) McAllister, 1990 (Salmoniformes: Salmonidae)	Evans (1974a)[a]
	Necrosis	*S. inermis* Plehn, 1905	Eurasion carp, *C. carpio* Linnaeus, 1758 (Cypriniformes: Cyprinidae)	Iqbal and Sommerville (1986)[b]; Lee (1990)[b]; Kirk and Lewis (1998)[a]
Other organs including kidney, liver, heart, brain	Granulomas around eggs	*S. inermis* Plehn, 1905	Eurasion carp, *C. carpio* Linnaeus, 1758 (Cypriniformes: Cyprinidae)	Iqbal and Sommerville (1986)[b]; Lee (1990)[b]; Kirk and Lewis (1998)[a]
		S. klamathensis Wales, 1958	Cutthroat trout, *O. clarkii* (Richardson, 1836) McAllister, 1990 (Salmoniformes: Salmonidae)	Evans (1974b)[a]
		S. lungensis Tang and Ling, 1975	Bighead carp, *H. nobilis* (Richardson, 1845) Okada, 1961 (Cypriniformes: Xenocyprididae); silver carp, *H. molitrix* (Valenciennes, 1844) Berg, 1949 (Cypriniformes: Xenocyprididae)	Tang and Ling (1975)[b]
Kidney	Hypertrophy, oedema, necrosis	*S. fontinalis* Hoffman, Fried, and Harvey, 1985	Brook trout, *Salv. fontinalis* (Mitchill, 1814) Okada, 1961 (Salmoniformes: Salmonidae)	Hoffman *et al.* (1985)[b]
		S. inermis Plehn, 1905	Eurasian carp, *C. carpio* Linnaeus, 1758 (Cypriniformes: Cyprinidae)	Lee (1990)[b], Kirk and Lewis (1998)[a]
		S. klamathensis Wales, 1958	Cutthroat trout, *O. clarkii* (Richardson, 1836) McAllister, 1990 (Salmoniformes: Salmonidae)	Evans (1974b)[a]

[a]Laboratory-infected fish; [b]wild or hatchery-infected fish.

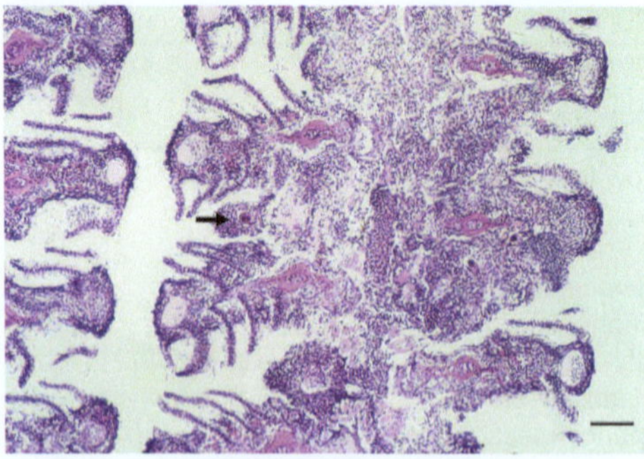

Fig. 16.6. *Sanguinicola inermis* eggs in the gills of a carp fingerling, note emigrating miracidium (arrowed). Haematoxylin and eosin section. Bar = 100 μm. (Author's own image.)

16.3. Protective and Control Strategies

16.3.1. Innate immunity

Most information is on immune responses in *C. carpio* infected with *S. inermis*. Eggs, adults and cercariae of *S. inermis* induce a cell-mediated response in carp. Ultrastructural studies by Richards *et al.* (1994a) show that granulomatous encapsulation around clusters of eggs in the mesonephric interstitial tissue commences with the aggregation of eosinophils around 0–1-week-old eggs (5 weeks pi). The eosinophils degranulate into an amorphous layer of cell debris around the eggs, possibly promoting infiltration by neutrophils and macrophages which surround 1–2-week-old eggs. Neutrophils and monocytes/macrophages phagocytose damaged tissues and are probably responsible for the breakdown of eggs and enclosed miracidia trapped within granulomas when eggs are 5–6 weeks old (9 weeks pi). The macrophages likely stimulate the deposition of collagenous and fibrotic connective tissue around the eggs as in schistosomiasis (Richards *et al.*, 1994a). Early events in the cell-mediated reaction to sequestered eggs in tissues and pathology in the gills are reflected by changes in the cellular composition of lymphoid organs between 5 and 9 weeks pi compared to uninfected control carp (Richards *et al.*, 1994b). Decreases in the numbers of pronephric and splenic eosinophils in this time period reflect their early involvement in the response to egg antigens and migration into associated sites of inflammation. Increases in splenic and pronephric macrophages and pronephric neutrophils occur when these cells predominate in the encapsulating granulomatous tissue around eggs. Levels of pronephric and splenic erythrocytes decrease between 5 and 9 weeks pi, probably due to haemorrhage in the gill tissue (Richards *et al.*, 1994b), while increasing numbers of splenic thrombocytes in infected carp are associated with subsequent coagulation processes (Richards *et al.*, 1994b).

Extracts of cercariae and adults have been shown to elicit proliferation of carp pronephric and splenic lymphocytes under *in vitro* conditions (Richards *et al.*, 1996a). Blastogenic response is dependent on temperature, host lymphoid organ and parasite stage. The highest levels of pronephric lymphocyte proliferation in response to cercariae and adult extracts occur at 20°C compared to 10°C. Adult worms are more mitogenic to splenic lymphocytes at 10°C than at 20°C. Adult extracts are more mitogenic than those of cercariae at both temperatures (Richards *et al.*, 1996a).

Humoral immune responses, probably mediated by pronephric lymphocytes, may be important in reducing fluke numbers in carp during the summer, but may not operate at lower temperatures. A reduced cell-mediated immune capacity may enable penetration of cercariae and survival of juveniles during spring and autumn and permit adult flukes to overwinter in carp (Richards *et al.*, 1996a). This hypothesis is supported by longevity data from experimental infections in which *S. inermis* adults survive up to 10 weeks pi at 20°C (Kirk and Lewis, 1996) and up to ~210 days at 15–18°C (Sommerville and Iqbal, 1991).

Live adults and cercariae induce polarization of pronephric neutrophils and eosinophils (Richards *et al.*, 1996b). Leucocytes readily attach to cercariae within 12 h and cause tegumental damage, but fewer leucocytes attach to post-penetration juveniles and adults. This suggests that transformation from cercariae to juveniles and adult stages may involve changes in the tegument that enable the adult flukes to evade the cellular immune response (Richards *et al.*, 1996c).

16.3.2. Adaptive immunity

There is evidence that *S. inermis* can elicit a humoral response which involves specific antibody production and non-specific complement activity. An ELISA developed by Roberts *et al.* (2005) showed that parasite-specific antibodies were detected in the serum of carp intraperitoneally injected with 150 live cercariae of *S. inermis* and maintained at 20 or 25°C, but not when exposed to 500 cercariae (Roberts *et al.*, 2005). Serum antibody levels peaked after 7 days at both temperatures and then remained at a constantly elevated titre for 63 days at 25°C. They declined at 20°C to below control levels, again emphasizing the influence of temperature on immune reactions to the parasite. The lack of an antibody response in carp naturally exposed to cercariae may be associated with the capability of *S. inermis* to bind host-like antibodies to its surface tegument or modulate antibody levels as part of an immune evasion/suppression strategy (Roberts *et al.*, 2005). Similar evasion strategies are demonstrated by mammalian adult schistosomes (reviewed in Schroeder *et al.*, 2009). Although immune evasion strategies may operate in *S. inermis*, they appear to offer limited protection since less than 7% of the original exposure dose survived to produce eggs in the vascular system of carp in experimental infections at 20°C (Richards *et al.*, 1994b; Kirk and Lewis, 1996). Deficiency in defence mechanisms may reduce pathogenicity in the host and therefore be advantageous for the parasite. Evidence for a partial acquired resistance in carp is indicated in studies by Roberts (1997) which show that when carp receive a challenge infection at 8 months post-primary infection (ppi), significantly fewer adult flukes established compared with the number present at 35 days pi in the primary infection. Numbers were not significantly decreased in a challenge infection administered at 13 months ppi.

Complement activity is induced by infection with cercariae of *S. inermis*. Fish intraperitoneally injected with 150 live cercariae and kept at 20 or 25°C displayed a peak in haemolytic complement activity at 3 weeks pi while those fish exposed to 500 cercariae and maintained at 20°C showed a peak in complement activity at 5 weeks pi, coincident with egg production, and then a decline to control levels (Roberts *et al.*, 2005). Elevated levels of complement activity probably result from increases in macrophages in the spleen and pronephros and other immune cells as complement in carp is associated with pronephric granulocytes and macrophages (Nakao *et al.*, 2003) and peripheral lymphocytes (Nakao *et al.*, 2004). The cercariae and eggs of *S. inermis* are potent inducers of complement activity.

16.3.3. Control measures

In a pond farm environment, an integrated approach involving parasite and snail control has been found to be effective in eliminating sanguinicoliasis from carp ponds. Selected ponds can be kept dry over the summer or winter as traditionally practised in Central Europe to interrupt transmission of *S. inermis* and other helminth parasites (Horák *et al.*, 2024). As snails can survive in the mud of drained ponds, compounds relatively harmless to the environment such as burnt lime can be applied to the surface. Application of molluscicides such as copper sulfate is not recommended due to their ecotoxicity (Horák *et al.*, 2024). Snails have been excluded from filled ponds and supply systems by wire-mesh traps and strategies for environmental management can include removal of snail biotopes like ditches and pits (Sapozhnikov, 1988). Vegetation can be removed from littoral zones where feasible and snail-eating fish can be introduced (Horák *et al.*, 2024).

Praziquantel (Droncit®) is one of the most effective broad-spectrum anthelmintics used for platyhelminth parasite control (Norbury *et al.*, 2022). It is the only medication that has been efficacious in controlling blood fluke infections in fish and is commercially used against marine blood flukes in farmed bluefin tuna and amberjacks (Widdicombe *et al.*, 2024). However, praziquantel for treatment of fish for human consumption is only registered for use by certain governments under restricted conditions, so application in aquaculture/food production is typically 'off label' under specific veterinary jurisdiction (Norbury *et al.*, 2022). Praziquantel is recommended for use against *Sanguinicola* in ornamental fish (Andrews *et al.*, 1988) but there is no specific treatment regimen, presumably due to a lack of recent drug efficacy studies.

Praziquantel has no significant effect on blood fluke eggs and viability of miracidia and does not prevent reinfection (Shirakashi *et al.*, 2012).

The optimum method of praziquantel delivery depends on the scale required, fish hosts and their willingness to feed, environmental setting, practicality and economics (Norbury *et al.*, 2022). Oral delivery is the most convenient and cost-effective method when combined with feed but needs uniform consumption in the treated population (Norbury *et al.*, 2022). Wildgoose and Lewbart (2001) recommend a praziquantel dose regimen of three treatments of 5–12 g/kg feed every 24 h for treating ornamental fish for digenean parasites. Praziquantel has very low palatability (Shirakashi *et al.*, 2012) so lower dietary inclusion levels will reduce problems with feeding, an important issue when treating fish with reduced appetites (Norbury *et al.*, 2022). Combination of praziquantel with fish (fresh or defrosted) will also encourage feeding (reviewed in Power *et al.*, 2020). Praziquantel baths ensure uniform treatment of fish and are suitable for a small number of fish but are labour-intensive in an aquaculture setting and can be stressful for fish. Disposal of large volumes of water containing praziquantel may result in negative environmental impacts for non-target species and possibly resistance development (Norbury *et al.*, 2022). Wildgoose and Lewbart (2001) recommend three treatments of 2–10 mg/l up to 4 h in duration repeated every 5 days for eliminating digenean infections from ornamental fish. Products containing praziquantel in a soluble formulation for closed water systems are widely available for aquarium and ornamental fish keepers. The discussed methods of control are not appropriate for extensive/recreational fisheries so regular monitoring of stocks and veterinary inspections prior to fish movements should be practised.

16.4. Conclusions and Suggestions for Future Studies

Species of Sanguinicolidae are pathogenic to their fish hosts due to the intense cellular response elicited by sequestered eggs leading to periovular granuloma formation, and mechanical damage caused by migrating juveniles, adults and miracidia. Pathophysiological impairment of organ systems due to freshwater sanguinicolids has been inadequately studied, but there is little incentive to fund studies now that effective interventions have been developed against the disease in cultured fish. However, the *S. inermis*–carp model shows great potential for the investigation of blood fluke immune evasion/suppression strategies and many aspects of the fish immune system including complement and helper T cell (Th2) type responses. The immunopathological response of carp hosts to *S. inermis* eggs shows a similarity to granuloma formation in schistosome-infected mice in which interleukin (IL-4) has a major role in driving the Th2 response to the eggs, including the inducement of alternative activation of macrophages (Sandor *et al.*, 2003). The *S. inermis*–carp model can, therefore, be used in the investigation of alternatively activated macrophages in fish immune systems (Joerink *et al.*, 2006). No anti-helminthic vaccines are available for fish, and their development would require considerable elucidation of key antigen targets and further insights into host responses to their parasites.

Recent research on fish blood flukes has largely concentrated on the discovery and description of new species, particularly within the Chimaerohemecidae and Aporocotylidae. However, with recent taxonomic revisions and the availability of nucleotide sequence data for several freshwater genera, there is a renewed opportunity, and need, to focus efforts on the Sanguinicolidae. Despite their significance, the species remain poorly understood. These taxa are especially challenging because they are small and delicate as well as the poor condition of type material and historically inadequate species descriptions. Future revisionary work will require new collections from type localities, though in many cases, these sites are now difficult or inaccessible places to work. While sequence data, particularly *28S* rDNA, has become the standard in modern species descriptions, there has been a growing trend towards a lack in morphological detail. This problem is likely to worsen as advancements in genomic sequencing become more available, potentially leading researchers to minimize morphological characterization altogether. To counter this, future research should emphasize robust morphological descriptions linked to museum voucher specimens supported with relevant sequence data (*28S*). This standard should also extend to life-cycle studies, particularly in the description and identification of larval stages, ensuring comprehensive and reproducible species diagnoses across all developmental stages.

References

Akhmerov, A.A. (1959) [A new trematode genus from fish.] *Trudy Gel'mintologicheskoi Laboratorii* 9, 45–48 (in Russian) (quoted from Yamaguti, 1971).

Akhmerov, A.A. (1960) [New trematodes from fish in the Amur River.] *Helminthologia* 2, 286–294 (in Russian; English, French and German summaries p. 294).

Andrews, C., Exell, A. and Carrington, N. (1988) *The Interpet Manual of Fish Health*. Interpet Publishing, London.

Bacha, W.J. (1966) Life history notes on *Sanguinicola occidentalis* Van Cleave and Mueller, 1932 (Trematoda: Sanguinicolidae) with a redescription of the adult. In: *Program and Abstracts, 41st Annual Meeting*. American Society of Parasitologists, Abstract No. 124.

Bauer, O.N. (1962) The ecology of parasites of freshwater fish. Parasites of freshwater fish and the biological basis for their control. *Bulletin of the State Scientific Research Institute of Lake and River Fisheries* 49, 3–215.

Bobiatynska-Ksok, E. (1964) Circulation cycle of *Sanguinicola* Plehn in the Dojlidy fish pond farm near Bialystok. *Wiadomosci Parazytologiczne* 10, 516–517 (in Polish).

Brewster, B. (2000) Disease management and control in carp fisheries in the United Kingdom. *Journal of the Fish Veterinary Society* (5), 57–63.

Bullard, S.A. and Dutton, H.R. (2022) Resolving the paraphyletic turtle blood flukes: revision of Spirorchiidae Stunkard, 1921 and proposal of Carettacolidae Yamaguti, 1958, Hapalotrematidae (Stunkard, 1921) Poche, 1926, Baracktrematidae n. fam., Plattidae n. fam., and Atamatamidae n. fam. *Journal of Parasitology* 108, 553–564.

Bullard, S.A., Jensen, K. and Overstreet, R.M. (2009) Historical account of the two family-group names in use for the single accepted family comprising the 'fish blood flukes'. *Acta Parasitologica* 54, 78–84.

Bullard, S.A., Roberts, J.R., Warren, M.B., Dutton, H.R. Whelan, N.V. *et al.* (2019) Neotropical turtle blood flukes: two new genera and species from the Amazon river basin with a key to genera and comments on a marine-derived parasite lineage in South America. *Journal of Parasitology* 105, 497–523.

Cutmore, S.C., Littlewood, D.T.J., Arellano-Martínez, M., Louvard, C. and Cribb, T.H. (2023) Evidence that a lineage of teleost-infecting blood flukes (Aporocotylidae) infects bivalves as intermediate hosts. *International Journal for Parasitology* 53, 13–25.

Davis, H.S., Hoffman, G.L. and Surber, E.W. (1961) Notes on *Sanguinicola davisi* (Trematoda: Sanguinicolidae) in the gills of trout. *Journal of Parasitology* 47, 512–514.

Dutton, H.R. and Bullard, S.A. (2020a) *Ruavermis mikebargeri* gen. et sp. n. (Digenea: Schistosomatoidea) infecting the yellow-headed temple turtle, *Heosemys annandalii* (Cryptodira: Geoemydidae), in Vietnam, including an updated phylogeny for the turtle blood flukes. *Folia Parasitologica* 67, 2020.013.

Dutton, H.R. and Bullard, S.A. (2020b) A new species and emendation of the seldom reported *Enterohaematotrema* Mehra, 1940 (Digenea: Schistosomatoidea), including a revised phylogenetic hypothesis for turtle blood flukes. *Systematic Parasitology* 97, 335–345.

Dutton, H.R., Warren, M.B. and Bullard, S.A. (2019) New genus and species of turtle blood fluke (Platyhelminthes: Digenea: Schistosomatoidea) infecting six-tubercled Amazon River turtles, *Podocnemis sextuberculata* (Pleurodira: Podocnemididae) from the Amazon River Basin (Peru). *Journal of Parasitology* 105, 671–685.

Ejsmont, L. (1926) Badania morfologiczne, systematyczne I rozwojowe nad gatunkami rodzaju *Sanguinicola* Plehn [Morphologische, systematische und entwicklungsgeschichtliche Untersuchungen an Arten des Genus *Sanguinicola* Plehn]. *Bulletin International de l'Academie Polonaise des Sciences et des Lettres, Serie B, Classe des Sciences Mathematiques et Naturelles, Sciences Naturelles* 9–10B, 877–966.

Erickson, D.G. and Wallace, F.G. (1959) Studies on blood flukes of the genus *Sanguinicola*. *Journal of Parasitology* 45, 310–322.

Evans, W.A. (1974a) Growth, mortality, and hematology of cutthroat trout experimentally infected with the blood fluke *Sanguinicola klamathensis*. *Journal of Wildlife Diseases* 10, 341–346.

Evans, W.A. (1974b) The histopathology of cutthroat trout experimentally infected with the blood fluke *Sanguinicola klamathensis*. *Journal of Wildlife Diseases* 10, 243–248.

Fischthal, J.H. (1949) *Sanguinicola huronis* n. sp. (Trematoda: Sanguinicolidae) from the blood system of the largemouth and smallmouth basses. *Journal of Parasitology* 35, 566–568.

Gomez-Bautista, M. and Simon-Martin, F. (1987) Haematological alterations in *Rutilus arcasi* (Cyprinidae) experimentally infected with *Sanguinicola* sp. (Digenea: Sanguinicolidae). *Revista Iberica de Parasitologia* Extraordinario, 189–193 (in Spanish).

Guidelli, G.M., Isaac, A. and Pavanelli, G.C. (2002) *Sanguinicola platyrhynchi* n. sp. (Digenea: Sanguinicolidae) parasite of visceral cavity of *Hemisorubim platyrhynchos* (Valenciennes, 1840) (Pisces: Pimelodidae) from the floodplain of the upper Paraná River, Brazil. *Brazilian Journal of Biology* 62, 801–806.

Herbert, B.W. and Shaharom-Harrison, F.M. (1995) A new blood fluke, *Parasanguinicola vastispina* gen. nov., sp. nov. (Trematoda: Sanguinicolidae), from sea bass *Lates calcarifer* (Centropomidae) cultured in Malaysia. *Parasitology Research* 81, 349–354.

Hlond, S., Kozlowski, F. and Szaryk, A. (1977) Gill necrosis in carp fry on the basis of trematode infection with *Sanguinicola inermis* Plehn. *Roczniki Nauk Rolniczych, Poland, Seria H* 98, 65–76 (in Polish).

Hoffman, G.L., Fried, B. and Harvey, J.E. (1985) *Sanguinicola fontinalis* sp. nov. (Digenea: Sanguinicolidae): a blood parasite of brook trout, *Salvelinus fontinalis* (Mitchill), and longnose dace, *Rhinichthys cataractae* (Valenciennes). *Journal of Fish Diseases* 8, 529–538.

Holliday, C.W. and Fried, B. (1986) Some physiological effects of *Sanguinicola fontinalis* (Trematoda: Sanguinicolidae) infection in the brook trout *Salvelinus fontinalis*. *Journal of Parasitology* 72, 189–190.

Horák, P., Bulatanová, J. and Mikeš, L. (2024) Other Schistosomatoidea and Diplostomoidea. In: Toledo, R. and Fried, B. (eds) *Digenetic Trematodes*, 3rd edn. Advances in Experimental Medicine and Biology, Vol. 1454. Springer, Cham, Switzerland, pp. 107–155.

Hu, C.Y., Long, S. and Lee, W.C. (1965) [On the seasonal incidence of the blood flukes of pond fish in Taihu, with a description of a new species of *Sanguinicola*.] *Acta Zoological Sinica* 17, 278–282 (in Chinese).

Imam, E.A., Marzouk, M.S.M., Hassan, A.A. and Itman, R.H. (1984) Studies on *Sanguinicola* sp. (Trematoda) of Nile fishes. *Veterinary Medical Journal* 32, 1–13.

Iqbal, N.A.M. and Sommerville, C. (1986) Effects of *Sanguinicola inermis* Plehn, 1905 (Digenea: Sanguinicolidae) infection on growth performance and mortality in carp, *Cyprinus carpio* L. *Aquaculture and Fisheries Management* 17, 117–122.

Ivasik, V.M. and Svirepo, B.G. (1971) *Sanguinicola inermis* in carp in the winter (Ukranian SSR). *Helminthologia Year 1969* 10, 103–105 (in Russian).

Joerink, M., Forlenza, M., Ribeiro, C.M.S., De Vries, B.J., Savelkoul, H.F.J. *et al.* (2006) Differential macrophage polarisation during parasitic infectins in common carp (*Cyprinus carpio* L.). *Fish and Shellfish Immunology* 21, 561–571.

Kirk, R.S. and Lewis, J.W. (1992) The laboratory maintenance of *Sanguinicola inermis* Plehn, 1905 (Digenea: Sanguinicolidae). *Parasitology* 104, 121–127.

Kirk, R.S. and Lewis, J.W. (1993) The life-cycle and morphology of *Sanguinicola inermis* Plehn, 1905 (Digenea: Sanguinicolidae). *Systematic Parasitology* 25, 125–133.

Kirk, R.S. and Lewis, J.W. (1994a) The distribution and host range of species of the blood fluke *Sanguinicola* in British freshwater fish. *Journal of Helminthology* 68, 315–318.

Kirk, R.S. and Lewis, J.W. (1994b) Sanguinicoliasis in cyprinid fish in the UK. In: Pike, A. and Lewis, J.W. (eds) *Parasitic Diseases of Fish*. Samara Publishing Ltd for the British Society for Parasitology and the Linnean Society of London, Dyfed, UK, pp. 101–117.

Kirk, R.S. and Lewis, J.W. (1996) Migration and development of the blood fluke *Sanguinicola inermis* Plehn, 1905 (Trematoda: Sanguinicolidae) in carp, *Cyprinus carpio* L. *Parasitology* 113, 279–285.

Kirk, R.S. and Lewis, J.W. (1998) Histopathology of *Sanguinicola inermis* infection in carp, *Cyprinus carpio*. *Journal of Helminthology* 72, 33–38.

Kirk, R.S. (2012) *Sanguinicola inermis* and related species. In: Woo. P.T.K. and Buchmann, K. (eds) *Fish Parasites: Pathobiology and Protection*. CAB International, Wallingford, UK, pp. 270–281.

Lee (Kirk), R.S. (1990) The development of *Sanguinicola inermis* Plehn, 1905 (Digenea: Sanguinicolidae) in the common carp (*Cyprinus carpio* L.). PhD thesis, University of London, London.

Li, L. (1980) [Studies on the agency of sanguinicoliasis of blunt-snout bream (*Megalobrama amblycephala*) and its control, with description of a new species.] *Journal of Fisheries of China* 4, 179–196 (in Chinese).

Lucky, Z. (1964) Contribution to the biology and pathogenicity of *Sanguinicola inermis* in juvenile carp. In: *Proceedings of the Symposium on Parasitic Worms and Aquatic Conditions*. Czechoslovak Academy of Sciences, Prague, pp. 153–157.

McMichael-Phillips, D.F., Lewis, J.W. and Thorndyke, M.C. (1992a) Ultrastructure of the egg of *Sanguinicola inermis* Plehn, 1905 (Digenea: Sanguinicolidae). *Journal of Natural History* 26, 895–904.

McMichael-Phillips, D.F., Lewis, J.W. and Thorndyke, M.C. (1992b) Ultrastructural studies on the miracidium of *Sanguinicola inermis* (Digenea: Sanguinicolidae). *Parasitology* 105, 435–443.

McMichael-Phillips, D.F., Lewis, J.W. and Thorndyke, M.C. (1994) Ultrastructure of the digestive system of adult *Sanguinicola inermis* Plehn, 1905 (Digenea: Sanguinicolidae). *Journal of Helminthology* 68, 149–154.

Meade, T.G. (1967) Life history studies on *Cardicola klamathensis* (Wales, 1958) Meade and Pratt, 1965 (Trematoda: Sanguinicolidae). *Proceedings of the Helminthological Society of Washington* 34, 210–212.

Meade, T.G. and Pratt, I. (1965) Description and life history of *Cardicola alseae* sp. n. (Trematoda: Sanguinicolidae). *Journal of Parasitology* 51, 575–578.

Moravec, F. (1984) Occurrence of endoparasitic helminths in carp (*Cyprinus carpio* L.) from the Macha lake fishpond system. *Vestnik Ceskoslovenske Spolecrosti Zooligicke* 48, 261–278.

Nakao, M., Fujiki, K., Konodo, M. and Yano, T. (2003) Detection of complement receptors on head kidney phagocytes of common carp *Cyprinus carpio*. *Fisheries Science* 65, 929–935.

Nakao, M., Miura, C., Itoh, S., Nakahara, M., Okumura, K. *et al.* (2004) A complement C3 fragment equivalent to mammalian C3d from the common carp (*Cyprinus carpio*): generation in serum after activation of the alternative pathway and detection of its receptor on the lymphocyte surface. *Fish and Shellfish Immunology* 16, 139–149.

Naumova, A.M. (1961) Seasonal dynamics of *Sanguinicola inermis* infections in carp. *Doklady Moskovskoĭ Sel'sko-Khozyaistvennoĭ Akademii imenika K.A. Timiryazeva* 69, 211–216 (in Russian).

Nolan, M.J. and Cribb, T.H. (2005) *Sanguinicola maritimus* n. sp. (Digenea: Sanguinicolidae) from Labridae (Teleostei: Perciformes) of southern Australian waters. *Systematic Parasitology* 61, 99–106.

Norbury, L.J., Shirakashi, S., Power, C., Nowak, B.F. and Bott, N.J. (2022) Praziquantel use in aquaculture – current status and emerging issues. *International Journal for Parasitology: Drugs and Drug Resistance* 18, 87–102. DOI: 10.1016/j.ijpddr.2022.02.001.

Odhner, T. (1911) *Sanguinicola* M. Plehn – a digenean trematode! With an appendum on previous observations of Prof. A. Looss, Kairo. *Zoologischer Anzeiger* 38, 33–45 (in German).

Odhner, T. and Woodland, W.N.F. (1924) Remarks on *Sanguinicola*. *Journal of Cell Science* 2, 403–411.

Olson, P.D., Cribb, T.H., Tkach, V.V., Bray, R.A. and Littlewood, D.T. (2003) Phylogeny and classification of the Digenea (Platyhelminthes: Trematoda). *International Journal for Parasitology* 33, 733–755.

Orélis-Ribeiro, R. and Bullard, S.A. (2015) Blood flukes (Digenea: Aporocotylidae) infecting body cavity of South American catfishes (Siluriformes: Pimelodidae): two new species from rivers in Bolivia, Guyana and Peru with a re-assessment of *Plehniella* Szidat, 1951. *Folia Parasitologica* 62, 2015.050.

Orélis-Ribeiro, R. and Bullard, S.A. (2016) Two new genera of fish blood flukes (Digenea: Aporocotylidae) from catfishes in the Peruvian Amazon. *Journal of Parasitology* 102, 357–368.

Orélis-Ribeiro, R., Arias, C.R., Halanych, K.M., Cribb, T.H. and Bullard, S.A. (2014) Diversity and ancestry of flatworms infecting blood of nontetrapod craniates 'fishes'. *Advances in Parasitology* 85, 1–64.

Paperna, I. (1964) Parasitic helminths of inland-water fishes in Israel. *Israel Journal of Zoology* 13, 1–26.

Plehn, M. (1905) *Sanguinicola armata* und *inermis* (n. gen. n. sp.) n. fam. Rhynchostomida. Endoparasitic turbellaria in the blood of cyprinids. *Zoologischer Anzeiger* 29, 244–252 (in German).

Plehn, M. (1908) Monozoic cestodes as blood parasites (*Sanguinicola armata* und *inermis* Plehn). *Zoologischer Anzeiger* 33, 427–440 (in German).

Poddubnaya, L.G., Warren, M.B. and Bullard, S.A. (2023) Foregut ultrastructure of adult *Sanguinicola volgensis* (Rašín, 1929) Mcintosh, 1934 (Digenea: Aporocotylidae). *Journal of Parasitology* 109, 27–34.

Power, C., Nowak, B.F., Cribb, T.H. and Bott, N.J. (2020) Bloody flukes: a review of aporocotylids as parasites of cultured marine fishes. *International Journal for Parasitology* 50, 743–753.

Rašín, K. (1929) *Janickia volgensis*. Gen. n. sp., krevnl motolice z ryby *Pelecus cultratus* (L.). *Biologicke Spisy Vysoke Skoly Zverolekarske* Brno 8, Art. 16, 21 pp. (in Czechoslovakian; German summary pp. 17–21).

Richards, D.T., Hoole, D., Lewis, J.W., Ewens, E. and Arme, C. (1994a) Ultrastructural observations on the cellular response of carp, *Cyprinus carpio* L., to eggs of the blood fluke *Sanguinicola inermis* Plehn, 1905 (Trematoda: Sanguinicolidae). *Journal of Fish Diseases* 17, 439–446.

Richards, D.T., Hoole, D., Lewis, J.W., Ewens, E. and Arme, C. (1994b) Changes in the cellular composition of the spleen and pronephros of carp *Cyprinus carpio* infected with the blood fluke *Sanguinicola inermis* (Trematoda: Sanguinicolidae). *Diseases of Aquatic Organisms* 19, 173–179.

Richards, D.T., Hoole, D., Lewis, J.W., Ewens, E. and Arme, C. (1996a) Stimulation of carp *Cyprinus carpio* lymphocytes *in vitro* by the blood fluke *Sanguinicola inermis* (Trematoda: Sanguinicolidae). *Diseases of Aquatic Organisms* 25, 87–93.

Richards, D.T., Hoole, D., Lewis, J.W., Ewens, E. and Arme, C. (1996b) *In vitro* polarization of carp leucocytes in response to the blood fluke *Sanguinicola inermis* Plehn, 1905 (Trematoda: Sanguinicolidae). *Parasitology* 112, 509–513.

Richards, D.T., Hoole, D., Lewis, J.W., Ewens, E. and Arme, C. (1996c) Adherence of carp leucocytes to adults and cercariae of the blood fluke *Sanguinicola inermis*. *Journal of Helminthology* 70, 63–67.

Roberts, M.L. (1997) The immune response of carp (*Cyprinus carpio* L.) to the blood fluke *Sanguinicola inermis* Plehn, 1905 (Trematoda: Sanguinicolidae). PhD thesis, Keele University, Keele, UK.

Roberts, M.L., Lewis, J.W., Wiegertjes, G.F. and Hoole, D. (2005) Interaction between the blood fluke, *Sanguinicola inermis* and humoral components of the immune response of carp, *Cyprinus carpio*. *Parasitology* 131, 261–271.

Sandor, M., Weinstock, J.V. and Wynn, T.A. (2003) Granulomas in schistosome and mycobacterial infections: a model of local immune responses. *Trends in Immunology* 24, 44–52.

Sapozhnikov, G.L. (1988) *Sanguinicola* infestation in carp and its control. *Veterinariya (Moscow, USSR)* 8, 36–38 (in Russian).

Schell, S.C. (1974) The life history of *Sanguinicola idahoensis* sp. n. (Trematoda: Sanguiniciolidae), a blood parasite of steelhead trout, *Salmo gairdneri* Richardson. *Journal of Parasitology* 60, 561–566.

Schroeder, H., Skelly, P.J., Zipfel, P.F., Losson, B. and Vanderplasschen, A. (2009) Subversion of complement by hematophagous parasites. *Developmental and Comparative Immunology* 33, 5–13.

Shaharom-Harrison, F., Seman, N.A. and Suhairi, M. (2011) Laboratory experimental infection of the freshwater snail experimental infection of the freshwater snail *Gyraulus convexiusculus* (Hutton, 1849) and the bighead carp *Aristichthys nobilis* (Richardson, 1845) with the blood fluke *Sanguinicola armata* Plehn, 1905. In: *Diseases in Asian Aquaculture VII*. Fish Health Section, Asian Fisheries Society, Selangor, Malaysia, pp. 63–71.

Shimazu, T. (2007) Digeneans (Trematoda) of freshwater fishes from Nagano Prefecture, Central Japan. *Bulletin of the National Museum of Nature and Science Series A* 33, 1–30.

Shimazu, T. (2013) Digeneans parasitic in freshwater fishes (Osteichthyes) of Japan. I. Aporocotylidae, Bivesiculidae, and Haploporidae. *Bulletin of the National Museum of Nature and Science Series A* 39, 167–184.

Shirakashi, S., Andrews, M., Kishimoto, Y., Ishimaru, K., Okada, T. *et al.* (2012) Oral treatment of praziquantel as an effective control measure against blood fluke infection in Pacific bluefin tuna (*Thunnus orientalist*). *Aquaculture* 326–329, 15–19. DOI: 10.1016/j.aquaculture.2011.10.035.

Simon-Martin, F., Rojo-Vazquez, F.A. and Simon-Vicente, F. (1987) *Sanguinicola rutili* n. sp. (Digenea: Sanguinicolidae) parasito del sistema circulatorio de *Rutilus arcasi* (Cyprinidae) en la provincia de Salamanca. *Revista Iberica de Parasitologia* 47, 253–261.

Smith, J.W. (1997a) The blood flukes (Digenea: Sanguinicolidae and Spirorchidae) of cold-blooded vertebrates. Part 1. A review of the published literature since 1971, and bibliography. *Helminthological Abstracts* 66, 255–294.

Smith, J.W. (1997b) The blood flukes (Digenea: Sanguinicolidae and Spirorchidae) of cold-blooded vertebrates. Part 2. Appendix I. Comprehensive parasite–host list; Appendix II: Comprehensive host–parasite list. *Helminthological Abstracts* 66, 329–344.

Sommerville, C. and Iqbal, N.A.M. (1991) The process of infection, migration, growth and development of *Sanguinicola inermis* Plehn, 1905 (Digenea: Sanguinicolidae) in carp, *Cyprinus carpio* L. *Journal of Fish Diseases* 14, 211–219.

Sweeting, R.A. (1979) *Sanguinicola* – a case study. *Proceedings of the Institute of Fisheries Management 10th Annual Study Course* 10, 217–220.

Szidat, L. (1951) Neue Arten der Trematoden familie Aporocotylidae aus dem Blut und der Leibeshole von Stisswasserfischen des Rio de la Plata. *Zeitschrift für Parasitenkunde* 15, 70–86 (Spanish summary p. 85).

Tang, C.C. and Ling, S.M. (1975) *Sanguinicola lungensis* sp. nov. and the outbreaks of sanguinicolosis in Lien-yü nursery ponds in South Fukien. *Journal of Xiamen University (Natural Science)* 2, 139–160 (in Chinese).

Truong, T.N. and Bullard, S.A. (2013) Blood flukes (Digenea: Aporocotylidae) of walking catfishes (Siluriformes: Clariidae): new genus and species from the Mekong River (Vietnam) with comments on related catfish aporocotylids. *Folia Parasitologica* 60, 237.

Van Cleave, H.J. and Mueller, J.F. (1932) Parasites of the Oneida Lake fishes. Part 1. Descriptions of new genera and new species. *Roosevelt Wild Life Annals* 3, 1–71.

Wales, J.H. (1958) Two new blood fluke parasites of trout. *California Fish and Game* 44, 125–136.

Wang, H. (1982) [Parasitic trematodes from fishes of Poyang Lake II. Four new species of the families Echinostomatidae, Gorgoderidae, and Sanguinicolidae.] *Acta Zootaxonomica Sinica* 7, 353–358 (in Chinese; English summary pp. 358–359).

Wang, H. (1983) [Parasitic trematodes from fishes of Poyang Lake VI. Descriptions of four new species of Opecoelidae and other families.] *Acta Zootaxonomica Sinica* 8, 337–344 (in Chinese; English summary pp. 343–344).

Warren, M.B. and Bullard, S.A. (2019) First elucidation of a blood fluke (*Electrovermis zappum* n. gen., n. sp.) life cycle including a chondrichthyan or bivalve. *International Journal for Parasitology: Parasites and Wildlife* 10, 170–183.

Warren, M.B. and Bullard, S.A. (2023) Systematic revision of the fish blood flukes with diagnoses of Chimaerohemecidae Yamaguti, 1971, Acipensericolidae n. fam., Sanguinicolidae poche, 1926, Elopicolidae n. fam., and Aporocotylidae Odhner, 1912. *Journal of Parasitology* 109, 401–418.

Warren, M.B., Bakenhaster, M.D., Dutton, H.R., Ksepka, S.P. and Bullard, S.A. (2021) Redescription of the type species of *Cardicola* Short, 1953 (Digenea: Aporocotylidae) and description of a new congener infecting yellowedge grouper, *Hyporthodus flavolimbatus* (Perciformes: Serranidae), from the Gulf of Mexico. *Journal of Parasitology* 107, 59–73.

Warren, M.B., Poddubnaya, L.G., Zhokhov, A.E., Reyda, F.B., Choudhury, A. *et al.* (2023) Revision of *Sanguinicola* Plehn, 1905 with redescription of *Sanguinicola volgensis* (Rašín, 1929) McIntosh, 1934, description of a new species, proposal of a new genus, and phylogenetic analysis. *Journal of Parasitology* 109, 296–321.

Warren, M.B., Jacobs, F., Dutton, H.R., Netherlands, E.C., DuPreez, L.H. *et al.* (2024) First report of a fish blood fluke from sub-Saharan Africa: *Nomasanguinicola dentata* (Paperna, 1964) Warren and Bullard, 2023 infecting African sharptooth catfish, *Clarias gariepinus* (Burchell, 1822) Teugles, 1982 in the Kavango River, Namibia, and a revised phylogeny for Sanguinicolidae Poche, 1926. *Parasitology International* 100, 102862.

Widdicombe, M., Coff, L., Nowak, B.F., Ramsland, P.A. and Bott, N.J. (2024) Understanding the host response of farmed fish to blood flukes (Trematoda: Aporocotylidae) for developing new treatment strategies. *Fish and Shellfish Immunology* 149, 109613. DOI: 10.1016/j.fsi.2024.109613.

Wildgoose, W.H. and Lewbart, G.A. (2001) Chapter 30 – Therapeutics. In: *BSAVA Manual of Ornamental Fish*, 2nd edn. British Small Animal Veterinary Association, Quedgeley, UK, pp. 237–258.

Woodland, W.N.F. (1923) *Sanguinicola* from the Sudan. *Journal of Cell Science* 2, 233–242.

17 *Schyzocotyle acheilognathi*

Roman Kuchta[1], Tomáš Scholz[1]* and Anindo Choudhury[2]

[1]*Institute of Parasitology, Biology Centre of the Academy of Sciences of the Czech Republic, České Budějovice, Czech Republic;* [2]*St. Norbert College, De Pere, Wisconsin, USA*

Abstract

Schyzocotyle acheilognathi (synonym *Bothriocephalus acheilognathi*), commonly known as Asian fish tapeworm (AFT), is a highly invasive cestode that infects a wide range of freshwater fish (>300 species), especially cyprinoids. Its pathobiology involves attachment to the intestinal mucosa, leading to inflammation, impaired nutrient absorption and, in severe cases, host mortality. The parasite poses a significant threat to aquaculture and the biodiversity of native fish worldwide. Effective protection strategies include strict biosecurity measures, routine parasitological screening and targeted treatment with anthelmintics. Environmental management and control of invasive fish species also play an important role in limiting its spread. Understanding host–parasite interactions and transmission dynamics is essential for the development of sustainable control programmes. Although the impact of AFT as a pathogen in Europe has declined in recent decades, it remains a problem for biodiversity and aquaculture, emphasizing the need for effective surveillance and biosecurity to control its spread.

17.1. Introduction

The Asian fish tapeworm, *Schyzocotyle acheilognathi* (Yamaguti, 1934) (synonym *Bothriocephalus acheilognathi* Yamaguti, 1934) (Cestoda: Bothriocephalidea), is the most important pathogenic cestode of cypriniform fish causing bothriocephalosis, and one of the most dangerous helminth parasites of farmed carp (Bauer *et al.*, 1977; Williams and Jones, 1994; Nie and Hoole, 2000; Scholz *et al.*, 2021). The parasite has also been detected in an extraordinarily large number of other freshwater teleosts, raising concerns about the disease in wild fish populations (Clarkson *et al.*, 1997; Heckmann, 2000; Kuchta *et al.*, 2018).

S. acheilognathi, hereafter referred to as AFT, has been reported under more than 20 different specific names, with *Bothriocephalus gowkongensis* Yeh, 1955 and *Bothriocephalus opsariichthydis* Yamaguti, 1934 being the most commonly used (for a list of synonyms, see Kuchta *et al.*, 2018; Marick *et al.*, 2024). Now, all reports of '*Bothriocephalus*' tapeworms from cyprinoids represent *S. acheilognathi* (with the exception of *Schyzocotyle nayarensis* in India; see Marick *et al.*, 2024).

AFT is most probably native to East Asia (see below) but spread rapidly worldwide with the fish trade in the second half of the 20th century (Kuchta *et al.*, 2018). The parasite has now been detected on all continents except Antarctica. The ability to successfully colonize new geographical

*Email: tscholz@paru.cas.cz

 Fish Parasites: Pathobiology and Protection, 2nd Edition (eds P.T.K. Woo and K. Buchmann)
DOI: 10.1079/9781800628748.0017

regions has been facilitated by its simple two-host life cycle and a broad range of fish hosts (Kuchta *et al.*, 2018). This has allowed AFT to establish itself in many new host species in areas where it has been introduced (Kuchta *et al.*, 2018). Once established, it can threaten native fish populations, including ecologically sensitive species and fish that are not closely related to the species in which it was introduced (Font and Tate, 1994; Dove and Fletcher, 2000).

AFT can have pronounced adverse effects on fish. These include severe damage to the digestive tract, physiological disturbances, reduced growth, loss of condition and death. Reports of 100% mortality in hatchery-reared common carp (*Cyprinus carpio*) illustrate the pathogenic potential of this parasite (Davydov, 1978; Hoole and Nisan, 1994).

17.1.1. Description

AFT is typically milky-white, elongate, actively motile and attached to the anterior and middle part of the intestine by a heart-shaped scolex. The worm is between 3.5 and 8 cm long and up to 4 mm wide (Yeh, 1955), although specimens of up to 1 m long have been observed (Baer and Fain, 1958; Granath and Esch, 1983a). Size is highly variable as it depends on: (i) ecological conditions (Nedeva and Mutafova, 1988); (ii) host size (Davydov, 1978); (iii) host species (Molnár and Murai, 1973; Granath and Esch, 1983a); (iv) host age; (v) intensity of infection (Davydov, 1978); (vi) host condition (Davydov, 1978); and (vii) fixation (Pool and Chubb, 1985). Upon relaxation, parasites can also increase in length by a factor of 1.5–2 (Pool, 1987). In contrast to earlier assumptions (Molnár and Murai, 1973), the size of the parasites is therefore not a valid characteristic that can be used for identification.

An important morphological feature is the heart-shaped scolex (in lateral view), with a weakly developed apical disc and a pair of deep, slit-like grooves (bothria) arranged dorsoventrally along the scolex (Fig. 17.1a and e, Fig. 17.2).

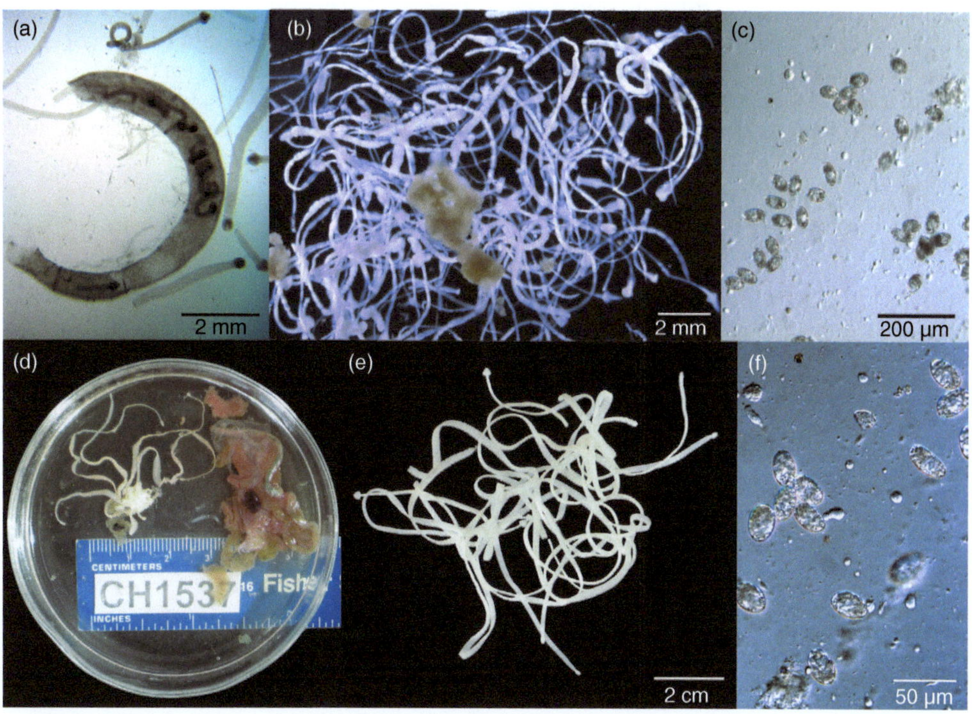

Fig. 17.1. Photomicrographs of *Schyzocotyle acheilognathi in situ*. (a) Immature tapeworms in and outside the intestine of green swordtail, *Xiphophorus helleri* (ornamental fish farm, Czech Republic); (b) immature tapeworms from blue discus fish, *Symphysodon aequifasciatus* (ornamental fish farm, Czech Republic); (c, f) eggs from *S. aequifasciatus* (ornamental fish farm, Czech Republic); (d) tapeworms from the gut of grass carp, *Ctenopharyngodon idella* (Lake Taihu, Wuxi, China); (e) tapeworms fixed with hot formalin. (Authors' own image.)

The scolex is much wider than the first proglottids. The strobila (body) consists of numerous proglottids (Fig. 17.1b), each containing a set of centrally arranged reproductive organs.

The shape of these proglottids varies according to maturity and contraction. Immature proglottids without developed reproductive organs are always wider than long, whereas more developed and gravid proglottids bearing eggs are square or longer than wide. However, the contraction and relaxation of the proglottids also leads to extreme variations in the length and width ratio of the strobila (Brandt *et al.*, 1981).

The male reproductive system of each proglottid consists of numerous spherical testes located in the medulla. A muscular cirrus-sac, located anterior to the ovary, opens on the dorsal side of the proglottids into a common genital atrium located along the midline of the body (Fig. 17.3).

The female reproductive system consists of a bilobed ovary located near the posterior margin of each proglottid. The vagina, which is short and slightly sinuous, opens into the common genital atrium posterior to the male genital pore. The vitelline follicles are very numerous, circumcortical and confluent between the proglottids. The uterus is sac-shaped, spherical to oval and opens on the ventral side in the anterior third of the proglottid (Fig. 17.3). The eggs are thick-walled, operculate (i.e. with a cap) at a narrow pole, about 50 μm long and usually unembryonated (without a formed embryo) when released into the water (Fig. 17.1c and f).

17.1.2. Life cycle and transmission

AFT uses two hosts; a planktonic copepod (Copepoda: Cyclopidae) serves as an intermediate host (Fig. 17.3). However, small fish (prey) can serve as paratenic hosts and thus accumulate juvenile worms in the gastrointestnal tract that can survive longer than larval stages (procercoids) in tiny planktonic copepods. Under favourable conditions, the life cycle can be completed in about 1 month. Eggs are released by adult worms into the intestinal lumen and then shed into the water with the faeces (Fig. 17.1c and f). Depending on the water temperature, an embryo (six-hooked oncosphere or hexacanth) forms inside the egg within a few days. A ciliated larva (coracidium) hatches and moves actively in the water column, attracting copepods (Crustacea: Copepoda) that eat them.

Several species of cyclopoid copepods (Copepoda: Cyclopoida) are suitable intermediate

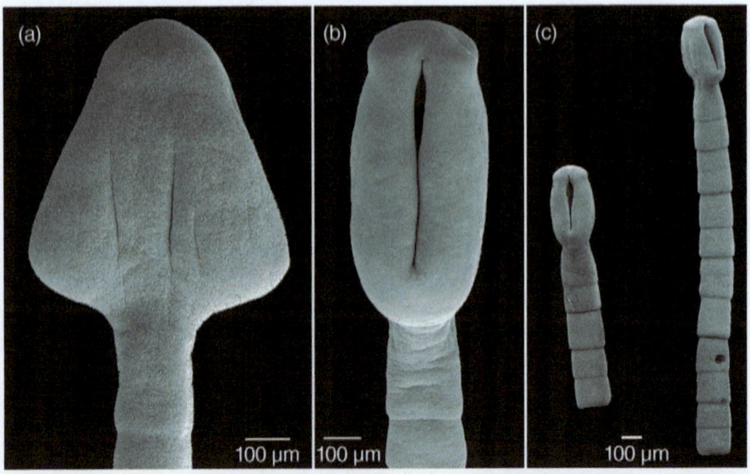

Fig. 17.2. Scanning electron micrographs of the scolex of *Schyzocotyle acheilognathi*. (a, b) Mature tapeworm from common carp, *Cyprinus carpio* (Czech Republic), showing lateral (a) and dorsoventral (b) view; (c) immature tapeworms from blue discus fish, *Symphysodon aequifasciatus* (ornamental fish farm, Czech Republic). (Author's own image.)

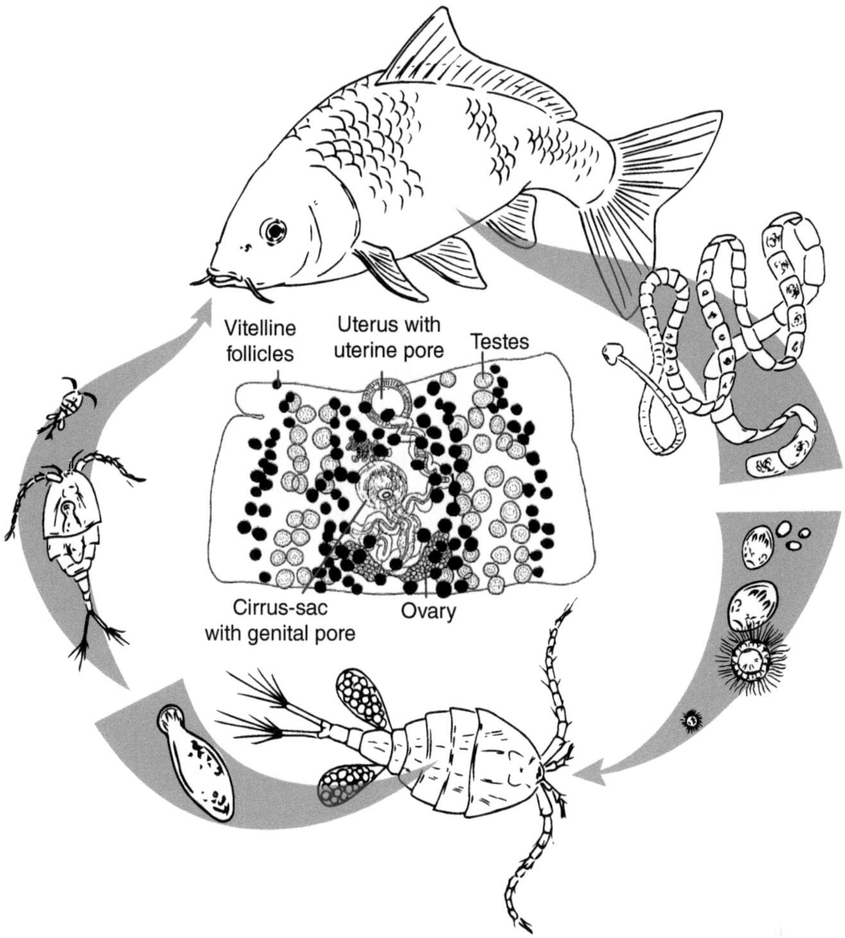

Fig. 17.3. Life cycle of *Schyzocotyle acheilognathi* including the first intermediate host (copepod), definitive host (carp) and mature proglottid in the centre. (Courtesy of Mona Luo.)

hosts under experimental and natural conditions (Pool, 1984; Marcogliese and Esch, 1989). However, other planktonic crustaceans, such as diaptomid copepods (Copepoda: Diaptomidae) and cladocerans (Cladocera), are not suitable intermediate hosts (Molnár, 1977).

After ingestion, the coracidium loses its ciliated covering and enters the body cavity of the copepod intermediate host, where it develops from an oncosphere into a procercoid (Fig. 17.3). Larval development is completed in a few weeks depending on the water temperature: within 21–23 days at 28–29°C (Liao and Shih, 1955), but 1.5–2 months at 15–22°C (Davydov, 1978). If the fish is infected in the autumn in temperate zones, the AFT does not reach maturity until the spring of the following year (Skachkov and Thakahova, 2018). The life cycle is completed when the fish ingests infected copepods, whereafter the tapeworm becomes sexually mature and produces eggs (but not in all hosts). Once established in the intestine of a suitable fish, egg production can begin in as little as 20 days (Liao and Shih, 1955). The lifespan of AFT ranges from several months to over a year (Davydov, 1978).

Transmission of adult parasites from fish to fish can occur through the predation of infected prey by piscivorous fish, a phenomenon known as post-cyclic transmission (Odening, 1976; Hansen *et al.*, 2007). Local spread by waterfowl such as *Anas platyrhynchos* and *Chlidonias niger* has been suggested based on experiments by

Prigli (1975) and field observations (detection of *S. acheilognathi* in *Ixobrychus minutus*) by Borgarenko (1981), but this mode of parasite spread remains to be verified. There is also evidence of that AFT may survive in an amphibian (axolotl, *Ambystoma dumerilii*; García-Prieto and Osorio-Sarabia, 1991), a snake (*Thamnophis melanogaster*; Pérez-Ponce de León *et al.*, 2001) and turtle (*Pelodiscus sinensis*) in Vietnam (T.T. Binh, Institute of Ecology and Biological Resources, Vietnamese Academy of Sciences, Hanoi, October 2010, personal communication), although these may be only incidental infections. Similarly, a single molecularly confirmed case of the eggs in human stool most likely represents an accidental infection or passage of tapeworms through the human digestive tract (Yera *et al.*, 2013).

17.1.3. Definitive (fish) hosts

The most suitable and frequently reported hosts of AFT are cyprinoids (mostly carp and minnows), in particular the common carp (*C. carpio*) and the grass carp (*Ctenopharyngodon idella*), which account for around 34% of the records (Kuchta *et al.*, 2018). However, AFT has also been reported in many freshwater and brackish-water fish and rarely in some amphibians, reptiles and birds (see above), which are most likely post-cyclic hosts. More than 310 species of freshwater fish from 40 families and 14 orders and 11 non-fish species have been reported as hosts (Kuchta *et al.*, 2018; R. Kuchta, 2025, unpublished results). Nevertheless, tapeworms mature only in a relatively small proportion of these fish species (Dove and Fletcher, 2000).

Holmes (1979) distinguishes three host categories according to their ability to enable the maturation of parasites: (i) 'required hosts'; (ii) 'suitable hosts'; and (iii) 'unsuitable hosts'. In 'required hosts' parasites usually reach full maturity. In 'suitable hosts' parasites can reach sexual maturity but are present only in small numbers, while in 'unsuitable hosts' parasites can establish themselves but do not reach sexual maturity. Consequently, while a parasite may infect many fish species, the maintenance of the parasite population may depend on a much narrower range in which reproduction occurs (Riggs *et al.*, 1987). In the case of AFT, this has serious epizootiological consequences.

Small fish are more frequently and intensively infected with AFT than large hosts (Leong, 1986). Brouder (1999) found a strong negative correlation between the size of the host and the intensity of AFT infection.

17.1.4. Geographical distribution

The AFT was originally described in a small cyprinid, *Acheilognathus rhombeus*, from Lake Ogura, Honshu, Japan (Yamaguti, 1934). This tapeworm was most likely originally distributed in Asia (China, Japan and the Amur River), but probably also in tropical Africa, where it was documented before the human introduction of cyprinids from Asia (Yeh, 1955; Dubinina, 1971; Kuchta *et al.*, 2018). The early translocation of AFT was closely related to the westward spread of common carp and grass carp from Far East Russia and China to the western part of the former USSR and to the eastern and central part of the USSR in the 1960s and 1970s (Minervini *et al.*, 1985).

The spread of AFT to most parts of the world is well documented (Bauer and Hoffman, 1976; Kuchta *et al.*, 2018) and represents one of the best examples of parasite translocation through human-assisted activities (Dove and Fletcher, 2000; Kuchta *et al.*, 2018). The rapid spread of this tapeworm has been facilitated by the trade of many cyprinoid species for: (i) aquaculture (Minervini *et al.*, 1985); (ii) the ornamental fish industry (Evans and Lester, 2001); (iii) aquatic weed control (Maitland and Campbell, 1992); (iv) mosquito control (Dove and Fletcher, 2000); and (v) the fish bait industry (Marcogliese *et al.*, 2016; Boonthai *et al.*, 2017).

The AFT was introduced to Europe (Ukraine) in 1954 through the uncontrolled import of grass carp and common carp from the Amur region and China. The tapeworm spread both in farmed carp and in a large number of wild fish (Malevitskaya, 1958; Radulescu and Georgescu, 1962; Bauer and Hoffman, 1976). The increasing importance of carp as food and weed control by grass carp led to a rapid spread of AFT throughout Europe (Kuchta *et al.*, 2018).

By 1970–1975, the AFT had colonized several countries in Central and Eastern Europe (Fig. 17.4). In the 1980s, the parasite became established in France (Denis *et al.*, 1983) and the

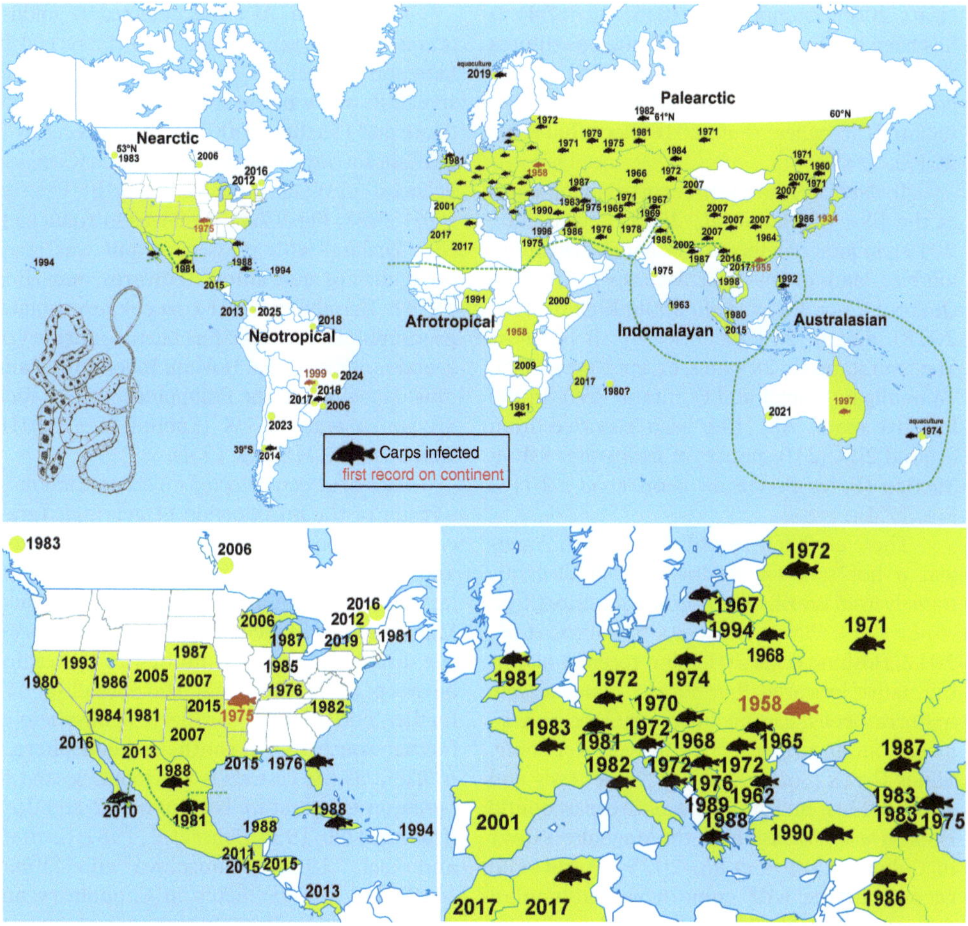

Fig. 17.4. Current geographic distribution of *Schyzocotyle acheilognathi* (in yellow), with the year of the first record in individual continents (in red) and countries (in black); yellow dots represent single records. (Updated from Kuchta *et al.*, 2018.)

UK (Andrews *et al.*, 1981) and was last detected in imported koi carp (*Cyprinus carpio*) in arctic Norway (Hansen and Alarcón, 2019).

However, the origin of African populations of AFT, which was first described as *Bothriocephalus* (*Clestobothrium*) *kivuensis* from barbels (*Barbus* spp.) by Baer and Fain (1958) in Zaire (now Democratic Republic of Congo) – the same year as the first report from Europe, has not been confirmed due to a lack of molecular data from Lake Kivu. AFT has since been reported from several countries across Africa (Ryšavý and Moravec, 1975; Brandt *et al.*, 1981; Kuchta *et al.*, 2018; Fig. 17.4).

AFT was first found in the New World in 1975 in introduced grass carp, native golden shiner (*Notemigonus crysoleucas*) and fathead minnow (*Pimephales promelas*) in Arkansas (Hoffman, 1980). The AFT was most likely first imported into the USA in 1963 along with grass carp in shipments of juvenile fish from Malaysia and Taiwan to the US Fish and Wildlife Federal Fish Hatcheries in Stuttgart, Arkansas and Auburn, Alabama, respectively (Choudhury and Cole, 2011; Kuchta *et al.*, 2018).

This invasive parasite is also well documented from Mexico, where grass carp was co-introduced from China in 1965 and AFT first detected in 1981 (Pérez-Ponce de León *et al.*, 2018), while only a few records are available from Canada (including British Columbia and Lake Winnipeg) (Hoffman, 1999; Choudhury *et al.*, 2006; Kuchta *et al.*, 2018; Fig. 17.4). It has been suggested that baitfish such as shiners are the main source of AFT infection in fish populations in the western USA and Great Lakes region (Marcogliese *et al.*, 2016; Boonthai *et al.*, 2017).

To date, AFT has been reported in 21 states in the USA (Kuchta *et al.*, 2018; Reyda *et al.*, 2019), in four provinces in Canada (British Columbia, Manitoba – Lake Winnipeg, Ontario, Quebec) (Choudhury *et al.*, 2006; Kuchta *et al.*, 2018), and in 214 localities in all but four Mexican states (in 28 states, except Nuevo León, Tamaulipas, Colima and Quintana Roo). In the last 40 years, AFT has been reported from around 22% (210 species) of freshwater fish in Mexico (Pérez-Ponce de León *et al.*, 2018; Fig. 17.4).

There are a few records from South America, a hot spot for freshwater fish diversity, namely from Brazil, mainly in aquaculture (Rego *et al.*, 1999; Piazza *et al.*, 2006; Santos *et al.*, 2017; Hoshino *et al.*, 2018) but recently also in the native loricariid *Rineloricaria pentamaculata* in Borrazópolis, Paraná and guppy *Poecilia reticulata* from an urban stream in Belo Horizonte, Minas Gerais (Souza *et al.*, 2018; de Assis and Pinto, 2024); and from the native parodontid *Parodon magdalenensis* from the Magdalena River in Colombia (Rave *et al.*, 2025). Additional records in the wild come from Patagonian Argentina, namely from introduced feral common carp and native creole perch *Percichthys trucha* (Waicheim *et al.*, 2014; Viozzi *et al.*, 2023; Fig. 17.4).

The first records of AFT from South Asia were in Sri Lanka in the 1960s from olive barb *Systomus sarana* (Fernando and Furtado, 1963). Later, several species, now considered *S. acheilognathi*, were described from various cyprinoids throughout Asia (Paperna, 1996; Kuchta *et al.*, 2018; Fig. 17.4).

Another tapeworm species, *S. nayarensis* (Malhotra, 1983), described from India, was confirmed as valid but only molecularly confirmed in trout barb (*Raiamas bola*) from West Bengal (Marick *et al.*, 2024). The occurrence of *S. acheilognathi* was also molecularly confirmed in India from Alghad snowtrout (*Schizothorax niger*) in Kashmir (Shah *et al.*, 2025). Therefore, both species may occur in India, but the actual distribution and host specificity of *S. nayarensis* should be molecularly confirmed.

In Australia, AFT was detected in goldfish (*Carassius auratus*) and koi carp (*C. carpio*) by Langdon (1992). The tapeworm is now widespread in many native fish in eastern Australia (Dove and Fletcher, 2000) and more recently in goldfish, koi carp and eastern gambusia (*Gambusia holbrooki*) in Western Australia (Perth) (Palermo *et al.*, 2021; Fig. 17.4). AFT was introduced to New Zealand with grass carp, but was eradicated during quarantine (Edwards and Hine, 1974). The ability of AFT to colonize isolated geographical locations has been confirmed on islands such as Cuba, Hawaii, Indonesia, Mauritius, Madagascar, the Philippines, Puerto Rico, Sri Lanka and the UK (Kuchta *et al.*, 2018; Scholz *et al.*, 2018; Fig. 17.4).

AFT has been detected on six continents as a result of the introduction of cyprinids (grass carp, carp) and guppies (mosquitofish – *Gambusia* and *Poecilia*) by humans to control mosquito larvae (Hoffman and Schubert, 1984; Salgado-Maldonado and Pineda-López, 2003). However, the distribution area is limited to the region between 61°N and 39°S. The spread of AFT further north in the northern hemisphere or further south in the southern hemisphere is unlikely, as the cestode is thermophilic and its optimum temperature is between 22 and 25°C (Liao and Shih, 1955; Bauer *et al.*, 1981; Granath and Esch, 1983a; Hanzelová and Žitňan, 1986; but see comments in Choudhury and Cole, 2011).

17.1.5. Importance of the disease

AFT is an important pathogen in aquaculture (Bauer *et al.*, 1981; Heckmann, 2009) and was listed as a 'Pathogen of Regional Concern' by the US Fish and Wildlife Service in 2010. Losses of juvenile fish with a mortality rate of up to 100% occurred in hatchery ponds, mainly before the 1980s (Liao and Shih, 1955; Mitchell, 2004). In commercial carp farms, fry (length 38–42 mm) can be infected 28–29 days after hatching (Hanzelová and Žitňan, 1986). The heavy infection of fry and fingerlings is probably because copepods make up a large part of the diet of these fish. The infection rate increases in juvenile fish with a peak at the end of summer and then decreases. Two-year-old fish are infected in spring and summer, but the infection rate is usually not high (Skachkov and Thakahova, 2018).

A high AFT infection intensity leads to intestinal obstruction and severe pathological changes affecting growth, condition and survival of fish (Scott and Grizzle, 1979; Granath and Esch, 1983b; Hoole and Nisan, 1994; Hansen *et al.*, 2006). Intestinal obstruction and reduced growth rate of fish occur with more than 12 tapeworms per fingerling, and death occurs with about 50 AFT per carp (Skachkov and Thakahova, 2018). AFT is also a problem in ornamental fish farms (Evans and Lester, 2001; Han *et al.*, 2010; Košuthová *et al.*, 2015; Hoshino *et al.*, 2018; Kuchta *et al.*, 2018).

Much less information is available on the effects of AFT in wild fish populations. The introduction of this alien tapeworm into new areas can endanger native fish species (Dove and Fletcher, 2000; Heckmann, 2000, 2009; Salgado-Maldonado and Pineda-López, 2003; Hansen *et al.*, 2006; Matey *et al.*, 2015). The potential effects of AFT were tested on the bonytail chub *Gila elegans* (Hansen *et al.*, 2006). The study included potential stress factors, such as a limited food base, and showed that infected fish had lower growth rates and higher mortality compared to uninfected individuals.

These results suggest that AFT poses a significant threat to native, naïve fish populations and should be considered in management decisions to conserve the local fish fauna, such as altered flow regimes and predation (Hansen *et al.*, 2006). This can be particularly serious for fish that reach only a small size at maturity, which can lead to reduced recruitment, growth, fitness and survival. However, an equilibrium between host and parasite can be established in a relatively short time, limiting the impact of the disease (Hoffman, 1999).

Recent data suggests that AFT was a serious veterinary issue in carp in Europe until the 1980s, when it was largely replaced by other Asian carp tapeworms, namely *Khawia sinensis* Hsü, 1935 first reported in Europe in the 1960s, and *Atractolytocestus huronensis* Anthony, 1958, which emerged in Europe in the 2000s and now dominates in Central European carp populations (Oros *et al.*, 2004, 2009). Assessing AFT impacts in wild fish remains difficult, as diseased individuals are rapidly removed by predators, water flow and necrophages (Blanc, 1997).

17.2. Diagnosis of the Infection and Clinical Signs

Infections can be readily detected at necropsy by recovering tapeworms (white in colour) with a characteristic heart-shaped scolex (Figs 17.1 and 17.2). Examination of faeces may reveal detached proglottids of adult tapeworms or eggs with an operculum at one end. The presence of AFT can also be detected using the squash plate method, which involves flattening the intestinal tract (or even whole small fishes up to 10 cm in length) between glass slides or plates and detecting the tapeworms under a dissecting stereomicroscope with transmitted light and low magnification (Fig. 17.1a).

Although mature AFT may be conspicuous in the intestine of infected fish and thus visible to the naked eye (Figs 17.1 and 17.5), the detection of light infections or the presence of juvenile parasites requires detailed microscopic examination. Although these infections may be of little

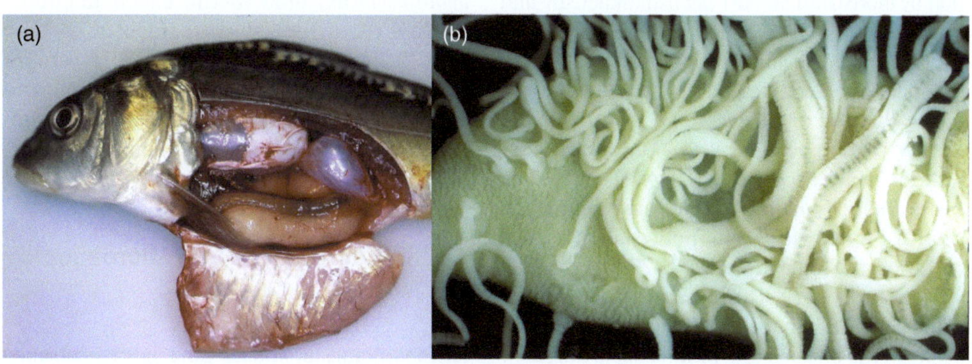

Fig. 17.5. Juvenile common carp (*Cyprinus carpio*) infected with *Schyzocotyle acheilognathi*. (a) Carp with opened body cavity; (b) opened intestine of carp with multiple tapeworms. (Author's own image.)

importance to the health of the infected hosts, detection can be crucial for effective disease control and limiting the spread of infection. In very small fish or those that are already heavily infected, the movement of AFT can be detected through the body wall prior to dissection.

In addition, AFT in the environment or in aquaculture could also be detected by non-invasive molecular methods such as environmental DNA (eDNA) – the detection of AFT DNA in water. Hofmeister *et al.* (2021) developed a sensitive and specific loop-mediated isothermal amplification (LAMP) method for the detection of AFT in less than 30 min from laboratory-prepared samples based on a variable region of the 18S ribosomal RNA gene of AFT, with detection and quantification of DNA on a real-time fluorometer with a limit of only two AFT eggs. The future application of this assay would be a cost-effective test for rapid and accurate detection of AFT DNA from environmental samples in the field, so that preventive measures can be taken to stop the spread of AFT through the movement of infected fish.

Infected fish can become sluggish and swim close to the water surface (Hoole, 1994). This may be accompanied by inappetence, slow growth, loss of condition, emaciation and signs of anaemia (Liao and Shih, 1955; Edwards and Hine, 1974; Scott and Grizzle, 1979; Hoole and Nisan, 1994; Sopinska and Guz, 1997). Exhaustion, anaemic gills and restricted movement are observed in infected 1-year-old fish. They cannot survive the winter in temperate zones of the northern hemisphere and die in mid-March or early April. Chronic inflammation of the intestinal mucosa is observed in infected 2-year-old carp, and death of carp fingerlings occurs with infection by more than 50 AFT per fish (Skachkov and Thakahova, 2018).

Infected fish may be more susceptible to secondary bacterial infections due to the debilitating effect of AFT (Clarkson *et al.*, 1997) and the destruction of the epithelial layer of the intestine (Bauer *et al.*, 1981). Heavy AFT loads can cause the body of infected fry, fingerlings and small fish species to become noticeably distended and swollen (Scott and Grizzle, 1979; Brandt *et al.*, 1981). However, Fu *et al.* (2022) found no significant difference in the condition factor of grass carp between the infected and uninfected groups.

The intestinal tract of infected fish is often greatly enlarged, has very thin walls and is obviously blocked. In such cases, the intestinal wall can be stretched to the point of transparency, so that the white-coloured tapeworms are visible and even individual proglottids of the parasites can be distinguished (Mitchell, 1989; Figs 17.1 and 17.5). The internal organs of infected hosts may be enlarged and the gallbladder swollen and distended. The parasites usually accumulate in the posterior part of the first loop of the intestine, posterior to the opening of the common bile duct. Small focal haemorrhages may be noted at the site of scolex attachment, which may progress to full haemorrhagic enteritis depending on severity (Hoole and Nisan, 1994; Pegg *et al.*, 2015). In extreme cases, intestinal perforation may occur if the intestinal tract ruptures (Scott and Grizzle, 1979; Heckmann, 2000).

Intensity of infection can range from 30 to 156 immature and mature worms per pond-reared carp (90–160 mm in length), and up to 20, although usually less than ten, in adult grass carp (Scott and Grizzle, 1979; Figs 17.1 and 17.3). The highest number in a single grass carp of about 10 cm in length was 467 tapeworms (Liao and Shih, 1955), but with no information on their size and their maturity. However, even a few large tapeworms can cause pronounced pathological changes, which suggests that the disease is due to the total mass of tapeworms, rather than the intensity of infection (Davydov, 1977).

The pathogenicity of AFT can also vary at different times of the year due to changes in the number of tapeworms, water temperature, metabolic rates, nutritional status of the host and duration of infection (Davydov, 1978; Scott and Grizzle, 1979; Pegg *et al.*, 2015). In a population of blue discus fish (*Symphysodon aequifasciatus*) bred in the Czech Republic, up to 41% of the fish were infected with up to 129 immature specimens of AFT per fish (Fig. 17.1b). AFT was the main cause of mortality in this population (R. Kuchta, 2023, unpublished results).

17.3. Macroscopic and Microscopic Lesions

Histopathological studies have been performed on a variety of fish species, including common carp (Sekretaryuk, 1983; Hoole and Nisan,

1994; Pegg *et al.*, 2015), grass carp (Liao and Shih, 1955; Scott and Grizzle, 1979; Fu *et al.*, 2022), spottail shiner *Notropis hudsonius*, fathead minnow *P. promelas*, woundfin *Plagopterus argentissimus* and roundtail chub *Gila robusta* (Heckmann, 2000). The pathology can generally be divided into damage caused by: (i) the scolex attachment; and (ii) the strobila in the intestinal lumen (Scott and Grizzle, 1979; Hoole and Nisan, 1994; Pegg *et al.*, 2015). Other organs such as liver, spleen or kidney of infected fish may also show signs of pathological changes (Balakhnin, 1979). Infected fish may show nutritional deficiency, with atrophy of hepatocytes in the liver (Davydov, 1977). In severe cases, these changes, such as destrobilization, are consistent with starvation (Davydov, 1978; Pegg *et al.*, 2015).

17.3.1. Pathological changes caused by the attachment of *Schyzocotyle acheilognathi*

The parasite attaches itself to the intestinal wall with its bothria, which wrap around the intestinal villi. This causes compression of the mucosal epithelium, focal pressure necrosis and haemorrhaging (Fig. 17.6a). Scolex attachment may also be associated with increased mucus production (Scott and Grizzle, 1979; Pegg *et al.*, 2015). Tapeworm attachment also elicits a local inflammatory response consisting mainly of lymphocytes. In severe infections, an increased number of lymphocytes can occur throughout the lamina propria.

Lesions associated with the scolex depend on the force exerted by the bothria to maintain attachment. The scolex is often pressed firmly against the intestinal wall, resulting in compression and the formation of localized pits that extend to the muscularis (Fig. 17.6). These attachment sites lead to pronounced thinning of the intestine at these points. Scolex attachment can also lead to a loss of the brush border and a general reduction in the thickness of the intestinal epithelium (Davydov, 1977; Hoole and Nisan, 1994). In advanced cases of infection, scolex attachment can lead to local ulceration. Desquamative catarrhal enteritis and proliferation of connective tissue around the scolex attachment site have also been observed (Bauer *et al.*, 1973; Pegg *et al.*, 2015).

Heckmann (2000) described penetration of the scolex throughout the host's intestine. Studies on woundfin and roundtail chub revealed severe pathology associated with penetration of the intestinal wall to the muscularis, resulting in a prominent inflammatory response, extensive haemorrhaging and necrosis. The scolex of some parasites even continued to penetrate the intestine wall into the body cavity, extending as far as the liver and gonads (Heckmann, 2000). This represents an unusual and rarely reported consequence of AFT infection.

Attachment of the scolex causes significant intestinal disruption, including: (i) destruction of the desmosomal junctions; (ii) loss of the intestinal microvillous border; (iii) detachment and loss of enterocytes; (iv) release of host-cell debris into the intestinal lumen; and (v) infiltration of leucocytes into the infected area. In small hosts (<4 cm in length), damage through

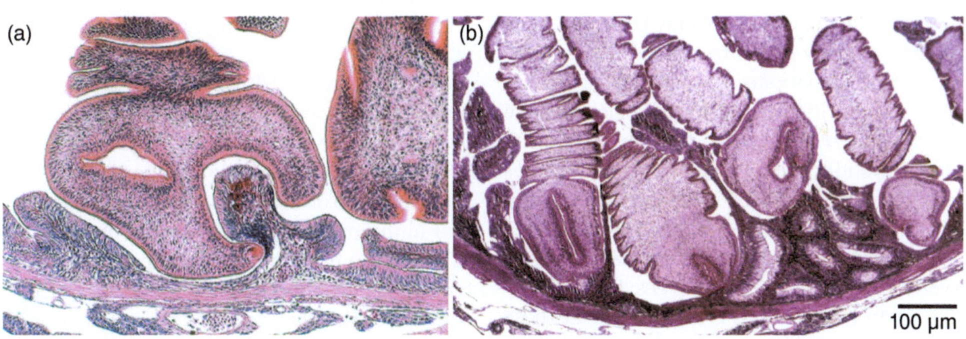

Fig. 17.6. Histology of the scolex of *Schyzocotyle acheilognathi* engulfing the intestinal mucosa of common carp (*Cyprinus carpio*) at the site of infection and causing compression. (a) Compression of the mucosa and localized haemorrhage; (b) marked thinning of the intestine, with formation of pits in the intestinal wall. (Author's own image.)

attachment can be extensive and is consistent with disruption of intestinal enzymes (Hoole and Nisan, 1994). In many places, the plasmalemma between the microtriches and the epithelial cells of the host intestine is absent, so that the matrix of the tegument is in direct contact with the cytoplasm of the host cells. Lysozomes have been detected surrounding the microtriches and embedded in the host cytoplasm (Smyth and McManus, 1989).

17.3.2. Pathological changes caused by the strobila of *Schyzocotyle acheilognathi*

The changes caused by the strobila generally exceed those associated with the scolex attachment. The extent and severity of this damage can vary depending on the size of the host, the size of the parasite and the intensity of the infection (Davydov, 1978; Hoole and Nisan, 1994). In small cyprinoids, the pathological changes are characterized by dilation of the intestine, compression of the intestinal folds and marked thinning of the intestinal wall (Fig. 17.6).

In very severe infections, distension may be accompanied by a complete loss of normal intestinal architecture, with occlusion of the intestine, congestion, compression, pressure necrosis, thinning and atrophy of the mucosa (Nakajima and Egusa, 1974a; Pegg *et al.*, 2015; Fig. 17.6). Detachment and degeneration of the epithelium may occur, with regions of complete epithelial loss. Lysis of large areas of the mucosa with necrotic changes has also been observed in heavily infected carp fry (Davydov, 1977; Sekretaryuk, 1983; Pegg *et al.*, 2015).

Inflammatory changes may be pronounced in heavy tapeworm burdens, with increased numbers of lymphocytes and eosinophilic granular cells occurring in the infected regions (Hoole and Nisan, 1994). Paradoxically, severe parasite infections and pronounced pathological changes have also been observed in apparently healthy fish (Scholz *et al.*, 2012). Nakajima and Egusa (1974a) described no signs of mortality, despite severe histopathological changes in common carp fry in Japan. What is rarely clear in these cases is the metabolic and physiological cost of these infections and the energetic or behavioural demands in the infected fish to maintain good condition.

17.4. Disease Mechanism

AFT causes a number of physiological changes in juvenile fish. These include: (i) protein deficiency; (ii) altered digestive enzyme activity; (iii) increased muscle fatigue in severely infected hosts; and (iv) mortality of juvenile fish (Liao and Shih, 1955; Davydov, 1978; Scott and Grizzle, 1979; Granath and Esch, 1983b; Brouder, 1999; Hansen *et al.*, 2006; Pegg *et al.*, 2015). Severe infections also reduce fat content and lead to a decrease in kidney, liver and spleen weight (Balakhnin, 1979; Žitňan and Hanzelová, 1982).

According to Clarkson *et al.* (1997), AFT infection in heavily infected hosts leads to a reduction in reproductive capacity, reduced swimming ability and increased muscle fatigue. Granath and Esch (1983b) also demonstrated a reduced ability of mosquitofish to adapt to changing water temperatures, which leads to the death of infected fish.

Relatively little is known about the relationship between the immune response of fish and AFT infections, although inflammation occurs in the gut of infected fish and leucocytes have been detected on the surface of the parasite (Hoole and Nisan, 1994; Nie and Hoole, 2000). The interaction between the parasite and the pronephric lymphocytes of carp was studied by examining the proliferation of lymphocytes isolated from both naïve fish and fish injected intraperitoneally with a cestode extract (Nie *et al.*, 1996). Parasite extracts increased antibody production and pronephric antibody-producing cells in the injected fish (Nie and Hoole, 1999) and stimulated the proliferation of pronephric lymphocytes *in vitro* (Nie *et al.*, 1996).

The effects of AFT infection on the intestinal microbiota, growth and immune responses of grass carp were investigated by Fu *et al.* (2022). AFT infection altered the composition of the intestinal microbiota but had no effect on microbial alpha diversity. The altered composition of intestinal bacteria by AFT, especially the increased relative abundance of *Turicibacter* spp., could have an effect on the lipid metabolism of grass carp. Finally, although the AFT infection activated the local intestinal mucosal immunity of the host, it had no effect on the growth of the grass carp (Fu *et al.*, 2022).

In infected young carp, a 25–30% reduction in haemoglobin and total blood volume has been reported, while the number of polymorphonuclear leucocytes and neutrophils increased (Kudryashova, 1970; Pár, 1978; Svobodová, 1978; Skachkov and Thakahova, 2018), but opinions differ on the intensity of infection required to cause these pathogenic effects. Kudryashova (1970) found these effects in fish with more than five tapeworms, while Svobodová (1978) found no significant effects on various physiological indices in fish with one to 21 tapeworms and attributed the increased leucocyte count to intestinal inflammation. According to Pár (1978), fish with one to 29 tapeworms showed an increased leucocyte count, and fish with more than 15 specimens showed significant damage to the intestine.

Biochemical studies revealed a reduction in the activities of enzymes such as alanine and aspartate aminotransferase, trypsin and chymotrypsin, amylase and acid phosphatase (Kudryashova, 1970; Matskási, 1984). In infected grass carp, a reduction in total proteins in the serum, impaired carbohydrate and protein metabolism and increased oxygen consumption were observed (Davydov, 1978). Morbidity and mortality in winter were attributed to changes in alanine and aspartate aminotransferase activities, which impaired protein synthesis (Lozinska-Gabska, 1981).

Inflammation of the intestine, severe catarrhal–haemorrhagic enteritis at the site of parasite attachment with proliferation of peripheral connective tissue and thinning of the intestinal wall were attributed to increased acid phosphatase activity during infection (Pár, 1978; Svobodová, 1978; Scott and Grizzle, 1979; Sekretaryuk, 1983).

There is some evidence that AFT secretes toxic substances of unknown composition that lead to intoxication of the host (Degger and Avenant-Oldewage, 2009) and damage to the epithelial mucosa (Hoole and Nisan, 1994). According to Bauer *et al.* (1981), intoxication of the entire host can cause degenerative processes in the organs. Hoole and Nisan (1994) demonstrated by ultrastructural investigations that electron-dense secretions are released from the surface of AFT, which may have a protective function for the parasite. Tapeworms that attach to the intestinal wall of the host injure the epithelial lining, produce and secrete toxic substances and impede the passage of intestinal contents (Bauer *et al.*, 1977).

17.5. Protective/Control Strategies

Due to the economic importance of AFT, its global distribution and its expanding host range, considerable efforts have been made to limit the impact of the disease. These include: (i) strict legal controls; (ii) comprehensive prophylaxis; (iii) veterinary examination of fish stocks; (iv) reduction of intensive stock management; and (v) active therapy (Weirowski, 1984).

Control of AFT can target either the copepod intermediate hosts (drainage of ponds in spring to remove planktonic invertebrates) or the fish stage of the life cycle, these measures being determined by economic and practical considerations. Fish ponds can be dried and disinfected with unslaked lime (Shcherban, 1965).

European fish farmers control bothriocephalosis by drying ponds annually or treating drained wet ponds with calcium chloride (approx. 70 kg/ha) or calcium hydroxide (approx. 2 t/acre, i.e. 0.81 t/ha) or calcium hypochlorite (HTH®) to kill the copepod intermediate host and treating fish with anthelmintics. Insecticides used as ectoparasiticides, such as Neguvon® (Masoten® or Dipterex® – at a concentration of 25 ppm, i.e. 25 g Masoten/t water) or similar compounds (Bromex®), can be used to reduce copepod populations in ponds (Hoffman, 1983). However, these agents are banned in many countries due to environmental and health concerns. In contrast, praziquantel (dose 20 μg/kg fish body mass) is approved for veterinary use in the European Union.

A wide range of chemotherapeutic agents have been used with varying degrees of success, including natural products such as: (i) tobacco dust (Avdosyev, 1973); (ii) lupine seeds (Balatskii *et al.*, 1976); (iii) needles of coniferous trees (Klenov, 1969a); and (iv) horseradish leaves (Klenov, 1969b). A number of compounds and insecticides have also been used (Molnár, 1970; Edwards and Hine, 1974; Fijan *et al.*, 1976; Pár *et al.*, 1977; Brandt *et al.*, 1981).

Comprehensive reviews of chemotherapeutic treatments for the control and eradication of AFT have been published by Bauer *et al.* (1981)

and Williams and Jones (1994). Skachkov and Thakahova (2018) and Skachkov and Safiullin (2021) conducted extensive trials of anthelmintics against AFT, including periods of preferential use in Russia. Mitchell (2004) tested the efficacy of praziquantel treatments against AFT in grass carp and found that AFT elimination occurred only at the maximum concentration of 1.5 mg/l when 88 g grass carp were stocked at a density of approximately 6 g/l. When fish density was raised to 60 g/l, the 1.5 mg/l treatment did not eliminate all AFT as four of 30 fish contained a single tapeworm (Mitchell, 2004).

Kline *et al.* (2009) investigated the effects of praziquantel on AFT eggs and found that praziquantel at 6 mg/l, which is a dose higher than the minimum recommended for complete AFT removal in 24 h, killed hundreds of adult AFT, and many ruptured and released eggs. These eggs were viable and produced thousands of coracidia over several days (Kline *et al.*, 2009). The authors warn fishery managers that even if fish receive the typically recommended praziquantel treatment regimen and all adult AFT are killed, viable eggs and coracidia may be present in the holding water.

The drugs are usually administered orally. Such preparations are often mixed in oil (corn, soybean and fish) and sprayed on pellets or mixed with feed. Efforts have focused on water-soluble chemotherapeutic agents that alleviate some of the problems associated with anorexia and dosing. It is important to distinguish between treatment to reduce the parasite load and treatment to completely eradicate the infection.

AFT can shed proglottids (destrobilization) under unfavourable conditions or in stressful situations, which regenerate when conditions become more favourable again (Davydov, 1978). Another important consideration is whether anthelmintics are ovicidal (i.e. kill the eggs of the tapeworms) (Kline *et al.*, 2009). This is necessary to prevent large numbers of infective eggs from being released into the environment when the worm is removed from the fish.

AFT eggs can be rapidly killed by drying, freezing and ultraviolet radiation. Of 11 chemicals tested for ovicidal activity, two chlorine-containing compounds were found to be effective: (i) 3.1 ppm sodium dichloroisocyanurate; and (ii) 9 ppm bleaching powder (Nakajima and Egusa, 1974b). However, there are very few chemical treatments currently approved for the treatment of AFT infections. Furthermore, the use of chemicals to control AFT in open waters can be very difficult, ineffective, harmful, expensive and illegal.

17.6. Conclusions and Suggestions for Future Studies

AFT is pathogenic to freshwater fish, especially young carp and smaller fish species, and can cause major economic losses in hatcheries and fish farms. It also has the extraordinary ability to colonize new regions and adapt to a wide range of native fish hosts. It is one of the most impressive, but also most unfortunate, examples of a parasite that is widely spread by the human-induced movement of fish. The speed of its geographical spread and the success of colonization have been facilitated by the cosmopolitan distribution of both intermediate and definitive hosts. However, the spread of AFT in many parts of the world is also the result of inadequate legislative controls, insufficient preventive measures and a lack of appropriate health-testing procedures prior to the introduction of fish (Hoffman, 1999; Heckmann, 2000; Kuchta *et al.*, 2018; Pérez-Ponce de León *et al.*, 2018).

The impact of AFT in Europe seems to have declined over the last decade. However, surveillance should be continued to prevent further spread to new areas. Efforts have been made to determine the resistance of the different strains of common carp used in European aquaculture. Hoole (1994) proposed the development of a vaccine against AFT, although practical and economic constraints continue to limit this approach. Exported fish, particularly carp and ornamental fish (such as guppies), should be inspected by veterinarians prior to movement to prevent further spread of AFT to new regions. Control measures, including treatment of infected fish, are generally effective, but the use of some anthelmintics is no longer permitted because of their negative effects on human health or the environment. Future work must therefore aim to develop new, effective and acceptable treatment methods to minimize economic losses.

Many aspects of the biology, ecology and pathology of AFT are well known and extensively documented. However, many of these observations are limited to farmed fish populations. As the host range and geographical distribution of AFT expand, the importance of the parasite to wild fish populations needs to be further investigated and documented. This is an important consideration given the global decline in biodiversity and increasing efforts to protect the aquatic environment. Comparative studies are needed to understand the differences in species' susceptibility and disease potential in newly infected hosts, as well as the consequences of the parasite's emergence in new environments. Early detection and eDNA methods will become critical for monitoring the spread of this tapeworm in the wild.

Sublethal effects of AFT on the growth, fitness, fecundity, behaviour or tolerance to environmental changes of the fish can also have important ecological effects. The physiological and bioenergetic costs of AFT under natural conditions also need to be clarified. This information is necessary to better understand future disease risks and to assess the role of this introduced AFT in the health and stability of fish populations.

References

Andrews, C., Coles, T. and Dearsley, A. (1981) *Bothriocephalus acheilognathi* Yamaguti, 1934 (Cestoda: Pseudophyllidea) in the British Isles. *Journal of Fish Diseases* 4, 89–93.

Assis, J.C.A. de and Pinto, H.A. (2024) Infection of guppies (*Poecilia reticulata*) with the Asian fish tapeworm *Schyzocotyle acheilognathi* in an urban stream in Brazil. *Revista Brasileira de Parasitologia Veterinaria* 33, e020323.

Avdosyev, B.S. (1973) The use of tobacco dust in the control of *Bothriocephalus gowkongensis* infection in carp. *Rybnoe Khozyaistvo* 1973, 109–118 (in Russian).

Baer, J.C. and Fain, A. (1958) *Bothriocephalus* (*Clestobothrium*) *kivuensis* n. sp., cestode parasite d'un barbel du Lac Kivu. *Annales de la Société Royale Zoologique de Belgique* 88, 287–302.

Balakhnin, I.A. (1979) Changes in the correlations between the intestinal organs of carp with bothriocephaliasis. *Gidrobiologicheskii Zhurnal* 15, 45–49 (in Russian).

Balatskii, K.P., Ivasik, V.P., Boyarchuk, V.M. and Novosad, N.L. (1976) *Bothriocephalus* infection in carp. *Veterinariya* 1976, 55 (in Russian).

Bauer, O.N. and Hoffman, G.L. (1976) Helminth range extension by translocation of fish. In: Page, L.A. (ed.) *Wildlife Diseases. Proceedings of the 3rd International Wildlife Disease Conference, Munich, 1975*. Plenum Press, New York, pp. 163–172.

Bauer, O.N., Musselius, V.A. and Strelkov, Y.A. (1973) *Diseases of Pond Fishes*. Program for Scientific Translations, Jerusalem.

Bauer, O.N., Musselius, V.A., Nikolaeva, V.M. and Strelkov, Y.A. (1977) *Ichthyopatologiya*. Izdatelsvo Pishchevaya Promyshlennost, Moscow, USSR, 431 pp. (in Russian).

Bauer, O.N., Musselius, V.A. and Strelkov, Yu.A. (1981) *Diseases of Freshwater Fish*. Legkaya i Pischevaya Promyshlenost, Moscow, USSR (in Russian).

Blanc, G. (1997) Introduced pathogens in European aquatic ecosystems: theoretical aspects and realities. *Bulletin Français de la Pêche et de la Pisciculture* 344–345, 489–513.

Borgarenko, L.F. (1981) Cestodes of the order Pseudophyllidea in birds in Tadzhikistan. *Izvestiya Akademii Nauk Tadzhikskoi SSR, Otdelenie Biologicheskikh Nauk* 1979, 99–100 (in Russian).

Boonthai, T., Herbst, S.J., Whelan, G.E., Van Deuren, M.G., Loch, T.P. and Faisal, M. (2017) The Asian fish tapeworm *Schyzocotyle acheilognathi* is widespread in baitfish retail stores in Michigan, USA. *Parasites & Vectors* 10, 618.

Brandt, F.W., Van As, J.G. and Hamilton-Attwell, V.L. (1981) The occurrence and treatment of bothriocephalosis in the common carp, *Cyprinus carpio* in fish ponds with notes on its presence in the large-mouth yellowfish *Barbus kimberleyensis* from the Vaal Dam, Transvaal. *Water SA* 7, 34–42.

Brouder, M.J. (1999) Relationship between length of roundtail chub and infection intensity of Asian fish tapeworm *Bothriocephalus acheilognathi*. *Journal of Aquatic Animal Health* 11, 302–304.

Choudhury, A. and Cole, R.A. (2011) The Asian fish tapeworm *Bothriocephalus acheilognathi*. In: Francis, R.A. (ed.) *A Handbook of Global Freshwater Invasive Species*. Routledge, London, pp. 389–404.

Choudhury, A., Charipar, E., Nelson, P., Hodgson, J.R., Bonar, S. and Cole, R.A. (2006) Update on the distribution of the invasive Asian fish tapeworm, *Bothriocephalus acheilognathi*, in the US and Canada. *Comparative Parasitology* 73, 269–273.

Clarkson, R.W., Robinson, A.T. and Hoffnagle, T.L. (1997) Asian tapeworm (*Bothriocephalus acheilognathi*) in native fishes from the Little Colorado River, Grand Canyon, Arizona. *Great Basin Naturalist* 57, 66–69.

Davydov, V.G. (1977) Host tissue reaction to different types of cestode attachment. *Biologiya Vnutrennikh Vod* 33, 45–48 (in Russian).

Davydov, O.N. (1978) Growth, development and fecundity of *Bothriocephalus gowkongensis* (Yeh, 1955), a parasite of cyprinid fish. *Gidrobiologicheskii Zhurnal* 14, 70–77 (in Russian).

Degger, N. and Avenant-Oldewage, A. (2009) Metal accumulation analysis within tissue of *Bothriocephalus acheilognathi*. *Journal of the South African Veterinary Association* 80, 127–128.

Denis, A., Gabrion, C. and Lambert, A. (1983) The presence in France of two parasites of East Asian origin: *Diplozoon nipponicum* (Monogenea) and *Bothriocephalus acheilognathi* (Cestoda) in *Cyprinus carpio*. *Bulletin Français de Pisciculture* 289, 128–134.

Dove, A.D.M. and Fletcher, A.S. (2000) The distribution of the introduced tapeworm *Bothriocephalus acheilognathi* in Australian freshwater fishes. *Journal of Helminthology* 74, 121–127.

Dubinina, M.N. (1971) Cestodes from fishes of the River Amur's basin. *Parazitologicheskii Sbornik* 25, 77–119 (in Russian).

Edwards, D.J. and Hine, P.M. (1974) Introduction, preliminary handling and diseases of grass carp in New Zealand. *New Zealand Journal of Marine and Freshwater Research* 8, 441–454.

Evans, B.B. and Lester, R.J.G. (2001) Parasites of ornamental fish imported into Australia. *Bulletin of the European Association of Fish Pathologists* 21, 51–55.

Fernando, C.H. and Furtado, J.I. (1963) A study of some helminth parasites of freshwater fishes in Ceylon. *Zeitschrift für Parasitenkunde* 23, 141–163.

Fijan, N., Kezic, N., Teskeredzic, E. and Kajgana, L. (1976) Treatment of carp bothriocephaliasis. *Veterinarski Arhiv* 46, 245–252 (in Russian).

Font, W.F. and Tate, D.C. (1994) Helminth parasites of native Hawaiian freshwater fishes: an example of extreme ecological isolation. *Journal of Parasitology* 80, 682–688.

Fu, P.P., Xiong, F., Wu, S.G., Zou, H., Li, M. *et al.* (2022) Effects of *Schyzocotyle acheilognathi* (Yamaguti, 1934) infection on the intestinal microbiota, growth and immune reactions of grass carp *Ctenopharyngodon idella*. *PLoS One* 17, e0266766.

García-Prieto, L. and Osorio-Sarabia, D. (1991) Distribución actual de *Bothriocephalus acheilognathi* en México. *Anales del Instituto de Biología, Universidad Nacional Autónoma de México, Serie Zoología* 62, 523–526.

Granath, W.O. and Esch, G.W. (1983a) Temperature and other factors that regulate the composition and infrapopulation densities of *Bothriocephalus acheilognathi* (Cestoda) in *Gambusia affinis* (Pisces). *Journal of Parasitology* 69, 1116–1124.

Granath, W.O. and Esch, G.W. (1983b) Survivorship and parasite-induced host mortality among mosquitofish in a predator-free, North Carolina cooling reservoir. *American Midland Naturalist* 110, 314–323.

Han, J.E., Shin, S.P., Kim, J.H., Choresca, C.H., Jun, J.W. *et al.* (2010) Mortality of cultured koi *Cyprinus carpio* in Korea caused by *Bothriocephalus acheilognathi*. *African Journal of Microbiology Research* 4, 543–546.

Hansen, H. and Alarcón, M. (2019) First record of the Asian fish tapeworm *Schyzocotyle* (*Bothriocephalus*) *acheilognathi* (Yamaguti, 1934) in Scandinavia. *Bioinvasions Records* 8, 437–441.

Hansen, S.P., Choudhury, A. and Cole, R.A. (2007) Evidence of experimental postcyclic transmission of *Bothriocephalus acheilognathi* in bonytail chub (*Gila elegans*). *Journal of Parasitology* 93, 202–204.

Hansen, S.P., Choudhury A., Heisey, D.M., Ahumada, J.A., Hoffnagle, T.L. and Cole, R.A. (2006) Experimental infection of the endangered bonytail chub (*Gila elegans*) with the Asian fish tapeworm (*Bothriocephalus acheilognathi*): impacts on survival, growth, and condition. *Canadian Journal of Zoology* 84, 1383–1394.

Hanzelová, V. and Žitňan, R. (1986) Embryogenesis and development of *Bothriocephalus acheilognathi* Yamaguti, 1934 (Cestoda) in the intermediate host under experimental conditions. *Helminthologia* 23, 145–155.

Heckmann, R.A. (2000) Asian tapeworm, *Bothriocephalus acheilognathi* Yamaguti, 1934, a recent cestode introduction into the western United States of America: control methods and effect on endangered fish populations. *Proceedings of Parasitology* 29, 1–24.

Heckmann, R.A. (2009) The fate of an endangered fish species (*Plagopterus argentissimus*) due to an invasive fish introduction (*Cyprinella lutrensis*) infected with Asian tapeworm (*Bothriocephalus argentissimus*): recovery methods. *Proceedings of Parasitology* 47, 43–52.

Hoffman, G.L. (1980) Asian tapeworm, *Bothriocephalus acheilognathi* Yamaguti, 1934, in North America. *Fisch Umwelt* 8 (Special), 69–75.

Hoffman, G.L. (1983) *Asian Fish Tapeworm,* Bothriocephalus opsariichthydis*, Prevention and Control*, revised edn. US Department of the Interior, Fish and Wildlife Service, Washington, DC.

Hoffman, G.L. (1999) *Parasites of North American Freshwater Fishes*. University of California Press, Berkeley, California.

Hoffman, G.L. and Schubert, G. (1984) Some parasites of exotic fishes. In: Courtenay, W.R. and Stauffer, J.R. (eds) *Distribution, Biology, and Management of Exotic Fishes*. John Hopkins University Press, Baltimore, Maryland, pp. 233–261.

Hofmeister, E., Georgousi, F., Lund, M., Roderick, C., Choudhury, A. *et al.* (2021) Loop-mediated isothermal amplification (LAMP) assay for detection of Asian fish tapeworm, *Schyzocotyle acheilognathi* (Yamaguti, 1934) syn. *Bothriocephalus acheilognathi*. *Journal of Parasitology* 107, 846–852.

Holmes, J.C. (1979) Parasite populations and host community structure. In: Nickol, B.B. (ed.) *Host–Parasite Interfaces. Proceedings of the Symposium at the University of Nebraska-Lincoln, 5–7 October*. Academic Press, London, pp. 27–46.

Hoole, D. (1994) Tapeworm infections in fish: past and future problems. In: Pike, A.W. and Lewis, J.W. (eds) *Parasitic Diseases of Fish*. Samara Publishing Limited, Tresaith, UK, pp. 119–140.

Hoole, D. and Nisan, H. (1994) Ultrastructural studies on the intestinal response of carp, *Cyprinus carpio* L. to the pseudophyllidean tapeworm, *Bothriocephalus acheilognathi* Yamaguti, 1934. *Journal of Fish Diseases* 17, 623–629.

Hoshino, É.M., Hoshino, M. and Tavares-Dias M. (2018) Parasites of ornamental fish commercialized in Macapá, Amapá State (Brazil). *Revista Brasileira de Parasitologia Veterinária* 27, 75–80.

Klenov, A.P. (1969a) Coniferous needles tested against *Bothriocephalus* in grass carp. *Veterinariya* 46, 65–67 (in Russian).

Klenov, A.P. (1969b) Testing 'phytoncides' (onion and leaves of horse-radish) against *Bothriocephalus* infection in grass carp. *Veterinariya* 46, 59 (in Russian).

Kline, S.J., Archdeacon, T.P. and Bonar, S.A. (2009) Effects of praziquantel on eggs of the Asian tapeworm *Bothriocephalus acheilognathi*. *North American Journal of Aquaculture* 71, 380–383.

Košuthová, L., Šmiga, L., Oros, M., Barčák, D. and Košuth, P. (2015) The pathogenic Asian fish tapeworm, *Bothriocephalus acheilognathi* Yamaguti, 1934 (Cestoda) in the red discus (*Symphysodon discus*). *Helminthologia* 52, 287–292.

Kuchta, R., Choudhury, A. and Scholz, T. (2018) Asian fish tapeworm: the most successful invasive parasite in freshwaters. *Trends in Parasitology* 34, 511–523.

Kudryashova, Y.V. (1970) The effect of *Bothriocephalus gowkongensis* on the hematological indicators of 2-year-old carp. *Doklady Moskovskoi Sel'skokhozyaistvennoi Akademii im. K.A. Timiryazeva* 164, 345–349 (in Russian).

Langdon, J.S. (1992) Major protozoan and metazoan parasitic diseases of Australian finfish. In: Munday, B. (ed.) *Fin Fish Workshop Refresher Course for Veterinarians.* Proceedings No. 182. Post Graduate Committee in Veterinary Science, University of Sydney, Sydney, Australia, pp. 1–27.

Leong, T.S. (1986) Seasonal occurrence of metazoan parasites of *Puntius binotatus* in an irrigation canal, Pulau Pinang, Malaysia. *Journal of Fish Biology* 28, 9–16.

Liao, H.-H. and Shih, L.-C. (1955) Contribution to the biology and control of *Bothriocephalus gowkongensis* Yeh, a tapeworm parasitic in young grass carp (*Ctenopharyngodon idellus* C. a. V.). *Acta Hydrobiologica Sinica* 1, 129–185 (in Chinese).

Lozinska-Gabska, M. (1981) Activity of aspartate and alanine aminotransferase in the alimentary canal of carp (*Cyprinus carpio* L.) infected with tapeworms *Bothriocephalus gowkongensis* Yeh, 1955 or *Khawia sinensis* Hsu, 1935. *Wiadomosci Parazytologiczne* 27, 717–743.

Maitland, P.S. and Campbell, R.N. (1992) *Freshwater Fishes of the British Isles*. HarperCollins, London.

Malevitskaya, M.A. (1958) On introduction of *Bothriocephalus gowkongensis*, a parasite with complex life cycle, during acclimatisation of Amur fish. *Doklady Akademii Nauk USSR* 123, 572–575 (in Russian).

Marcogliese, D.J. and Esch, G.W. (1989) Experimental and natural infection of planktonic and benthic copepods by the Asian tapeworm, *Bothriocephalus acheilognathi*. *Proceedings of the Helminthological Society of Washington* 56, 151–155.

Marcogliese, D.J., Gendron, A.D., Forest, J.J.H., Li, W., Boyce, K. *et al.* (2016) Range expansion and molecular confirmation of the Asian fish tapeworm in the lower Great Lakes and St. Lawrence River with notes on infections in baitfish. *Journal of Great Lakes Research* 42, 819–828.

Marick, J., Choudhury, A., Scholz, T., Biswas, R. and Ash, A. (2024) Taxonomic summary of *Schyzocotyle* (Cestoda: Bothriocephalidae) with a redescription of *Schyzocotyle nayarensis* (Malhotra, 1983) from India. *Journal of Helminthology* 98, e73, 1–14.

Matey, V.E., Ervin, E.L. and Hovey, T.E. (2015) Asian fish tapeworm (*Bothriocephalus acheilognathi*) infecting a wild population of convict cichlid (*Archocentrus nigrofasciatus*) in Southwestern California. *Bulletin of the Southern California Academy of Sciences* 114, 89–97.

Matskási, I. (1984) The effect of *Bothriocephalus acheilognathi* infection on the protease and α-amylase activity in the gut of carp fry. In: Olaha, J. (ed.) *Fish, Pathogens and Environment in European Polyculture* (Proceedings of an International Seminar, 23–27 June 1981, Szarvas). *Symposia Biologica Hungarica* 23, 119–125.

Minervini, R., Lombardi, F. and Cave, D. (1985) L'introduzione di *Bothriocephalus acheilognathi* Yamaguti, 1934, in Italia: osservazioni su popolazioni naturali e di allevamento di carpa (*Cyprinus carpio*). *Rivista Italiana di Piscicultura e Ittiopatogia* 20, 27–32.

Mitchell, A.J. (1989) Squash-plate technique for detecting Asian tapeworms in fish. *Journal of Aquatic Animal Health* 1, 243–244.

Mitchell, A.J. (2004) Effectiveness of praziquantel bath treatments against *Bothriocephalus acheilognathi* in grass carp. *Journal of Aquatic Animal Health* 16, 130–136.

Molnár, K. (1970) An attempt to treat fish bothriocephalosis with devermin. Toxicity for the host and anti-parasitic effect. *Acta Veterinaria Academiae Scientiarum Hungaricae* 20, 325–331.

Molnár, K. (1977) On the synonyms of *Bothriocephalus acheilognathi* Yamaguti, 1934. *Parasitologia Hungarica* 10, 61–62.

Molnár, K. and Murai, E. (1973) Morphological studies on *Bothriocephalus gowkongensis* Yeh, 1955 and *B. phoxini* Molnár, 1968 (Cestoda, Pseudophyllidea). *Parasitologia Hungarica* 6, 99–108.

Nakajima, K. and Egusa, N. (1974a) *Bothriocephalus opsariichthydis* Yamaguti (Cestoda: Pseudophyllidea) found in the gut of cultured carp, *Cyprinus carpio* (Linne) – I. Morphology and taxonomy. *Fish Pathology* 9, 31–39 (in Japanese).

Nakajima, K. and Egusa, N. (1974b) *Bothriocephalus opsariichthydis* Yamaguti (Cestoda: Pseudophyllidea) found in the gut of cultured carp, *Cyprinus carpio* (Linne) – III. Anthelmintic effects of some chemicals. *Fish Pathology* 9, 46–49 (in Japanese).

Nedeva, I. and Mutafova, T. (1988) On the morphology of *Bothriocephalus acheilognathi* Yamaguti, 1934 (Bothriocephalidae). *Khelmintologiya* 26, 39–46 (in Bulgarian).

Nie, P. and Hoole, D. (1999) Antibody response of carp, *Cyprinus carpio* to the cestode, *Bothriocephalus acheilognathi*. *Parasitology* 118, 635–639.

Nie, P. and Hoole, D. (2000) Effects of *Bothriocephalus acheilognathi* on the polarization response of pronephric leucocytes of carp, *Cyprinus carpio*. *Journal of Helminthology* 74, 253–257.

Nie, P., Hoole, D. and Arme, C. (1996) Proliferation of pronephric lymphocytes of carp, *Cyprinus carpio* induced by extracts of *Bothriocephalus acheilognathi*. *Journal of Helminthology* 70, 127–131.

Odening, K. (1976) Conception and terminology of hosts in parasitology. *Advances in Parasitology* 14, 1–93.

Oros, M., Hanzelová, V. and Scholz, T. (2004) The cestode *Atractolytocestus huronensis* (Caryophyllidea) continues to spread in Europe: new data on the helminth parasite of the common carp. *Diseases of Aquatic Organisms* 62, 115–119.

Oros, M., Scholz T. and Hanzelová, V. (2009) Tapeworm *Khawia sinensis*: review of the introduction and subsequent decline of a pathogen of carp, *Cyprinus carpio*. *Veterinary Parasitology* 164, 217–222.

Palermo, C.J., Morgan, D.L., Beatty, S.J., Elliot, A. and Greay, T.L. (2021) The Asian fish tapeworm *Schyzocotyle acheilognathi* discovered in Western Australia may pose a threat to the health of endemic native fishes. *Journal of Helminthology* 95, e60.

Paperna, I. (1996) *Parasites, Infections and Diseases of Fishes in Africa: An Update*. CIFA Technical Paper No. 31. Food and Agriculture Organization of the United Nations, Rome.

Pár, O. (1978) Low-intensity invasion by tapeworm *Bothriocephalus gowkongensis*, as acting on the physiological and condition parametres of the health state of the carp. *Bulletin VÚRH Vodňany* 14, 26–33.

Pár, O., Párová, J. and Prouza, A. (1977) Mansonil – an effective anthelminthic for the treatment of botriocephalosis in the carp. *Bulletin VÚRH Vodňany* 1, 17–25.

Pegg, J., Andreou, D., Williams, C.F. and Britton, J.R. (2015) Temporal changes in growth, condition and trophic niche in juvenile *Cyprinus carpio* infected with a non-native parasite. *Parasitology* 142, 1579–1587.

Pérez-Ponce de León, G., Jiménez-Ruiz, F.A., Mendoza-Garfias, B. and García-Prieto, L. (2001) Helminth parasites of garter snakes and mud turtles from several localities of the Mesa Central of Mexico. *Comparative Parasitology* 68, 9–20.

Pérez-Ponce de León, G., Lagunas-Calvo, O., García-Prieto, L., Briosio-Aguilar, R. and Aguilar-Aguilar, R. (2018) Update on the distribution of the co-invasive *Schyzocotyle acheilognathi* (*Bothriocephalus acheilognathi*), the Asian fish tapeworm, in freshwater fishes of Mexico. *Journal of Helminthology* 92, 279–290.

Piazza, R.S., Martins, M.L., Guiraldelli, L. and Yamashita, M.M. (2006) Parasitic diseases of freshwater ornamental fishes commercialized in Florianópolis, Santa Catarina, Brazil. *Boletim do Instituto de Pesca* 32, 51–57.

Pool, D. (1984) A scanning electron microscope study of the life cycle of *Bothriocephalus acheilognathi* Yamaguti, 1934. *Journal of Fish Biology* 25, 361–364.

Pool, D.W. (1987) A note on the synonymy of *Bothriocephalus acheilognathi* Yamaguti, 1934, *B. aegyptiacus* Ryšavý and Moravec, 1975 and *B. kivuensis* Baer and Fain, 1958. *Parasitology Research* 73, 146–150.

Pool, D.W. and Chubb, J.C. (1985) A critical scanning electron microscope study of the scolex of *Bothriocephalus acheilognathi* Yamaguti, 1934, with a review of the taxonomic history of the genus *Bothriocephalus* parasitizing cyprinid fishes. *Systematic Parasitology* 7, 199–211.

Prigli, M. (1975) The role of aquatic birds in spreading *Bothriocephalus gowkongensis* Yeh, 1955 (Cestoda). *Parasitologia Hungarica* 8, 61–62.

Radulescu, I. and Georgescu, R. (1962) Contributii la cunoasterea parasitofaunei speciei *Centropharyngodon idella* in primul an de aclimatizare in R.P. Romina. *Buletinul Institutului de Cercetari si Proiectari Piscicole* 21, 85–91.

Rave, A., Lopez Osorio, S, Uribe M, Hermosilla, C.R. and Chaparro-Gutiérrez J.J. (2025) First record of the Asian fish tapeworm *Schyzocotyle acheilognathi* (Cestoda: Bothriocephalidae) in the native freshwater fish *Parodon magdalenensis* from Colombia. *Frontiers in Veterinary Science* 12, 1614531.

Rego, A.A., Chubb, J.C. and Pavanelli, G.C. (1999) Cestodes in South American freshwater teleost fishes: keys to genera and brief description of species. *Revista Brasileira de Zoologia* 16, 299–367.

Reyda, F.B., Pommelle, C.P. and Doolin, M.L. (2019) Asian fish tapeworm (*Schyzocotyle acheilognathi*) found in New York State for the first time after a long-term fish-parasite survey. *Comparative Parasitology* 86, 108–113.

Riggs, M.R., Lemly, A.D. and Esch, G.W. (1987) The growth, biomass, and fecundity of *Bothriocephalus acheilognathi* in a North Carolina cooling reservoir. *Journal of Parasitology* 73, 893–900.

Ryšavý, B. and Moravec, F. (1975) *Bothriocephalus aegyptiacus* sp. n. (Cestoda: Pseudophyllidea) from *Barbus bynni*, and its life cycle. *Věstník Československé Společnosti Zoologické* 39, 68–72.

Salgado-Maldonado, G. and Pineda-López, R.F. (2003) The Asian fish tapeworm *Bothriocephalus acheilognathi*: a potential threat to native freshwater fish species in Mexico. *Biological Invasions* 5, 261–268.

Santos, M.A., Jerônimo, G.T., Cardoso, L., Tancredo, K.R., Medeiros, P.B. *et al.* (2017) Parasitic fauna and histopathology of farmed freshwater ornamental fish in Brazil. *Aquaculture* 470, 103–109.

Scholz, T., Kuchta, R. and Williams, C. (2012) *Bothriocephalus achelognathi*. In: Woo, P.T.K. and Buchmann, K. (eds) *Fish Parasites: Pathobiology and Protection*. CAB International, Wallingford, UK, pp. 282–297.

Scholz, T., Šimková, A., Rasamy Razanabolana, J. and Kuchta, R. (2018) The first record of the invasive Asian fish tapeworm (*Schyzocotyle acheilognathi*) from an endemic cichlid fish in Madagascar. *Helminthologia* 55, 84–87.

Scholz, T., Kuchta, R. and Oros, M. (2021) Tapeworms as pathogens of fish: a review. *Journal of Fish Diseases* 44, 1883–1900.

Scott, A.L. and Grizzle, J.M. (1979) Pathology of cyprinid fishes caused by *Bothriocephalus gowkongensis* Yeh, 1955 (Cestoda: Pseudophyllidea). *Journal of Fish Diseases* 2, 69–73.

Sekretaryuk, K.V. (1983) Morphohistochemistry study of the intestine of carp in bothriocephalosis. *Parazitologiya* 17, 203–208 (in Russian).

Shah, I.M., Maqbool, N., Nazir, J., Khurshid, I., Ahmad, F. and Ahmad, S.M. (2025) Helminth infection of *Schizothorax niger* in Kashmir, India: morphological and molecular characterization. *Molecular Biology Reports* 52, 118.

Shcherban, M.P. (1965) *Cestode Infections of Carp*. Izdatelstvo Urozhai, Kiev, USSR (in Russian).

Skachkov, D.P. and Safiullin, R.T. (2021) Bothriocephalids of carp in a warm-water tank farm under natural conditions of fish keeping (dynamics of infection, therapeutic and preventive measures). *IOP Conference Series: Earth and Environmental Science* 677, 052064.

Skachkov, D.P. and Thakahova, A.A. (2018) *Bothriocephalus* spp. infection of Cyprinidae: epizootiology, clinical features and pathogenesis, diagnostics, therapeutic and prophylactic measures. *AGROFOR* 3, 91–96.

Smyth, J.D. and McManus, D.P. (1989) *The Physiology and Biochemistry of Cestodes*. Cambridge University Press, Cambridge.

Sopinska, A. and Guz, L. (1997) Fenbendazole treatment against *Bothriocephalus acheilognathi* in carp, *Cyprinus carpio*. *Bulletin of the European Association of Fish Pathologists* 17, 86–87.

Souza, G.A., Moresca, V.O., Teixeira, G.M., Jerep, F.C. and Aguiar, A. (2018) First record of the invasive tapeworm, *Schyzocotyle acheilognathi* (Pseudophyllidea; Bothriocephalidae) in native freshwater fish, Brazil. *Anais da Academia Brasileira de Ciências* 90, 2845–2849.

Svobodová, Z. (1978) Values of some conformation, condition and physiological parameters of two-year-old carp invaded by the tapeworm *Bothriocephalus gowkongensis*. *Bulletin VÚRH Vodňany* 3, 21–25.

Viozzi, G., Rauque, C., Flores, V., Vega, R. and Waicheim, A. (2023) A regional scale study of parasites in *Percichthys trucha*, an endemic fish of southern South America: insights on diversity and distribution from two decades of field surveys. *Parasitology Research* 122, 2667–2689.

Waicheim, A., Blasetti, G., Cordero, P., Rauque, C. and Viozzi, G. (2014) Macroparasites of the invasive fish, *Cyprinus carpio*, in Patagonia, Argentina. *Comparative Parasitology* 81, 270–275.

Weirowski, F. (1984) Occurrence, spread and control of *Bothriocephalus acheilognathi* in the carp ponds of the German Democratic Republic. In: Olaha, J. (ed.) *Fish, Pathogens and Environment in European Polyculture* (Proceedings of an International Seminar, 23–27 June, Szarvas). *Symposia Biologica Hungarica* 23, 149–155.

Williams, H. and Jones, A. (1994) *Parasitic Worms of Fish*. Taylor & Francis, London.

Yamaguti, S. (1934) Studies on the helminth fauna of Japan. Part 4. Cestodes of fishes. *Japanese Journal of Zoology* 6, 1–112.

Yeh, I.S. (1955) On a new tapeworm *Bothriocephalus gowkongensis* n. sp. (Cestoda: Bothriocephalidae) from freshwater fish in China. *Acta Zoologica* 7, 69–74 (in Chinese).

Yera, H., Kuchta, R., Brabec, J., Peyron, F. and Dupouy-Camet, J. (2013) First identification of eggs of the Asian fish tapeworm *Bothriocephalus acheilognathi* (Cestoda: Bothriocephalidea) in human stool. *Parasitology International* 62, 268–271.

Žitňan, R. and Hanzelová, V. (1982) Negative effects of bothriocephalosis on weight gains in carp. *Folia Veterinaria* 26, 173–181.

18 *Anisakis* Species

Arne Levsen*, Miguel Bao and Paolo Cipriani
Institute of Marine Research, Bergen, Norway

Abstract

Anisakis spp. third-stage larvae infecting fish generally have low pathogenicity. Disease outbreaks are rare and they are often linked to specific environmental conditions. Thus, the red vent syndrome in Atlantic salmon (*Salmo salar*) has been generally associated with rising *Anisakis* intensities in wild salmon returning to rivers in North-Eastern Europe. The severity of *Anisakis* infections varies with immune responses in the fish host and age; for example, Atlantic mackerel (*Scomber scombrus*) seems to exhibit enhanced immunity with age, allowing it to reduce *Anisakis* infections over time. While heavily infected fish often appear healthy, intense infestations in the liver and stomach can cause significant tissue damage. *Anisakis* infections in wild fish may affect growth and reproduction, while in farmed fish, prevalence is low, with no associated disease.

18.1. Introduction

The members of the nematode genus *Anisakis* (order Ascaridida, family Anisakidae), commonly known as the herring or whale worm, occur worldwide (except in strictly Antarctic waters) as third larval stage in numerous marine teleost fish species. Several of the commonly infected fish host species are among the most valuable fisheries resources. Historically, only very few species were recognized within the genus *Anisakis* (Davey, 1971), with *Anisakis simplex* as the most widespread and consequently the most intensively studied. However, based on recent multilocus phylogenetic revisions, there are now six nominal *Anisakis* species within three clades. The first clade contains the members of the *A. simplex* (*sensu lato*) (*s.l.*) complex, i.e. *A. simplex* (*sensu stricto*) (*s.s.*), *Anisakis pegreffii* and *Anisakis berlandi*. The second clade includes *Anisakis ziphidarum* and *Anisakis nascettii* while a third clade comprises *Anisakis typica* (*s.l.*) likely consisting of two distinct sister species, indicated as *A. typica* sp. A and *A. typica* sp. B by Cipriani *et al.* (2022). However, all species share the larval morphology known as *Anisakis* Type I (*sensu* Berland, 1961). The species possessing morphotype II, III and IV characters (*sensu* Berland, 1961; Shiraki, 1974; Murata *et al.*, 2011), as adults primarily infecting cetaceans of the Physeteridae and Kogiidae families and placed within clade 3 (*sensu* Mattiucci *et al.*, 2018), were recently moved to genus *Skrjabinisakis*, i.e. *Skrjabinisakis physeteris*, *Skrjabinisakis brevispiculata* and *Skrjabinisakis paggiae*. This reclassification was based on analyses of the partial large subunit (LSU) and

*Email: arne.levsen@hi.no

 Fish Parasites: Pathobiology and Protection, 2nd Edition (eds P.T.K. Woo and K. Buchmann)
DOI: 10.1079/9781800628748.0018

internal transcribed spacer (ITS) rDNA sequences, as well as the *cox*2 mtDNA sequence (Safonova *et al.*, 2021; Bao *et al.*, 2022; Takano and Sata, 2022; Bao *et al.*, 2023).

A. simplex (*s.s.*) is the most studied and it occurs circumpolarly in subarctic, temperate and subtropical waters in the northern hemisphere. It has been recorded in both the western and eastern Atlantic and Pacific Oceans with its southern limit at around 30°N latitude. A comprehensive review of the molecular epidemiology of the genus *Anisakis* (*s.l.*) is provided by Mattiucci *et al.* (2018).

Anisakis species have indirect, complex life cycles which mainly involve various whale species as definitive hosts while planktonic or pelagic crustaceans act as first intermediate or paratenic hosts, and fish and squid as second intermediate or paratenic hosts. The adult worms live in the stomach of various cetaceans such as dolphins and porpoises (Odontoceti) or baleen whales (Mysticeti). Notably, the harbour seal (*Phoca vitulina*) has recently been reported as an alternative definitive host for *A. simplex* (*s.s.*), confirming that the parasite may successfully complete its life cycle in at least one pinniped host species (Cipriani *et al.*, 2025a; Kumas *et al.*, 2025). After the final two moults, maturation and copulation, the female worms shed eggs which, with the definitive host's faeces, are voided into the sea. There they embryonate producing tiny third-stage larvae (Køie *et al.*, 1995), which are ingested by small crustaceans such as copepods or euphausiids (krill) in which they grow within the haemocoel. Fish or squid become infected by eating crustaceans containing third-stage larvae which bore through the wall of the digestive tract into the viscera, body cavity and/or body musculature followed by host-induced encapsulation. When an infected fish is eaten by another fish the encapsulated larvae become free, thus repeating the larval fish host cycle. This is important from an epidemiological perspective since the repeated transmission of larvae between fishes may result in extensive accumulation. Some large and older piscivorous fish sometimes harbour hundreds or thousands of encapsulated larvae. The definitive hosts become infected by eating crustaceans, fish or squid containing larvae. The generalized life cycle of *Anisakis* species is shown in Fig. 18.1.

The majority of *A. simplex* larvae are typically encapsulated as flat, tight spirals (measuring 4–5 mm across) in and on the visceral organs. However, a smaller number of larvae may migrate from the abdominal cavity into the flesh. This eventually results in worms in fillets, which again may draw the attention of consumers and food safety authorities. Most of the flesh-invading larvae reside in the belly flaps but some may penetrate deeply into the dorsal musculature of the fish host. However, due to their small size and transparency, most *Anisakis* larvae in the fish flesh may remain undetected during industrial processing and are, hence, still present when the final product reaches the market. When liberated from the capsule, the worm, 20–30 mm long, moves vigorously. The third-stage larvae of *Anisakis* spp. and the other frequently occurring anisakids in fish (e.g. *Phocanema* spp. and *Contracaecum* spp.) have a projecting boring tooth on their head which may act as a piercing device during their migration across the gut wall. However, enzymes secreted from gland cells in the oesophagus, released through the excretory pore located anteriorly to the nerve ring and ventral to the boring tooth, are probably important in facilitating the larvae's migration from the gut into the body cavity. As the encapsulated larvae may live for years in the fish hosts, it is possible that the boring tooth lacerates the inner capsule wall permitting body growth and access to host cells (see Berland, 2006). *Anisakis* sp. third-stage larvae are clearly distinguished from those of the other anisakid species by a comparatively broad and elongate oesophageal ventricle which in live worms is clearly visible at low magnification due to its somewhat opaque appearance (Fig. 18.2).

During the past three decades there has been a huge increase in research activities on anisakid nematodes and *A. simplex* (*s.l.*) in particular, consequently resulting in a vast body of literature. Numerous studies focus on the quality-reducing or actual consumer health hazardous properties of the parasite. These efforts have been accompanied or supported by the extensive research and development in methodology and insights regarding the taxonomy, molecular systematics and co-evolutionary host–parasite relationships of this group of nematodes. Partly due to the popularity of Asian or South American-inspired seafood such as sashimi, sushi or ceviche, based on semi-processed or raw fish meat, increasing numbers of 'anisakiasis' cases

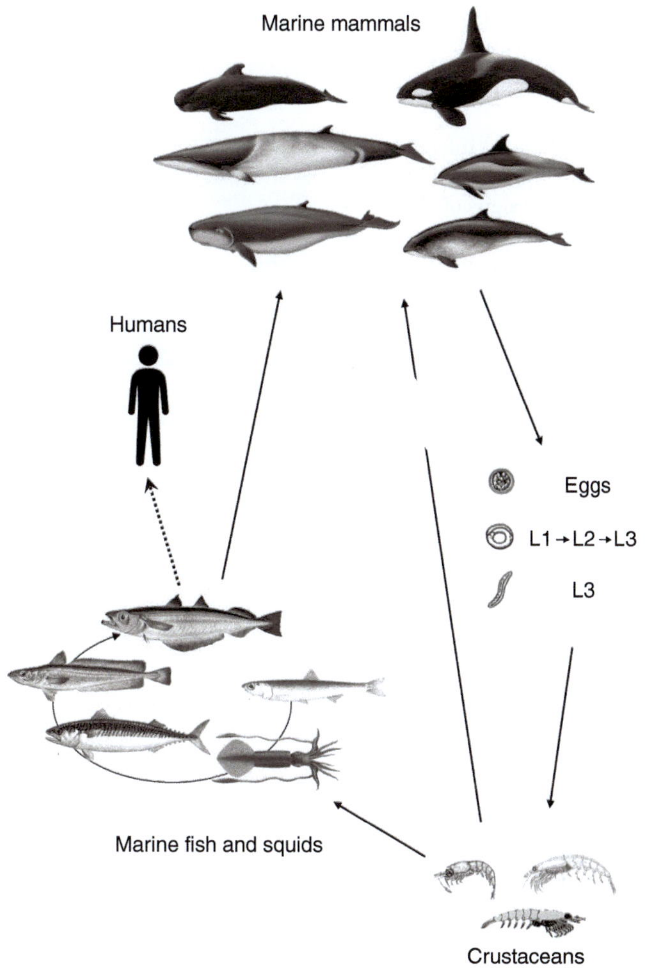

Fig. 18.1. Generalized life cycle of *Anisakis* species. L, larval stage. (Author's own image.)

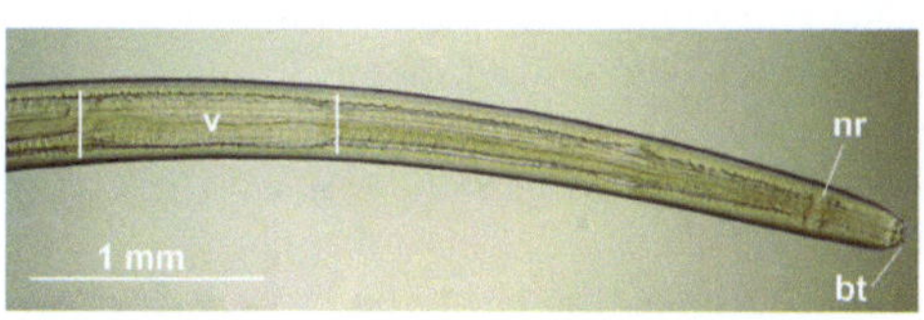

Fig. 18.2. Anterior body of *Anisakis simplex* (*s.l.*) third-stage larva. Note the boring tooth (bt), nerve ring (nr) and oesophageal ventricle (v). (Author's own image.)

in humans have been reported worldwide in the past few years. Moreover, various studies have demonstrated that *A. simplex* larvae, both dead and alive, may cause allergic reactions after consumption of infected seafood (see Audicana *et al.*, 2017; González-Fernández *et al.*, 2024; Hamada *et al.*, 2024).

In contrast to the many studies on the consumer health implications, systematics and ecology of *Anisakis* species, there are comparatively few published studies on the detrimental effects of these worms on the health, condition or fitness of the fish. Thus, this chapter discusses some key pathobiological features or effects of *Anisakis* species, with emphasis on *A. simplex* (*s.l.*), on various economically important fish species including Atlantic salmon (*Salmo salar*), Atlantic cod (*Gadus morhua*), blue whiting (*Micromesistius poutassou*), European hake (*Merluccius merluccius*), Atlantic mackerel (*Scomber scombrus*) and bluefin tuna (*Thunnus thynnus*).

18.2. Pathobiology

18.2.1. Macroscopic appearance

Fish that is more or less heavily infected with *Anisakis* sp. larvae usually appears healthy. The intensity or any macroscopic signs of the infection become obvious on visual examination of the visceral organs, mesenteries and peritoneal linings. Depending on various factors such as fish host species, host size and infection intensity, the larvae may occur scattered singly or in clusters, with sometimes hundreds of worms, on the organs and mesenteries of the visceral cavity (Fig. 18.3). The larvae are typically surrounded by a fibrous connective tissue capsule generated by the host. Especially in heavy infections, host connective tissue capsules may also be formed around clusters of larvae (Fig. 18.4). Each capsule consists of at least three layers. The inner layer mostly consists of host-cell debris with traces of pycnosis and surrounds each coil of the larva. The middle layer has a denser fibrous appearance due to the presence of fibroblastic elements, while the outermost is dominated by blood vessels, large fibroblasts and extravascular erythrocytes and their remnants (Margolis, 1970). The capsule thickness seems to depend on the infection site (abundance of connective tissue) and the age of infection. Older capsules may gradually decrease in size, the connective tissue layers become more compact, sometimes accompanied by deposition of calciferous granules. Another frequently observed feature of infections with *Anisakis* sp. is the presence of melanomacrophage aggregates around larval infection sites on the liver (Fig. 18.5). The nature of these aggregates and their role in fish pathology were reviewed by Agius and Roberts (2003), who suggested that the melanomacrophage centres develop focally in association with late-stage chronic inflammations due to various pathogens including parasites. However, the presence of macrophage aggregates (MAs) in the vicinity of encapsulated *A. simplex* larvae on the surface or in the parenchyma of the liver of flounder (*Platichthys flesus*) (Dezfuli *et al.*, 2007) and Atlantic salmon (Murphy *et al.*, 2010) is apparently not associated with any significant tissue damage. Clusters of hundreds of *A. simplex* (*s.l.*) larvae have been observed in the viscera of fish species such as European hake (Fig. 18.3), allis shad (*Alosa alosa*) and Atlantic herring (*Clupea harengus*) (Bao *et al.*, 2015, 2017; Pascual *et al.*, 2018; Cipriani *et al.*, 2025b). In European hake, the clustered larvae were connected by degraded host tissue and infiltrated with leucocytes, including macrophages. Granulation tissue layers were observed encasing many of the larvae, further indicating the chronic nature of these lesions (Pascual *et al.*, 2018). The mechanisms behind this *A. simplex* (*s.l.*) clustering behaviour remain unknown.

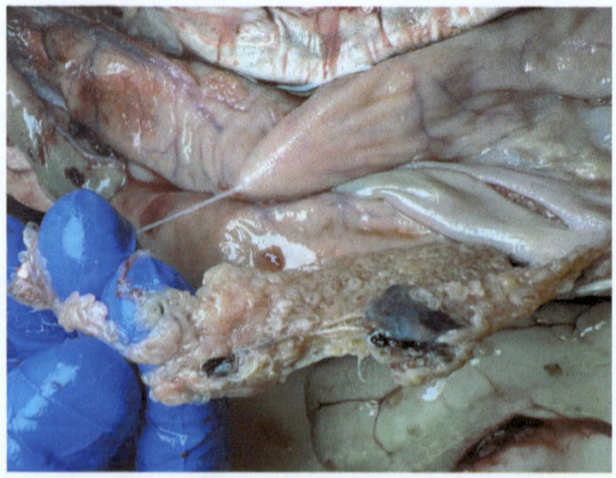

Fig. 18.3. Massive infection of *Anisakis simplex* (*s.l.*) third-stage larvae on the mesenteries surrounding the visceral organs of Atlantic hake (*Merluccius merluccius*). (Author's own image.)

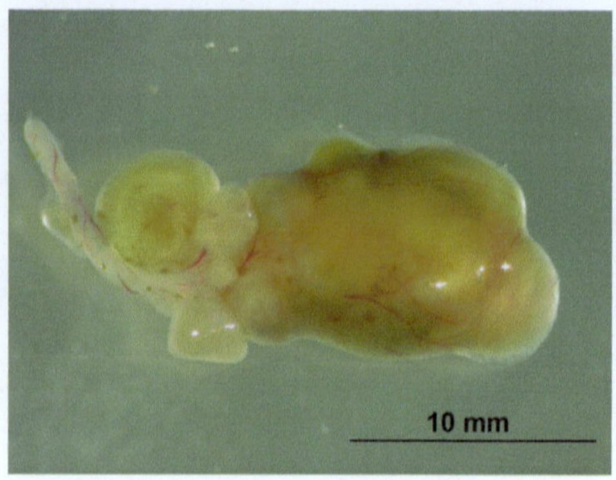

Fig. 18.4. Host-induced connective tissue capsule around a cluster of *Anisakis simplex* (*s.l.*) third-stage larvae in the visceral cavity of saithe (*Pollachius virens*) from western Norway. Note blood vessels in the outer tissue layer of the capsule. (Author's own image.)

While *Anisakis* sp. seems to be by far the most prevalent anisakid in pelagic or semi-pelagic fish species such as blue whiting, herring, mackerel or saithe (*Pollachius virens*), mixed infections

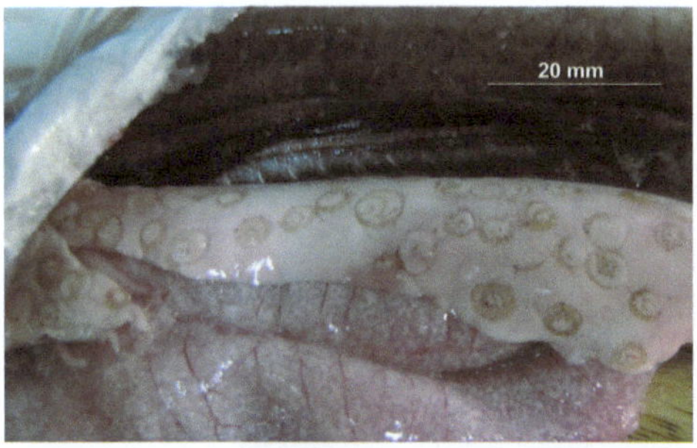

Fig. 18.5. *Anisakis simplex* (*s.l.*) third-stage larvae on the liver of blue whiting (*Micromesistius poutassou*). Numerous melanomacrophage aggregates appear as tiny black spots on or around the encapsulated larvae. (Author's own image.)

with the larvae of two or more anisakid species (e.g. *Anisakis* sp., *Phocanema* sp. and *Contracaecum* sp.) are commonly observed in demersal fish such as cod or monkfish (*Lophius* spp.) from offshore or coastal waters (Levsen *et al.*, 2018, 2022). Thus, the primary cause of lesions or other detrimental effects in mixed infections may not always be obvious since the actual anisakid species may interact.

18.2.2. Gross pathology and host-tissue damage

As with many other parasitic infections, the ability and extent to which *Anisakis* sp. larvae may pathologically affect the fish host appear to depend largely upon the intensity of infection and the infection site (e.g. lots of larvae in or on vital organs such as the liver are more likely to induce more tissue damage than would clusters of worms on the mesenteries). Thus, heavy infections of *Anisakis* sp. larvae have been reported to cause severe damage to the liver in several species of fish. For example, heavily infected livers of cod and hake may be flaccid and reddish-brown with local haemorrhages or even appear green due to the destruction of bile ducts (Margolis, 1970, and references therein). The latter may occur in cases where larvae have penetrated deeply into the liver parenchyma (Kahl, 1938; A. Levsen, 2005, unpublished results). In the liver of blue whiting from the North-East (NE) Atlantic, infections with *A. simplex* (*s.s.*) larvae seem often to co-occur with the coccidian *Goussia* sp. In these cases, macrophages and MAs were abundant around encapsulated *Anisakis* larvae, and inside the MAs, the presence of engulfed *Goussia* sp. oocysts was frequent. Moreover, in co-infected liver tissue, hepatocytes with cytoplasmic rarefaction and acute cell swelling were observed (Dezfuli *et al.*, 2021).

18.2.2.1. The 'stomach crater syndrome' of cod and tuna

The 'stomach crater syndrome' was frequently observed in larger cod (> 5 kg) caught at the spawning grounds off the Lofoten Islands, northern Norway (Berland, 1981). The stomach wall of heavily infected fish was very thick, up to 1 cm, and had in its mucosa several craters or pits from which the tails of numerous *A. simplex* (*s.l.*) larvae were protruding, their heads penetrating deeply into the pits (Fig. 18.6). Apparently, these fish had repeatedly been infected by new larvae over the years which gradually resulted in extensive accumulation. Thus, sections of the stomach wall revealed the presence of densely packed larvae (Fig. 18.7) causing tissue deformation and fibrosis within the mucosa. Rapid onset of host immunological processes, including capsule formation, subsequently stopped the larvae halfway in their tracks. The syndrome appeared to reach a peak in 1974–1975 when more than 50% of the cod stomachs investigated (n = 300–500 annually over a 12-year period) showed this condition. Any possible long-term pathobiological implications of the disease on affected cod or the local cod population were not investigated. The underlying reasons for the apparent sudden rise in prevalence of the syndrome in 1969, and its marked decrease 12 years later, also remain unclear.

In five large adult Atlantic bluefin tuna caught off western Norway during autumn of 2022 and 2023, crater-like ulcers in the mucosa of the stomach wall were observed (Bao *et al.*, 2025). Similarly to the observations in cod, most of the ulcers contained clusters of living third-stage *A. simplex* (*s.l.*) larvae with their head-ends deeply embedded in the wall and their tails protruding into the lumen (Fig. 18.8). Additionally, old healing lesions, featuring what appeared to be reabsorbed dead larvae, were noted as well. Some of the ulcerative lesions emitted a putrid odour, suggesting the presence of necrosis and decaying tissue.

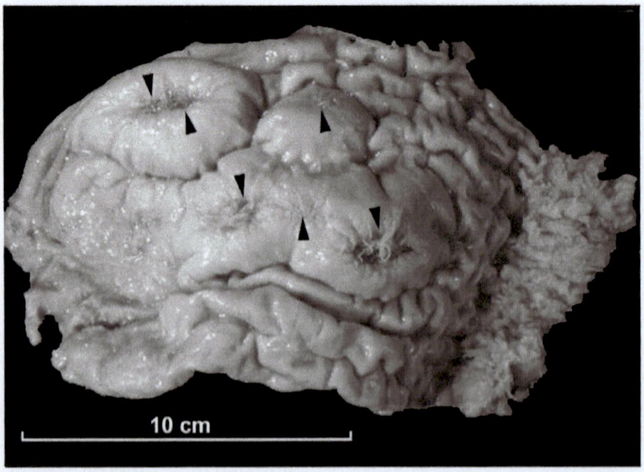

Fig. 18.6. Gross appearance of the 'stomach crater syndrome' in Atlantic cod (*Gadus morhua*), with arrowheads pointing at stomach craters filled with *Anisakis* larvae. (Author's own image.)

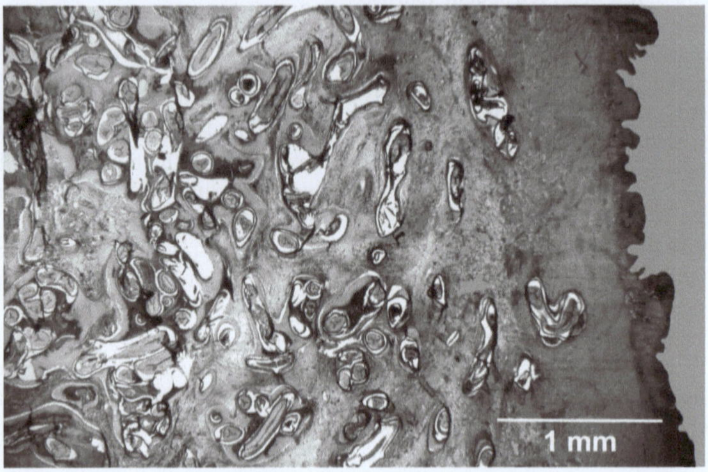

Fig. 18.7. *Anisakis simplex* third-stage larvae in the stomach wall ('stomach crater syndrome') of Atlantic cod (*Gadus morhua*). (Author's own image.)

Crater-like ulcers associated with *Anisakis* larvae in the stomach of bluefin tuna have not been previously reported. The condition seems primarily to occur in large, old fish with thick stomach walls (Berland, 2006). While the impact on affected fish is unclear, the presence of old, healing ulcers suggests that bluefin tuna may respond immunologically to *A. simplex* larvae by killing and reabsorbing them. Indeed, Mladineo *et al.* (2011) found that the prevalence of *Anisakis* sp. in wild-caught juvenile tuna declined from 33 to 17% after 1.5 to 2 years of fattening in sea cages, suggesting larval death and subsequent reabsorption. Moreover, gastric nodular lesions caused by massive infections with *A. pegreffii* were described in the yellowmouth barracuda (*Sphyraena viridensis*) (De Benedetto *et al.*, 2021).

18.2.2.2. The 'red vent syndrome' (RVS) of wild Atlantic salmon

During the early summer of 2006 and 2007, many wild Atlantic salmon returning to rivers in Scotland, England and Wales had bleeding, swollen

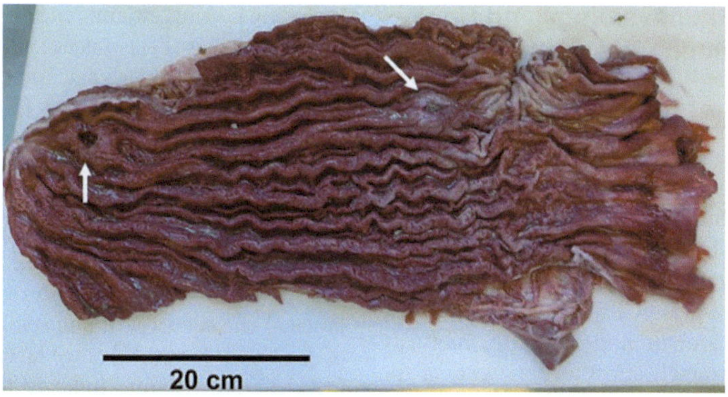

Fig. 18.8. Crater-like ulcers (white arrows) associated with clustered *Anisakis simplex* (*s.l.*) larvae in the stomach wall of Atlantic bluefin tuna (*Thunnus thynnus*). (Author's own image.)

and haemorrhagic vents. This condition, popularly named 'red vent syndrome' (RVS), was subsequently attributed to large numbers of *A. simplex* (*s.s.*) third-stage larvae in the tissues surrounding the vent and urogenital papilla (Beck *et al.*, 2008; Noguera *et al.*, 2009). RVS occurred mainly in adult one-sea-winter salmon of both sexes, although it was also recorded from some two-sea-winter salmon and sea trout (*Salmo trutta*). By the end of 2007, most major salmon rivers in mainland England, Scotland and Wales had confirmed records of affected fish. Moreover, the condition was also reported from Atlantic salmon returning to rivers in Iceland in 2007 and Norway and Quebec, Canada, in 2008.

External clinical signs include a swollen, protruding and haemorrhagic vent, sometimes accompanied by erosion of the skin, scale loss and moderate to severe bleedings in affected tissue areas. Histologically, affected vent regions showed gross lesions around lots of unencapsulated *A. simplex* larvae, with haemorrhages and moderate to severe inflammation dominated by eosinophilic granular cells and melanomacrophages. There was apparently no correlation between larval intensity in the organs and mesenteries of the body cavity, and the numbers of larvae found in the discrete area of the vent and urogenital papilla. It was noted, however, that independent of the severity of the lesions, affected fish were generally in good overall condition. Moreover, there was no evidence of RVS-induced wild salmon mortality or any other pathogenic viral or primary bacterial infections (Beck *et al.*, 2008; Noguera *et al.*, 2009). It also turned out that the extent of the lesions differed depending on how long fish had been in fresh water since salmon captured after they had spent some time upstream in the rivers showed signs of recovery.

The causative reason for RVS has as yet not been fully elucidated. Noguera *et al.* (2009) hypothesized that climate-driven spatial or temporal changes in the NE Atlantic pelagic ecosystem may have influenced the physiological stage of the fish. This was supported by the findings of strong eosinophilic inflammatory responses predominantly in early-summer fish still in the pre-spawning phase.

However, several studies on *Anisakis* occurrence in returning salmon off coastal Scotland and Norway (Senos *et al.*, 2013; Noguera *et al.*, 2015; Kent *et al.*, 2020; Mo *et al.*, 2021) suggest that generally rising intensities of *A. simplex* (*s.l.*) over the past 50 years have contributed significantly to the infection of the perianal musculature and the emergence of RVS in Atlantic salmon populations. Indeed, Scottish salmon have shown an almost fourfold increase in mean intensity from 2009 to 2015. This was accompanied by a significant increase in the number of *Anisakis* in the musculature surrounding the vent (Kent *et al.*, 2020). However, salmon returning to Norwegian rivers did not show this increase, which may explain why RVS is only rarely reported in Norway. Thus, and similar to the stomach crater syndrome in Atlantic cod, the RVS seemed to disappear as quickly as it appeared in Atlantic salmon returning to Norwegian rivers (Mo *et al.*, 2021).

18.3. Pathophysiology and Host Immune Responses

18.3.1. Pathophysiology

No information seems to exist regarding any direct pathophysiological effect of *Anisakis* sp. infections in fish. There are indications, however, that heavy larval infections may – at least in some pelagic or semi-pelagic fish species – indirectly impede body growth and/or sexual maturity and, hence, adversely affect the fecundity of the actual hosts.

18.3.2. Host immune responses

Although *Anisakis* sp. larvae appear to be generalists at the fish host level, different fish species represent different microhabitats, each characterized by specific physiological properties which may also be expressed as different immune responses to the parasite. Several commercially important pelagic and demersal fish species including herring, Atlantic cod and Atlantic hake show an increase in prevalence and abundance of *Anisakis* sp. larvae with age and size (Petrie and Wootten, 2009; Levsen and Lunestad, 2010; Levsen *et al.*, 2018, 2022; Kumas *et al.*, 2024; Cipriani *et al.*, 2025b). However, in Atlantic mackerel from the North Sea and southern Norwegian Sea, a somewhat different infection pattern seems to occur (Levsen and Midthun, 2007). Thus, results from an ongoing surveillance of the occurrence and spatial distribution of *A. simplex* (*s.l.*) third-stage larvae in mackerel from the NE Atlantic indicate that there is a slight trend towards higher larval intensity in smaller fish (< 500 g) compared with larger mackerel (> 500 g) (A. Levsen, 2019, unpublished results). Such a trend was observed in NE Atlantic mackerel examined in 2018–2019 ($n = 393$) and is illustrated in Fig. 18.9. The infection pattern suggests that at least smaller and younger mackerel are capable of reducing the infection immunologically. This is supported by frequent findings of dead larvae, and what appear to be disintegrated capsules, on the visceral organs and the fillets, especially in mackerel weighing < 500 g (Fig. 18.10).

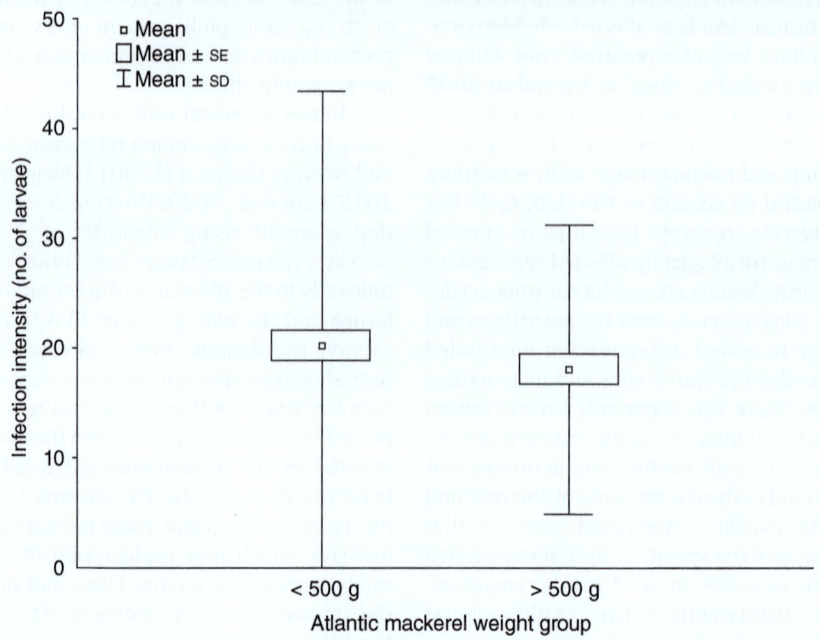

Fig. 18.9. Intensity of *Anisakis simplex* (*s.l.*) third-stage larvae in two weight groups of Atlantic mackerel (*Scomber scombrus*) from the North Sea and southern Norwegian Sea in 2018–2019. Number of mackerel examined $n = 393$; larval prevalence = 97%. (Author's own image.)

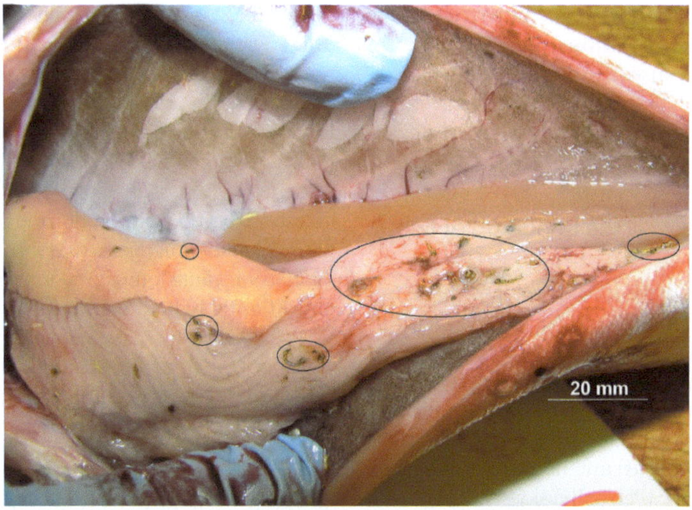

Fig. 18.10. Dead *Anisakis simplex* (*s.l.*) third-stage larva and disintegrated capsules (encircled) on the viscera of Atlantic mackerel (*Scomber scombrus*) from the northern North Sea. (Author's own image.)

Basically the same trend in *A. simplex* (*s.l.*) infection pattern has been found in saithe from the NE Atlantic (Priebe *et al.*, 1991). In this species, smaller and younger fish (3–4 years old) showed a significantly higher intensity of *A. simplex* (*s.l.*) larvae in the body musculature (fillets and belly flaps) compared with saithe older than 5 years. However, and somewhat in contrast to mackerel, up to 10% of the larvae in the muscle of older saithe were dead while only living larvae were found in the flesh of younger fish. Subsequent indirect ELISA analysis of various serum samples of the different age groups revealed a moderate correlation between antibody titre level and the age of underfeeding saithe (post-spawning), and a close correlation in fish caught during feeding periods (pre-spawning). The authors concluded that the migration ability and lifetime of the muscle-lodging larvae in saithe are influenced by a specific immune response which increases with age of the fish.

Differences in immune response to the same parasite species are known from several more-or-less closely related fish host species. For example, the plerocercoids of the pseudophyllidean cestode *Ligula intestinalis* provoke a pronounced cellular response in European roach (*Rutilus rutilus*) including massive infiltration of various leucocytes into the body cavity, often accompanied by extensive deposition of connective tissue fibres. In gudgeon (*Gobio gobio*), another frequently occurring cyprinid species in Europe, no cellular response to *L. intestinalis* is ever found (Arme, 1997). Although European *Ligula* populations apparently consist of two genetically distinct lineages maintained in sympatry (Bouzid *et al.*, 2008), various host factors including immunological responses may account for the different response patterns in these two cyprinid fish hosts, as well (Arme, 1997; Stefka *et al.*, 2009). Basically the same phenomenon is known from infections of different salmonid fish species with the ectoparasitic copepod *Lepeophtheirus salmonis*. Thus, while there is little evidence of host-tissue responses in Atlantic salmon at the parasite's feeding or attachment sites, coho salmon (*Oncorhynchus kisutch*) show strong tissue responses to *L. salmonis*, characterized by pronounced epithelial hyperplasia and inflammation (Wagner *et al.*, 2008).

These observations support the hypothesis that the *A. simplex* (*s.l.*) infection pattern, at least in some pelagic or semi-pelagic fish species, is not only related to specific life-history traits (e.g. the feeding habits and size/age of the actual fish host) but may also be influenced by host- and/or age-specific immunological characteristics. Consequently, in heavily infected smaller mackerel there may be a trade-off in metabolic energy use between the necessity to cope with the infection and the need to grow and to optimize fecundity. However, further investigations are needed in order to elucidate the possible impact of heavy *A. simplex* (*s.l.*) infections on body growth, fecundity and, consequently, the fitness of individual mackerel, or even on the robustness and recruitment of the NE Atlantic mackerel stock.

18.3.3. Effect on the condition of fish

Several workers have studied the possible effect of *Anisakis* sp. larvae on the condition factor of various wild fish host species such as sculpin (*Myoxocephalus scorpius*), Baltic herring, allis shad, twaite shad (*Alosa fallax*), European hake, haddock (*Melanogrammus aeglefinus*), whiting (*Merlangius merlangus*) and horse mackerel (*Trachurus trachurus*) (Petrushevsky and Kogteva, 1954, cited by Margolis, 1970; Podolska and Horbowy, 2003; Bao *et al.*, 2015; Pascual *et al.*, 2018; Roca-Geronés *et al.*, 2020; Macchioni *et al.*, 2021). A few studies reported increasing condition coefficient with increasing intensity of *Anisakis* sp., while in others an inverse relationship was found, even when investigating the same fish species. Additionally, co-infections with other parasites complicate the picture. Therefore, it may not always be possible to pinpoint any specific effects of *Anisakis* sp. on fish host condition. It was also hypothesized that a better condition at high larval prevalence may reflect good feeding conditions and, therefore, a higher chance of infection. However, this perspective may be oversimplistic, as it does not consider the potential negative effects of the larvae on the fish host, as demonstrated in hake (see Pascual *et al.*, 2018). Thus, further research is required to better understand this complex topic.

18.4. *Anisakis* Larvae and Farmed Fish

The larvae of *Anisakis* sp. have no significance as disease-causing parasites in cultured fish. A number of studies from different countries or areas have shown that several sea-caged salmonid fish species including Atlantic salmon, coho salmon and rainbow trout (*Oncorhynchus mykiss*) do not carry *Anisakis* larvae (Pacific North America – Deardorff and Kent, 1989; France – Angot and Brasseur, 1993; Japan – Inoue *et al.*, 2000; Norway – Lunestad, 2003; Levsen and Maage, 2016; Roiha *et al.*, 2020; Chile – Sepúlveda *et al.*, 2004; Denmark – Skov *et al.*, 2009). The occurrence of *Anisakis* sp. in the most relevant farmed fish species in the European Union/European Free Trade Association was recently reviewed (EFSA BIOHAZ Panel *et al.*, 2024). There was no evidence of *Anisakis* sp. infections in market-quality Atlantic salmon, marine rainbow trout, gilthead seabream (*Sparus aurata*), turbot (*Scophthalmus maximus*), meagre (*Argyrosomus regius*) and Atlantic halibut (*Hippoglossus hippoglossus*), while the parasite was reported from European sea bass (*Dicentrarchus labrax*), Atlantic bluefin tuna and cod. A recent study reported the occurrence of *A. simplex* (*s.s.*) in 2.5% of market-size farmed cod in Norway, with one fish carrying a single encapsulated larva in the flesh (Bao *et al.*, 2025). Overall, the probability of market-quality farmed fish being infected with *Anisakis* sp. appears to be low or very low. However, some of the farmed rainbow trout and cod examined had remains of small fish in their stomach. These findings suggest that opportunistic feeding on wild organisms occasionally entering the cages may represent an important transmission route of *Anisakis* sp. in the fish (Skov *et al.*, 2009; Bao *et al.*, 2025). Thus, case-by-case and continuous monitoring for *Anisakis* sp. in sea-caged farmed fish is recommended, although absolute absence may not be achievable in open marine farming facilities. It is important to note, however, that none of the reported *Anisakis* sp. infections in farmed fish were associated with any disease or pathologies in the fish.

18.5. Protective and Control Strategies

The effect of eight different anthelmintics (mebendazole, flubendazole, parbendazole, triclabendazole, piperazine dihydrochloride, netobimin, trichlorfon and nitroscanate) on the survival and post-treatment development of *Anisakis simplex* (*s.l.*) third-stage larvae in experimentally infected rainbow trout was investigated by Tojo *et al.* (1994). They found that none of the drugs showed any larvicidal activity nor did they affect the ability of the larvae to undergo ecdysis to the fourth larval stage. Dziekonska-Rynko *et al.* (2002) and Arias-Diaz *et al.* (2006) investigated the *in vitro* survival of *A. simplex* third-stage larvae upon treatment with ivermectin and albendazole. Both drugs reduce the survival of the larvae, but their effect appears to depend on the duration and dosage of the treatment, as well as the pH condition of the aqueous culture solution. For example, all *A. simplex* larvae were killed after 48 h exposure to ivermectin or albendazole 1 μg/ml at pH 7.0. At pH 2.0, however, 100% lethality was observed only at ivermectin and albendazole concentrations ≥ 50 μg/ml and ≥ 200 μg/ml, respectively (Dziekonska-Rynko *et al.*, 2002). In another study, the *in vitro* effect of various monoterpenic derivatives from different essential oils on *A. simplex* (*s.l.*) third-stage larvae was investigated by Navarro *et al.* (2008), who found that α-pinene, ocimene and cineole had high larvicidal activity at a concentration of 125 μg/ml for 48 h while only α-pinene and ocimene were active at 62.5 μg/ml. It must be emphasized, however, that all the above *in vitro* trials were conducted at high temperatures (36–37°C) since they were primarily aimed at exploring the applicability of the drugs or compounds against human anisakiasis. A recommended drug against intestinal nematodes such as *Oxyuris* spp., *Capillaria* spp. and *Camallanus cotti* parasitizing ornamental freshwater fishes is levamisole hydrochloride (Sanford, 2007). Recently, Donzeli Pereira *et al.* (2025) documented that wood creosote concentration of 6.7 mg/ml killed *A. simplex* (*s.l.*) larvae in *in vitro* studies. However, the possible effect of the drug on encapsulated nematode larvae in the visceral cavity of fish has yet to be investigated.

The effects of physical (e.g. heating, freezing, high-pressure processing, drying) and chemical treatments (e.g. salting, marinating, use of natural compounds) for the killing of *Anisakis* spp. in fishery products have recently been reviewed by EFSA BIOHAZ Panel *et al.* (2024).

18.5.1. Management procedures in fisheries and processing plants

Evisceration, whether performed on board or at processing plants, significantly reduces the parasite load in fishery products and prevents the potential post-mortem tissue migration of *A. simplex* (*s.l.*) from the viscera to the muscle (Cipriani *et al.*, 2024; Kumas *et al.*, 2024; Arrebola-Casañas *et al.*, 2025). Notably, a technological device designed to inactivate *A. simplex* (*s.l.*) present in fish offal before discarding into the sea was tested on a fishing vessel operating in the Grand Sole fishing area. This inactivation process, if adopted by the fleet, could theoretically lead to a substantial reduction in the number of infective larvae released back into the marine ecosystem, thereby potentially fostering the parasite's life cycle (Gonzalez *et al.*, 2018). Additionally, trimming the belly flaps can effectively reduce the *Anisakis* load in the fillets (Levsen *et al.*, 2022). In some particularly valuable fish species such as Atlantic cod, manual removal of visible anisakid larvae from the fillets on a candling table is commonly practised by the Norwegian fish-processing industry. However, this process is labour-intensive, time-consuming and costly. In response, efforts are underway to automatically detect and remove nematodes from fillets using hyperspectral imaging and deep learning techniques, along with water cutting and robotics (Syed *et al.*, 2024; https://www.fhf.no/prosjekter/prosjektbasen/901897/, accessed 28 November 2025).

Finally, fish farmed in closed recirculating aquaculture systems or flow-through facilities that utilize filtered water intake and are fed heat-treated feed are free from *Anisakis* sp. (EFSA BIOHAZ Panel *et al.*, 2024). However, as mentioned above, fish farmed in open sea cages may be exposed to the parasite.

18.6. Conclusions and Suggestions for Future Studies

The third-stage larvae of *Anisakis* spp. must be considered as parasites of low pathogenicity and virulence in fishes. Some more-or-less detrimental *Anisakis*-related disease outbreaks (e.g. the RVS in Atlantic salmon) appear to be geographically or temporarily isolated events, presumably induced by a chain of concurrent environmental changes at a particular time or locality. In general, the effects of heavy infections of *Anisakis* sp. larvae in fish seem to be governed by factors that are linked to the actual host individual or species rather than to the parasite itself. For example, considerable differences seem to exist between fish species with respect to their ability to respond immunologically against the larvae. Thus, at least some stages or age groups of Atlantic mackerel appear to be capable of reducing the

A. simplex infection by immunological means. Since the latter fish species is among the most valuable fish stocks in the North Atlantic, further studies on the significance of heavy *A. simplex* infections on the growth and fecundity of Atlantic mackerel should be carried out. Considering the predicted rise in average water temperature in the northern hemisphere, *Anisakis* sp. in Atlantic mackerel may provide a useful model for studying the dynamics or adaptability of a discrete pelagic fish host–parasite system during changing environmental conditions.

References

Agius, C. and Roberts, R.J. (2003) Melano-macrophage centres and their role in fish pathology. *Journal of Fish Diseases* 26, 499–509.

Angot, V. and Brasseur, P. (1993) European farmed Atlantic salmon (*Salmo salar* L.) are safe from anisakid larvae. *Aquaculture* 118, 339–344.

Arias-Diaz, J., Zuloaga, J., Vara, E., Balibrea, J. and Balibrea, J.L. (2006) Efficacy of albendazole against *Anisakis simplex* larvae *in vitro*. *Digestive and Liver Disease* 38, 24–26.

Arme, C. (1997) Ligulosis in two cyprinid hosts: *Rutilus rutilus* and *Gobio gobio*. *Helminthologia* 34, 191–196.

Arrebola-Casañas, F.J., Garrido, M., Adroher, F.J., Benítez, R. and Morales-Yuste, M. (2025) First insights from on-board fish gutting into the zoonotic nematode burden of pouting (*Trisopterus luscus*) at the point of sale to the consumer. *Pathogens* 14, 252. DOI: 10.3390/pathogens14030252.

Audicana, M., Girao, I. and Longo, N. (2017) *Anisakis simplex*, a new hero in the anaphylaxis scene. *SM Emergency Medicine and Critical Care* 1, 1008.

Bao, M., Mota, M., Nachón, D.J., Antunes, C., Cobo, F. *et al.* (2015) *Anisakis* infection in allis shad, *Alosa alosa* (Linnaeus, 1758), and twaite shad, *Alosa fallax* (Lacépède, 1803), from Western Iberian Peninsula rivers: zoonotic and ecological implications. *Parasitology Research* 114, 2143–2154. DOI: 10.1007/s00436-015-4403-5.

Bao, M., Strachan, N.J.C., Hastie, L.C., MacKenzie, K., Seton, H.C. and Pierce, G.J. (2017) Employing visual inspection and magnetic resonance imaging to investigate *Anisakis simplex* s.l. infection in herring viscera. *Food Control* 75, 40–47. DOI: 10.1016/j.foodcont.2016.12.030.

Bao, M., Olsen, K.M., Levsen, A., Cipriani, P., Giulietti, L. *et al.* (2022) Characterization of *Pseudoterranova ceticola* (Nematoda: Anisakidae) larvae from meso/bathypelagic fishes off Macaronesia (NW Africa waters). *Scientific Reports* 12, 17695. DOI: 10.1038/s41598-022-22542-0.

Bao, M., Giulietti, L., Levsen, A. and Karlsbakk, E. (2023) Resurrection of genus *Phocanema* Myers, 1959, as a genus independent from *Pseudoterranova* Mozgovoĭ, 1953, for nematode species (Anisakidae) parasitic in pinnipeds and cetaceans, respectively. *Parasitology International* 97, 102794. DOI: 10.1016/j.parint.2023.102794.

Bao, M., Cipriani, P., Giulietti, L. and Levsen, A. (2025) Occurrence of *Anisakis simplex* in Norwegian farmed Atlantic cod (*Gadus morhua*). *Aquaculture* 609, 742814. DOI: 10.1016/j.aquaculture.2025.742814.

Beck, M., Evans, R., Feist, S.W., Stebbing, P., Longshaw, M. and Harris, E. (2008) *Anisakis simplex sensu lato* associated with red vent syndrome in wild adult Atlantic salmon *Salmo salar* in England and Wales. *Diseases of Aquatic Organisms* 82, 61–65.

Berland, B. (1961) Nematodes from some Norwegian marine fishes. *Sarsia* 2, 1–50.

Berland, B. (1981) Massenbefall von *Anisakis simplex*-Larven am Magen des Kabeljaus (*Gadus morhua* L.). In: *IV. Wissenschaftliche Konferenz zu Fragen der Physiologie, Biologie und Parasitologie von Nutzfischen*. Wilhelm-Pieck-Universität, Rostock, Germany, pp. 125–128.

Berland, B. (2006) Musings on nematode parasites. *Fisken og Havet* 11, 1–26.

Bouzid, W., Lek, S., Mace, M., Ben Hassine, O., Etienne, R. *et al.* (2008) Genetic diversity of *Ligula intestinalis* (Cestoda: Diphyllobothriidea) based on analysis of inter-simple sequence repeat markers. *Journal of Zoological Systematics and Evolutionary Research* 46, 289–296. DOI: 10.1111/j.1439-0469.2008.00471.x.

Cipriani, P., Giulietti, L., Shayo, S.D., Storesund, J.E., Bao, M. *et al.* (2022) Anisakid nematodes in *Trichiurus lepturus* and *Saurida undosquamis* (Teleostea) from the South-West Indian Ocean: genetic evidence for the existence of sister species within *Anisakis typica* (s.l.), and food-safety considerations. *Food and Waterborne Parasitology* 28, e00177. DOI: 10.1016/j.fawpar.2022.e00177.

Cipriani, P., Giulietti, L., Bao, M., Palomba, M., Mattiucci, S. and Levsen, A. (2024) *Post-mortem* tissue migration of *Anisakis simplex* (s.s.) larvae (Nematoda: Anisakidae) in three commercially harvested fish species from the Northeast Atlantic: the role of storage time and temperature. *Food Control* 157, 110162. DOI: 10.1016/j.foodcont.2023.110162.

Cipriani, P., Giulietti, L., Palomba, M., Rodriguez Fernandez, V., Mattiucci, S. *et al.* (2025a) Anisakid biodiversity in two young harbour seals (*Phoca vitulina* L.) from coastal South-West Norway. *Parasitology Research* 124, 110. DOI: 10.1007/s00436-025-08559-0.

Cipriani, P., Bao, M., Giulietti, L., Storesund, J.E., Staby, A. and Levsen, A. (2025b) Anisakid parasites (Nematoda: Anisakidae) in European hake (*Merluccius merluccius*) from Norwegian waters: considerations on food safety and host population ecology. *Food Control* 171, 111097. DOI: 10.1016/j.foodcont.2024.111097.

Davey, J.T. (1971) A revision of the genus *Anisakis* Dujardin, 1845 (Nematoda: Ascaridida). *Journal of Helminthology* 45, 51–72.

De Benedetto, G., Giannetto, A., Riolo, K., Iaria, C., Brianti, E. and Gaglio, G. (2021) *Anisakis pegreffii* larvae in *Sphyraena viridensis* and description of granulomatous lesions. *Animals* 11, 3449. DOI: 10.3390/ani11123449.

Deardorff, T.L. and Kent, M.L. (1989) Prevalence of larval *Anisakis simplex* in pen-reared and wild-caught salmon (Salmonidae) from Puget Sound, Washington. *Journal of Wildlife Diseases* 25, 416–419.

Dezfuli, B.S., Pironi, F., Shinn, A.P., Manera, M. and Giari, L. (2007) Histopathology and ultrastructure of *Platichthys flesus* naturally infected with *Anisakis simplex* s.l. larvae (Nematoda: Anisakidae). *Journal of Parasitology* 93, 1416–1423.

Dezfuli, B.S., Simoni, E., Bosi, G., Palomba, M., Mattiucci, S. *et al.* (2021) Immunohistopathological response against anisakid nematode larvae and a coccidian in *Micromesistius poutassou* from NE Atlantic waters. *Journal of Helminthology* 95, 1–10.

Donzeli Pereira, C., Shimokawa, C., Sugiyama, H., Shiroyama, M. and Miura, T. (2025) Effects of wood creosote on anisakiasis: a Japanese traditional medicine as a potential tool against *Anisakis* larva infection. *Parasitology International* 108, 103077. DOI: 10.1016/j.parint.2025.103077.

Dziekonska-Rynko, J., Rokicki, J. and Jablonowski, Z. (2002) Effects of ivermectin and albendazole against *Anisakis simplex in vitro* and in guinea pigs. *Journal of Parasitology* 88, 395–398.

EFSA BIOHAZ Panel (European Food Safety Authority Panel on Biological Hazards), Koutsoumanis, K., Allende, A., Alvarez-Ordóñez, A., Bover-Cid, S. *et al.* (2024) Re-evaluation of certain aspects of the EFSA Scientific Opinion of April 2010 on risk assessment of parasites in fishery products, based on new scientific data. Part 1: ToRs1–3. *EFSA Journal* 22(4), e8719. DOI: 10.2903/j.efsa.2024.8719.

González, A.F., Gracia, J., Miniño, I., Romón, J., Larsson, C. *et al.* (2018) Approach to reduce the zoonotic parasite load in fish stocks: when science meets technology. *Fisheries Research* 202, 140–148. DOI: 10.1016/j.fishres.2017.08.016.

González-Fernández, J., Ullate, L., Fernández-Fígares, V., Rodero, M., Daschner, A. and Cuéllar, C. (2024) Serum IgA contributes to the comprehension of *Anisakis simplex* associated chronic urticaria. *International Immunopharmacology* 129, 111602. DOI: 10.1016/j.intimp.2024.111602.

Hamada, Y., Nakatani, E., Watai, K., Iwata, M., Nakamura, Y. *et al.* (2024) Effects of raw seafood on the risk of hypersensitivity reaction recurrence in patients with an *Anisakis* allergy: a retrospective observational study in Japan. *Allergology International* 73, 171–173. DOI: 10.1016/j.alit.2023.08.002.

Inoue, K., Oshima, S.-I., Hirata, T. and Kimura, I. (2000) Possibility of anisakid larvae infection in farmed salmon. *Fisheries Science* 66, 1049–1052.

Kahl, W. (1938) Nematoden in Seefischen. II. Erhebungen über den Befall von Seefischen mit Larven von *Anacanthocheilus rotundatus* (Rudolphi) und die durch diese Larven hervorgerufenen Reaktionen des Wirtsgewebes. *Zeitschrift für Parasitenkunde* 10, 513–534.

Kent, A.J., Pert, C.C., Briers, R.A., Diele, K. and Rueckert, S. (2020) Increasing intensities of *Anisakis simplex* third-stage larvae (L3) in Atlantic salmon of coastal waters of Scotland. *Parasites and Vectors* 13, 62. DOI: 10.1186/s13071-020-3942-5.

Køie, M., Berland, B. and Burt, M.D.B. (1995) Development to third-stage larvae occurs in the eggs of *Anisakis simplex* and *Pseudoterranova decipiens* (Nematoda, Ascaridoidea, Anisakidae). *Canadian Journal of Fisheries and Aquatic Sciences* 52(Suppl. 1), 134–139.

Kumas, K., Al-Jubury, A., Kania, P.W., Abusharkh, T. and Buchmann, K. (2024) Location and elimination of *Anisakis simplex* third stage larvae in Atlantic herring *Clupea harengus* L. *International Journal of Parasitology: Parasites and Wildlife* 24, 100937. DOI: 10.1016/j.ijppaw.2024.100937.

Kumas, K., Gonzalez Fernadez, C.M., Kania, P.W. and Buchmann, K. (2025) Gastrointestinal parasites of harbour seal (*Phoca vitulina* L.) in Danish marine waters: prevalence, abundance, intensity and reproductive potential. *International Journal of Parasitology: Parasites and Wildlife* 27, 101066. DOI: 10.1016/j.ijppaw.2025.101066.

Levsen, A. and Lunestad, B.T. (2010) *Anisakis simplex* third stage larvae in Norwegian spring spawning herring (*Clupea harengus* L.), with emphasis on larval distribution in the flesh. *Veterinary Parasitology* 171, 247–253.

Levsen A. and Maage A. (2016) Absence of parasitic nematodes in farmed, harvest quality Atlantic salmon (*Salmo salar*) in Norway – results from a large-scale survey. *Food Control* 68, 25–29. DOI: 10.1016/j.foodcont.2016.03.020.

Levsen, A. and Midthun, E. (2007) Occurrence and spatial distribution of *Anisakis* sp. in three commercially important pelagic fish stocks from the NE Atlantic, with comments on the significance to consumer safety. *Parassitologia* 49(Suppl. 2), 402–403.

Levsen, A., Svanevik, C.S., Cipriani, P., Mattiucci, S., Gay, M. *et al.* (2018) A survey of zoonotic nematodes of commercial key fish species from major European fishing grounds – introducing the FP7 PARASITE exposure assessment study. *Fisheries Research* 202, 4–21. DOI: 10.1016/j.fishres.2017.09.009.

Levsen, A., Cipriani, P., Palomba, M., Giulietti, L., Storesund, J.E. and Bao, M. (2022) Anisakid parasites (Nematoda: Anisakidae) in three commercially important gadid fish species from the southern Barents Sea, with emphasis on key infection drivers and spatial distribution within the hosts. *Parasitology* 149(14), 1942–1957. DOI: 10.1017/S0031182022001305.

Lunestad, B.T. (2003) Absence of nematodes in farmed Atlantic salmon (*Salmo salar* L.) in Norway. *Journal of Food Protection* 66, 122–124.

Macchioni, F., Tedesco, P., Cocca, V., Massaro, A., Sartor, P. *et al.* (2021) Anisakid and Raphidascaridid parasites in *Trachurus trachurus*: infection drivers and possible effects on the host's condition. *Parasitology Research* 120, 3113–3122. DOI: 10.1007/S00436-021-07200-0.

Margolis, L. (1970) Nematode diseases of marine fishes. In: Snieszko, S.F. (ed.) *A Symposium on Diseases of Fishes and Shellfishes*. American Fisheries Society, Washington, DC, pp. 190–208.

Mattiucci, S., Cipriani, P., Levsen, A., Paoletti, M. and Nascetti, G. (2018) Molecular epidemiology of *Anisakis* and Anisakiasis: an ecological and evolutionary road map. *Advances in Parasitology* 99, 93–263. DOI: 10.1016/bs.apar.2017.12.001.

Mladineo, I., Segvić, T. and Petrić, M. (2011) Do captive conditions favor shedding of parasites in the reared Atlantic bluefin tuna (*Thunnus thynnus*)? *Parasitology International* 60, 25–33. DOI: 10.1016/j.parint.2010.09.007.

Mo, T.A., Fossøy, F. and Poppe, T.T. (2021) Increasing intensities of *Anisakis simplex* (Rudolphi, 1809 det. Krabbe, 1878) larvae with weight and sea age in returning adult Atlantic salmon, *Salmo salar* L., of coastal waters of Norway. *Journal of Fish Diseases* 44, 1075–1089. DOI: 10.1111/jfd.13369.

Murata, R., Suzuki, J., Sadamasu, K. and Kai, A. (2011) Morphological and molecular characterization of *Anisakis* larvae (Nematoda: Anisakidae) in *Beryx splendens* from Japanese waters. *Parasitology International* 60, 193–198. DOI: 10.1016/j.parint.2011.02.008.

Murphy, T.M., Berzano, M., O'Keeffe, S.M., Cotter, D.M., McEvoy, S.E. *et al.* (2010) Anisakid larvae in Atlantic salmon (*Salmo salar* L.) grilse and post-smolts: molecular identification and histopathology. *Journal of Parasitology* 96, 77–82.

Navarro, M.C., Noguera, M.A., Romero, M.C., Montilla, M.P., González de Selgas, J.M. and Valero, A. (2008) *Anisakis simplex* s.l.: larvicidal activity of various monoterpenic derivatives of natural origin against L3 larvae *in vitro* and *in vivo*. *Experimental Parasitology* 120, 295–299.

Noguera, P., Collins, C., Bruno, D., Pert, C., Turnbull, A. *et al.* (2009) Red vent syndrome in wild Atlantic salmon *Salmo salar* in Scotland is associated with *Anisakis simplex sensu stricto* (Nematoda: Anisakidae). *Diseases of Aquatic Organisms* 87, 199–215.

Noguera, P., Pert, C., Collins, C., Still, N. and Bruno, D. (2015) Quantification and distribution of *Anisakis simplex* sensu stricto in wild, one sea winter Atlantic salmon, *Salmo salar*, returning to Scottish rivers. *Journal of the Marine Biological Association of the United Kingdom* 95, 391–399. DOI: 10.1017/S0025315414001374.

Pascual, S., Rodríguez, H., Pierce, G.J., Hastie, L.C. and González, A.F. (2018) The NE Atlantic European hake: a neglected high exposure risk for zoonotic parasites in European fish markets. *Fisheries Research* 202, 69–78. DOI: 10.1016/j.fishres.2017.12.008.

Petrie, A.B. and Wootten, R. (2009) A survey of *Anisakis* and *Pseudoterranova* in Scottish fisheries and the efficacy of current detection methods. *Report of the Food Standards Agency – Project S14008*. Food Standards Agency Scotland, Aberdeen, UK.

Petrushevsky, G.K. and Kogteva, E.P. (1954) Effect of parasitic diseases on condition of fish. *Zoologicheskii Zhurnal* 33, 395–405 (in Russian).

Podolska, M. and Horbowy, J. (2003) Infection of Baltic herring (*Clupea harengus membras*) with *Anisakis simplex* larvae, 1992–1999: a statistical analysis using generalized linear models. *ICES Journal of Marine Science* 60, 85–93.

Priebe, K., Huber, C., Märtlbauer, E. and Terplan, G. (1991) Nachweis von Antikörpern gegen Larven von *Anisakis simplex* beim Seelachs *Pollachius virens* mittels ELISA. *Journal of Veterinary Medicine B* 38, 209–214.

Roca-Geronès, X., Segovia, M., Godínez-González, C., Fisa, R. and Montoliu, I. (2020) *Anisakis* and *Hysterothylacium* species in Mediterranean and North-East Atlantic fishes commonly consumed in Spain: epidemiological, molecular and morphometric discriminant analysis. *International Journal of Food Microbiology* 325, 108642. DOI: 10.1016/j.ijfoodmicro.2020.108642.

Roiha, I.S., Maage, A. and Levsen, A. (2020) Farmed rainbow trout (*Oncorhynchus mykiss*) in Norway are at low risk of carrying anisakid nematodes. *Journal of applied Aquaculture* 33, 279–290. DOI: 10.1080/10454438.2020.1785368.

Safonova, A.E., Voronova, A.N. and Vainutis, K.S. (2021) First report on molecular identification of *Anisakis simplex* in *Oncorhynchus nerka* from the fish market, with taxonomical issues within Anisakidae. *Journal of Nematology* 53, e2021–e2023. DOI: 10.21307/jofnem-2021-023.

Sanford, S. (2007) Levamisole Hydrochloride – Its Application and Usage in Freshwater Aquariums. *Loaches Online*. Available at: https://www.loaches.com/Members/shari2/levamisole-hydrochloride-1 (accessed 28 November 2025).

Senos, M., Poppe, T.T., Hansen, H. and Mo, T.A. (2013) Tissue distribution of *Anisakis simplex* larvae (Nematoda; Anisakidae) in wild Atlantic salmon, *Salmo salar*, from the Drammenselva river, south-east Norway. *Bulletin of the European Association of Fish Pathologists* 33, 111–117.

Sepúlveda, F., Marín, S.L. and Carvajal, J. (2004) Metazoan parasites in wild fish and farmed salmon from aquaculture sites in southern Chile. *Aquaculture* 235, 89–100.

Shiraki, T. (1974) Larval nematodes of family Anisakidae (Nematoda) in the northern Sea of Japan as a causative agent of eosinophilic phlegmone of granuloma in the human gastro-intestinal tract. *Acta Medica et Biologica* 22, 57–98.

Skov, J., Kania, P.W., Olsen, M.M., Lauridsen, J.H. and Buchmann, K. (2009) Nematode infections of maricultured and wild fishes in Danish waters: a comparative study. *Aquaculture* 298, 24–28.

Stefka, J., Hypsa, V. and Scholz, T. (2009) Interplay of host specificity and biogeography in the population structure of a cosmopolitan endoparasite: microsatellite study of *Ligula intestinalis* (Cestoda). *Molecular Ecology* 18, 1187–1206.

Syed, S., Ortega, S., Anderssen, K.E., Nilsen, H.A. and Heia, K. (2024) Hyperspectral imaging and deep learning for parasite detection in white fish under industrial conditions. *Scientific Reports* 14, 27426. DOI: 10.1038/s41598-024-76808-w.

Takano, T. and Sata, N. (2022) Multigene phylogenetic analysis reveals non-monophyly of *Anisakis* s. l. and *Pseudoterranova* (Nematoda: Anisakidae). *Parasitology International* 91, 102631. DOI: 10.1016/j.parint.2022.102631.

Tojo, J.L., Santamarina, M.T., Leiro, J.L., Ubeira, F.M. and Sanmartin, M.L. (1994) Failure of antihelmintic treatment to control *Anisakis simplex* in trout (*Oncorhynchus mykiss*). *Japanese Journal of Parasitology* 43, 301–304.

Wagner, G.N., Fast, M.D. and Johnson, S.C. (2008) Physiology and immunology of *Lepeophteirus salmonis* infections of salmonids. *Trends in Parasitology* 24, 176–183.

19 *Lernaea cyprinacea* and Related Species

Annemariè Avenant-Oldewage*
Department of Zoology, University of Johannesburg, South Africa

Abstract

The lernaeids or 'anchor worms' are ectoparasites on the skin and/or gills of various fish and amphibian species. Post-metamorphosed females attach on their hosts and cuticular outgrowths form anchors that penetrate the hosts' muscles. The parasites cause unsightly sores and/or scars which impact on marketability of the fish, cause blindness when they attach to the eyes or death in young fish when they penetrate organs. They have a direct life cycle, and an inseminated female produces many eggs that protrude in two egg sacks from the hind body. The eggs hatch into free-living larvae. The parasite is frequently introduced during fish trade and subsequently infects indigenous species. Post-metamorphosed females attach and grow into the dermis of hosts, causing large, inflamed sores with severe haemorrhagic pits and aggregations of melanin in the epidermis. After a few days a connective tissue capsule is deposited around the parasite causing lesions on the host. Partial immunity is acquired and reinfection results in a lower number of parasite eggs being produced. Various treatment strategies are discussed although many have not been registered for use in aquaculture and are also detrimental to the environment. The chapter concludes by highlighting suggested future research areas.

19.1. Introduction

The lernaeids are commonly referred to as 'anchor worms', a misleading term for these mesoparasitic crustaceans. The vernacular name is derived from the body shape of the gravid adult female that has a highly metamorphosed thorax (Figs 19.1, 19.2 and 19.3). The post-metamorphosis female *Lernaea* Linnaeus, 1758 has an elongated, tubular body that is separated into three tagmata: a cephalothorax, thorax and abdomen (Harding, 1950). The thorax enlarges disproportionally along with the ovaries after copulation and attachment, while the remainder of the body and appendages retain their larval sizes and are, therefore, minute in comparison to the thorax (Figs 19.3 and 19.4). All other life stages and adult males are not permanently attached to a host and resemble free-living copepods in size and shape. In adult females the cephalothorax typically consists of a head with two or three pointed or protruding anchors/'horns', two pairs of antennae, the mandibles, two pairs of maxillae as well as the first pair of maxillipeds (Robinson and Avenant-Oldewage, 1996; Dalu *et al.*, 2012) (Fig. 19.2a and b). The thorax contains the ovaries and bears five pairs of swimming legs and two conspicuous egg-filled sacs that hang

*Email: aoldewage@uj.ac.za

 Fish Parasites: Pathobiology and Protection, 2nd Edition (eds P.T.K. Woo and K. Buchmann)
DOI: 10.1079/9781800628748.0019

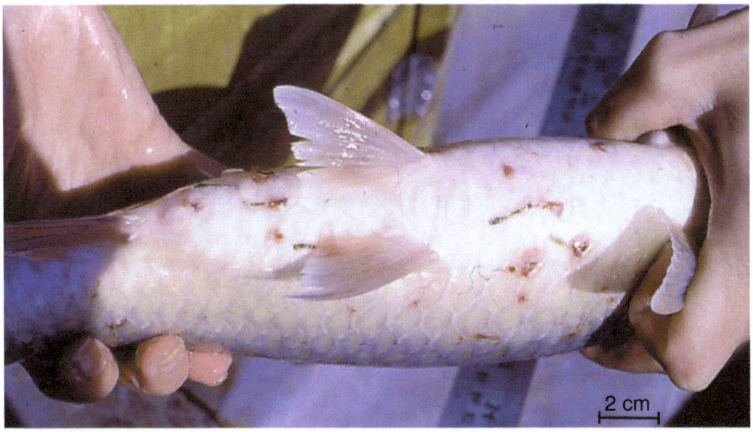

Fig. 19.1. *Lernaea cyprinacea* Linnaeus, 1758 post-metamorphosis female *in situ* on rednose labeo, *Labeo rosae* Steindachner, 1894; ventral view of fish. Active parasitic infections and lesions occur interspersed over the host body. (Author's own image.)

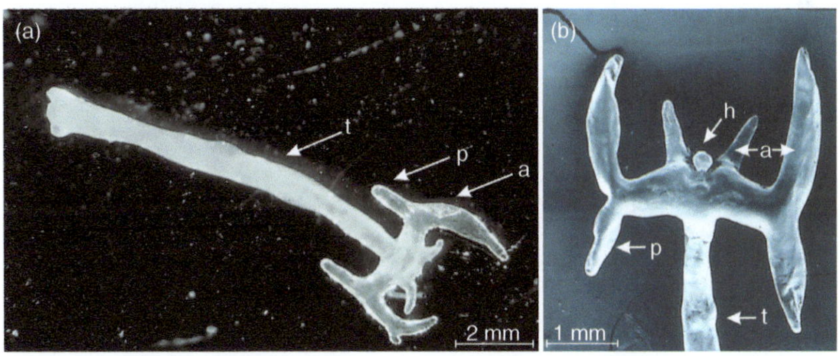

Fig. 19.2. (a) *Lernaea cyprinacea* post-metamorphosis female after detachment from the host and removing the host capsule to expose the attachment structures and head. (b) Scanning electron micrograph of the head of *L. cyprinacea* female, the anterior end bears the minute head and the huge attachment structures/anchors. a, anterior process of the anchor; h, head; p, posterior process of the anchor; t, thorax. (Author's own image.)

from two openings in the posterior end of the thorax, referred to as the genital somite. The genital somite also bears the genital openings. Adult females reach a length of 12–16 mm excluding the egg sacs, which may add up to 6 mm to the length (Figs 19.1 and 19.5).

Larval *Lernaea* are not attached to a host and late-stage copepodids, cyclopodids and mature stages frequent the gills. After insemination adult females attach permanently, and the anterior part of their body is mostly lodged in the host's musculature. Cephalic outgrowths of the cuticle extend into the host tissue and secure the parasite where the epizootics cause unsightly red sores on the host (Fig. 19.1). Old lesions (lacking a parasite) occur interspersed between active infections. In severe cases or in small fish or fry, the infection causes death of the host (Innal and Avenant-Oldewage, 2012) or impairment of movement (Fig. 19.5). Barson *et al.* (2008) reported a 100% prevalence, coupled with a mean intensity of up to 149 parasites per fish, in two *Oreochromis* species in impoundments in the south-eastern lowveld of Zimbabwe. The unsightly sores in edible fish cause consumer resistance (Marina *et al.*, 2008).

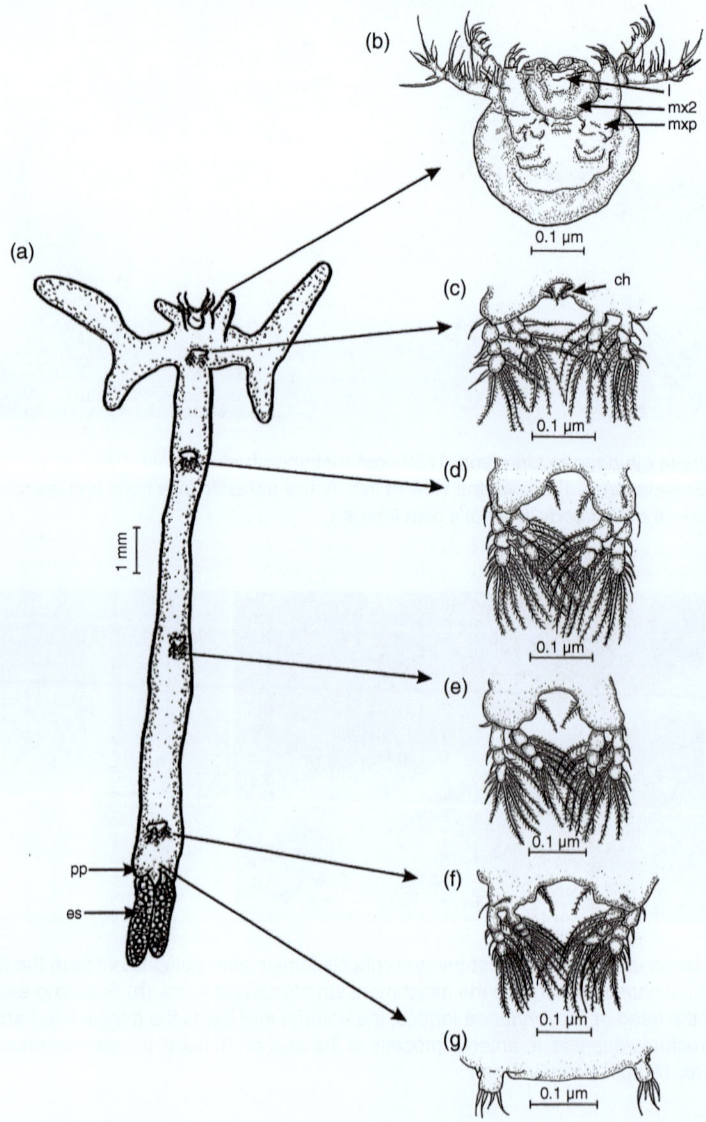

Fig. 19.3. Line drawing of *Lernaea cyprinacea* post-metamorphosis female: (a) mature ovigerous female; (b) cephalothorax with appendages; (c) first pair of biramous thoracopods; (d) second pair of biramous thoracopods; (e) third pair of biramous thoracopods; (f) fourth pair of biramous thoracopods; (g) fifth pair of thoracopods (uniramous). ch, chitinized hook; es, egg sack; l, lower lip; mx2, second maxilla; mxp, maxilliped; pp, pregenital prominence. (Redrawn from Robinson and Avenant-Oldewage, 1996 with permission.)

19.1.1. Host range

Lernaeids occur in freshwater fishes in natural water systems (Kularatne *et al.*, 1994a; Barson *et al.*, 2008) and are a pest in aquaculture environments. They have a direct life cycle (Fig. 19.4); therefore an inseminated female can lead to infection of resident fish. They are notorious killers, specifically of small fishes (Woo and Shariff, 1990; Innal *et al.*, 2017), and cause great economic loss (Kabata, 1985; Shariff and Roberts, 1989; Hoffman, 1999; Piasecki *et al.*, 2004; Hemaprasanth *et al.*, 2008). Local fishermen in Zimbabwe may discard infected fish (Dalu *et al.*,

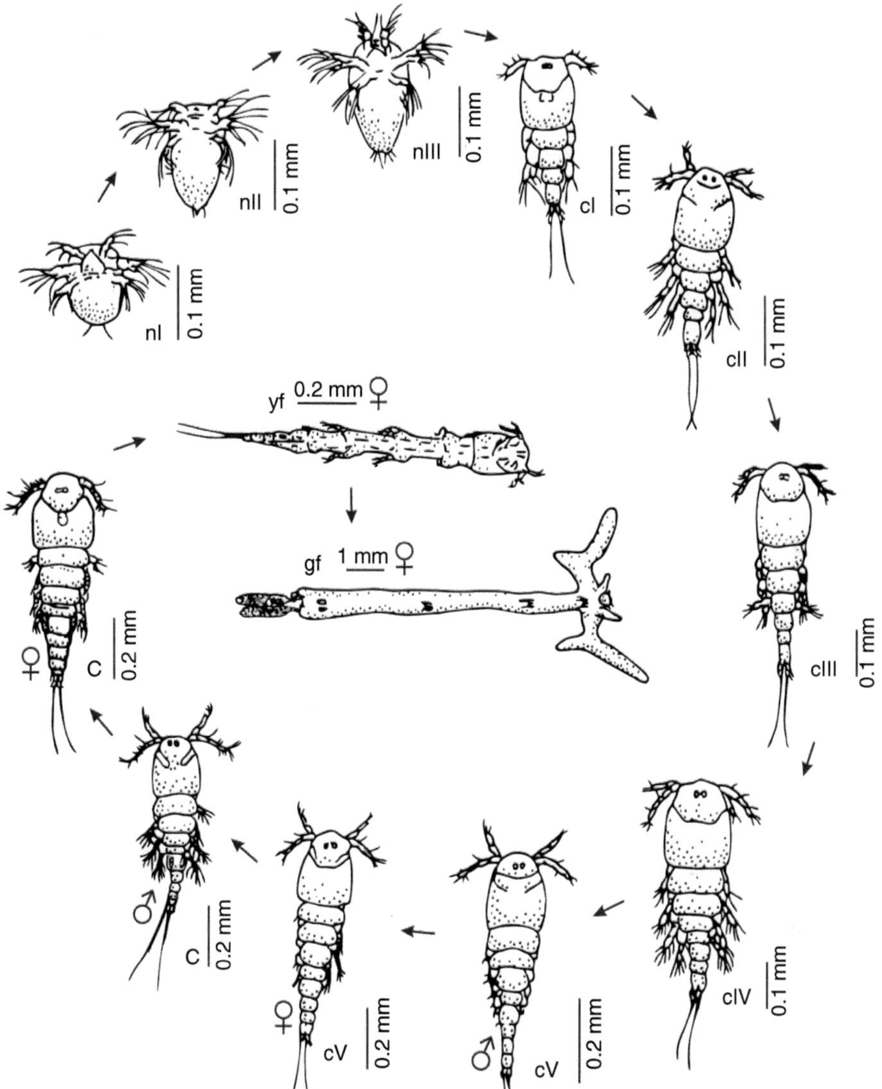

Fig. 19.4. Line drawing of life cycle of *Lernaea cyprinacea*. nI, nauplius I; nII, nauplius II; nIII, nauplius III; cI, copepodite I; cII, copepodite II; cIII, copepodite III; cIV, copepodite IV; cV, copepodite V; C, cyclopoid; yf, young female; gf, gravid female (nI–yf, redrawn from Grabda, 1963; yf, redrawn from Kasahara, 1962). Note the big difference in scale bars between larval and mature specimens. (Author's own image.)

2012) as the sores and/or scars cause consumer resistance. They are, furthermore, suspected of transmitting viruses and/or bacteria that result in secondary infections (Noga, 1986; Woo and Shariff, 1990).

L. cyprinacea was described from Crucian carp *Carassius carassius* (Linnaeus, 1758) collected in Sweden (Linnaeus, 1758). There are currently 57 valid *Lernaea* species listed in the World of Copepods database with many *species inquirenda* (Walter and Boxshall, 2025). This is probably linked to applying the shape of the anchors as a distinguishing feature. Fryer (1961) already reported that the anchor shapes differ between

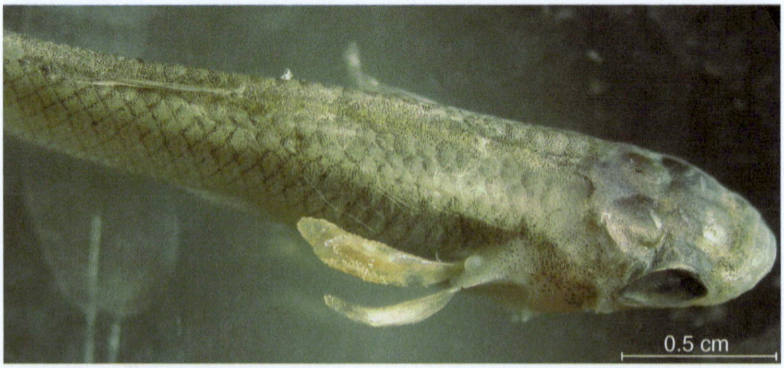

Fig. 19.5. *Lernaea cyprinacea in situ* at the base of the fin on eastern mosquitofish, *Gambusia holbrooki* Girard, 1859. (Image courtesy of Deniz Innal.)

specimens of the same species and cautioned that this plasticity may influence accurate identification when it is based on only this characteristic. Tasawar *et al*. (2009) reported a mixed infection containing four *Lernaea* species on the grass carp *Ctenopharyngodon idella* (Valenciennes, 1844). Poddubnaâ (1973), however, reported that when different host species were infected by larvae from a single batch of *Lernaea elegans* (a synonym of *Lernaea cyprinacea* Linnaeus, 1758), adult parasites exhibited varying anchor characteristics, some of which corresponded to other species of *Lernaea*. Pallavi *et al*. (2017) assigned four species to *Lernaea* specimens collected in nature and aquaculture based on their morphology but reported that analyses of 18S and 28S ribosomal DNA markers confirmed that all morphotypes were *L. cyprinacea*. However, using morphology Hua *et al*. (2019) identified *Lernaea cruciata* (Lesueur, 1824) from eastern mosquitofish *Gambusia holbrooki* Girard, 1859 and *L. cyprinacea* from goldfish *Carassius auratus* (Linnaeus, 1758). The fishes were collected from nature and from aquaculture, but when both species were infected in the laboratory with *L. cyprinacea* offspring, the parasites from both fish species conformed to *L. cyprinacea* based on molecular data. Thus, these two species are conspecific, and the morphological differences are host induced. Similarly, Zhu *et al*. (2021) reported a huge variety of anchor shapes from fishes in Australia but reported the genetic characterization confirmed that all specimens were *L. cyprinacea*.

The application of molecular identification of *Lernaea* is gaining traction, particularly the use of ribosomal DNA markers (18S and 28S) (Pallavi *et al*., 2017; Soares *et al*., 2018; Hua *et al*., 2019; Zhu *et al*., 2021; Shah *et al*., 2025), but mitochondrial DNA (CO1, cytochrome c oxidase subunit I) is not informative at species level in this genus (Pallavi *et al*., 2017).

Lernaea occurs on all continents, but most species occur in Africa (Piasecki *et al*., 2004; Piasecki and Avenant-Oldewage, 2008; Walter and Boxshall, 2025). *L. cyprinacea* has a cosmopolitan distribution, frequently as an introduced parasite, and infects a variety of hosts (Kabata, 1979; Shariff *et al*., 1986; Paperna, 1996). Some *Lernaea* species have restricted host ranges (Shariff *et al*., 1986; Paperna, 1996) as parasites of freshwater teleosts, specifically cyprinids, but also infect salmonids and other fishes such as tilapia (Kabata, 1979; Shariff *et al*., 1986; Paperna, 1996; Robinson and Avenant-Oldewage, 1996; Barson *et al*., 2008; Shinn *et al*., 2023). Fryer (1966) and Thurston (1969) reported *Lernaea barnimiana* (Hartmann, 1865) and *L. cyprinacea* on *Bagrus*, and adult females on tilapia species. Dalu *et al*. (2012) found that African sharptooth catfish *Clarias gariepinus* (Burchell, 1822), tigerfish *Hydrocynus vittatus* Castelnau, 1861 and the tank goby *Glossogobius giuris* (Hamilton, 1822) were not infected, although all other fish species in an isolated dam in Zimbabwe were infected.

Lernaeids have also been recorded from: (i) foothill yellow-legged frog, *Rana boylii* Baird, 1854 (Kupferberg *et al*., 2009); (ii) unidentified tadpoles in North America (Baldauf, 1961; Tidd and Shields, 1963; Kupferberg *et al*., 2009), South America (Martins and Souza, 1996;

Alcalde and Batistoni, 2005) and Asia (Ming, 2001); and (iii) axolotl, *Ambystoma mexicanum* (Shaw and Nodder, 1798), (Carnevia and Speranza, 2003; Melidone *et al.*, 2004). Furthermore, the copepodids (late-stage larvae) of *Lernaea* have been reported from the gills of many freshwater fish species (Shields and Tidd, 1974) and from the gills of *Rana* frogs (Fryer, 1966; Shields and Tidd, 1974). Thus, lernaeids do not appear to be strictly host specific.

19.1.2. Life cycle

Lernaea has a direct life cycle, commonly involving a single host. However, Wilson (1917) reported *Lernaea variabilis* (Wilson, 1916) copepodids from short-nosed gar *Lepistomus platostomus* Rafinesque, 1820, whereas their adult females occurred on the bluegill.

The life cycle consists of three nauplius stages and five copepodid stages, of which the last stage gives rise to male and female cyclopoids (Fig. 19.4). During copulation, two spermatophores are attached on the two sperm receptacles situated dorsally on the genital somite of females. After copulation the males die and inseminated females attach permanently to a host (Piasecki and Avenant-Oldewage, 2008). The naupliar stages are free-swimming and non-feeding (Shields and Tidd, 1974). The third stage moults into the first copepodid stage. The rate of development of larvae is determined by the ambient temperature. At 22–25°C the life cycle from egg to mature adult is completed in 13–14 days (Al-Hamed and Hermiz, 1973).

Copepodids of both sexes are frequently encountered on the host's gills and apparently feed on epidermal and dermal tissues (Shields and Tidd, 1974; Goodwin, 1999). They are not permanently attached, and periods of attachment are interspersed with bouts of energetic swimming in the vicinity of the gill filaments. After insemination, females attach permanently to the host by burrowing with the aid of the head appendages into the host tissue. The direction of growth is initially forwards beneath a scale and after the initial establishment it grows in a plane parallel to the flank of the fish, and they become tightly secured between scales (Fryer, 1961). This process is further enhanced by the secretion of what appears to be digestive or histolytic enzymes (Shields and Goode, 1978; Shariff and Roberts, 1989). They then undergo metamorphosis of the cephalic region to form lateral processes, the anchors (Fig. 19.2), which grow into the parasite in soft host tissue, usually in the superficial layer of the skin, although they have also been reported from the gills and the buccal cavity (McNeil, 1961; Fryer, 1966; Ghittino, 1987). The shape of the anchors differs between species (simple anchors or anchors with branches) but also between specimens in the same species (similar branching but different size or orientation) and is also affected by the consistency of the surrounding tissue (Fryer, 1968). After attachment the thorax expands disproportionately to form the main part of the parasite body.

In post-metamorphosed females, the anterior end is embedded in host tissue while the thorax and abdomen remain on the surface of the host allowing the parasite access to feeding on host tissue while the eggs are released into the egg sack. Eggs sacks are produced within 4 days after attachment (Al-Hamed and Hermiz, 1973).

19.1.3. Distribution

19.1.3.1. On the host

Parasites attach to all exterior parts of the host body, inside the mouth, and gill chambers (Noga, 1986; Barson *et al.*, 2008). Occasionally they are on gill filaments or even in the eye of fish (Woo and Shariff, 1990) in stagnant or slow-flowing water. In fast-flowing water they are found on protected areas such as behind the fins. Parasite intensity increases in dry seasons due to the reduced volume of the water (Robinson and Avenant-Oldewage, 1996; Manna *et al.*, 1999; Medeiros and Maltchik, 1999) and consequently infection increases further because of immunosuppression caused by environmental stress (Plaul *et al.*, 2010).

Larger fish are prone to higher parasite prevalence and intensities (Noga, 1986; Tamuli and Shanbhogue,1996a; Gutiérrez-Galindo and Lacasa-Millán, 2005; Pérez-Bote, 2010), but Tasawar *et al.* (2009) found that *Lernaea* was significantly more prevalent on grass carp smaller than 15 cm.

19.1.3.2. Geographical distribution

L. cyprinacea was described from Sweden by Linnaeus in 1758 and thereafter recorded by many authors from Europe (Harding, 1960). It now has a cosmopolitan distribution, and five subspecies are recognized (Walter and Boxshall, 2025). However, according to Piasecki *et al.* (2004) and Figueira and Ceccarelli (1991), it was introduced into North and South America and Australia (Lymbery *et al.*, 2010) along with imported cyprinids. It has spread to many states in the USA. In a *Lernaea* outbreak in Arkansas, most of the channel catfish *Ictalurus punctatus* (Rafinesque, 1818) on a farm died (Goodwin, 1999). In Bulgaria it became widespread, presumably after human introduction (Daskalov and Georgiev, 2001). Similarly, in Egypt, *L. cyprinacea* was reported to infect native Nile tilapia *Oreochromis niloticus* (Linnaeus, 1758) and common carp *Cyprinus carpio* Linnaeus, 1758 after the introduction of goldfish *Carassius auratus* (Linnaeus, 1758) (cf. Mahmoud *et al.*, 2009), and it was also introduced into central and southern Africa (Fryer, 1968; Viljoen, 1986; Paperna, 1996; Robinson and Avenant-Oldewage 1996; Boane *et al.*, 2008; Barson *et al.*, 2008; Welicky *et al.*, 2017). In South America, it was introduced into Brazil (Silva-Souza *et al.*, 2000; Gallio *et al.*, 2007), Uruguay (Carnevia and Speranza, 2003) and Argentina (Vanotti and Tanzola, 2005; Soares *et al.*, 2018) where most of the imported cyprinid species became infected. It has also been reported from Japan (Nagasawa *et al.*, 2012; Yoshimine *et al.*, 2015), Indonesia (Muchlisin *et al.*, 2014), India (Mandal *et al.*, 2016), Pakistan (Dawar *et al.*, 2015; Shah *et al.*, 2025), Iran (Bozorgnia *et al.*, 2012) and from 40 fish species in Turkey (Koyun and Atici, 2018).

The occurrence and development rate of the parasite are dependent on temperature. In temperate regions it occurs mostly during late summer, the optimal temperature is between 25 and 30°C (Shields and Tidd, 1968; Noga, 1986; Marcogliese, 1991; Hoffman, 1998) and more than one life cycle may be completed per season. It is therefore rare in cooler regions, the life cycle is interrupted when the temperature of the water drops below 14°C and inseminated females may overwinter on hosts (Grabda, 1963). It is prevalent in slow-flowing water and therefore intensive culture conditions or man-made lakes provide ideal environments (Pérez-Bote, 2010). In temperate regions metamorphosed females overwintered on the hosts (Shields and Tidd, 1968).

19.1.4. Impact on production

Infected fishes have a significantly lower condition factor (mass per length ratio) than non-parasitized fishes and their haematocrit value was also lower (Kabata, 1985; Pérez-Bote, 2010). As few as six parasites can cause the death of fingerlings (Daskalov *et al.*, 1999; Innal *et al.*, 2017).

19.2. Diagnosis of the Infection

19.2.1. Host behaviour

Only 4 days post-infection with *Lernaea polymorpha*, Yü, 1938 naïve fish displayed swift, agitated movements, interspersed with periods of resting. Soon thereafter they rubbed their bodies against the gravel substrate or against other fish in the tank (Shields and Goode, 1978; Woo and Shariff, 1990), while fish with severe parasitaemia eventually became sluggish and mortality occurred (Shariff and Roberts, 1989; Tamuli and Shanbhogue, 1996a). Similar behaviour was reported in kissing gourami *Helostoma temminckii*, Cuvier, 1829 infected by *L. cyprinacea* (Woo and Shariff, 1990).

19.2.2. Clinical signs

Adult female parasites can be observed macroscopically, and the attachment sites are surrounded by a haemorrhagic area on the skin (Fig. 19.1). The parasite thorax and abdomen extend from the wound, and it is not unusual to observe two egg sacs attached to the posterior end of the parasite's genital somite (Fig. 19.1). An area of up to 1 cm in diameter surrounding the parasite is red and inflamed. Lesions without parasites are also common (Berry *et al.*, 1991) (Fig. 19.1), which may be old lesions.

Larval (copepodid) infections occur on the gills and skin. The larvae are small (0.6 mm) and can be better detected with a dissection microscope or magnifying glass. Furthermore, the larvae are only temporarily attached to the gills and attachment is interspersed with periods of erratic activity; thus larvae may therefore easily go unnoticed, particularly by an untrained eye. Infected fish may display respiratory difficulty (Kabata, 1985) as the larvae feed on the gills.

19.3. External/Internal Lesions (Macroscopic and Microscopic)

19.3.1. Larvae

Larvae (copepodids) do not permanently attach to the gills but cause disruption and necrosis and even the death of the host (Khalifa and Post, 1976). Copepodids in high intensities on the gills of channel catfish resulted in epithelial hyperplasia, telangiectasis, haemorrhage and death (Goodwin, 1999).

19.3.2. Adults

In naïve fish, adult females penetrate the host at an angle by sliding between overlapping scales (Shariff and Roberts, 1989). They penetrate via the epidermis to the dermis, causing necrosis and punctuate haemorrhages measuring up to 5 mm in diameter (Khalifa and Post, 1976). These lesions are detectable by the naked eye (Figs 19.1 and 19.5) and in *L. polymorpha*, they are visible 8–24 h after metamorphosis of the cyclopoid stage (Shariff and Roberts, 1989). Haemorrhage occurs when the female's head penetrates the host tissue, which is followed by an acute inflammatory response in the immediately surrounding area (Joy and Jones, 1973; Innal *et al.*, 2017) (Fig. 19.6b). Haemorrhaging also occurs along the path of entry, under the scales and between muscle bands resulting in pockets of subepithelial erythrocytes and large aggregations of melanin within the dermal layer. In *L. polymorpha* these aggregations of melanin melanosomes occur in the epidermal layer and are sometimes released to the surface (Shariff and Roberts, 1989). Metamorphosed females feed on host erythrocytes and tissue debris resulting from the damage they cause while burrowing for attachment (Shariff and Roberts, 1989).

Necrosis of the host's muscles occurs at the anterior end of the parasite, which is surrounded by infiltrating leucocytes and giant cells (Daskalov *et al.*, 1999). Blood from severed blood vessels may ooze into the water behind the parasite. Behind the parasite's head, epidermal cells form an irregular cumulus in an apparent attempt to seal the lesion off from the environment (Shariff and Roberts, 1989).

When acute inflammation sets in, blood vessels become congested with leucocytes and oedematous swelling of the surrounding tissue occurs. Myofibres adjacent to the parasite

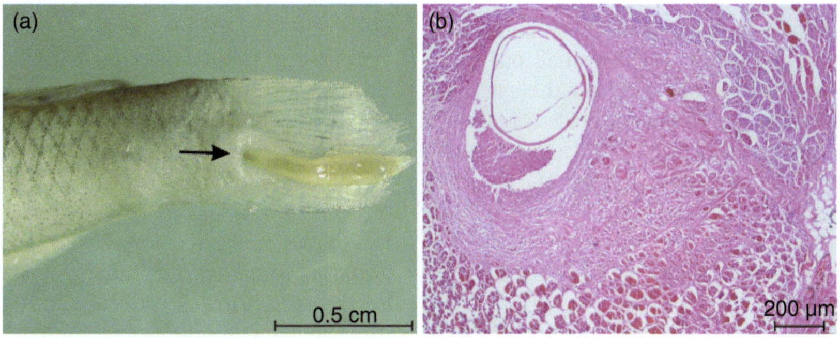

Fig. 19.6. *Lernaea cyprinacea*: (a) parasite *in situ* on the eastern mosquitofish, *Gambusia holbrooki* Girard, 1859, showing chronic granulomatous fibrosis that forms a collar around the parasite (arrowed); (b) a section through the parasite attachment area in Burdur loach, *Oxynoemacheilus anatolicus* Erk'akan, Özeren and Nalbant, 2008, to show inflammatory pathology and chronic granulomatous fibrosis that encapsulates the parasite. Haematoxylin and eosin staining. (Image (a) courtesy of Deniz Innal; image (b) courtesy of Özlem Özmen.)

anchors show necrosis of the sarcoplasm (Shariff and Roberts, 1989).

Approximately 3 days after infection, neutrophils and monocytes, interspersed with exudates, are present at the sites of penetration and the point of entry becomes blocked by a nodule resulting from inflammatory exudates. Vessels surrounding the lesion become congested with mononuclear cells. An increase in vascularization of the area occurs with large clumps of melanin in the dermis and beneath the epidermis among fragmented dermal layers. At 5 days post-infection, degeneration of the inflammatory cells occurs, damaged muscle fibres start to degenerate, the fragmented dermis thickens, and a mesh of collagen forms adjacent to the inserted parasite head and anchors. Ten days after infection mononucleated and club cells are abundant and spongiosis is present. Three weeks after attachment, eosinophilic granule cells (EGCs) and cells resembling lymphocytes were reported in largemouth black bass *Micropterus salmoides* (Lacepède, 1802) infected with *L. polymorpha* (cf. Noga, 1986; Shariff and Roberts, 1989).

Chronic inflammation results in a layer of vascular chronic granulomatous fibrosis that encapsulates the part of the parasite embedded in the fish (Fig. 19.6a and b) and even extends out from the fish to form a collar (Khalifa and Post, 1976; Shields and Goode, 1978; Berry *et al.*, 1991; Innal *et al.*, 2017). The capsule is more prominent towards the anterior horns of the anchor (Shariff and Roberts, 1989). Blindness occurs when the eyes are infected (Uzman and Rayner, 1958; Shariff, 1981).

In recovered fishes, lesions differ markedly as the epidermal breach is relatively small, but extensive haemorrhaging occurs below the epidermis and around the scale beds. The epidermis around the edges of the lesion is thickened and spongiotic with many EGCs and lymphocytes. The dermis is also oedematous with distended blood vessels with EGCs with lymphocytes around them (Noga, 1986; Shariff and Roberts, 1989). Noga (1986) observed remnants of recently metamorphosed *L. cruciata* females in the lesions and that the wounds were secondarily infected with *Aeromonas* (bacteria) and fungi. Furthermore, in kissing gourami previously exposed to *L. cyprinacea*, the number of parasites that successfully mature and the number of eggs per parasite were reduced in a second exposure (Woo and Shariff, 1990).

In small fish the anchor of the parasite frequently extends into the internal organs and the traumatic damage to vital organs results in death (Otte, 1965; Khalifa and Post, 1976; Shariff and Roberts, 1989; Innal *et al.*, 2017). Manual removal of the parasite is complicated by the collar and frequently the parasite breaks when an attempt is made to pull it from the host. Removal is more successful when the scale anterior to the parasite is lifted or removed and the parasite is then carefully pulled by the thorax with a tweezer, dislodging both parasite and collar. Since the parasite is removed with the connective tissue collar, the collar should be removed, preferably prior to fixation, because the shape of the anchors is an important taxonomic feature. Remove the collar by inserting two Dumont tweezers into the opening of the collar; pull the tweezers in opposite directions to tear the collar to release the parasite undamaged. It should preferably be preserved in 96% v/v ethanol/dH_2O to allow for genetic characterization to confirm the species identification as various studies showed that morphological characteristics, particularly the shape of the anchors, are not conclusive.

19.4. Pathophysiology

Kurovskaya (1984) reported that the weight and size of infected carp fry were not affected by lernaeosis, although alkaline phosphatase activity was reduced and the activities of amylase and protease increased, indicating that parasites affect the fish's nutritional status. However, various other researchers reported weight loss. Infected fishes had a significantly lower condition factor than non-parasitized fishes (Kabata, 1985; Faisal *et al.*, 1988; Pérez-Bote, 2010) and Shariff and Sommerville (1986) noted that infested carp were up to 35% lighter. In infected fish the haematocrit count is lower, and fish may display respiratory difficulty (Kabata, 1985). Furthermore, Silva-Souza *et al.* (2000) indicated that the haematocrit displayed intense lymphocytopenia and neutrophilia as well as a very high number of immature leucocytes.

Parasites cause open wounds, allowing opportunistic microbial infections in and on the host (Noga, 1986). They also cause fluid, protein and ion losses, due to disruption of the host integument. Even though the epidermal cells form a collar, a complete plug is not achieved due to constant movement of the distal parts of the parasite's body, and the inflammatory exudate and the underlaying tissue are therefore constantly exposed to the environment.

Tadpoles of the American bullfrog *Lithobates catesbeianus* (Shaw, 1802) infected by *L. cyprinacea* showed retarded growth, a lower health status as expressed by the body condition, a higher frequency of both mature and immature lymphocytes, and a higher haematocrit compared to uninfected individuals. The wounds provided optimal conditions for secondary infections that in turn caused retarded growth and behavioural changes, which eventually reduced the size of the population (Salinas *et al.*, 2019).

19.4.1. Host immune response

Silva-Souza *et al.* (2000) reported lymphocytopenia and a significant increase in neutrophils in the anastomid fish *Schizodon intermedius* Garavello and Britski, 1990, both in hosts with lesions and those currently infected by *Lernaea*. Recovered bighead carp *Aristichthys nobilis* (Richardson, 1845) and silver carp *Hypophthalmichthys molitrix* (Valenciennes, 1844) are more resistant (immune) to *L. polymorpha* reinfections (Pan *et al.*, 1979).

Lesions on immune fish differed from those on naïve fish. In naïve bighead carp infected with *L. polymorpha*, the epidermis had a relatively small opening but the underlying tissue exhibited very extensive haemorrhaging. Aggregation of melanin occurred in the epidermal layer and melanosomes were in some instances released to the surface. The edges of the ulcer were greatly thickened and spongiotic, with an infiltration of ECGs and lymphocytes, distended blood vessels and oedematous dermis (Shariff and Roberts, 1989). In the later stages of infection, a reduction in the number of parasites occurred, probably due to a cellular immune response (Shields and Goode, 1978; Noga, 1986; Shariff and Roberts, 1989; Woo and Shariff, 1990). Fish that recovered from lernaeosis were resistant to the copepods, indicating a protective immunity due to an anamnestic response elicited by memory cells as reported by Woo and Shariff (1990) in recovered kissing gourami. Protection was complete in some recovered fish provided the challenge dose was low. However, if the number of larvae the fish were exposed to was high, the fish were still susceptible to infection. The fecundity of the parasites was suppressed presumably due to immunological starvation of parasites, and those on recovered fish lost more egg sacks and the eggs did either not hatch or were non-infective even to naïve fish (Woo and Shariff, 1990). Lesions contained remnants of recently metamorphosed females (Noga, 1986).

Protective immunity was not obtained in silver barb *Puntius gonionotus* (Bleeker, 1849) infected by *Lernaea minuta*, Kuang, in Kuang and Qian, 1983 (*taxon inquirendum*) and this was attributed to the fact that the pathology in this species is less severe (Kularatne *et al.*, 1994b).

19.5. Protective/Control Strategies

19.5.1. Host immunity

The piscine immune system is well developed, plays a vital role in controlling diseases and can be exploited against pathogens. Woo and Shariff (1990) reported that only 50% of the eggs produced by *Lernaea* from recovered hosts were viable, whereas 100% of the eggs from naïve hosts hatched, indicating a reduction in parasite fecundity, probably due to immunological lesion starvation, which would also affect parasite longevity. Noga (1986) reported that in their study only 2% of lesions contained visible females while the remainder of lesions contained remnants of dead *L. cruciata* parasites, due to the immune response. Therefore, if no naïve fish are introduced into a pond, there will, after a period, be no infective larvae and the system will be safe for restocking. In this regard, Shields (1978) recommended increasing the frequency of water changes, while Shariff and Sommerville (1986) suggested that at 25–29°C all fish should be removed from a pond for a minimum of 7–9 days as this would cause all nauplii and copepodids to hatch and subsequently die from starvation due to a lack of hosts.

19.5.2. Chemotherapy

Inorganic chemicals and/or toxic organophosphates are still used to treat lernaeosis (Abbas *et al.*, 2014), but these have severe negative effects on the environment as they are non-specific, kill non-target organisms and cause residues that potentially affect human health. Many of these products are therefore not registered for use in aquaculture. Withdrawal of treatment with organophosphates is required to make sure that the pesticide residue is removed and Ghittino (1987) recommends that treatment should be terminated at least 1 month before eels are marketed. The primary mechanism of action of organophosphate pesticides is by inhibiting carboxyl ester hydrolases, particularly acetylcholinesterase. Effective elimination of the embedded lernaeid females (from a pond) usually requires treatment over an extended period to interrupt the life cycle as embedded parasites are mostly not susceptible to treatment.

To eradicate adult females Shariff *et al.* (1986) recommend the use of the organophosphate insecticides trichlorphon (Dipterex®) (0.16 ppm) and propoxur (Unden®, a carbamate ester) at a dosage of 0.16 ppm with weekly intervals for 5 weeks, because both are biodegradable. However, fish treated with trichlorphon tend to fast for the full period of treatment, with a resultant effect on their condition. Furthermore, after the fourth treatment copepodids also became resistant to propoxur. Ghittino (1987) also applied trichlorphon (0.25–0.3 ppm) in 3 to 6 weekly treatments in eels and stopped the treatment 1 month before harvesting. It is furthermore recommended to treat ponds to eradicate free-living larvae with trichlorphon (Dipterex, Nevugon® and Masoten®) at 0.25 ppm. Treatments should be repeated to mimic the duration of larval metamorphosis, which is temperature dependent. Recommended intervals for the treatment of *L. cyprinacea* copepodids are: 12 days at 20°C, 9 days at 25°C, 7 days at 30°C and 5 days at 35°C. Below 20°C, monthly treatment suffices (Sarig, 1971; Paperna, 1996). Although a single treatment of trichlorphon at 0.25 ppm kills the copepodid stages, it needs to be repeated against the nauplii or adults (Kabata, 1985) (see previous paragraph about treatment of adults), whereas naled (Bromex®, a dimethyl-1,2-bromo-2,2-dichloroethylphosphate) at 0.12–0.15 ppm kills both nauplii and copepodids (Sarig, 1971). Malathion at 0.01–0.02% repeated three times with 10-day intervals killed lernaeids (Manal *et al.*, 1995).

The insecticide diflubenzuron (Dimilin®), an insect growth regulator, is effective against adult females at concentrations of 0.03–0.05 ppm (Hoffman and Lester, 1987). Burtle and Morrison (1987) reported with diflubenzuron (10–30 μg/l) that complete and lasting eradication of lernaeosis was not achieved, but another treatment 10 days after the first was effective. This insecticide has not been approved for use with food fish. Furthermore, its degradation in the environment is slow, and contaminated water should not be released until at least 30 days after treatment.

Another insecticide, benzene hexachloride (Lindane®) at 10 ppm for 72–96 h every 2 weeks eradicated *Lernaea* on rainbow trout *Oncorhynchus mykiss* (Walbaum, 1792) with varying success (McNeil, 1961). The author furthermore reported that treatment of empty ponds with 5 ppm effectively sterilized the ponds and killed all life stages. In many countries this insecticide is not registered for use in fisheries in many countries.

Dipping of fish in a powerful oxidizer such as potassium permanganate ($KMnO_4$) at 20–25 ppm for 2–3 h, or the application of an 8 ppm concentration to ponds, effectively kills attached female lernaeids (Sarig, 1971; Kabata, 1985; Faisal *et al.*, 1988; Vulpe *et al.*, 2000) but the fish become severely distressed and the eggs and free-living stages of the parasite remain viable (Tamuli and Shanbhogue, 1996a). Great caution should be exercised because the effective concentrations are very close to toxic levels (safety index 1.7–2.0). The treatment is suitable only for fish of over 25 g, and tolerance will vary with species. Increased aeration of the ponds is suggested as $KMnO_4$ reduces the oxygen-binding potential of water. Tamuli and Shanbhogue (1996b) found that brushing concentrated $KMnO_4$ on to each individual parasite was less stressful for the fish and killed female *Lernaea* effectively. Alternatively, they recommend clipping the female parasites off the fish and report that it is very effective. This method is not viable on a large-scale fish farm. Sodium percarbonate, at 100 mg/l, is effective against *L. cyprinacea* (Pavlov and Nikolov, 2007).

Doramectin (Dectomax®; Pfizer), a chloride-channel activator affecting the nervous system and a fermentation-derived endectocidal agent of the avermectin class, in pelleted feed at 1 mg/kg body weight cured young fringed-lipped peninsula carp *Labeo fimbriatus* and fingerlings of *L. cyprinacea* within 18 days, as opposed to 42 days for untreated fish. A decrease in number of eggs per egg sac was observed. The treatment had the additional benefit that wound healing was augmented (Hemaprasanth *et al.*, 2008). However, the safety testing of this drug in aquatic organisms has not been completed and it was previously reported to cause the death of fish (Palmer *et al.*, 1997; Katoch *et al.*, 2003) and other sediment-dwelling organisms (Davies *et al.*, 1997, 1998).

Sodium chlorite is a non-residual alternative (Dempster *et al.*, 1988) that, when applied at a concentration of 20–40 mg/l at a pH above 6, killed *L. cyprinacea* in a commercial aquarium but at the same time killed the bacteria in the biological filter. Therefore, the water needs to be exchanged for at least 2 weeks after treatments to reduce the ammonia and nitrite levels until the chlorite-resistant bacteria in the filters recuperate sufficiently to become biologically active again.

Herbal remedies are gaining traction. Toro *et al.* (2003) found that steamed *Pinus* resin fractions were effective in treatment of lernaeosis in the anostomid fish, *Leporinus piau* Fowler, 1941. Fatma (2014) reported eradication of almost 90% of *Lernaea* after treatment of infected common carp fry with a mixture of carvacrol and cymene plant extracts applied in a water bath for 96 h.

Chitosan–silver nanocomposites at 5.495 ppm for 1 h caused the *L. cyprinacea* females to dislodge from their hosts. Subsequent scanning electron microscopy of the parasites showed that the particles adsorbed on the parasite's cuticle where they caused severe pathological changes to the cuticle. This treatment, furthermore, enhanced healing of the wound formed at the parasite attachment site in the experimental goldfish in aquaria (Abu-Elala *et al.*, 2018). The enhanced healing was probably due to the add-on effect of effective eradication of bacteria reported by Dananjaya *et al.* (2016). However, consumer safety of fishes following nanosilver treatment has not been established and it has been shown that the silver accumulates in the exposed as well as other organs (Ferdous and Nemmar, 2020).

19.5.3. Biological control

Welicky *et al.* (2017) reported the complete eradication of *L. cyprinacea* from a natural water body that dried completely during a drought period. This suggests that eggs were not able to resist desiccation and the unfortunate natural disaster may indicate that deliberate drying out of ponds in aquaculture may be considered a biosafe method of control of repeated outbreaks.

Kabata (1985) found that the copepod *Mesocyclops* Sars, 1914 feeds on free-swimming *Lernaea* larvae and suggested predation as an alternative treatment. It was also observed that goldfish removed maturing parasites from each other (Shields, 1978) and Mozambique tilapia, *Oreochromis mossambicus* (Peters, 1852), effectively reduced the number of parasites in tanks where catla, *Labeo catla* (Hamilton, 1822), with *Lernaea* occurred (Tamuli and Shanbhogue, 1995). Ashraf *et al.* (2008) reported that an increase in vitamin C in the diet of the fish reduced the parasite numbers.

19.6. Conclusions and Suggestions for Future Studies

The plasticity in the anchor morphology of mature females implies that all *Lernaea* species currently listed will have to be confirmed using molecular techniques, particularly using ribosomal DNA markers (18S and 28S) as mitochondrial DNA (CO1) is not informative at species level in this genus. This exercise will require collection of fresh specimens from the type hosts at the type localities and fixation in 96% v/v ethanol/dH_2O. It would be prudent to simultaneously collect specimens for light and scanning electron microscopic study to describe the fine detail of morphological features that may have been overlooked in previous studies. The number of species will most likely be reduced further.

Mechanical removal of parasites appears to be effective and Tamuli and Shanbhogue (1996b) clipped the female parasites from fish; however, this is not sustainable on fish farms due to the cost of labour. Future studies may consider evaluating the development and application of facial recognition software with the intention to use robots to apply treatment directly on attached parasites or to damage the attached parasites without harming the fish.

The possibility of vaccination should be evaluated in future studies. It is well documented that the immune response in chronic infections effectively reduces the number of eggs produced as well as the viability of the eggs in subsequent generations (Noga, 1986; Shariff and Roberts, 1989), although Kularatne *et al.* (1994b) reported that immunity did not develop in Javanese carp. Furthermore, probiotic *Aliivibrio* spp. Urbanczyk, Ast, Higgins, Carson and Dunlap, 2007 was used to treat sea lice *Lepeophtheirus salmonis* (Krøyer, 1837) infection on Atlantic salmon, *Salmo salar* Linnaeus, 1758, with a fair amount of success (Dobloug *et al.*, 2023) and this could be tested against *Lernaea*, too.

Rotational farming practices should be considered where pond utilization is rotated between three or four ponds to include a period where each pond will be lacking fish. The effect will be that eggs will hatch in fish-free ponds and starvation of larvae will occur. Fish should be returned to the pond before all parasites have died so that the fish will receive an immunological challenge, which will provide immunological protection against disastrous parasite outbreaks.

Kabata's (1985) suggestion of using *Mesocyclops* for biological control could also be investigated further. As biological control seldom causes complete eradication it would allow resistance to develop in the fish population while preventing disastrous outbreaks.

Fatma (2014) suggested that the addition of a mixture of carvacrol and cymene in food needs to be investigated. Such a study should include evaluation of accumulation and possible transfer of chemicals to the edible parts of fish and the resulting food safety concerns.

Parasites are valuable information units on environmental conditions; their presence or absence informs about host ecology, food web interactions, biodiversity and environmental stressors (Avenant-Oldewage, 2003; Almeida *et al.*, 2008; Gilbert and Avenant-Oldewage, 2021; Latief *et al.*, 2024). Some pollutants cause an increase in the intensity of parasites due to the stress they induce on the hosts' immune response or due to the increase in organic matter (such as from sewage) providing sustenance for the free-living stages of the parasites or for their intermediate hosts. Other pollutants such as metals, pharmaceuticals or pesticides eradicate parasites either directly or by destroying their habitat or that of their intermediate hosts. Parasites play an integral and valuable part in any healthy natural environment, and their free-living stages make up a meaningful part of the food available to other organisms. Care should, therefore, be taken when treatment regimens are planned.

Although there is currently very little information available about the use of any *Lernaea* species as a bioindicator of environmental health, results from various studies on *Lamproglena clariae* Fryer, 1956, a close relative in the Lernaeidae, shows that this species can make a sensitive sentinel. In polluted environments it produces the stress hormone metallothionein in higher concentrations per gram of tissue than its respective fish hosts (Ndaba *et al.*, 2022). *L. clariae* furthermore accumulates metals to higher concentrations than its hosts (Latief *et al.*, 2023; Pretorius *et al.*, 2025). In laboratory exposure experiments *L. clariae* larvae hatch but die soon after leaving the protective covering of the egg and egg sack when exposed to environmentally relevant concentrations of aluminium (Pretorius and Avenant-Oldewage, 2023), explaining their extirpation at polluted sites in natural systems (Pretorius and Avenant-Oldewage, 2022). Similar studies could be done on *Lernaea* to gain an understanding of the effect of anthropogenic activities on their occurrence and biodiversity in general.

Climate change impacts water temperature, pH, dissolved oxygen and salinity that may have a ripple effect on the transmission and survival/multiplication of parasites. Temperature affects the rate of completion of the *Lernaea* life cycle. Preliminary results led Kupferberg *et al.* (2009) to speculate that global warming may be responsible for an increase in *Lernaea* parasitaemia in northern California, USA in near-threatened foothill yellow-legged frog. However, in the subtropical conditions in Zimbabwe, Dalu *et al.* (2012) reported a negative correlation between parasite intensity and increased temperature but a positive relationship with increased dissolved oxygen and pH. It is possible that the optimal temperature for *Lernaea* was exceeded in Zimbabwe, as these authors reported a mean temperature above 30°C during late summer. Welicky *et al.* (2017) reported that drought (a side effect of global warming) caused increased hypersalinity in a pan in South Africa and that hypersalinity correlated with a reduction in the *Lernaea* infection when comparing two consecutive years.

Fishes are also exposed to anthropogenic changes to the environment, and these stressors negatively impact on their immune response.

It is already well known that fishes develop immunity against *Lernaea* infection (Noga, 1986; Shariff and Roberts, 1989) but in fish with a compromised immunity the response will be suboptimal. The presence and effect of pollutants on hosts should therefore be considered when studying fish immunity against *Lernaea*.

The low species specificity and opportunistic global spreading of *L. cyprinacea* threaten extinction of the endangered foothill yellow-legged frog (Kupferberg *et al.*, 2009) and the endemic Eastern Cape rocky kurper, *Sandelia bainsii* Castelnau, 1861 (Chakona *et al.*, 2019). Accurate parasite identification, integrating light and scanning electron microscopy with appropriate markers for molecular study and storage of hologenophores in museums should take priority. The distribution of the infections should be reported diligently and parasite-free refugia for endangered species should be erected and maintained.

References

Abbas, F., Ashraf, M., Hafees-ur-Rehman, M.H., Iqbal, K.J., Abbas, S. and Javid, A. (2014) *Lernaea* susceptibility, infestation and its treatment in indigenous major and exotic Chinese carps under polyculture system. *Pakistan Journal of Zoology* 46(5), 1215–1222.

Abu-Elala, N.M., Attia, M.M. and Abd-Elsalam, R.M. (2018) Chitosan–silver nanocomposites in goldfish aquaria: a new perspective in *Lernaea cyprinacea* control. *International Journal of Biological Macromolecules* 111, 614–622.

Alcalde, L. and Batistoni, P. (2005) *Hyla pulchella cordobae* (Cordoba treefrog). *Herpetological Review* 36, 302.

Al-Hamed, M. and Hermiz, L. (1973) Experiments on the control of anchor worm (*Lernaea cyprinacea*). *Aquaculture* 2, 45–51.

Almeida, D., Almodóvar, A., Nicola, G.C. and Elvira, B. (2008) Fluctuating asymmetry, abnormalities and parasitism as indicators of environmental stress in cultured stocks of goldfish and carp. *Aquaculture* 279, 120–125.

Ashraf, M., Ayub, M. and Rauf, A. (2008) Effect of vitamin C on growth, survival and resistance to *Lernaea* infection in mrigal (*Cirrhinus mrigala*) fingerlings. *Pakistan Journal of Zoology* 40, 165–170.

Avenant-Oldewage, A. (2003) *Lamproglena* and *Lernaea* as possible indicators of environmental deterioration in a river in South Africa. *Journal of the South African Veterinary Association* 74, 96.

Baldauf, R.J. (1961) Another case of parasitic copepods in amphibians. *Journal of Parasitology* 47, 195.

Barson, M., Mulonga, A. and Nhiwatiwa, T. (2008) Investigation of a parasitic outbreak of *Lernaea cyprinacea* Linnaeus (Crustacea: Copepoda) in fish from Zimbabwe. *African Zoology* 43, 175–183.

Berry, C.R., Babey, G.J. and Shrader, T. (1991) Effect of *Lernaea cyprinacea* (Crustacea: Copepoda) on stocked rainbow trout (*Oncorhynchus mykiss*). *Journal of Wildlife Diseases* 27, 206–213.

Boane, C., Cruz, C. and Saraiva, A. (2008) Metazoan parasites of *Cyprinus carpio* L. (Cyprinidae) from Mozambique. *Aquaculture* 284, 59–61.

Bozorgnia, A., Youssefi, M.R., Barzegar, M. Hosseninifard, S.M. and Ebrahimpour, S. (2012) Biodiversity of parasites of fishes in Gheshlagh (Vahdat) Reservoir, Kurdistan Province, Iran. *World Journal of Fish and Marine Sciences* 4(3), 249–253.

Burtle G. and Morrison, J. (1987) Dimilin for control of *Lernaea* in golden shiner ponds. *Journal of the Arkansas Academy of Science* 41, 17–19.

Carnevia, D. and Speranza, G. (2003) First report of *Lernaea cyprinacea* L., 1758 in Uruguay, introduced by goldfish, *Carassius auratus* (L., 1758) and affecting axolotl *Ambystoma mexicanum* (Shaw, 1798). *Bulletin of the European Association of Fish Pathologists* 23, 255–256.

Chakona, A., Rennie, G., and Kadye, K.W. (2019) First record of *Lernaea cyprinacea* (Copepoda: Lernaeidae) on an imperilled endemic anabantid, *Sandelia bainsii* (Teleostei: Anabantidae), from the Eastern Cape province, South Africa. *African Journal of Aquatic Science* 44(2), 183–187. DOI: 10.2989/16085914.2019.1619513.

Dalu, T., Nhiwatiwa, T., Clegg, B. and Barson, M. (2012) Impact of *Lernaea cyprinacea* Linnaeus 1758 (Crustacea: Copepoda) almost a decade after an initial parasitic outbreak in fish of Malilangwe Reservoir, Zimbabwe. *Knowledge and Management of Aquatic Ecosystems* 406, 03. DOI: 10.1051/kmae/2012020.

Dananjaya, S.H.S., Godahewa, G.I., Jayasooriya, R.G.P.T., Lee, J. and De Zoysa, M. (2016) Antimicrobial effects of chitosan silver nano composites (CAgNCs) on fish pathogenic *Aliivibrio (Vibrio) salmonicida*. *Aquaculture* 450, 422–430.

Daskalov, C. and Georgiev, L. (2001) Research on diagnosis, therapy and prophylaxis of lernaeosis on carp. *Zhivotnov dni Nauki* 38, 50–52.

Daskalov, H., Stoikov, D. and Grozeva, N. (1999) A preliminary hygienic view in case of lernaeosis in the common carp (*Cyprinus carpio* L.) based on clinical and pathomorphological observations. *Bulgarian Journal of Veterinary Medicine* 2, 59–64.

Davies, I.M., McHenery, J.G. and Rae, G.H. (1997) Environmental risk from dissolved ivermectin to marine organisms. *Aquaculture* 158, 263–275.

Davies, I.M., Gillibrand, P.A., McHenery, J.G. and Rae, G.H. (1998) Environmental risk of ivermectin to sediment dwelling organisms. *Aquaculture* 163, 29–46.

Dawar, F.U., Khan, M.F. Kamal, R. and Ullah, S. (2015) Prevalence of parasites in freshwater pond fishes from district D.I. Khan, Pakistan. *The Journal of Zoological Studies* 2(2), 47–50.

Dempster, R.P., Morales, P. and Glennon, F.X. (1988) Use of sodium chlorite to combat anchor worm infestation of fish. *The Progressive Fish-Culturist* 50, 51–55.

Dobloug, M.S., Skagen-Sandvik C., Evensen, Ø., Gadan, K., Jørgensen Bakke, M. *et al.* (2023) Reduced infestation levels of *Lepeophtheirus salmonis* in Atlantic salmon (*Salmo salar*) following immersion exposure to probiotic *Aliivibrio* spp. *Applied Microbiology* 3(4), 1339–1354. DOI: 10.3390/applmicrobiol3040090.

Faisal, M., Easa, M., Shalaby, S.I. and Ibrahim, M.M. (1988) Epizootics *of Lernaea cyprinacea* (Copepoda: Lernaeidae) in imported cyprinids to Egypt. *Tropenlandwirt* 89, 131–141.

Fatma, M.M. (2014) Lernaeosis affecting hatchery reared common carp (*Cyprinus carpio*) fries and a novel approach for its treatment. *Global Journal of Fisheries and Aquaculture Research* 1(2), 173–189.

Ferdous, A. and Nemmar, A. (2020) Health impact of silver nanoparticles: a review of the biodistribution and toxicity following various routes of exposure. *International Journal of Molecular Sciences* 21, 2375. DOI: 10.3390/ijms21072375.

Figueira, L.B. and Ceccarelli, P.S. (1991) Observaçoes sobre a presença de ectoparasitas em piscicultyras de interior (CEPTA e Regiao). *Boletim Técnico do CEPTA* 4, 57–65 (in Portuguese).

Fryer, G. (1961) Variation and systematic problems in a group of lernaeid copepods. *Crustaceana* 2(4), 275–285.

Fryer, G. (1966) Habitat selection and gregarious behaviour in parasitic crustaceans. *Crustaceana* 10, 199–209.

Fryer, G. (1968) The parasitic Crustacea of African freshwater fishes, their biology and distribution. *Journal of Zoology (London)* 156, 45–95.

Gallio, M., da Silva, A.S. and Monteiro, S.G. (2007) Parasitismo por *Lernaea cyprinacea* em *Astyanax bimaculatus* provenientes de um acude no municipio de Antonio Prado, Rio Grande do Sul. *Acta Scientiae Veterinariae* 35, 209–212 (in Portuguese).

Ghittino, C. (1987) Positive control of buccal lernaeosis in eel farming. *Rivista Italiana di Piscicoltura e Ittiopatologia* 22, 26–29.

Gilbert, B.M. and Avenant-Oldewage, A. (2021) Monogenea as bioindicators: a meta-analysis of effect size of contaminant exposure toward Monogenea (Platyhelminthes). *Ecological Indicators* 130, 1080602. DOI: 10.1016/j.ecolind.2021.108062.

Goodwin, A.E. (1999) Massive *Lernaea cyprinacea* infestation damaging the gills of channel catfish polyculture with bighead carp. *Journal of Aquatic Animal Health* 11, 406–408.

Grabda, J. (1963) Life cycle and morphogenesis of *Lernaea cyprinacea* L. *Acta Parasitologica Polonica* 11, 169–198.

Gutiérrez-Galindo, J.F. and Lacasa-Millán, M.I. (2005) Population dynamics of *Lernaea cyprinacea* (Crustacea: Copepoda) on four cyprinid species. *Diseases of Aquatic Organisms* 67, 111–114.

Harding, J.P. (1950) On some species of *Lernaea* (Crustacea: Copepoda) freshwater parasites of fish. *Bulletin of the British Museum of Natural History (Zoology)* 1, 1–27.

Hemaprasanth, K.P., Raghavendra, A., Sing, R., Sridhar, N. and Raghunath, M.R. (2008) Efficacy of doramectin against natural and experimental infections of *Lernaea cyprinacea* in carps. *Veterinary Parasitology* 156, 261–269.

Hoffman, G.L. (1998) *Parasites of North American Freshwater Fishes*. Cornell University Press, Ithaca, New York.

Hoffman, G. (1999) *Parasites of North American Freshwater Fishes*, 2nd edn. University of California Press, Berkeley, California.

Hoffman, G.L. and Lester, R.J.G. (1987) Workshop 4F: crustacean parasites of fish. *International Journal for Parasitology* 17, 1030–1031.

Hua, C.J., Zhang, D., Zou, H., Li, M., Jakovlić, I. *et al.* (2019) Morphology is not a reliable taxonomic tool for the genus *Lernaea*: molecular data and experimental infection reveal that *L. cyprinacea* and *L. cruciata* are conspecific. *Parasites and Vectors* 12, 579. DOI: 10.1186/s13071-019-3831-y.

Innal, D. and Avenant-Oldewage, A. (2012) Occurrence of *Lernaea cyprinacea* on mosquito fish (*Gambusia affinis*) from Kundu Estuary System (Antalya–Turkey). *Bulletin of the European Association of Fish Pathologists* 32(4), 140–147.

Innal, D., Avenant-Oldewage, A., Dogangil, B., Stavrescu-Bedivan, M.M., Ozmen, O. and Macruk, S. (2017) Susceptibility of endemic and non-indigenous fish to *Lernaea cyprinacea* (Copepoda: Lernaeidae): a case study from Drüger Spring Creek (Burdur– Turkey). *Bulletin of the European Association of Fish Pathologists* 37(3), 100–109.

Joy, J.E. and Jones, L.P. (1973) Observations on the inflammatory response within the dermis of a white bass, *Morone chrysops* (Rafinesque), infected with *Lernaea cruciata* (Copepoda: Caligidea). *Journal of Fish Biology* 5, 21–23.

Kabata, Z. (1979) *Parasitic Copepoda of British Fishes*. The Ray Society, London.

Kabata, Z. (1985) *Parasites and Diseases of Fish Cultured in Tropics*. Taylor and Francis, London, 302 pp.

Kasahara, S. (1962) Studies on the biology of the parasitic copepod *Lernaea cyprinacea* Linnaeus and the method for controlling this parasite in fish-culture ponds. *Contributions of the Fisheries Laboratory, Faculty of Agriculture University of Tokyo* 3, 103–196.

Katoch, R., Khurana, S.R., Chatterjee, S., Telang, R.S. and Agnihotri, R.K. (2003) Ivermectin toxicity in fish: a controlled trial. *Journal of Veterinary Parasitology* 17, 79–80.

Khalifa, K.A. and Post, G. (1976) Histopathological effect of *Lernaea cyprinacea* (a copepod parasite) on fish. *The Progressive Fish-Culturist* 38, 110–113.

Koyun, M. and Atici, A.A. (2018) First record of *Lernaea cyprinacea* (Crustacea: Copepoda) on *Capoeta capoeta* (Actinopterygii: Cyprinidae) from Karasu Creek (Van) Eastern Anatolia. *Biharean Biologist* 12(2), 70–72.

Kularatne, M., Shariff, M. and Subasinghe, R.P. (1994a) Comparison of larval morphometrics of *Lernaea minuta*, a copepod parasite of *Puntius gonionotus* from Malaysia, with those of *L. cyprinacea* and *L. polymorpha*. *Crustaceana* 67, 288–295.

Kularatne, M., Subasinghe, R.P. and Shariff, M. (1994b) Investigations on the lack of acquired immunity by the Javanese carp, *Puntius gonionotus* (Bleeker), against the crustacean parasite, *Lernaea minuta* (Kuang). *Fish and Shellfish Immunology* 4, 107–114.

Kupferberg, S.J., Catenazzi, A., Lunde, K., Lind, A.J. and Palen, W.J. (2009) Parasitic copepod (*Lernaea cyprinacea*) outbreaks in foothill yellow-legged frogs (*Rana boylii*) linked to unusually warm summers and amphibian malformations in northern California. *Copeia* 3, 529–537.

Kurovskaya, L.Y. (1984) The influence of parasite infection of carp fry on the activity of their intestinal enzymes. *Sbornik Nauchnykh Trudov Vsesoyuznogo Nauchno-Issledovatel'skogo Instituta Prudovogo Rybnogo Khozyaistva* 40, 68–73.

Latief, L., Gilbert, B.M. and Avenant-Oldewage, A. (2023) Biomineralisation and metal sequestration in a crustacean ectoparasite infecting the gills of a freshwater fish. *Journal of Comparative Physiology B.* 193, 271–279. DOI: 10.1007/s00360-023-01489-2.

Latief, L. Gilbert, B.M. and Avenant-Oldewage, A. (2024) Effects of water quality on fish parasite biodiversity and physiological responses in the host fish *Clarias gariepinus* from a eutrophic lake subjected to acid mine drainage in South Africa. *Integrated Environmental Assessment and Management* 20, 1539–1553. DOI: 10.1002/ieam.4885.

Linnaeus, C. (1758) Systema Naturae per regna tria naturae, secundum classes, ordines, genera, species, cum characteribus, differentiis, synonymis, locis [The system of nature through the three kingdoms of nature, according to classes, orders, genera, species, with characters, differences, synonyms, places]. *Impensis Direct. Laurentii Salvii. Holmiae [Stockholm]* 1(10) [iii], 824 pp. Available at: https://biodiversitylibrary.org/page/726886 (accessed 3 December 2025).

Lymbery, A.J., Hassan, M., Morgan, D.L., Beatty, S.L. and Doupé, R.G. (2010) Parasites of native and exotic freshwater fishes in south-western Australia. *Journal of Fish Biology* 76, 1770–1785.

Mahmoud, M.A., Aly, S.M., Diab, A.S. and John, G. (2009) The role of ornamental goldfish *Carassius auratus* in transfer of some viruses and ectoparasites to cultured fish in Egypt: comparative ultrapathological studies. *African Journal of Aquatic Science* 34, 111–121.

Manal, E.M.A.A., Oifat, M.A. and El, S.E.M. (1995) Lernaeosis outbreak in cultured freshwater fish fingerlings at Kafr El Sheikh governorate, Egypt. *Egyptian Journal of Comparative Pathology and Clinical Pathology* 8, 109–121.

Mandal, B., Dubey S.K., Dasgupta, P., Mahapatra, B.J. and Chand, B.K. (2016) A preliminary survey on parasitic occurrence in indigenous climbing perch, *Anabas testudineus* (Bloch, 1972) from West Bengal state of India. *Journal of Coastal Life Medicine* 4(8), 592–596.

Manna, A.K., Paria, T. and Ghosh, S. (1999) Incidence and intensity of anchor worm *Lernaea* infection on the Asiatic rice fish *Oryzias metastigma*. *Environment and Ecology* 17, 73–75.

Marcogliese, D.J. (1991) Occurrence of *Lernaea cyprinacea* in fishes in Belews Lake, North Carolina. *Journal of Parasitology* 77, 326–327.

Marina, H., Beatty, S., Morgan, D., Doupé, R. and Lymbery, A. (2008) An introduced parasite, *Lernaea cyprinacea* L., found on native freshwater fishes in the south west of Western Australia. *Journal of the Royal Society of Western Australia* 91, 149–153.

Martins, M.L. and Souza, F.L.D. (1996) Experimental infestations of *Rana catesbiana* Shaw tadpoles by copepodids *Lernaea cyprinacea* Linnaeus (Copepoda, Lernaeidae). *Revista Brasileira de Zoologia* 12, 619–625.

McNeil, P.L. (1961) The use of benzene hexachloride as a copepodicide and some observations on lernaean parasites in trout rearing units. *The Progressive Fish-Culturist* 23, 127–133.

Medeiros, S.F. and Maltchik, L. (1999) The effects of hydrological disturbance on the intensity of infestation of *Lernaea cyprinacea* in an intermittent stream fish community. *Journal of Arid Environments* 43, 351–356.

Melidone, R., Chow, J.A. and Principato, M. (2004) *Lernaea cyprinacea* infestation in an axolotl. *Exotic DVM* 6, 24–25.

Ming, L.T. (2001) Parasitic copepods responsible for limb abnormalities? *Froglog* 46, 3.

Muchlisin, Z.A., Munazir, A.M., Fuady, Z., Winaruddin, W., Sugianto, S. *et al.* (2014) Prevalence of ectoparasites on mahseer fish (*Tor tambra* Valenciennes, 1842) from aquaculture ponds and wild population of Nagan Raya District, Indonesia. *HVM Bioflux* 6(3), 148–152.

Nagasawa, K., Morimoto, S., Asai, T., Kitagawa T. and Hosoya, K. (2012) A checklist of the parasites of medaka (*Oryzias latipes*) of Japan (1929–2012), with new records of *Lernaea cyprinacea* (Copepoda: Lernaeidae) in wild populations of medaka in Japan. *Bulletin of the Biogeographical Society of Japan* 67, 1–13 (in Japanese).

Ndaba, J., Gilbert, B.M. and Avenant-Oldewage, A. (2022) Metallothionein expression in a parasitic crustacean, *Lamproglena clariae* (Crustacea: Copepoda), on *Clarias gariepinus* (Teleostei: Clariidae) corresponds to water quality. *Journal of Parasitology* 108(1), 10–20. DOI: 10.1645/21-62.

Noga, E.J. (1986) The importance of *Lernaea cruciata* (Le Sueur) in the initiation of skin lesions in large-mouth bass, *Micropterus salmoides* (Lacépède), in Chowan River, North Carolina, USA. *Journal of Fish Diseases* 9, 295–302.

Otte, E. (1965) An observed heavy infection of rainbow trout (Osteichthyes) with a previously unknown *Lernaea* species, new species *Lernaea minima* (Copepoda). *Wien Tierärtzliche Monatsschrift* 5, 21–25.

Pallavi, B., Shankar, K.M., Abhiman, P.B. and Ahmed, I. (2017) Molecular identification of the fish parasite *Lernaea*. *Indian Journal of Fisheries* 64, 76–82.

Palmer, R., Coyne, R., Davey, S. and Smith, P. (1997) Case notes on adverse reaction associated with ivermectin therapy of Atlantic salmon. *Bulletin of the European Association of Fish Pathologists* 17, 62–67.

Pan, J., Yang, T. and Xu, G. (1979) Studies on the biology of the parasitic copepod *Lernaea polymorpha* of silver carp (*Hypophthalmichthys molitrix*) and big-head carp (*Aristichthys nobilis*) and its control. *Acta Hydrobiologica Sinica* 6, 377–370 (in Chinese).

Paperna, I. (1996) *Parasites, Infections and Diseases of Fishes in Africa. An Update.* Committee for Inland Fisheries of Africa (CIFA) Technical Paper No. 31. Food and Agriculture Organization of the United Nations, Rome.

Pavlov, A. and Nikolov, G. (2007) Investigation of sodium percarbonate as a means to fight with *Lernaea cyprinacea* in some freshwater fish. *Journal of Agriculture and Forest Science* 6, 21–23.

Pérez-Bote, J.L. (2010) *Barbus comizo* infestation by *Lernaea cyprinacea* in the Guandiana River, south-western Spain. *Journal of Applied Ichthyology* 26, 592–595.

Piasecki, W. and Avenant-Oldewage, A. (2008) Diseases caused by Crustacea. In: Eiras, J. Segner, H., Wahli, T. and Kapoor, B.G. (eds) *Fish Diseases*. Science Publishers, Enfield, New Hampshire, pp. 1115–1200.

Piasecki, W., Goodwin, A.E., Eiras, J.C. and Nowak, B.F. (2004) Importance of Copepoda in freshwater aquaculture. *Zoological Studies* 43, 193–205.

Plaul, S.E., Garcia Romero, N. and Barbeito, C.G. (2010) Distribution of the exotic parasite, *Lernaea cyprinacea* (Copepoda, Lernaeidae) in Argentina. *Bulletin of the European Association of Fish Pathologists* 30, 65–73.

Poddubnaâ, A.V. (1973) Variability and specificity of *Lernaea* from pond fishes. *Trudy vsesoûznogo naučno-issledovatel'skogo Instituta ozer'nogo rybnogo hozâjstva* 22, 159–173 (in Russian).
Pretorius, M. and Avenant-Oldewage, A. (2022) Parasites as biological indicators: the impact of environmental quality on the infections of *Lamproglena clariae* (Crustacea) on *Clarias gariepinus* along the Vaal River, South Africa. *Biological Trace Element Research* 200(6), 2937–2947. DOI: 10.1007/s12011-021-02899-5.
Pretorius, M.M. and Avenant-Oldewage, A. (2023) Hatchability and survival of *Lamproglena clariae* Fryer, 1956 exposed to increasing concentrations of aqueous aluminium. *Applied Sciences* 13, 2145. DOI: 10.3390/app13042145.
Pretorius, M.M., Gradwohl, A., Windisch, J., Jirsa, F. and Avenant-Oldewage, A. (2025) Bioaccumulation of selected metals in *Lamproglena clariae* Fryer, 1956 infecting *Clarias gariepinus* (Burchell, 1822) collected from six sampling sites along the Vaal River, South Africa. *Water Environment Research* 97, e70037. DOI: 10.1002/wer.70037.
Robinson, J. and Avenant-Oldewage, A. (1996) Aspects of the morphology of the parasitic copepod *Lernaea cyprinacea* Linnaeus, 1758 and notes on its distribution in Africa. *Crustaceana* 69, 610–626.
Salinas, ZA, Babini, M.S., Grenat, P.R., Biolé, F.G., Martino, A.L. and Salas, N.E. (2019) Effect of parasitism of *Lernaea cyprinacea* on tadpoles of the invasive species *Lithobates catesbeianus*. *Heliyon* 5, e01834. DOI: 10.1016/j.heliyon.2019.e01834.
Sarig, S. (1971) *The Prevention and Treatment of Diseases of Warmwater Fish Under Subtropical Conditions, With Special Emphasis on Intensive Fish Farming*. T.F.H. Publications Inc., Jersey City, New Jersey.
Shah, S.Q.A., Mahmood, K., Rashid, M.I., Naz, H., Sohail, M.L. *et al.* (2025) Prevalence, morphological and molecular characterization of *Lernaea cyprinacea* from major carps of Southern Punjab, Pakistan. *Pakistan Veterinary Journal* 45, 422–427. DOI: 10.29261/pakvetj.2024.308.
Shariff, M. (1981) The histopathology of the eye of big head carp *Aristichthys nobilis* (Richardson) infested with *Lernaea piscinae* Harding, 1950. *Journal of Fish Diseases* 4, 161–168.
Shariff, M. and Roberts, R.J. (1989) The experimental histopathology of *Lernaea polymorpha* Yu, 1938, infection in naïve *Aristichthys nobilis* (Richardson) and a comparison with the lesion in naturally infected clinically resistant fish. *Journal of Fish Diseases* 12, 405–414.
Shariff, M. and Sommerville, C. (1986) Effects of *Lernaea polymorpha* on the growth of big head carp, *Aristichthys nobilis*. In: *International Congress of Parasitology (ICOPA) VI Handbook*. Australian Academy of Sciences, Canberra, Abstract no. 598, p. 227.
Shariff, M., Kabata, Z. and Sommerville, C. (1986) Host susceptibility to *Lernaea cyprinacea* L. and its treatment in a large aquarium system. *Journal of Fish Diseases* 9, 393–401.
Shields, R.J. (1978) Procedures for the laboratory rearing of *Lernaea cyprinacea* L. (Copepoda). *Crustaceana* 35, 259–264.
Shields, R.J. and Goode, R.P. (1978) Host rejection of *Lernaea cyprinacea* L. (Copepoda). *Crustaceana* 35, 301–307.
Shields, R.J. and Tidd, W.M. (1968) Effect of temperature on the development of larval and transformed females of *Lernaea cyprinacea* L. (Lernaeidae). *Crustaceana* 1, 87–95.
Shields, R.J. and Tidd, W.M. (1974) Site selection on hosts by copepods of *Lernaea cyprinacea* L. (Copepoda). *Crustaceana* 27, 225–230.
Shinn, A., Avenant-Oldewage, A., Bondad-Reantaso, M., Cruz-Laufer, A. García Vásquez, A. *et al.* (2023) A global review of problematic and pathogenic parasites of farmed tilapia. *Reviews in Aquaculture* 15(Suppl. 1), 92–153. DOI: 10.1111/raq.12742.
Silva-Souza, A.A., Almeida, S.C. and Machado, P.M. (2000) Effect of the infestation by *Lernaea cyprinacea* Linnaeus, 1758 (Copepoda, Lernaeidae) on the leucocytes of *Schizodon intermedius* Garavello and Britski, 1990 (Osteichthyes, Anostomidae). *Revista Brasileira de Biología* 60, 217–220.
Soares, I.A., Salinas, V., Del Ponti, O. Mancini, M.A. and Luque, J.L. (2018) First molecular data for *Lernaea cyprinacea* (Copepoda: Cyclopoida) infesting *Odontesthes bonariensis* a commercially important freshwater fish in Argentina. *Brazilian Journal of Veterinary Parasitology* 27(1), 105–108. DOI: 10.1590/s1984-29612018005.
Tamuli, K.K. and Shanbhogue, S.L. (1995) Biological control of *Lernaea* L. infection employing *Oreochromis mossambica*, Peters. *Journal of the Assam Science Society* 37, 123–128.
Tamuli, K.K. and Shanbhogue, S.L. (1996a) Incidence and intensity of anchor worm *Lernaea bhadraensis* infection on cultivated carps. *Environment and Ecology* 14, 282–288.
Tamuli, K.K. and Shanbhogue, S.L. (1996b) Acquired immunity of Indian major carp *Catla catla* to infection of the anchor worm *Lernaea bhadraensis*. *Environment and Ecology* 14, 518–523.

Tasawar, Z., Zafar, S., Lashari, M.H. and Hayat, C.S. (2009) The prevalence of lernaeid ectoparasites in grass carp (*Ctenopharyngodon idella*). *Pakistan Veterinary Journal* 29, 95–96.

Thurston, J.P. (1969) The biology of *Lernaea barnimiana* (Crustacea: Copepoda) from Lake George, Uganda. *Revue de Zoologie et de Botanique Africaines* 60, 15–33.

Tidd, W.M. and Shields, R.J. (1963) Tissue damage inflicted by *Lernaea cyprinacea* Linnaeus, a copepod parasitic on tadpoles. *Journal of Parasitology* 49, 693–696.

Toro, R.M., Gessner, A.A.F., Furtado, N.A.J.C., Ceccarelli, P.S., de Albuquerque, S. and Bastos, J.K. (2003) Activity of the *Pinus elliottii* resin compounds against *Lernaea cyprinacea in vitro*. *Veterinary Parasitology* 118, 143–149.

Uzman, J.R. and Rayner, H.J. (1958) Record of the parasitic copepod *Lernaea cyprinacea* L. in Oregon and Washington fishes. *Journal of Parasitology* 44, 452–453.

Vanotti, M.D. and Tanzola, R.D. (2005) Relación entre la craga parasiaria total yalgunos parámetros hematologicos de *Rhamdia* sap oval. (Pisces) en condiciones naturals. *Biología Acuática* 22, 247–256.

Viljoen, B.C.S. (1986) A seasonal investigation of the genus *Lernaea* (Crustacea: Copepoda) on cyprinid fish in Boskop Dam, Transvaal, South Africa. *South African Journal of Wildlife Research* 16(1), 27–31.

Vulpe, V., Năstasă, V. and Cura, P. (2000) Studies about the therapeutic modalities in parasitoses of the fish of culture. *Lucrăi Ştiinifice – Medicină Veterinară Universitatea de Ştiinţe Agricole şi Medicină Veterinară 'Ion Ionescu de la Brad' Iaşi, Romania* 43(2), 376–379.

Walter, T.C. and Boxshall, G.A. (2025) World of Copepods Database. Available at: http://www.marinespecies.org/copepoda (accessed 17 January 2025).

Welicky, R.L., De Swardt, J., Gerber, R., Netherlands, E.C. and Smit, N.J. (2017) Drought-associated absence of alien invasive anchor worm, *Lernaea cyprinacea* (Copepoda: Lernaeidae), is related to changes in fish health. *International Journal for Parasitology: Parasites and Wildlife* 6, 430–438.

Wilson, C.B. (1917) North American parasitic copepods belonging to the lernaeidae with a revision of the entire family. *Proceedings of the US National Museum* 53, 1–150.

Woo, P.T.K. and Shariff, M. (1990) *Lernaea cyprinacea* L. (Copepoda: Caligidae) in *Helostoma temmincki* Cuvier and Valenciennes: the dynamics of resistance in recovered and naïve fish. *Journal of Fish Diseases* 13, 485–494.

Yoshimine, Y. Isshkihi, T. Aino, S., Tun, K.L. and Yoshinaga, T. (2015) Occurrence of *Lernaea cyprinacea* (Copepoda) in wild ayu *Plecoglossus altivelis* and several other fishes in the Shonai River, Japan. *Fish Pathology* 50(2), 81–84.

Zhu, X., Barton, D.P., Wassens, S. and Shamsi, S. (2021) Morphological and genetic characterisation of the introduced copepod *Lernaea cyprinacea* Linnaeus (Cyclopoida: Lernaeidae) occurring in the Murrumbidgee catchment, Australia. *Marine and Freshwater Research* 72, 876–886. DOI: 10.1071/MF20145.

20 *Argulus* and Related Species

Annemariè Avenant-Oldewage*
Department of Zoology, University of Johannesburg, South Africa

Abstract

Argulidae are ectoparasites of fishes and amphibia in fresh, brackish and marine environments. In aquaculture and sometimes in nature they reach high numbers. They cause damage to the skin of their hosts by rasping the epidermis off with serrated mandibles and feed on the blood and epidermis of their hosts, and high intensities may cause host death. Open wounds caused by feeding and attachment are susceptible to secondary fungal and bacterial infections. Furthermore, Skrjabillanidae nematodes are transmitted by *Argulus* sp. and *Molnaria erythrophthalmi* by *Argulus foliaceus*. Treatment regimens are discussed but few of these are registered for use in aquaculture and prevention of infection is best practice. Suggestions for future research are provided, including a request for holistic approaches for species descriptions including light and scanning electron microscopy and genetic characterization to address the existing confusion with species identification due to incomplete descriptions as well as a call for alternative treatment strategies.

20.1. Introduction

The Branchiura (family Argulidae) is a Crustacea group parasitizing primarily freshwater fishes (Piasecki and Avenant-Oldewage, 2008; Neethling and Avenant-Oldewage, 2016). They have also been collected from brackish and marine fishes, sharks, tadpoles and alligators (Schram *et al.*, 2005; Neethling and Avenant-Oldewage, 2016). They are referred to as 'fish lice'. The family includes only four genera: (i) *Argulus* Müller, 1785 (more than 60 species) which has a cosmopolitan distribution; (ii) *Dolops* Audouin, 1837 (ten species) occurring in South America (eight species), Africa (one species) and Tasmania (one species); (iii) *Chonopeltis* Thiele, 1900 (12 species) which is endemic in Africa; and (iv) *Dipteropeltis* Calman, 1912 (three species) endemic in South America (WoRMS Editorial Board, 2025). These parasites are not permanently attached to their hosts. It is well known that larval and adult *Argulus* and *Dolops* are ardent swimmers and they are frequently present in the plankton samples (Neethling and Avenant-Oldewage, 2016, table I, III, IV, V, IX). Adult *Chonopeltis* is unable to swim (Fryer, 1956). When removed from the host, they lift the corners of the carapace and use the second maxillae first and second thoracic legs as oars, but this effort does not lift them (Fryer, 1956). When inserted at the top of an aquarium they float through the water column while feebly

*Email: aoldewage@uj.ac.za

DOI: 10.1079/9781800628748.0020

moving their second maxillae, first and second thoracopods (A. Avenant-Oldewage, 1985, unpublished results). On a host they relocate with movements resembling reverse 'walking'. These are accomplished by alternating attachment of the suckers (first maxillae) and swinging the thorax from side to side (Fryer, 1956). Similarly, *Dipteropeltis longicaudatus* Gaboardi, Reeves, Morey, Stanton and Carney, 2023 adults, once removed from their hosts, are not able to move at all (Gaboardi *et al.*, 2023) although their larvae can swim erratically (Gaboardi *et al.*, 2023, supplementary video 4). Most Branchiura are transparent, resembling a speck of mucus with a greenish tinge, and they are easily overlooked (Neethling and Avenant-Oldewage, 2016) and therefore probably under-reported (Fig. 20.1a–d). Two pigmented compound eyes assist to spot them on a host, particularly the larvae. A blood-filled intestine in feeding, or recently fed, adult organisms further aids spotting the parasites (Fig. 20.2a–i). They are not strictly host specific, although some species are more frequent on some fish families (Neethling and Avenant-Oldewage, 2016; Van As *et al.*, 2017). Host death has not been reported for species infected with *Dolops*, but Avenant-Oldewage (1994) described loss of the epidermis and bleeding lesions on fish infected by *Dolops ranarum* (Stuhlmann, 1891). In nature, *Dolops* infection intensity is usually low; a single report documents an isolated instance where an African sharptooth catfish *Clarias gariepinus* (Burchell, 1822) was collected with 35 specimens (Avenant and Van As, 1985; Tavares-Dias *et al*, 2007). Recently, Gonzales *et al.* (2024) reported they found high prevalence (100%) of *Dolops carvalhoi* Lemos de Castro, 1949 in some species but that the mean intensities vary between 1.6 and 15 parasites per fish. Tavares-Dias *et al.* (2007) reported that blood parameters changed in fishes infected with *D. carvalhoi*. Møller and Olesen (2012) reported larval *D. carvalhoi* on gulper catfish *Asterophysis batrachus* Kner, 1858 in Japan, following the import of the fish for aquaculture from the Madeira River, a tributary of the Amazon River (South America), to Japan. It was an isolated incident and no further reports of this introduction to Japan exist.

In *Chonopeltis*, a thesis reports that *Chonopeltis australis* Boxshall, 1976 scrapes mucus off its hosts (Van Niekerk, 1984) and the author assumed that the parasites feed on the mucus. No reports of outbreaks or host deaths exist for *Chonopeltis*, and prevalence and intensity are generally low (Neethling and Avenant-Oldewage, 2020).

However, argulosis outbreaks are frequently reported. Hosts become emaciated and die, both in holding facilities and in nature (Kruger *et al.*, 1983). Severe outbreaks, with fish mortality, are mostly linked to three species: *Argulus foliaceus* (Linnaeus, 1758); *Argulus japonicus* Thiele, 1900; and *Argulus coregoni* Thorell, 1865. Introduced *A. japonicus* reach high intensities in natural impoundments (Kruger *et al.*, 1983; Avenant-Oldewage, 2001) in South Africa and in south-western Bangladesh (Jahan *et al.*, 2025). High intensities of *A. foliaceus* infections occurred in still-water trout facilities in the UK (Taylor *et al.*, 2009) and an aquarium in Denmark (Møller *et al.*, 2008). The parasites are exceptionally good travellers, and it is suspected that they have been introduced along with imported fish hosts.

20.2. Morphology

The morphology of some species of the genus *Argulus* is well studied, especially the widespread species which include *A. foliaceus*, *A. japonicus* and *A. coregoni* (Leydig, 1889; Wilson, 1902; Thiele, 1904; Monod, 1928; Tokioka, 1936; Meehan, 1940; Rushton-Mellor, 1992; Avenant-Oldewage and Swanepoel, 1993; Møller *et al.*, 2007; Everts and Avenant-Oldewage, 2009; Tam and Avenant-Oldewage, 2009a,b; Kaji *et al.*, 2011; Nagasawa *et al.*, 2024).

Branchiura vary in size, larvae are less than 0.5 mm, mature individuals vary between species from *Chonopeltis minutus* Fryer, 1977 (3.9 mm ♀, 2.5 mm ♂) (Van As and Van As, 1999) to *Dipteropeltis campanaformis* Neethling, Malta and Avenant-Oldewage, 2014 (20 mm ♀) (Neethling *et al.*, 2014) (Fig. 20.2e). Males are smaller than females of the same species (Pasternak *et al.*, 2004b). All branchiurans are dorsoventrally flattened and their body comprises: (i) a fused head with five cephalic appendages connected to (ii) a thorax bearing four pairs of biramous thoracopods which are used for swimming; and (iii) an unsegmented bilobed abdomen with furcal rami (Fig. 20.2a–i).

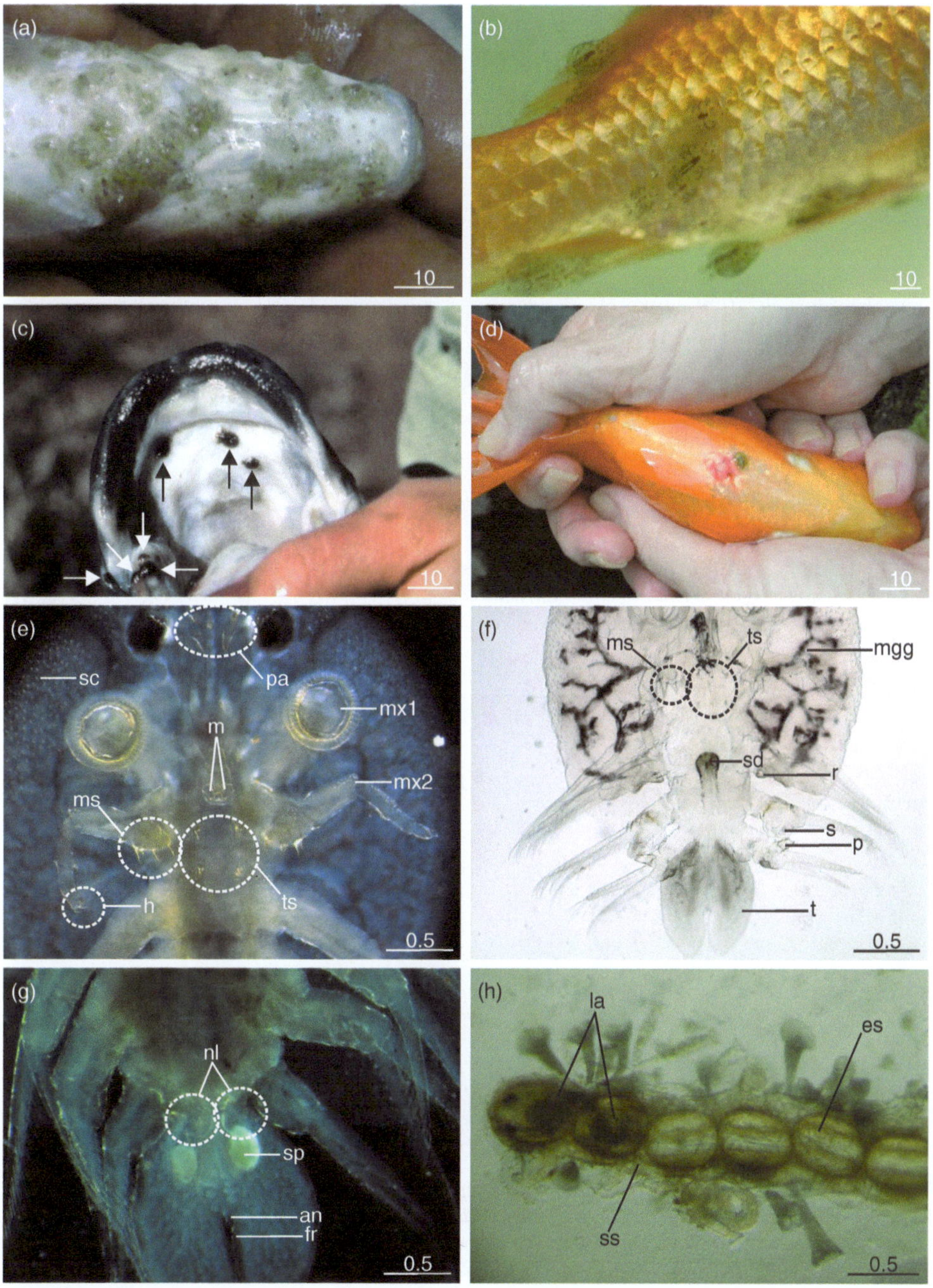

Fig. 20.1. (a) *Argulus japonicus* on *Labeo capensis*; (b) *A. japonicus* on *Carassius auratus*; (c) *Dolops ranarum* in *Oreochromis mossambicus* buccal cavity, arrows show parasites; (d) *A. japonicus* on *C. auratus* showing haemorrhage at attachment site; (e) *A. japonicus* ventral; (f) *A. japonicus* male dorsal; (g) *A. japonicus* female ventral; (h) *A. japonicus* eggs string, with opportunistic unicellular organisms. an, anus; es, empty shell; fr, furcal ramus; h, hook; la, larvae; m, mandible; mgg, midgut gland; ms, maxillar spine; mx1, first maxilla; mx2, second maxilla; nl, natatory lobe; p, peg; pa, post-antennal spine; r, scale covered concavity; s, socket; sc, scale; sd, sperm ducts; sp, spermatheca; ss, sticky substance; t, testis; ts, thoracic spine. Scale bars = cm. (Images (a, c) courtesy of Johan Theron; image (b) courtesy Lourelle Neethling; with permission. All others are author's own.)

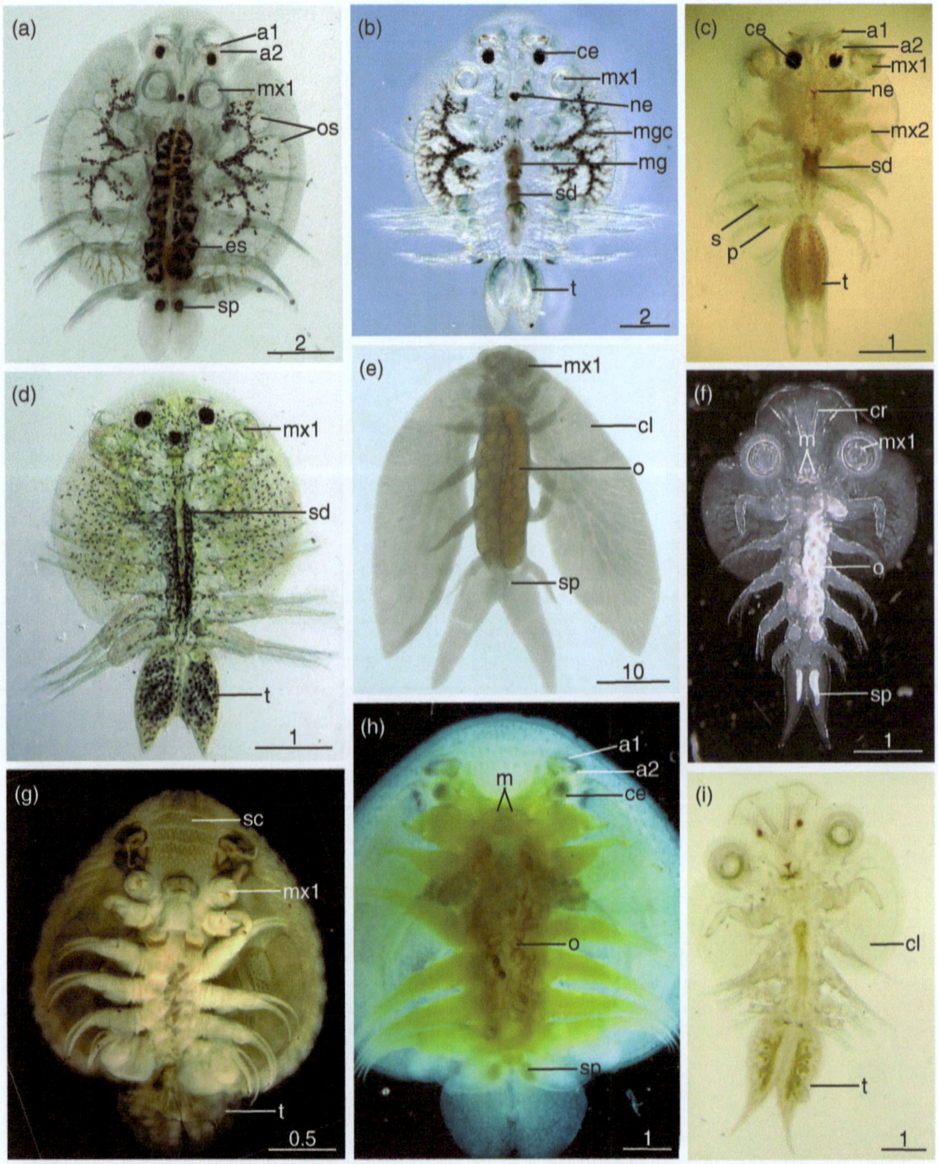

Fig. 20.2. (a) *Argulus japonicus* female dorsal; (b) *A. japonicus* male dorsal; (c) *Argulus personatus* male dorsal; (d) *Dolops ranarum* male dorsal; (e) *Dipteropeltis campanaformis* female dorsal; (f) *Chonopeltis australis* female ventral; (g) *Dolops intermedia,* male ventral; (h) *Dolops discoidalis* female ventral; (i) *Chonopeltis inermis* male ventral. a1, first antenna; a2, second antenna; ce, compound eye; cl, carapace lobe; cr, chitinous rod; es, egg sack; m, mandible; mg, midgut; mgc, midgut caeca; mx1, first maxilla; mx2, second maxilla; ne, nauplius eye; o, oocyte; os, osmoregulatory area; p, peg; s, socket; sd, semen duct; sc, scale/s; sp, spermatheca; t, testis. Scale bars = mm. (Image (c) courtesy of Quinton Tam; image (e) courtesy of Lourelle Neethling; image (g) courtesy of Riccardo Mugnai; with permission. All others are author's own.)

Dorsally are two large, dark compound eyes with many ocelli (Meyer-Rochov *et al.*, 2001) and slightly posterior to them, a smaller median nauplius eye consisting of three pigment cups (Fig. 20.2b and c). A carapace covers the body dorsally; in *Chonopeltis* the anterior lobe of the carapace has four chitin rods (Fig. 20.2f and i) in all species apart from *Chonopeltis flaccifrons* Fryer, 1960 where these structures are absent, as the species name suggests ('soft face'). The cephalic lobes extend posteriorly as two large shields, covering the legs on either side of the thorax (Fig. 20.2a–i). In some species, the carapace lobes extend far enough to cover the abdomen (Yamaguti, 1963; Cressey, 1972; Thatcher, 1991) and their shapes and lengths are used for identification purposes. The carapace lobes contain two highly branched midgut caeca, on either side of the midgut (Fig. 20.2a and b), well described in *D. ranarum* by Avenant-Oldewage and Van As (1990), in *C. australis* by Avenant-Oldewage *et al.* (1994) and in *A. japonicus* by Tam and Avenant-Oldewage (2009a, b).

On the ventral side, the carapace lobes bear specialized areas, with a thinner cuticle for osmoregulation (Haase, 1975), sometimes (wrongly) referred to as 'respiratory areas' (Fig. 20.2a). The shape and placement of the 'respiratory areas' are also often used for species determination (Grobben, 1908; Rushton-Mellor, 1994; Boxshall, 2005). In *Argulus* there are usually two smaller areas anterior and two larger kidney-shaped areas posterolateral to the smaller areas (Fig. 20.2a). *In vivo*, *Argulus* is relatively transparent and resembles a speck of mucus, with a greenish hue and with two compound eyes. In gravid females yellow/whitish oocytes are visible in the egg sack (Tokioka, 1936; Ikuta and Makioka, 1997) (Fig. 20.2a, e, f and h), and in males white to yellowish testes (in the abdomen) and sperm vesicles, ejaculatory ducts and prostate glands occur in the thorax (Fig. 20.1f; Fig. 20.2b, c, d, g and i).

Five pairs of cephalic appendages occur on *Argulus*, *Dolops* and *Dipteropeltis*: the small first antenna which has a large hook laterally (on the first podomere) (Fig. 20.2a, c, g and h) and post-antennal hooks between the antennae (Fig. 20.1e); the second antennae with sensory setae and small hooks terminally (Fig. 20.2a, c and h). In *Chonopeltis* the first pair of antennae is absent throughout all life stages (Van Niekerk and Kok, 1989). In *Argulus*, *Chonopeltis* and *Dipteropeltis* the first maxillae become modified during larval development from appendages with a terminal hook into large sucker cups adorned with discs on the rims (Fig. 20.2a, b, e, f and i; Fig. 20.3a). Ontogeny was described by Kaji *et al.* (2011). *Dolops* retain the neotenic first maxillae, with a terminal hook, into adulthood (Fig. 20.2c, d, g and h; Fig. 20.3d). The second maxilla bears three posteriorly directed stout 'maxillar teeth' on the basal podomere (Fig. 20.1e and f) and two small hooks apically (Fig. 20.1e). Maxillar teeth (Fig. 20.3a) vary in shape and size from narrow to wide, blunt to sharp, short to long, and their placing varies from even to clustered. Therefore, the shape, size and spacing of the maxillar teeth are used to distinguish between species, an extreme example being *Dolops bidentata* (Bouvier, 1899) that has only two teeth (Silva-Souza, *et al.*, 2011). A mouth cone occurs between the first maxilla. The mouth cone is a proboscis and bears an opening at the tip, the opening is enclosed by a labrum (dorsally) and labium (ventrally) (Fig. 20.1e; Fig. 20.3a and b). The proboscis contains two sickle-shaped mandibles in the buccal cavity. The mandibles are crescent shaped and serrated proximally (Fig. 20.1e; Fig. 20.3b and c), the serrations differ between genera. The mouth tube is very short in larval and mature *Dolops*, and short in larvae of *Argulus* and *Chonopeltis* but of varying length in adults. It is long in adults in all three *Dipteropeltis* species (Neethling *et al.*, 2014; Gaboardi *et al.*, 2023). The proboscis is completely fused into a tube in all Branchiura (Martin, 1932; Gresty *et al.*, 1993) (Fig. 20.3a and b). The mandibles can rotate in and out of the buccal cavity and along each other; they are also used to scrape host tissue into the buccal cavity and the abrasive action can eventually sever blood vessels in the host dermis. On the buccal cavity floor between the mandibles two buccal spines occur, these contain the openings of ducts from glands (Swanepoel and Avenant-Oldewage, 1992). A pre-oral spine or stylet is situated anterior to the mouth cone, this cuticular outgrowth is very manoeuvrable and can be retracted (Fig. 20.3a). Two ducts open into the apical tip of the pre-oral spine (Swanepoel and Avenant-Oldewage, 1992). The spine tip is protected by a small flap (apron) which lifts to expose the openings of the two ducts (Swanepoel and Avenant-Oldewage, 1992). These ducts are connected to various glands situated at the base of the spine and in the carapace; their precise function is still debated (Swanepoel and Avenant-Oldewage, 1992; Gresty *et al.*, 1993) although lysis of host tissue and vasodilation of blood vessels have not been

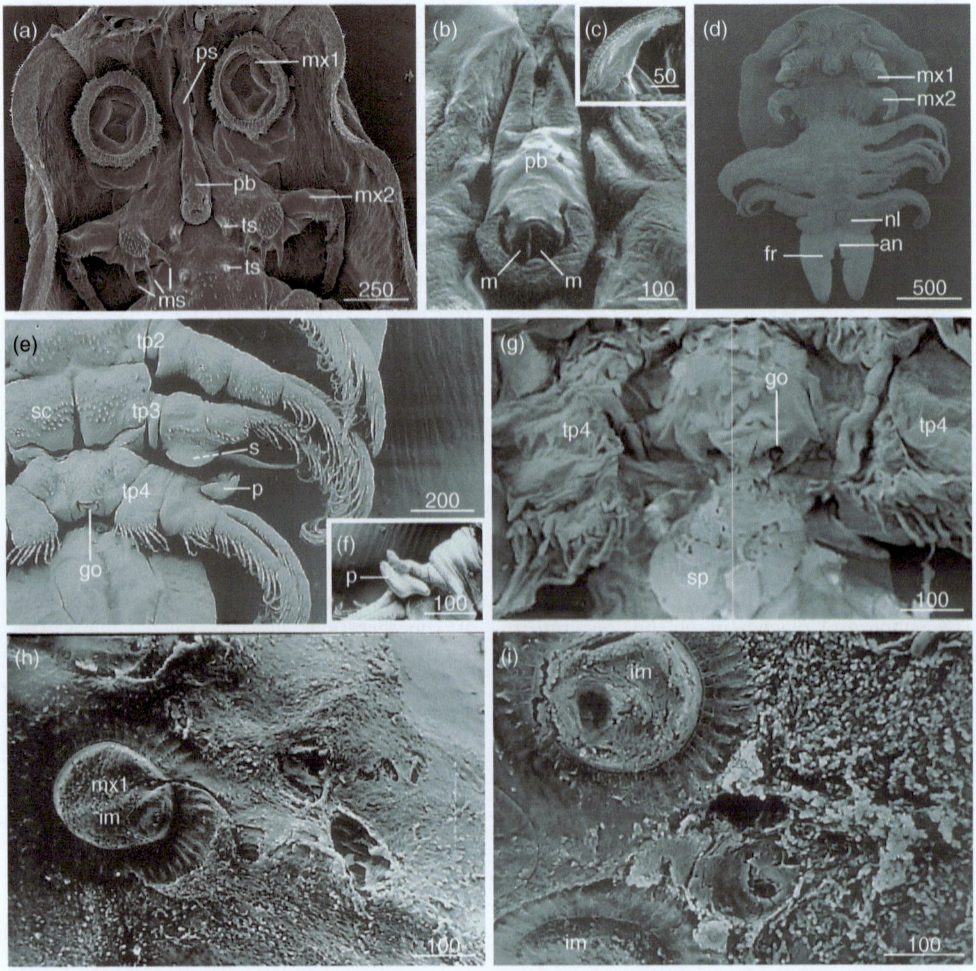

Fig. 20.3. Scanning electron micrographs of: (a) *Argulus japonicus* anterior, ventral view; (b) proboscis of *A. japonicus*; (c) mandible of *Dolops ranarum*; (d) *D. ranarum* ventral view; (e) *A. japonicus* posterior, ventral view; (f) *A. japonicus* dorsal view, peg on fourth thoracopod; (g) *A. japonicus* ventral view, spermatophore; (h) *Clarias gariepinus* skin with *A. japonicus* lesions; (i) *C. gariepinus* skin with *A. japonicus* lesions. an, anus; fr, furcal ramus; go, genital opening; im, imprint; m, mandible; ms, maxillar spine; mx1, first maxilla; mx2, second maxilla; nl, natatory lobe; p, peg; pb, proboscis; ps, pre-oral spine; s, socket; sc, scale/s; sp, spermatophore; ts, thoracic spine; tp, thoracopod. Scale bars = µm. (Image (d) courtesy of Quinton Dos Santos; image (g) from Avenant-Oldewage and Everts, 2010; with copyright permission. All others are author's own.)

ruled out. The ventral aspect of the carapace is adorned with scales packed on the circumference of the carapace and the ventral surface of the thoracopods (Fig. 20.1e; Fig. 20.3a and e). Four thoracic spines occur between the first two pairs of thoracopods (Fig. 20.1e and f; Fig. 20.3a).

All the various hooks (first antennae, post-antennular spines, maxillar teeth, thoracic spines, hooks on the tips of the second maxillae) and scales are directed to the posterior of the parasite and assist in secondary attachment to the host. The modified first maxillae (suckers or hooks) are the primary attachment structures. The suckers are also used for locomotion on the host, by alternating releasing and reattaching in the required direction, imitating walking. Two large cephalic lobes extend to cover the thoracopods dorsally. The length and shape of the carapace lobes vary between genera and species, therefore being used for identification. The most remarkable is *Dipteropeltis hirundo* Calman, 1912, where the lobes are almost double the length of the organism (Neethling *et al.*, 2014) – the species name aptly captures their resemblance to a swallow. The thorax bears four pairs of biramous thoracopods (swimming legs) (Fig. 20.2a–i; Fig. 20.3d). The first two pairs each bear a shorter flabellum dorsally, that rotates consistently and circulates water between the thoracopods and the carapace. In male specimens, secondary reproductive structures occur on the second, third and fourth thoracopods in *Argulus* and *Chonopeltis* (Van As and Van As, 1999; Neethling and Avenant-Oldewage, 2016). The protrusion on the fourth leg is referred to as a 'peg' and the structure on the third leg the 'socket' (Figs 20.1f and 20.3e). Only a small protrusion was reported on the third thoracopods in *D. ranarum* by Avenant *et al.* (1989a), but in *D. bidentata* and *Dolops intermedia* Silva, 1978, males bear protrusions on the second leg and a peg and socket on the third and fourth thoracopods, respectively (Silva-Souza *et al.*, 2011; Mugnai *et al.*, 2022). Females have enlarged proximal segments on the fourth thoracopods (Fig. 20.1g; Fig. 20.3d and e): these structures are referred to as the natatory lobes and assist in placement of eggs while depositing them; they also cover the spermathecal spines and partly cover the spermatophore when it is present.

The abdomen is bilobed, the anterior part is fused to the level of the anus (Fig. 20.2a–i), the shape and length of the abdomen vary greatly between species, even within the same genus (compare Fig. 20.2a and Fig. 20.2c). The length of the abdomen, the ratio of the abdomen versus the body length as well as the shape of the lobes are therefore also useful diagnostic features for species identification. Two furcal rami bearing setae occur on the inner margin of the abdominal split (anterior to the anus) (Fig. 20.1g; Fig. 20.3d) and their length and shape vary between genera and species, thus their morphology is also used for species identification. The testes and spermathecae occur in the abdomen of males and females, respectively (Fig. 20.1f and g; Fig. 20.2a–i).

Females are distinguished from males by the absence of the secondary copulatory structures on the thoracopods, the presence of two round, cuticle-lined spermathecae in the abdomen, and in mature specimens, oocytes in the thorax (Fig. 20.1g; Fig. 20.2a, e, f and h). Males have reproductive structures on the second, third and fourth thoracopods, sperm ducts (seminal vesicle, ejaculatory ducts, prostate duct) in the thorax and the two testes in the abdomen (Avenant-Oldewage and Everts, 2010; Neethling and Avenant-Oldewage, 2015) (Fig. 20.1f; Fig. 20.2b, c, d, g and i). The testes are elongated and reach into the abdominal lobes and vary between species; for example, in *D. ranarum* and *D. intermedia* the testes are three-lobed (Fig. 20.2d and g), while they are crenulated in *Chonopeltis meridionalis* Fryer, 1964 and *Chonopeltis inermis* Thiele, 1900 (Fig. 20.2i) (Fryer, 1956; Avenant *et al.*, 1989a; Neethling and Avenant-Oldewage, 2015; Van As *et al.*, 2017; Mugnai *et al.*, 2022). Males have not been described in *Dipteropeltis*.

In *Dolops* the morphology of newly hatched larvae has been described for *D. ranarum* by Avenant *et al.* (1989b) and for an immature *D. carvalhoi* by Møller and Olesen (2012). In *C. australis*, newly hatched larvae were described by Van Niekerk and Kok (1989), and late-stage juveniles of *D. longicaudatus* by Gaboardi *et al.* (2023). In all instances, the larvae resemble the adults, the mandibles are crescent shaped with serrations on the outer periphery, and the larvae have well-developed thoracopods enabling them to swim. Newly hatched *Argulus*, *Chonopeltis* and *Dolops* larvae bear a hook on the terminal segment of the first maxillae (Shimura, 1981; Avenant *et al.*, 1989b; Van Niekerk and Kok, 1989; Rushton-Mellor and Boxshall, 1994; Lutch and Avenant-Oldewage, 1995). These hooks transform during ontogeny to cup-shaped suckers (see summary in Kaji *et al.*, 2011). In *Dolops* the hooks are retained into adulthood, but the morphology of this appendage in newly hatched or early-stage larvae of *Dipteropeltis* is still unknown.

Later-stage *Argulus* and *Dolops* larvae are obligatory micropredators of fish, feeding opportunistically on host mucus, tissue and blood (Gilbert *et al.*, 2025), in males and females, and the meal includes whole erythrocytes (Walker *et al.*, 2011).

20.3. Life Cycle

Copulation in *Argulus* takes place on, as well as off, the host (Clark, 1902; Wilson, 1902; Avenant-Oldewage and Everts, 2010); similarly in

D. ranarum and *C. australis* (A. Avenant-Oldewage, 1985, unpublished results). Fryer (1960) was the first to observe a spermatophore in Branchiura and reported a spermatophore on *D. ranarum* females and mentioned that it resembles a pearl in shape and lustre. Many years later, Avenant-Oldewage and Everts (2010) observed copulation in *A. japonicus* and reported that a spermatophore also occurs in this genus albeit a flimsy spermatophore (Fig. 20.3g). Thereafter, Neethling and Avenant-Oldewage (2015) observed a spermatophore being transferred also in *C. australis*. The spermatophore is transferred via the peg and socket structures on the third and fourth thoracopods and placed on the spermathecal spines on the female abdomen. A scaled concavity on the second thoracopod (Fig. 20.1f; Fig. 20.3e) is used to trap and hold the female's thoracopods between the second and third thoracopods of the male during copulation (Avenant-Oldewage and Everts, 2010). Sperm enters the spermathecae (on the female abdomen) via spermathecal spines and ducts. Avenant *et al.* (1989b) reported they observed the spermathecal spines in *D. ranarum* also being used to penetrate shelled oocytes as they are released. The spine penetrates an oocyte, and sperm is injected into the shelled oocytes, when the abdomen contracts Wingstrand (1972) described that *A. foliaceus* has filiform sperm. Eggs are deposited in rows (Fig. 20.1h) and are cemented to stones, rocks, the glass sides and bottom of aquaria, air stones, wood structures and even on plant material in shallow brinks to as deep as 8.5 m (Walker *et al.*, 2004; Harrison *et al.*, 2006; Piasecki and Avenant-Oldewage, 2008). The number of eggs per batch varies from a few to several hundred eggs. In extreme instances, multiple layers of eggs are deposited on top of each other in *A. coregoni* in fishponds (Mikheev *et al.*, 2001). Hatching rates are consistently very high (>90%) (Hakalahti and Valtonen, 2003; Hakalahti *et al.*, 2003). Egg development and time to hatching depend on temperature. Shafir and Van As (1986) exposed *A. japonicus* eggs in the laboratory to temperatures varying between 10 and 35°C with 5°C increments and reported that eggs in the same batch hatched randomly, not correlated to their position or the order in which they were laid. The optimal temperature, when the highest percentage of eggs hatched in the shortest period, was 20–25°C which is commensurate with summer water temperatures in South Africa. Some eggs, randomly scattered in a batch, did not hatch at all and eggs at 10°C did not develop beyond colour change, which the authors suggested was due to the eggs possibly overwintering. Hindle (1949) noticed that *A. foliaceus* eggs, laid in autumn, hatched in spring after resting for 5–7 months. Similarly, Mikheev *et al.* (2001) reported uneven and extended hatching and coined the phrase 'hedging your bets'. This strategy has since been reported for *Argulus* by various authors (Fenton and Hudson, 2002; Hakalahti and Valtonen, 2003; Hakalahti *et al.*, 2003, 2004, 2005; Taylor, 2004; Bandilla *et al.*, 2007; Mikheev *et al.*, 2007; Lynn *et al.*, 2020). Eggs of *Dolops discoidalis* Bouvier, 1899 hatch unevenly but within days of each other (17–22 days at 28°C) (Oliveira *et al.*, 2021); *D. ranarum* larvae hatch after 27–35 days (Fryer, 1964) to 57 days at 20°C (Avenant *et al.*, 1989b).

The life cycle of *Argulus* is well studied (cf. Shimura, 1981 for *A. coregoni*; Rushton-Mellor and Boxshall, 1994 for *A. foliaceus*), but the same cannot be said of the other genera. Females deposit between a few to a few hundred eggs in rows in *Dolops*, *Argulus* and *Chonopeltis* (Shafir and Van As, 1986; Avenant *et al.*, 1989b; Møller and Olesen, 2012). The eggs are deposited along with a sticky substance that hardens soon after egg depositing. Eggs hatch after various days, depending on the temperature (see previous paragraph) and larvae are mobile as soon as they leave the eggs (Shafir and Van As, 1986; Avenant *et al.*, 1989b). In *Argulus*, *Dolops* and *Chonopeltis* larvae, the mouth tube is short and contains tiny mandibles, presumably inadequate to penetrate fish skin (Avenant *et al.*, 1989b; Van Niekerk and Kok, 1989; Tam and Avenant-Oldewage, 2006). Stable isotope analysis confirmed that larvae of *A. japonicus* are not feeding during the first larval stage (Gilbert *et al.*, 2025). The eggs are telolecithal and newly hatched larvae derive sustenance from the yolk.

Both sexes leave their hosts; females, to deposit eggs on a substrate and males to deposit a spermatophore (Fig. 20.3g) (confirmed in *Argulus* and *Dolops*) to a female (Fryer, 1960; Avenant-Oldewage and Everts, 2010). Sperm is stored in the spermathecae until the oocytes are ready for fertilization (Fig. 20.1g; Fig. 20.2a, e and h).

20.4. Hosts and Host Finding

Mature parasites switch between hosts; females remain stationary for longer periods to feed and increase in body size and fecundity, but males leave their hosts to search for a new partner (Bandilla *et al.*, 2008). This behaviour is risky as they may succumb to starvation and/or predation (Mikheev *et al.*, 2015). Poulin and Fitzgerald (1988) observed a male-dominated population in *Argulus canadensis* Wilson, 1916; similarly in *A. japonicus* the male to female ratio is 3:1 (Shafir and Oldewage, 1992) and in *Argulus bengalensis* Ramakrishna, 1952 it is 2:1 (Guha *et al.*, 2013). This oversupply suggests that not all males are able to relocate a host. However, successful return to a different host provides an opportunity to transfer secondary parasites between hosts (see Section 20.7 for more details).

A. foliaceus responds to light and dark cues and showed preference for a silver flash that could resemble the body of a potential host (Mikheev *et al.*, 1998). They have compound eyes, and Meyer-Rochov *et al.* (2001) reported 60 ommatidia per eye in *A. foliaceus* and up to 90 in *A. coregoni*. Mikheev *et al.* (2000) furthermore described that those parasites kept in lit environments hover at an incline in an 'ambush' strategy, but in the dark, they would swim faster and locate a host. In experiments, *A. foliaceus* responded to fish odour and also located a mate through chemotaxis (Bandilla *et al.*, 2007). *Argulus* exhibits a circadian rhythm and responds to different light sources, with preference given in the order blue, yellow, green and red (Yoshizawa and Nogami, 2008).

Both *A. foliaceus* and *A. japonicus* are not strictly host specific and have been found on many freshwater fishes as well as in brackish-water fishes. Hosts include: the small stickleback, *Gasterosteus aculeatus* L., 1758; rudd, *Scardinius erythrophthalmus* L., 1758; perch, *Perca fluviatilis* L., 1758; carp, *Cyprinus carpio* (L., 1758); carp bream, *Abramis brama* L., 1758; tench, *Tinca tinca* L., 1758; eel, *Anguilla anguilla* L., 1758; large pike, *Esox lucius* L., 1758; trout, *Salmo trutta* L., 1758; rainbow trout, *Oncorhynchus mykiss* Walbaum, 1792; largescale yellowfish, *Labeobarbus marequensis* (Smith, 1841); moggel, *Labeo umbratus* (Smith, 1841); African sharptooth catfish, *C. gariepinus*; freshwater minnow, *Opsariichthys platypus* (Cyprinidae); and largemouth bass, *Micropterus salmoides* (cf. Kollatsch, 1959; Menezes *et al.*, 1990; Paperna, 1991, 1996; Buchmann and Bresciani, 1997; Evans and Matthews 2000; Avenant-Oldewage, 2001; Taylor *et al.*, 2009; Nagasawa, 2017, 2019, 2021). When the scaleless, African sharptooth catfish is kept with cyprinids, *A. japonicus* occurs in very low numbers on the catfish (A. Avenant-Oldewage, 1985, unpublished results) implying preference for cyprinids. The same phenomenon occurs in nature (Kruger *et al.*, 1983; Avenant-Oldewage, 2001). In aquaria, attachment of *A. japonicus* on the catfish is temporary and they switch host as soon as another species is introduced (A. Avenant-Oldewage, 1985, unpublished results).

A. coregoni prefers salmonids (Bandilla *et al.*, 2004; Pasternak *et al.*, 2004a; Mikheev *et al.*, 2007). Later, Everts and Avenant-Oldewage (2009) reported it from the holding facility of a restaurant in Malaysia on (presumably) red belly tilapia; and recently, Nagasawa and Nishimura (2025) reported it in Japan in a small stream that originates on a mountain. It was found on two cypriniform fishes, the fat minnow *Rhynchocypris lagowskii steindachneri* (Sauvage, 1883) (Leuciscidae) and the dark chub *Nipponocypris temminckii* (Temminck and Schlegel, 1846) (Xenocyprididae), even when salmonids were present at the site.

A. foliaceus, *A. japonicus* and *A. coregoni* have spread widely, probably through transport of live fish for aquaculture, recreational fisheries and the pet industry (Menezes *et al.*, 1990; Rushton-Mellor, 1992; Paperna, 1996; Northcott *et al.*, 1997; Bandilla *et al.*, 2004; Hakalahti *et al.*, 2004; Catalano and Hutson, 2010). All three species exhibit low species specificity and are probably under-reported. The high variation in genetic data on gene repositories for *Argulus* identified as *A. japonicus* suggests that some specimens may have been misidentified even among researchers. It is therefore suggested that recent updates in descriptions of species be consulted when identifications are done. These appear in papers by Nagasawa and Nishimura (2025) for *A. viridis*, by Nagasawa (2021) for *A. japonicus*, by Møller and Olesen (2012) for *A. foliaceus* and for *Argulus personatus* Cunnington, 1913 by Tam *et al.* (2005). There are also various comprehensive reports for the South American Branchiura (Thatcher, 1991; Malta and Varella, 2009; Mugnai *et al.*, 2022; Bonfirm *et al.*, 2025).

20.5. Diagnosis of Infection and Clinical Signs of the Disease

Mature *Argulus* is easily spotted on fish, whereas larvae are small and transparent and therefore more challenging to detect on a host. The best visual cues are the two dark compound eyes. Typically, parasites attach to the skin, and the preferred attachment site is at the base of fins (Kollatsch, 1959; Schlüter, 1978; Mikheev *et al.*, 1998). In some host fish, *A. foliaceus* is also commonly found in the mouth cavity and under the gill covers (e.g. in pike) (Møller and Olesen, 2012). In extreme infections, more than 250 adults and more than 1500 juvenile *Argulus* have been reported from a single fish specimen (Kruger *et al.*, 1983; Northcott *et al.*, 1997). Such heavy infections result in severe damage to the integument of the host, which leads to high mortality (Walker *et al.*, 2004), but even small numbers of parasites can cause mortality in fish larvae (Poulin, 1999). Early in infection, there is an increase in fish jumping (Taylor *et al.*, 2006); later, fish are lethargic, show erratic swimming behaviour and flashing (Yildiz and Kumantas, 2002) and their appetite is suppressed, which causes emaciation and retarded growth (Kabata, 1985; Singhal *et al.*, 1990). As infection progresses, infected sites become haemorrhagic (Fig. 20.1d) and sometimes infected with secondary fungal and bacterial infections and large-scale mortalities may occur (Poulin, 1999; Taylor *et al.*, 2006). Various reports observed changes in shoal behaviour (summarized by Taylor *et al.*, 2006) and active avoidance of parasitized conspecifics was shown in sticklebacks (Poulin and FitzGerald, 1989; Dugatkin *et al.*, 1994; Poulin, 1999; Barber *et al.*, 2000). Fish lose scales and this, coupled with their reduced appetite and emaciation, caused consumer resistance in recreational fishing in trout farms in Scotland which then resulted in financial losses (Taylor *et al.*, 2006).

20.6. Macroscopic and Microscopic Lesions

In *Argulus* and *Dolops* a wound is caused by the opposing scything motion of the serrated mandibles (Fig. 20.1e; Fig. 20.3b and c). Subsequently, the tissue is moved towards the buccal cavity. During feeding, the labrum and labium together seal the tip of the mouth cone on the host, and sustenance is sucked into the midgut (intestine) when the oesophageal muscles dilate (Tam and Avenant-Oldewage, 2006). During this time, the pre-oral spine and buccal spines (Fig. 20.3a and b) are in contact with the surface and releasing substances of glandular origin on the surface (Swanepoel and Avenant-Oldewage, 1992). Walker *et al.* (2011) reported that whole (not macerated or predigested) erythrocytes occur in the intestine of mature *A. japonicus*, proving that the parasites consume the cells.

Feeding in larval *A. japonicus* has been a topic of discussion for a considerable time and particularly their ability to feed on host blood. Tam and Avenant-Oldewage (2006) reported that the proboscis (approximately 50 μm long) and the mandibular blades (approximately 15 μm long) inside the proboscis are probably insufficient in length to reach blood vessels in the host dermis as the typical cyprinid epidermis is thicker and suggested that the larvae may not be blood feeders. Walker *et al.* (2011) later confirmed that whole blood cannot be consumed by larvae as the erythrocytes from carp are typically around 12–13 μm in diameter and that the proboscis aperture is not wide enough to allow the ingestion of whole erythrocytes. They could also not find any erythrocytes in squash preparations of larval parasites. The debate was concluded in a recent study by Gilbert *et al.* (2025) who, using stable isotope analysis, showed that the first larval stages are neither feeding on fish (mucus, epithelia or blood) nor on algae, and concluded that maternal yolk (derived from telolecithal eggs) is their only source of energy that is then utilized to find a host off which they will feed from the second larval stage onwards.

Shimura and Inoue (1984) injected an extract derived from *A. coregoni* into rainbow trout and found that it induced a haemorrhagic response, which could facilitate haematophagy in *A. coregoni*.

Feeding causes local trauma to the host integument, and the damaged epithelium is prone to secondary infections (Walker *et al.*, 2004; Boxshall, 2005; Piasecki and Avenant-Oldewage, 2008) (Fig. 20.3h and i). Spring viraemia (carp virus), infamous for killing many cyprinids, is spread by *A. foliaceus* (cf. Pfeil-Putzien, 1977; Ahne, 1985; Walker *et al.*, 2004) (as *Rhabdovirus carpio*, cf. Pfeil-Putzien and Baath, 1978). Bacteria and *Saprolegnia* (a fungus) occur in wounds caused by *Argulus* (cf. Singhal *et al.*, 1990). Fish infected with *Flavobacterium columnare* Davis (1922) and *A. coregoni* had a reduced survival rate compared to fish infected with only the bacterium, so it was concluded that *Argulus* increases the fish's susceptibility to bacterial infection (Bandilla *et al.*, 2006). Furthermore, several authors reported the presence of larval Skrjabillanidae nematodes in *Argulus* (cf. Tikhomirova, 1983; Molnár and Moravec, 1997; Molnár and Székely, 1998). *Molnaria erythrophthalmi* Molnár, Eszterbauer, Marton, Cech and Székely, 2009 was reported in *A. foliaceus* and its transmission confirmed in three of 79 fish species in the Elbe River basin in what was then Czechoslovakia (Moravec, 1978; Molnár and Szekely, 1998). Later, Moravec *et al.* (1999) reported transmission of a daniconematid nematode, *Mexiconema cichlasomae* Moravec, Vidal and Salgado-Maldonado, 1992, by an unidentified *Argulus* sp. in Mexico.

20.7. Pathophysiology

Fish infected by *Argulus* are weak and clinical signs include suppression of appetite, emaciation, growth cessation and ultimately death (Shimura, 1983; Kabata, 1985; Tavares-Dias *et al.*, 1999; Piasecki and Avenant-Oldewage, 2008). Changes to the haematological parameters of infected fish include increased monocyte and granulocyte counts indicating an immune response; and depending on the intensity of infection and a longer period of exposure, a general decrease in haemoglobin and haematocrit (erythrocyte and leucocyte) values can occur (Shimura, 1983; Tavares-Dias *et al.*, 1999, 2007; Piasecki and Avenant-Oldewage, 2008). A specific immune response to *A. foliaceus* antigens was reported in rainbow trout by Ruane *et al.* (1995), and Walker *et al.* (2004) summarized data from other investigations showing increased expression of the interleukin-1 and tumour necrosis factor-α genes in response to *Argulus* infections. Typical histopathological changes include hypertrophy of the epithelia at the wound margins and damage to the stratum compactum (Walker *et al.*, 2004). Ultimately, osmoregulation became compromised in severely infected killifish *Fundulus heteroclitus* (Linnaeus, 1766) and the authors were able to relate it directly to the severity of tissue damage (Marshall *et al.*, 2008). Furthermore, the parasites move around on the host, creating multiple wounds (Fig. 20.3h and i). The role of argulids as stress inducers was reviewed by Walker *et al.* (2004) who concluded that only high infection rates induce any detectable stress responses such as elevated cortisol levels in the hosts.

Parasites of the genus *Dolops* attach by inserting the hooks on the first maxillae into the dermis, which causes punctiform lesions that are exacerbated by feeding with a proboscis with mandibles (Thatcher, 1991; Avenant-Oldewage, 1994; Malta and Varella, 2009). In *C. gariepinus* infected with *D. ranarum*, loss of epidermis was related to feeding and haemorrhaging wounds deep in the dermis and thereby to insertion of the hooks. The wounds healed and scar tissue formed (Avenant-Oldewage, 1994). In *D. carvalhoi* on hybrid tambacu *Colossoma macropomum* Cuvier, 1818 × pacu *Piaractus mesopotamicus* Holmberg, 1887 fish, no macroscopic lesions were reported in a mild infection (mean intensity of 19 parasites per fish). The fish had lower haematocrit and magnesium levels and increased mean corpuscular haemoglobin concentration (MCHC), plasma glucose, serum protein, sodium and chloride levels compared to uninfected fish in natural infections. There was also an increase in the number of monocytes as well as the number of PAS (periodic acid–Schiff)-positive granulocytes (Tavares-Dias *et al.*, 2007).

20.8. Protective/Control Strategies

Methods for control of *Argulus* infections need to take cognisance of the opportunistic nature of the branchiurans displayed by, among others, the following life strategies: females deposit many eggs in various batches that hatch over an extended period (hedging); larvae, males and females are excellent swimmers that could re/locate a host; the population consists of more males than females to counterbalance losses incurred during host switching; spermatophores are produced and sperm is stored in spermathecae until the oocytes are ready for insemination; one sperm is injected per oocyte (frugal); first-stage larvae acquire sustenance from yolk. Preventing egg development is probably the most effective and environmentally responsible strategy. Although draining of aquaria and scrubbing of glass walls to remove all eggs is effective, it is labour-intensive, and drying aquaculture ponds and treating them with lime (Chen, 1933), even if effective, is not practical.

Hakalahti *et al.* (2004) and Gault *et al.* (2002) recommended that use of alternative egg-depositing surfaces, which could then be removed and destroyed, was effective to treat the spreading of lice, but Taylor *et al.* (2006) recorded that farmers from 77 sites were not using these, even during massive outbreaks. Instead, they noticed that dropping the water level by 30 cm in summer was more effective.

Organochlorine and organophosphate pesticides have proved to be effective against *Argulus* infections at concentrations of 2.5 mg/l and 0.25 ppm in other cases (summarized in Walker *et al.*, 2004; Piasecki and Avenant-Oldewage, 2008). Tavares-Dias *et al.* (1999) applied the chlorinated organophosphate trichlorphon at 0.4 mg/500 l water. Ranzani-Paiva *et al.* (1987) observed that organophosphate treatment decreased mean corpuscular volume (MCV), MCHC, leucocyte, neutrophil and granulocytic cells and monocyte numbers, and a later report (Tavares-Dias *et al.*, 2007) confirmed reduced red blood cell count (RBC) and haemoglobin values in fish. Both groups of chemicals affect the nervous system (Niesink *et al.*, 1996) and their use is generally discouraged and banned in the European Union (Paperna, 1991, 1996; Piasecki and Avenant-Oldewage, 2008).

Hakalati-Sirén *et al.* (2008) evaluated various integrated pest management approaches for sustainable prevention and reported that 100% mortality of juveniles and adults of *A. coregoni* was achieved with potassium permanganate treatments (0.01 g/l) whereas treatments with formalin (0.6 ml/l), sodium chloride (20 g/l) or malachite green/formalin were not effective. They also noticed that shaking infected fish in a hand net detached parasites and caused >80% decrease in parasite numbers. For eggs, drying over a minimum period of 24 h and formalin treatments (120 ml/l) caused significantly higher mortality. Other treatments, such as baths in potassium permanganate (1 g/l) or sodium chloride (50 g/l), did not significantly affect the viability of eggs.

Pyrethroids (Na^+-ion channel activators) are less toxic to humans (LD_{50}, the lethal concentration for 50% of the population, is estimated at *c.*1 g/kg) but more toxic to aquatic invertebrates and have also been used with relative success against branchiuran infections at 20–200 ppm (Piasecki and Avenant-Oldewage, 2008). Various other substances with less acute human toxicity have also been applied in branchiuran infection control. For example, in-feed treatments with emamectin benzoate, a γ-aminobutyric acid (GABA)-receptor-binding Cl^--channel activator, derived from an actinomycete secondary metabolite and used as an insecticide, was successful in controlling *A. coregoni* at 50 mg/kg fish (Hakalahti *et al.*, 2004). Alkaloid plant derivatives such as pellitorine (amides group) at 5 mg/ml cause detachment of 80% of *Argulus* spp. from goldfish *Carassius auratus* (Linnaeus, 1758) and Boopathi *et al.* (2024) reported that the treatment enhanced the host immune response by promoting superoxide dismutase (SOD) and catalase (CAT) production. They furthermore reported that treatment with pellitorine caused the formation of reactive oxygen species (ROS) which caused cellular damage in the parasite. *In vitro* effects of the treatment still require confirmation in practice. Similarly, 100% eradication (*in vivo*) was achieved of an unidentified *Argulus* with piperine. Stock solution was prepared from commercial Piperine EC 97% (Sigma, USA) by adding 1.0 g piperine to 2 ml organic solvent (dimethylsulfoxide) and filled to 100 ml with distilled water. Thereafter, a working solution was prepared in borehole water at 9.0 mg/l after 48 h exposure (Kumar *et al.*, 2012). Banerjee *et al.* (2014) reported a reduction in the number of previtellogenic, vittelogenic and post-vittelogenic oocytes in the ovary of females after treatment with neem, *Azadirachta indica* Juss. Neem leaf dust extract was freshly prepared daily (see Banerjee *et al.*, 2014 for the extraction procedure). The neem treatment (120 ppm and 250 ppm azadirachtin) impacted the number of eggs deposited as well as hatching success. However, *in vitro* treatment of eggs after deposition was only successful if the treatment was applied within 70 min after the eggs had been deposited; if this optimal period was missed the eggs developed normally (Banerjee *et al.* 2014).

Lynn *et al.* (2020) experimented with the effect of salinity on *A. canadensis* and reported that initially more embryos and hatched larvae were present in fresh water, but that at an increase in salinity to 17 ppt, unhatched embryos were dead/dying at the end of the trial. Eggs did not even develop at 34 ppt, suggesting that a salt bath would be effective for the treatment of aquaria.

Nanoparticles have gained interest in medicine, and this was also tested against *Argulus*. Iron nanoparticles (FeNPs) effectively eradicated *Argulus siamensis* Wilson, 1926: after 6 h exposure (1.75 mg/ml on juveniles; 2.0 mg/l on adults) 100 and 87% mortality was achieved, respectively. The authors caution that the treatment still needs to be evaluated in ponds (Brahmchari *et al.*, 2023).

Tadpoles of the river frog *Lithobates heckscheri* (Wright, 1924) in South Carolina were successfully treated with diflubenzuron (Wolfe *et al.*, 2001). The authors used lufenuron (tablets crushed and added as a suspension in water) to a final concentration of 15 mg/l for 3 weeks with weekly water changes (50%) followed by redosing. The treatment was supplemented by sodium chloride at 3 g/l in water. Argulosis was eradicated and all frogs developed normally following the treatment. The authors highlight that diflubenzuron is less toxic to fish than organophosphates but 25,000 times more toxic to aquatic invertebrates than to fishes, and its use is restricted in wetlands and water bodies in the USA.

20.9. Conclusions and Suggestions for Future Studies

Argulus infections rarely cause serious impacts to wild fish populations. However, their impact can be severe in populations of farmed and aquarium fish populations. Various secondary infections are transmitted and the risk of spring viraemia infections transmission remains problematic. *Argulus* and *Dolops* cause physiological stress in the fish, the damage from their feeding activity can be serious and infections remain under-reported. Furthermore, when it is done at all, the 'culprit' species is frequently not identified to species level.

Unfortunately, many species descriptions are incomplete or type specimens not available, and some have not been updated since the work of Wilson (1902). Some species have been reported only once and type specimens were either not allocated or not submitted to a reputable museum, they may be missing from the storing institution, not labelled properly, not well preserved or all of the previous together (see, for instance, Neethling *et al.*, 2014). Many museums switched to storing specimens in methanol or other combinations of chemicals that spoils them for currently available genetic profiling techniques. As description of most species requires a revisit and application of current techniques such as scanning electron microscopy (SEM) and genetic characterization, new material needs to be collected. Furthermore, host identifications are frequently absent or questionable. Future studies should include surveys to collect and describe species. A holistic approach, using light and scanning electron microscopy and genetic characterization with various markers for both the parasite and host, should be followed. Material should be fixed and preserved with a variety of fixatives that will allow an array of techniques. Type specimens, hologenophores (in 90–100% v/v ethanol in dH_2O for additional/alternative future extractions) and host tissue samples (in 90–100% v/v ethanol in dH_2O) to confirm host identifications should be deposited in various (at least three) international museums. The recent bloom of research papers on Branchiura from South America is encouraging because these add to the number of species and information on host response but description of a male *Dipteropeltis* is still outstanding.

The distribution of *A. foliaceus*, *A. japonicus* and *A. coregoni*, the species that are responsible for outbreaks in aquaculture, should be documented in reputable journals to gain understanding of their natural range. This is a prerequisite for prevention of parasitic infections and the pathogens they transmit from spreading from natural to farmed and aquarium trade fish stocks, and vice versa. Specific host reactions, such as the response to *Argulus* infections, are still poorly known in comparison with, for instance, the salmon and salmon louse interface. Detailed studies on cause/effect on hosts and parasites are still required at the individual and population levels. A lot of knowledge can be gained from understanding the development of resistance in the salmon lice saga.

Prevention, including studies on immune responses, are preferable over treatment as environmental and consumer health concerns have not been resolved and cause consumer resistance. Promising results have been obtained with chitosan–silver nanocomposites in another crustacean, *Lernaea* Linnaeus, 1758, and this appears to constitute a promising future treatment (Abu-Elala *et al.*, 2018). Nano-silver has a suppressive effect on bacteria and enhanced wound healing has been reported, with its use having been accepted for human application such as in socks or wound dressings. Experimental work on the use of nano-silver or other nano products for their efficacy and safety should be conducted on Branchiura infections. Studies should also report on bioaccumulation of the product/s in Branchiura and the effect of the treatment on unintended biota. A recent study on *A. japonicus* reported that it effectively bioaccumulates a variety of metals (Gilbert and Avenant-Oldewage, 2018) to much higher levels than its hosts, suggesting its usefulness as an indicator of environmental pollution. The study applied fluorescence stains and used fluorescence microscopy to locate the presence of metals in the parasite body. It was followed by SEM coupled with energy-dispersive X-ray spectroscopy (EDS) and reported accurate identification and quantification of metals. These techniques could be applied in other studies using metals, metalloids or nanometal products.

References

Abu-Elala, N.M., Attia, M.M. and Abd-Elsalam, R.M. (2018) Chitosan–silver nanocomposites in goldfish aquaria: a new perspective in *Lernaea cyprinacea* control. *International Journal of Biological Macromolecules* 111, 614–622.

Ahne, W. (1985) *Argulus foliaceus* (L.) and *Piscicola geometra* L. as mechanical vectors of spring viraemia of carp virus (SVCV). *Journal of Fish Diseases* 8, 241–242.

Avenant, A and Van As, J.G. (1985) Occurrence and distribution of *Dolops ranarum* (Stuhlmann), ectoparasite of freshwater fish in the Transvaal, South Africa. *Journal of Fish Biology* 27, 403–416.

Avenant, A., Loots, G.C. and Van As, J.G. (1989a) A description of *Dolops ranarum* (Stuhlmann 1891) (Crustacea: Branchiura). *Systematic Parasitology* 13, 141–151.

Avenant, A., Van As, J.G. and Loots, G.C. (1989b) On the hatching and morphology of *Dolops ranarum* larvae (Crustacea: Branchiura). *Journal of Zoology* 217, 511–519.

Avenant-Oldewage, A. (1994) Integumental damage caused by *Dolops ranarum* (Stuhlmann, 1891) (Crustacea: Branchiura) to *Clarias gariepinus* (Burchell), with reference to normal histology and wound-inflicting structures. *Journal of Fish Diseases* 17, 641–647.

Avenant-Oldewage, A. (2001) *Argulus japonicus* in the Olifants River system – possible conservation threat? *South African Journal of Wildlife Research* 31, 59–63.

Avenant-Oldewage, A. and Everts, L. (2010) *Argulus japonicus*: sperm transfer by means of a spermatophore on *Carassius auratus* (L). *Experimental Parasitology* 126, 232–238.

Avenant-Oldewage, A. and Swanepoel, J.H. (1993) The male reproductive system and mechanism of sperm transfer in *Argulus japonicus* (Crustacea: Branchiura). *Journal of Morphology* 215, 51–63.

Avenant-Oldewage, A. and Van As, J.G. (1990) The digestive system of the fish ectoparasite *Dolops ranarum* (Crustacea: Branchiura). *Journal of Morphology* 204, 103–112.

Avenant-Oldewage, A., Swanepoel, J.H. and Knight, E. (1994) Histomorphology of the digestive tract of *Chonopeltis australis* (Crustacea: Branchiura). *South African Journal of Zoology* 29(1), 74–81.

Bandilla, M., Hakalahti, T., Hudson, P.J. and Valtonen, E.T. (2004) Aggregation of *Argulus coregoni* (Crustacea: Branchiura) on rainbow trout (*Oncorhynchus mykiss*): a consequence of host susceptibility or exposure? *Parasitology* 130, 169–176.

Bandilla, M., Valtonen, E.T., Suomalainen, L.-R., Aphalo, P.J. and Hakalahti, T. (2006) A link between ectoparasite infection and susceptibility to bacterial disease in rainbow trout. *International Journal for Parasitology* 36, 987–991.

Bandilla, M., Hakalahti-Sirén, T. and Valtonen, E.T. (2007) Experimental evidence for a hierarchy of mate- and host-induced cues in a fish ectoparasite, *Argulus coregoni* (Crustacea, Branchiura). *International Journal for Parasitology* 37, 1343–1349.

Bandilla, M., Hakalahti-Sirén, T. and Valtonen, E.T. (2008) Patterns of host switching in the fish ectoparasite *Argulus coregoni*. *Behavioral Ecology and Sociobiology* 62, 975–982.

Banerjee, A., Manna, S. and Saha, S.H. (2014) Effect of aqueous extract of *Azadirachta indica* A. Juss (neem) leaf on oocyte maturation, oviposition, reproductive potentials and embryonic development of a freshwater fish ectoparasite *Argulus bengalensis* Ramakrishna, 1951 (Crustacea: Branchiura). *Parasitology Research* 113, 4641–4650. DOI: 10.1007/s00436-014-4155-7.

Barber, I., Hoare, D. and Krause, J. (2000) Effects of parasites on fish behaviour: a review and evolutionary perspective. *Reviews in Fish Biology and Fisheries* 10, 131–165.

Bonfirm, V.C.d., Manoel, L.d.O., Parra, A.B., Ramos, I.P. and Franceshini, L. (1925) Host–parasite relationships between *Dolops* spp. (Crustacea: Branchiura) and freshwater fish from the Neotropical Region. *Acta Parasitologica* 70, 76–85. DOI 10.1007/s11686-025-01008-z.

Boopathi, S., Kevavan, D., Sudhakaran, G. Priya, P.S., Haridevamuthu, B. *et al.* (2024) Exploring the efficacy of pellitorine as an antiparasitic agent against *Argulus*: impacts on antioxidant level and immune responses in goldfish (*Carassius auratus*). *Acta Parasitologica* 69, 734–746. DOI: 10.1007/s11686-024-00792-4.

Boxshall, G.A. (2005) Crustacean parasites: Branchiura. In: Rohde, K. (ed.) *Marine Parasitology*. CSIRO Publishing, Melbourne, Australia, pp. 145–147.

Brahmchari, R.K., Kumari, P., Kumar, S., Sharma, R., Prasad, K.P. *et al.* (2023) Antiparasitic effect of biogenic iron nanoparticle against the fish ectoparasite *Argulus siamensis*: *in vitro* study. *Indian Journal of Fisheries* 70(3), 107–115. DOI: 10.21077/ijf.2023.70.3.132524-14.

Buchmann, K. and Bresciani, J. (1997) Parasitic infection in pond-reared rainbow trout *Oncorhynchus mykiss* in Denmark. *Diseases of Aquatic Organisms* 28, 125–138.

Catalano, S.R. and Hutson, K.S. (2010) Harmful parasitic crustaceans infecting wild arripids: a potential threat to southern Australian finfish aquaculture. *Aquaculture* 303, 101–104.

Chen, T. (1933) A study on the methods of prevention and treatment of fish lice in pond culture. *Lignan Science Journal* 12, 241–244.

Clark, F.N. (1902) *Argulus foliaceus*. A contribution to the life history. *Proceedings of the South London Entomological and Natural History Society*, 12–21.

Cressey, R.F. (1972) *The Genus Argulus (Crustacea: Branchiura) of the United States*. Biota of Freshwater Ecosystems Identification Manual, No. 2. Project # 18050 ELD. Environmental Protection Agency, Washington, DC, pp. 1–14.

Dugatkin, L.A., FitzGerald, G.J. and Lavoie, J. (1994) Juvenile three-spined sticklebacks avoid parasitized conspecifics. *Environmental Biology of Fishes* 39, 215–218.

Evans, D.W. and Matthews, M.A. (2000) First record of *Argulus foliaceus* on the European eel in the British Isles. *Journal of Fish Biology* 57, 529–530.

Everts, L.A.M. and Avenant-Oldewage, A. (2009) First record of *Argulus coregoni* a fish ectoparasitic crustacean from Malaysia and additional notes on the morphology. *Malaysian Applied Biology* 38(2), 61–71.

Fenton, A. and Hudson, P.J. (2002) Optimal infection strategies: should macroparasites hedge their bets? *Oikos* 96, 92–101.

Fryer, G. (1956) A report on the parasitic Copepoda and Branchiura of the fishes of Lake Nyasa. *Proceedings of the Zoological Society of London* 127, 293–344. DOI: 10.1111/j.1096-3642.1956.tb00473.x.

Fryer, G. (1960) The spermatophores of *Dolops ranarum* (Crustacea: Branchiura): their structure, formation, and transfer. *Quarterly Journal of Microscopical Science* 101, 407–432.

Fryer, G. (1964) Further studies in the parasitic Crustacea of African freshwater fishes. *Proceedings of the Zoological Society of London* 143, 79–102.

Gaboardi, L.M., Reeves, L.E., Morey, G.A.M., Stanton, D.L. and Carney, R.M. (2023) A new species of the fish louse genus *Dipteropeltis* Calman, 1912 (Crustacea: Branchiura) from Peru. *Zootaxa* 5315(2), 101–121. DOI: 10.11646/zootaxa.5315.2.1.

Gault, N.F.S., Kilpatrick, D.J. and Stewart, M.T. (2002) Biological control of the fish louse in a rainbow trout fishery. *Journal of Fish Biology* 60, 226–237.

Gilbert, B.M. and Avenant-Oldewage, A. (2018) Trace element biomineralisation in the carapace in male and female *Argulus japonicus*. *PLoS One* 13(6), e0197804. DOI: 10.1371/journal.pone.0197804.

Gilbert, B.M., Nachev, M., Sures, B. and Avenant-Oldewage, A. (2025) Dietary shifts among the developmental stages of the ectoparasite, *Argulus japonicus* (Crustacea; Branchiura), mirror ontogeny as shown through differences in stable isotope ratios of carbon (δ^{13}C) and nitrogen (δ^{15}N). *Ecology and Evolution* 15, e70652. DOI: 10.1002/ece3.70652.

Gonzales, A.F., Babilonia, J., Paredes, M., Delgado, P.M., Oliveira, M.S.B. and Fernández-Méndez, C. (2024) The first record of *Dolops carvalhoi* (Crustacea: Branchiura) parasitizing three farmed fish species of the Peruvian Amazon. *Aquaculture International* 32, 7997–8007. DOI: 10.1007/s10499-024-01551-y.

Gresty, K.A., Boxshall, G.A. and Nagasawa, K. (1993) The fine structure and function of the cephalic appendages of the branchiuran parasite, *Argulus japonicus* Thiele. *Philosophical Transactions of the Royal Society of London* 339, 119–135.

Grobben, K. (1908) Beitrage zur Kenntnis des Baues und der systematischen Stellung der Arguliden. *Sitzungsberichte der kaiserlichen Akademie der Wissenschaften in Wien* 117, 191–233.

Guha, A., Aditya, G. and Samar Saha, K. (2013) Survivorship and fecundity of *Argulus bengalensis* (Crustacea; Branchiura) under laboratory conditions. *Invertebrate Reproduction & Development* 57, 301–308. DOI:10.1080/07924259.2013.793217.

Haase, W. (1975) Ultrastruktur und Funktion der Carapaxfelder von *Argulus foliaceus* (L.) (Crustacea, Branchiura). *Zeitschrift für Morphologie der Tiere* 81, 161–189.

Hakalahti, T. and Valtonen, E.T. (2003) Population structure and recruitment of the ectoparasite *Argulus coregoni* Thorell (Crustacea: Branchiura) on a fish farm. *Parasitology* 127, 79–85.

Hakalahti, T., Pasternak, A.F. and Valtonen, E.T. (2003) Seasonal dynamics of egg laying and egg-laying strategy of the ectoparasite *Argulus coregoni* (Crustacea: Branchiura). *Parasitology* 128, 655–660.

Hakalahti, T., Lankinen, Y. and Valtonen, E.T. (2004) Efficacy of emamectin benzoate in the control of *Argulus coregoni* (Crustacea: Branchiura) on rainbow trout *Oncorhynchus mykiss*. *Diseases of Aquatic Organisms* 60, 197–204.

Hakalahti, T., Bandilla, M. and Valtonen, E.T. (2005) Delayed transmission of a parasite is compensated by accelerated growth. *Parasitology* 131, 647–656.

Hakalahti-Sirén, T., Mikheev, V.N. and Valtonen, T.E. (2008) Control of freshwater fish louse *Argulus coregoni*: a step towards an integrated management strategy. *Diseases of Aquatic Organisms* 82, 67–77. DOI: 10.3354/dao01971.

Harrison, A.J., Gault, N.F.S. and Dick, J.T.A. (2006) Seasonal and vertical patterns of egg-laying by the freshwater fish louse *Argulus foliaceus* (Crustacea: Branchiura). *Diseases of Aquatic Organisms* 68, 167–173.

Hindle, E. (1949) Notes on the treatment of fish infected with *Argulus*. *Proceedings of the Zoological Society of London* 119, 79–81.

Ikuta, K. and Makioka, T. (1997) Structure of the adult ovary and oogenesis in *Argulus japonicus* Thiele (Crustacea: Branchiura). *Journal of Morphology* 231, 29–39.

Jahan, F., Rahman, H., Ahammad, B., Mohammed, K., Rahman, Z. *et al.* (2025) *Argulus japonicus*: a concerning health issue for *Channa punctata* in southwestern Bangladesh. *Veterinary Medicine and Science* 11, e70250. DOI: 1002/vms3.70250.

Kabata, Z. (1985) Branchiura. In: *Parasites and Diseases of Fish Cultured in the Tropics*. Taylor and Francis, London, pp. 255–265.

Kaji, T., Møller, O.S. and Tsukagoshi, A. (2011) A bridge between original and novel states: ontogeny and function of 'suction discs' in the Branchiura (Crustacea). *Evolution & Development* 13, 119–126.

Kollatsch, D. (1959) Untersuchungen uber die Biologie und Okologie der Karpfenlaus (*Argulus foliaceus* L.). *Zoologische Beitrage* 5, 1–36.

Kruger, I., van As, J.G. and Saayman, J.E. (1983) Observations on the occurrence of the fish louse *Argulus japonicus* Thiele, 1900 in the western Transvaal. *South African Journal of Zoology* 18, 408–410.

Kumar, A., Raman, R.P., Kumar, K., Pandey, P.K. and Kumar, S. (2012) Antiparasitic efficacy of piperine against *Argulus* spp. on *Carassius auratus* (Linn. 1758): *in vitro* and *in vivo* study. *Parasitology Research* 111, 2071–2076. DOI: 10.1007/s00436-012-3054-z.

Leydig, F. (1889) Ueber *Argulus foliaceus*. Neue Mittheilung. *Archiv für mikroskopische Anatomie* 33, 1–51.

Lutch, E. and Avenant-Oldewage, A. (1995) The ultrastructure of the newly hatched *Argulus japonicus* Thiele, 1900 larvae (Branchiura). *Crustaceana* 68, 329–340.

Lynn, T.J., Jeong, J.-W. and Duffy, M.S. (2020) Bet hedging and cold-temperature termination of diapause in the life history of the Atlantic salmon ectoparasite *Argulus canadensis*. *Parasitology* 147, 1774–1785. DOI: 10.1017/S0031182020001766.

Malta, J.C.O. and Varella, A.M.B. (2009) Branchiura. In: Fonseca, C.R.V., Magalhães, C.U., Rafael, J.A. and Franklin, E. (eds) *A fauna de Artrópodes da reserva florestal Ducke*. INPA, Manaus, Brasil, pp. 17–20 (in Portuguese).

Marshall, W.S., Cozzi, R.R.F. and Strapps, C. (2008) Fish louse *Argulus funduli* (Crustacea: Branchiura) ectoparasites of the euryhaline teleost host, *Fundulus heteroclitus*, damage the ion-transport capacity of the opercular epithelium. *Canadian Journal of Zoology* 86, 1252–1258.

Martin, M.F. (1932) On the morphology and classification of *Argulus* (Crustacea). *Proceedings of the Zoological Society of London* 102, 771–806.

Meehan, O.L. (1940) A review of the parasitic Crustacea of the genus *Argulus* in the collections of the United States National Museum. *Proceedings of the United States National Museum* 88, 459–522.

Menezes, J., Ramos, M.A., Pereira, T.G. and da Silva, A.M. (1990) Rainbow trout culture failure in a small lake as a result of massive parasitosis related to careless fish introduction. *Aquaculture* 89, 123–126.

Meyer-Rochov, V.B., Au, D. and Keskinen, E. (2001) Photoreception in fishlice (Branchiura); the eyes of *Argulus foliaceus* Linne, 1758 and *A. coregoni* Thorell, 1865. *Acta Parasitologia* 46(4), 321–331.

Mikheev, V.N., Valtonen, E.T. and Rintamaki-Kinnunen, P. (1998) Host searching in *Argulus foliaceus* (L.) (Crustacea: Branchiura): the role of vision and selectivity. *Parasitology* 116, 425–430.

Mikheev, V.N., Mikheev, A.V., Pasternak, A.F. and Valtonen, E.T. (2000) Light-mediated host searching strategies in a fish ectoparasite, *Argulus foliaceus* L. (Crustacea: Branchiura). *Parasitology* 120, 409–416.

Mikheev, V.N., Pasternak, A.F., Valtonen, E.T. and Lankinen, Y. (2001) Spatial distribution and hatching of overwintered eggs of a fish ectoparasite, *Argulus coregoni* (Crustacea: Branchiura). *Diseases of Aquatic Organisms* 46, 123–128.

Mikheev, V.N., Pasternak, A.F. and Valtonen, E.T. (2007) Host specificity of *Argulus coregoni* (Crustacea: Branchiura) increases at maturation. *Parasitology* 134, 1767–1774.

Mikheev, V.N., Pasternak, A. and Valtonen, E.T. (2015) Behavioural adaptations of argulid parasites (Crustacea: Branchiura) to major challenges in their life cycle. *Parasites and Vectors* 8, 394. DOI: 10.1186/s13071-015-1005-0.

Møller, O.S. and Olesen, J. (2012) First description of larval stage 1 from a non-African fish parasite *Dolops* (Branchiura). *Journal of Crustacean Biology* 32(2), 231–238.

Møller, O.S., Olesen, J. and Waloszek, D. (2007) Swimming and cleaning in the free-swimming phase of *Argulus* larvae (Crustacea, Branchiura) – appendage adaptation and functional morphology. *Journal of Morphology* 268, 1–11.

Møller, O.S., Olesen, J., Avenant-Oldewage, A., Thomsen and Glenner, P.F. (2008) First maxillae suction discs in Branchiura (Crustacea): development and evolution in light of the first molecular phylogeny of Branchiura, Pentastomida, and other 'Maxillopoda'. *Arthropod Structure and Development* 37, 333–346. DOI: 10.1016/j.asd.2007.12.002.

Molnár, K. and Moravec, F. (1997) *Skrjabillanus cyprinid* n. sp. (Nematioda: Racunculoidea) from the scales of common carp *Cyprinus carpio* (Pisces) from Hungary. *Systematic Parasitology* 38, 147–151.

Molnár, K. and Szekely, C.S. (1998) Occurrence of skrjabillinid nematodes in fishes in Hungary and in the intermediate hosts, *Argulus foliaceus* L. *Acta Veterinaria Hungarica* 46, 451–463.

Monod, T. (1928) Les Argulides du Musee du Congo. *Revue de Zoologie et de Botanique Africaines* 16, 242–274.

Moravec, F. (1978) First record of *Molnaria erythrophthalmi* larvae in the intermediate host in Czechoslovakia. *Folia Parasitologica* 25, 141–142.

Moravec, F., Vidal-Martínez, V. and Aguirre-Macedo, L. (1999) Branchiurids (*Argulus*) as intermediate hosts of the daniconematid nematode *Mexiconema cichlasomae*. *Folia Parasitologica* 46, 79.

Mugnai, R., Santos-Reis, M.R. and Avenant-Oldewage, A. (2022) Additional information on *Dolops intermedia* Silva, 1978 (Crustacea: Argulidae) and its occurrence on fishes in northeastern Brazil. *Comparative Parasitology* 89(1), 1–8. DOI: 10.1654/1525-2647-89.1.1.

Nagasawa, K. (2017) *Argulus japonicus* (Branchiura: Argulidae) parasitic on a freshwater minnow, *Opsariichthys platypus* (Cyprinidae): the second record from Shikoku, western Japan. *Biogeography* 19, 50–52.

Nagasawa, K. (2019) Survival of *Argulus japonicus* (Branchiura: Argulidae) on a cyprinid in drought-induced brackish waters in a Japanese lake. *Crustacean Research* 48, 99–103.

Nagasawa, K. (2021) *Argulus japonicus* (Branchiura: Argulidae) parasitic on largemouth bass *Micropterus salmoides* in Japan, with the morphology of the adult female of the argulid. *Crustacean Research* 50, 119–129.

Nagasawa, K. and Nishimura, H. (2025) Infection of cypriniform fishes with *Argulus coregoni* (Crustacea: Branchiura: Argulidae) in a low-elevation stream, central Japan. *Species Diversity* 30, 1–9. DOI: 10.12782/specdiv.30.1.

Nagasawa, K., Nitta, M. and Azuma, N. (2024) New records of a freshwater fish parasite *Argulus japonicus* (Branchiura: Argulidae) from northern Honshu, Japan, with a note on its occurrence in a brackish water lake. *Crustacean Research* 53, 1–8. DOI: 10.18353/crustacea.53.0_1.

Neethling, L.A.M. and Avenant-Oldewage A. (2015) *Chonopeltis australis* (Crustacea) male reproductive system morphology; sperm transfer and review of reproduction in Branchiura. *Journal of Morphology* 276, 209–218. DOI: 10.1002/jmor.20334.

Neethling, L.A.M. and Avenant-Oldewage, A. (2016) Branchiura – a compendium of the geographical distribution and a summary of their biology. *Crustaceana* 89, 1243–1446.

Neethling, LA.M. and Avenant-Oldewage, A. (2020) Host selection and notes on the distribution of *Chonopeltis australis* Boxshall, 1976 in southern Africa. *African Journal of Aquatic Science* 45, 500–508. DOI: 10.2989/16085914.2020.1757401.

Neethling, L.A.M., Malta, J.C.O. and Avenant-Oldewage, A. (2014) Additional morphological information on *Dipteropeltis hirundo* Calman, 1912, and a description of *Dipteropeltis campanaformis* n. sp. (Crustacea: Branchiura) from two characiform benthopelagic fish hosts from two Northern rivers of the Brazilian Amazon. *Zootaxa* 3755, 179–193. DOI: 10.11646/zootaxa.3755.2.4.

Niesink, R.J.M., de Vries, J. and Hollinger, M.A. (1996) *Toxicology: Principles and Applications*. CRC Press, Boca Raton, Florida.

Northcott, S.J., Lyndon, A.R. and Campbell, A.D. (1997) An outbreak of freshwater fish lice, *Argulus foliaceus* (L.), seriously affecting a Scottish stillwater fishery. *Fisheries Management and Ecology* 4, 73–75.

Oliveira, E.C., Pereira, E.C., Cajado R.A., da Silva L.V.F. and Corrêa L.L. (2021) Description of the life cycle of *Dolops discoidalis* (Bouvier, 1899) (Branchiura: Argulidae), a parasite of the fish species *Rhytiodus argenteofuscus* (Kner, 1858) from the Brazilian Amazon. *Annals of Parasitology* 67, 473–482. DOI: 10.17420/ap6703.360.

Paperna, I. (1991) Diseases caused by parasites in the aquaculture of warm water fish. *Annual Review of Fish Diseases* 1991, 155–194.

Paperna, I. (1996) Parasitic crustacea. In: *Parasites, Infections and Diseases of Fishes in Africa. An Update*. CIFA Technical Paper No. 31. Food and Agriculture Organization of the United Nations, Rome, pp. 179–204.

Pasternak, A.F., Mikheev, V.N. and Valtonen, E.T. (2004a) Growth and development of *Argulus coregoni* (Crustacea: Branchiura) on salmonid and cyprinid hosts. *Diseases of Aquatic Organisms* 58, 203–207.

Pasternak, A., Mikheev, V.N., Mikheev, E. and Valtonen, E.T. (2004b) Adaptive significance of the sexual size dimorphism in a fish ectoparasite *Argulus coregoni* (Crustacea: Branchiura). *Doklady Biological Sciences* 399, 477– 480. DOI: 10.1007/s10630-005-0017-x.

Pfeil-Putzien, C. (1977) New results in the diagnosis of spring viremia of carp caused by experimental transmission of *Rhabdovirus carpio* with carp louse (*Argulus foliaceus*). *Bulletin de l'Office International des Epizooties* 87, 457.

Pfeil-Putzien, and Baath, C.H. (1978) Isolation of the *Rhabdovirus carpio* from carp and carp lice (*Argulus foliaceus*). *Berliner und Münchener Tierätztliche Wochenschrift* 91, 445–447.

Piasecki, W. and Avenant-Oldewage, A. (2008) Diseases caused by crustacea. In: Eiras, J.C., Segner, H., Wahli, T. and Kapoor, B.G. (eds) *Fish Diseases*. Science Publishers, Enfield, New Hampshire, pp. 1115–1200.

Poulin, R. (1999) Parasitism and shoal size in juvenile sticklebacks: conflicting selection pressures from different ectoparasites? *Ethology* 105, 959–968.

Poulin, R. and Fitzgerald, G. (1988) Male-biased sex ratio in *Argulus canadensis* Wilson, 1916 (Crustacea: Branchiura) ectoparasitic on sticklebacks. *Canadian Journal of Zoology* 67, 2078–2080.

Poulin, R. and FitzGerald, G.J. (1989) A possible explanation for the aggregated distribution of *Argulus canadensis* Wilson, 1916 (Crustacea: Branchiura) on juvenile sticklebacks (Gasterosteidae). *Journal of Parasitology* 75, 58–60.

Ranzani-Paiva, M.J., Ishikawa, C.M., Portella, M.C. and Celiberto, R.J. (1987) Hematologia da carpa comum I, infestada por *Argulus* sp. e após um tratamento com fosfato de 0,0-dimetil-oxi-2,2,2,-tricloroetilo (Neguvon) [Hematology of carp, *Cyprinus carpio*, infested by *Argulus* sp and after treatment with 0,0-dimethyl-oxy-2 phosphonate, 2,2,2,-trichloroethyl (Neguvon)]. *Bulletin of the Fisheries Institute, Sao Paulo* 14, 83–92 (in Portuguese).

Ruane, N.M., McCarthy, T.K. and Reilly, P. (1995) Antibody response to crustacean ectoparasites in rainbow trout, *Oncorhynchus mykiss* (Walbaum), immunized with *Argulus foliaceus* L. antigen extract. *Journal of Fish Diseases* 18, 529–537.

Rushton-Mellor, S.K. (1992) Discovery of the fish louse, *Argulus japonicus* Thiele (Crustacea: Branchiura), in Britain. *Aquaculture and Fisheries Management* 23, 269–271.

Rushton-Mellor, S.K. (1994) The genus *Argulus* (Crustacea: Branchiura) in Africa: identification keys. *Systematic Parasitology* 28, 51–63.

Rushton-Mellor, S.K. and Boxshall, G.A. (1994) The developmental sequence of *Argulus foliaceus* (Crustacea: Branchiura). *Journal of Natural History* 28, 763–785.

Schlüter, U. (1978) Observations about host attacking by the common fish louse *Argulus foliaceus* L. (Crustacea, Branchiura). *Zoologischer Anzeiger* 200, 85–91.

Schram, T.A., Iversen, L., Heuch, P.A. and Sterud, E. (2005) *Argulus* sp. (Crustacea: Branchiura) on cod, *Gadus morhua* from Finmark, northern Norway. *Journal of the Marine Biological Association of the United Kingdom* 85, 81–86.

Shafir, A. and Oldewage, W.H. (1992) Dynamics of fish ectoparasite populations: opportunistic parasitism in *Argulus japonicus* (Crustacea: Branchiura). *Crustaceana* 62, 50–64.

Shafir, A. and Van As, J.G. (1986) Laying, development and hatching of eggs of the fish ectoparasite *Argulus japonicus* (Crustacea: Branchiura). *Journal of Zoology* 210, 401–414.

Shimura, S. (1981) The larval development of *Argulus coregoni* Thorell (Crustacea: Branchiura). *Journal of Natural History* 15, 331–348. DOI: 10.1080/00222938100770251.

Shimura, S. (1983) SEM observations on the mouth tube and preoral sting of *Argulus coregoni* Thorell and *Argulus japonicus* Thiele (Crustacea: Branchiura). *Fish Pathology* 18, 151–156.

Shimura, S. and Inoue, K. (1984) Toxic effects of extract from the mouth-parts of *Argulus coregoni* Thorell (Crustacea: Branchiura). *Bulletin of the Japanese Society of Scientific Fisheries* 50, 729.

Silva-Souza, A.T., Abdallah, V.D., de Azevedo, R.K., da Silva, F.A. and Luque, J.L. (2011) Expanded description of *Dolops bidentata* (Bouvier, 1899) (Branchiura: Argulidae) based on specimens collected on *Pygocentrus nattereri* Kner, 1858 (Characiformes) from Poconé Wetland, MT, Brazil. *Brazilian Journal of Biology* 71, 145–149.

Singhal, R.N., Reet, S. and Davies, E.W. (1990) The effects of argulosis–saprolegniases on the growth and production of *Cyprinus carpio*. *Hydrobiologia* 202, 27–31.

Swanepoel, J.H. and Avenant-Oldewage, A. (1992) Comments on the morphology of the pre-oral spine in *Argulus* (Crustacea: Branchiura). *Journal of Morphology* 212, 155–162.

Tam, Q. and Avenant-Oldewage, A. (2006) The digestive system of larval *Argulus japonicus* (Branchiura). *Journal of Crustacean Biology* 26, 447–454.

Tam, Q. and Avenant-Oldewage, A. (2009a) The ultrastructure of the digestive cells of *Argulus japonicus*, Thiele 1900 (Crustacea: Branchiura). *Arthropod Structure & Development* 38, 45–53. DOI: 10.1016/j.asd.2008.07.003.

Tam, Q. and Avenant-Oldewage, A. (2009b) The effect of starvation on the ultrastructure of the digestive cells of *Dolops ranarum* (Stuhlmann, 1891) (Crustacea: Branchiura). *Arthropod Structure & Development* 38, 391–399. DOI: 10.1016/j.asd.2009.03.002.

Tam, Q., Avenant-Oldewage, A. and Williams, E.H. (2005) An ultrastructural investigation of *Argulus personatus* Cunnington, 1913 (Crustacea: Branchiura) from Lake Tanganyika, northern Zambia. *African Zoology* 40(2), 301–308.

Tavares-Dias, M., Martins, M.L. and Kronka, S.N. (1999) Evaluation of the haematological parameters in *Piaractus mesopotamicus* Holmberg (Osteichthyes, Characidae) with *Argulus* sp. (Crustacea, Branchiura) infestation and treatment with organophosphate. *Revista Brasileira de Zoologia* 16, 553–555. DOI:10.1590/S0101-81751999000200019.

Tavares-Dias M., Moraes, F.R., Onaka, E.M. and Rezende, C.B. (2007) Changes in blood parameter of hybrid tambacu fish parasitized by *Dolops carvalhoi* (Crustacea, Branchiura), a fish louse. *Veterinarski Archiv* 77, 353–363.

Taylor, N.G.H. (2004) The epidemiology and population ecology of *Argulus* spp. infections in UK stillwater trout fisheries. PhD thesis, University of Stirling, Stirling, UK.

Taylor, N.G.H., Sommerville, C. and Wootten R. (2006) The epidemiology of *Argulus* spp. (Crustacea: Branchiura) infections in stillwater trout fisheries. *Journal of Fish Diseases* 29, 193–200.

Taylor, N.G.H., Wootten, R. and Sommerville, C. (2009) The influence of risk factors on the abundance, egg laying habits and impact of *Argulus foliaceus* in stillwater trout fisheries. *Journal of Fish Diseases* 32, 509–519.

Thatcher, V.E. (1991) Amazon fish parasites. *Amazoniana* 11, 263–572.

Thiele, J. (1904) Beiträge zur Morphologie der Arguliden. *Mitteilungen aus dem Zoologischen Museum für Naturkunde Berlin* 2(4), 5–51 (in German).

Tikhomirova, V.A. (1983) On nematodes of the family Skrjabillanidae (Nematoda: Camellanata). *Parazitologiia* 14, 258–262 (in Russian with English summary).

Tokioka, T. (1936) Larval development and metamorphosis of *Argulus japonicus*. *Memoirs of the College of Science, Kyoto Imperial University, Series B* 12, 93–114.

Van As, L.L. and Van As, J.G. (1999) Aspects of the morphology and a review of the taxonomic status of three species of the genus *Chonopeltis* (Crustacea: Branchiura) from the Orange-Vaal and South West Cape River Systems, South Africa. *Folia Parasitologica* 46, 221–228.

Van As, L., Smit, N. and Van As, J.G. (2017) Rediscovery of *Chonopeltis meridionalis* Fryer, 1964 (Crustacea: Branchiura) from *Labeo rosae* Steindachner in the River Olifants, Mpumalanga, and the taxonomic status of *C. victori* Avenant-Oldewage, 1991 and *C. koki* Van As, 1992. *Systematic Parasitology* 94, 797–807. DOI: 10.1007/s11230-017-9737-1.

Van Niekerk, J.P. (1984) Die biologie van die genus *Chonopeltis* Thiele, 1900 (Crustacea: Branchiura) uit die Oranje-Vaal opvanggebied [The biology of the genus *Chonopeltis* Thiele, 1900 (Crustacea: Branchiura) from the Orange-Vaal catchment area]. PhD thesis, University of the Orange Free State, Bloemfontein, South Africa (in Afrikaans).

Van Niekerk, J.P. and Kok, D.J. (1989) *Chonopeltis australis* (Branchiura): structural, developmental and functional aspects of the trophic appendages. *Crustaceana* 57, 51–56.

Walker, P.D., Flik, G. and Bonga, S.E.W. (2004) The biology of parasites from the genus *Argulus* and a review of the interactions with its host. In: Wiegertjes, G.F. and Flik, G. (eds) *Host–Parasite Interactions*. Garland Science/BIOS Scientific Publishers (Taylor and Francis), Abingdon, UK, pp. 107–129.

Walker, P.D., Russon, I.J., Haond, C., Van Der Velde, G., Sjoerd, E. and Wendelaar-Bonga, S.E. (2011) Feeding in adult *Argulus japonicus* Thiele, 1900 (Maxillopoda, Branchiura), an ectoparasite on fish. *Crustaceana* 84(3), 307–318. DOI: 10.1163/001121610X551881.

Wilson, C.B. (1902) North American parasitic copepods of the family Argulidae, with a bibliography of the group and a systematic review of all known species. *Proceedings of the United States National Museum* 25, 635–742.

Wingstrand, K.G. (1972) Comparative spermatology of a pentastomid, *Raillietiella hemidactyli*, and a branchiuran crustacean, *Argulus foliaceus*, with a discussion of pentastomid relationships. *Det Kongelige Danske Videnskabernes Selskab, Biologiske Skrifter* 19, 1–72.

Wolfe, B.A., Harms, C.A., Groves, J.D. and Loomis, M.R. (2001) Treatment of *Argulus* sp. infestations of river frogs. *Contemporary Topics in Laboratory Animal Science* 40, 35–36.

WoRMS Editorial Board (2025) World Register of Marine Species. Available at: https://www.marinespecies.org at VLIZ (accessed 2 July 2025). DOI: 10.14284/170.

Yamaguti, S. (1963) *Parasitic Copepoda and Branchiura of Fishes*. Interscience Publishers, New York.

Yildiz, K. and Kumantas, A. (2002) *Argulus foliaceus* infection in a goldfish (*Carassius auratus*). *Israel Journal of Veterinary Medicine* 57, 118–120.

Yoshizawa, K.S. and Nogami, S. (2008) The first report of phototaxis of fish ectoparasite *Argulus japonicus*. *Research on Veterinary Science* 85, 128–130.

21 *Caligus rogercresseyi*, the Sea Louse Affecting Farmed Salmonids in the Southern Hemisphere

Margarita P. González-Gómez[1]* and Sandra L. Marín[2]
[1]*Escuela de Medicina Veterinaria, Facultad de Medicina Veterinaria, Universidad San Sebastián, Puerto Montt, Chile;* [2]*Instituto de Acuicultura y Medio Ambiente, Universidad Austral de Chile, Puerto Montt, Chile*

Abstract

This chapter explores relevant features related to the parasite *Caligus rogercresseyi*, currently the most important pathogen affecting the salmon industry of Chile, being a permanent threat. Its geographic distribution ranges from southern Chile to Argentina, being present in salmonid and native fishes of both countries. In Chile, it is also common on *Eleginops maclovinus*, which is a native fish that interacts closely with the salmon in farms, perpetuating infestations. Physical damage on fish produced by the parasite is characterized by skin injuries, loss of the integrity of the skin, peeling and petechial haemorrhage, among other injuries. This chapter updates the knowledge about this parasitosis, addressing the life cycle, transmission and distribution, parasite diagnosis, pharmacological and non-pharmacological tools and economic impact.

21.1. Life Cycle and Morphological Traits

Caligus rogercresseyi belongs to the phylum Arthropoda, class Copepoda, order Siphonostomatoida and family Caligidae. It affects native fishes in both marine and estuarine waters.

The life cycle of this parasite includes eight stages: two nauplii; an infestive stage called a copepodid; four attached parasitic stages called chalimus I, II, III and IV, respectively; and the adult stage (male or female) (González and Carvajal, 2003) (Fig. 21.1).

Adults present a flattened body adapted for attachment and possess antennules and maxillipeds modified for host adhesion. They are transparent to greyish in coloration, making detection challenging. Females (5–8 mm), with paired egg sacs, are larger than males (3–5 mm).

According to González and Carvajal (2003), the planktonic nauplius I is about 425 μm long and nauplius II measures about 463 μm. The copepodid is about 658 μm in length. The parasitic stage begins with chalimus I up to chalimus IV, ending in the adult females and males (Fig. 21.1). Chalimus stages are characterized by having a flat cephalothorax with rounded posterior margins and a frontal filament with a rounded base, in which a new lobe is added after each moult.

Fecundation occurs inside the genital segment of females where spermatozoa transferred by the male are kept in the spermatheca. Eggs

*Email: margarita.gonzalez@uss.cl

 Fish Parasites: Pathobiology and Protection, 2nd Edition (eds P.T.K. Woo and K. Buchmann)
DOI: 10.1079/9781800628748.0021

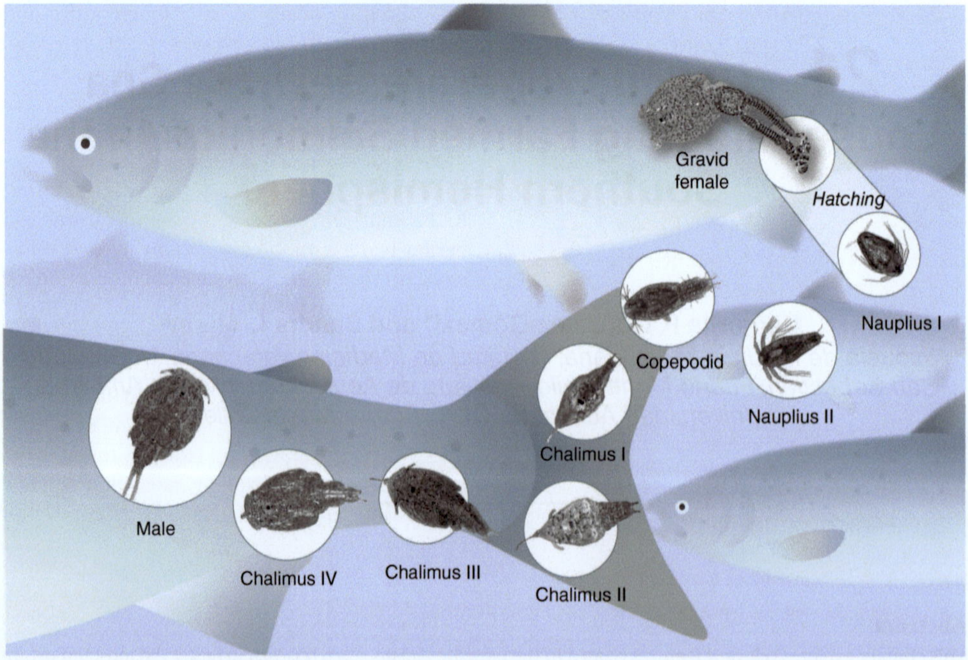

Fig. 21.1. Life cycle of the ectoparasite *Caligus rogercresseyi*. (From Marín and Fast, 2021.)

are extruded into two strings where development takes place until the hatching of nauplius I (Schram, 2000). A female may develop up to 11 pairs of egg strings during its life (Bravo, 2010). Reproduction occurs throughout the year. Reports of average fecundity among females collected from farmed salmon vary between 85 (González, 2006), 35 (Bravo, 2010), 45 (Bravo *et al.*, 2009) and 19 to 80 eggs per string on Atlantic salmon (*Salmo salar*), and 19 to 95 eggs per string on rainbow trout (*Oncorhynchus mykiss*) (González *et al.*, 2012). Meanwhile, fecundity in the native fish, the Patagonian blenny *Eleginops maclovinus* (Valenciennes), varies between 12 and 56 eggs per string (González *et al.*, 2012). Fecundity of *C. rogercresseyi* varies from season to season (Bravo *et al.*, 2009). However, the fecundity of females from farmed salmon and native fish has been positively correlated with female size, and differences in fecundity are explained by differences in the body size of the females collected in different months of the year (González *et al.*, 2012).

The naupliar stages (free-living) do not feed, instead using the yolk sac reserves in the larvae (González and Carvajal, 2003). The free-living infestive stage (copepodid) can survive for a maximum of 12 days by using its energy reserves (Bravo *et al.*, 2008b). Within this period of time, copepodids must attach to a host to ensure their survival. Pino-Marambio *et al.* (2007) suggested that male adults of *C. rogercresseyi* are able to respond to chemical cues released from the host. Once the settlement site has been selected, the extrusion of the frontal filament occurs through three different phases, described as early, advanced (Piasecki and MacKinnon, 1993) and extruded (Farias, 2005; González, 2006). The filament adheres to the host surface, allowing the development of the attached stages of the parasite. The last attached stage, chalimus IV, moults into the adult stage (González and Carvajal, 2003).

Research into settlement under controlled conditions indicates that more than 77.6% of attachments were on the pectoral, dorsal and caudal fins when fish were exposed to infestation pressure of 50, 100 and 150 copepodids per fish (Araya *et al.*, 2012). However, the ventral surface and the post-anal area were also reported as zones of high concentrations of parasite attachment under experimental conditions and on farms (Treasurer and Bravo, 2011).

21.2. Environmental Drivers of the Life Cycle

Factors, such as temperature and salinity, affect life-history traits and population parameters. The life cycle of *C. rogercresseyi* is temperature dependent, where higher temperatures accelerate the development rate of the parasite, resulting in shorter generation times than those for parasites living at lower temperatures (González and Carvajal, 2003; Marín *et al.*, 2009). The minimum development temperature threshold is 4.2°C (González and Carvajal, 2003). Salinity affects survival during the larval and adult stages (González and Carvajal, 2003; Bravo *et al.*, 2008a, 2009). Field data indicate that temperature and salinity are important factors in explaining variations in the abundance of the parasite (Zagmutt-Vergara *et al.*, 2005; Kristoffersen *et al.*, 2013; Arriagada *et al.*, 2017).

Water temperature, water salinity and current velocity of waters are the most important variables that limit the geographical distribution of *C. rogercresseyi* (Lepe-López *et al.*, 2021). The combination of salinity and temperature affects the hatching and survival time of *C. rogercresseyi* (Montory *et al.*, 2018), with a salinity tolerance threshold of 20 ppt and lower salinities negatively affecting the parasite (Bravo *et al.*, 2008a). In addition, previous studies have indicated that the combination of temperature and carbon dioxide pressure (pCO_2) affects the physiological and developmental rates of the parasite, with lower temperatures increasing both the copepodid survival rate and the nauplius II development time (Montory *et al.*, 2020); information that agrees with evidence from the sea louse, *Lepeophtheirus salmonis*, which has mechanisms like energy reserves to compensate the increase in pCO_2 and populations that will be tolerant in projected future ocean acidification scenarios (Thompson *et al.*, 2019). Regarding oxygen conditions, *C. rogercresseyi* larvae do not survive at an oxygen saturation lower than 60%, with survival improving at oxygen saturations higher than 90%, which apparently is the optimal oxygen conditions for the parasite (Mardones *et al.*, 2019). Moreover, environmental variables such as water temperature and oxygen can enhance reproduction, abundance of juveniles and the rate of development of *C. rogercresseyi* (González-Gómez *et al.*, 2020).

Based on available data, temperature and salinity affect the life cycle of *C. rogercresseyi*. Jeong *et al.* (2022) estimated parameter values for the developmental, survival and fertility rates of *C. rogercresseyi* at each life stage. Based on the models developed by these authors: (i) the copepodid developmental period was not found to be markedly affected by temperature, the period being estimated to be on average 3.07 days; (ii) the background survival proportion for all chalimus stages could be estimated as 0.9652 according to salinity-independent survival proportion of 0.965 for chalimus I and II grouped and for chalimus III and IV grouped; and (iii) salinity-independent survival was found to differ significantly between males and females, the average period until death for adult males and females was estimated to be 17.83 and 33.66 days, respectively.

21.3. Geographical Distribution and Host Range

This parasite was first reported in Chile on farmed salmon in 1992 (González, 1994) and, according to Carvajal *et al.* (1998), the parasite was transmitted from the native fishes *E. maclovinus* and Chilean silverside *Odontesthes regia* (Humboldt) while visiting cages and feeding on food given to salmon (Sepúlveda *et al.*, 2004). It is known that the parasite's swimming capacity during its mobile stages allows it to switch fish and that the copepodid, during its infestive stage, can be spread via water currents by up to 30 km (Kristoffersen *et al.*, 2014).

C. rogercresseyi has been found in different native and introduced fish species in Chile (Carvajal *et al.*, 1998). The geographical distribution of *C. rogercresseyi* includes Chile and Argentina (Bravo *et al.*, 2006). In Chile, it has been reported on the three introduced salmonid species being farmed in the administrative regions of Los Lagos and Aysén and Magallanes (Arriagada *et al.*, 2019). Atlantic salmon is considered the most susceptible to high parasite loads and the development of severe pathologies.

It has also been reported on native non-salmonid fishes, such as Patagonian blenny, Chilean silverside and small-eyed flounder, *Paralichthys microps* (Günther) (Sepúlveda *et al.*, 2004; Muñoz and Olmos, 2007). Under experimental conditions it was demonstrated that the parasite can infest the native salmonid *Galaxias maculatus* (Jenyns, 1842), the common jollytail (Marín *et al.*, 2009).

In Argentina, *C. rogercresseyi* is found in the Río Gallegos estuary (51°46′53″S 69°6′14″W) infesting brown trout (*Salmo trutta* (Linné, 1758)), rainbow trout, the native fish species *E. maclovinus*, the Argentinian silverside (*Odonthestes nigricans*), the parona leatherjacket (*Parona signata*) and the Patagonian sprat (*Sprattus fueguensis*) (Bravo *et al.*, 2006).

21.4. Disease, Clinical Signs and Pathogenesis

This disease caused by the copepod ectoparasite *C. rogercresseyi* is called caligidosis. The State of Chile has classified this disease as high risk, putting it on List 2 (Exempt Resolution 1741). Its inclusion on List 2 means that: (i) it is not included on the Office International des Epizooties (OIE; now the World Organisation for Animal Health) list of notifiable diseases; (ii) its presence was detected before it was declared a high-risk disease; and (iii) it is geographically distributed over an extensive area of national territory (Decree 319). Its classification as a high-risk disease allowed the Chilean State to formulate a protection, control and eradication programme. Under this regulatory framework, the specific sanitary surveillance and control programme for caligidosis was established in 2007 (Exempt Resolution No. 1789). The latest version of this has been in force since 2022 (Sernapesca, 2022).

Caligidosis affects fish by producing skin injuries, loss of continuity of the skin, peeling, petechial haemorrhage, ecchymosis, lacerations and occasionally ocular injuries. Diagnosis of this disease is made by visual inspection and counting the parasites present on the fish surface (Sernapesca, 2015, 2022). There are more detailed descriptions of the clinical signs of damage to fish caused by the caligid parasite species affecting both farmed and wild salmon in the northern hemisphere, *L. salmonis*. The damage is characterized as large open ulcers and lesions (MacKinnon, 1998), bleeding on the back of the head, subepidermal erosion and haemorrhage in the perianal region (Wootten *et al.*, 1982; Johnson *et al.*, 1996), as well as reduction of mucus production, which can cause death by osmoregulatory failure (Fast *et al.*, 2002).

Parasite pathogenicity varies as a product of host factors, such as age, stage of development and species, as well as intrinsic factors, like the number and state of development of the parasite (Johnson *et al.*, 1996; Wagner *et al.*, 2008).

The size/age of fish is an important variable determining the pathological effect of the parasite. Smaller fish are more susceptible to damage caused by the sea louse *L. salmonis* because of their overall body surface. Although higher absolute numbers of sea lice occur on larger fish, the heaviest intensities (number of lice per cm^2) occur on the smallest fish (Tucker *et al.*, 2002).

During the development of *C. rogercresseyi* it has been reported that attached copepodids and chalimus stages can cause physical and/or biochemical damage that can be attributed to their adhesion and feeding activities (Johnson *et al.*, 2004), since they feed on the mucus and skin of fish (González *et al.*, 2000). This damage increases as the parasite develops from chalimus I to chalimus IV (Jones *et al.*, 1990).

In Chile, the disease has been reported on the three introduced salmonid species: rainbow trout, Atlantic salmon and coho salmon (*Oncorhynchus kisutch*) (González *et al.*, 2000). However, the three species show different susceptibility to infestation by copepodids, with Atlantic salmon and rainbow trout being similar in susceptibility and coho salmon the least susceptible based on farm parasite abundance (Zagmutt-Vergara *et al.*, 2005; Yatabe *et al.*, 2011; Hamilton-West *et al.*, 2012).

The low abundance of the parasite in coho salmon could be due to a non-specific tissue response mechanism similar to that observed against *L. salmonis* (Fast *et al.*, 2002; Wagner *et al.*, 2008), but also to a lower preference of *C. rogercresseyi* for this species. Adult males exhibit an avoidance behaviour in the presence of coho salmon-conditioned water, whereas they exhibit an attractant response in rainbow trout- or Atlantic salmon-conditioned water, suggesting that these differences are mediated by different chemical cues released by different host species (Pino-Marambio *et al.*, 2007).

Biological effects in the host caused by *C. rogercresseyi* have been described, mainly on host physiology. González *et al.* (2015a) reported that when fish faced an infestation of a single cohort, the plasma glucose, protein, amino acid and triglyceride levels of Atlantic salmon decreased as early as 1 day post-infestation. However, they also reported that glucose levels rose with increasing copepodid load, suggesting that this parasite induces a stress response at the beginning of the infestation. Hyperglycaemia (Heath, 1995; Ellis *et al.*, 2012) and high cortisol levels have been described as useful indicators of stress in fish (Barton, 2000). The initial parasite infestation probably produced an adjustment, or acute stressor response, on Atlantic salmon. Furthermore, these authors found that increasing loads of *C. rogercresseyi* diminished the levels of glucose, amino acids and triglycerides when fish faced the chalimus I and II stages, and of glucose and proteins when they faced the chalimus III and IV stages, suggesting the fish used these substrates to cope with the energy demand. In addition, infestations with 24 chalimus III and IV, or seven adults of *C. rogercresseyi* produced a stress response in Atlantic salmon, as suggested by the high cortisol levels observed at those levels of abundance.

González *et al.* (2016a) found that long infestations (56 days post-infestation) with low numbers of adult *C. rogercresseyi* did not have an apparent impact on plasma energy substrates or cortisol in Atlantic salmon. They observed a local response evidenced by elevated numbers of small mucous cells in the skin of infested fish. However, when fish faced a second and heavy infestation with *C. rogercresseyi* copepodids, an acute stress response with a rise in plasma cortisol levels along with low plasma levels of glucose and triglycerides was observed. These results indicate that *C. rogercresseyi* induces a local response on skin when the infestation is prolonged, but when high infestation pressure occurs, a new stress response occurs in fish in order to cope with the infestation. The local response was corroborated by González *et al.* (2015a,b), which indicates that prolonged and also advanced chalimus stages infestation by *C. rogercresseyi* led to an augment of the number of small skin mucous cells on Atlantic salmon, reducing the cell size with the increase in parasite loads. The increase in the number of skin mucous cells could be a permanent response to an adverse condition (i.e. the *C. rogercresseyi* infestation). Furthermore, González *et al.* (2016b) found in Atlantic salmon that the presence of both the bacterium *Piscirickettsia salmonis* and *C. rogercresseyi* increased haematocrit, plasma glucose and pCO_2 levels but decreased haemoglobin and pO_2 levels, suggesting that a stress response and hypercapnia occur in fish when faced by infestations under farm conditions, corroborating the laboratory results described above.

Previously, coho salmon has been described as less susceptible to infestation by *C. rogercresseyi* (González *et al.*, 2000). A comparative study was performed by Vargas-Chacoff *et al.* (2016) who concluded that the amino acid and carbohydrate catabolism enzymes activated sooner in coho salmon than in Atlantic salmon, specifically at the beginning of the infestation with the parasite. This makes the energy substrates available earlier in coho salmon than Atlantic salmon and contributes to them coping earlier with the increased energy demand imposed by the infestation. Both species react to the infestation by increasing the lactate response via an energy metabolism pathway in the liver and muscle, indicating that fish need more energy to respond to increased infestation (Vargas-Chacoff *et al.*, 2017).

Vera-Bizama *et al.* (2015) found that genes associated with oxidative stress responses were upregulated in both Atlantic and coho salmon, suggesting that this response could modulate the sea louse antioxidant system. Atlantic salmon evidenced an upregulation of trypsins and serpins which was higher than that in coho salmon. Moreover, these authors revealed an inverse time-dependent pattern based on the different responses of *C. rogercresseyi* infecting both salmon species, where Atlantic salmon strongly modulated the transcriptome responses at earlier infection stages; meanwhile the coho salmon revealed a less marked modulation, increasing the transcription activity during the infection process.

Boltaña *et al.* (2016b) showed that when Atlantic salmon were infested by *C. rogercresseyi*, an activation of the pro-inflammatory and type 1 helper T cell (Th1) immune responses occurred. In addition, these authors observed differential macrophage responses between fish with high and low infestation rates. Specifically, the highly infested group showed a macrophage response in the skin and an upregulation of genes encoding antioxidants, suggesting high oxidative stress levels. Moreover, the mRNAs identified in relation to each type of parasitic load (i.e. high and low) were differentially associated with immunological processes, being higher in the highly infested fish group than in the less infested fish group, suggesting higher activity levels in relation to the Th1 immune system, the inflammatory response and/or macrophage activation (e.g. *T-bet, stat4, cd83* and *mmp13*). Also, an increase of *cox2* expression in the skin was observed for the highly infested fish but not in the less infested fish, suggesting that highly infested fish produce strong inflammatory responses.

Comparative immunological studies on Atlantic and coho salmon have been undertaken. Valenzuela-Muñoz *et al.* (2016) indicated that from global transcriptome analysis, both Atlantic and coho salmon showed similar tissue-specific transcription patterns, with modulations in the skin during early sea lice infestation stages and in the head kidney during late-stage parasitism. Furthermore, Atlantic salmon showed acute transcriptome responses of immune genes, whereas coho salmon showed the highest differentially expressed transcript at 14 days post-infestation. Coho salmon presented an increased Th1 response during *C. rogercresseyi* infestation, which decreased their mucus production. This is advantageous as it helps them deal with the infestation by decreasing the food available to *C. rogercresseyi*. Additionally, Toll-like receptors (TLRs) were found to play a possible role in the immune response to sea lice. Valenzuela-Muñoz *et al.* (2017) described differences in the regulation of genes associated with the pro-inflammatory response, with a high regulation of these genes in coho salmon. Also, these authors indicated changes in the regulation of iron transport genes, with iron availability being higher in Atlantic salmon during *C. rogercresseyi* infestation. For these reasons, they concluded that Atlantic salmon evidenced a nutritional immunity response, strongly modulating haem biosynthesis/degradation pathways and iron transport proteins. However, these responses did not apparently occur in coho salmon during *C. rogercresseyi* infestation.

21.5. Spatial and Temporal Trends of the Disease and Parasite

21.5.1. Introduction and spread of the disease

As mentioned previously, the original hosts for the parasite correspond to endemic fishes in Chile, in which no clinical signs associated with this infection have been reported (Bravo *et al.*, 2006). As *C. rogercresseyi* colonizes susceptible farmed salmon species the prevalence and infestation intensity increase, and so clinical signs are reported for farmed fish. Differences in the manifestation of the disease between native and farmed fishes are probably due to the higher intensity of infection in farmed salmon than in native fishes (Sepúlveda *et al.*, 2004). The high density of fish-farming stock facilitates the spread of pathogens. There is a strong association between sea lice levels and the abundance of fish hosts in the surrounding area (Jansen *et al.*, 2012).

C. rogercresseyi infests its farmed host species during the growth phase of the production cycle in areas where salinity and temperature are in the range it can tolerate; it can be found in both sea water and estuarine waters. The infestation is present all year round on farmed salmon (Molinet *et al.*, 2011). On native fishes, the presence of the parasite may be interrupted for those fish species that migrate to estuarine waters, such as *E. maclovinus* (Licandeo *et al.*, 2006).

Salmon farming began in the Los Lagos and Aysén regions during the 1980s. However, the production volume and intensity, as well as farm density, were higher in the Los Lagos region than in the Aysén region until 2007 (Intesal, 2014). In addition, in the Aysén region the salinity was lower than in the Los Lagos region, which naturally limited the population growth of this parasite. These conditions kept the parasite abundance at low levels. Since 1999 the Salmon Technical Institute (Intesal) has conducted a private parasite monitoring programme in southern Chile but, unfortunately, because of the low abundance of the parasite in the Aysén region, there was no *C. rogercresseyi* monitoring there until 2007, when the increase in *Caligus* abundance in the region began to be obvious (Intesal, 2014).

The disease caused by *C. rogercresseyi* in salmonids in Chile did not cause mortalities or significant loss of growth until 2004. This is probably because, at that time, once fish reached the threshold abundance of five parasites per fish, they were persistently treated. It is also due to the availability of effective treatments (Rozas and Ascencio, 2007). Results from the Intesal monitoring programme reported a number of adult parasites per fish of 3.28 for the period 1999 to 2002 (Zagmutt-Vergara *et al.*, 2005). However, between 2004 and 2007, an increase in the number of infested cages and parasite abundance was described. The abundance (juveniles and adults) in 2004 was five, ten and three parasites per fish in Atlantic salmon, rainbow trout and coho salmon, respectively. In 2007 these numbers increased to 20, 34 and 29, respectively (Rozas and Ascencio, 2007). Possible causes listed by these authors for this higher abundance were: (i) increased production volumes in geographic zones with optimal conditions for the parasite; (ii) the predominance of favourable environmental conditions for the parasite (e.g. salinity); and (iii) the discontinuation of associative, coordinated work in executing a strategic plan to control the parasite. In addition, from 2000 onwards, the only chemical agent used to control *C. rogercresseyi* was emamectin benzoate.

Given the increase in parasite abundance in both regions, the National Fisheries and Aquaculture Service (Sernapesca) implemented an official surveillance programme. Its first activity was to carry out a general diagnostic regarding the abundance of the parasite on all active farms during August of 2007.

In Argentina, *C. rogercresseyi* was first reported in 1998 in brown trout in the Río Gallegos estuary. Since then, the parasite has spread and become established in the area, showing an increase in both the number of parasites per fish and host species (Bravo *et al.*, 2006). According to these authors no severe effect by the parasite has been observed in wild fish. However, they indicated that severe physical damage was observed on the infested fish in areas with high concentrations of adult parasites between the dorsal and caudal fins (petechial haemorrhages in tissues). It may be possible that the fish introduced are those exhibiting the damage.

21.5.2. Understanding the temporal and spatial dynamics of infestation

The first comprehensive analysis of temporal and spatial variations in *C. rogercresseyi* infestations for the three farmed salmon species was carried out with data from December 1999 to April 2002 and was focused on the Los Lagos region (Zagmutt-Vergara *et al.*, 2005). This analysis was conducted during the adult stages of the parasite for the period prior to 2004–2007, during which the abundance of *C. rogercresseyi* mainly increased (Rozas and Ascencio, 2007).

Variations in adult parasite abundance at the regional level were explained by the variables fish species, water temperature and salinity, fish weight, juvenile parasite count, avermectin treatment the previous month, and the interaction between treatments during the current and previous months (fixed effect). This is to be expected, as high temperatures accelerate the generation time of the parasite, lower salinities affect the survival of the larval stages of the parasite, and fish weight has been indicated as a proxy of age, representing hosts that have been exposed to the parasite for longer periods of time than smaller fish (Saksida *et al.*, 2007). The juvenile parasite count is closely related to adult abundance, as they will build the adult population on fish. Fish treatment with avermectins in the previous month was associated with the lowest abundance of the adult parasites compared to fish that had not been treated or had been treated with other products.

The significance of the farm random factors could indicate that any high variability in parasite abundance not explained by the fixed factors may be explained by the influence of environmental and genetic factors that are not uniform among farms and stressors varying in a pen over time (bacterial and viral infections, transport, stock densities, handling and crowding). Water temperature and salinity variations over time are traditionally associated with variations in parasite abundance. However, the significant interaction between date and cage indicates that changes in parasite abundance at the pen level over time can be explained by other factors besides fixed factors like temperature and salinity. As a consequence, the date effect may be associated with the previously mentioned stressors.

After this study, the data gathered by the official surveillance programme implemented by Sernapesca was grouped at two levels of spatial scale. One of the analyses included a smaller spatial scale in which salmon farms operating in the Los Lagos and Aysén regions were grouped into ten and 11 productive–environmental zones, respectively (Yatabe *et al.*, 2011). The other study grouped the information according to ten productive–ecological macrozones defined by Intesal including the Los Lagos and Aysén regions (Hamilton-West *et al.*, 2012).

In the first analysis Yatabe *et al.* (2011) reported that geographic zone, fish species, treatment one month before sampling, stocking density, fish weight and water salinity were significantly associated with total parasite abundance. Treatment two or three months before sampling, use of photoperiods and water temperature were not significant. There was a considerable level of unexplained variation at all the aggregation levels (zones, farm and cage), with the farm having the highest level of variation. By that time, the study was able to identify two major productive–environmental zones: the Los Lagos region was associated with higher infestation levels and the Aysén region with lower infestation levels. The authors attributed the higher densities on farms in the Los Lagos region than on those in Aysén to zone differences, and the differences between species to the differential susceptibility of farmed salmon species in Chile, as indicated previously. Regarding treatments, the authors inferred that although treatment applied one month before sampling reduced parasite abundance, the reduction was not enough to reduce the high loads observed in fish that were about to be treated, compared to fish that did not require treatment. Stocking density is an important factor affecting fish welfare; fish farmed at high densities exhibit higher stress levels, which in turn increases their susceptibility to sea lice (Jansen *et al.*, 2012). With regard to fish weight, the results of this study coincide with those from previous studies indicating that larger fish have a higher absolute number of parasites than smaller fish, as they have been exposed to parasites for a longer time (Henriksen *et al.*, 2023). The lack of significance of water temperature in this study seems to be an effect of the study design that included a very specific and restricted period of the year, with a narrow temperature range (90% of the observations took place at between 8.2°C and 10.8°C) (Yatabe *et al.*, 2011). Several factors may be responsible for the high variation among farms: the effect on fish stress caused by different husbandry practices, local oceanographic conditions, different sanitary status among farms and genetic differences in the fish populations among farms or fish-farming companies.

In the second analysis, Hamilton-West *et al.* (2012) found that the prevalence among fish farms and at the cage level was highest in the north of the region, specifically Seno de Reloncaví, and lowest in the south of the region, in Puerto Aysén. The average sea lice abundance per fish was 11.8 and was statistically different between macrozones. Seno de Reloncaví, Hornopirén and North Chiloé had the highest abundance, and the lowest levels were found on Puerto Aysén and Puerto Cisnes. Abundance of ovigerous females showed the same variation pattern. Thus, *C. rogercresseyi* infestation was widespread across the Los Lagos and Aysén regions and geographic differences were explained by differences in environmental factors, such as temperature and salinity, as well as management practices.

A third study was carried out using data collected from the sea lice electronic monitoring programme conducted by the Chilean salmon farmers' association (SalmonChile) from January 2009 to April 2012 (Kristoffersen *et al.*, 2013). The main objective of this study was to understand the sources of sea lice (internal–farm and external–regional) and the factors affecting lice infection pressure on salmon farms in Chile to improve mitigation efforts. The response variable in the study was the number of juvenile parasites, since it represents the earliest stage of infection. The internal source of parasites was the farm itself, and it was estimated as the number of ovigerous females two weeks prior. The potential external sources of parasites were holding facilities at processing plants, neighbouring farms and shellfish farms. The environmental factors included were water salinity and temperature and geographical area (Los Lagos and Aysén regions). The management factors and fish characteristics analysed were the number of fish on the farm, the mean weight of the fish, fish species, sea lice treatment and the number of juveniles the week prior. The results indicated that of the external potential sources of parasites, shellfish were not significant. Proximity to holding facilities and neighbouring farms were significant however, with neighbouring farms being the most important, presumably because of the high number of fish managed on each farm. Distance was important since the closer the studied farm was to holding facilities and/or a neighbouring farm, the higher was the number of juveniles per fish on the studied farm. The association between the level of ovigerous female parasites on neighbouring farms and a farm's abundance of juvenile parasites two weeks later was a function of the neighbourhood size. According to the model implemented by the authors the optimal neighbourhood size would be 30 km.

Pressure from neighbouring farms was also more important than internal sources. This was explained by the authors as an effect of the current dispersing larval stages from the source farm during the development of the infestive stage period, and/or due to a relatively good control of adult parasites by the farmer but poorer control by neighbouring farmers. The positive association between treatment and juvenile abundance suggested that, on average, treatments were not effectively controlling this stage. This is to be expected considering that the treatment most frequently used at that time did not prevent infestation from external sources, since their target was the adult parasites. The effects of water salinity and temperature, fish species and fish weight were similar to those reported by previous studies (Yatabe *et al.*, 2011; Hamilton-West *et al.*, 2012). With regard to the zone effect, the results of this study also supported the differences reported in previous studies, indicating that in average locations in the Aysén region sea lice are less likely to be present, and that on average the Aysén region presents a lower abundance of juvenile lice than farms in the north.

On a smaller spatial scale, during the period July 2008–July 2009 in Codigue Bay in the Los Lagos region, the variability of ovigerous females was significantly explained by salmon biomass, chemical treatment and host species (Molinet *et al.*, 2011). These authors reported that the continuous presence of ovigerous females during the year explained the continuous presence of larval stages of the parasite, which was higher during the summer. The circulation pattern of the prevailing current in the study area suggested that most of the infestation pressure for the farms inside the bay would be generated by the bay itself since it leads to a retention of larvae, facilitating the host–parasite encounter. The authors suggested that it would be difficult to reduce parasite abundance without first reducing the fish biomass in the bay.

Mancilla-Schulz *et al.* (2019) compared the effect of farming, sanitary practices and environmental variables on the abundance of gravid females (GF) and juveniles (JUV) of *C. rogercresseyi* on Atlantic salmon in three Salmon Neighbourhood Areas (SNAs) in the Los Lagos region, southern Chile (SNA10a, 10b and 17a). Linear mixed-effects models of the negative binomial distribution were used to evaluate the effect of the different explanatory variables on GF and JUV. The results indicated that the abundance of both GF and JUV can be explained by common variables (SNA, year class, company, average fish weight, bath treatments, number of fish per site, salinity), while some unique variables help explain GF (JUV itself has an important impact) and JUV abundance levels are explained by oral treatment and temperature. Given the significant effect of the number of fish on a farm in explaining JUV abundance, it is suggested that self-infestation could be important on these farms because the number of fish on the farm was positively associated with the abundance of JUV on the farm. The results of autocorrelation functions (ACFs) for regular spaced time series on JUV stages were highly significant during YC12 (year class 12), revealing regular cycles lasting around 5 weeks in the three SNAs, despite the different patterns of abundance observed among SNAs. The relevance of SNA in both GF and JUV models can be explained by the contribution of SNA10b to the juvenile populations of neighbouring areas, specifically SNA10a. Both SNAs appear to be unique areas in terms of the population dynamics of *C. rogercresseyi*, where JUV plays an important role in the persistence of the disease at the sites and is therefore relevant to GF abundance.

The results from this study suggest that temperature played a minor role compared with the productive variables in explaining JUV abundance in the system but was significant enough to explain the differences in the persistence of JUV between SNAs. SNA17a reported the highest water temperatures during the study period, which contributed to maintaining the JUV for 86 weeks. The authors concluded that *C. rogercresseyi* is not controlled and JUV are persistent in the three SNAs; specifically, sanitary practices are not controlling the dissemination of the parasite among sites and environmental variables had a low impact on sea lice abundance.

Lepe-López *et al.* (2021) carried out a multivariate spatial scan statistic to identify geographic areas and times of *C. rogercresseyi* infestation and to estimate the factors associated with such patterns. The authors used the monitoring data that the Chilean authority manages at the farm level, with a set of 13 covariates, to provide adjustment within the analyses. The analyses were carried out for a period of 5 years (2012–2016) and included three fish species (Atlantic salmon, rainbow trout and coho salmon) in order to assess the consistency of the identified clusters. A retrospective multinomial, spatial and temporal scan test was implemented to identify farm clusters of any of the different categories of *C. rogercresseyi*-infested farms: baseline, medium and high, based on the control chemical threshold established by the health authority (three ovigerous females). The baseline represents adequate farm performance against *C. rogercresseyi* infestation. Then, production and environmental factors of the medium- and high-infestation farms were compared with the baseline using regression techniques. The results revealed a total of 26 clusters ($P < 0.001$), of which 12 correspond to baseline, one to medium, and the remaining 13 to high-infestation clusters. In general, baseline clusters are detected in a latitudinal gradient on estuarine areas, with increasing relative risks to complex island water systems. There is a spatial structure in specific sites, north of Los Lagos region and central in Aysén region, with high infestation clusters and epidemic peaks during 2013. Average weight, salmon species, chemotherapeutants, latitude, temperature, salinity and year category are factors associated with these *C. rogercresseyi* patterns. Recommendations for an integrated parasite management plan are provided, along with a discussion that considers the involvement of stock density thresholds of salmon species and the spatial structure of the efficacy of chemical control, both intended to avoid the advance of resistance and to minimize environmental residues.

The previous studies include data from 1999 to 2020 and all of them revealed that there are factors that have been significant to explain spatial and temporal variations of *C. rogercresseyi* – particularly fish species, fish weight, temperature, salinity and treatment – the latter being more important when the juvenile's stages are the target, as they maintain the populations on fish. In fact, the abundance of juveniles significantly explains the abundance of the mobile populations. When treatments target adults the effect of treatment is less significant. It is worth noting that the significance of the number of fish may be indicating self-infestation. This means that copepodids infesting fish in each farm came from the parasite population of the same farm. These results should be considered to analyse the present regulation that aims to control this parasitosis, focusing on the target of available treatments as well as the fish stocking.

21.6. Preventive and Control Strategies

21.6.1. Pharmacological treatments

In Chile, there are eight pharmaceutically active chemical compounds used for the control of *C. rogercresseyi*, namely: emamectin benzoate, diflubenzuron, lufenuron, hexaflumuron, hydrogen peroxide, deltamethrin, cypermethrin and azamethiphos (Sernapesca, 2022; González-Gómez *et al.*, 2023, 2025). These commercially available treatments are categorized into four classes: benzoylureas (diflubenzuron, lufenuron and hexaflumuron); pyrethroids (deltamethrin and cypermethrin); avermectins (emamectin benzoate); and organophosphates (azamethiphos) (González-Gómez *et al.*, 2025).

21.6.1.1. Benzoylureas

Of the benzoylureas, diflubenzuron and lufenuron are applied by feed, and hexaflumuron is applied by bath treatment. These compounds are chitin synthesis inhibitors (CSIs), which interfere with the moulting process and chitin formation (Sun *et al.*, 2015). Chitin is a polymer of *N*-acetylglucosamine, being one of the major components of the exoskeleton of arthropods (Harðardóttir *et al.*, 2019). The synthesis of a new exoskeleton takes place as the old exoskeleton is partially degraded (Harðardóttir *et al.*, 2019). Benzoylureas interfere with chitin biosynthesis and interact with sulfonylurea receptors which mediate chitin vesicle transport (Douris *et al.*, 2016). CSIs interfere with chitin formation in the procuticle and the deposition of epicuticle, resulting in abortive moult and death (Gangishetti *et al.*, 2009). CSIs have been shown to affect the structure and composition of the exoskeleton (Binnington, 1985; Harðardóttir *et al.*, 2019) and have also been demonstrated to inhibit egg fertility and hatching in insects (Perez-Farinos *et al.*, 1998). Studies on *C. rogercresseyi* are scarce; however, in *L. salmonis*, Harðardóttir *et al.* (2019) indicated that nauplius I and II were affected following exposure, and the authors indicate it is possible that an inhibition of the enzyme chitin synthase (LsCHS1) may be happening. Parasites shed the old exoskeleton and the few larvae that completed the moult to copepodids appeared to have a more flexible and transparent exoskeleton than the control larvae (Harðardóttir *et al.*, 2019).

21.6.1.2. Pyrethroids

Pyrethroids are synthetic insecticides derived from pyrethrum, that contains active compounds called pyrethrins, a natural insecticide extracted from *Chrysanthemum* flowers (Hassaan and El Nemr, 2020). They are widely used to control pests in agriculture, public health and households. In Chile two pharmaceuticals are authorized, which are deltamethrin and cypermethrin. These compounds are direct stimulators of sodium channels in neuronal cells, which causes fluctuations in the dynamics of sodium cation channels in the membrane of the nerve cell leading to an increase in the time of opening of the sodium channels (Hassaan and El Nemr, 2020), where they induce rapid depolarization and spastic paralysis leading to death of parasites (Burka *et al.*, 2012). The effect is specific to the parasite since the drugs are only slowly absorbed by the host and rapidly metabolized once absorbed (Burka *et al.*, 2012). Currently, cypermethrin is no longer being used in Chile, unlike deltamethrin. Deltamethrin (AlphaMax™) was authorized for use to control sea lice in 2007 (Bravo *et al.*, 2014) and induces a lower effect on juveniles than on mobile stages (Arriagada *et al.*, 2014). Through an RNA-sequencing analysis in conjunction with heatmap hierarchical clustering, Chavez-Mardones and Gallardo-Escárate (2015) indicated that these compounds modify the ectoparasitic transcriptome in adults, altering processes associated with the nervous system, cuticle formation, oxidative stress, reproduction and metabolism, among others, being a sex-related response in *C. rogercresseyi*. Also, deltamethrin modulates the antioxidant system gene expression in *C. rogercresseyi*, promoting the generation of free radicals for the biodegradation of the insecticide (Chavez-Mardones and Gallardo-Escárate, 2014).

21.6.1.3. Avermectins

Emamectin benzoate is the only representative of the avermectin chemical group approved for use in Chile, which was granted in 2000 (Bravo *et al.*, 2008b). It has neurotoxic properties, it selectively opens glutamate-gated chloride channels in arthropod neuromuscular tissues to cause hyperpolarization and flaccid paralysis leading to death (Burka *et al.*, 2012). Bravo *et al.* (2008b) evaluated parasite sensitivity in 18 salmon farms in Chile. The results, expressed as EC_{50} values (effective concentration to immobilize 50% of the parasites), revealed a generalized loss of sensitivity. During summer, EC_{50} values ranged from 57 to 203 ppb, while in winter they increased dramatically, reaching ranges between 202 and 870 ppb. Comparing these data with a reference value of 34 ppb – obtained from a sensitive strain of *Lepeophtheirus mugiloidis* – it was observed that this value is 4.2 times lower than the average EC_{50} of *C. rogercresseyi* (142 ppb) collected at the centres during the summer. In addition, Bravo *et al.* (2010) mentioned that this trend is persistent during at least seven generations of *C. rogercresseyi* cultivated in the laboratory, showing no changes in EC_{50} values across time. In addition, a difference in susceptibility between genders was described by Agusti *et al.* (2016), who indicated that males tended to be less susceptible than females to emamectin benzoate when sensitivity decreased.

21.6.1.4. Organophosphates

Organophosphates are acetylcholinesterase inhibitors and cause excitatory paralysis leading to death of sea lice after a bath treatment (Burka *et al.*, 2012). Azamethiphos is the only chemical authorized in Chile from this group. Marín *et al.* (2015) indicated that there is a spatial variability of parasite sensitivity to antiparasitics (including azamethiphos), and Solano and Pontigo (2024) mentioned that susceptibility to this compound has been reduced over time in Chile. However, temperature could influence the response of the parasite to azamethiphos treatment, since sensitivity to this organophosphate decreases with temperature (González-Gómez *et al.*, 2023). Regarding resistance mechanisms in *C. rogercresseyi*, Valenzuela-Miranda and Gallardo-Escárate (2016) mentioned that exposure of this parasite to azamethiphos induces an overexpression of genes related to cytochrome P450 and its receptors, and also receptors of acetylcholine. More recently, Sáez-Vera *et al.* (2022) indicated that a differential expression of genes related to cytochrome P450, long non-coding RNAs (lncRNAs) 8967 and 532, were observed after azamethiphos exposure and mentioned that these genes could be good candidate biomarkers for drug sensitivity testing.

21.6.2. Non-chemical approaches

There are several methods in experimental and on-farm conditions that are identified as good tools to control *C. rogercresseyi* in Chile. These tools include the use of cleaner fish, thermal treatment, hyposaline water, natural oils, electromagnetic pulses, ultrasound, ultrasonic cavitation and functional diets, among others. Some of these tools are described below, since literature about these treatments is scarce.

21.6.2.1. Cleaner fish

The use of *E. maclovinus* as a cleaner fish for *C. rogercresseyi* control was evaluated; however, efficacies varied among experiments. An efficacy of 93.6% was described in tanks with parasitized Atlantic salmon cohabitating with *E. maclovinus* under controlled experimental conditions, and 47.2% efficacy in fish cohabitating in an experiment under field conditions (Sánchez *et al.*, 2018). Some troubles have been identified with this tool, like culture density, salmon size, environmental conditions, pathogens and feeding behaviour of *E. maclovinus*, which can be fed with salmon pellets (Mora, 2025).

21.6.2.2. Thermal treatment

Thermal treatment relies primarily on the application of hot water for a short period of time, which causes the parasites to detach and become inactive (Mora, 2025). This technique is feasible because salmon can withstand brief exposures to temperatures between 30 and 34°C (Elliott and Elliott, 1995). Although lice have a similar thermal threshold, their smaller size means they cannot withstand these high temperatures for as long as fish (Grøntvedt *et al.*, 2015). Literature regarding the application of this treatment in Chile is scarce. However, González-Gómez *et al.* (2022) indicated efficacies over 90% for 2021, along with some negative issues regarding animal welfare.

21.6.2.3. Hyposaline water

Hyposaline water treatments exploit the osmotic change due to differences in salinity, lowering the survival by killing the parasite or inducing its detachment, especially of adult parasites (Mc Dermott *et al.*, 2021; Borchel *et al.*, 2023; Guttu *et al.*, 2024). Some biological studies regarding the effects of variations in salinity on *C. rogercresseyi* have been done. Bravo *et al.* (2015) have demonstrated that fresh water affected 100% of adult *C. rogercresseyi* following a 30 min exposure; however, once returned to sea water, 93% of the males and 73% of the ovigerous females were able to recover. In a second study by the same authors, the time of exposure was extended, inducing 100% effect in adult parasites, without any recovery. In the early stages of the parasite infestation, salinities lower than 14 ppt reduced hatching success at different temperatures, and no nauplius I and II survival was observed at this salinity (Montory *et al.*, 2018). This evidence suggests that *C. rogercresseyi* is highly sensitive to low-salinity water and that time is an important factor which should be considered during freshwater treatments.

21.6.2.4. Natural oils

Among the non-pharmacological strategies for the control of *C. rogercresseyi*, two alternatives are used in Chile which stand out for their natural composition and validated efficacy; these are Lyptus Plus® and Rosseus® (both from Sudvet). According to this company, the antiparasitic solutions act by interfering with the parasite's sensory mechanisms, with good efficacy and minimal impact on animal welfare. However, there are no published scientific studies indicating the biological effects, mechanisms of action, or effects on salmon welfare.

Scientific information regarding these kinds of treatments and their effect on *C. rogercresseyi* and the salmon host is scarce in Chile. It is hoped that within the next few years this will be resolved to gain a deeper understanding of the impact of these treatments on parasitosis, animal welfare and environmental impacts.

21.7. Evidence of Resistance to Antiparasitic Treatments

Loss of sensitivity or susceptibility is defined as 'the development of a variant or strain capable of surviving the lethal dose compared to most individuals in a normal population' (Ffrench-Constant and Roush, 1990). Considering this definition, evidence has been described indicating that *C. rogercresseyi* has lost sensitivity to different antiparasitic drugs. Regarding pyrethroids, it has been mentioned that a reduction in phenotypic susceptibility to deltamethrin from 2008 to 2012 occurred in Chile (Helgesen *et al.*, 2014), which has potentially caused loss of efficacy of field treatments (Bravo *et al.*, 2013). Moreover, a loss in azamethiphos and deltamethrin phenotypic sensitivity has been reported in this parasite from different salmon farms across southern Chile since 2018 (González-Gómez, 2021; Solano-Iguarán, 2022). From a phenotypic point of view, it was mentioned that the sensitivity to azamethiphos, deltamethrin and cypermethrin of *C. rogercresseyi* varied among different geographic zones into which the farms are organized (Marín *et al.*, 2015), concentrating the resistant variant in the Los Lagos region of Chile (Agusti *et al.*, 2016), a region that contains a large proportion of the farms of the Chilean salmon industry. In addition, azamethiphos susceptibility showed variation across the seasons with a higher frequency of moderate and non-susceptible variants in autumn and winter, when environmental and water temperatures are lower (González-Gómez, 2021). In a recent study, a temperature of 9°C induced lower azamethiphos susceptibility than temperatures above 12°C (González-Gómez *et al.*, 2023), suggesting that temperature could have a relevant effect on susceptibility to this antiparasitic.

From a molecular point of view, several genes of different enzymes have been described in the resistance mechanism of *C. rogercresseyi*. LncRNAs were associated with resistance to azamethiphos and pyrethroids (Núñez-Acuña *et al.*, 2020), and also differential expression of three genes of cytochrome P450 (Valenzuela-Muñoz and Gallardo-Escárate, 2016; Sáez-Vera *et al.*, 2022), 8967 lncRNA and 532 lncRNA (Sáez-Vera *et al.*, 2022), as well as trypsin, chymotrypsin and bantam microRNA (Núñez-Acuña *et al.*, 2021), was described for resistant variants. In addition, it has been described that acetylcholinesterase genes are involved in the organophosphates resistance mechanism of *C. rogercresseyi* (Agusti *et al.*, 2016; Valenzuela-Muñoz and Gallardo-Escárate, 2016) and P-glycoprotein could be involved in detoxification of pyrethroids (Valenzuela-Muñoz *et al.*, 2014), as also could activating mRNA of the NOTCH signalling pathway and of ABC genes (Boltaña *et al.*, 2016a). Regarding hydrogen peroxide, Chávez-Mardones *et al.* (2017) mentioned that a differential antioxidant response from males and females was observed, being CrPRX2, CrGST1, CrGST-like and CrGST-κ1 augment in the expression for males, and CrPHGP1, CrCAT, CrSOD, CrSe-GPX and CrFERR for females. This evidence shows that the *C. rogercresseyi* parasite is showing a loss of sensitivity and that it also possesses different mechanisms to detoxify itself and confront antiparasitic drugs.

21.8. Economic Impact

Dresdner *et al.* (2019) estimated the impact of the *C. rogercresseyi* treatments on the unit cost in salmon farms located in areas different regarding salinity (marine, estuarine). The results indicated that the main effect is the presence of *C. rogercresseyi* itself, and that it should not be correct to indicate that the unitary cost of salmon production increases significantly by treatment. It would be more precise to indicate that the total costs of producing salmon have increased on the farms due to the necessity to deal with it.

The unit cost in a situation of no *C. rogercresseyi* is different across the study farms as well as the impact of this parasite, where the less impact was estimated in estuarine areas and the larger in marine areas. The increase in cost in the situation of presence of *C. rogercresseyi* with respect to a situation with no parasite is estimated as $US1.4 per kilogram, and it is not different from the situation of presence of the parasite and treatment.

The average cost of production increases due to the presence of *C. rogercresseyi* because of the negative effect that the parasite has on salmon growth and productivity. As salmon grow slower, the unit cost per production cycle increases. Then, applying treatments produces an increase in the volume of biomass at the end of the production cycle, but this increase is compensated by the high cost of the bath treatments, which in turn results in there being no difference in unit cost between the presence of the parasite and no treatment, and the situation in which *C. rogercresseyi* is treated.

21.9. Conclusions and Suggestions for Future Studies

C. rogercresseyi remains a critical pathogen in southern hemisphere aquaculture, demanding region-specific management strategies. Different studies across time have demonstrated that management practices such as farmed fish species, fish weight and number of fish per farm, and environmental variables such as temperature and salinity, remain being significant to explain the spatial and temporal distribution of the abundance of this parasite. It seems that this parasitosis is not yet controlled and the treatment focus should be on juveniles to interrupt the parasite cycle on the fish. This is especially important in the context of climate change due to expected changes in water temperature and salinity as well as acidification, which will not be the same across geographic areas. Geographical differences in parasite response to management practices and environmental variables suggest that regulations should take into consideration these differences. Sustainable control requires a combination of chemical, biological and husbandry innovations, alongside ongoing surveillance for resistance. The pathology associated with this parasite is severe, affecting the health, welfare and productivity of farmed fish. Although advances have been made in non-pharmacological control strategies and integrated management, the adaptability of the parasite and the development of resistance to conventional treatments demand continuous innovation. Research focused on parasite and host genomics, the development of new therapeutic and preventive tools (including vaccines and functional diets) and the optimization of management strategies at the ecosystem scale are essential to ensure the long-term sustainability of salmon farming in the region and mitigate the profound impact of this ectoparasite. Collaboration between academia, industry and the public sector is crucial to address this complex health problem.

References

Agusti, C., Bravo, S., Contreras, G., Bakke, M.J., Helgesen, K.O. *et al.* (2016) Sensitivity assessment of *Caligus rogercresseyi* to anti-louse chemicals in relation to treatment efficacy in Chilean salmonid farms. *Aquaculture* 458, 195–205.

Araya, A., Mancilla, M., Lhorente, J.P., Neira, R. and Gallardo, J.A. (2012) Experimental challenges of Atlantic salmon *Salmo salar* with incremental levels of copepodids of sea louse *Caligus rogercresseyi*: effects on infestation and early development. *Aquaculture Research* 43, 1904–1908.

Arriagada, G.A., Stryhn, H., Campistó, J.L., Rees, E.E., Sanchez, J. *et al.* (2014) Evaluation of the performance of pyrethroids on different life stages of *Caligus rogercresseyi* in southern Chile. *Aquaculture* 426–427, 231–237.

Arriagada, G., Stryhn, H., Sanchez, J., Vanderstichel, R., Campistó, J.L. *et al.* (2017) Evaluating the effect of synchronized sea lice treatments in Chile. *Preventive Veterinary Medicine* 136, 1–10.

Arriagada, G., Valenzuela-Muñoz, V., Arriagada, A.M., Núñez-Acuña, P., Brossard, M. *et al.* (2019) First report of the sea louse *Caligus rogercresseyi* found in farmed Atlantic salmon in the Magallanes region, Chile. *Aquaculture* 512, 734386.

Barton, B. (2000) Salmonid fishes differ in their cortisol and glucose responses to handling and transport stress. *North American Journal of Aquaculture* 62, 12–18.

Binnington, K.C. (1985) Ultrastructural changes in the cuticle of the sheep blowfly, *Lucilia*, induced by certain insecticides and biological inhibitors. *Tissue and Cell* 17, 131–140.

Boltaña, S., Chávez-Mardones, J., Valenzuela-Muñoz, V. and Gallardo-Escárate, C. (2016a) Evidence for the induction of key components of the NOTCH signaling pathway via deltamethrin and azamethiphos treatment in the sea louse *Caligus rogercresseyi*. *International Journal of Molecular Sciences* 17, 304.

Boltaña, S., Sanchez, M., Valenzuela, V. and Gallardo-Escárate, C. (2016b) Density-dependent effects of *Caligus rogercresseyi* infestation on the immune responses of *Salmo salar*. *Fish and Shellfish Immunology* 59, 365–374.

Borchel, A., Heggland, E.I. and Nilsen, F. (2023) Without a pinch of salt: effect of low salinity on eggs and nauplii of the salmon louse (*Lepeophtheirus salmonis*). *Parasitology Research* 122, 1893–1905.

Bravo, S. (2010) The reproductive output of sea lice *Caligus rogercresseyi* under controlled conditions. *Experimental Parasitology* 125, 51–54.

Bravo, S., Perroni, M., Torres, E. and Silva, M. (2006) Report of *Caligus rogercresseyi* in the anadromous brown trout (*Salmo trutta*) in the Rio Gallegos estuary, Argentina. *Bulletin of the European Association of Fish Pathologists* 26, 186–196.

Bravo, S., Pozo, V. and Silva, M. (2008a) The tolerance of *Caligus rogercresseyi* to salinity reduced in southern Chile. *Bulletin of the European Association of Fish Pathologists* 28, 197–204.

Bravo, S., Sevatdal, S. and Horsberg, T.E. (2008b) Sensitivity assessment of *Caligus rogercresseyi* to emamectin benzoate in Chile. *Aquaculture* 282, 7–12.

Bravo, S., Erranz, F. and Lagos, C. (2009) A comparison of sea lice, *Caligus rogercresseyi*, fecundity in four areas in southern Chile. *Journal of Fish Diseases* 32, 107–113.

Bravo, S., Sevatdal, S. and Horsberg, T. (2010) Sensitivity assessment in the progeny of *Caligus rogercresseyi* to emamectin benzoate. *Bulletin of the European Association of Fish Pathologists* 30, 99–105.

Bravo, S., Nuñez, M. and Silva, M.T. (2013) Efficacy of the treatments used for the control of *Caligus rogercresseyi* infecting Atlantic salmon, *Salmo salar* L., in a new fish-farming location in Region XI, Chile. *Journal of Fish Diseases* 36, 221–228.

Bravo, S., Sepulveda, M., Silva, M.T. and Costello, M.J. (2014) Efficacy of deltamethrin in the control of *Caligus rogercresseyi* (Boxshall and Bravo) using bath treatment. *Aquaculture* 432, 175–180.

Bravo, S., Pozo, V. and Silva, M.T. (2015) Evaluación de la efectividad del tratamiento con agua dulce para el control del piojo de mar *Caligus rogercresseyi* Boxshall & Bravo, 2000. *Latin American Journal of Aquatic Research* 43, 322–328.

Burka, J.F., Fast, M.D. and Revie, C.W. (2012) *Lepeophtheirus salmonis* and *Caligus rogercresseyi*. In: Woo, P.T.K. and Buchmann, K. (eds) *Fish Parasites: Pathobiology and Protection*. CAB International, Wallingford, UK, pp. 350–370.

Carvajal, J., González, L. and George-Nascimento, M. (1998) Native sea lice (Copepoda: Caligidae) infestation of salmonids reared in netpen systems in southern Chile. *Aquaculture* 166(3–4), 241–246.

Chavez-Mardones, J. and Gallardo-Escárate, C. (2014) Deltamethrin (AlphaMax™) reveals modulation of genes related to oxidative stress in the ectoparasite *Caligus rogercresseyi*: implications on delousing drug effectiveness. *Aquaculture* 433, 421–429.

Chavez-Mardones, J. and Gallardo-Escárate, C. (2015) Next-generation transcriptome profiling of the salmon louse *Caligus rogercresseyi* exposed to deltamethrin (AlphaMax): discovery of relevant genes and sex-related differences. *Marine Biotechnology* 17, 793–810.

Chávez-Mardones, J., Asencio, G., Latuz, S. and Gallardo-Escárate, C. (2017) Hydrogen peroxide modulates antioxidant system transcription, evidencing sex-dependent responses in *Caligus rogercresseyi*. *Aquaculture Research* 48, 969–978.

Douris, V., Steinbach, D., Panteleri, R., Livadaras, I., Pickett, J.A. *et al.* (2016) Resistance mutation conserved between insects and mites unravels the benzoylurea insecticide mode of action on chitin biosynthesis. *Proceedings of the National Academy of Sciences USA* 113, 14692–14697.

Dresdner, J., Chávez, C., Quiroga, M., Jiménez, D., Artacho, P. and Tello, A. (2019) Impact of *Caligus* treatments on unit costs of heterogeneous salmon farms in Chile. *Aquaculture Economics & Management* 23, 1–27.

Elliott, J. and Elliott, J. (1995) The effect of the rate of temperature increase on the critical thermal maximum for parr of Atlantic salmon and brown trout. *Journal of Fish Biology* 47, 917–919.

Ellis, T., Yildiz, H.Y., Lopez-Olmeda, J., Spedicato, M.T., Tort, L., Overli, O. and Martins, C.I. (2012) Cortisol and finfish welfare. *Fish Physiology and Biochemistry* 38, 163–188.

Farias, D. (2005) Aspectos biológicos y conductuales del estadio infectante de Caligus rogercresseyi Boxshall & Bravo 2000 (Copepoda: Caligidae), en peces nativos y de cultivo de Chile. Tesis de Grado para optar al Título de Biólogo Marino, Universidad Austral de Chile, Valdivia, Chile, p. 47.

Fast, M.D., Ross, N.W., Mustafa, A., Sims, D.E., Johnson, S.C. *et al.* (2002) Susceptibility of rainbow trout *Oncorhynchus mykiss*, Atlantic salmon *Salmo salar* and coho salmon *Oncorhynchus kisutch* to experimental infection with sea lice *Lepeophtheirus salmonis*. *Diseases of Aquatic Organisms* 52, 57–68.

Ffrench-Constant, R. and Roush, R. (1990) Resistance detection and documentation: the relative roles of pesticidal and biochemical assays. In: Roush, R.T. and Tabashnik, B.E. (eds) *Pesticide Resistance in Arthropods*. Springer, Boston, Massachusetts, pp. 4–38.

Gangishetti, U., Breitenbach, S., Zander, M., Saheb, S.K., Müller, U. *et al.* (2009) Effects of benzoylphenylurea on chitin synthesis and orientation in the cuticle of the *Drosophila* larva. *European Journal of Cell Biology* 88, 167–180.

González, L. (1994) Parásitos en los cultivos marinos de salmónidos en el sur de Chile. *Investigición Pesquera (Chile)* 38, 87–96.

González, L. and Carvajal, J. (2003) Life cycle of *Caligus rogercresseyi,* (Copepoda: Caligidae) parasite of Chilean reared salmonids. *Aquaculture* 220, 101–117.

González, L., Carvajal, J. and George-Nascimento, M. (2000) Differential infectivity of *Caligus flexispina* (Copepoda, Caligidae) in three farmed salmonids in Chile. *Aquaculture* 183, 13–23.

González, M. (2006) Selectividad del copepodito de *Caligus rogercresseyi* Boxshall & Bravo, 2000 (Copepoda: Caligidae) frente a diferentes hospederos. Tesis de Grado para optar al Título de Biólogo Marino, Universidad Austral de Chile, Valdivia, Chile, p. 60.

González, M.T., Molinet, C., Arenas, B., Asencio, G. and Carvajal, J. (2012) Fecundity of the sea louse *Caligus rogercresseyi* on its native host *Eleginops maclovinus* captured near salmon farms in southern Chile. *Aquaculture Research* 43, 853–860.

González, M., Marín, S. and Vargas-Chacoff, L. (2015a) Effects of *Caligus rogercresseyi* (Boxshall and Bravo, 2000) infestation on physiological response of host *Salmo salar* (Linnaeus 1758): establishing physiological thresholds. *Aquaculture* 438, 47–54.

Gonzalez, M., Marin, S. and Vargas-Chacoff, L. (2015b) Stress response of *Salmo salar* (Linnaeus 1758) facing low abundance infestation of *Caligus rogercresseyi* (Boxshall & Bravo 2000), an object in the tank, and handling. *Journal of Fish Diseases* 39, 853–865.

González, M., Vargas-Chacoff, L. and Marín, S. (2016a) Stress response of *Salmo salar* (Linnaeus 1758) when heavily infested by *Caligus rogercresseyi* (Boxshall & Bravo 2000) copepodids. *Fish Physiology and Biochemistry* 42, 263–274.

González, M., Muñoz, J., Valerio, V. and Vargas-Chacoff, L. (2016b) Effects of the ectoparasite *Caligus rogercresseyi* on *Salmo salar* blood parameters under farm conditions. *Aquaculture* 457, 29–34.

González-Gómez, M. (2021) *Informe final: Vigilancia de la resistencia de Caligus rogercresseyi a antiparasitarios aplicados en la salmonicultura nacional (Etapa IV)*. Instituto de Fomento Pesquero, Puerto Montt, Chile, p. 154.

González-Gómez, M.P., Ovalle, L., Spinetto, C., Oyarzo, C., Oyarzún, R. *et al.* (2020) Experimental transmission of *Caligus rogercresseyi* between two different fish species. *Diseases of Aquatic Organisms* 141, 127–138.

González-Gómez, M.P., Solano, J., Pontigo, F. and Contreras-Lynch, S. (2022) Estado del arte de los métodos de tratamiento no farmacológicos para la Caligidosis, evaluación de sus ventajas y desventajas y sus posibles aplicaciones en Chile *(CUI 2020-39-DAC-9)*. Instituto de Fomento Pesquero, Puerto Montt, Chile, p. 183.

González-Gómez, M.P., Spinetto, C., Oyarzo, C., Álvarez, D., Oyarzún, R. and Rivas, M. (2023) Effects of temperature on azamethiphos sensitivity profile of *Caligus rogercresseyi*. *Aquaculture* 575, 739824.

González-Gómez, M.P., Campanini-Salinas, J., Olmos-Iturrieta, P., Peralta, A., Espinoza, M. and Mancilla-Schulz, J. (2025) Antiparasitic effect of imidacloprid on the copepodite and adult stages of *Caligus rogercresseyi*. *Aquaculture* 596, 741878.

Grøntvedt, R.N., Nerbøvik, I.-K.G., Viljugrein, H., Lillehaug, A., Nilsen, H. and Gjevre, A.-G. (2015) *Thermal De-licing of Salmonid Fish – Documentation of Fish Welfare and Effect*. Report Series 13-2015. Norwegian Veterinary Institute, Oslo.

Guttu, M., Gaasø, M., Båtnes, A.S. and Olsen, Y. (2024) The decline in sea lice numbers during freshwater treatments in salmon aquaculture. *Aquaculture* 579, 740131.

Hamilton-West, C., Arriagada, G., Yatabe, T., Valdés, P., Hervé-Claude, L.P. and Urcelay, S. (2012) Epidemiological description of the sea lice (*Caligus rogercresseyi*) situation in southern Chile in August 2007. *Preventive Veterinary Medicine* 104, 341–345.

Harðardóttir, H.M., Male, R., Nilsen, F. and Dalvin, S. (2019) Effects of chitin synthesis inhibitor treatment on *Lepeophtheirus salmonis* (Copepoda, Caligidae) larvae. *PLoS One* 14, e0222520.

Hassaan, M.A. and El Nemr, A. (2020) Pesticides pollution: classifications, human health impact, extraction and treatment techniques. *Egyptian Journal of Aquatic Research* 46, 207–220.

Heath, A.G. (1995) *Water Pollution and Fish Physiology.* CRC Press, Boca Raton, Florida.

Helgesen, K., Bravo, S., Sevatdal, S., Mendoza, J. and Horsberg, T. (2014) Deltamethrin resistance in the sea louse *Caligus rogercresseyi* (Boxhall and Bravo) in Chile: bioassay results and usage data for antiparasitic agents with references to Norwegian conditions. *Journal of Fish Diseases* 37, 877–890.

Henriksen, E.H., Frainer, A., Poulin, R., Knudsen, R. and Amundsen, P.A. (2023) Ectoparasites population dynamics are affected by host body size but not host density or water temperature in a 32-year long time series. *Oikos* 2023, e09328.

Intesal (2014) *Compendio la caligidosis en salmónideos de cultivo, resultados del programa de monitoreo Caligus rogercresseyi. Vigilancia y control de Intesal. Período octubre 2007 a diciembre 2009.* Intesal–SalmonChile, Puerto Varas, Chile, p. 124.

Jansen, P.A., Anja B.K., Hildegunn, V., Daniel, J., Magne, A. and Audun, S. (2012) Sea lice as a density-dependent constraint to salmonid farming. *Proceedings of the Royal Society B: Biological Sciences* 279, 2330–2338.

Jeong, J., McEwan, G.F., Arriagada, G., Gallardo-Escárate, C. and Revie, C.W. (2022) Quantifying key parameters related to the life cycle of *Caligus rogercresseyi*. *Journal of Fish Diseases* 45, 219–224.

Johnson, S.C., Blaylock, R.B., Elphick, J. and Hyatt, K.D. (1996) Disease induced by the sea louse (*Lepeophteirus salmonis*) (Copepoda: Caligidae) in wild sockeye salmon (*Oncorhynchus nerka*) stocks of Alberni Inlet, British Columbia. *Canadian Journal of Fisheries and Aquatic Sciences* 53, 2888–2897.

Johnson, S.C., Treasurer, J., Bravo, S., Nagasawa, K. and Kabata, Z. (2004) A review of the impact of parasitic copepods on marine aquaculture. *Zoological Studies* 43, 229–243.

Jones, M.W., Sommerville, C. and Bron, J. (1990) The histopathology associated with the juvenile stages of *Lepeophtheirus salmonis* on the Atlantic salmon, *Salmo salar* L. *Journal of Fish Diseases* 13, 303–310.

Kristoffersen, A.B., Rees, E.E., Stryhn, H., Ibarra, R., Campisto, J.L. *et al.* (2013) Understanding sources of sea lice for salmon farms in Chile. *Preventive Veterinary Medicine* 111, 165–175.

Kristoffersen, A.B., Jimenez, D., Viljugrein, H., Grøntvedt, R., Stien, A. and Jansen, P.A. (2014) Large scale modelling of salmon lice (*Lepeophtheirus salmonis*) infection pressure based on lice monitoring data from Norwegian salmonid farms. *Epidemics* 9, 31–39.

Lepe-López, M., Escobar-Dodero, J., Rubio, D., Alvarez, J., Zimin-Veselkoff, N. and Mardones, F.O. (2021) Epidemiological factors associated with *Caligus rogercresseyi* infection, abundance, and spatial distribution in southern Chile. *Frontiers in Veterinary Science* 8, 595024.

Licandeo, R.R., Barrientos, C.A. and González, M.T. (2006) Age, growth rates, sex change and feeding habits of notothenioid fish *Eleginops maclovinus* from the central–southern Chilean coast. *Environmental Biology of Fishes* 77, 51–61.

Mackinnon, B.M. (1998) Host factors important in sea lice infections. *ICES Journal of Marine Science* 55, 188–192.

Mancilla-Schulz, J., Marín, S.L. and Molinet, C. (2019) Dynamics of *Caligus rogercresseyi* (Boxshall & Bravo, 2000) in farmed Atlantic salmon (*Salmo salar*) in southern Chile: are we controlling sea lice? *Journal of Fish Diseases* 42, 357–369.

Mardones, A., Gajardo, V., Pizarro, M.I., Augsburger, A., Vega, R. *et al.* (2019) Evaluation of survival and metamorphosis of larvae of *Caligus rogercresseyi* (Boxshall and Bravo, 2000) (Crustacea, Copepoda) in Chile, depending on temperature, salinity and oxygen. *Brazilian Journal of Biology* 79, 174–179.

Marín, S.L. and Fast, M.D. (2021) *Caligus rogercresseyi* and caligid sea lice species. In: Sitjà-Bobadilla, A., Bron, J., Wiegertjes, G. and Piazzon, M.C. (eds) *Fish Parasites: A Handbook of Protocols for their Isolation, Culture and Transmission*. CAB International, Wallingford, UK, pp. 330–350.

Marín, S.L., Carvajal, J., Manríquez, A. and Mancilla, M. (2009) Effects of experimental infection by *Caligus rogercresseyi* (Copepoda: Caligidae) on the common jollytail, *Galaxias maculatus* (Osmeriforme: Galaxiidae) (Jenyns, 1842) in Chile. *Aquaculture* 295, 138–141.

Marín, S., Ibarra, R., Medina, M.H. and Jansen, P.A. (2015) Sensitivity of *Caligus rogercresseyi* (Boxshall and Bravo 2000) to pyrethroids and azamethiphos measured using bioassay tests – a large scale spatial study. *Preventive Veterinary Medicine* 122, 33–41.

McDermott, T., D'Arcy, J., Kelly, S., Downes, J.K., Griffin, B. *et al.* (2021) Novel use of nanofiltered hyposaline water to control sea lice (*Lepeophtheirus salmonis* and *Caligus elongatus*) and amoebic gill disease, on a commercial Atlantic salmon (*Salmo salar*) farm. *Aquaculture Reports* 20, 100703.

Molinet, C., Cáceres, M., Gonzalez, M.T., Carvajal, J., Asencio, G. *et al.* (2011) Population dynamic of early stages of *Caligus rogercresseyi* in an embayment used for intensive salmon farms in Chilean inland seas. *Aquaculture* 312, 62–71.

Montory, J.A., Cumillaf, J.P., Cubillos, V.M., Paschke, K., Urbina, M.A. and Gebauer, P. (2018) Early development of the ectoparasite *Caligus rogercresseyi* under combined salinity and temperature gradients. *Aquaculture* 486, 68–74.

Montory, J.A., Cumillaf, J.P., Gebauer, P., Urbina, M., Cubillos, V.M. *et al.* (2020) Early development and metabolic rate of the sea louse *Caligus rogercresseyi* under different scenarios of temperature and pCO_2. *Marine Environmental Research* 162, 105154.

Mora, V. (2025) Revisión bibliográfica acerca de tratamientos alternativos y medidas de prevención para la caligidosis. Memoria de Título para optar al Título de Médico Veterinario, Universidad San Sebastián, Puerto Montt, Chile.

Muñoz, G. and Olmos, V. (2007) Revisión bibliográfica de especies ectoparásitas y hospedadoras de sistemas acuáticos de Chile. *Revista de Biología Marina y Oceanografía* 42, 89–148.

Núñez-Acuña, G., Sáez-Vera, C., Valenzuela-Muñoz, V., Valenzuela-Miranda, D., Arriagada, G. and Gallardo-Escárate, C. (2020) Tackling the molecular drug sensitivity in the sea louse *Caligus rogercresseyi* based on mRNA and lncRNA interactions. *Genes* 11, 857.

Núñez-Acuña, G., Valenzuela-Muñoz, V., Carrera-Naipil, C., Sáez-Vera, C., Benavente, B.P. *et al.* (2021) Trypsin genes are regulated through the miRNA bantam and associated with drug sensitivity in the sea louse *Caligus rogercresseyi*. *Non-Coding RNA* 7, 76.

Perez-Farinos, G., Smagghe, G., Marco, V., Tirry, L. and Castañera, P. (1998) Effects of topical application of hexaflumuron on adult sugar beet weevil, *Aubeonymus mariaefranciscae*, on embryonic development: pharmacokinetics in adults and embryos. *Pesticide Biochemistry and Physiology* 61, 169–182.

Piasecki, W. and MacKinnon, B.M. (1993) Changes in structure of the frontal filament in sequential developmental stages of *Caligus elongatus* von Nordmann, 1832 (Crustacea, Copepoda, Siphonostomatoida). *Canadian Journal of Zoology* 71, 889–895.

Pino-Marambio, J., Mordue, A.J., Birkett, M., Carvajal, J., Asencio, G. *et al.* (2007) Behavioural studies of host, non-host and mate location by the sea louse, *Caligus rogercresseyi* Boxshall & Bravo, 2000 (Copepoda: Caligidae). *Aquaculture* 271, 70–76.

Rozas, M. and Ascencio, G. (2007) Evaluación de la situación epidemiológica de caligidiasis en Chile: hacia una estrategia de control efectiva. *Salmociencia* 2, 43–49.

Sáez-Vera, C., Núñez-Acuña, G. and Gallardo-Escárate, C. (2022) Sensitivity assessment to azamethiphos by time-to-response bioassay and biomarkers in the sea louse *Caligus rogercresseyi*. *Aquaculture* 546, 737340.

Saksida, S., Karreman, G.A., Constantine, J. and Donald, A. (2007) Differences in *Lepeophtheirus salmonis* abundance levels on Atlantic salmon farms in the Broughton Archipelago, British Columbia, Canada. *Journal of Fish Diseases* 30, 357–366.

Sánchez, J.C., Mancilla, J., Hevia, M. and Saez, P.J. (2018) The Patagonian blenny (*Eleginops maclovinus*): a Chilean native fish with potential to control sea lice (*Caligus rogercresseyi*) infestations in salmonids. In: Treasurer, J. (ed.) *Cleaner Fish Biology and Aquaculture Applications*. CAB International, Wallingford, UK, pp. 468–480.

Schram, T. (2000) The egg string attachment mechanism in salmon lice *Lepeophtheirus salmonis* (Copepoda: Caligidae). *Contributions to Zoology* 69, 21–29.

Sepúlveda, F., Marín, S.L. and Carvajal, J. (2004) Metazoan parasites in wild fish and farmed salmon from aquaculture sites in southern Chile. *Aquaculture* 235, 89–100.

Sernapesca (2015) Establece programa sanitario específico de vigilancia y control de caligidosis (psevc-caligidosis). Deja sin efecto resolución N° 1141 Exenta, de 2012. In: *Resolución 013 EXENTA*. Ministerio de Economía, Fomento y Turismo; Subsecretaría de Pesca; Servicio Nacional de Pesca, Valparaíso, Chile.

Sernapesca (2022) Aprueba programa sanitario específico de vigilancia y control de caligidosis. Deja sin efecto resolución Número 13 exenta de 2015 del Servicio Nacional de Pesca y Acuicultura In: *Resolución 60*

EXENTA. Ministerio de Economía, Fomento y Turismo; Subsecretaría de Pesca y Acuicultura; Servicio Nacional de Pesca y Acuicultura; Dirección Nacional, Valparaíso, Chile.

Solano-Iguarán, J. (2022) *Informe final: Vigilancia de la resistencia de Caligus rogercresseyi a antiparasitarios aplicados en la salmonicultura nacional (Etapa V)*. Instituto de Fomento Pesquero, Puerto Montt, Chile, p. 195.

Solano, J. and Pontigo, F. (2024) *Determinación y vigilancia de la resistencia de Caligus rogercresseyi a antiparasitarios aplicados en la salmonicultura nacional. Etapa VII, 2023–2024*. Instituto de Fomento Pesquero, Puerto Montt, Chile, p. 122.

Sun, R., Liu, C., Zhang, H. and Wang, Q. (2015) Benzoylurea chitin synthesis inhibitors. *Journal of Agricultural and Food Chemistry* 63, 6847–6865.

Thompson, C.R.S., Fields, D.M., Bjelland, R.M., Chan, V.B.S., Durif, C.M.F. *et al.* (2019) The planktonic stages of the salmon louse (*Lepeophtheirus salmonis*) are tolerant of end-of-century pCO_2 concentrations. *PeerJ* 7, e7810.

Treasurer, J.W. and Bravo, S. (2011) The spatial distribution patterns of *Caligus rogercresseyi* and *C. elongatus* on Atlantic salmon hosts (*Salmo salar*). *Aquaculture* 320(3–4), 154–158.

Tucker, C.S., Sommerville, C. and Wootten, R. (2002) Does size really matter? Effects of fish surface area on the settlement and initial survival of *Lepeophtheirus salmonis*, an ectoparasite of Atlantic salmon *Salmo salar*. *Diseases of Aquatic Organisms* 49, 145–152.

Valenzuela-Miranda, D. and Gallardo-Escárate, C. (2016) *Caligus rogercresseyi* serine proteases: transcriptomic analysis in response to delousing drugs treatments. *Aquaculture* 465, 65–77.

Valenzuela-Muñoz, V. and Gallardo-Escárate, C. (2016) Transcriptome mining: multigene panel to test delousing drug response in the sea louse *Caligus rogercresseyi*. *Marine Genomics* 25, 103–113.

Valenzuela-Muñoz, V., Nuñez-Acuña, G. and Gallardo-Escárate, C. (2014) Molecular characterization and transcription analysis of P-glycoprotein gene from the salmon louse *Caligus rogercresseyi*. *Journal of Aquaculture Research & Development* 5, 1000236.

Valenzuela-Muñoz, V., Boltaña, S. and Gallardo-Escárate, C. (2016) Comparative immunity of *Salmo salar* and *Oncorhynchus kisutch* during infestation with the sea louse *Caligus rogercresseyi*: an enrichment transcriptome analysis. *Fish and Shellfish Immunology* 59, 276–287.

Valenzuela-Muñoz, V., Boltaña, S. and Gallardo-Escárate, C. (2017) Uncovering iron regulation with species-specific transcriptome patterns in Atlantic and coho salmon during a *Caligus rogercresseyi* infestation. *Journal of Fish Diseases* 40, 1169–1184.

Vargas-Chacoff, L., Muñoz, J.L.P., Hawes, C., Oyarzún, R., Pontigo, J.P. *et al.* (2016) Atlantic salmon (*Salmo salar*) and Coho salmon (*Oncorhynchus kisutch*) display differential metabolic changes in response to infestation by the ectoparasite *Caligus rogercresseyi*. *Aquaculture* 464, 469–479.

Vargas-Chacoff, L., Muñoz, J.L.P., Hawes, C., Oyarzún, R., Pontigo, J.P. *et al.* (2017) Ectoparasite *Caligus rogercresseyi* modifies the lactate response in Atlantic salmon (*Salmo salar*) and coho salmon (*Oncorhynchus kisutch*). *Veterinary Parasitology* 243, 6–11.

Vera-Bizama, F., Valenzuela-Muñoz, V., Gonçalves, A.T., Marambio, J.P., Hawes, C. *et al.* (2015) Transcription expression of immune-related genes from *Caligus rogercresseyi* evidences host-dependent patterns on Atlantic and coho salmon. *Fish and Shellfish Immunology* 47, 725–731.

Wagner, G.N., Fast, M.D. and Johnson, S.C. (2008) Physiology and immunology of *Lepeophtheirus salmonis* infections of salmonids. *Trends in Parasitology* 24, 176–183.

Wootten, R., Smith, J.W. and Needham, E.A. (1982) Aspects of the biology of the parasitic copepods *Lepeophtheirus salmonis* and *Caligus elongatus* on farmed salmonids, and their treatment. *Proceedings of the Royal Society of Edinburgh. Section B: Biological Science* 81, 185–197.

Yatabe, T., Arriagada, G., Hamilton-West, C. and Urcelay, S. (2011) Risk factor analysis for sea lice, *Caligus rogercresseyi*, levels in farmed salmonids in southern Chile. *Journal of Fish Diseases* 34, 345–354.

Zagmutt-Vergara, F., Tim, E.C., Thomas, B.F. and Ronald, P.H. (2005) Spatial and temporal variations in sea lice (Copepoda: Caligidae) infestations of three salmonid species farmed in net pens in southern Chile. *Diseases of Aquatic Organisms* 64, 163–173.

22 *Lepeophtheirus salmonis*

Mark D. Fast[1]* and Dylan Michaud[2]

[1]Atlantic Veterinary College, University of Prince Edward Island, Charlottetown, Canada; [2]Pacific Biological Station, Fisheries and Oceans, Canada, Nanaimo, British Columbia, Canada

Abstract

This chapter is an update on the review by Burka and colleagues in the first edition of this book. In the time since the last review our understanding of *Lepeophtheirus salmonis* has increased manyfold. This chapter builds on the foundational review from 2012, with a newly modified life cycle of the parasite and newly defined subspecies in the North Atlantic and Pacific Oceans, with their own genotypic and phenotypic singularities. The chapter covers updated information on morphological development, new integrated pest management strategies, and medicinal and non-medicinal targets for control. New understanding on the parasite's pathobiology and its interactions with the host have also driven new immunological strategies, and all are combined into new integrated pest management portfolios that attempt to reduce drug resistance and parasite impacts on farmed and wild fish worldwide.

22.1. Introduction

Sea lice are parasitic copepods in the order Siphonostomatoida, family Caligidae. Recent revisions within the family have reduced it to 27 recognized genera, which include approximately 124 *Lepeophtheirus* von Nordmann, 1832, and 276 *Caligus* species, which together make up over 75% of the total 503 species (Bernot *et al.*, 2025). *Lepeophtheirus salmonis* and various *Caligus* species are adapted to salt water and are major ectoparasites of farmed and wild Atlantic salmon, *Salmo salar* (Linnaeus, 1758). They feed on mucus, epidermal tissue and blood of host fish. *L. salmonis* is the primary sea louse of concern in the northern hemisphere, where two different subspecies exist in the Atlantic (*Lepeophtheirus salmonis salmonis*) and Pacific Oceans (*Lepeophtheirus salmonis oncorhynchii*). Similarly, *Caligus rogercresseyi* is recognized as a significant pathogen on salmon farms in Chile (Chapter 21, this volume), primarily rainbow trout, *Oncorhynchus mykiss* (Walbaum, 1792), and Atlantic salmon (González and Carvajal 2003; Marín *et al.*, 2015a,b). This chapter reviews *L. salmonis*.

22.2. Diversity and Hosts: Sea Lice on Wild Fish

L. salmonis (two subspecies: *L. salmonis salmonis* located in the North Atlantic Ocean and *L. salmonis oncorhyhnci* subsp. novo located in the North Pacific Ocean), the salmon louse, has high

*Email: mfast@upei.ca

DOI: 10.1079/9781800628748.0022

specificity for salmonids, most importantly the widely farmed Atlantic salmon (*Salmo salar*). It is found on all other salmonid species in marine environments, including brown trout (sea trout: *Salmo trutta*), Arctic char (*Salvelinus alpinus*) and all species of Pacific salmon (*Oncorhynchus* spp.). Coho (*Oncorhynchus kisutch*) and pink salmon (*Oncorhynchus gorbuscha*) have strong tissue responses and reduced infection levels in laboratory exposures compared to more susceptible species such as Atlantic salmon (Johnson and Albright 1992a,b; Braden *et al.*, 2023; Salisbury *et al.*, 2024; Sveen *et al.*, 2025). However, wild adult pink, chum (*Oncorhynchus keta*) and sockeye salmon (*Oncorhynchus nerka*) maintain significantly higher infections of *L. salmonis oncorhynchii* than coho and Chinook salmon (*Oncorhynchus tshawytscha*) (Beamish *et al.*, 2005), suggesting possible behavioural, ecological and age-associated immunological differences resulting in more complex interactions in wild populations. Further, *L. salmonis oncorhynchii* also develops on the three-spined stickleback (*Gasterosteus aculeatus*) (Jones *et al.*, 2006); although high numbers of lice develop through the attached chalimus stages on this non-salmonid, it appears that mobile pre-adult/adult stages do not develop or at least do not remain on sticklebacks. A very different interaction occurs with its hosts for *L. salmonis salmonis* in the Atlantic Ocean. The major host for this subspecies is farmed Atlantic salmon, with smaller populations of wild Atlantic salmon and sea trout being negatively impacted by *L. salmonis salmonis* linked to significant contributions of lice from farmed fish (Vollstet *et al.*, 2014; Serra-Llinarez *et al.*, 2020). Although prevalence and abundance of *L. salmonis oncorhynchii* can be high on three-spined stickleback, *L. salmonis salmonis* is only rarely found on non-salmonid hosts including the three-spine stickleback (Pietrak *et al.*, 2019).

Zooplankton often show either positive or negative phototaxis, and *L. salmonis* (Heuch *et al.*, 1995) and *Caligus elongatus* (MacKinnon, 2011) migrate upwards in the water column towards light, likely increasing interactions with potential hosts. Chemical cues in the water column are also important in host finding and recognition and both light and chemical traps have been investigated for their use in attracting and removing infectious stages of lice in the farm environment (Mordue and Birkett, 2009; Krasnov *et al.*, 2024; McGowan *et al.*, 2025).

Dispersal of infectious stages has been modelled for *L. salmonis* throughout their Atlantic and Pacific ranges, to improve our understanding of site connectivity and enhance the success of implemented mitigation strategies (Samsing *et al.*, 2016; Parent *et al.*, 2024a). Connectivity is an epidemiological concept in which movement of a pathogen/parasite between geographical locations is facilitated or impeded by its environment. As an example, areas in Eastern Canada (Bay of Fundy) with few wild Atlantic salmon result in salmon farms serving as parasite 'habitat patches', and the seaway distance or coastal currents that move between these patches significantly impact the transmission of *L. salmonis* between sites and hence the degree of connectivity between these farms (Parent *et al.*, 2024a). Areas with greater coastal/currents or wild salmon populations would potentially increase the connectivity between further afield sites, whereas river outflows or freshwater incursions could act as a barrier. Effective dispersal of the parasite results from movement of planktonic stages from one release point, through water currents to successful parasitism of salmon at another location. In some places this can be as high as 30–40 km; in others such as Bay of Fundy, Canada this has been estimated to be 7–10 km (Parent *et al.*, 2024a,b).

22.3. Morphology and Development: Possible Targets for Integrated Management

All species of sea lice have free-swimming (planktonic) and parasitic life stages, and these stages are separated by moults (Johnson and Albright, 1991a,b; Schram, 1993). Development time is directly related to temperature, and equations for the development rate based on temperature have been generated for both subspecies (Hamre *et al.*, 2019; Jeong *et al.*, 2021). *L. salmonis* has eight stages, each separated by a moult (Hamre *et al.*, 2013; Eichner *et al.*, 2014). Nauplius I larvae are the first life stage hatched from maternal egg strings. These are planktonic and unable to self-navigate but passively drift while adjusting their vertical depth within the water column. They are characterized as primarily translucent where the yolk and bands of longitudinal muscle are visible, along with two pigmented areas (Schram, 1993). Black pigments are notable around the developing eyespots, while brown pigmentation is in the middle of the body distributed on either side of the intestinal tract. Nauplius I larvae are approximately 0.5 mm in length and 0.2 mm in width (Schram, 1993) and developmental time frames, as with all copepods, are largely temperature dependent, where at 5°C the stage lives approximately 52 h and at 15°C approximately 9 h (Hamre *et al.*, 2019). The nauplius II stage is quite similar to the previous stage; however, it is longer (average length of 0.6 mm) with a slight increase in width (0.205 mm), and the swimming appendages are on average two to three times the size (Schram, 1993). These larval stages are dependent on maternally acquired energy in the form of yolk stores (Pike and Wadsworth, 1999). The free-swimming copepodid is the first infective stage and on average is 0.7 mm long and 0.2 mm wide.

Copepodids continue to rely on maternal yolk stores; however, as these are consumed, with age a decline in successful host settlement can be observed, significantly at 5 days post-moult to copepodid (Tucker *et al.*, 2000, 2002). Settling upon a host, copepodids use the maxillae and maxilliped to grip the host surface and specialized antennae to further hook on to the epithelium. Crucially a frontal filament, which pierces beneath the epithelial layer, is developed, securely anchoring the louse to the host's surface (Bron *et al.*, 1991). This filament is suspected to be developed by three different groups of cells generating two distinct secretions, one of which forms the basal plate of the filament while the other becomes the stem (Gonzalez-Alanis *et al.*, 2001). Chalimus I and II are sessile remaining attached at a fixed point via the frontal filament, have an average length of 1.1 mm and width of 0.5 mm and length of 1.3 mm and width of 0.5 mm, respectively, and the armature of all appendages is substantially reduced in overall length (Schram, 1993). Previously *L. salmonis* were thought to have four chalimus stages, as is the case with several copepod species, however astute observations of discrete moulting events by Hamre *et al.* (2013) determined that only two stages exist. Furthermore, the current earliest reliable detection point for sexual dimorphism has been developed by Eichner *et al.* (2014) in which differences in cephalothorax length during the chalimus II stage can determine sex and cephalothorax-to-body-length ratio at the instar age. At 10°C chalimus I tend to develop at 6 days post-infection (dpi), while chalimus II males emerge at approximately 11 dpi and females at 13 dpi (Hamre *et al.*, 2019). The succeeding pre-adult and adult stages importantly see the emergence of mobility across the host's surface and often relocation to preferred anatomical sites such as the head and ventral surface, and to positions posterior to the dorsal and anal fins, can be observed. At these stages, differences between males and females are more easily discerned due to morphological differences between the genital segments (Ritchie *et al.*, 1996). Developmental sexually dimorphic trends continue through these remaining life stages characterized by faster male maturation compared to females (at 10°C: ~17 dpi males, ~20 dpi females, pre-adult I; ~23 dpi males, ~28 dpi females, pre-adult II) (Hamre *et al.*, 2019). Furthermore, adult male *L. salmonis* exhibit divergent behaviours compared to their female counterparts such as increased host-switching frequencies, mate-searching behaviours driven by ionotropic receptors facilitating chemotaxis to semiochemical cues, and pre-/post-copulatory mate-guarding/-pairing formations characterized by the direct physical establishment over the female genital segment (Ritchie *et al.*, 1996; Hull *et al.*, 1998; Pike and Wadsworth, 1999; Ingvarsdóttir *et al.*, 2002; Stephenson, 2012). These copulatory positions are predominately taken up with pre-adult II or virgin adult females in which males hold their respective mating partners around the fourth pedigerous segment using the antennae. Copulation generally occurs post-moult to adults in which male lice use maxillipeds to manipulate and raise the female genital segment and transfer a spermatophore to the seminal receptacles via the copulatory ducts; the spermatophore can be held for multiple weeks and inseminate numerous clutches. Heuch *et al.* (2000) reported that fertilized *L. salmonis* can produce a dozen egg-string pairs following a single mating, and Ritchie *et al.* (1996) indicated that a single mating is sufficient to fertilize all eggs produced in the lifetime of a female *L. salmonis*. However, loss of spermatophores, sperm competition and polyandry have been reported to occur for *L. salmonis* and the potential for assortative mating has also been proposed due to enhanced survival rates of copepodids from parents with similar recombination rates (Todd *et al.*, 2005; Danzmann *et al.*, 2018).

Salinity below 30 ppt results in decreased development of *L. salmonis* eggs to the copepodid stage (Johnson and Albright, 1991b). Despite the stress of lower salinity on all stages of *L. salmonis*, adults have been described on returning wild salmon, and laboratory studies have shown that females can survive up to 19 days (>190 degree-days) in fresh water when attached to a host (Finstad *et al.*, 1995; Ghanei-Motlagh *et al.*, 2025a).

Upon reaching adulthood reproduction, two egg strings are produced averaging about 285 eggs per egg string for *L. salmonis* (Heuch *et al.*, 2000). They darken with maturation and are approximately the same length as the female's body. The first egg strings produced by a female are always shorter than subsequent strings and one female can produce between six and 11 pairs of egg strings in a lifetime of approximately 7 months (Heuch *et al.*, 2000; Mustafa *et al.*, 2001). Egg strings are longer and contain more eggs in sea lice from areas of lower salinity as well as in the winter, although eggs at colder temperatures are smaller and less viable (Heuch *et al.*, 2000). Development of egg strings also takes four times longer at 7°C than at 12°C and the time between extrusion of egg strings doubles at the colder temperature (Heuch *et al.*, 2000). Thus temperature has a direct influence on egg development. In response to fresh water, *L. salmonis* females have been observed to release egg strings within < 4 h, and this freshwater exposure prevents development of nauplii (Ghanei-Motlagh *et al.*, 2025a).

The importance of ecdysis in parasites such as *L. salmonis* cannot be overstated, as a moult separates each developmental stage ($n = 8$). Chitin, which is a polymer of *N*-acetylglucosamine, provides the structural support in the exoskeleton of arthropods, and is synthesized, metabolized and recycled throughout the moulting process. Poley *et al.* (2018) described the chitin synthesis pathway for *L. salmonis* by matching contiguous sequences with the well-described *Drosophila melanogaster*, elucidating for the first time important molecular signals (novel chitin-binding and C-type lectins) linked to formation and metabolism of the louse cuticle. This was further updated by Braden *et al.* (2020) (Fig. 22.1) and led to several studies functionally characterizing individual components within the chitin synthesis pathway. In *Caligus rogercresseyi*, Michaud *et al.* (2019) were able to show the strong negative correlation over time between glucosamine:fructose-6-phosphate aminotransferase (LsGFAT), a rate-limiting enzyme in the hexosamine pathway, and phosphoacetylglucamine mutase (LsAGM) expression, where LsGFAT increased through the copepodid moult period and LsAGM decreased (also observed through the moult in nauplii II of *L. salmonis*; Harðardóttir *et al.*, 2019). Knockdown (KD) studies in *L. salmonis* (Braden *et al.*, 2020) also showed the importance of these molecules in moulting and development. Post-transcriptional silencing of LsGFAT in *L. salmonis* nauplii resulted in strong inhibition of this gene by the copepodid stage, followed by a subsequent induction in the chitinase degradation pathway and a significant inhibition of chitin synthase 1 (LsCHS1) (Braden *et al.*, 2020). Whereas inhibition of LsCHS1 resulted in induction in UDP-*N*-acetylglucosamine pyrophosphorylase (LsAUP) encoding the enzyme directly preceding LsCHS1 in the chitin biosynthesis pathway (Fig. 22.1), KD of LsAUP resulted in the opposite effect on LsCHS1. LsCHS1, LsGFAT and LsCHS1+CHS2 double KD, as well as KD of chitin deacetylase (LsCDA5969) all resulted in abnormal exoskeletal formation in copepodids and abrogated infection potential, resulting in no development through to chalimus II when exposed to naïve Atlantic salmon hosts (Braden *et al.*, 2020). When RNA interference (RNAi) was applied to pre-adult I stage *L. salmonis*, KD of LsCHS1 resulted in lethal phenotypes with deformed cuticle, ovaries and oocytes in adult lice (Harðardóttir *et al.*, 2021). These studies have laid the foundation for understanding how moulting inhibitors can impact development and survival of sea lice on their farmed hosts, providing key therapeutic targets for control as discussed further below.

22.4. Pathophysiology

22.4.1. Feeding habits

Attached copepodid, chalimus, pre-adult and adult stages feed on mucus, epidermis and blood

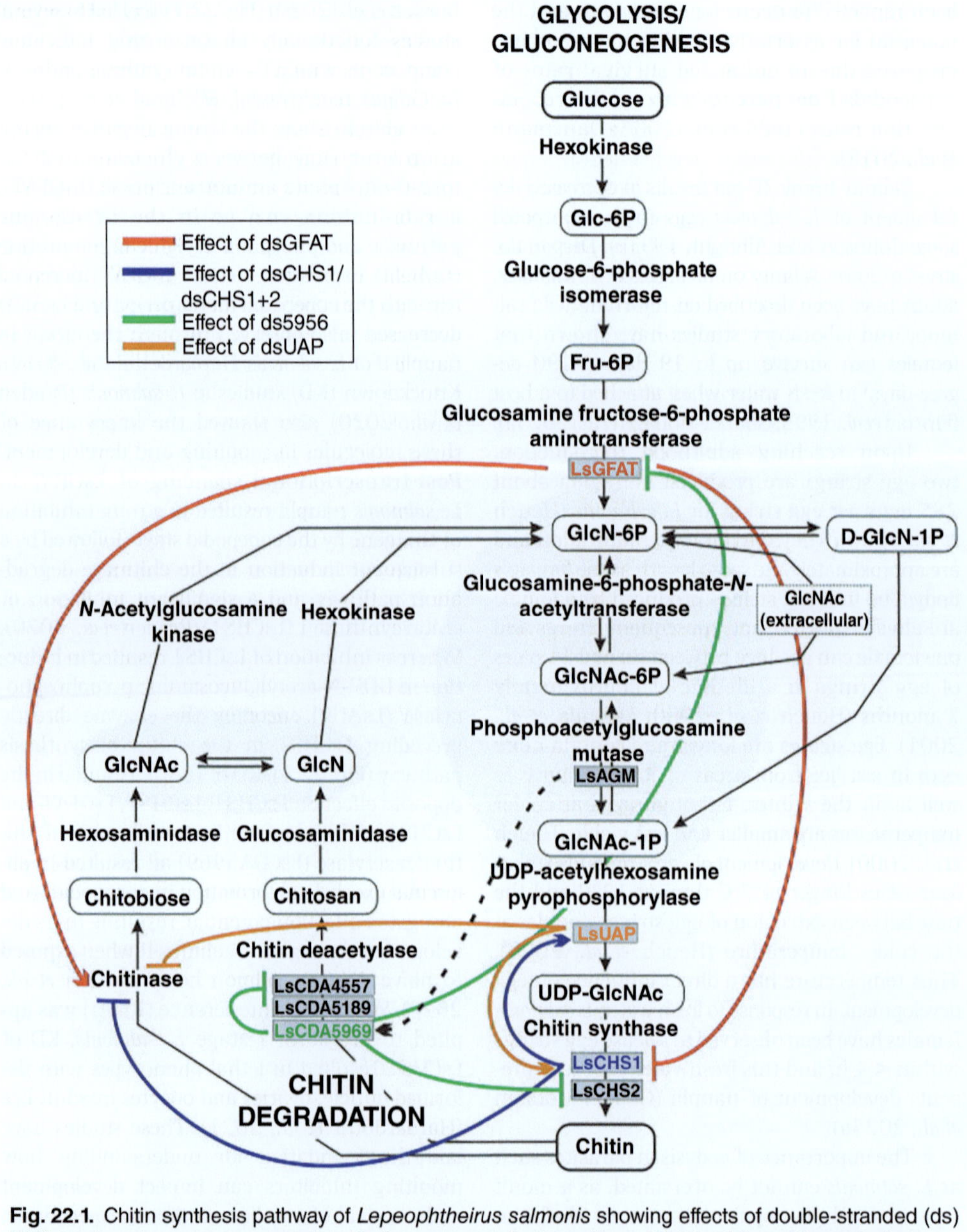

Fig. 22.1. Chitin synthesis pathway of *Lepeophtheirus salmonis* showing effects of double-stranded (ds) RNA treatments on gene expression of other enzymes in the pathway. Points of the pathway that are within grey shaded areas are assumed to be less sensitive to perturbations as evidenced by a normal phenotype after RNAi (Braden *et al.*, 2020). Glc-6P, glucose-6-phosphate; Fru-6P, fructose-6-phosphate; GlcN-6P, glucosamine-6-phosphate; GlcNAc-6P, *N*-acetyl-D-glucosamine 6-phosphate; GlcNAc-1P, *N*-acetyl-D-glucosamine 1-phosphate; UDP-GlcNAc, uridine diphosphate *N*-acetylglucosamine; D-GlcN-1P, D-glucosamine-*N*-1-phosphate; GlcNAc, *N*-acetylglucosamine; GlcN, glucosamine. (Reproduced with permission from Braden *et al.*, 2020.)

of the host (Kabata, 1970; Brandal *et al.*, 1976; Bron *et al.*, 1993), the result of which includes skin lesions, elevated stress responses (Fast *et al.*, 2006a,b), and reduced growth rates and feeding activities (Godwin *et al.*, 2015). Due to their small size, damage by copepodids and chalimus is minor and limited to the area immediately adjacent to their point of attachment, where they can erode the epidermis (Fig. 22.2), sometimes characterized by melanized spots (Bron *et al.*, 1991; Grimnes and Jakobsen, 1996). However the pre-adult and adult developmental stages are larger and mobile and the damage associated with these stages is often more severe (greater haematophagous feeding activity) and widespread, with areas of skin erosion (Fig. 22.2), haemorrhaging, altered host mucus consistency and generalized host stress response mediated by cortisol (Wootten *et al.*, 1982; Grimnes and Jakobsen, 1996; Nolan *et al.*, 1999; Bowers *et al.*, 2000; Ross *et al.*, 2000; Burka *et al.*, 2012; Fast and Dalvin, 2020). More recent literature has questioned the importance of blood in the meal of *L. salmonis*. Work by Heggland *et al.* (2020) confirmed earlier anecdotal evidence of slower development through chalimus stages in lice that have settled on gill filaments compared to those on the fins, coupled with significant alteration in their transcriptome, involving elevation of pro-oxidative molecules, haem, digestive and detoxification enzymes, all with potential roles in clot prevention. Premature onset of blood feeding or its greater contribution to the parasite meal could have anti-nutritional and even stress-inducing impacts. Bricknell and Pietrak (2023) also identified a high pH and high osmolality of the louse gut more similar to that of its seawater environment, and highlighted appendages associated with the mouth/feeding as more adept at grazing on skin and mucus and only opportunistically on blood.

Serious infestations may lead to open lesions in which the epidermis is breached and the underlying tissues are exposed, increasing blood loss or consumption (Johnson and Albright, 1991a; Jónsdóttir *et al.*, 1992). As mucus and epithelial layers are eroded, subsequent secondary infections become increasingly problematic and frequent (Johnson and Albright, 1992b). Furthermore, mortalities may occur directly as a result of extremely heavy infestations via loss of physiological homeostasis including osmotic stress, anaemia and hypoproteinaemia (Wootten *et al.*, 1982; Fast *et al.*, 2006a). Swimming performance has also been shown to be reduced by up to 22% when infection levels average only 0.1 lice/g fish compared to uninfected fish (Wagner *et al.*, 2003). For further information on how specific infection densities impact stress, cortisol induction and morbidity, the reader is directed to the earlier reviews of Johnson and Fast (2004) and Wagner *et al.* (2008).

22.4.2. Sea louse–host interactions

Host resistance to *L. salmonis* varies between different salmonid species but does not appear to be

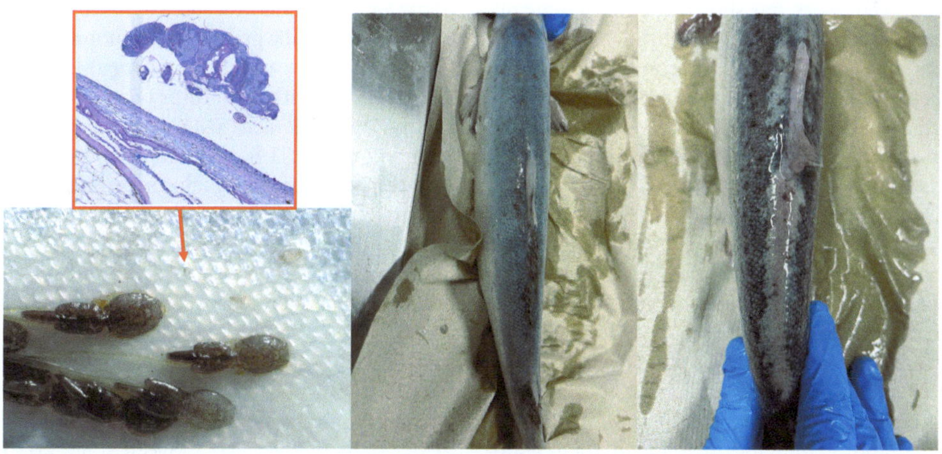

Fig. 22.2. *Lepeophtheirus salmonis* infection in Atlantic salmon, with multiple life stages showing: (left) infection of adult females alongside immature stages, with copepodid stage identified by the red arrow and magnified to show minor histological impact at attachment site (left upper); (middle) Atlantic salmon infected along its dorsum by adult male and female lice; (right) adult male and female lice removed and evidence of epithelial erosion and haemorrhage from lice feeding. (Author's own image.)

affected by subspecies of *L. salmonis*. For example, coho salmon are the most resistant species, while intermediate resistance has been demonstrated for pink salmon, Chinook salmon and rainbow trout. Highly susceptible species include chum salmon, sockeye salmon, brown trout and Atlantic salmon (Johnson and Albright, 1992b; Fast *et al.*, 2002; Braden *et al.*, 2020). This profile appears to be unchanged when laboratory studies have been conducted on multiple salmonid host species involving either *L. salmonis salmonis* or *L. salmonis oncorhynchii* (Johnson and Albright 1992b; Fast *et al.*, 2002; Jones *et al.*, 2007; Sveen *et al.*, 2025). Pro-inflammatory responses concomitant with epithelial hyperplasia appear to characterize a successful immune response to both sea lice subspecies. The most recent literature has demonstrated granulomatous infiltrate and epithelial hyperplasia associated with the anterior end of attached *L. salmonis* on the skin of coho salmon, surrounding the embedded frontal filament and concurrent with the moult from copepodid to chalimus I (Braden *et al.*, 2023). Granulomas are aggregations of macrophages and other immune cells which form in response to chronic inflammation. Braden *et al.*'s (2023) study revealed that granulomas engulf larval *L. salmonis* as infections progress: by 10 dpi, *L. salmonis* are fully encased and present grossly as an opaque mass on the host surface. Responses to lice infection in coho salmon occur quickly; in fact recent work has shown that proteomic differences in the skin occur within 12 and 36 h and involve neutrophil degranulation (Sveen *et al.*, 2025). Using spatial transcriptomics at the attachment site, Sveen *et al.* (2025) also showed local upregulation of inflammatory genes and that the large-scale inflammatory response was driven by neutrophils in the first 48 h post-infection. Salisbury *et al.* (2024) were able to characterize the importance of keratinocytes in the hyperplastic response of coho salmon by using single nuclei transcriptomics (SNT). They observed strong and rapid upregulation of genes associated with cell proliferation, cell motility, and extracellular matrix strengthening in keratinocytes and a dramatic increase in their abundance at the infection site. In fact, three different types of keratinocytes were identified and proposed to serve different functions: superficial keratinocytes playing a sentinel role in detection of lice and attraction of immune cells, whereas intermediate keratinocytes, lying between superficial and basal keratinocytes, rapidly increase in abundance at >48 h post-infection with sea lice and are likely responsible for the observed thickening of the skin. Finally, the basal keratinocytes were proposed to regulate cell motility and proliferation of the upper layers of keratinocytes and strengthen the epidermal basement membrane. These latter two studies show the rapidity, complexity and integration of the cellular responses in coho salmon to lice.

Immune transcripts upregulated in these studies consistently involve inflammation/type 1 helper T cell (Th1) response (caspase (*casp1*), interleukins (*il12b, il17d, il18, il1r2*)), cellular recruitment (*clec4, il8*, CC chemokine ligands (*ccl2, ccl10*)) and complement (*c5ar1*, complement factors (*cfJ, cfh*)), the latter likely involved in protection against secondary bacterial infection (Braden *et al.*, 2023; Salisbury *et al.*, 2024). Braden *et al.* (2023) also suggest the aggressive inflammatory cascade resembles an allergic reaction, which may in part be due to tissue-resident macrophages sensing chitin and/or carbohydrate pathogen-associated molecular patterns (PAMPs). These molecules interact with pattern recognition receptors (PRRs) such as mannose-binding macrophage receptor 1 (mrc1), a C-type lectin receptor (CLR), to initiate pro-inflammation effector molecules and cellular recruitment. Such responses are proposed to occur for coho salmon where significant expression of *mrc1*, acidic mammalian chitinase (*chia*), *il2b*, tumour necrosis factor-α (*tnfa*), *ccl2* and *il18*, together with signatures of macrophages, natural cytotoxic cells (NCCs) and cytotoxic T lymphocytes (CTLs), potentiates the initial Th1-response driven by chitin sensing. Thus, successful immunity of coho salmon is now thought to occur due to a multipronged response to parasite-derived carbohydrates, chitin-like molecules and/or secreted/excreted proteins (Fast *et al.*, 2003, 2005, 2007; Braden *et al.*, 2023).

While the coho salmon response can prevent >90% of settled copepodids from developing through the chalimus life stages (Fast *et al.*, 2002; Braden *et al.*, 2023; Sveen *et al.*, 2025), variability in resistance to *L. salmonis* exists in Atlantic salmon, just not to the same degree of effectiveness. Comparison of susceptible versus relatively resistant Atlantic salmon families highlighted expression differences in several immune response and pattern recognition genes against *C. rogercresseyi* (Robledo *et al.*, 2018). Similarly, family-based RNA sequencing studies in Atlantic salmon have shown immune-inflammatory response, tissue repair, apoptosis, cell adhesion and heat-shock responses are linked to differential family infection rates with *L. salmonis*, across multiple thermal regimes (Ghanei-Motlagh *et al.*, 2025b). This variation in family-based responses to sea lice infection has resulted in considerable effort to examine breeding resistance to sea lice in Atlantic salmon brood stock programmes. While brood stock genetics differ between company and farming region, heritability of resistance to sea lice has generally been estimated to be around 0.22, with studies ranging from as low as 0.1 to as high as 0.3 (Onabanjo *et al.*, 2024). Significant genome-wide quantitative trait loci (QTLs) associated with reduced lice load have also been variable across studies, with strong signals in European Atlantic salmon being associated with chromosomes Ssal 2, 5, 11 and 25 (Aslam *et al.*, 2023), whereas studies on North American Atlantic salmon have identified regions on chromosomes Ssal 4, 14 and 20 (Holborn *et al.*, 2019), and finally chromosomes Ssal 8 and 9 with *L. salmonis* resistance at 10°C, whereas chromosomes Ssal2 and 10 were identified with *L. salmonis* resistance at 20°C (Allen *et al.*, 2023). Across these studies QTLs have not been field validated over multiple year classes and differences exist in sample size, population of salmon studied, species and population structure of the louse, and whether the challenges were completed in land-based laboratories or sea cages. While improvement to lice resistance in Atlantic salmon breeding programmes will continue in all major salmon-farming regions, a major opposing force to any gains is the versatility of the parasite and its ability to immunomodulate its host.

Critical physiological and immunological disruption of the salmon host is created by sea lice, and these differ across parasitic life stage (Johnson and Fast, 2004; Wagner *et al.*, 2008). Uncontrolled and persistent inflammation, dampened/dysregulated immune responses and impaired tissue repair at attachment sites are all amplified by the adult life stage in comparison to chalimus stages, regardless of family background and potential reduced lice load (Ghanei-Motlagh *et al.*, 2025b). As with many other ectoparasitic species, *L. salmonis* secrete a suite of bioactive molecules highly evolved to manipulate the circulatory and immune system of their hosts, inhibiting or suppressing cellular immunity, blood clotting and wound healing and thereby contributing to successful parasitism of the host (Johnson *et al.*, 2002; Fast *et al.*, 2003, 2004, 2007; Kvamme *et al.*, 2004; Braden *et al.*, 2017; Heggland *et al.*, 2019). Multiple trypsin-like proteases have been identified in the mucus of *L. salmonis*-infected Atlantic salmon and studies by Fast *et al.* (2003, 2007) and Firth *et al.* (2000) were the first to identify and suggest that lice were secreting these proteins upon the host during infection. Since these initial characterizations, several hundred secretory/excretory proteins (SEPs) have been identified including serine-type endopeptidases, carboxypeptidases and cathepsins (Hamilton *et al.*, 2018). Two cathepsins, cathepsin L1 and L2, were identified in *L. salmonis* and are suggested to be involved in the digestion of host tissue, immunoevasion and successful establishment of the parasite on the host (McCarthy *et al.*, 2012). Furthermore, *L. salmonis* SEPs have even been demonstrated to have direct anti-chemotactic activity and inhibitory effects on the recruitment of immune cells at the site of attachment (Piesz *et al.*, 2020). These previous characterizations of SEPs for *L. salmonis* generated a list of putative virulence factors which share homology with other ectoparasitic species, supporting their putative roles and functions (Ribeiro, 1987; Ramachandra and Wikel, 1992; Firth *et al.*, 2000; Fast *et al.*, 2003, 2004, 2005, 2007; Braden *et al.*, 2017). Following up on an excellent characterization of the exocrine glands of *L. salmonis* by Øvergård *et al.* (2016), Øvergård *et al.* (2022) and Midtbø *et al.* (2024a,b) have since characterized several labial gland proteins with immune-dampening and even apoptotic activity against salmon leucocytes, with potential as vaccine candidates. Similarly, *C. elongatus*, which appears to induce an even greater immune-dampening impact than *L. salmonis*, has been shown to express multiple labial gland proteins orthologous to those in *L. salmonis* (Øvergård *et al.*, 2025). Further to these direct louse protein–host ligand/cell interactions, infection by *L. salmonis* has also been shown to drive upregulation of *socs3* (suppressor of cytokine signalling 3) and other *socs* orthologues, both in Atlantic salmon skin and head kidney transcriptomes (Salisbury *et al.*, 2024). In general, SOCS3 is described in other vertebrate host–pathogen interactions to have an inflammation-dampening impact (Carow and Rottenberg, 2014) and, alongside host cortisol induction described upon development to pre-adult/adult life stages, may contribute another indirect modification the louse induces to the host immune system.

22.4.3. Sea lice as vectors/contributors to other diseases

Sea lice have been a common parasite on farmed salmon, and as such have been associated with other infectious diseases affecting these hosts. As mentioned earlier (Section 22.4.2), infection with *L. salmonis* can have drastic impacts on the immunophysiology of the host, and this impacts downstream response to other infecting organisms. Microorganisms (*Aeromonas*, *Tenacibaculum*, *Pseudomonas* and *Vibrio*) have been cultured from internal and external surfaces of *L. salmonis* (Barker *et al.*, 2009). Other bacterial species that impact cultured salmon, such as *Moritella viscosa*, have been shown to be exacerbated by *L. salmonis* infection. Carvalho *et al.* (2020) showed increased impacts of co-infection of *L. salmonis* and *M. viscosa* with increasing lice load, and Parrish *et al.* (2019) showed that order of infection with these two common salmon pathogens impacted survival outcomes. Initial infection with *L. salmonis* significantly increased mortality when the secondary pathogen was *M. viscosa*, compared to *M. viscosa*-infected fish alone, or when initial infection was caused by *M. viscosa* then followed by *L. salmonis*. In all cases, inflammation was strongly induced in the skin of co-infected animals, and transcription levels of multiple CLRs (i.e. C-type lectin domain family 1 member A, B, E (*clec1a*, *clec1b*, *clec4e*) and C type 1 (*mrc1*)) were also significantly elevated in all co-infected groups (Cai *et al.*, 2022, 2024) and in sea lice-infested Atlantic salmon intraperitoneally injected with formalin-killed *Aeromonas salmonicida* (Caballero-Solares *et al.*, 2022). This suggests that it is an important immune pathway in Atlantic salmon skin in response to lice and *M. viscosa* infection and a target for immunotherapy.

Chang *et al.* (2023) also recently identified 32 previously unknown RNA viruses from *L. salmonis*, *Caligus clemensi* and *C. rogercresseyi*, which encompassed all existing phyla of RNA viruses. Virus-derived small RNAs contained highly conserved patterns, consistent with those infecting other arthropods, yet less than 2% of the transcripts in *C. clemensi* were assigned to other eukaryotes. The potential for these to emerge as fish pathogens needs further studies. Infectious salmon anaemia virus (ISAV) is listed by the World Organisation for Animal Health as it has frequently been associated with *L. salmonis* infection in Atlantic salmon, causing major disruptions to the salmon aquaculture industry. Laboratory examination of this relationship by Barker *et al.* (2019) showed the process of infestation by *L. salmonis* prior to ISAV exposure significantly increased the mortality and death rates of Atlantic salmon and was consistent across both Pennobscot and Saint John River Atlantic salmon strains. However, related work in *L. salmonis* was not able to confirm it acting as a vector or passively transporting the virus to naïve fish. The virus is easily passed through contaminated water, coprophagy and cohabitation with infected individuals, making the vector status of sea lice largely irrelevant, and a major risk due to the impact of lice infection on antiviral responses, both systemically and in the skin (Cai *et al.*, 2022; Zhong *et al.*, 2023). Finally, although multiple functional feeds exist that are able to successfully reduce lice loads, Carvalho *et al.* (2024) have shown in some cases these result in poor survival of co-infection, due to the immunological status induced.

22.5. Protective/Control Strategies

22.5.1. Non-medicinal control

Non-medical interventions have been increasingly pursued as resistance to current therapeutics becomes more prevalent. Barrett *et al.* (2020a) proposed two categories of preventive methods, the first of which is reducing encounters. The intention is to reduce encounters between the salmon and the infective copepodid stage, and the measures include, but are not limited to, the following. First, the designation of hydrographic and area management zones during a production cycle (Bron *et al.*, 1993); the effects of fallowing have been considerably underestimated and effective fallowing of farm sites in the same hydrographic or management area can delay the need for sea lice treatment within the first production year (Bron *et al.*, 1993). Physical barrier methods aim to exploit the behaviours of copepodids, which are often present within the first 2 m of the water column. Surface layers and a skirt made from permeable plankton mesh can be applied to pens to prevent copepodids from easily accessing the pen (Jónsdóttir *et al.*, 2023; Stien *et al.*, 2018); however, oxygen levels have been reported to decline when skirts are applied and require monitoring and management (Grøntvedt *et al.*, 2018). Furthermore, behavioural manipulation of the salmon has also been explored in hopes of maintaining salmon deeper in the pens and away from surface copepodids (Dempster *et al.*, 2009). The first of these approaches utilizes deep lighting regimes to promote activity and time spent deeper in the pens, the second involves the release of feed through specialized feeders deep within the pen (Hevrøy *et al.*, 2003; Barrett *et al.*, 2020a), and a further approach involves use of a 'snorkel cage' which utilizes a layer of netting below the surface to physically maintain salmon deep within the pens but still with access to an enclosed tube extending to the water surface to enable salmon to continue to reach the surface to take in air and fill the swim bladder (Oppedal *et al.*, 2019). Another behaviour exploitation method involves sea lice traps containing pheromone or other chemoattractant compounds to lure copepodids away from pens and capture them, although this method has not been assessed extensively or successful deployed yet (Ingvarsdóttir *et al.*, 2002). A more elaborate system is to prevent salmon–copepodid interactions while still at sea and involves fully enclosed cages, where water is filtered or pumped from deep sea water (Nilsen *et al.*, 2017). This closed containment system has the potential to eradicate lice settlement but is an expensive system to deploy and maintain with potential welfare issues. Novel and/or experimental barrier strategies include electrical fencing (Seafarm Pulse Guard system) which consists of vertical cables surrounding the pen and disruptive power pulses emitted throughout the adjacent waters (Barrett *et al.*, 2020a). Another novel method involves a barrier of air bubbles at the bottom of the net which disrupts copepodids from entering the pen (Barrett *et al.*, 2020a). Lastly, land-based aquaculture has been proposed, which would eliminate any interactions with sea lice or predators and provide a highly controlled environment; however, enormously high operating and investment costs, as well as potentially large carbon footprint and environmental impacts, leave such an operation currently unviable from an economic standpoint (Martin *et al.*, 2021).

The second preventive category to reduce infection is targeted at post-settlement survival. Many wild salmonids have evolved an anadromous life cycle, returning to freshwater rivers to spawn, but also returning to brackish water intermittently to reduce lice burdens (Thorstad *et al.*, 2015). As discussed earlier (Section 22.3), the tight ideal salinity range for *L. salmonis* makes use of freshwater baths an option in several salmon-farming regions. Administration of bath treatments will be further discussed below, but essentially freshwater bath treatments can run from 4 to 24 h, largely reflective of logistical issues with the longer treatments (Bui *et al.*, 2023). Bui *et al.* (2023) found that single freshwater bath treatments and freshwater baths combined with other treatments had the greatest delousing efficacy, in comparison to thermal or mechanical treatments. Recent findings by Ghanei-Motlagh *et al.* (2025a) have also shown lack of development of egg strings after just a 4 h bath in fresh water, with no impact of selection towards freshwater tolerance after five generations of selection. While *L. salmonis* removed from the host cannot survive more than a few hours in fresh water (Ghanei-Motlagh *et al.*, 2025a), survival at mid-level or brackish-water salinities (<35 ppt but >0 ppt) needs further studies (Groner *et al.*, 2019).

Biological control involves cohabitation with 'cleaner fish' that consume the adult lice on salmon (Brooker *et al.*, 2018; Barrett *et al.*, 2020b). In Norway, salmon farms have historically relied on five main species of cleaner fish: (i) corkwing wrasse, *Symphodus melops*; (ii) goldsinny wrasse, *Ctenolabrus rupestris*; (iii) ballan wrasse, *Labrus bergylta*; (iv) rock cook or small-mouthed wrasse, *Centrolabrus exoletus*; and (v) Atlantic lumpfish, *Cyclopterus lumpus*. Ballan wrasse and Atlantic lumpfish were the two most commonly used fish species for cleaner fish management in salmonid farming. The number of wrasses used in the farms increased dramatically to over 21 million in 2016 from only a few million in the early 2000s (Gonzalez and de Boer, 2017). Poor fisheries landings and ability to produce a greater number of lumpfish through culture caused a shift to greater usage of lumpfish in Norway, from 10 million individuals in 2015 to almost 43 million in 2019. This was gradually reduced to 27 million in 2021. The decline was because of growing concern about their welfare and survival (e.g. cold winter temperatures, predation by salmon, stress/disease) in commercial salmon cages. The smaller wrasse species (goldsinny and rock cook) were preferred during the early salmon post-smolt phase, while the larger corkwing and especially ballan wrasse were large enough to delouse salmon during their second year in net pens, as smaller goldsinny and rock cook would be eaten by salmon. While lumpfish are used in Canada and the UK, these concerns remain alongside biosecurity risks.

Mechanical management strategies have the most success in managing sea lice infections post-settlement. The hydrolicer was introduced in 2018 to the Canadian Pacific coast and has since become the second most predominant strategy for sea lice mitigation behind in-feed treatments (DFO, 2020), whereas non-medicinal intervention in Norway has been the most common strategy since 2015. The hydrolicer systems are installed on barges and operate by pumping salmon from net pens into a treatment zone where pressured water and turbulence are generated to detach lice from the host surface before being returned to the net pen. The water is then filtered to prevent lice from being rereleased into the adjacent waters. Due to the limited release of industry data regarding this management strategy, details on the efficacy, impact on salmon welfare and mortalities are scarce. However, hydrolicer representatives have reported an impressive 82–100% removal of mobile lice. Currently, the impacts of this treatment on salmon health and welfare indicate reductions in short-term growth and sex-dependent effects on the diversity of the skin microbiome which may impact host health after farming manipulations (Walde *et al.*, 2022; Casadei *et al.*, 2023). Two other mechanical treatments similar to the hydrolicer system are available. These treatment technologies require the fish to be crowded and pumped into the treatment system for mechanical louse removal. Currently, the most is known about the FLS system where delousing efficiency was 81–100% removal of mobile lice according to a report by the Norwegian Veterinary Institute (Gismervik *et al.*, 2017). Thermal delousing is similar to the mechanical systems but is based on the disruption of lice after short exposures to warm water (Grøntvedt *et al.*, 2015; Nilsson *et al.*, 2023) compared to the robustness of salmonids at the same temperatures (Elliott and Elliott, 1995). There are two systems for thermal treatments: the Thermolicer® and the Optilicer®. In both systems, salmon are again crowded before being pumped into a thermal bath of sea water or fresh water, up to 36°C for between 20 and 30 s. Thermal treatments are often associated with greater salmon mortality when compared to similar management strategies. Another new commercially available control measure is optical or laser delousing. It is an innovation which utilizes an optical beam to directly target a louse. The automated camera system uses machine learning to recognize and target sea lice to kill them with a laser pulse. This does not impact the skin of salmon (Frenzl, 2017). Since this is new technology, there is little evidence on efficiency. However, in one study there was no difference in lice abundance on fish in cages with or without lasers after 54 days (Bui *et al.*, 2020).

22.5.2. Immunostimulation

Aside from genomic and pedigree-based selective breeding, gene editing of salmon has become an attractive tool to reduce the time to produce resistant Atlantic salmon. A solution would be to manipulate Atlantic salmon to mount an immune response similar to those in other resistant salmonids (e.g. coho salmon). By characterizing the genes important in coho salmon resistance, global research consortia (e.g. CRISPResist) are focusing on editing both species to determine the feasibility of knocking out/reducing or knocking in/inducing gene expression that promotes lice rejection in Atlantic salmon (Robinson *et al.*, 2022). Through understanding the functional mechanisms involved in lice rejection, better breeding strategies and potentially future farming of edited fish may become a reality. Ethical and environmental concerns of using edited fish in the open cage environment must be considered, but solutions in this realm are still some years away.

Functional feeds aim to utilize immunostimulant additives to better prime the mucosal-associated lymphoid tissues of Atlantic salmon against sea lice and other pathogens and would be an easily administered management strategy (Eslamloo *et al.*, 2017; Martin and Król, 2017; Xue *et al.*, 2019; Cai *et al.*, 2022). These feeds often include compounds aimed to stimulate the general innate or inflammation immune pathways in Atlantic salmon and have reduced *L. salmonis* abundancies. However, lack of additional evidence regarding the efficacy of available or novel functional feeds and variations in costs associated with production have hindered full deployment. Feeds that reduce lice cannot be considered in isolation from other pathogens and while studies have shown up to 30–50% reductions in lice numbers in some cases, these reductions need to be assessed in concert with the potential for increased risk of other diseases (e.g. ISAV).

One strategy which has been pursued for three decades would be development of a viable vaccine against *L. salmonis*. Sea louse vaccine development efforts began in the mid-1990s, and the majority were pilot investigations of crude whole louse preparations; however, no commercial vaccine is currently on the market (Grayson *et al.*, 1995; Roper *et al.*, 1995; reviewed in Woo, 1997). Benefits of vaccination of Atlantic salmon against *L. salmonis* compared to administration of anti-sea-louse medications include sustained action and no period of withdrawal or residual chemicals within the salmon flesh. Vaccines are often designed to directly target the parasites and have the advantage of being unlikely induce resistance; or, if it does occur, it can be counteracted through modification or inclusion of a new antigenic component(s).

Gut antigens used in the cattle tick vaccines have provided the proof-of-concept (Rodriguez-Mallon, 2023) and provide an alternative pathway to circumvent issues in obtaining natural immunity; however, this has yet to be done successfully. This has been used to develop novel *L. salmonis* vaccines for several years, investigating potential antigens within the digestive tract of the louse (Raynard *et al.*, 2002; Carpio *et al.*, 2011; Casuso *et al.*, 2019). However, no antigens identified in sea lice were able to produce results as successful as those against the cattle tick. It has been suggested the lack of success is due to differences in the gut environment of sea lice compared to their terrestrial counterparts. The gut-antigen approach requires sufficient similarity to their mammalian haematophagous parasite counterparts to ensure sufficient antigen and antibody contact occurs. Cattle ticks take substantial blood meals at multiple times per day, while salmon lice only tend to feed on blood at the pre-adult/adult stages and blood makes up only a portion of their diet. Thus, this calls into question whether sufficient antibodies would be taken up by the louse to elicit a protective response or whether a critical gut-associated antigen capable of producing the desired immune response can be identified at low concentrations of antibody.

Currently, one gut-associated vaccine has demonstrated a negative correlation between adult lice counts and antigen-specific immunoglobulin M (IgM) levels in Atlantic salmon plasma in a dose-dependent manner after vaccination (Tartor *et al.*, 2021). P33 is the targeted lice-gut antigen expressed as a recombinant protein and used to vaccinate Atlantic salmon in the laboratory, providing support that despite the challenges associated with the louse gut environment there may still be potential for exploiting the haematophagous nature of the louse if the correct antigen can be identified. While overall reductions in adult lice burdens were negatively correlated post-vaccination for this antigen, further investigation would be beneficial on whether the reduction translates into any biological relevance in the field. Other studies such as Rodríguez *et al.* (2025) have examined other recombinant virulence and development targets for *L. salmonis*, with efficacy demonstrated in the laboratory, and the potential for next-phase field studies. However, there is still no current commercial vaccine against sea lice in aquaculture.

22.5.3. Medicinal treatment

Initially, treatment of sea lice relied on a group of approved chemotherapeutics which belong to five chemical classes: pyrethroids, avermectins, organophosphates, benzoylphenyl ureas (BPUs) and hydrogen peroxide. Resistance to commonly used chemotherapeutics has become increasingly problematic. This led to the emergence of non-medicinal interventions (Sections 22.5.1 and 22.5.2). The 'development of an ability, in a strain of insects, to tolerate doses of toxicants which would prove lethal to the majority of individuals in a normal population of the same species' is a common definition used to define resistance to insecticides. For an excellent review on sea lice treatments and resistance development, the reader should consult Aaen *et al.* (2015) and Aldrin *et al.* (2023). Below, the history of commonly used and approved (either full approval or emergency release medication) chemotherapeutics applied in aquaculture, their putative mechanisms of action and proposed resistance mechanisms, as well as resistance reports for lice populations, are briefly detailed.

The first chemicals to control sea lice infections of salmon involved organophosphates (azamethiphos: Salmosan®, dichlorvos: Nuvan®, metrifonate or trichlorfon: Neguvon®) and have been used historically since 1974 in Norway, 1979 in Scotland, 1981 in Chile, 1990 in Canada and 1997 in the Faroe Islands (Aaen *et al.*, 2015), trichlorfon in Norway and dichlorvos in Scotland (Rae, 2002). These were the earliest chemotherapeutics used, administered as a bath treatment, often using full tarpaulins to gather salmon and enclose the whole of the treatment volume, and were highly successful. The mechanism of action involves the inhibition of acetylcholinesterase (AChE) in cholinergic synapses, preventing the termination of synaptic transmission and leading to overexcitation, paralysis and eventual death of the organism (Smissaert, 1964; Roth *et al.*, 1996). Mutations in the AChE gene have been attributed to resistance to these compounds in arthropods, with reports dating back to the 1960s (Denholm *et al.*, 2002), and a comparable mutation (missense Phe362Tyr) has been reported for one of the genes encoding AChE (*ace1a*) in *L. salmonis* populations in the North Atlantic (Kaur *et al.*, 2015). Trichlorfon is administered at 0.25 ppm for 1 h, dichlorvos is administered at 1 ppm for 1 h and azamethiphos is administered at 100 ppb for 30 min.

Another class of bath-administered chemotherapeutics are pyrethroids (cypermethrin: Excis® or Betamax®, deltamethrin: Alpha Max®), which have been used globally in aquaculture as early as 1994 in Norway, 1997 in the Faroe Islands and Scotland, 2006 in Ireland, 2007 in Chile and the emergency drug release for 2009–2010 in Canada (Aaen *et al.*, 2015). This chemical class disrupts neural signals through interference of voltage-dependent sodium channels, which results in depolarization caused by a prolonged influx of sodium ions during neural excitation leading to subsequent paralysis. Resistance in arthropods and non-target aquatic species has been reported, primarily achieved through enhanced drug metabolic functioning (Ffrench-Constant *et al.*, 2016). Overexpression of enzymes such as cytochrome P450 (CYP), glutathione *S*-transferase, superoxide dismutase and reduced cuticle penetration have all been linked to pyrethroid resistance in several arthropods (Rinkevich *et al.*, 2013; Weston *et al.*, 2013; Xu *et al.*, 2013). Similar resistance mechanisms to pyrethroids are suspected in sea lice (Sevatdal *et al.*, 2005; Marín *et al.*, 2015a). Pyrethroids are administered as baths in aquaculture: deltamethrin is administered at 0.2 ppb for 30 min and cypermethrin is administered at 15 ppb for 30 min. Environmental footprint and impact on non-target species have hampered use of pyrethroids in areas such as Canada, due to potential impacts on the American lobster (*Homarus americanus*), whereas the use of hydrogen peroxide baths has a much-reduced ecological risk.

Hydrogen peroxide (Interox Paramove 50®) has been utilized to treat *L. salmonis* infestations in Norway (1993–1997, 2009 to date), Scotland (1993–1999, 2009 to date), the Faroe Islands (1991–1992), Chile (2007 to date), Ireland (1987–2000) and Canada (2014 to date), and is often administered in baths at a dose of 1500 ppm for 20 min. Although the mechanism of action has not been fully elucidated, it has been proposed that gas bubbles formed within the haemolymph of the louse result in detachment from the host surface (Bruno and Raynard, 1994). As with the other bath treatments, reduced efficacy of hydrogen peroxide has been detected in multiple farming regions (Helgesen *et al.*, 2015; Van Iderstine *et al.*, 2020).

The above treatments are all administered as baths either through tarps surrounding cages, or through pumping fish into well-boats, which provides greater control of treatment dose and exposure time.

Macrocyclic lactones (emamectin benzoate: SLICE®, ivermectin: Ivomec®) include one of the newer additions to treatment rotations, emamectin benzoate, and its earliest use was in 1998 in Norway, since 1999 in Canada, Chile and the Faroe Islands, and since 2000 in Scotland (Aaen *et al.*, 2015). These compounds are administered in-feed and operate through activation of glutamate- and γ-aminobutyric acid (GABA)-gated chloride channels, resulting in reduced cell excitability and suppression of muscle contraction (Geary and Moreno, 2012; Wolstenholme and Kaplan, 2012). Resistance reported in arthropods and lice is attributed to overexpression of similar detoxification enzymes as with pyrethroids, as well as some evidence for changes in glutamate- and histidine-gated ion channel genes (Igboeli *et al.*, 2012; Carmichael *et al.*, 2013; Poley *et al.*, 2015; Sutherland *et al.*, 2015). Ivermectin is administered at 0.07 mg/kg fish for 3 weeks, while emamectin benzoate is administered at 50 mg/kg fish per day for 7 days. Reduced efficacy of emamectin benzoate became evident in different farming regions initially in 2006–2008. Besnier *et al.* (2014) and Messmer *et al.* (2018) have identified regions in chromosome 5 associated with this resistance in both subspecies of *L. salmonis*, in the Atlantic and Pacific, respectively. Diagnostic tests continue to be pursued for emamectin benzoate resistance, among other treatment resistance targets, to provide the global industry with better understanding of drug resistance spread and areas where treatments can still be used.

BPUs (teflubenzuron: Calicide™, diflubenzuron: Lepsidon™, lufenuron: Imvixa™, hexaflumuron: Alpha Flux™) are chemicals which inhibit chitin synthesis, often resulting in abnormal utilization, production and deposition of chitin resulting in the inability of an organism to successfully detach from the exuvium during moulting (Merzendorfer, 2013). Currently, BPUs are the only chemical class used to treat sea lice to which no resistance has been reported, although resistance in terrestrial arthropods has been associated with both overexpression of CYPs or polymorphisms associated with the chitin synthase 1 gene (Douris *et al.*, 2016). Hexaflumuron is administered as an immersion treatment on well-boats often at 2 ppm for 2 h. Teflubenzuron and diflubenzuron are administered in-feed at a dose of 10 mg/kg fish per day for 7 days and 6 mg/kg fish per day for 14 days, respectively. These feeds are top coated with either compound but have relatively poor absorption across the gastrointestinal tract of salmonids. Thus, uneaten medicated pellets, particulate waste spread to surrounding water, and sediment or spillover during bath immersions have led to ecological concerns for non-target species such as king crab, shrimp and lobsters, especially if moulting is imminent (Olsvik *et al.*, 2015; Samuelsen *et al.*, 2015; Parsons *et al.*, 2021). Teflubenzuron has been used in Scotland (2007–2013), Ireland (2006–2012), the Faroe Islands (1997, 2011 to date) and Norway (1996–2001, 2009 to date), while diflubenzuron has been used in the Faroe Islands (1997, 2011 to date), Norway (1996–2000, 2009 to date) and Chile (2009 to date). Lufenuron is the latest BPU to be introduced in Chilean aquaculture and is administered in-feed at a dose of 5 mg/kg fish per day for 7 days. Currently, use is limited to freshwater hatcheries prior to seawater transfer with a minimum 7-day holding period to remove residual particulates and provide long-term protection against larval stages of sea lice (Poley *et al.*, 2018; Olsvik *et al.*, 2024).

Ectosan® (containing imidacloprid), is a neonicotinoid and received market authorization in Norway in 2021, the first medicinal treatment with an active substance from a new chemical class that has been present in the Norwegian market for more than 20 years (Aldrin *et al.*, 2023). This new bath treatment is used in conjunction with a water purification system (CleanTreat®) to prevent environmental release of the compound, which can have strong non-target species toxicity. The mechanism of action of imidacloprid is unknown in sea lice but it is expected to bind to the nicotinic receptor and block nerve impulses. In *L. salmonis* the median lethal concentration value (LC_{50}) has been estimated to be 0.06 ppm (based on 30 min and 24 h exposure bioassays). Although being relatively new, imidacloprid has shown good efficacy in controlling adult sea lice with a mortality rate > 98% (Aldrin *et al.*, 2023). According to Aaen and Horsberg (2016), the effective dose is 50 ppm for a 30 min exposure and 5 ppm over 24 h, whereas in *C. rogercresseyi* the concentrations to immobilize 100% of adults are lower (González-Gómez *et al.*, 2025).

Resistance of *L. salmonis* to medicinal intervention has emerged as a major challenge in aquaculture following decades of reliance on chemotherapeutics across multiple chemical classes. Early treatments such as organophosphates and pyrethroids, while initially effective, lost efficacy as lice populations developed resistance through target-site mutations, enhanced detoxification and reduced cuticle penetration. As the industry has grown, so have options for treatment but macrocyclic lactones like emamectin benzoate also faced rapid, declining effectiveness, while hydrogen peroxide – though ecologically safer – has also shown reduced efficacy in several farming regions. BPUs, which inhibit chitin synthesis, remain the only chemical class without confirmed resistance in sea lice, though similar resistance has been observed in terrestrial arthropods; and the introduction of neonicotinoids such as imidacloprid represents a new chemical tool with high efficacy, though long-term resistance outcomes remain uncertain. Interconnected populations of *L. salmonis* across international borders adds difficulty in ensuring proper rotation and coordinated use of medicinal therapies. However, the repeated development of resistance highlights the evolutionary adaptability of sea lice, despite diversified treatment strategies, and the need for cautious use of new medicines and their integrated control across borders.

22.5.4. Implementation of integrated control strategies

In the northern hemisphere, Norway has the most stringent baseline thresholds for reporting and treatment of *L. salmonis*; requiring less than 0.2 adult lice per fish during the sensitive period (i.e. the time span juvenile wild salmonids are out-migrating from rivers to sea and at their most vulnerable stage, often 1 May – 31 June). Furthermore, in 2017 Norway adopted a new, area-based management system that regulates aquaculture biomass based on sea lice infestation levels in the wild, known as the 'Traffic Light System'. The coastline of Norway was split into 13 production areas and risk assessments for wild salmon mortality based on a combination of hydrodynamic dispersion models, which predict the spread of lice larvae from production sites based on lice levels, sea temperature and water currents, and data from the national surveillance programme for salmon lice on wild salmon. Dependent on risk level (green, yellow or red) this system determines the number of salmon allowed in a given production area. While policies in Norway are driven by potential impacts on wild populations of salmon, in other countries treatment thresholds often lack scientific consensus regarding the impact farm sites may have on wild populations and policy is driven based on both reducing the impacts on wild salmonids and the welfare of the cultured salmon. Ireland and the Faroe Islands require implementation of reporting and treatment when mature lice exceed 0.5 per fish, while in Canada (British Columbia) lice burden cannot exceed 3.0 motile lice (equivalent to approximately 0.9 adult female lice) per fish in the sensitive period. This is a threshold value and if the value is higher, the farm must implement measures to reduce lice levels below 3.0 within 42 days. Scotland requires fewer than 2.0 lice per fish and has begun to implement a similar traffic light system inspired by that of Norway. Currently, Scotland has no requirements concerning the sensitive period. The Aquaculture Stewardship Council requires any participant aquafarmers to maintain fewer than 0.1 lice per fish as an absolute requirement; however, this obligation is quite strict and often not easily attained, as several aquafarmers have had to request exemptions, and consideration to move away from this threshold must be discussed.

While conducting consistent monitoring of fish health status/lice loads and ensuring treatment thresholds are adhered to, integrated pest management control of sea lice in any region involves several factors. Fallowing between production cycles and stocking, along with integration of preventive tools (skirts, snorkels and other innovative cage designs) with cleaner fish and/or hatchery administration of protective medicines like lufenuron, can help prevent initial settlement and infection levels at the beginning of grow-out. Application of non-medicinal and medicinal treatments, alongside functional feeds with proven effect, needs to be synchronized and coordinated within the Area Bay Management (ABM). As new tools for control such as resistant strains of salmon, reduced grow-out periods at sea or vaccination become available, these too need to be integrated into a plan for the particular ABM.

References

Aaen, S.M. and Horsberg, T.E. (2016) A screening of multiple classes of pharmaceutical compounds for effect on preadult salmon lice *Lepeophtheirus salmonis*. *Journal of Fish Diseases* 39, 1213–1223. DOI: 10.1111/jfd.12463.

Aaen, S.M., Helgesen, K.O., Bakke, M.J., Kaur, K. and Horsberg, T.E. (2015) Drug resistance in sea lice: a threat to salmonid aquaculture. *Trends in Parasitology* 31(2), 72–81. DOI: 10.1016/j.pt.2014.12.006.

Aldrin, M., Huseby, R.B., Stige, L.C. and Helgesen, K.O. (2023) Estimated effectiveness of treatments against salmon lice in marine salmon farming. *Aquaculture* 574, 739749.

Allen, M., Danzmann, R., Rise, M.L., Gamperl, A.K., Garber, A. and Fast, M.D. (2023) Genomic architecture of sea lice resistance in Atlantic salmon at different thermal profiles. Presented at *Aquaculture Association of Canada Meeting*, 7–10 May, Victoria, British Columbia, Canada.

Aslam, M.L., Boison, S.A., Baranski, M., Norris, A., Gonen, S. *et al.* (2023) GWAS reveals multiple QTLs for sea lice resistance in Atlantic salmon (*Salmo salar*). In: *Aquaculture Europe 2023: Balanced Diversity in Aquaculture Development.* Spinger, Vienna, pp. 78–79.

Barker, D.E., Braden, L.M., Coombs, M.P. and Boyce, B. (2009) Preliminary studies on the isolation of bacteria from sea lice, *Lepeophtheirus salmonis*, infecting farmed salmon in British Columbia, Canada. *Parasitology Research* 105, 1173–1177.

Barker, S.E., Bricknell, I.R., Covello, J., Purcell, S., Fast, M.D. *et al.* (2019) Sea lice, *Lepeophtheirus salmonis* (Kroyer 1837), infected Atlantic salmon (*Salmo salar* L.) are more susceptible to infectious salmon anemia virus. *PLoS One* 14, e0209178.

Barrett, L.T., Oppedal, F., Robinson, N. and Dempster, T. (2020a) Prevention not cure: a review of methods to avoid sea lice infestations in salmon aquaculture. *Reviews in Aquaculture* 12(4), 2527–2543. DOI: 10.1111/raq.12456.

Barrett, L.T., Overton, K., Stien, L.H., Oppedal, F. and Dempster, T. (2020b) Effect of cleaner fish on sea lice in Norwegian salmon aquaculture: a national scale data analysis. *International Journal for Parasitology* 50(10–11), 787–796. DOI: 10.1016/j.ijpara.2019.12.005.

Beamish, R.J., Neville, C.M., Sweeting, R.M. and Ambers, N. (2005) Sea lice on adult Pacific salmon in the coastal waters of central British Columbia, Canada. *Fisheries Research* 76, 198–208.

Bernot, J.P., Boxshall, G.A., Kihara, T.C. and Arbizu, P.M. (2025) An updated key to the genera of Caligidae (Copepoda: Siphonostomatoida). *Journal of Parasitology* 111, 10–25.

Besnier, F., Kent, M., Skern-Mauritzen, R., Lien, S., Malde, K. *et al.* (2014) Human-induced evolution caught in action: SNP-array reveals rapid amphi-Atlantic spread of pesticide resistance in the salmon ecotoparasite *Lepeophtheirus salmonis*. *BMC Genomics* 15(1), 937. DOI: 10.1186/1471-2164-15-937.

Bowers, J.M., Mustafa, A., Speare, D.J., Conboy, G.A., Brimacombe, M. *et al.* (2000) The physiological response of Atlantic salmon, *Salmo salar* L., to a single experimental challenge with sea lice, *Lepeophtheirus salmonis*. *Journal of Fish Diseases* 23(3), 165–172. DOI: 10.1046/j.1365-2761.2000.00225.x.

Braden, L.M., Sutherland, B.J.G., Koop, B.F. and Jones, S.R.M. (2017) Enhanced transcriptomic responses in the Pacific salmon louse *Lepeophtheirus salmonis oncorhynchi* to the non-native Atlantic Salmon *Salmo salar* suggests increased parasite fitness. *BMC Genomics* 18(1), 110. DOI: 10.1186/s12864-017-3520-1.

Braden, L.M., Michaud, D., Igboeli, O.O., Dundrop, M., Hamre, L. *et al.* (2020) Identification of critical enzymes in the salmon louse synthesis pathway as revealed by RNAi-mediated abrogation of infectivity. *International Journal for Parasitology* 50(10–11), 873–889. DOI: 10.1016/j.ijpara.2020.06.007.

Braden, L.M., Michaud, D., Groman, D., Byrne, P., Hori, T.S. and Fast, M.D. (2023) Rejection of *Lepeophtheirus salmonis* driven in part by chitin sensing is not impacted by seawater acclimitization in coho salmon (*Oncorhynchus kisutch*). *Scientific Reports* 13(1), 9685. DOI: 10.1038/s41598-023-36632-0.

Brandal, P.O., Egidius, E. and Romslo, I. (1976) Host blood: a major food component for the parasitic copepod *Lepeophtheirus salmonis* Kroyeri, 1838 (Crustacea: Caligidae). *Norwegian Journal of Zoology* 24(4), 341–343.

Bricknell, I. and Pietrak, M. (2023) A glimpse into the bio-physical environment of the sea louse (*Lepeophtheirus salmonis* (Krøyer 1837)) digestive tract. *Aquaculture* 562, 738744. DOI: 10.1016/j.aquaculture.2022.738744.

Bron, J.E., Sommerville, C., Jones, M. and Rae, G.H. (1991) The settlement and attachment of early stages of the salmon louse, *Lepeophtheirus salmonis* (Copepoda: Caligidae) on the salmon host *Salmo salar*. *Journal of Zoology* 224, 201–212.

Bron, J.E., Sommerville, C., Wootten, R. and Rae, G.H. (1993) Fallowing of marine Atlantic salmon, *Salmo salar* L., farms as a method for the control of sea lice, *Lepeophtheirus salmonis* (Krøyer, 1837). *Journal of Fish Diseases* 16, 487–493.

Brooker, A.J., Papadopoulou, A., Gutierrez, C., Rey, S., Davie, A. and Migaud, H. (2018) Sustainable production and use of cleaner fish for the biological control of sea lice: recent advances and current challenges. *Veterinary Record* 183(12), 383. DOI: 10.1136/vr.104966.

Bruno, D.W. and Raynard, R.S. (1994) Studies on the use of hydrogen peroxide as a method for the control of sea lice on Atlantic salmon. *Aquaculture International* 2(1), 10–18. DOI: 10.1007/BF00118529.

Bui, S., Geitung, L., Oppedal, F. and Barrett, L.T. (2020) Salmon lice survive the straight shooter: a commercial scale sea cage trial of laser delousing. *Preventive Veterinary Medicine* 181, 105063. DOI: 10.1016/j.prevetmed.2020.105063.

Bui, S., Skern, R., Saito, T. and Thompson, C. (2023) *Optimising Delousing Strategies: Developing Best Practice Recommendations for Maximal Efficacy and Positive Welfare*. Report commissioned by FHF on Project 15769. FHF (Norwegian Seafood Research Fund), Oslo.

Burka, J.F., Fast, M.D. and Revie, C.W. (2012) *Lepeophtheirus salmonis* and *Caligus rogercresseyi*. In: Woo, P.T.K and Buchmann, K. (eds) *Fish Parasites: Pathobiology and Protection*. CAB International, Wallingford, UK, pp. 350–370.

Caballero-Solares, A., Umasuthan, N., Xue, X., Katan, T., Kumar, S. *et al.* (2022) Interacting effects of sea louse (*Lepeophtheirus salmonis*) infection and formalin-killed *Aeromonas salmonicida* in Atlantic salmon skin transcriptome. *Frontiers in Immunology* 13, 804987. DOI: 10.3389/fimmu.2022.804987.

Cai, W., Kumar, S., Navaneethaiyer, U., Caballero-Solares, A., Carvalho, L.A. *et al.* (2022) Transcriptome analysis of Atlantic salmon (*Salmo salar*) skin in response to sea lice and infectious salmon anemia virus co-infection under different experimental functional diets. *Frontiers in Immunology* 12, 787033. DOI: 10.3389/fimmu.2021.787033.Cai, W.C., Zhong, L., Parrish, K., Kumar, S., Whyte, S.K. *et al.* (2024) Effects of single infection and different scenarios of co-infection with sea lice (*Lepeophtheirus salmonis*) and the bacteria *Moritella viscosa* on Atlantic salmon (*Salmo salar*): insights from global transcriptome analysis of the skin. *Aquaculture* 591, 741115.

Carmichael, S.N., Bron, J.E., Taggart, J.B., Ireland, J.H., Bekaert, M. *et al.* (2013) Salmon lice (*Lepeophtheirus salmonis*) showing varying emamectin benzoate susceptibilities differ in neuronal acetylcholine receptor and GABA-gated chloride channel mRNA expression. *BMC Genomics* 14(1), 408. DOI: 10.1186/1471-2164-14-408.

Carow, B. and Rottenberg, M.E. (2014) SOCS3, a major regulator of infection and inflammation. *Frontiers in Immunology* 5, 58.

Carpio, Y., Basabe, L., Acosta, J., Rodríguez, A., Mendoza, A. *et al.* (2011) Novel gene isolated from *Caligus rogercresseyi*: a promising target for vaccine development against sea lice. *Vaccine* 29(15), 2810–2820. DOI: 10.1016/j.vaccine.2011.01.109.

Carvalho, L.A., Whyte, S.K., Braden, L.M., Purcell, S.L., Manning, A.J. *et al.* (2020) Impact of co-infection with *Lepeophtheirus salmonis* and *Moritella viscosa* on inflammatory and immune responses of Atlantic salmon (*Salmo salar*). *Journal of Fish Diseases* 43(4), 459–473. DOI: 10.1111/JFD.13144.

Carvalho, L.A., Whyte, S.K., Purcell, S.L., Hay, T., Taylor, R.G. *et al.* (2024) Impacts of functional feeds on Atlantic salmon (*Salmo salar*) systemic immune responses to high and low levels of sea lice infection (*Lepeophtheirus salmonis*) and co-infection of sea lice and infectious salmon anemia virus. *Comparative Immunology Reports* 6, 2000147.

Casadei, E., Mani, A., Cisco, M., Vågnes, Ø., Salinas, I. and Patel, S. (2023) Sex-dependent effects of mechanical delousing on the skin microbiome of broodstock Atlantic salmon (*Salmo salar* L.). *Scientific Reports* 13(1), 10824. DOI: 10.1038/s41598-023-37670-4.

Casuso, A., Núñez-Acuña, G., Valenzuela-Muñoz, V., Leal, Y. and Gallardo-Escárate, C. (2019) Identification of peritrophins as potential vaccine candidates against sea lice: a reverse vaccinology approach. *Fish and Shellfish Immunology* 91, 393. DOI: 10.1016/j.fsi.2019.04.081.

Chang, T., Hunt, B.P.V., Hirai, J. and Suttle, C.A. (2023) Divergent RNA viruses infecting sea lice, major ectoparasites of fish. *PLoS Pathogens* 19(6), e1011386. DOI: 10.1371/journal.ppat.1011386.

Danzmann, R.G., Norman, J.D., Rondeau, E.B., Leong, J.S., Messmer, A.M. *et al.* (2018) A genetic linkage map for the salmon louse (*Lepeophtheirus salmonis*) evidence for high male:female recombination rates and assortative mating. *Molecular Genetics and Genomics* 294(2), 343–363. DOI: 10.1007/s00438-018-1513-7.

Dempster, T., Korsoen, O., Folkedal, O. Juell, J-E. and Oppedal, F. (2009) Submergence of Atlantic salmon (*Salmo salar* L.) commercial cale sea-cages: a potential short-term solution to poor surface conditions. *Aquaculture* 288, 254–263.

Denholm, I., Devine, G.J., Horsberg, T.E., Sevatdal, S., Fallang, A. *et al.* (2002) Analysis and management of resistance to chemotherapeutants in salmon lice, *Lepeophtheirus salmonis* (Copepoda: Caligidae). *Pest Management Science* 58(6), 528–536. DOI: 10.1002/ps.482.

DFO (2020) *Regulating and Monitoring British Columbia's Marine Finfish Aquaculture Facilities*. Catalogue No. Fs141-3E-PDF. Fisheries and Oceans, Nanaimo, British Columbia, Canada.

Douris, V., Steinbach, D., Panteleri, R., Livadaras, I., Pickett, J.A. *et al.* (2016) Resistance mutation conserved between insects and mites unravels the benzoylurea insecticide mode of action on chitin biosynthesis. *Proceedings of the National Academy of Sciences USA* 113(51), 14692–14697. DOI: 10.1073/pnas.1618258113.

Eichner, C., Hamre, L.A. and Nilsen, F. (2014) Instar growth and molt increments in *Lepeophtheirus salmonis* (Copepoda: Caligidae) chalimus larvae. *Parasitology International* 64(1), 86–96. DOI: 10.1016/j.parint.2014.10.006.

Elliott, J.M. and Elliott, J.A. (1995) The effect of the rate of temperature increase on the critical thermal maximum for parr of Atlantic salmon and brown trout. *Journal of Fish Biology* 47(5), 917–919. DOI: 10.1111/j.1095-8649.1995.tb06014.x.

Eslamloo, K., Xue, X., Hall, J.R., Smith, N.C., Caballero-Solares, A. *et al.* (2017) Transcriptome profiling of antiviral immune and dietary fatty acid dependent responses of Atlantic salmon macrophage-like cells. *BMC Genomics* 18(1), 706. DOI: 10.1186/s12864-017-4099-2.

Fast, M.D. and Dalvin, S. (2020) Lepeophtheirosis (*Lepeophtheirus salmonis*). In: Woo, P.T.K., Leong, J.-A. and Buchmann, K. (eds) *Climate Change and Infectious Fish Diseases*. CABI International, Wallingford, UK, pp. 471–498.

Fast, M.D., Ross, N.W., Mustafa, A., Sims, D.E., Johnson, S.C. *et al.* (2002) Susceptibility of rainbow trout *Oncorhynchus mykiss*, Atlantic salmon *Salmo salar* and coho salmon *Oncorhynchus kisutch* to experimental infection with sea lice *Lepeophtheirus salmonis*. *Diseases of Aquatic Organisms* 52, 57–68.

Fast, M.D., Burka, J.F., Johnson, S.C. and Ross, N.W. (2003) Enzymes released from *Lepeophtheirus salmonis* in response to mucus from different salmonids. *Journal of Parasitology* 89, 7–13.

Fast, M.D., Ross, N.W., Craft, C.A., Locke, S.J., MacKinnon, S.L. and Johnson, S.C. (2004) *Lepeophtheirus salmonis*: characterization of prostaglandin E_2 in secretory products of the salmon louse by RP-HPLC and mass spectrometry. *Experimental Parasitology* 107, 5–13.

Fast, M.D., Ross, N.W. and Johnson, S.C. (2005) Prostaglandin E_2 modulation of gene expression in an Atlantic salmon (*Salmo salar*) macrophage-like cell line (SHK-1). *Developmental and Comparative Immunology* 29, 951–963.

Fast, M.D., Muise, D.M., Easy, R.E., Ross, N.W. and Johnson, S.C. (2006a) The effects of successive *Lepeophtheirus salmonis* infections on the immunological status of Atlantic salmon (*Salmo salar*). *Fish and Shellfish Immunology* 21, 228–241.

Fast, M.D., Ross, N.W., Muise, D.M. and Johnson, S.C. (2006b) Differential gene expression in Atlantic salmon, *Salmo salar*, infected with *Lepeophtheirus salmonis* (Copepoda: Caligidae). *Journal of Aquatic Animal Health* 18, 116–127.

Fast, M.D., Johnson, S.C., Eddy, T.D., Pinto, D. and Ross, N.W. (2007) *Lepeophtheirus salmonis* secretory/excretory products and their effects on salmonid immune gene regulation. *Parasite Immunology* 29, 179–189.

Ffrench-Constant, R.H., Williamson, M.S., Davies, T.G.E. and Bass, C. (2016) Ion channels as insecticide targets. *Journal of Neurogenetics* 30(3–4), 163–177. DOI: 10.1080/01677063.2016.1229781.

Firth, K.J., Johnson, S.C. and Ross, N.W. (2000) Characterization of proteases in the skin mucus of Atlantic salmon (*Salmo salar*) infected with the salmon louse (*Lepeophtheirus salmonis*) and in whole-body louse homogenates. *Journal of Parasitology* 86, 1199–1205.

Finstad, B., Bjørn, P.A. and Nilsen, S.T. (1995) Survival of salmon lice, *Lepeophtheirus salmonis* Krøyer, on Arctic charr, *Salvelinus alpinus* (L.), in fresh water. *Aquaculture Research* 26(10), 791–795. DOI: 10.1111/j.1365-2109.1995.tb00871.x.

Frenzl, B. (2017) Lasers against parasites: revolutionizing the control of sea louse in Atlantic farmed salmon. *The Journal of Ocean Technology* 12, 92–93.

Geary, T.G. and Moreno, Y. (2012) Macrocyclic lactone anthelmintics: spectrum of activity and mechanism of action. *Current Pharmaceutical Biotechnology* 13(6), 866–872. DOI: 10.2174/138920112800399077.

Ghanei-Motlagh, R., Whyte, S.K., Soto-Davila, M., Fajei, E., Guevara, M. *et al.* (2025a) Salinity tolerance is not impacted in *Lepeophtheirus salmonis* over 5 generations of treatment selection. Presented at *Workshop on Freshwater and Combination Treatment Against Lice*, 20 February, Trondheim, Norway.

Ghanei-Motlagh, R., Garber, A., Cai, W.C., Poley, J.D., Whyte, S.K. *et al.* (2025b) Sea lice (*Lepeophtheirus salmonis*) life stage impacts Atlantic salmon transcriptomic responses under different thermal profiles. *Frontiers in Genetics* 16, 1633603. DOI: 10.3389/fgene.2025.1633603.

Gismervik, K., Nielsen, K.V., Lind, M.B. and Viljugrein, H. (2017) *Mekanisk avlusing med FLS-avlusersystem (Mechanical Delousing with the FLS Delousing System)*. Rapport 6 – 2017. Norwegian Veterinary Institute, Ås, Norway.

Godwin, S.C., Dill, L.M., Reynolds, J.D. and Krkošek, M. (2015) Sea lice, sockeye salmon, and foraging competition: lousy fish are lousy competitors. *Canadian Journal of Fisheries and Aquatic Sciences* 72(7), 1113–1120. DOI: 10.1139/cjfas-2014-0284.

González, E.B. and de Boer, F. (2017) The development of the Norwegian wrasse fishery and the use of wrasse as cleaner fish in the salmon aquaculture industry. *Fisheries Science* 83, 661–670.

González, L. and Carvajal, J. (2003) Life cycle of *Caligus rogercresseyi*, (Copepoda: Caligidae) parasite of Chilean reared salmonids. *Aquaculture* 220(1–4), 101–117.

González-Alanis, P., Wright, G.M., Johnson, S.C. and Burka, J.F. (2001) Frontal filament morphogenesis in the salmon louse *Lepeophtheirus salmonis*. *Journal of Parasitology* 87, 561–574.

González-Gómez, M.P., Campanini-Salinas, J., Olmos-Iturrieta, P., Peralta, A., Espinoza, M. and Mancilla-Schulz, J. (2025) Antiparasitic effect of imidacloprid on the copepodite and adult stages of *Caligus rogercresseyi*. *Aquaculture* 596(2), 741878.

Grayson, T.H., John, R.J., Wadsworth, S., Greaves, K., Cox, D. *et al.* (1995) Immunization of Atlantic salmon against the salmon louse: identification of antigens and effects on louse fecundity. *Journal of Fish Biology* 47(sA), 85–94. DOI: 10.1111/j.1095-8649.1995.tb06046.x.

Grimnes, A. and Jakobsen, P.J. (1996) The physiological effects of salmon lice infection on post-smolt of Atlantic salmon. *Journal of Fish Biology* 48(6), 1179–1194. DOI: 10.1111/j.1095-8649.1996.tb01813.x.

Groner, M.L., Laurin, E., Stormoen, M., Sanchez, J., Fast, M.D. and Revie, C.W. (2019) Evaluating the potential for sea lice to evolve freshwater tolerance as a consequence of freshwater treatments in salmon aquaculture. *Aquaculture Environment Interactions* 11, 507–519.

Grøntvedt, R.N., Nervikbø, I., Viljugrein, H., Lillehaug, A., Nilsen, H. and Gjevre A. (2015) *Thermal De-licing of Salmonid Fish – Documentation of Fish Welfare and Effect*. Rapport 13–2015. Norwegian Veterinary Institute, Oslo, p. 32.

Grøntvedt, R.N., Kristoffersen, A.B. and Jansen, P.A. (2018) Reduced exposure of farmed salmon to salmon louse (*Lepeophtheirus salmonis* L.) infestation by use of plankton nets: estimating the shielding effect. *Aquaculture* 495, 865–872. DOI: 10.1016/j.aquaculture.2018.06.069.

Hamilton, S., McLean, K., Monaghan, S.J., McNair, C., Inglis, N.F. *et al.* (2018) Characterisation of proteins in excretory/secretory products collected from salmon lice, *Lepeophtheirus salmonis*. *Parasites and Vectors* 11(1), 294. DOI: 10.1186/s13071-018-2885-6.

Hamre, L.A., Eichner, C., Caipang, C.M.A., Dalvin, S.T., Bron, J.E. *et al.* (2013) The salmon louse *Lepeophtheirus salmonis*) (Copepoda: Caligidae) life cycle has only two chalimus stages. *PLoS One* 8(9), e73539. DOI: 10.1371/journal.pone.0073539.

Hamre, L.A., Bui, S., Oppedal, F., Skern-Mauritzen, R. and Dalvin, S. (2019) Development of the salmon louse *Lepeophtheirus salmonis* parasitic stages in temperatures ranging from 3 to 24°C. *Aquaculture Environment Interactions* 11, 429–443. DOI: 10.3354/aei00320.

Harðardóttir, H.M., Male, R., Nilsen, F., Eichner, C., Dondrup, M. and Dalvin, S. (2019) Chitin synthesis and degradation in *Lepeophtheirus salmonis*: molecular characterization and gene expression profile during synthesis of a new exoskeleton. *Comparative Biochemistry and Physiology Part A: Molecular & Integrative Physiology* 227, 123–133.

Harðardóttir, H.M., Male, R., Nilsen, F. and Dalvin, S. (2021) Chitin synthases are critical for reproduction, molting, and digestion in the salmon louse (*Lepeophtheirus salmonis*). *Life* 11(1), 47.

Heggland, E.I., Eichner, C., Støve, S.I., Martinez, A., Nilsen, F. and Dondrup, M. (2019) A scavenger receptor B (CD36)-like protein is a potential mediator of intestinal heme absorption in the hematophagous ectoparasite *Lepeophtheirus salmonis*. *Scientific Reports* 9(1), 4218. DOI: 10.1038/s41598-019-40590-x.

Heggland, E.I., Dondrup, M., Nilsen, F. and Eichner, C. (2020) Host gill attachment causes blood-feeding by the salmon louse (*Lepeophtheirus salmonis*) chalimus larvae and alters parasite development and transcriptome. *Parasites and Vectors* 13, 225.

Helgesen, K.O., Romstad, H., Aaen, S.M. and Horsberg, T.E. (2015) First report of reduced sensitivity towards hydrogen peroxide found in the salmon louse *Lepeophtheirus salmonis* in Norway. *Aquaculture Reports* 1, 37–42. DOI: 10.1016/j.aqrep.2015.01.001.

Heuch, P.A., Parsons, A. and Boxaspen, K. (1995) Diel vertical migration: a possible host finding mechanism in salmon lice (*Lepeophtheirus salmonis*) copepodids? *Canadian Journal of Fisheries and Aquatic Sciences* 52, 681–689.

Heuch, P.A., Nordhagen, J.R. and Schram, T.A. (2000) Egg production in the salmon louse [*Lepeophtheirus salmonis* (Krøyer)] in relation to origin and water temperature. *Aquaculture Research* 31, 805–814.

Hevrøy, E.M., Boxaspen, K., Oppedal, F., Taranger, G.L. and Holm, J.C. (2003) The effect of artificial light treatment and depth on the infestation of the sea louse *Lepeophtheirus salmonis* on Atlantic salmon (*Salmo salar* L.) culture. *Aquaculture* 220(1–4), 1–14. DOI: 10.1016/S0044-8486(02)00189-8.

Holborn, M.K., Rochus, C.M., Ang, K.P., Elliott, J.A.K., Leadbeater, S. *et al.* (2019) Family-based genome wide association analysis for salmon lice (*Lepeophtheirus salmonis*) resistance in North American Atlantic salmon using a 50 K SNP array. *Aquaculture* 517, 734215.

Hull, M.Q., Pike, A.W., Mordue (Luntz), A.J. and Rae, G.H. (1998) Patterns of pair formation and mating in an ectoparasitic caligid copeopod *Lepeophtheirus salmonis* (Krøyer, 1837): implications for its sensory and mating biology. *Philosophical Transactions of the Royal Society of London B* 353, 753–764.

Igboeli, O.O., Fast, M.D., Heumann, J. and Burka, J.F. (2012) Role of P-glycoprotein in emamectin benzoate (SLICE®) resistance in sea lice, *Lepeophtheirus salmonis*. *Aquaculture* 344–349, 40–47. DOI: 10.1016/j.aquaculture.2012.03.026.

Ingvarsdottir, A., Birkett, M.A., Duce, L., Genna, R.L., Mordue, W. *et al.* (2002) Role of semiochemicals in mate location by parasitic sea louse, *Lepeophtheirus salmonis*. *Journal of Chemical Ecology* 28, 2107–2117.

Jeong, J., Stormoen, M., Thakur, K.K. and Revie, C.W. (2021) Imperfect estimation of *Lepeophtheirus salmonis* abundance and its impact on salmon lice treatment on Atlantic salmon farms. *Frontiers in Marine Science* 8, 763206. DOI: 10.3389/fmars.2021.763206.

Johnson, S.C. and Albright, L.J. (1991a) The developmental stages of *Lepeophtheirus salmonis* (Krøyer, 1837) (Copepoda: Caligidae). *Canadian Journal of Zoology* 69, 929–950.

Johnson, S.C. and Albright, L.J. (1991b) Development, growth, and survival of *Lepeophtheirus salmonis* (Copepoda: Caligidae) under laboratory conditions. *Journal of the Marine Biological Association of the United Kingdom* 71, 425–436.

Johnson, S.C. and Albright, L.J. (1992a) Comparative susceptibility and histopathology of the host response of naïve Atlantic, Chinook, and coho salmon to experimental infection with *Lepeophtheirus salmonis* (Copepoda: Caligidae). *Diseases of Aquatic Organisms* 14, 179–193.

Johnson, S.C. and Albright, L.J. (1992b) Effects of cortisol implants on the susceptibility and the histopathology of the responses of naive coho salmon *Oncorhynchus kisutch* to experimental infection with *Lepeophtheirus salmonis* (Copepoda: Caligidae). *Diseases of Aquatic Organisms* 14, 195–205.

Johnson, S.C. and Fast, M.D. (2004) Interactions between sea lice and their hosts. In: Wiegertjes, G.F. and Flik, G. (eds) *Host–Parasite Interactions*. BIOS Scientific Publishers, Oxford, pp. 131–161.

Johnson, S.C., Ewart, K.V., Osborne, J.A., Delage, D., Ross, N.W. and Murray, H.M. (2002) Molecular cloning of trypsin cDNAs and trypsin gene expression in the salmon louse *Lepeophtheirus salmonis* (Copepoda: Caligidae). *Parasitology Research* 88, 789–796.

Jones, S.R.M., Prosperi-Porta, G., Kim, E., Callow, P. and Hargreaves, N.B. (2006) The occurrence of *Lepeophtheirus salmonis* and *Caligus clemensi* (Copepoda: Caligidae) on threespine stickleback *Gasterosteus aculeatus* in coastal British Columbia. *Journal of Parasitology* 92, 473–480.

Jones, S.R.M., Fast, M.D., Johnson, S.C. and Groman D.B. (2007) Differential rejection of salmon lice by pink and chum salmon: disease consequences and expression of proinflammatory genes. *Diseases of Aquatic Organisms* 75, 131–161.

Jónsdóttir, H., Bron, J.E., Wootten, R. and Turnbull, J.F. (1992) The histopathology associated with the pre-adult and adult stages of *Lepeophtheirus salmonis* on the Atlantic salmon, *Salmo salar* L. *Journal of Fish Diseases* 15(6), 521–527. DOI: 10.1111/j.1365-2761.1992.tb00684.x.

Jónsdóttir, K.E., Misund, A.U., Sunde, L.M., Schrøder, M.B. and Volent, Z. (2023) Lice shielding skirts through the decade: efficiency, environmental interactions, and rearing challenges. *Aquaculture* 562, 738817. DOI: 10.1016/j.aquaculture.2022.738817.

Kabata, Z. (1970) *Crustacea as Enemies of Fishes*. Fisheries Research Board of Canada, Nanaimo, British Columbia, Canada.

Kaur, K., Helgesen, K.O., Bakke, M.J. and Horsberg, T.E. (2015) Mechanism behind resistance against the organophosphate azamethiphos in salmon lice (*lepeophtheirus salmonis*). *PLoS ONE* 10(4), e0124220. DOI: 10.1371/journal.pone.0124220.

Krasnov A., Birkett, M., Caulfield, J., Foster, S., Fields, D.M. *et al.* (2024) Chemical communication between the host and salmon louse. Presented at *Aquaculture Europe*, 26–30 August, Copenhagen, Denmark.

Kvamme, B.O., Skern, R., Frost, P. and Nilsen, F. (2004) Molecular characterisation of five trypsin-like peptidase transcripts from the salmon louse (*Lepeophtheirus salmonis*) intestine. *International Journal for Parasitology* 34, 823–832.

MacKinnon, B.M. (2011) Response of the copepodid larvae of *Caligus elongatus* to light, and the ultrastructure of the eyes. *Canadian Journal of Fisheries and Aquatic Sciences* 50, 793–799.

Marín, S.L., Ibarra, R., Medina, M.H. and Jansen, P. (2015a) Sensitivity of *Caligus rogercresseyi* (Boxshall & Bravo 2000) to pyrethroids and azamethiphos measured using bioassay tests – a large scale spatial study. *Preventive Veterinary Medicine* 122, 33–41. DOI: 10.1016/j.prevetmed.2015.09.017.

Marín, S.L., Martin, R. and Lewis, R. (2015b) Effects of *Caligus rogercresseyi* (Boxshall & Bravo 2000) chalimus stage condition (dead, moribund, live) on the estimates of cypermethrin BETAMAX® efficacy. *Aquaculture Research* 46(1), 30–36.

Martin, S.A.M. and Król, E. (2017) Nutrigenomics and immune function in fish: new insights from omics technologies. *Developmental and Comparative Immunology* 75, 86–98. DOI: 10.1016/j.dci.2017.02.024.

Martin, S.J., Mather, C., Knott, C., Bavington, D. (2021) 'Landing' salmon aquaculture: ecologies, infrastructures and the promise of sustainability. *Geoforum* 123, 47–55. DOI: 10.1016/j.geoforum.2021.04.025.

McCarthy, E., Cunningham, E., Copley, L., Jackson, D., Johnston, D. *et al.* (2012) Cathepsin L proteases of the parasitic copepod, *Lepeophtheirus salmonis*. *Aquaculture* 356–357, 264–271. DOI: 10.1016/j.aquaculture.2012.05.007.

McGowan, M.J., Bron, J.E., Bekaert, M., Fields, D., Browman, H. *et al.* (2025) Free-swimming copepodids salmon lice (*Lepeophtheirus salmonis*) undergo a transcriptomic shift when exposed to salmonid host cues. Presented at *International Conference for Diseases of Fish and Shellfish*, 1–4 September, Heraklion, Greece.

Merzendorfer, H. (2013) Chitin synthesis inhibitors: old molecules and new developments. *Insect Science* 20(2), 121–138. DOI: 10.1111/j.1744-7917.2012.01535.x.

Messmer, A.M., Leong, J.S., Rondeau, E.B., Mueller, A., Despins, C.A. *et al.* (2018) A 200K SNP chip reveals a novel Pacific salmon louse genotype linked to differential efficacy of emamectin benzoate. *Marine Genomics* 40, 45–57. DOI: 10.1016/j.margen.2018.03.005.

Michaud, D., Poley, J.D. and Fast, M.D. (2019) Expression and evolution of sex-biased genes in salmon lice (*Lepeophtheirus salmonis*). *FACETS* 4, 254–274.

Midtbø, H.M.D., Borchel, A., Morton, H.C., Paley, R., Monaghan, S. *et al.* (2024a) Cell death induced by *Lepeophtheirus salmonis* labial gland protein 3 in salmonid fish leukocytes: a mechanism for disabling host immune responses. *Fish and Shellfish Immunology* 154, 109992. DOI: 10.1016/j.fsi.2024.109992.

Midtbø, H.M.D., Eichner, C., Hamre, L.A., Dondrup, M., Flesland, L. *et al.* (2024b) Salmon louse labial gland enzymes: implications for host settlement and immune modulation. *Frontiers in Genetics* 14, 1303898. DOI: 10.3389/fgene.2023.1303898.

Mordue (Luntz), A.J. and Birkett, M.A. (2009) A review of host finding behaviour in the parasitic sea louse, *Lepeophtheirus salmonis* (Caligidae: Copepoda). *Journal of Fish Diseases* 32, 3–13.

Mustafa, A., Conboy, G.A. and Burka, J.F. (2001) Life-span and reproductive capacity of sea lice, *Lepeophtheirus salmonis*, under laboratory conditions. *Aquaculture Association of Canada Special Publication* 4, 113–114.

Nilsen, A., Nielsen, K.V., Biering, E. and Bergheim, A. (2017) Effective protection against sea lice during the production of Atlantic salmon in floating enclosures. *Aquaculture* 466, 41–50. DOI: 10.1016/j.aquaculture.2016.09.009.

Nilsson, J., Barrett, L.T., Mangor-Jensen, A., Nola, V., Harboe, T. and Folkedal, O. (2023) Effect of water temperature and exposure duration on detachment rate of salmon lice (*Lepeophtheirus salmonis*); testing the relevant thermal spectrum used for delousing. *Aquaculture* 562, 738879. DOI: 10.1016/j.aquaculture.2022.738879.

Nolan, D.T., Reilly, P. and Bonga, S.W. (1999) Infection with low numbers of the sea louse *Lepeophtheirus salmonis* induces stress-related effects in postsmolt Atlantic salmon (*Salmo salar*). *Canadian Journal of Fisheries and Aquatic Sciences* 56(6), 947–959. DOI: 10.1139/f99-021.

Olsvik, P.A., Samuelsen, O.B., Agnalt, A.-L. and Lunestad, B.T. (2015) Transcriptional responses to teflubenzuron exposure in European lobster (*Homarus gammarus*). *Aquatic Toxicology* 167, 143–156. DOI: 10.1016/j.aquatox.2015.07.008.

Olsvik, P.A., Brokke, K.E., Samuelsen, O.B. and Hannisdal, R. (2024) Lufenuron treatment temporarily represses gene expression and affects the SUMO pathway in liver of Atlantic salmon. *Journal of Fish Diseases* 47(2), e13880. DOI: 10.1111/jfd.13880.

Onabanjo, O., Meuwissen, T., Aslam, M.L., Schmitt, A.O. and Dagnachew, B. (2024) Use of whole-genome sequence data for fine mapping and genomic prediction of sea louse resistance in Atlantic salmon. *Frontiers in Genetics* 15, 1381333. DOI: 10.3389/fgene.2024.1381333.

Oppedal, F., Bui, S., Stien, L., Overton, K. and Dempster, T. (2019) Snorkel technology to reduce sea lice infestations: efficacy depends on salinity at the farm site, but snorkels have minimal effects on salmon production and welfare. *Aquaculture Environment Interactions* 11, 445–457. DOI: 10.3354/aei00321.

Øvergård, A.C., Hamre, L.A., Harasimczuk, E., Dalvin, S., Nilsen, F. and Grotmol, S. (2016) Exocrine glands of *Lepeophtheirus salmonis* (Copepoda: Caligidae): distribution, developmental appearance and site of secretion. *Journal of Morphology* 277, 1616–1630.

Øvergård, A.C., Midtbø, H.M.D., Hamre, L.A., Dondrup, M., Bjerga, G.E.K. *et al.* (2022) Small, charged proteins in salmon louse (*Lepeophtheirus salmonis*) secretions modulate Atlantic salmon (*Salmo salar*) immune responses and coagulation. *Scientific Reports* 12, 7995. DOI: 10.1038/s41598-022-11773.

Øvergård, A.C., Borchel, A., Eichner, C., Hjertaker, S., Nagata, J. *et al.* (2025) The generalist *Caligus elongatus* is better at dampening the Atlantic salmon immune response than the salmonid specialist *Lepeophtheirus salmonis*. *Fish and Shellfish Immunology* 160, 110225.

Parent, M.I., Stryhn, H., Hammell, K.L., Fast, M.D., Grant, J. and Vanderstichel, R. (2024a) Predicting the dispersal of *Lepeophtheirus salmonis* in the Bay of Fundy, New Brunswick. *Journal of Aquatic Animal Health* 36(4), 355–373. DOI: 10.1002/aah.10235.

Parent, M.I., Stryhn, H., Hammell, K.L., Grant, J. and Vanderstichel, R. (2024b) Estimation and comparison of connectivity measures for the dispersal of *Lepeophtheirus salmonis* sea lice among Atlantic salmon farms in New Brunswick, Canada. *Journal of Experimental Marine Biology and Ecology* 572, 151992.

Parrish, K.S., Purcell, S.L., Whyte, S.K., Manning, T., Taylor, R.G. *et al.* (2019) The effects of *Lepeophtheirus salmonis* and *Moritella viscosa* co-infection in Atlantic salmon physiology. Presented at *Ocean Frontiers Institute Researchers Workshop*, 18 November 2019, St. John's, Newfoundland, Canada.

Parsons, A.E., Samuelsen, O.B., Johnsen, I.A., Hannisdal, R., Tjensvoll, T. and Husa, V. (2021) Distribution and persistence of diflubenzuron and teflubenzuron in the marine environment around salmonid aquaculture facilities. *Frontiers in Marine Science* 8, 694577. DOI: 10.3389/fmars.2021.694577.

Piesz, J.L., Barker, S.E. and Bricknell, I.R. (2020) Anti-chemotactic activity in the secretory/excretory products of *Lepeophtheirus salmonis*. *Fish and Shellfish Immunology* 98, 296–300. DOI: 10.1016/j.fsi.2020.01.023.

Pietrak, M., Jensen, A., Zydlewksi, G.B. and Bricknell, I.R. (2019) The three-spined stickleback, *Gasterosteus aculeatus* Linnaeus 1758, plays a minor role as a host of *Lepeophtheirus salmonis* (Kroyer 1837) in the Gulf of Maine. *Journal of Fish Diseases* 42, 985–989.

Pike, A.W. and Wadsworth, S.L. (1999) Sealice on salmonids: their biology and control. *Advances in Parasitology* 44, 233–337.

Poley, J.D., Igboeli, O.O. and Fast, M.D. (2015) Towards a consensus: multiple experiments provide evidence for constitutive expression differences among sexes and populations of sea lice (*Lepeophtheirus salmonis*) related to emamectin benzoate resistance. *Aquaculture* 448, 445–450. DOI: 10.1016/j.aquaculture.2015.06.026.

Poley, J.D., Braden, L.M., Messmer, A.M., Igboeli, O.O., Whyte, S.K. *et al.* (2018) High level efficacy of lufenuron against sea lice (*Lepeophtheirus salmonis*) linked to rapid impact on moulting processes. *International Journal for Parasitology: Drugs and Drug Resistance* 8(2), 174–188. DOI: 10.1016/j.ijpddr.2018.02.007.

Rae, G.H. (2002) Sea louse control in Scotland, past and present. *Pest Management Science* 58(6), 515–520. DOI: 10.1002/ps.491.

Ramachandra, R.N. and Wikel, S.K. (1992) Modulation of host-immune responses by ticks (Acari: Ixodidae): effect of salivary gland extracts on host macrophages and lymphocyte cytokine production. *Journal of Medical Entomology* 29(5), 818–826. DOI: 10.1093/jmedent/29.5.818.

Raynard, R.S., Bricknell, I.R., Billingsley, P.F., Nisbet, A.J., Vigneau, A. and Sommerville, C. (2002) Development of vaccines against sea lice. *Pest Management Science* 58(6), 569–575. DOI: 10.1002/ps.474.

Ribeiro, J. (1987) Role of saliva in blood-feeding by arthropods. *Annual Review of Entomology* 32(1), 463–478.

Rinkevich, F.D., Du, Y. and Dong, K. (2013) Diversity and convergence of sodium channel mutations involved in resistance to pyrethroids. *Pesticide Biochemistry and Physiology* 106(3), 93–100. DOI: 10.1016/j.pestbp.2013.02.007.

Ritchie, G., Mordue (Luntz), A.J., Pike, A.W. and Rae, G.H. (1996) Observations on mating and reproductive behaviour of *Lepeophtheirus salmonis*, Krøyer (Copepoda: Caligidae). *Journal of Experimental Marine Biology and Ecology* 201(1–2), 285–298. DOI: 10.1016/0022-0981(96)00008-1.

Robinson, N.A., Robledo, D., Sveen, L., Ruiz-Daniels, R., Krasnov, A. *et al.* (2022) Application of genetic technologies to combat infectious diseases in aquaculture. *Reviews in Aquaculture* 15(2), 491–535. DOI: 10.1111/raq.12733.

Robledo, D., Gutiérrez, A.P., Barría, A., Yáñez, J.M. and Houston, R.D. (2018) Gene expression response to sea lice in Atlantic salmon skin: RNA sequencing comparison between resistant and susceptible animals. *Frontiers in Genetics* 9, 287. DOI: 10.3389/fgene.2018.00287.

Rodríguez, A., Gadan, K., Perez, L., Evensen, Ø., Estrada, M.P. and Carpio, Y. (2025) Prime-boost vaccination with chimeric antigens adjuvanted in Montanide™ ISA50 V2 confers protection against experimental *Lepeophtheirus salmonis* infestation in Atlantic salmon (*Salmo salar* L.). *Frontiers in Immunology* 16, 1570948. DOI: 10.3389/fimmu.2025.1570948.

Rodriguez-Mallon, A. (2023) The Bm86 discovery: a revolution in the development of anti-tick vaccines. *Pathogens* 12, 231.

Roper, J., Grayson, T.H., Jenkins, P.G., Hone, J.V., Wrathmell, A.B. *et al.* (1995) The immunocytochemical localisation of potential candidate vaccine antigens from the salmon louse *Lepeophtheirus salmonis* (Kroyer 1837). *Aquaculture* 132(3–4), 221–232. DOI: 10.1016/0044-8486(94)00402-A.

Ross, N.W., Firth, K.J., Wang, A., Burka, J.F. and Johnson, S.C. (2000) Changes in hydrolytic enzyme activities of naive Atlantic salmon (*Salmo salar*) skin mucus due to infection with the salmon louse (*Lepeophtheirus salmonis*) and cortisol implantation. *Diseases of Aquatic Organisms* 41, 43–51.

Roth, M., Richards, R.H., Dobson, D.P. and Rae, G.H. (1996) Field trials on the efficacy of the organophosphorus compound azamethiphos for the control of sea lice (Copepoda: Caligidae) infestation of farmed Atlantic salmon (*Salmo salar*). *Aquaculture* 140, 217–239.

Salisbury, S.J., Ruiz Daniels, R., Monaghan, S., Bron, J.E., Vallamayor, P.R. *et al.* (2024) Keratinocytes drive the epithelial hyperplasia key to sea lice resistance in coho salmon. *BMC Biology* 22, 160.

Samsing, F., Oppedal, F., Dalvin, S., Johnsen, I., Vagseth, T. and Dempster, T. (2016) Salmon lice (*Lepeophtheirus salmonis*) development times, body size, and reproductive outputs follow universal models of temperature dependence. *Canadian Journal of Fisheries and Aquatic Sciences* 73, 1841–1851.

Samuelsen, O.B., Lunestad, B.T., Hannisdal, R., Bannister, R., Olsen, S. *et al.* (2015) Distribution and persistence of the anti sea-lice drug teflubenzuron in wild fauna and sediments around a salmon farm, following a standard treatment. *Science of the Total Environment* 508, 115–121. DOI: 10.1016/j.scitotenv.2014.11.082.

Schram, T.A. (1993) Supplementary descriptions of the developmental stages of *Lepeophtheirus salmonis* (Krøyer, 1837) (Copepoda: Caligidae). In: Boxshall, G.A. and Defaye, D. (eds) *Pathogens of Wild and Farmed Fish: Sea Lice*. Ellis Horwood, Chichester, UK, pp. 30–47.

Serra-Llinarez, R.M., Bohn, T., Karlsen, O., Nilsen, R., Freitas, C. *et al.* (2020) Impacts of salmon lice on mortality, marine migration distance and premature return in sea trout. *Marine Ecology Progress Series* 635, 151–168.

Sevatdal, S., Magnusson, Å., Ingebrigtsen, K., Haldorsen, R. and Horsberg, T.E. (2005) Distribution of emamectin benzoate in Atlantic salmon (*Salmo salar* L.). *Journal of Veterinary Pharmacology and Therapeutics* 28, 101–107.

Smissaert, H.R. (1964) Cholinesterase inhibition in spider mites susceptible and resistant to organophosphate. *Science* 143(3602), 129–131. DOI: 10.1126/science.143.3602.129.

Stephenson, J.F. (2012) The chemical cues of male sea lice *Lepeophtheirus salmonis* encourage others to move between host Atlantic salmon *Salmo salar*. *Journal of Fish Biology* 81(3), 1118–1123. DOI: 10.1111/j.1095-8649.2012.03347.x.

Stien, L.H., Lind, M.B., Oppedal, F., Wright, D.W. and Seternes, T. (2018) Skirts on salmon production cages reduced salmon lice infestations without affecting fish welfare. *Aquaculture* 490, 281–287. DOI: 10.1016/j.aquaculture.2018.02.045.

Sutherland, B.J.G., Poley, J.D., Igboeli, O.O., Jantzen, J.R. *et al.* (2015) Transcriptomic responses to emamectin benzoate in Pacific and Atlantic Canada salmon lice *Lepeophtheirus salmonis* with differing levels of drug resistance. *Evolutionary Applications* 8(2), 133–148. DOI: 10.1111/eva.12237.

Sveen, L., Fast, M.D., Tengs, T., Timmerhaus, G., Vaadal, M. *et al.* (2025) Local inflammation at the salmon louse (*Lepeophtheirus salmonis salmonis*) attachment site contributes to copepodid rejection in coho salmon (*Oncorhynchus kisutch*). *Cell and Tissue Research* 401(2), 181–211. DOI: 10.1007/s00441-025-03976-0.

Tartor, H., Karlsen, M., Skern-Mauritzen, R., Monjane, A.L., Press, C.M. *et al.* (2021) Protective immunization of Atlantic salmon (*Salmo salar* L.) against salmon lice (*Lepeophtheirus salmonis*) infestation. *Vaccines* 10(1), 16. DOI: 10.3390/vaccines10010016.

Thorstad, E.B., Todd, C.D., Uglem, I., Bjørn, P.A., Gargan, P.G. *et al.* (2015) Effects of salmon lice *Lepeophtheirus salmonis* on wild sea trout Salmo trutta: a literature review. *Aquaculture Environment Interactions* 7(2), 91–113. DOI: 10.3354/aei00142.

Todd, C., Stevenson, R., Reinardy, H. and Ritchie, M. (2005) Polyandry in the ectoparasitic copepod *Lepeophtheirus salmonis* despite complex precopulatory and postcopulatory mate-guarding. *Marine Ecology Progress Series* 303, 225–234. DOI: 10.3354/meps303225.

Tucker, C.S., Sommerville, C. and Wootten, R. (2000) An investigation into the larval energetics and settlement of the sea louse, *Lepeophtheirus salmonis*, an ectoparasitic copepod of Atlantic salmon, *Salmo salar. Fish Pathology* 35(3), 137–143. DOI: 10.3147/jsfp.35.137.

Tucker, C.S., Norman, R., Shinn, A.P., Bron, J.E., Sommerville, C. and Wootten, R. (2002) A single cohort time delay model of the life-cycle of the salmon louse *Lepeophtheirus salmonis* on Atlantic salmon *Salmo salar*. *Fish Pathology* 37(3), 107–118.

Van Iderstine, C.R., Poley, J.D., Whyte, S.K., Purcell, S.L. and Fast, M.D. (2020) Hydrogen peroxide treatment and its impacts on *Lepeophtheirus salmonis* originating from the Bay of Fundy, Canada. *Journal of Fish Diseases* 44(6), 757–769. DOI: 10.1111/jfd.13299.

Vollstet, K.W., Barlaup, B.T., Skoglund, H., Normann, E.S. and Skilbrei, O.T. (2014) Salmon lice increase the age of returning Atlantic salmon. *Biology Letters* 10(1), 20130896. DOI: 10.1098/rsbl.2013.0896.

Wagner, G.N., McKinley, R.S., Bjørn, P.A. and Finstad, B. (2003) Physiological impact of sea lice on swimming performance of Atlantic salmon. *Journal of Fish Biology* 62(5), 1000–1009. DOI: 10.1046/j.1095-8649.2003.00091.

Wagner, G.N., Fast, M.D. and Johnson, S.C. (2008) Physiology and immunology of *Lepeophtheirus salmonis* infections of salmonids. *Trends in Parasitology* 24, 176–183.

Walde, C.S., Stormoen, M., Pettersen, J.M., Persson, D., Røsæg, M.V. and Bang Jensen, B. (2022) How delousing affects the short-term growth of Atlantic salmon (*Salmo salar*). *Aquaculture* 561, 738720. DOI: 10.1016/j.aquaculture.2022.738720.

Weston, D.P., Poynton, H.C., Wellborn, G.A., Lydy, M.J., Blalock, B.J. *et al.* (2013) Multiple origins of pyrethroid insecticide resistance across the species complex of a nontarget aquatic crustacean, *Hyalella azteca*. *Proceedings of the National Academy of Sciences USA* 110(41), 16532–16537. DOI: 10.1073/pnas.1302023110.

Wolstenholme, A.J. and Kaplan, R.M. (2012) Resistance to macrocyclic lactones. *Current Pharmaceutical Biotechnology* 13(6), 873–887. DOI: 10.2174/138920112800399239.

Woo, P.T. (1997) Immunization against parasitic diseases of fish. *Developments in Biological Standardization* 90, 233–241.

Wootten, R., Smith, J.W. and Needham, E.A. (1982) Aspects of the biology of the parasitic copepods *Lepeophtheirus salmonis* and *Caligus elongatus* on farmed salmonids, and their treatment. *Proceedings of the Royal Society of Edinburgh. Section B: Biological Sciences* 81(3), 185–197. DOI: 10.1017/S0269727000003389.

Xu, L., Wu, M. and Han, Z. (2013) Overexpression of multiple detoxification genes in deltamethrin resistant *Laodelphax striatellus* (Hemiptera: Delphacidae) in China. *PLoS One* 8(11), e79443. DOI: 10.1371/journal.pone.0079443.

Xue, X., Woldemariam, N.T., Caballero-Solares, A., Umasuthan, N., Fast, M.D. *et al.* (2019) Dietary immunostimulant CpG modulates microRNA biomarkers associated with immune responses in Atlantic salmon (*Salmo salar*). *Cells* 8(12), 1592. DOI: 10.3390/cells8121592.

Zhong, L., Carvalho, L.A., Gao, S., Whyte, S.K., Purcell, S.L. *et al.* (2023) Transcriptome analysis revealed immune response in the head kidney of Atlantic salmon (*Salmo salar*) co-infected with sea lice and infectious salmon anemia virus. *Fish and Shellfish Immunology* 143, 109210.

Index

Note: Page numbers in **bold** type refer to **figures;** page numbers in *italic* type refer to *tables.*